management of
PERIPHERAL NERVE PROBLEMS

GEORGE E. OMER, JR., M.D., M.Sc. *(Orthopaedic Surgery)*
Professor of Orthopaedics,
Chairman, Department of Orthopaedics;
Professor of Surgery,
Chief, Division of Hand Surgery;
Professor of Anatomy;
School of Medicine, The University of New Mexico,
Albuquerque, New Mexico

MORTON SPINNER, M.D.
Clinical Professor of Orthopaedic Surgery,
Albert Einstein College of Medicine, New York;
Chief of the Hand Surgical Service,
Department of Orthopaedic Surgery,
Brookdale Hospital Medical Center,
Brooklyn, New York

1980
W. B. SAUNDERS COMPANY
Philadelphia • London • Toronto

W. B. Saunders Company: West Washington Square
                          Philadelphia, PA   19105

                          1 St. Anne's Road
                          Eastbourne, East Sussex BN21 3UN, England

                          1 Goldthorne Avenue
                          Toronto, Ontario M8Z 5T9, Canada

Management of Peripheral Nerve Problems

ISBN   0-7216-6975-1

Last digit is the print number: 9   8   7   6   5   4   3   2   1

Dedicated to our wives,
WENDIE *and* PAULA

and to our children,
ERIC, MICHAEL,
JEFFREY, ROBERT *and* STEVEN.

Contributors

ADEL R. ABADIR, M.D.

Clinical Professor of Anesthesiology, New York University Medical Center; Director of Anesthesiology, Brookdale Hospital Medical Center; Attending Anesthesiologist, Bellevue Hospital Center, New York, New York.

Diagnostic Nerve Blocks. Therapeutic Nerve Blocks for the Relief of Chronic Pain.

IRVING M. ARIEL, M.D.

Professor of Clinical Surgery, New York Medical College and State University of New York at Stony Brook, Senior Surgeon, Pack Medical Foundation, Attending Surgeon, Flower and Fifth Avenue Hospital, Metropolitan Hospital, New York Hospital, Bird S. Coler Hospital, New York, New York.

Current Concepts in the Management of Peripheral Nerve Tumors

A. GRISWOLD BEVIN, M.D.

Associate Professor of Surgery (Plastic), Chief, Division of Plastic and Reconstructive Surgery and Surgery of the Hand, University of North Carolina at Chapel Hill School of Medicine, Chief, Plastic Surgery, North Carolina Memorial Hospital, Director, Hand Rehabilitation Center, University of North Carolina, Chapel Hill, North Carolina.

Burn Induced Peripheral Nerve Injury. (With Roger E. Salisbury.)

MONICA C. BISCHOFF

Research Assistant, Albert Einstein College of Medicine, New York, New York.

Contemporary Morphological Techniques for Evaluating Peripheral Nerves. (With Peter S. Spencer.)

PAUL W. BRAND, M.B., B.S., F.R.C.S. (England)

Clinical Professor of Surgery and Orthopedic Surgery, Louisiana State University Medical School; Chief, Rehabilitation Branch, U.S. Public Health Service Hospital, Carville, Louisiana.

Management of Sensory Loss In the Extremities.

RICHARD M. BRAUN, M.D.

Associate Clinical Professor of Orthopaedic Surgery, University of California at San Diego Medical School, Consultant in Upper Extremity Surgery, Rancho Los Amigos Hospital, Consultant in Hand Surgery, U.S. Navy Medical Center, San Diego, California.

Epineurial Nerve Repair.

DONALD S. BRIGHT, M.D.

Assistant Professor of Orthopaedic Surgery, Duke University Medical Center, Durham, North Carolina.

The Relationship of Blood Flow to Pain, and Assessment of Cold Tolerance.
(With J. Leonard Goldner.)

HARRY J. BUNCKE, M.D.

Associate Clinical Professor of Surgery, University of California Medical School, San Francisco; Plastic Surgical Staff, Ralph K. Davies Medical Center, San Francisco; Peninsula Hospital, Burlingame; Mills Hospital, San Mateo, California.

Sensory Rehabilitation of the Hand Utilizing Free Microneurovascular Flaps from the Foot.
(With Berish Strauch.)

WILLIAM E. BURKHALTER, M.D.

Professor of Orthopaedics, University of Miami School of Medicine; Chief, Division of Hand Surgery, Jackson Memorial Hospital, Miami, Florida.

Tendon Transfers as Internal Splints.

BERNARD R. CAHILL, M.D.

Adjunct Professor of Sports Medicine, Illinois State University, Normal, Illinois; Assistant Professor of Clinical Surgery, Peoria School of Medicine; Medical Director, Great Plains Sports Medicine Foundation, Peoria, Illinois.

Quadrilateral Space Syndrome.

RAYMOND M. CURTIS, M.D.

Chief, Division of Hand Surgery, Union Memorial Hospital, Associate Professor of Plastic Surgery and Associate Professor of Orthopaedic Surgery, Johns Hopkins University, Baltimore, Maryland, Consultant in Hand Surgery to the Surgeon General of the Army.

Sensory Re-education After Peripheral Nerve Injury. (With A. Lee Dellon.)

ROLLIN K. DANIEL, M.D., F.R.C.S. (Canada)

Assistant Professor of Surgery (Plastic Surgery), McGill University, Chief of Plastic Surgery, Royal Victoria Hospital, Montreal, Quebec, Canada.

Intraoperative Assessment of Nerve Lesions with Fascicular Dissection and Electrophysiological Recordings. (With Julia K. Terzis and H. Bruce Williams.)

EDWARD F. DELAGI, M.D.

Professor, Albert Einstein College of Medicine; Clinical Director of Rehabilitation Medicine, Bronx Municipal Hospital Center; Attending Physician, The Hospital of the Albert Einstein College of Medicine, New York.

Electrodiagnosis in Peripheral Nerve Lesions.

A. LEE DELLON, M.D.

Instructor, Johns Hopkins Hospital; Attending Hand Surgeon, Union Memorial Hospital, Consultant, Johns Hopkins Hospital, Union Memorial Hospital, and Childrens Hospital, Baltimore, Maryland.

Sensory Re-education in the Upper Extremity. (With Raymond M. Curtis.)
The Evaluation of Sensibility by Microhistological Studies. (With Michael E. Jabaley.)

THOMAS B. DUCKER, M.D.

Professor and Head, Division of Neurosurgery, University of Maryland School of Medicine, Baltimore, Maryland.

Pathophysiology of Peripheral Nerve Trauma.

RICHARD G. EATON, M.D.

Associate Clinical Professor of Surgery, Columbia University College of Physicians and Surgeons; Co-Chief, Hand Service, Roosevelt Hospital, New York, New York.

Painful Neuromas.

CARL DAMIAN ENNA, M.D.

Associate Clinical Professor, Department of Anatomy, Louisiana State University School of Medicine, New Orleans; Chief, Department of Surgery, U.S. Public Health Service Hospital (National Leprosarium), Carville, Louisiana.

The Management of Leprous Neuritis.

H. MARTIN FRIZELL, M.D.

Assistant Professor, Department of Neurobiology, University of Göteborg; Clinical Neurologist, Sahlgren's Hospital, Göteborg, Sweden.

Axonal Transport Studies. (With A. Johan Sjöstrand and W. Graham McLean.)

GARY K. FRYKMAN, M.D.

Assistant Professor of Orthopedic Surgery and Rehabilitation, Loma Linda University School of Medicine, Loma Linda; Active Staff, Loma Linda University Medical Center, Riverside General Hospital–University Medical Center, Jerry L. Pettis Memorial Veterans Administration Hospital, California.

Automated Nerve Fiber Counting in Complex Animal Nerves. (With Virchel E. Wood and Ernest L. Hall.)

FRED GENTILI, M.Sc., M.D.

Chief Resident, Neurosurgery, University of Toronto, St. Michael's Hospital, Toronto, Ontario, Canada.

Peripheral Nerve Injection Injury. (With Alan R. Hudson and David G. Kline.)

PHILIP L. GILDENBERG, M.D., Ph.D.

Professor and Chief, University of Texas Medical School (Division of Neurosurgery); Chief, Neurosurgery Service, Hermann Hospital, Houston, Texas.

Central Surgical Procedures for Pain of Peripheral Nerve Origin.

J. LEONARD GOLDNER, M.D.

Professor and Chairman, Division of Orthopaedic Surgery, Duke University Medical Center, Durham, North Carolina.

Pain: Extremities and Spine—Evaluation and Differential Diagnosis, The Effect of Extremity Blood Flow on Pain and Cold Tolerance. (With Donald S. Bright.) *Electrical Stimulation of Peripheral Nerves with Micro-electrical Implants for Pain Relief.* (With Blaine Nashold and Donald S. Bright.)

ERNEST L. HALL, Ph.D.

Associate Professor of Electrical Engineering, University of Tennessee, Knoxville, Tennessee.

Automated Nerve Fiber Counting in Complex Animal Nerves. (With Gary K. Frykman and Virchel E. Wood.)

MARK HALLETT, M.D.

Assistant Professor of Neurology, Harvard Medical School; Director of Neurophysiology Laboratories, Peter Bent Brigham Hospital; Consultant in Neurology, Robert Breck Brigham Hospital, Boston, Massachusetts.

Neurological Involvement of the Extremities Associated with Rheumatoid Arthritis. (With Lewis H. Millender.)

JAMES C. HARKIN, M.D.

Professor of Pathology, Tulane University School of Medicine, New Orleans, Louisiana.

Differential Diagnosis of Peripheral Nerve Tumors.

ALAN R. HUDSON, M.B., Ch.B., F.R.C.S. (Edinburgh) F.R.C.S. (Canada)

Associate Professor and Chairman, Division of Neurosurgery, University of Toronto, Neurosurgeon-in-Chief, St. Michael's Hospital, Toronto, Ontario, Canada.

Peripheral Nerve Injection Injury. (With David G. Kline and Fred Gentili.)

YOSHIKAZU IKUTA, M.D.

Associate Professor of Orthopedic Surgery, Hiroshima University School of Medicine; Attending Physician, Hiroshima University Hospital, Hiroshima, Japan.

Microsurgical Muscle Free Transplantation.

ALLAN E. INGLIS, M.D.

Clinical Professor of Anatomy, Clinical Professor of Surgery, Cornell University Medical College; Attending Orthopaedic Surgeon, The New York Hospital, The Hospital for Special Surgery, New York, New York.

Surgical Exposure of Peripheral Nerves.

MICHAEL E. JABALEY, M.D.

Professor and Chairman, Plastic Surgery Department, University of Mississippi Medical Center; Consultant in Plastic Surgery, Mississippi Baptist Medical Center and Mississippi Methodist Rehabilitation Center, Jackson, Mississippi.

The Evaluation of Sensibility by Microhistological Studies. (With A. Lee Dellon.)

EMANUEL B. KAPLAN, M.D.

Clinical Professor of Orthopedic Surgery, New Jersey School of Medicine and Dentistry, Newark, Emeritus Associate Professor of Anatomy, Columbia University College of Physicians and Surgeons, New York, Consultant, Hospital for Joint Diseases, New York.

Normal and Anomalous Innervation Patterns in the Upper Extremity. (With Morton Spinner.)

HAROLD E. KLEINERT, M.D.

Clinical Professor of Surgery, University of Louisville School of Medicine and Indiana University School of Medicine, Indianapolis, Indiana.

Surgical Sympathectomy — Upper and Lower Extremity. (With Hans Norberg and John J. McDonough.)

DAVID GELLINGER KLINE, M.D.

Professor and Head, Department of Neurosurgery, Louisiana State University School of Medicine and Charity Hospital; Staff, Charity Hospital, Baptist Hospital, Hotel Dieu Hospital, and Touro Infirmary; Academic Staff, Ochsner Hospital; Consultant, Veterans Administration Hospital, U.S. Public Health Service Hospital, and Biloxi Air Force Base Hospital.

Evaluation of the Neuroma in Continuity. Operative Experience with Lower Extremity Lesions, Including the Lumbosacral Plexus and the Sciatic Nerve. Peripheral Nerve Injection Injury. (With Alan R. Hudson and Fred Gentili.) *Primate Laboratory Models for Peripheral Nerve Repair.*

HARVEY P. KOPELL, M.D.

Clinical Professor of Orthopedic Surgery, New York University School of Medicine; Chief, Orthopedic Surgery, Castle Point Veterans Administration Medical Center.

Lower Extremity Lesions.

L. LEE LANKFORD, M.D.

Clinical Professor of Orthopaedic Surgery, The University of Texas Health Science Center at Dallas, Founding Director, Hand Clinic, Parkland Memorial Hospital, Dallas, Member, Teaching Service, Department of Orthopaedic Surgery, Baylor University Medical Center, Dallas, Texas.

Reflex Sympathetic Dystrophy.

ROBERT D. LEFFERT, M.D.

Associate Professor of Orthopaedic Surgery, Harvard Medical School; Chief of the Surgical Upper Extremity Rehabilitation Unit and Department of Rehabilitation Medicine, Massachusetts General Hospital, Boston, Massachusetts.

Thoracic Outlet Syndrome. Reconstruction of the Shoulder and Elbow Following Brachial Plexus Injury.

ROBERT W. LIPKE, M.D.

Former Fellow in Hand Surgery, Massachusetts General Hospital, Boston, Massachusetts.

Surgical Treatment of Peripheral Nerve Tumors of the Upper Limb. (With Richard J. Smith.)

GÖRAN LUNDBORG, M.D., Ph.D.

Associate Professor of Hand Surgery, University of Götesborg; Division of Hand Surgery, Department of Orthopedic Surgery, Sahlgren Hospital, Göteborg, Sweden.

Intraneural Microcirculation and Peripheral Nerve Barriers: Techniques for Evaluation— Clinical Implications.

LENNART MANNERFELT, M.D.

Associate Professor of Orthopaedic Surgery, University of Tübingen, West Germany; Former Assistant Professor in Orthopaedic and Hand Surgery, University of Lund, Sweden; Head of Hand Unit, Goldenbühl Hospital, Villingen West Germany.

Motor Function Testing.

JOHN J. MCDONOUGH, M.D.

Associate Professor of Surgery, University of Cincinnati College of Medicine, Cincinnati, Ohio.

Surgical Sympathectomy—Upper and Lower Extremity. (With Harold Kleinert and Hans Norberg.)

W. GRAHAM MCLEAN, Ph.D.

Department of Pharmacology, School of Pharmacy, Liverpool Polytechnic, Liverpool, England.

Axonal Transport Studies. (With Å. Johan Sjöstrand and Martin Frizell.)

JOSEPH E. MILGRAM, M.D., Sc.D.

Professor Emeritus of Clinical Orthopaedic Surgery, Albert Einstein College of Medicine, New York, Director Emeritus, Orthopaedic Surgery, Hospital for Joint Diseases, New York, Lecturer in Orthopaedics, Mount Sinai College of Medicine, New York, Orthopaedic Surgeon, Bronx Municipal Hospital, Consulting Orthopaedist, Jewish Hospital of Brooklyn and Kingsbrook Jewish Medical Center, Brooklyn, New York.

Morton's Neuritis and Management of Post-Neurectomy Pain.

LEWIS H. MILLENDER, M.D.

Assistant Clinical Professor of Orthopaedic Surgery, Harvard Medical School; Assistant Chief, Hand Service, Robert Breck Brigham Hospital; Attending Staff, Peter Bent Brigham Hospital, Beth Israel Hospital, and New England Baptist Hospital, Boston, Massachusetts.

Neurological Involvement of the Extremities Associated with Rheumatoid Arthritis. (With Mark Hallett.)

HANNO MILLESI, M.D.

Professor of Plastic and Reconstructive Surgery, University of Vienna; Head of Plastic and Reconstructive Surgery Unit, I. Chirurgische Universitatsklinik; Head, Ludwig Boltzmann Institute for Experimental Plastic Surgery, Vienna, Austria.

Nerve Grafts: Indications, Techniques, and Prognosis. Trauma Involving the Brachial Plexus.

BLAINE S. NASHOLD, JR., M.D.

Professor of Neurosurgery, Duke University School of Medicine; Attending Staff, Duke University Hospital, Durham, North Carolina.

Electrical Stimulation: Transcutaneous and Implant Techniques. (With J. Leonard Goldner.)

HANS NORBERG, M.D.

Former Christine Kleinert Fellow in Hand Surgery, University of Louisville School of Medicine, Louisville, Kentucky.

Surgical Sympathectomy—Upper and Lower Extremity. (With Harold E. Kleinert and John J. McDonough.)

JOSÉ OCHOA, M.D., Ph.D.

Associate Professor of Neurology, Dartmouth Medical School; Attending Neurologist, Dartmouth-Hitchcock Medical Center, Hanover, New Hampshire.

Nerve Fiber Pathology in Acute and Chronic Compression.

GEORGE E. OMER, JR., M.D., M.Sc.

Professor of Orthopaedics and Chairman, Department of Orthopaedics, Professor of Surgery and Chief, Division of Hand Surgery, Professor of Anatomy, School of Medicine, The University of New Mexico, Albuquerque, New Mexico.

Sensibility Testing. Continuous Peripheral Epineurial Infusion for the Treatment of Acute Pain. The Evaluation of Clinical Results Following Peripheral Nerve Suture. The Results of Untreated Traumatic Injuries. Neurovascular Cutaneous Island Pedicle Flaps. Tendon Transfers for Reconstruction of the Forearm and Hand Following Peripheral Nerve Injuries. Tendon Transfers as Reconstructive Procedures in the Leg and Foot.

MICHAEL G. ORGEL, M.D., M.Sc.

Associate Professor of Surgery (Plastic Surgery) and Chief, Division of Plastic Surgery, University of New Mexico School of Medicine, Attending Plastic Surgeon, Bernalillo County Medical Center and Veterans Administration Hospital, Albuquerque, New Mexico.

Coordination of Axon Neurophysiology and Axon Counting Techniques for Nerve Regeneration. (With Julia K. Terzis.)

LAWRENCE PRUTKIN, Ph.D.

Associate Professor of Anatomy, Department of Cell Biology, New York University School of Medicine, New York, New York.

Normal and Anomalous Innervation Patterns in the Lower Extremity.

ROGER E. SALISBURY, M.D.

Associate Professor of Surgery and Director, Burn Center and Burn Research Laboratory, University of North Carolina School of Medicine; Consultant in Plastic Surgery, Veterans Hospital, Fayetteville, and Womack Army Hospital, Fort Bragg, North Carolina.

Burn Induced Peripheral Nerve Injury. (With A. Griswold Bevin.)

MADJID SAMII, M.D.

Professor of Neurosurgery, Johannes Gutenberg Universitat, Mainz; Director, Norstadt Krankenhaus, Hanover Neurosurgical Hospital.

Nerves of the Head and Neck.

ROBERT J. SCHULTZ, M.D.

Professor and Chairman, Department of Orthopaedic Surgery, New York Medical College; Attending Orthopaedic Surgeon, Westchester County Medical Center, Metropolitan Hospital Center, New York.

Acupuncture. Management of Nerve Gaps.

Å. JOHAN B. SJÖSTRAND, M.D., Ph.D.

Assistant Professor, Department of Ophthalmology, University of Göteborg; Clinical Ophthalmologist, Sahlgren's Hospital, Göteborg, Sweden.

The Application of Axonal Transport Studies to Peripheral Nerve Problems. (With Martin Frizell and W. Graham McLean.)

RICHARD J. SMITH, M.D.

Clinical Professor of Orthopedic Surgery, Harvard Medical School; Chief, Hand Surgery, Department of Orthopaedic Surgery, Massachusetts General Hospital, Boston, Massachusetts.

Surgical Treatment of Peripheral Nerve Tumors of the Upper Limb. (With Robert W. Lipke.)

CLIFFORD CHARLES SNYDER, M.D.

Professor and Chairman, Division of Plastic Surgery, University of Utah College of Medicine; Chief, Surgical Service, Veterans Administration Hospital, Salt Lake City, Utah.

The History of Nerve Repair.

PETER S. SPENCER, Ph.D.

Associate Professor of Neuroscience, Albert Einstein College of Medicine, New York, New York.

Contemporary Morphological Techniques for Evaluation of Peripheral Nerves. (With Monica C. Bischoff.)

MORTON SPINNER, M.D.

Clinical Professor of Orthopaedic Surgery, Albert Einstein College of Medicine, New York; Chief, Hand Surgical Service, Department of Orthopaedic Surgery, Brookdale Hospital Medical Center, Brooklyn, New York.

Normal and Anomalous Innervation Patterns in the Upper Extremity. (With Emanuel B. Kaplan.) *Nerve Compression Lesions of the Upper Extremity.*

ALFRED J. SPIRO, M.D.

Professor of Neurology and Pediatrics, Albert Einstein College of Medicine; Attending in Neurology and Pediatrics, Hospital of the Albert Einstein College of Medicine and Bronx Municipal Hospital, Bronx, New York.

Contemporary Muscle Morphology as Related to Nerve Pathology.

BERISH STRAUCH, M.D.

Associate Professor and Chief, Division of Plastic Surgery, Albert Einstein College of Medicine and Montefiore Hospital and Medical Center; Attending Plastic Surgeon, Montefiore Hospital and Medical Center, Hospital of the Albert Einstein College of Medicine, The North Central Bronx Hospital, and Bronx Municipal Hospital Center, Bronx, New York.

Sensory Rehabilitation of the Hand Utilizing Free Microneurovascular Flaps from the Foot. (With Harry J. Buncke.)

JULIA K. TERZIS, M.D., F.R.C.S. (Canada)

Assistant Professor of Surgery (Plastic Surgery), McGill University; Assistant Director, Microsurgical Research Laboratories; Attending Plastic Surgeon, Royal Victoria Hospital, Montreal, Canada.

Intraoperative Assessment of Nerve Lesions with Fascicular Dissection and Electrophysiological Recordings. (With Rollin K. Daniel and H. Bruce Williams.) *Coordination of Axon Neurophysiology and Axon Counting Techniques for Nerve Regeneration.* (With Michael G. Orgel.)

PETER TSAIRIS, M.D.

Associate Professor of Clinical Neurology, Cornell Medical College; Director of Neurology and Muscle Disease Clinic, Hospital for Special Surgery; Associate Attending Neurologist, The New York Hospital, New York, New York.

Differential Diagnosis of Peripheral Neuropathies.

KENYA TSUGE, M.D.

Professor and Chairman, Department of Orthopaedic Surgery, Hiroshima University School of Medicine, Hiroshima, Japan.

Special Surgical Techniques.

JACK WILLIAM TUPPER, M.D.

Associate Clinical Professor, University of California at San Francisco; Director, Hand Clinic, Highland Alameda County Hospital; Attending Staff, Samuel Merritt Hospital, Children's Hospital of Northern California, Oakland, California.

Fascicular Nerve Repair.

E. F. SHAW WILGIS, M.D.

Assistant Professor of Orthopaedic Surgery and Assistant Professor of Plastic Surgery,

The Johns Hopkins Hospital, Attending Hand Surgeon, Union Memorial Hospital, Baltimore, Maryland.

Special Diagnostic Studies.

H. Bruce Williams, M.D.

Associate Professor of Surgery (Plastic Surgery), McGill University, Chief of Plastic Surgery, Montreal General Hospital, Montreal, Quebec, Canada.

Intraoperative Assessment of Nerve Lesions with Fascicular Dissection and Electrophysiological Recordings. (With Julia K. Terzis and Rollin K. Daniel.)

Virchel E. Wood, M.D.

Associate Professor, Orthopedic Surgery and Rehabilitation, Loma Linda University Medical Center; Active Staff, Loma Linda University Medical Center, Riverside General Hospital–University Medical Center, San Bernardino County Medical Center, Riverside, California.

Automated Nerve Fiber Counting in Complex Animal Nerves. (With Gary K. Frykman and Ernest L. Hall.)

Foreword

The problems of management of peripheral nerve afflictions are complicated and require the participation of experts in a variety of fields. Clinical experience and a knowledge of precise morphological anatomy and physiology are essential.

The contributions of Sterling Bunnell, Sir Herbert Seddon, Sir Sydney Sunderland, and Erik Moberg in this century brought attention to the problems of peripheral nerve injuries. Their methods and techniques have spread throughout the world. They have encouraged others to investigate and study the application of the improved methods and principles which are developed in the present text.

The authors who have contributed to this edition have added distinct contributions to the surgery of peripheral nerves. It was not intended to present an encyclopaedic treatise but a practical and valuable text for general application and understanding. The purpose of this book is to indicate how to solve specific clinical problems. In addition, experimental methods to study particular aspects of the basic physiology and internal morphology of the peripheral nerves are presented. The book will be of great assistance to all who have taken up the challenge of the management of afflictions of the peripheral nervous system.

I have known the editors, George Omer and Morton Spinner, for more than 25 years. I have encouraged and enjoyed their excellent progress and contributions in the area of understanding and treatment of the complicated problems that are observed in derangements of the peripheral nervous system, and I am pleased to have had a part in their development.

This work brings together experts with national and international reputations in this field. The contributors successfully present the contemporary status of the art of management of peripheral nerve problems.

EMANUEL B. KAPLAN, M.D.

Preface

Peripheral nerve injuries are seen in large numbers, with major complications, during military campaigns. Our clinical interest in these devastating conditions was stimulated by surgical experience gained during the early 1950's in the Medical Corps of the United States Army. Military professional and administrative assignments during the 1960's provided an overview of the chronicity of these problems and the difficult rehabilitation process faced by these patients. The management of the civilian with a peripheral nerve injury should be individualized, but the basic professional principles remain the same during peace or war. During the 1970's, we have shared our continuing surgical experience through applied teaching, such as an ongoing Instructional Course on Peripheral Nerve Testing and Suture Techniques for the annual meetings of the American Academy of Orthopaedic Surgeons, and many Symposia on varied peripheral nerve conditions for the American Society for Surgery of the Hand. This book is the result of our accumulated experience and continuing interest in the complex clinical problems associated with peripheral nerve injury. We intend that this volume will present the current state of the art for those professionals actively involved with the management of these complex problems.

There has been a tremendous expansion in techniques and innovative concepts for the management of peripheral nerve problems that can be attributed to the practical use of microsurgery, computer technology, and the electron microscope. This makes it impossible for the individual surgeon to evaluate all available research and clinical studies; yet he must make practical decisions based on pertinent data from these sources. In an attempt to meet his need, we have selected a limited number of contributors who are recognized as being in the vanguard of research and clinical activities related to peripheral nerve disorders. We believe these contributors represent well the great number of specialists who have evolved in this complex field of medicine. We have limited the subjects for discussion to a representative cross section of the common peripheral nerve problems confronting the clinical surgeon.

For individualized reference, the book has been arranged into sections related to clinical problems. The laboratory section was designed to indicate the future for current clinical techniques and concepts.

We are indebted to our colleagues who have contributed to this book; and to Doctors Emanuel B. Kaplan, Leo Mayer, Erik Moberg, and Daniel Riordan, who have been our mentors in orthopaedics and hand surgery and peripheral nerve techniques and concepts. Our gratitude to Marleece Kendrick and Jean Fertel for their administrative assistance, and to Hugh Thomas and George Thomas for their artistic contributions. We extend credit to Doctors Mooyoung Jun and Irwin R. Cohen for editorial assistance with some specific chapters; and we recognize the research assistance of Mrs. Ada Gams and Mr. Denis Gafney of the Library of the New York Academy of Medicine. We are thankful to our wives and children for their encouragement and tolerance under the stress of many hours forfeited from family activities to this project. We also want to acknowledge the assistance and contributions of the editorial staff of W. B. Saunders Company, especially George Vilk, Carroll Cann, Charles Graham, and Andrew J. Piernock, Jr.

GEORGE E. OMER, JR., M.D.
MORTON SPINNER, M.D.

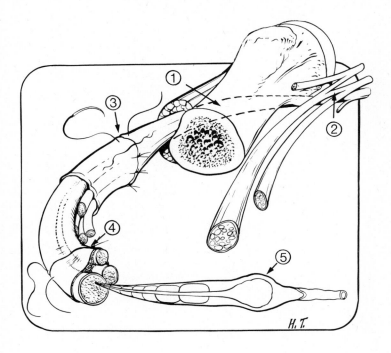

The logo on the book cover is a composite representation which was designed by Mr. Hugh Thomas of New York. In addition, Mr. Thomas has illustrated several chapters. In this logo, the radial nerve (1) is seen traversing its anatomical course posterior to the humerus. Details of the infraclavicular portion of the brachial plexus (2) are stylized medial to the humerus. An epineurial repair (3) of the radial nerve is depicted. A funicular group repair is represented at (4). From this repair site, the growing axon cone (5), an ultrastructure, is demonstrated. We selected this particular logo from many choices because it seemed to typify the major themes of the book. All of the subject areas are discussed in detail in the appropriate chapters of this text.

Contents

PART III — ANATOMICAL EXPOSURES

PART IV — SUTURE TECHNIQUES

PART V — TRAUMA: MISSILES, LACERATIONS, COMPRESSION, INJECTIONS, TRACTION, AND FRICTION

PART VI – SPECIAL PROBLEMS

PART VII – REHABILITATION

Introduction

Although Paul of Aegina (625–690) was the first to attempt nerve repair by approximation of the nerve stumps when closing a wound, for many centuries following, surgeons did not dare to touch the nerve stumps, being afraid that they would cause convulsions in the patient by such a maneuver. Approximation of nerve ends was achieved indirectly, *cum carne,* by approximation of the remaining soft tissue (Avicenna, 980–1037). These rules were obeyed even until the middle of the last century (Baudens, 1836; von Langenbeck, 1854).

With the introduction of the epineural nerve suture (Hueter, 1871, 1873), a new era began. Hueter suggested primary nerve repair, and Nelaton (1864) secondary nerve repair. The problem of tension at the suture site was recognized, and Mikulicz in 1882 introduced tension-relieving sutures. Loebke (1884) performed bone shortening by osteotomy to achieve coaptation without tension. Albert in 1876 grafted nerve defects, and Gluck (1880) and Büngner (1891) were pioneers in tubulization of the suture site.

The reader should be aware that all the problems discussed today had been perceived a century ago. The main contributions of modern times are microsurgery, which permits surgery within the nerve without too much punishment resulting from tissue reaction, and a more biologic approach rather than a mechanistic one. There is still no magic solution, and different situations require different attitudes and approaches. To help the practicing surgeon select the proper technique, a survey of the complete problem of peripheral nerve surgery is an ultimate necessity.

George Omer and Morton Spinner accepted the challenge to edit a volume that surveys the many problems facing the surgeon who deals with peripheral nerves. Both men are eminently qualified for this enterprise. Each is a distinguished surgeon with an outstanding scientific and professional career, and each has made remarkable contributions to the field of peripheral nerve surgery. They have succeeded in enlisting a large number of authors for the task who have risen to the challenge admirably. The 63 chapters in this book cover the problems of peripheral nerve surgery comprehensively and authoritatively.

The great experience of the editors, their excellent grasp of the subject matter, and their perceptive selection of contributors virtually ensure that the book will fulfill its task; that is, be a useful guide for the surgeon confronted with the problems of peripheral nerve surgery.

PROF. DR. HANNO MILLESI

xxvii

Diagnostic Techniques
and
Innervation Patterns

I

1

SENSIBILITY TESTING

GEORGE E. OMER, JR.

The human nervous system is bombarded simultaneously by a multitude of stimuli. The afferent input is limited by the inconstant threshold of the peripheral nerve endings and the specialized receptor organs associated with them. Sensation is the acceptance and activation of impulses in the afferent nerve fibers of the nervous system.

The brain receives and elaborates a continuously changing flood of sensations. Varied sensations are synthesized into three-dimensional experiences. Central neural mechanisms, such as memory storage and introspection, influence the conscious perception of the external and internal environment. Sensibility is the conscious appreciation and interpretation of the stimulus that produced sensation.

ANATOMICAL CONSIDERATIONS

A sensory unit is a single first-order afferent neuron including all peripheral and central branches. Five elementary qualities of sensibility can be evoked: (1) touch–pressure, (2) warmth, (3) cold, (4) pain, and (5) movement and position. Sensation for these qualities depends upon many factors; some involving the sensory unit are: (1) the diameter of the first-order afferent neuron, (2) the properties of the sensory receptors, (3) the size and population of the receptive field, and (4) the threshold for the entire sensory unit.

Axons are classified in three groups: A (with subgroups alpha, beta, and delta), B, and C. The A axons are the largest, up to 20 μ in diameter, while C axons may be less than 1 μ in diameter. The larger the diameter of an axon, the more rapid the conduction rate and the lower its threshold to electrical stimulation. The larger myelinated afferents (alpha and beta groups, A axons) are specialists in touch — pressure and movement — position. Small myelinated afferents (delta group, A axons) conduct acute pricking pain, cold and warmth, and deep pressure. Single unit analysis of unmyelinated afferents (C axons) reveals that they conduct the total range of qualitative sensations. All major

3

somesthetic sensations (pressure, pain, cold, and warmth) are conducted by the small myelinated afferents (delta group, A axons) and the smaller unmyelinated afferents (C axons); these two systems indicate the multiple functional duplication in the peripheral nervous system. A property of any group of axons is that they transmit an identical impulse no matter how they are excited; different sensations occur through the combinations of axons transmitting impulses. The frequency and sequence of the impulses are determined by the peripheral receptors.

The peripheral branches of sensory units may terminate in complex receptor organs composed in part of non-neural tissue, such as the hair follicle or pacinian corpuscles. These receptors initiate the depolarization of the afferent neuron through their generator potential. The generator potential is not conducted, but can be increased both temporally and spatially to invade adjacent regions of the parent axon. Receptors vary in their rate of adaptation to continued stimuli (Table 1–1). Most of the receptor organs with non-neural tissue are mechanoreceptive afferents. The form, number, and distribution of specialized receptor organs vary with age, region of the body, and occupation. Free nerve endings can be differentially sensitive in the absence of a specialized receptor organ.

The receptor fields of ectodermal sensory units vary greatly in population and size. The population of the isolated cutaneous spots for temperature sensitivity is an example: cold spots are more numerous than warm spots by ratios of 4:1 to 10:1, and both types of cutaneous spots are more common on the hands and face than elsewhere on the body (Mountcastle, 1974). The smaller the receptive field is in size, the greater the number of sensory units into a given body area and the greater the representation of that body part at the cerebral cortex. The superficial tissues of the hand are densely innervated compared to more proximal cutaneous areas of the upper extremity, and may have as many as 2500 nerve endings in one square millimeter of tissue (Montcastle, 1974). The peripheral branches of one ectodermal sensory unit overlap with the branches of

Table 1–1 Sensibility and Receptor Organs

STIMULUS OF SENSATION	MODALITY OF SENSIBILITY	RECEPTOR STRUCTURE	ADAPTABILITY OF RECEPTOR
Mechanical force	Light touch and vibration	Free nerve endings (A and C)	Slow
		Pacinian corpuscles	Fast
		Meissner corpuscles	Fast
Mechanical force	Pressure	Free nerve endings (A and C)	Slow
		Merkel disk-hair follicles	Slow
Mechanical force	Deep pressure	Free nerve endings (A and C)	Slow
	Movement-rate direction	Cylinders of Ruffini	Fast
		Muscle spindles-flower spray annulospiral	Slow
	Position-posture		Slow
		Golgi–Mazzoni corpuscles	Fast
Temperature change	Warmth (24–45°C)	Free nerve endings (A and C)	Slow
	Cold (12–37°C)	Arteriolar diameter change	Slow
Extremes of mechanical force or temperature change; presence of chemicals or electrical energy	Pain	Free nerve endings	
		Pricking pain—delta group, A axons	Fast
		Burning pain—C axons	Slow

adjacent sensory units, so that the activity of sensory units gradually changes with a moving stimulus. Consequently, sensibility is very accurate for a light pressure or moving position stimulus to the volar tip of the fingers. Discrimination of light touch on the volar finger pulp, as two points and not one, is normally accurate between 3 to 5 millimeters. In contrast, two-point discrimination of light touch proximal to the elbow is between 65 and 75 millimeters (Werner and Omer, 1970).

Sensibility for body position and movement results from stimulation of proprioceptors in mesodermal tissues, such as muscles, tendons, joints, and periosteum as well as of cutaneous receptors (Moberg, 1965). Impulses generated in muscle–tendon units and joints assist in guiding action in such diverse performances as hand grip, lever manipulation, estimating hardness of compliant materials, and spanning an object with the fingers. The preciseness of proprioception is the reverse of exteroception for the proximal and distal portions of the extremities. In the shoulder joint, less than one degree of passive movement can be recognized, and a given position can be reproduced within two degrees. An interphalangeal joint requires five to 10 degrees of movement for recognition (Cohen, 1958). The precise sense of position and direction of extremity movement is related to the receptors found about joints, and proximal joints are more densely populated than distal joints (Stopford, 1921–1922).

The mesodermal receptors with the highest threshold to stretch are the Golgi organs within tendons. These afferents connect into a disynaptic reflex arc that influences both synergists and antagonists of the involved muscle (Omer and Vogel, 1965). The flower-spray nerve endings (beta and gamma groups, A axons) and the annulospiral nerve endings (alpha group, A axons) are afferents found in the muscle spindle. The annulospiral nerve endings have the lowest threshold to stretch. In addition to the afferent receptors, small motor nerves termed gamma efferents terminate in the muscle spindle. The gamma efferents can tense the muscle spindle even when the total muscle is relaxed. This causes the annulospiral alpha afferents to discharge even though the total muscle continues relaxed. This double stimulation mechanism maintains the myostatic reflex while the muscle is either contracted or relaxed. The motor neurons for these spinal reflex arcs come from a competing pool of afferent impulses that includes cutaneous and central stimulation. The central pathways are inhibitory to protect the muscle from overload by preventing damaging contraction against strong stretch. When central impulses are uncoordinated, as in cerebral palsy, the alpha afferents and gamma efferents are always imbalanced. As the afferent pool is increased, the sphere of influence involves additional synergistic and antagonistic muscles.

First order sensory afferent impulses are conducted centrally by at least two systems. The larger myelinated afferents (alpha and beta groups, A axons) connect with large myelinated fibers in the dorsal horn of the spinal cord and traverse the ipsilateral dorsal column. The impulse is then projected, via the medial lemiscus, upon the contralateral ventrobasal thalamic complex and finally to the postcentral gyrus of the sensory cortex. The distinguishing feature of this system is that information concerning location, shape, quality, and temporal sequence of stimuli is transmitted with great fidelity at each synaptic station (Mountcastle, 1974). Small myelinated afferents (delta group, A axons) and unmyelinated afferents (C axons) also connect by the interneuronal system of the dorsal horn. Some cross to the contralateral side in the spinothalamic tract and others remain ipsilateral to continue centrally in the anterolateral columns. Compared to the lemniscal system, these tracts are phylogenetically older and less precise. Their cortical representation is less exact. Little is known about how messages coded by the activity of ensembles of peripheral neurons are integrated by centrally located neurons. However, it is this process that ultimately leads to the conscious recognition termed sensibility.

THRESHOLD FACTORS

The thresholds of sensory units vary for many reasons (Table 1–2). The sensorimotor system works best at the level to which it is adapted, and unexperienced variations in threshold will influence the interpretation by the individual. For example, temperature change will produce a mechanoreceptive illusion, in that weights feel heavier when cold than when warm. Sensibility is affected also by sensory cortex storage. Almost all patterns of information are converted into a recorded form that preserves the topographical representation of the periphery in the sensory cortex. One example is the reaction of patients with neurovascular cutaneous island pedicle transfers. The patient can be trained to interpret a sensory experience into the spatial pattern of the recipient site of the pedicle transfer, but in an emergency the training will be lost (Omer et al. 1970). Thus, a patient will first move the donor ring finger when a cigarette burns the thumb that is the recipient of the pedicle transfer.

QUANTITATIVE EXAMINATION

The electrical conduction velocity study for sensory nerves is the only quantitative technique for measuring sensation. The range of conduction veloci-

Table 1–2   Threshold Variables for Sensibility

A. Receptors: somatic, peripheral
   1. Age of individual
   2. Condition of overlying epithelium – occupation
   3. Circulation in area of receptor
   4. Intensity of stimulation energy
   5. Time (duration) of stimulation
   6. Number of receptors or receptive fields stimulated
     a. region of body
   7. Temperature in area of receptor
   8. Specific morphology and adaptability
   9. Central influence on receptor system
     a. spinal reflex arcs, such as muscle spindle
     b. activity facilitated by autonomic efferents
B. Afferent pathway systems
   1. Both inhibitory and facilitory effect on transmission and summation
C. Sensory cortex
   1. Attention and concentration of individual
   2. Spatial–temporal pattern of impulse input
   3. Stored memory and experience
   4. Coordination with vision, smell, hearing
   5. Selection and erasure of irrelevant information

Table 1–3   Quantitative Sensibility

SENSIBILITY MODALITY	TECHNIQUE AND NORMALS
Touch-pressure	von Frey hair pressure, with point localization between 2.44 and 2.83
	Weber two-point discrimination distance of 3 to 5 mm. in the digital autonomous zone of cutaneous nerve in the hand
	Ridged aesthesiometer, with recognition of keel depth at 3/8 mm. or less
Body movement–position	5 to 10 degrees of movement at an interphalangeal joint, 1 degree at shoulder or hip joint
Pain	Algesimeter (5 gm. pressure) should be localized within 2 cm.
Temperature	Copper test tubes, with recognition between 20° and 35° C.
Vibration	200 to 250 cps
Protective sensibility	Conscious appreciation of pain, cold, warmth, or pressure before tissue damage results from the stimulus

ty is 45 to 75 meters per second (Juul-Jensen and Mayer, 1966). Regardless of the nature of the stimulus, the form of the action potential is remarkably constant. The combination of receptor organ and diameter of the myelinated afferent axon might provide some specificity to sensation, but this specificity cannot be expressed in the form of the action potential.

Attempts have been made to examine sensibility in quantitative terms (Table 1–3), but the response is subjective, not objective (Omer, 1971). For example, there is no correlation between sensory nerve conduction velocity and two-point discrimination following surgical repair of a peripheral nerve. Sensibility for light touch usually returns in the young patient after nerve suture, while sensory nerve conduction velocity does not recover (Almquist and Eeg-Olofsson, 1970).

Testing the skin with a pin for pain, with cotton wool for touch, or with test-tube contact for warmth or cold is unsatisfactory for estimating functional loss. It is impossible to duplicate these tests periodically with comparable quantitative results, and only protective sensibility is evaluated (Moberg, 1958). In fact, most tests for sensibility cannot differentiate between paresthesia and good quality sensation (Brand and Ebner, 1969).

Only a few tests are useful:

Von Frey Pressure Test

In 1898 von Frey attempted to standardize the stimuli for testing the subjective sense of light touch by using a series of horsehairs of varying thickness and stiffness (Von Frey, 1922). Weinstein used nylon monofilaments mounted in Lucite rods as substitutes for the hairs (Weinstein, 1962). The Weinstein–Semmes pressure aesthesiometer consists of a series of 20 probes marked 1.65 to 6.65. The number represents the logarithm of 10 times the force in milligrams required to bow the monofilament (Levan, Pearsall, and Ruderman, 1978.) Clinical testing techniques were developed by Werner and Omer (1970) and every other probe provides adequate information for clinical evaluation.

The room temperature should be comfortable for the patient without excess humidity to affect stiffness of the monofilaments. The monofilament is applied perpendicular to the body surface, and pressure is increased until the monofilament bends. The very light monofilaments (1.65 to 3.84) should be "bounced off" the skin for adequate stimulation. When using heavier monofilaments (4.08 to 6.65) the monofilament is applied in one motion. The patient closes his eyes while the examiner touches the skin with the monofilament. If the patient feels the pressure, he opens his eyes and localizes the touch point with a small wooden dowel 3/8 inch in diameter and several inches long. When using monofilaments 1.65 through 4.08, the monofilament should be applied three times. If the patient misses the same monofilament twice in the same area, a larger number monofilament is selected. When using 4.17 through 6.65, only one stimulation is used and must be recognized the first time by the patient.

Testing should begin with the uninvolved extremity. This allows the patient to become familiar with the testing procedure and the examiner to establish the patient's normal sensibility (Table 1–4). Higher values may be considered normal when the results of testing the uninvolved extremity are higher than established normals.

When the involved hand is tested, it should be marked off into seven zones (Fig. 1–1). Testing is begun at the more sensitive pulp tip, zone 7, and is continued proximally, either all the way proximally on each digit or all across the hand at each level. Localization is a major factor in the von Frey test and can be either point or area identification. Point localization should be used in the hand because it requires more precise sensibility. If the patient cannot localize the exact indentation point by bringing the wooden dowel in contact with the point stimulated, the identification should be considered a miss (Fig. 1–2). Area localization is the ability to recognize stimulation but not the exact point within the tested skin zone. On occasion, the patient will miss the indentation point in a zone but then will precisely cover that same point when the next more proximal zone is stimulated. This "summation" usually happens just before protective sensibility is regained (Omer, 1968). Finally, the speed of the patient's response is indicative of sensibility. The normal response to the stimulation is immediate "bull's-eye" point localization.

Normal sensibility localizes pressure between 2.44 and 2.83 at the distal end of the extremities, but normal pressure is between 4.08 and 4.17 at the proximal portion of the extremities. Sensibility over 6.10 is only protective and is lost when 6.65 is unrecognized. Children recognize the same pressure as adults, but will not localize as well, even when cooperating. Judged by the von Frey test, some

Table 1–4   Von Frey Pressure Sensibility in the Hand

CALCULATED PRESSURE (gm/mm²)	AESTHESIOMETER	INTERPRETATION	CALCULATED FORCE (gm)
3.25–4.86	2.44–2.83	Normal light touch	0.0276–0.068
11.1–47.3	3.22–4.56	Diminished light touch – point localization intact	0.166–3.64
68.0–243	4.74–6.10	Minimal light touch – area localization intact	5.51–126.0
243–439	6.10–6.65	Sensation, but without localization	126–448

Point localization: the dowel is in contact with the skin point stimulated

Area localization: the dowel is in contact with any point inside the zone of the area being tested

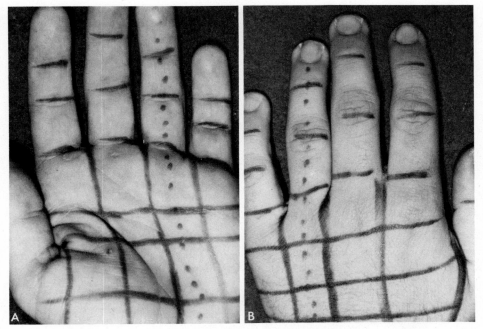

Figure 1–1 The hand is divided into seven zones for testing: creases for the interphalangeal joints, the interdigital skin margin, and palmar creases are utilized for zone margins. Testing is begun at the more sensitive volar pulp tip. *A*, Volar; *B*, dorsal.

patients who do not regain motor function do develop minimal light touch several months after a traumatic nerve injury.

Weber Two-Point Discrimination Distance

This test was introduced by Weber in 1835 (Weber, 1835). The object is to determine if the patient can discriminate between being touched with one or two points and the minimum distance at which two points touching the skin are recognized. Clincal testing techniques were developed by Moberg (1958, 1962) for the hand. The test should be demonstrated while the patient is watching the procedure. Several areas on the uninvolved hand should be checked because some patients have congenitally abnormal two-point discrimination.

The testing instrument can be a Boley gauge, a blunt eye caliper, or an ordinary paper clip (Fig. 1–3) (Moberg, 1965). Testing is begun distally and proceeds proximally. The points of the caliper are set at 10 millimeters and progressively brought together as accurate responses are obtained. The pressure from the testing instrument should not produce an ischemic area on the skin. When two points are applied, they make contact simultaneously, and the line between the points is in the longitudinal axis of the finger. The patient closes his eyes, but he indicates immediately if he feels one or two points. An interval of three to five seconds should be allowed between application of the points. A series of one or two points is applied with varied sequence in each finger zone (see Fig. 1–1). The procedure is done three times; if the patient does not record

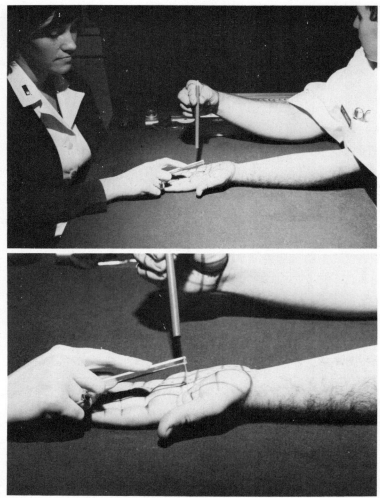

Figure 1–2   Von Frey testing. Sensibility should be recorded as "point accuracy" or "zone accuracy." In the hand, normal sensibility should be localized to the point of stimulation, and is abnormal if the patient only touches the zone of stimulation.

two of the three correctly, the result is considered a failure at that test distance. If the patient correctly identifies the number of points applied, the testing distance is decreased by 5 millimeters. Omer uses this three-application technique throughout the extremity (Omer, 1968; Werner and Omer, 1970), but Moberg uses a different system in the hand: there are 10 applications of two points and 10 applications of one point at random. The total of incorrect one-point applications is subtracted from the total of correct two-point applications. An answer of five or more is considered a "pass" (Lister, 1977).

The normal threshold for two-point discrimination distance for the volar surface of the hand varies according to the zone being tested (Table 1–5). The threshold for the dorsal surface is higher in all zones: normal is 7 to 12 mm.,

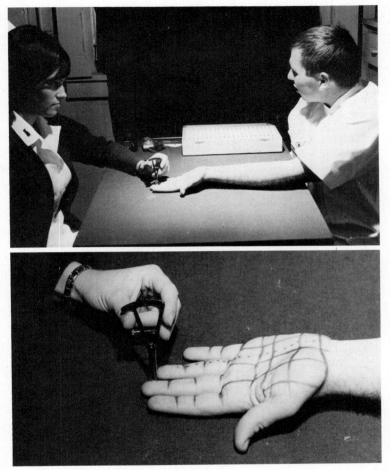

Figure 1–3 Weber two-point discrimination distance. Testing is begun distally and proceeds proximally. Both the examiner and patient should be comfortable.

diminished is 13 to 20 mm., and absent is greater than 20 mm. Below elbow and below knee two-point discrimination distance is normal between 40 to 50 mm., diminished between 55 and 80 mm., and absent above 80 millimeters. Above elbow and above knee two-point discrimination distance is normal between 65 to 75 mm., diminished between 80 and 100 mm., and absent above 100 mm. (Omer, 1971). Abnormal skin texture, such as heavy scales or calluses, has a marked influence on the test results. Testing can be done in the presence of edema or infection, but the result demonstrates the sensibility present, which may not be the true status of the nerve.

Picking-Up Test

Although two-point discrimination distance correlates with constant touch, such as various pinch or grip positions, it does not assess tactile gnosis, which

Table 1–5   Two-Point Discrimination Distance
Volar Surface of Hand

	HAND ZONE	DISTANCE IN MILLIMETERS		
		Normal	*Diminished*	*Absent*
Between fingertip and D-I-P joint	7	3–5	6–10	10+
Between D-I-P joint and P-I-P joint	6	3–6	7–10	10+
Between P-I-P joint and finger web	5	4–7	8–10	10+
Between web and distal palmar crease	4	5–8	9–20	20+
Between distal crease and central palm	3	6–9	10–20	20+
Base of palm and wrist	1–2	7–10	11–20	20+

requires movement (Wynn-Parry and Salter, 1976). The sensation generated by moving the fingertips across something is mediated by the quickly adapting receptors (Dellon et al., 1972, 1974), and Dellon has developed a moving two-point discrimination distance test. In 1958, Moberg published the picking-up test as a technique for determining the functional value of sensibility in the hand: ". . . pick up a number of small objects on a table and put them as quickly as he can into a small box, first with one hand and then with the other. After he has done this a few times he is asked to do the same thing blindfolded. It is then studied how rapidly and efficiently he picks up the objects; comparison is made between his right and left hands. The test with blindfolding can be made harder by asking him to identify the objects as he picks them up" (Moberg, 1958). Moberg demonstrated the abnormal functional pattern in a hand with median cutaneous sensibility loss. The picking-up test is used only in patients with median or combined median and ulnar nerve injuries.

Seddon states that the precursor of the picking-up test is the coin test, as described by Riddoch in 1940 (Seddon, 1975). The patient, whose eyes must be closed, is given a coin and asked to identify it. (See Figure 1–4).

Omer quantitated the picking-up test by choosing nine objects of different size and shape (Omer, 1968). A "normal" result is considered to be five to eight seconds for young adult males, but a better normal is the time required by the uninvolved hand. The objects can include such things as a key, marble, small square piece of wood, nut and bolt, paper clip, short pencil or safety pin.

The picking-up test is done first with the uninvolved hand and then with the injured hand, first with the eyes open and then with them closed. The patient should attempt to identify the objects when his eyes are closed. The functional aptitude of the patient for picking up the objects is noted by the examiner. Sometimes a piece of chalk is substituted for one of the objects so that a trail of functional surfaces will remain on the hand. The patient is timed with a stopwatch each time he performs the test, and comparison of periodic tests indicates the changing status of function. Normal tactile gnosis requires motion and power as well as cutaneous sensibility.

Tinel's Sign

Tinel described a "formication sign" that indicates the presence of axons in the process of regeneration: "When percussion is lightly applied to the injured nerve trunk, we find in the cutaneous region of the nerve a creeping sensation usually compared by the patient to that caused by electricity" (Tinel, 1918). The percussion should be done with a tuning fork and should begin at the distal

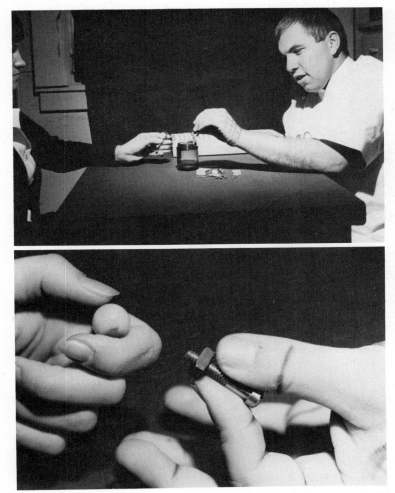

Figure 1–4 Timed picking-up test. The patient should attempt to identify each object, then is timed while transferring all objects from the table to the jar.

portion of the extremity to delay the patient's discomfort until the final point of the test. The point of maximum response is measured from bony prominences. The reaction to percussion appears approximately six weeks after injury or surgery (Henderson, 1948). A nerve response that remains fixed at one level for several months probably indicates frustrated nerve regeneration, but an advancing level of response does not assure a sufficient quantity of fibers for clinical function. In addition, there is no measurement of quality, so that the response may indicate paresthesia rather than useful sensibility.

The Wrinkled Finger Test

O'Riain (1973) has recorded a common but unappreciated observation: the skin of denervated fingers does not wrinkle or shrivel as normal skin does when

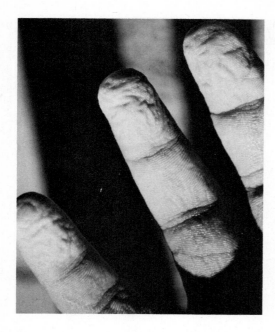

Figure 1–5   Normal fingertip wrinkling after immersion in warm water.

immersed in warm water. This objective test can be performed without the patient's concentration or cooperation, and is particularly indicated in small children. Shriveling of the skin returns progressively with recovery of nerve function. O'Riain recommends immersion in water at approximately 40° C. for a period of 30 minutes. Smooth skin indicates loss of sensibility. (See Figure 1–5).

Body Position – Movement

The precision of sensibility for body position or movement is the reverse of that of cutaneous sensibility for the proximal and distal portion of the extremity. The patient can identify the position and directional change in a finger or toe when passive movements of the interphalangeal joints are performed. An interphalangeal joint requires five to 10 degrees of passive movement for recognition, but in the shoulder joint less than one degree of passive movement can be recognized, and a given position can be reproduced within two degrees.

SENSIBILITY FOLLOWING NERVE LOSS

Children recover protective sensibility without education. Patients under 35 years of age often recover protective sensibility for pain, warmth, cold, position, movement, and pressure without localization following traumatic injury and suture of a single peripheral cutaneous nerve (Omer,1974). This level of sensibility returns nine to 12 months after injury. However, two-point discrimination distance remains at least 12 to 15 millimeters in most young adults with repaired nerve injuries. This pattern of sensibility would seem to indicate increased responsibility for the unmyelinated afferents and a changed priority of information for sensory cortex interpretation.

Sensibility return is limited when multiple nerves are injured, resulting in decreased motor activity and functional loss. There are many clinical observations suggesting that sensibility depends upon total extremity homeostasis and activity. Techniques for the reeducation of sensibility are discussed in Chapter 47.

REFERENCES

Almquist, E., and Eeg-Olofsson, O.: Sensory-nerve-conduction velocity and two-point discrimination in sutured nerves. J. Bone Joint Surg. *52A*:791, 1970.

Brand, P. W., and Ebner, J. D.: Pressure sensitive devices for denervated hands and feet. J. Bone Joint Surg. *51A*:109, 1969.

Cohen, L. A.: Analysis of position sense in human shoulder. J. Neurophysiol. *21*:550, 1958.

Dellon, A. L., Curtis, R. M., and Edgerton, M. T.: Evaluating recovery of sensation in the hand following nerve injury. Johns Hopkins Med. J. *130*:235, 1972.

Dellon, A. L., Curtis, R. M., and Edgerton, M. T.: Reeducation of sensation in the hand after nerve injury and repair. Plast. Reconstr. Surg. *53*:297, 1974.

Henderson, W. R.: Clinical assessment of peripheral nerve injuries: Tinel's test. Lancet *2*:801, 1948.

Juul-Jensen, P. and Mayer, R. F.: Threshold stimulation for nerve conduction studies in man. Arch. Neurol. *15*:410, 1966.

Levin, S., Pearsall, G., and Ruderman, R. J.: von Frey's method of measuring pressure sensibility in the hand; an engineering analysis of the Weinstein-Semmes pressure aesthesiometer. J. Hand Surg. *3*:211, 1978.

Lister, G.: The Hand: Diagnosis and Indications. Edinburgh, Churchill Livingstone, 1977.

Moberg, E.: Objective methods for determining the functional value of sensibility in the hand. J. Bone Joint Surg. *40B*:454, 1958.

Moberg, E.: Criticism and study of methods for examining sensibility of the hand. Neurology *12*:8, 1962.

Moberg, E.: Relation of touch and deep sensation to hand reconstruction. Am. J. Surg. *109*:353, 1965.

Moberg, E.: Correspondence letter, The American Society for Surgery of the Hand, December 5, 1969.

Mountcastle, V. B.: Medical Physiology, 13th ed. Saint Louis, C. V. Mosby Company, 1974.

Omer, G. E. Jr.: Evaluation and reconstruction of the forearm and hand after acute traumatic peripheral nerve injuries. J. Bone Joint Surg. *50A*:1454, 1968.

Omer, G. E. Jr.: The Assessment of Peripheral Nerve Injuries. In Cramer, L. M., and Chase, R. A.: Symposium on the Hand. Educ. Found. Am. Soc. Plast. Reconstr. Surg. Saint Louis, C. V. Mosby Company, 1971, Vol. 3, p. 1.

Omer, G. E. Jr.: Sensation and sensibility in the upper extremity. Clin. Orthop. *104*:30, 1974.

Omer, G. E. Jr., and Vogel, J. A.: Determination of physiological length of a reconstructed muscle-tendon unit through muscle stimulation. J. Bone Joint Surg. *47A*:304, 1965.

Omer, G. E. Jr., Day, D. J., Ratliff, H. and Lambert, P.: The neurovascular cutaneous island pedicles for deficient median nerve sensibility. New technique and results of serial functional tests. J. Bone Joint Surg. *52A*:1181, 1970.

O'Riain, S.: New and simple test of nerve function in the hand. Br. Med. J. *3*:615, 1973.

Seddon, H.: Surgical Disorders of the Peripheral Nerves. 2nd ed., New York, Churchill Livingstone, 1975.

Stopford, J. S. B.: The nerve supply of the interphalangeal and metacarpo-phalangeal joints. J. Anat. *56*:1–11, 1921.

Tinel, J.: Nerve Wounds: Symptomatology of Peripheral Nerve Lesions Caused by War Wounds. (Translated by F. Rothwell, edited by C. A. Joll.) New York, William Wood and Company, 1918.

von Frey, M.: Zur Physiologic der Juckempfindung. Arch. Neerl. de Physiologie *7*:142, La Haye, 1922.

Weber, E. H.: Veber den Tastsinn. Arch. Anat. Physiol. Wissensch. Med. p. 152, 1835.

Weinstein, S.: Tactile sensitivity of the phalanges. Percept. Mot. Skills *14*:351, 1962.

Werner, J. L., and Omer, G. E. Jr.: Evaluating cutaneous pressure sensation of the hand. Am. J. Occup. Ther. *24*:347, 1970.

Wynn-Parry, C. B., and Salter, M: Sensory re-education after median nerve lesions. Hand *8*:250, 1976.

2

MOTOR FUNCTION TESTING

LENNART MANNERFELT

Brachial Plexus
Axillary Nerve
Radial Nerve
Musculocutaneous Nerve
Median Nerve
Ulnar Nerve
Obturator Nerve
Femoral Nerve
Sciatic Nerve

GENERAL CONSIDERATIONS

The five main nerves of the upper extremity and the three main nerves of the lower extremity are all mixed; that is, they are both motor and sensory.

The state of a damaged mixed nerve, therefore, must be investigated by testing both its key muscles *and* its own sensory area. An example of this is radial nerve damage in fracture of the humerus: Although complete motor paralysis exists, some degree of sensation can be elicited on the dorsal aspect of the thumb. This indicates a partial lesion or neuropraxia with continuity of the radial nerve. Therefore, when examining a damaged peripheral mixed nerve always integrate adequate sensory testing with motor function testing.

To examine a complex peripheral nerve lesion is sometimes a challenge. The investigation must be logical and systematic, going from a proximal to a distal direction, and is based on a thorough knowledge of anatomy. In fresh, acute cases, as well as in old ones, there are several problems and questions to be solved and answered. The following check list should be followed:

1. Is the lesion closed or open?
2. Is more than one nerve injured?

3. Is the lesion total or partial?
4. What is the level of the lesion?
5. Is the nerve injured at more than one level? — multiple skin wounds.
6. Based on knowledge or diagnostic blocks, are there signs of nerve anomalies or double innervation?
7. In old cases, a) is some degree of reinnervation present? b) are trick movements present?

In answering these questions, the motor function is used as an instrument, and, in recording the state of each muscle tested, the following system* is suggested:

0 = No contraction.
1 = Flicker or trace of contraction.
2 = Active movement, with gravity eliminated.
3 = Active movement against gravity.
4 = Active movement against gravity and some resistance.
5 = Normal power.

When testing motor function, it is imperative that the examiner look for and feels the contraction of the specific muscle. Palpate the relaxed muscle; is it smooth or fibrosed? Pain, whatever its origin, always has an adverse effect on muscle testing. Blocking a neuroma or a painful point can sometimes help the examiner to better evaluate the function of the tested muscle. Finally, because muscle and sensory testing is tiresome for the patient, always explain the nature and object of the examination to him or her. Perform the examination in a quiet room, and pause if the patient becomes tired or lacks concentration.

Motor function testing can be qualitative, semiquantitative (0 to 5 system), or quantified with the aid of dynamometers such as the Collins, Bechtol-Jamar Vigorimeter or Intrinsicmeter.

The Use of Reflexes

The tendon hammer is used in the study of reflexes while the muscle is contracted against resistance. In lower motor neuron disorders, such as division or severe damage of a peripheral nerve, the reflexes are absent. Reflexes are significantly exaggerated when upper motor neuron damage, division, or disease is present.

UPPER EXTREMITY

Brachial Plexus Lesions (C5–T1)

If possible, injuries to the brachial plexus should be differentiated by zones: Zone I lesions are those that occur proximal to the rami communicantes grisei (preganglionic). Zone II lesions occur distal to Zone I and proximal to the clavicle. Zone III injuries are those that occur distal to the clavicle (Fig. 2–1).

---

*Medical Research Council: Aids to the examination of the peripheral nervous system. Memorandum No. 45, London: Her Majesty's Stationery Office, 1976.

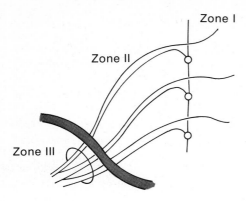

Zone I

Zone II

Zone III

Figure 2–1 Levels of brachial plexus injury.

Total Brachial Plexus Injuries, Zone I

A flail arm with paralysis of all the muscles of the hand is observed. There is no sensation, but the sudoriferic function — sweating — is intact. Thus, without sensation, the Ninhydrin test will show full representation of the sweat points in the hand.

Upper Plexus Paralysis (C5–C6), Erb-Duchenne Type

In this disorder, there is paralysis of the biceps, deltoid, brachialis, supraspinatus, infraspinatus, and rhomboids. When the sixth cervical branch is involved, there is also weakness in the triceps, pectoralis major, and the two radial carpal extensor muscles as well. The position of the extremity is classic: the arm hangs adducted, internally rotated at the shoulder, the elbow extended, and the forearm pronated in the so-called "waiter's tip" position. The elbow cannot be flexed and, because of paralysis of the infraspinous muscle, external rotation of the shoulder is lost. Wrist extension is impaired only in C6 lesions. Most finger movements are intact. The biceps reflex is absent.

Lower Plexus Paralysis (C8–T1), Dejerine-Klumpke Type

Here, the first dorsal nerve (T1) is usually the only one damaged, but C8 may be involved. All the intrinsic muscles of the hand are paralyzed. When C8 is involved, there is weakness of the flexor carpi ulnaris and flexor digitorum profundus of the little finger. Sometimes Horner's syndrome (ptosis, miosis, enophthalmos) is concomitant, thus indicating an avulsion of the T1 root from the spinal cord.

Key muscles to be tested are the intrinsic muscles of the hand (see under Ulnar and Median nerves), the flexor carpi ulnaris, and the flexor digitorum profundus of the little finger.

Axillary Nerve (C5–C6)

The key muscle to be tested is the deltoid. When testing the motor function of this muscle the examiner should stand behind the patient and firmly grip the scapula. Ask the patient to actively abduct the arm from the hanging position; the palm of the hand should point downward. Against resistance, look for and feel the muscle contraction. *Trick movements* to be concerned with are that the long head of the biceps, coracobrachialis, and/or trapezium can imitate shoulder abduction. The *sensory area* corresponds roughly to the shape of the muscle itself.

Radial (Musculospiral) Nerve (C5–T1)

Branches and Key Muscles*

1. *Common branch*
     *1.1 Triceps
     *1.2 Brachioradialis
     *1.3 Extensor carpi radialis longus and brevis
2. *Posterior Interosseous Nerve*
     2.1 Superficial muscle layer
       *2.1.1 Extensor digitorum communis II-V
       *2.1.2 Extensor digiti quinti proprius
       *2.1.3 Extensor carpi ulnaris
     2.2 Deeper muscle layer
       2.21 Abductor pollicis longus
       2.2.2 Extensor pollicis brevis
       *2.2.3 Extensor pollicis longus
       *2.2.4 Extensor indicis proprius
       2.2.5 Sensory branch to wrist joint
3. *Superficial Radial Nerve — sensory dorsally to the thumb.*

MOTOR FUNCTION TESTING OF KEY MUSCLES

1.1 Triceps. The patient is standing. The arm is held horizontally and fully abducted at the shoulder; the forearm is flexed 90 degrees. The patient is asked to actively extend the forearm at the elbow. While resistance is exerted, the examiner sees and feels the contraction of the muscle. When this technique is used, trick movements are avoided.

1.2 Brachioradialis. Test active elbow flexion against resistance. See and palpate the muscle belly contracting in the proximal, radial part of the forearm. Note that the biceps, brachialis (musculocutaneous nerve), and pronator teres (median nerve) have similar action.

1.3 Extensor Carpi Radialis Longus and Brevis. With the patient's forearm fully pronated on a table, active dorsal and dorsal-radial extension of the wrist joint against resistance is evaluated. Note that the extensor carpi ulnaris extends the wrist joint in ulnar abduction.

A special test can be done to evaluate regeneration of the extensor carpi radialis longus and brevis. Let the patient grasp a dynamometer to measure the force of the grip. If the extensor carpi radialis longus and brevis are weak, the measured force will be low, and the wrist will tend to go into flexion. As regeneration proceeds, the measured value rises, and the patient can hold the wrist in extension. Record the dynamometer value together with the wrist position, in degrees, in flexion, in neutrality, and in extension.

2.1.1 Extensor Digitorum Communis II-V. The forearm is pronated on the table with the wrist joint extended. The four ulnar fingers are flexed in a fist. In this position, the patient should be able to fully extend the fingers at the metacarpophalangeal joints. *Trick movements*: In active tenodesis brought about by paresis of the radial nerve the four ulnar fingers passively extend when the wrist drops in a flexion position. It is important to keep the wrist in extension throughout the evaluation of the extensor digitorum communis.

2.1.2 Extensor Digiti Quinti Proprius. The patient assumes the same position as in test 2.1.1. After making a fist the patient should extend the little finger only. He is not allowed to grasp the three radial fingers with the thumb.

2.1.3 Extensor Carpi Ulnaris. Test ulnar deviation and dorsoulnar extension of the wrist joint against resistance.

2.2.3 Extensor Pollicis Longus. Both forearms are on a table, in mid-position between pronation and supination, and the elbows are in 90 degree flexion. The wrist is in mid-position between extension and flexion. The four ulnar fingers are totally extended, the palms facing each other. The patient adducts both thumbs to the volar aspect of the index fingers. He or she is asked to fully extend (not abduct) the thumbs. Look for difference in extension. Strength can be evaluated by fixing the basal phalanx of the thumb and testing active extension of the distal phalanx against resistance. *Trick movement:* Intrinsics (abductor pollicis brevis, median nerve, and adductor pollicis-ulnar nerve) take part in extension of the distal phalanx of the thumb, but never with force and never to a position of hyperextension.

2.2.4 Extensor Indicis Proprius. Use the same technique as for 2.1.2, but request extension of the index finger.

Sensory Area

The total distal dorsal aspect of the thumb is innervated by the superficial radial nerve. The radial-dorsal part of the hand and the basal phalanx of the index and middle finger can also be supplied by this nerve.

Differential Diagnosis and Pitfalls

A wrist drop could be seen in rheumatoid arthritis because of rupture of all three carpal extensors. Also in rheumatoid arthritis, a defect in finger extension (mostly on the dorsal-ulnar aspect) is obvious in the so-called ulnar-head, or Vaughan-Jackson, syndrome — attrition ruptures of the extensor digitorum communis IV and V and extensor digiti quinti (Bäckdahl, 1963). In this same disease, rupture of the extensor pollicis longus is common. This tendon rupture is also seen in connection with (and sometimes following) Colles' fracture. Lead poisoning, diabetes, and some virus diseases involve the radial nerve, causing wrist drop or finger drop, or both, without sensory disturbance. Hysterical paresis with wrist drop is known, and can be clinically and electrically distinguished.

Important Clinical Syndrome

Posterior interosseous-nerve paralysis, refer to Chapters 34 and 52.

Musculocutaneous Nerve (C5-C6)

The key muscles are the biceps and the brachialis.

Branches and Key Muscles

1. Biceps
2. Brachialis
   MOTOR FUNCTION TESTING OF KEY MUSCLES. The forearm is in active flexion at the elbow. The examiner applies resistance and sees and feels the two muscle bellies contracting. The examiner must always test and observe the co-action of the brachioradial muscle (radial nerve). Supination of the forearm minimizes the action of this muscle. *Trick movement:* The pronator teres (median nerve) also takes part in elbow flexion.
   SENSORY AREA.   This nerve terminates with a sensible area more or less in the distal volar radial aspect of the forearm, and it sometimes innervates the thenar skin area.

Differential Diagnosis and Pitfalls

The radial nerve sometimes takes part in the innervation of the brachialis muscle.

Ulnar Nerve (C8–T1)

Branches and Key Muscles*

1. *Common branch*
   *1.1 Flexor carpi ulnaris
   *1.2 Flexor digitorum profundus of the ring and little fingers
2. *Deep branch*
   *2.1 Abductor digiti quinti
   2.2 Flexor digiti quinti brevis
   2.3 Opponens digiti quinti
   2.4 Lumbrical IV
   *2.5 Third and fourth dorsal and volar interosseous
   2.6 Lumbrical III
   *2.7 Second web space dorsal and volar interosseous
   *2.8 Adductor pollicis
   *2.9 First web space – First dorsal interosseous
   2.10 Flexor pollicis brevis – deep head

3. *Sensory — ulnar 1½ digits*

MOTOR FUNCTION TESTING OF KEY MUSCLES

1.1 Flexor Carpi Ulnaris. With the patient's forearm fully supinated, place resistance on the palm of the hand and ask the patient to flex his or her wrist joint. Palpate the contracted tendon of the muscle. Allow the patient to relax so that the muscle tendon is easily movable from side to side. Note that volar flexion also is supported by the flexor carpi radialis and the palmaris longus (median nerve), but that these two muscles do not abduct in the ulnar direction. *Trick movement*: In cases of complete ulnar and median lesions, sometimes a wrist flexion elicited by the abductor pollicis longus can be seen. This is due to the gradual shifting of the abductor pollicis longus tendon to the volar aspect of the radioulnar axis of the wrist joint.

1.2 Flexor Digitorum Profundus of the Ring and Little Fingers. With the patient's hand fully supinated on the table, support the middle phalanx of the fourth and fifth finger. Ask the patient to flex the end phalanges against resistance. The ring finger flexor digitorum profundus is sometimes doubly innervated from the median nerve. *Trick movement*: Adhesions of all profundus muscles in/or proximal to the carpal tunnel in ulnar paralysis could give some action also in the flexor digitorum profundus of the little finger.

2.1 Abductor Digiti Quinti. With the wrist in a zero degree position, the patient is asked to abduct the little finger against the examiner's resistance. Visualize and feel the muscle belly. Palpate the relaxed muscle. *Trick movements*: In longstanding cases of low ulnar nerve injuries with intact innervation of the flexor carpi ulnaris, this muscle can — via the pisiform and a fibrosed abductor digiti quinti — simulate ulnar abduction of the little finger. Palpation of the muscle belly (hard and fibrosed) confirms the condition. Note that forced finger extension with the ulnar extrinsic extensors can also deviate the little finger ulnarward.

2.5 Third and Fourth Web Space Dorsal and Volar Interosseous Muscles. The examiner holds the little and middle fingers of the affected hand apart and fixed. The patient is asked to perform side to side movements of the ring finger. In addition, the middle finger should abduct ulnarly well against resistance. Similarly, the little should adduct well. Test for intrinsic contracture. The finger to be tested is blocked in hyperextension at the metacarpophalangeal joint. Then passive flexion of the proximal interphalangeal joint is tested. If the proximal interphalangeal joint can be flexed fully there is no intrinsic contracture.

2.7 Second Web Space Volar and Dorsal Interosseus Muscles. Test side to side movements of the middle finger. The technique is similar to that in test 2.5. In addition, adduction of the index finger against resistance should be tested. Test for intrinsic contracture. *Trick movement*: Ulnar abduction of the index finger can be performed by action of the extensor indicis proprius.

2.8 Adductor Pollicis. The patient's elbow is flexed and the forearm is in midposition between pronation and supination, with the wrist joint in zero degree position and all four ulnar fingers extended. From the fully abducted (pronated) position, the thumb goes into palmar adduction and "lands" at the volar aspect of the base of the extended index finger. In this position the thumbnail should be at right angles to the other finger nails. Test for strength by pulling the thumb away from the index finger. *Trick movement*: The extensor pollicis longus ("extensor pollicis adducens" of Fick, 1845) can adduct the thumb, but only with limited force. Look for Froment's sign. In maximal volar flexion of the wrist joint the axis of motion shifts, and the extensor pollicis longus produces no adduction movement of the thumb.

2.9 First Dorsal Interosseous Muscle. Assume the same starting position as in test 2.8. Test the abducted index finger against resistance. Look for and palpate the muscle. This muscle can sometimes be doubly innervated by the median nerve. *Trick movement:* In cases of complete ulnar nerve paralysis the extensor digitorum communis of the index finger can sometimes abduct the index finger.

Sensory Area

The whole *dorsal* area of the little finger is innervated by the ulnar nerve (dorsal cutaneous branch), which is important when determining levels of lacerations in the distal ulnar volar forearm. In the volar aspect, the entire little finger and the ulnar half of the ring finger are usually supplied by the ulnar nerve.

Differential Diagnosis and Pitfalls

Rarely, all intrinsic hand muscles are innervated by the branches of the median nerve. In some instances of complete high laceration of the ulnar nerve, the radial intrinsics (adductor pollicis and first dorsal interosseous) may still function, the only sign of an ulnar lesion being total loss of sensation in the little finger and paralysis of the more ulnar located intrinsics (abductor digiti quinti, opponens V, flexor brevis V, and the ulnar dorsal and volar interosseous muscles). The reason for this is the important so-called Martin-Gruber anastomosis

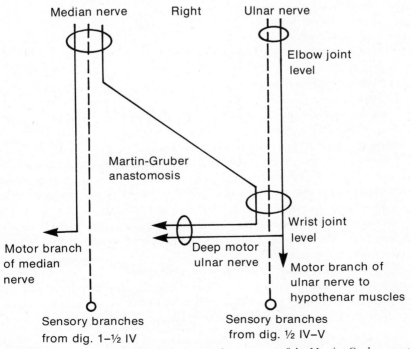

Figure 2–2   Schematic drawing to demonstrate the entrance of the Martin–Gruber anastomosis in the distal ulnar nerve.

between the median and ulnar nerves in the forearm. This neural connection supplies fibers for the radial intrinsic muscles via the median nerve to the ulnar nerve distal to the laceration (Figure 2–2).

Important Clinical Syndromes

These are the cubital tunnel syndrome and compressions in Guyon's canal; compressions of the ulnar nerve due to aneurysms of the ulnar artery or a ganglion in or distal to Guyon's canal and lesions of the deep motor branch of the ulnar nerve in connection with fractures of the hook of the hamate.

Median Nerve (C5-T1)

Branches and Key Muscles*

1. *Common branch after union of components from the lateral and medial cords*
   *1.1 Pronator teres
   *1.2 Flexor carpi radialis
    1.3 Palmaris longus
   *1.4 Flexor digitorum superficialis of the digits—II–V
2. *Anterior interosseous nerve*
   *2.1 Flexor pollicis longus
   *2.2 Flexor digitorum profundus of the index and long fingers
    2.3 Pronator quadratus
    2.4 Sensory (wrist joint)
3. *Palmar cutaneous nerve*
    3.1 *Sensory—median palmar cutaneous branch*
4. *Motor branch*
   *4.1 Abductor pollicis brevis
    4.2 Opponens pollicis
    4.3 Flexor pollicis brevis, superficial head
5. *Sensory—radial 3½ digits*

MOTOR FUNCTION TESTING OF KEY MUSCLES

1.1 Pronator Teres.   The patient stands with the arm in contact with the trunk, the elbow flexed to 90 degrees, and the forearm in full supination. The examiner holds the patient's arm fixed at the cubital fossa, and grasps the patient's hand with the other hand. The patient is asked to pronate, and to draw his or her arm and hand inward. Test the strength and palpate the muscle. Let the patient relax the muscle. Note that the pronator quadratus (median nerve) also takes part in the pronation.

1.2 Flexor Carpi Radialis.   The forearm is fully supinated on a table. Against resistance, test palmar flexion of the wrist. Note that the flexor carpi ulnaris and palmaris longus also take part in wrist flexion. *Trick movement*: With total ulnar and median paralysis the abductor pollicis longus can act as a wrist flexor.

1.4 Flexor Digitorum Superficialis of the Digits. When testing, for example, the flexor digitorum superficialis of the long finger, the examiner fully extends the patient's index, ring, and little fingers by holding them beyond the distal interphalangeal joints, thus locking the flexor digitorum profundus muscle mass. The examiner then asks the patient to flex the middle finger. This will be accomplished at the proximal interphalangeal joint (Apley's sign [Apley, 1956]). The same test can be applied to the flexor digitorum superficialis of the ring finger. Sometimes the flexor superficialis of the index finger can be tested this way, as occasionally can the flexor superficialis of the little finger, but the test is not as accurate for these digits.

2.1 Flexor Pollicis Longus. Hold the proximal phalanx of the thumb in a fixed position. While placing resistance with the other hand, test the force of the muscle as the patient flexes the terminal phalanx.

2.2 Flexor Digitorum Produndus II and III. Fix the middle phalanx. While applying pressure to the terminal phalanx, ask the patient to flex. Test the force of the flexion.

4.1 Abductor Pollicis Brevis. The forearm is on the table, in midposition between supination and pronation. The wrist joint is in zero degree position, and the four ulnar fingers are fully extended. The ulnar aspect of the thumb touches the volar aspect of the index finger. The thumbnail should now be at right angles to the other finger nails. From this position the patient is asked to perform an antipalmar abduction (antipulsion). This is a combination of abduction and pronation of the thumb. Test the strength in this position. Look for and palpate the muscle. Then, let the patient relax, and palpate the muscle once again.

4.2 Opponens Pollicis. Ask the patient to pinch hard with the thumb against the pulp of the little finger. Put your middle finger in the "O" formed, draw your finger through, and evaluate the strength of the pinch.

Sensory Area

The palmar branch innervates the skin of the thenar eminence. This nerve is diagnostically important when evaluating level problems in median nerve injury proximal to the carpal tunnel. A lesion in which the sensibility of the thenar area is intact indicates the level distal to the origin of this sensory branch. Furthermore, the radial three and a half digits are usually innervated by the median nerve.

Differential Diagnosis and Pitfalls

In rheumatoid arthritis and in some rare cases of pronounced arthrosis deformans of the wrist, sharp bony prominences and spiculae penetrate the floor of the carpal tunnel. Rupture of the flexor pollicis and flexor digitorum profundus of the index finger, which simulates an anterior interosseous syndrome, has been known to occur (Mannerfelt and Norman, 1969).

LOWER EXTREMITY

Obturator Nerve (L2-L4)

The key muscles are the adductors of the hip.

MOTOR FUNCTION TESTING. The patient, while in a supine position, adducts his limb against resistance. The examiner palpates the adductor muscle bellies (adductor magnus, brevis, and longus).

SENSORY AREA. The proximal, medial, and dorsomedial aspects of the thigh are affected.

Femoral Nerve (L2-L4)

The key muscle is the quadriceps femoris.

MOTOR FUNCTION TESTING. The patient lies supine on the examining table, with his or her hip and knee flexed. Against resistance, the patient extends the leg. The examiner looks for and palpates the quadriceps femoris muscle belly (Figure 2–3).

Sensory Area

This is the anterior aspect of the thigh, with proximal and distal variations, through the terminal saphenous branch to the medial aspect of the leg and foot.

Differential Diagnosis and Pitfalls

In cases of femoral nerve injuries, the patients can, to some extent, with the aid of the tensor fascia lata (the superior gluteal nerve), extend the knee (Seddon, 1972).

Sciatic Nerve (L4-S3)

Branches and Key Muscles*

1. *Common branch*
    1.1 Semitendinosus
   *1.2 Biceps, long and short heads
    1.3 Semimembranosus
2. *Posterior tibial nerve*
   *2.1 Gastrocnemius, medial and lateral heads
    2.2 Soleus
   *2.3 Tibialis posterior
   *2.4 Flexor digitorum longus
   *2.5 Flexor hallucis longus
   *2.6 Medial and lateral plantar nerves to intrinsic muscles of foot

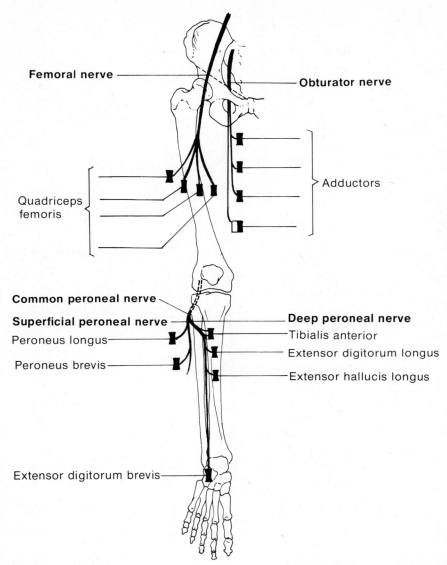

Femoral nerve

Obturator nerve

Quadriceps
femoris

Adductors

Common peroneal nerve

Superficial peroneal nerve

Peroneus longus

Peroneus brevis

Deep peroneal nerve

Tibialis anterior

Extensor digitorum longus

Extensor hallucis longus

Extensor digitorum brevis

Figure 2–3 Diagram of the anterior aspect of lower limb and muscles. Modified from: Medical Research Council: Aids to the examination of the peripheral nervous system. Memorandum No. 45, London: Her Majesty's Stationery Office, 1976.

3. *Common peroneal nerve*
   3.1 *Superficial peroneal nerve*
      *3.1.1 Peroneus longus
      *3.1.2 Peroneus brevis
   3.2 *Deep peroneal nerve*
      *3.2.1 Tibialis anterior
      3.2.2 Extensor digitorum longus
      *3.2.3 Extensor hallucis longus

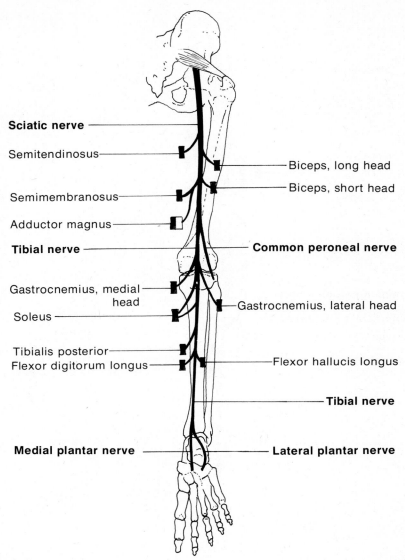

Figure 2–4   Diagram of nerves on posterior aspect of lower limb, and muscles. Modified from: Medical Research Council: Aids to the examination of the peripheral nervous system. Memorandum No. 45, London: Her Majesty's Stationery Office, 1976.

MOTOR FUNCTION TESTING IN KEY MUSCLES (Figure 2–4)

1.2 Biceps.   The patient lies prone, with the leg flexed at the knee. He or she tries to maintain this leg position while the examiner exerts pressure against the position. The biceps tendon can be seen and felt laterally.

2.1 Gastrocnemius.   The patient, who is lying on his side, tries to plantar flex his foot against resistance. The knee should be stretched. See and palpate the muscle. The soleus and tibialis posterior both take part in this movement. The peronei (superficial peroneal nerve) also are involved, but weakly.

2.3 Tibialis Posterior. The patient actively turns the foot inward (inversion) against resistance. The tendon can be felt just behind the medial malleolus. Note that the tibialis anterior (deep peroneal nerve) also takes part in this movement.

2.5 Flexor Hallucis Longus. This is the last extrinsic muscle innervated by the posterior tibial nerve, and is most easily tested against resistance. Plantar flexion of the great toe is a function of this muscle.

3.1.1 and 3.1.2 Peronei. The patient tries to evert the foot against resistance. Both tendons, in action, can be seen and felt behind and distal to the lateral malleolus.

3.2.1 Tibialis Anterior. The tibialis anterior muscle, together with the extensor digitorum longus, dorsiflexes the foot. The muscle belly of the tibialis anterior is seen to contract, and can be palpated.

3.2.3 Extensor Hallucis Longus. The patient extends the great toe against resistance. The tendon is well seen and palpable. A good trick, here, to evaluate strength is to counteract its extension by repeated stretchings in the plantar direction and to compare strength and tenacity with those of the other great toe.

Sensory Area

The usual area of loss of cutaneous sensation in lesion of the sciatic nerve consists of the lateral and posterolateral aspects of the leg and foot.

REFERENCES

Apley, A. C.: Test for the power of the flexor digitorum sublimis. Brit. Med. J. *1*:6, 1956.
Bäckdahl, M.: The caput ulnae syndrome in rheumatoid arthritis. A study of the morphology, abnormal anatomy and clinical picture. Acta Rheumatol. Scand. Suppl. 5:1, 1963.
Daniels, L. and Worthingham, C.: Muscle Testing. 3rd Ed., Philadelphia, W. B. Saunders Company, 1972.
Fick, L.: Physiologische Anatomie des Menschen. Verlag von Christian Ernst Kollmann, Leipzig, 1845:1.
Haymaker, W., and Woodhall, B.: Peripheral Nerve Injuries, Principles of Diagnosis. 2nd Ed., Philadelphia, W. B. Saunders Company, 1953.
Lister G.: The Hand: Diagnosis and Indications. London, Churchill Livingstone, 1977.
Mannerfelt, L.: Studies on the hand in ulnar nerve paralysis. Acta Orthop. Scand., Suppl. 87, 1966.
Mannerfelt, L., and Norman, O.: Attrition ruptures of flexor tendons in rheumatoid arthritis caused by bony spurs in the carpal tunnel. J. Bone Joint Surg., (Brit.) *51*:270, 1969.
Medical Research Council: Aids to the examination of the peripheral nervous system. Memorandum No. 45, London: Her Majesty's Stationery Office, 1976.
Mumenthaler, M., and Schliack, H.: Läsionen peripherer Nerven, Diagnostik und Therapie. Stuttgart, Georg Thieme Verlag, 1977.
Seddon, H. J.: Peripheral Nerve Injuries. Medical Research Council Special Report Series No. 282, London: Her Majesty's Stationery Office, 1954.
Seddon, H. J.: Surgical Disorders of the Peripheral Nerves. London, Churchill Livingstone, 1972.
Spinner, M.: Injuries to the Major Branches of Peripheral Nerves of the Forearm. 2nd Ed. Philadelphia, W. B. Saunders Company, 1978.

3

ELECTRODIAGNOSIS IN PERIPHERAL NERVE LESIONS

EDWARD F. DELAGI

Electrodiagnosis makes a significant contribution to the management of nerve lesions by offering data as to the nature, location, and degree of nerve involvement and the viability of the involved muscle. It should be considered as an extension of the clinical examination and not purely a laboratory procedure because of the many nerves and muscles which may or may not require examination in a specific case and the many possible modalities of examination, most of which are uncomfortable and time consuming. The physician performing the electrodiagnostic tests must precede them with a thorough neurological and kinesiological examination so that he may apply the appropriate modalities and examine the relevant nerves and muscles. It also requires a dialogue between the referring physician and the electrodiagnostician, in which the referring physician shares all pertinent information and formulates specific questions to which he wishes specific answers, and the physician–electrodiagnostician, in turn, reports not only the answers to such questions but any other diagnostic possibilities raised by his examination.

The physician who manages peripheral nerve injuries requires a basic knowledge of the common modalities of electrodiagnosis. These are electromyography, nerve conduction studies, and electrical muscle stimulation studies.

Other modalities, such as skin resistance to delineate areas of sympathetic denervation, single muscle fiber studies, and repetitive stimulation to uncover myoneural junction dysfunction, as in myasthenia gravis and Eaton-Lambert syndrome, can also make a valuable contribution when indicated.

ELECTROMYOGRAPHY

Electromyography is the diagnostic evaluation of the electrical potentials produced by muscle tissue.

These potentials arise from muscle fibers normally organized into motor units, each motor unit consisting of a single anterior horn cell (motor neuron), its axon cylinder, the unmyelinated axon twigs, motor end plates, and all the muscle fibers it innervates.

A particular motor neuron may innervate from 15 to 2000 muscle fibers, depending on the function of the muscle. Muscles requiring precise movement, such as the extraocular muscles of the eye and the opponens pollicis of the thumb have less muscle fibers per motor unit than those which subserve strength, such as the antigravity muscles. For instance, the superior rectus muscle has about 23 muscle fibers per motor unit and the opponens pollicis 13, while the anterior tibial has 610 and the gastrocnemius over 2000. This is of importance in electromyography, since the number of muscle fibers and their spatial arrangement in a particular motor unit will influence the amplitude and duration of the electrical potential it produces when it is activated.

The excitation and depolarization of the muscle fiber membrane is the source of the electrical potential we study by means of the electromyograph. This is similar to the process of propagation of the nerve impulse in nervous tissue. There is a difference in resting potential between the interior of the muscle cell and the exterior of the membrane in the order of about 60–80 mV. With depolarization at the motor end plate a "wave of negativity" traverses the length of the muscle fiber. This propagated electrical potential, or so-called "action potential," is made visible and audible by the electromyograph. From certain characteristics of these potentials inferences can be made as to the physiological state of the muscle itself and that of the nerve innervating it.

The patient is grounded to the apparatus, a needle electrode is inserted into the muscle, and the muscle is examined in four conditions: (1) on electrode insertion, (2) with the muscle at rest, (3) on minimum contraction, and (4) on maximum contraction (Fig. 3–1).

Response to Electrode Insertion

Normally, there is a short burst of activity on electrode insertion that lasts for only a few milliseconds. In conditions in which there has been some change in the stability of the muscle membrane, such as beginning denervation, there is a prolongation of the response to insertion or there may be characteristic very prolonged discharges, as in myotonia and pseudomyotonia. In myotonia there is a high frequency discharge that rapidly changes in frequency and amplitude. This gives rise to a sound that has been likened to a diving airplane and is spoken of as "the dive bomber" effect. This is found in all forms of myotonia.

Pseudomyotonia is also a high frequency discharge but lacks the waxing and waning of the myotonic discharge. The sound of this discharge has been likened to the sound of a sawmill in that it is a steady, continuous sound with no change in pitch or amplitude. This phenomenon may be found in any condition that produces muscle membrane instability, such as muscular dystrophy or denervation due to anterior horn cell disease or neuropathy.

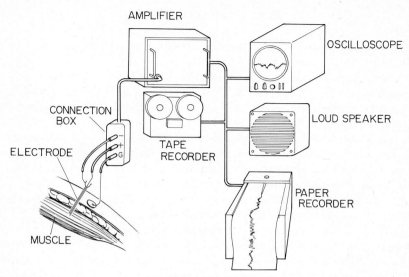

Figure 3–1   Block diagram of a typical electromyographic scheme demonstrating the intramuscular coaxial electrode, display, and recording equipment.

The electromyographer may become aware of fibrotic changes taking place in the muscle he is studying by noting the amount of force needed to penetrate it with the intramuscular electrode.

At Rest

A normal muscle is electrically silent and no potentials are visible or audible except if the electrode is inserted in the vicinity of the end plate zone, in which case we hear and see end plate potentials.

End plate potentials produce a rushing sound in the loudspeaker and many small amplitude high frequency deflections on the screen of the oscilloscope. Because the sound is similar to that heard when one places one's ear to a conch shell, it is referred to as "seashell." If one explores further in this region one is likely to see negative spike potentials of one to two msec. duration. These can be differentiated from true fibrillation potentials (see below) by their location in the vicinity of a "seashell" discharge and by the fact that their initial deflection is negative in polarity.

Other types of spontaneous activity in resting muscle are as follows.

Fasciculations are spontaneous, nonvoluntary contractions of the muscle fibers of an entire motor unit. They are arrhythmic in occurrence, and the parameters of the potential may be those of the normal or abnormal motor unit producing it. Fasciculations are frequently found in pathological conditions involving the anterior horn cells (amyotrophic lateral sclerosis and progressive muscular atrophy), less frequently in nerve root compression and neuropathies. Occasionally, fasciculations are reported as an isolated finding without any other indication of nerve pathology and are referred to as benign fasciculations.

Myokymia is the spontaneous synchronous discharge of several motor units at one time. They are considered to be benign, occurring frequently in fatigued muscles.

Fibrillations are spontaneous, nonvoluntary discharges of single muscle fibers and are usually considered to be pathognomonic of denervation, although they have been occasionally described as occurring in certain upper neuron lesions during the period of diaschisis of spinal shock or cerebrovascular accident, and in myopathies. These potentials are of short duration (0.5 to 3 msec), are small in amplitude (50–150 μV), and are both rhythmic and arrhythmic in frequency. They produce a high pitched clicking sound in the loudspeaker of the electromyograph.

Positive sharp waves are spontaneous, nonvoluntary potentials that have a rapid positive phase with a gradual return to the baseline and then a small negative phase with a slow return to the baseline. They are from 10 to 100 msec in duration and 50 μV to 1 mV in amplitude.

Although the exact mechanism for the production of these potentials is not known, they have the same clinical significance as fibrillation, and they are usually accepted as evidence of denervation.

Minimum Voluntary Contraction

On minimum voluntary contraction the normal muscle produces motor unit potentials that represent a summation of all the electrical activity produced by all the muscle fibers of the motor unit. Depending on the size of the motor unit and the spatial arrangement of its muscle fibers, potentials have a duration of 3 to 15 msec and an amplitude of 200 to 500 μV. These potentials are triphasic with an initial positive phase.

Dystrophic potentials are shorter in duration and smaller in amplitude, having a duration of less than 3 msec. in muscles which normally have motor unit potentials of 5 to 15 msec in duration. These may have the exact parameters of fibrillations but occur only on volition and not at rest. Polyphasic potentials having an amplitude of 50 to 200 μV and a duration of 5 to 12 msec are usually considered evidence of primary muscle disease such as muscular dystrophy or polymyositis, although they have also been described as occurring in some phases of denervation.

Large polyphasic potentials are usually 15 to 20 msec in duration, markedly polyphasic, and very high in amplitude (up to 10,000 μV). These are considered to be the product of collateral reinnervation and are found frequently in partially denervated muscles and in chronic, slowly denervating conditions such as the anterior horn cell disease of amyotrophic lateral sclerosis, progressive spinal atrophy, or longstanding radiculopathy.

Nascent potentials are small amplitude, short duration potentials found in previously denervated muscle, and are usually the first sign of reinnervation.

Maximum Voluntary Contraction

On maximum voluntary contraction a normal muscle produces a pattern of activity that covers the face of the oscilloscope, and the baseline cannot be distinguished. There is a roaring sound produced in the loudspeaker. This is called an *interference pattern*. It occurs when considerable resistance is given to the muscle being tested.

A *partial interference pattern*, in which the baseline is not completely obliterated, indicates some weakness of the muscle involved, if we can be assured that the patient is making a maximum effort. This pattern is sometimes inhibited because of pain either due to a pre-existing condition or to the intramuscular electrode. The gastrocnemius is notable for being able to produce only a partial interference pattern because it is difficult to give sufficient resistance manually with the patient in the recumbent position.

Isolated potentials, or "picket fence" pattern, are seen in the marked weakness of severely denervated muscle.

Early interference, or early recruitment, the development of an interference pattern on relatively slight effort, is seen in primary muscle disease.

Noting the pattern of denervation as revealed by electromyography makes it possible to localize lesions to specific levels of peripheral nerve, plexus, root, or anterior horn cell.

If the lesion is proximal to the bifurcation of the anterior primary and the posterior divisions, we are likely to find denervation potentials in the paravertebral muscles and limb muscles. If distal to this point, we will only find evidence of denervation in the limb muscles.

Nerve Conduction

The conduction characteristics of a motor or sensory nerve can reveal important information regarding the location and nature of peripheral nerve lesions.

In motor nerve conduction studies the nerve is stimulated and the evoked response produced in a muscle it innervates is observed as to shape, latency, amplitude, and duration. Such latency includes not only the time the propagated impulse took to traverse the nerve but the time it took to pass through the unmyelinated axon twigs, the myoneural junction, and the depolarization of the muscle fibers. If we wish to calculate the nerve conduction velocity, we must stimulate the nerve at another point and subtract the distal latency from the proximal latency, and divide the remainder into the distances between the points of stimulation (Fig. 3–2).

$$\frac{\text{Distance between points of stimulation (mm)}}{\text{Proximal latency (msec)} - \text{distal latency (msec)}} =$$

nerve conduction velocity in m/sec

Motor nerve conduction studies are also very useful in uncovering anomalous innervations, particularly of the intrinsic muscles of the hand where they occur so frequently, and in demonstrating nerve crossovers in the forearm, such as in the Martin–Gruber anomaly.

In sensory nerve conduction it is possible to record the evoked response in either the orthodromic or antidromic direction. Since it has been established that the propagated impulse travels at the same speed in either direction, and since it

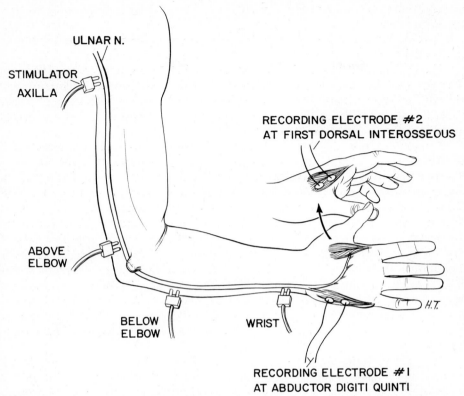

ULNAR N.

STIMULATOR
AXILLA

RECORDING ELECTRODE #2
AT FIRST DORSAL INTEROSSEOUS

ABOVE
ELBOW

BELOW
ELBOW

WRIST

RECORDING ELECTRODE #1
AT ABDUCTOR DIGITI QUINTI

Figure 3–2 Segmental motor conduction study of ulnar nerve. Study may include more proximal portion by stimulating at Erbs Point (not shown). The elbow is flexed to take up the slack of the nerve, and the measurement is made along the course of the nerve through the ulnar groove. The recording is from the abductor digiti quinti for the superficial branch: from the first dorsal interosseous for the deep branch.

is usually technically much easier to record from the distal portion of the sensory nerve because it is more superficial, most determinations are made in the antidromic direction.

Since we record the sensory evoked response directly from the nerve, we can calculate the nerve conduction velocity in meters/second by measuring the distance from the point of stimulation to the active recording electrode in millimeters and dividing by the latency in milliseconds.

Sensory nerve conduction is useful in localizing root lesions. Since the cell body nourishing the sensory axon is in the posterior ganglion in lesions proximal to this point, the patient has loss of sensation on clinical examination but has a normal sensory evoked response in the periphery. Loss of sensation and no sensory evoked response, or a delayed or low amplitude response, indicates that the lesion is distal to the posterior ganglion.

In the upper extremity the sensory evoked response is very useful in diagnosing carpal tunnel entrapment of the median nerve, since in many cases the sensory fibers of the nerve are involved before there is any evidence of motor deficit.

In the lower extremity the most common nerve studied for sensory function is the sural nerve, since this is frequently involved very early in the sensory neuropathies.

Two methods of studying nerve conduction in its more proximal segments are by use of the Hoffmann reflex or the F response.

The Hoffmann, or "H," reflex is normally only consistently obtainable in the S-I portion of the tibial nerve and is usually recorded from the soleus muscle, although it is sometimes seen in other nerves. In patients with upper neuron lesions it is found in those muscles manifesting spasticity and has been used as a measure of the "central excitatory state."

It depends upon the fact that the 1A afferent nerve fibers are more easily stimulated in the mixed tibial nerve in the popliteal fossa than the motor or efferent nerve fibers. This results in a monosynaptic reflex stimulation of the motor neuron at a lesser intensity than that required to stimulate the motor axon directly. Consequently, if one gradually increases the intensity of the stimulation, the first response seen at the lowest intensity is the reflex stimulation of the muscle. When recorded from the soleus on stimulation in the popliteal fossa, it normally occurs about 32 msec after the stimulus. With increasing intensity of the stimulus, the motor axon becomes excited, and the muscle is directly stimulated through the motor axon and the H-wave disappears. With supramaximal stimulation, the H-wave is no longer present; however, a late-appearing variable wave can usually be detected at this time — the F-wave. This is thought to represent retrograde stimulation of the anterior horn cell and not to be a reflex response.

The H-wave and the F-wave can be used to study the conduction in the proximal nerve, the nerve root, and the reflex arc. Normal latency values for these responses vary with the patient's age and limb length. In unilateral lesions, it is best to perform these studies on both the normal and involved sides. An increase in latency of 1 msec for the H reflex or 2 msec for the F-wave on the involved side is considered to be significant.

Muscle Stimulation

Although we refer to this modality as muscle stimulation, we must be aware that we only stimulate a muscle directly when it is denervated. As long as the muscle is innervated the response to stimulation at the motor point will be through the nerve, since the nerve is more sensitive to electrical stimulation than the muscle fibers themselves. Under muscle stimulation we usually consider the following factors:

1. *Reaction to degeneration* — the inability of denervated muscle to respond to faradic, or rapidly alternating, current, while responding with a slow, wormlike contraction to galvanic, or long-acting direct, current.

2. *Galvanic–tetanus/twitch ratio.* In normal muscle, stimulation with galvanic, or direct, current results in a visible twitch at threshold intensity, and with an increase in intensity the muscle goes into tetany or a sustained contraction. In normal muscle there is a considerable difference between these two values so that tetanus/twitch ratio is 3.5–6.5; with increasing denervation this value approaches unity. In a completely denervated muscle it is 1.0.

3. *Strength–duration curve.* By graphing on semi-log paper the amount of

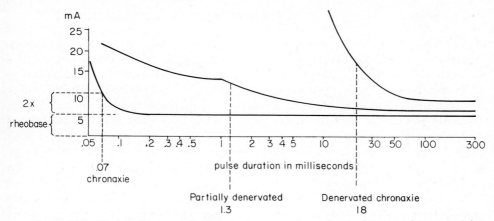

Figure 3–3 Typical SD (strength-duration) curves of completely denervated (upper right), reinnervating (middle), and normally innervated (lower) muscle, with chronaxie values indicated below.

current of decreasing duration applied to the motor point of a muscle which produces a minimal visible contraction, we produce a curve which can give us a measure of the degree of denervation of a specific muscle. Serial studies of such curves can reveal either progressive reinnervation or denervation (Fig. 3–3).

On such a curve we can identify specific values frequently used in electrodiagnosis, such as rheobase and chronaxie.

Rheobase is the amount of current of infinite duration required to cause a minimal contraction, and is reported in millivolts or milliamperes.

Chronaxie is the length of time required for current two times the rheobase in intensity to produce a minimal contraction, and is reported in milliseconds. The chronaxie varies in different muscles from a low of .07 millisecond in the rectus femoris to a high of .25 in the peroneus longus.

In a completely denervated muscle the SD curve is far to the right and the chronaxie is 100 times normal. A common rule of thumb is that a chronaxie of 1 msec or less is probably normal. Above that value the degree of denervation increases until at about 18 msec it is considered to be complete.

Strength-duration curves are helpful in following patients for reinnervation, since a characteristic "kink" that develops in the curve is frequently the earliest sign of reinnervation.

Muscle stimulation is also useful in demonstrating the continuity of a specific muscle-tendon complex. This is most helpful in traumatic cases where the question arises as to whether the functional loss is due to muscle denervation or tendon laceration, or both. It is also useful in distinguishing the common tendon ruptures in rheumatoid arthritis, which on casual examination frequently appear to be due to peripheral nerve injuries.

It must be remembered that if the muscle being tested is completely denervated, we must use galvanic, or direct, current stimulation to produce an adequate contraction of the muscle so that we can assess the continuity of the tendon by observing either its increased prominence or movement of the distal segment into which it is inserted.

Denervation

A muscle fiber is not truly physiologically denervated until wallerian degeneration has taken place. This requires from 10 to 14 days from when the discontinuity of the axon or death of the anterior horn cell has occurred. Up until that time electromyography will not be very revealing, although there may be some indication of membrane instability, as demonstrated by an increase in insertion potentials, and the strength-duration curve may be abnormal. Once wallerian degeneration has taken place, fibrillations and positive sharp waves appear that are considered to be pathognomonic of denervation. In anterior horn cell disease this may be preceded by and accompanied with fasciculation and bizarre high frequency discharges.

As regards viability of muscle, the finding of numerous fibrillations and positive sharp waves indicates not only denervation but also the presence of viable muscle fibers that have the potential to become functional with reinnervation.

On the other hand, the finding of electrical silence with "fibrotic" resistance to electrode insertion would indicate lack of viable muscle, and any surgery aimed at increasing innervation would be fruitless.

A nerve distal to a complete lesion may conduct normally up to 20 hours after an injury. In proximal lesions, distal latencies may be obtainable up to one week, but more proximal nerve conduction is lost. Therefore, normal nerve conduction two or more days after injury in the face of clinical paralysis indicates a neurapraxia. In such a condition, where physiologic block to conduction is present, conduction distal to the block will be normal, while conduction across the block may be absent or slowed.

In complete lesions, whether axonotmetic or neurotmetic, there is no conduction below the lesion after wallerian degeneration of the axons has taken place.

In partial lesions there will be conduction across the lesion unless the anatomically intact portion of the nerve is neurapraxic. The degree of partiality of the lesion will determine how closely the evoked response approaches normal.

The strength-duration curve will reflect the degree of involvement by the amount of shift to the right and the numerical value of the chronaxie.

In completely denervated muscle the reaction to degeneration will be positive and the galvanic twitch/tetanus ratio will be unity.

Reinnervation

Where complete denervation of a muscle has existed the first indication of reinnervation is a decrease in the number of fibrillation potentials, followed by so-called nascent motor potentials, and, finally, normal motor potentials under voluntary control. These potentials are at first polyphasic, but gradually, as the innervating axons and axon twigs mature, they approach the parameters of normal motor unit potentials. The patient is at first able to produce isolated potentials on maximum effort and with the increase in innervated motor units an interference pattern will gradually develop.

In partial lesions reinnervation does not have to wait on regrowth of the injured axon, since most of it will occur as a result of collateral reinnervation, a process by which the terminal twigs of the axons of the intact motor units branch and innervate the denervated muscle fibers of the involved motor units. This causes a more rapid reinnervation and the production of larger than normal motor units which produce high amplitude, long duration polyphasic potentials on volition.

When a muscle demonstrates large polyphasic potentials without any fibrillations after a partial nerve injury, we can assume that it has attained maximum reinnervation of the previously denervated muscle fibers by collateral reinnervation and, therefore, a procedure to increase innervation would not be indicated.

The first sign of reinnervation on the strength duration curve is the development of a "kink." This can precede clinical evidence of recovery by five to six weeks. As recovery takes place the curve approaches normal (see Fig. 3–3).

Electrodiagnostic Finding in Some Common Nerve Lesions

Anterior Horn Cell Disease

Electromyography reveals fasciculations, fibrillations, positive sharp waves, and giant complex potentials. Occasionally, we see bizarre high frequency discharges.

Nerve conduction studies are usually normal except that the evoked response may be somewhat lower than normal in amplitude. In advanced disease there may be moderate slowing of motor conduction. Sensory conduction studies are entirely normal.

The strength-duration curve reflects the degree of denervation.

Root Lesions Proximal to Posterior Ganglion
(Avulsions)

ELECTROMYOGRAPHY. In complete lesions fibrillations and positive sharp waves are found in limb and paravertebral muscles. No motor unit potentials are seen on volition. In incomplete lesions, in addition to the fibrillations and positive sharp waves, we would find large complex potentials and partial interference or isolated potentials depending on the severity of the lesion.

NERVE CONDUCTION. In complete lesions after wallerian degeneration has taken place, there would be no motor conduction. In partial lesions the evoked motor response would be normal in latency; however, there would be a decrease in amplitude proportional to the degree of completeness of the lesion. In both complete and incomplete lesions the sensory evoked response would be normal in amplitude and latency. The H reflex and F-waves would be absent in complete lesions or, if present in incomplete lesions, reduced in amplitude and increased in latency.

MUSCLE STIMULATION. The strength-duration curve will reflect the degree of completeness of the lesion, as would chronaxie ranging from 1 msec in a mild partial lesion to 18 msec in a complete lesion.

Root Lesions Distal to Origin of Posterior Primary Ramus

ELECTROMYOGRAPHY. Fibrillations and positive sharp waves are found in limb muscles innervated by the involved segments, but normal findings are found in the paravertebral muscles.

All muscles (except the rhomboids) are innervated by multiple roots. Therefore, in complete lesions of a single root the muscles subserved by the involved segment will be only partially denervated and, therefore, will demonstrate positive sharp waves, fibrillations at rest, complex and normal motor unit potentials on minimum effort, and partial interference on maximum effort.

In complete lesions of multiple roots the muscle may be completely denervated and, therefore, may not produce any voluntary potentials.

NERVE CONDUCTION. Motor nerve conduction of peripheral nerves in a complete single root lesion usually is normal with a decrease in the amplitude of the evoked response in proportion to the contribution made by the involved segment to the muscle studied.

In root compression syndromes in which axonotmesis has not taken place, use of the H-reflex in suspected first sacral root lesions may be useful. An increase in msec latency on the involved side as compared to the uninvolved side is considered evidence of slowing across the root if we have ruled out a peripheral nerve lesion.

In other segments, where the H-reflex is not obtained, we may use the F-wave in the same manner, but, since this phenomenon is somewhat more variable, an increase in latency of more than 2 msec is considered suggestive of a proximal compressive lesion.

Peripheral Neuropathy

The EMG findings may be meager and frequently do not reflect the degree of clinical involvement. In the face of severe muscle weakness there may be findings of only a decrease in interference pattern on maximum voluntary effort, a few fibrillation potentials, an occasional fasciculation, and some increase in complex potentials.

Nerve conduction studies are much more revealing.

In conditions producing segmental demyelination (diabetes, vasculitis, compression) there is usually slowing of motor and sensory conduction only in the segments involved, with relatively normal values in all other segments.

When the involvement is mainly axonal, as in the toxic neuropathies (alcohol, heavy metals, etc.), the slowing of conduction is most marked in distal segments. This results in a considerable lengthening of the distal latencies of the involved nerves.

It is possible to have a neuropathy that involves mainly either the sensory or motor axons. Therefore, it is important to test both motor and sensory conduction in all suspected cases.

Cubital Tunnel Syndrome

ELECTROMYOGRAPHY. Depending on severity, the findings include fibrillation potentials and complex potentials in all ulnar-innervated muscles distal to the point of compression. Where the compression has not yet produced axonotmesis, motor and sensory nerve conduction would be normal above and below the point of compression and slowed across the point of compression.

Because the ulnar nerve is slack when the elbow is extended, it is preferable to perform this test with the elbow flexed to 90 degrees, and when measuring the distance between points of stimulation to measure along the course of the nerve (see Fig. 3–2). A value across the elbow 10 m/sec below the forearm segment would indicate compression in this region. Because of possible entrapment in the arcade of Struthers, it is best to compare the midarm-to-above-elbow segment with the other segments rather than just the segment running across the ulnar groove.

Guyon-Tunnel Syndrome (Deep Palmar Branch Entrapment)

ELECTROMYOGRAPHY.   Here, EMG reveals normal responses from the abductor digiti minimi, whereas the interosseus muscles will demonstrate denervation potentials if the lesion is severe enough to produce axonotmesis: that is, complex potentials, fibrillations, positive sharp waves, and less than a normal interference pattern.

Nerve conduction studies will demonstrate normal sensory conduction to the fifth digit and a normal motor latency from the wrist to the abductor digiti minimi but a prolongation of the motor latency to the first dorsal interosseus muscle. A difference in latency of over 1 msec is considered significant, indicating a slowing in the deep branch of the ulnar nerve consistent with Guyon-tunnel syndrome.

Anterior Interosseous Syndrome

If axonotmesis has occurred we find fibrillation and complex potential in all muscles innervated by the anterior interosseus nerve on electromyography.

Motor conduction studies recorded from the abductor pollicis brevis are normal, as are sensory conduction studies.

Motor conduction from the elbow to the pronator quadratus will be slowed and the amplitude of the evoked response decreased in proportion to the severity of the lesion.

Carpal Tunnel Syndrome

ELECTROMYOGRAPHY.   If axonotmesis has occurred, the opponens and abductor pollicis brevis will reveal fibrillation, positive sharp waves and complex potentials on minimum effort, and a less than normal interference pattern on maximum effort.

Whether axonotmesis has occurred or not the nerve conduction studies will be helpful.

The motor latency from the wrist to the abductor pollicis brevis is prolonged (over 4 msec), while motor conduction of the forearm segment of the nerve is normal. There is some evidence that a severe entrapment can cause slowing of the forearm segment because of retrograde degeneration; however, in that case, one can rule out a more proximal lesion by the lack of denervation potentials in the median innervated forearm muscle.

Sensory conduction from the wrist to the first three digits is slowed. By stimulating the sensory nerve to the second digit in the wrist and in the palm we can calculate the speed of conduction across the carpal tunnel. If axonotmesis has taken place the conduction will be slowed in both segments and the amplitude will be lower than normal. If the block is mainly physiological we will have slowing of conduction across the carpal tunnel with a low amplitude response (less than 20 microvolts), while on stimulation in the palmar region we will have normal conduction with an amplitude of evoked response that approaches normal (greater than 30 microvolts).

Posterior Interosseus Syndrome

ELECTROMYOGRAPHY.   If axonotmesis has taken place we will find fibrillation potentials and positive sharp waves in muscles innervated by the posterior interosseus nerve.

NERVE CONDUCTION.   Whether or not axonotmesis has occurred, there will be a prolongation of latency on stimulation of the radial nerve at the elbow, recording from the extensor indicis proprius. Because it is not always possible to percutaneously stimulate the posterior interosseus nerve in its more distal portion, it is necessary to stimulate with a needle inserted in the vicinity of the nerve if one wishes to determine the nerve velocity across the usual point of entrapment.

The antidromic sensory response from 11 cm above the first metacarpophalangeal joint will be normal in latency and amplitude.

Sciatic Nerve Lesions

Injuries to the tibial division are easily differentiated from more distal lesions by finding fibrillations and positive sharp waves in the hamstring muscles. However, peroneal division injuries, which are by far more frequent, can only be differentiated from the very common peroneal palsy due to compression at the fibula neck by exploration of the short head of the rectus femoris, which is the only muscle above the knee innervated by the peroneal division.

Peroneal Nerve Compression at Fibular Neck

ELECTROMYOGRAPHY.   If axonotmesis has occurred, denervation potentials will be found in anterior compartment muscles and in the extensor digitorum brevis.

NERVE CONDUCTION.   Whether or not axonotmesis has occurred, motor nerve conduction across the fibula neck will be slowed.

Tarsal Tunnel Syndrome

This consists of compression of the posterior tibial nerve in the region of the medial malleolus. Here we can have prolongation of motor latency to the abductor hallucis through the medial plantar nerve (greater than 6.5 msec) or to the abductor digiti quinti through the lateral plantar nerve (greater than 7 msec), or both.

If axonotmesis has occurred we will find fibrillation potentials in the abductor hallucis or the abductor digiti quinti, or in both.

REFERENCES

Desmedt, J. E. (ed.): New Developments in Electromyography and Clinical Neurophysiology. New York, S. Karger, 1973.

Goodgold, J., and Eberstein, R.: Electrodiagnosis of Neuromuscular Diseases. Baltimore, Williams & Wilkins, 1978.

Lenman, J., and Ritchie, A. E.: Clinical Electromyography. 2nd. ed., Philadelphia, J. B. Lippincott, 1977.

Licht, S. (ed.): Electrodiagnosis and Electromyography. 3rd ed., New Haven, Conn., E. Licht, Publisher, 1971.

Smorto, M. P., and Basmajian, J. K.: Electrodiagnosis. A Hand Book for Neurologists. New York, Harper & Row, 1977.

4

DIAGNOSTIC NERVE BLOCKS

ADEL R. ABADIR

Diagnostic nerve blocks are useful procedures in the evaluation and localization of pain. They can also serve to predict the outcome of permanent denervation by section of a neuropathway in a given patient. In any discussion on the role of diagnostic and prognostic nerve blocks, an understanding of the types of pain and their causative mechanisms is essential for proper selection and application.

Pain may be either acute or chronic. Acute pain is usually caused by noxious stimuli traveling along neuropathways to the brain, where they are perceived as nociception. Noxious stimuli trigger specialized pain receptors known as nociceptors (Bonica, 1974, 1976; Burgess, 1974); these are located in skin, subcutaneous tissue, viscera, muscle, and deep structures, and are characterized by high threshold (Bonica, 1974, 1976; Perl, 1971; Burgess, 1974). They transmit a persistent discharge in response to a suprathreshold stimulus along small A delta and C fibers (Bonica, 1976; Burgess, 1974; Hollin, 1974; Iggo, 1972). Impulses travel along these fibers to the dorsal horn cells where they are modulated by a highly developed process of selection, integration, and abstraction (Melzack, 1965; Wall, 1967). Further modulation and selection also occurs in the ascending tracts of the spinal cord and in the midbrain (Bonica, 1977). The stimulus finally reaches the primary somato-sensory cortex. The somato-cortex, through its discriminative function, and probably by regulating subcortical activity, will further modulate nociception (Bonica, 1977). However, the brain, through the descending neural systems, can influence transmission in the thalamus, reticular formation, dorsal column of the spinal cord (Fetz, 1968; Taub, 1964; Wall, 1967), and trigeminal system (Sessle, 1976).

Since pain is an emotional experience, psychological factors play a great role in the patient's total pain experience (Chapman, 1977; Merskey, 1967; Sternbach, 1968). Neocortical processes modulate cognitive and psychological factors such as anxiety, prior conditioning, experience, and emotional and cultural background (Melzack, 1965, 1968). Causes of pain are generally accepted as 1)

44

nociception, 2) central pain states, 3) psychological factors, and 4) behavioral phenomena (Murphy, 1977).

Singly or in combination, the causes listed above can be responsible for pain. Certainly, nociception may play the primary role in acute pain. However, when pain is chronic, psychological factors become more important (Chapman, 1977; Melzack, 1974), and still persist after the cessation of nociception.

Central pain states (Noordenbos, 1974; Pagni, 1974) may be secondary to a lesion within the central nervous system; for example, tumor, herpes virus, trauma, or other CNS disease states (Bonica, 1977). However, in a great number of cases, no specific causative lesion is identifiable.

ROLE OF DIAGNOSTIC AND PROGNOSTIC NERVE BLOCKS

1. To localize the area where noxious stimuli are produced.
2. To define neuro-pathways where noxious stimuli may be transmitted.
3. To determine if transection of the nerve or root could be successful in eliminating pain. In this particular role, diagnostic nerve blocks play a definite role in subsequent patient management.
4. To evaluate patients' acceptance of prolonged denervation. Many patients find anesthesia more objectionable than the original pain.
5. To assess long term nerve blocks with alcohol or phenol as to the possible occurrence of permanent dysesthesia. To avoid permanent nerve damage, low concentrations of phenol are recommended, as denervation is not always reversible when high concentrations of phenol are used.

PREPARATION OF A PATIENT FOR NERVE BLOCK

In acute pain, simple interruption of the appropriate neuropathway will provide relief. At this point, patients are not usually addicted to any medication, and psychological factors do not usually play a major role. After a complete physical and neurological examination, one or more provisional diagnoses are usually arrived at. One of two approaches can be chosen at this point.

1. If the etiology of the pain is relatively clear, the block is expected to confirm the provisional diagnosis. There is no need for screening blocks; for example, spinal, epidural, or caudal. It is far less traumatic and disruptive to the patient to proceed with the least invasive technique. For instance, if a myofascial syndrome is suspected, simple local infiltration of the involved muscle or fascial plane will be the block of choice. More extensive blocks will only be resorted to if local infiltration fails. This would probably indicate that the causative mechanism may not be a simple myofascial syndrome limited to the particular area of infiltration.
2. If the nature of the pain is very indefinite and poorly localized, screening blocks can be helpful. For example, if a lumbar epidural with complete anesthesia below T12–L1 spinal dermatomes fails to alleviate leg pain, it is rather obvious that the pain will not be interrupted by blocking any neuro-

pathway in the lower limbs. A different mechanism for nociception in that leg should be searched for. If, however, the screening block is successful in eliminating the pain, then more distal blocks will be necessary to further localize the neuro-pathway involved.

In chronic pain states, patients often present for treatment at such a late stage that most of them have already been subjected to large amounts of narcotics, sedatives, and tranquilizers. These patients have become drug dependent and it is impossible to differentiate whether most of their pain symptoms are actually indirect requests for medication or demonstrate true nociception. Sudden cessation of addictive drugs may produce severe withdrawal symptoms and even worse pain; therefore, gradual withdrawal of the drugs, with the help of qualified psychiatric assistance, is the most expedient approach. In the meantime, other methods for alleviating pain, such as continuous epidural block or percutaneous nerve stimulation, as well as any appropriate physical therapy during the period of drug withdrawal, should be employed. Only when the patient is no longer drug dependent can one proceed with diagnostic blocks.

Psychiatric evaluation prior to blocks should be required in all chronic pain problems even if the patient presents with valid reasons for his chronic pain. Screening tests, such as the Minnesota Multiphasic Personality Inventory (MMPI) and many other psychological tests are very helpful in defining the psychological component.

Weaning patients off narcotics, psychiatric evaluation, and supportive therapy are tedious and time consuming. However, unless ample time as well as effort is allocated, arriving at a correct diagnosis and initiation of therapy may be impossible. When a nerve block is finally selected, the patient is asked to abstain from analgesics for a few hours, after which the pain should be reassessed as to its degree, nature, duration, and triggering mechanisms. When the pain is paroxysmal or intermittent, it is very difficult to assess the value of the block, if, at the time of the block, the patient has been free of pain. Long duration blocks with an indwelling catheter may be necessary. If pain does not recur within a few days it is safe to assume that the involved neuro-pathway has been interrupted.

KEY POINTS FOR EFFECTIVE DIAGNOSTIC BLOCKS

1. Success of a block should not be in doubt. It is imperative to be absolutely sure that the block is fully in effect by evaluating sensory deficits, signs of sympathetic blockade (e.g., Horner syndrome in head or neck), increases in skin temperature, or loss of motor power. Monitoring limb temperature by a sensitive thermocouple before and after a block would detect any change in temperature secondary to vasodilation of skin vessels when sympathetic hyperactivity is interrupted.
2. Blocks should be performed with minimal paresthesia and nerve damage. Repeated puncture of nerves may produce iatrogenic pain.
3. Several drugs of varying duration and placebos should be used to evaluate chronic pain. It may be wise not to inform the patient of the normal therapeutic duration of the drug utilized. During assessment of the block the patient should report on the duration and degree of relief.

ASSESSMENT OF BLOCK

DEGREES OF PAIN RELIEF. The patient is asked to evaluate the degree of relief in percentages; if no or poor relief of pain is experienced, the patient should be asked to stimulate trigger points, if any, or to perform any movement or activity that is known to elicit pain, and then the amount of relief should be reassessed. Many patients will be surprised to find that they can perform many activities or movements that they were unable to perform prior to the block without eliciting a degree of pain sufficient to interrupt the activity.

DURATION OF RELIEF. This is important in assessing the value of the block. The usual responses from patients when asked about the duration of relief are as follows:

1. Duration of relief exceeds anesthetic duration of the drug. This is a common occurrence, the reasons for which are not quite understood at the moment, probably by prolonging the refractory period of the nerve (Condouris, 1966), thereby modulating neuro-information. This is typical also of causalgic pain, wherein patients sometimes report relief for 24 hours or longer. However, if the same effect is also obtained after a placebo, psychogenic factors should be suspected to be the actual causative mechanism; true central pain is rarely helped consistently by placebos. Several blocks with agents of different anesthetic duration may be necessary to differentiate between pain of psychogenic nature and true nociception.
2. Duration of anesthesia produced by nerve block far exceeds relief. The amount of relief obtained is adequate, but only for a very short period and far less than the duration of sensory block; in such cases, the psychological component of pain may be the predominant factor. In some patients, drug addiction may play a role, especially if the patient demands the usual dose of narcotics to which he has been accustomed.
3. Duration of relief equals the anesthetic duration of the drug. This is typical of nociception, and these patients are proper candidates for permanent denervation if the permanent anesthesia that will develop is acceptable.
4. No relief at all is obtained. This can be attributed to an unsuccessful block, to nociception transmitted through a different neuro-pathway, to central pain states, or to pain of psychological origin. Screening blocks that would anesthetize large segments of the body are of value in this situation. If these screening blocks are unsuccessful in interrupting pain, further search of the true pathways should be made.

TYPES OF NERVE BLOCKS

Sympathetic

These are primarily designed to interrupt sympathetic innervation to regions where sympathetic hyperactivity may be the causative mechanism of pain. Sympathetic hyperactivity (sympathetic reflex dystrophy) usually presents with burning pain, coldness, pallor, trophic changes of the skin, and excessive sweating (hyperhydrosis) (Doupe, 1944). Stellate and lumbar sympathetic blocks can provide pure sympathetic block, while spinal, epidural, caudal, or plexus blocks with low concentration of local anesthetics can produce a differential sympathetic block, owing to the fact that sympathetic fibers are very small and unmyelinated, and the minimum concentration (CM) required to block these fibers will hardly affect the larger sensory and motor fibers. For this reason, 0.25 per cent lidocaine, 0.5 per cent procaine or chloroprocaine and 0.125 per cent bupivicaine may be successful in producing a true sympathetic differential block. Continuous blocks with an indwelling catheter will assess results of sympathetic blockade up to four days. If the patient has complete relief for a few days with an indwelling catheter placed at the stellate or lumbar sympathetic chain, relief with a permanent chemical or surgical sympathectomy should be expected.

Sensory

1. Trigger point injections — local infiltration of trigger points in myofascial syndromes with the usual concentrations of anesthetics used for local infiltration is sufficient to provide pain relief. Long acting anesthetics are preferable, although short acting anesthetics or, at times, even placebos can be of value. These injections are used to determine if pain is due to a reflex mechanism triggered by local pathology.
2. Somatic nerve blocks are some of the most useful diagnostic tools available for pain syndromes. They range from large screening blocks (spinal, epidural, caudal, or plexus) to blocks involving individual small nerves.
3. Differential sensory nerve blocks are of value in achieving anesthesia without any major interruption of motor activity.
4. Placebo blocks are particularly helpful in assessing pain that appears to be psychosomatic in nature.
5. Motor nerve blocks are used if pain results from spasm of a muscle or group of muscles. These are usually prognostic and are done prior to surgery to determine if spasm in involved muscles can be relieved by interruption of the motor nerve supply.

LOCAL ANESTHETIC DRUGS

For the safe use of local anesthetics, the following rules should be observed:
1. Use the minimum dose and concentration necessary to produce adequate anesthesia. Increasing the concentration of the local anesthetic is not an efficient way of prolonging the block. Anesthetic solutions containing epinephrine should be used instead.
2. Aspirate carefully. Avoid intravascular injection; most toxic reactions occur when this simple precaution is neglected.
3. If a larger dose for a large area is needed, it is preferable to inject the drugs in divided doses.
4. For nerve blocks, place the needle carefully; with accurate placement of the anesthetic, smaller doses can be used.
5. Use nerve blocks instead of local infiltration when large areas are to be anesthetized.
6. Avoid injecting into any infected area.

7. Deposit anesthetic solution around the nerve. Do not puncture the nerve unnecessarily.
8. Allow sufficient time for the anesthetic agent to work.

A comprehensive description of these drugs is beyond the scope of this chapter, and the reader is advised to refer to the appropriate texts (Moore, 1965; Covino, 1974; Collins, 1976). A brief description of the most commonly used drugs will be included. Local anesthetic drugs can be divided into two major groups; namely, amides and esters. The pertinent differences in their pharmacological properties are:

1. Ester groups are generally of shorter duration of action, except tetracaine, which is the only compound of considerable duration.
2. Allergic reactions are more common in the esters group. Most complications with the amide group are due to either toxicity from overdosage or intravascular injection.
3. Onset of action is usually shorter in the ester compounds.
4. Esters are detoxified in the bloodstream by pseudocholinesterases and, therefore, the duration of action is considerably shorter if mixed with blood. Amides are detoxified mainly in the liver and the effect of blood will not alter the duration of these compounds.

The most commonly used ester compounds are procaine (Novacaine) and 2-3-chloroprocaine (Nesacaine), and their pharmacological characteristics are listed above. Concentrations commonly used are 0.5 to 2 per cent for procaine and 1 to 3 per cent for chloroprocaine. They may be mixed with 1/100,000 to 1/200,000 epinephrine solution to increase duration and reduce systemic absorption. Duration with no epinephrine added is approximately 30 minutes for 2-chloroprocaine and up to 45 minutes for procaine. If epinephrine is added the duration can be increased by 50 to 100 per cent, depending on the vascularity of the area being infiltrated. Maximum dose should not exceed 15 mg per kg for single injection.

In the amide group, lidocaine (Xylocaine), mepivacaine (Carbocaine), bupivicaine (Marcaine), and etidocaine (Duranest) are commonly used.

Lidocaine and mepivacaine are clinically similar and can be used in these concentrations:

1. For infiltration anesthesia, sympathetic differential nerve block 0.25–0.5 per cent.
2. For block of small nerves and sensory differential nerve block: 1.0 per cent.
3. For block of large nerves: 1.5 per cent.
4. For spinal (Lidocaine): 2.0 per cent.
5. For epidural (Lidocaine): 1.5 to 2.0 per cent.

Their duration of action ranges from 45 to 90 minutes. Addition of 1/100,000 to 1/200,000 epinephrine solution may increase the duration 50 to 100 per cent.

Bupivicaine is similar in structure to mepivacaine but is three to four times more potent; it owes its long duration of anesthesia to its binding property to tissue proteins. The duration of anesthesia is three to four hours, depending on the vascularity of the region. The concentrations used are:
1. For sympathetic blocks: 0.12 to 0.25 per cent

2. For small sensory nerve and sensory differential nerve blocks: 0.25 per cent
3. For large nerve blocks: 0.5 per cent
4. For spinal and epidural blocks: 0.25 to 0.75 per cent

Bupivicaine produces excellent differential blocks in smaller concentrations, as it has a particular affinity for sensory fibers. The onset of action is rather slow, and addition of epinephrine does not increase the duration of the drug to any appreciable degree. The maximum dose for a single injection is approximately 250 mg, although 400 mg have been used extensively and without any undesirable effects (Moore, 1975).

Etidocaine is a new drug similar in properties to bupivicaine. The concentration used is about twice that of bupivicaine. It affects the motor fibers more than bupivicaine (Moore, 1975), and would not be suitable for differential blocks.

TECHNIQUES OF MOST FREQUENTLY USED
DIAGNOSTIC BLOCKS
Head and Neck Region

Infraorbital Nerve Block

The infraorbital nerve supplies the lower eyelid, the lower third of the lateral surface of the nose, the upper lip (including mucous membrane), the columella and the upper two incisors (Fig. 4–1*A* and *C*).

The infraorbital foramen can be very easily palpated below the infraorbital ridge, which is on the same line as the pupil when the eyes are looking straight forward (Fig. 4–1*B*). Three or four ml of a low concentration local anesthetic injected into the infraorbital foramen provides immediate anesthesia. Paresthesia is usually elicited as the needle is advanced along the infraorbital canal, which runs posteriorly, superiorly, and outward.

Mental Nerve Block

The mental nerve supplies the chin and lower lip, including the mucous membrane and the lower cheek. It can be blocked at the mental canal or as it emerges from the mental foramen (Fig. 4–1 *A* and *C*).

The mental foramen lies below the second bicuspid tooth about midway between the upper and lower borders of the lower mandible. With age, in the edentulous patient, and with the progressive atrophy of the alveolar ridge, the foramen comes closer to the upper border of the mandible until it lies close to the very upper margin. The alveolar foramen can be entered with the needle pointing downward medially and forward. Paresthesia should be elicited to insure a good block.

Supraorbital Nerve Block

The supraorbital nerves can be blocked at the supraorbital notch, which is located one inch lateral to the midline at the inferior edge of the supraorbital

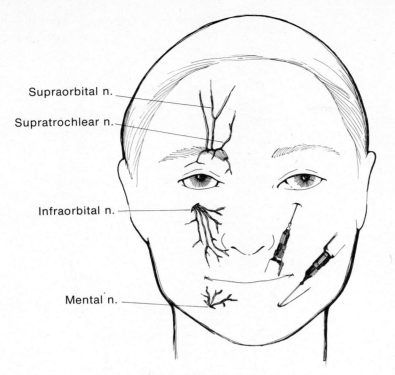

Supraorbital n.

Supratrochlear n.

Infraorbital n.

Mental n.

Figure 4–1A

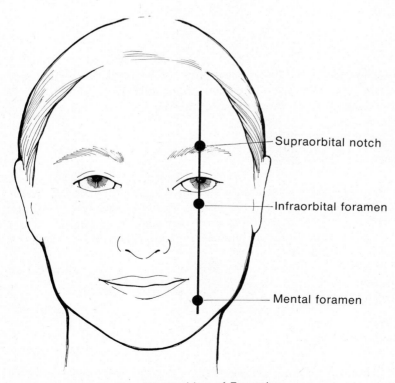

Supraorbital notch

Infraorbital foramen

Mental foramen

Figure 4–1B   Line of Foramina

51

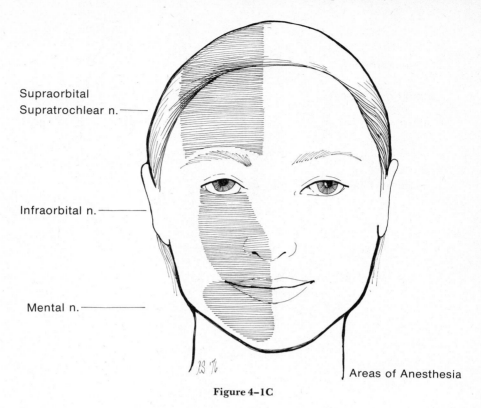

Supraorbital
Supratrochlear n.

Infraorbital n.

Mental n.

Areas of Anesthesia

Figure 4–1C

ridge (Fig. 4–1*A* and *C*). The supraorbital notch can be easily palpated with the finger; 3 ml of a local anesthetic agent deposited at the notch inferior to the supraorbital ridge will render complete anesthesia for the corresponding half of the forehead.

Supratrochlear Nerve Block

The supratrochlear nerve exists from the orbit halfway between the supraorbital notch and the pulley of the superior oblique muscle. It emerges lateral to the medial border of the orbit to curve upward. It supplies the lower part of the forehead and the bridge of the nose. Paresthesia should be elicited if alcohol or phenol is used (Fig. 4–1*A* and *C*).

For blocks of maxillary nerves or its branches, readers should refer to the excellent descriptions by H. S. Kramer Jr. and W. H. Schmidt, 1977, and by D. C. Moore, 1965.

Cervical Plexus Block

The patient is in the dorsal supine position, without a pillow, his arms at his sides, and his head turned to the side opposite the side being blocked. One half inch posterior to a line connecting the tip of the mastoid process and Chassaignac's tubercle, palpate the second, third, and fourth transverse process (Fig. 4–1D). Landmarks can be easily checked by locating Chassaignac's tubercle and counting the transverse processes in the cephalad direction. Skin wheals are raised over the second, third, and fourth transverse processes. The 2 inch, 22 gauge needles are inserted perpendicular to the skin wheal, tilted slightly caudad until they meet the transverse processes of the second, third, and fourth cervical vertebrae. Should stimulation of the second or third cervical nerves occur, pain radiating to the back of the head will be felt. To better position the needle on the transverse process, the needle is withdrawn to the subcutaneous layer and redirected a few degrees caudad and cephalad.

The needle is "walked" over the tip of the transverse process anteriorly until it is advanced a quarter of an inch anterior to the tip of the process. Further advancement of the needle may puncture the vertebral artery. If the artery is penetrated, withdraw the needle a few millimeters and aspirate until no blood returns. Each needle is held against the transverse process and connected to a 10 cc syringe that is filled with local anesthetic agent. After careful aspiration for CSF or blood, or both, 7 ml of anesthetic solution is injected; the remaining 3 ml is injected while withdrawing the needle.

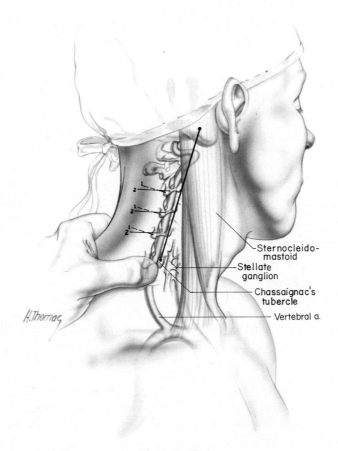

Sternocleido-
mastoid

Stellate
ganglion

Chassaignac's
tubercle

Vertebral a.

Figure 4–1D

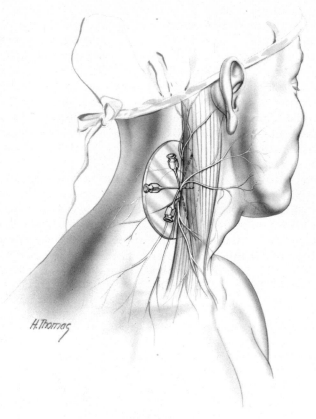

Figure 4–1E

For superficial cervical plexus block, a 5 cm needle is inserted through the skin wheal over the third cervical transverse process and a dose of 10 to 15 ml of suitable local anesthetic agent is deposited to a distance of 3 centimeters, both cephalad and caudad along the posterior inferior border of the sternocleidomastoid muscle (Fig. 4–1E).

Stellate Ganglion Block

The patient is in the supine position and his head is tilted backward with neck full extension. A skin wheal is made over the seventh cervical transverse process and along the medial border of the sternocleidomastoid muscle, to a breadth of approximately two fingers above the clavicle and two fingers lateral to the jugular notch. The carotid sheath and the sternocleidomastoid muscle are pulled laterally (Fig. 4–2). The carotid pulsation should be felt at the lateral side of the depressing fingers. The needle is then introduced through the skin wheal perpendicular to the skin and advanced downward until it contacts the sixth

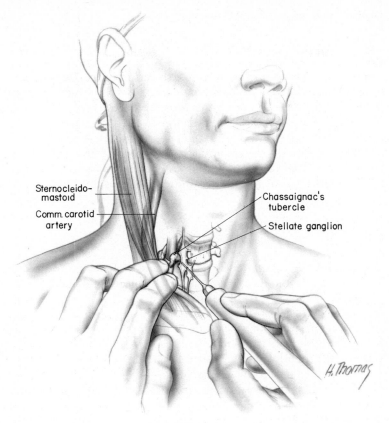

Sternocleido-
mastoid

Comm. carotid
artery

Chassaignac's
tubercle

Stellate ganglion

H. Thomas

Figure 4–2

cervical transverse process. The depression of the skin by the index and middle
fingers and the physique of the patient will determine the depth of the tip of the
transverse process. After the needle contacts the sixth cervical transverse process, it should be withdrawn 2 to 3 mm. After careful aspiration, 12 ml of the local
anesthetic solution is deposited.

Upper Extremity

The commonly used nerve blocks are the axillary plexus, median nerve,
radial nerve, ulnar nerve, and transmetacarpal. Median, ulnar and radial nerves
can be blocked at any point along their course in the forearm. It is preferable not
to block any nerve that is in immediate contact with periosteum or when it is
enclosed in rigid fascial compartments, as the possibility of damage to the nerve
is high; for example, the ulnar nerve preferably should not be injected behind
the medial epicondyle (Bonica, J. J., 1953).

Interscalenous Block of Brachial Plexus

The patient is in the supine position with his head turned to the side opposite the one being blocked. The patient is then instructed to take a maximum deep breath and hold it a few seconds; in this manner the lateral border of anterior scalenus muscle may be easily palpated. A skin wheal is raised at the lateral border of the anterior scalenus muscle at the level of Chassaignac's tubercle. The needle is inserted perpendicular to the skin wheal and redirected slightly laterally until paresthesias are elicited that are felt radiating to the shoulder or upper arm. If paresthesias do not occur, the needle should be withdrawn and redirected fanwise caudad and cephalad. As soon as paresthesia is elicited, 25 to 30 ml of local anesthetic solution is deposited.

Axillary Plexus Block

The axillary artery is palpated at the apex of the axilla, and a skin wheal raised. A four-inch intravenous catheter-needle combination is advanced, directing it as close to the artery as possible, until paresthesia in any part of the hand or forearm is elicited. After careful aspiration the needle is withdrawn. A full syringe of the appropriate local anesthetic is attached. The catheter is advanced while injecting the solution until it is fully inserted. It is necessary to inject simultaneously with the advancement of the catheter to prevent kinking of the plastic sheath. If the axillary artery is inadvertently punctured, simple withdrawal of the catheter while maintaining pressure on the artery for a few minutes will prevent hematoma formation. The procedure can then be repeated. It is usually necessary to inject 30 to 40 ml of the drug to establish a complete block. This total amount may be administered in 10 ml fractional doses to prevent overdosage. Signs of toxicity are extremely rare; usually, intravascular injection is responsible for most complications. Anesthesia is usually complete in 10 to 30 minutes, depending on the drug used and the accuracy of placement.

Ulnar Nerve Block at Wrist

A skin wheal is raised 1½ inches above the distal crease of the anterior aspect of the wrist joint, at the approximate border of the ulnar bone, and the needle is advanced diagonally across the medial border of the ulnar, almost touching the periosteum (Fig. 4–3). While advancing the needle, carefully aspirate, and inject 7 to 8 cc of local anesthetic. Keep advancing the needle until the tip is almost felt by a finger placed at the back of the forearm. Paresthesia is not necessary for a successful block. Onset of anesthesia is within five to ten minutes.

Radial Nerve Block at Wrist

The same technique used in ulnar nerve block may be used at the lateral border of the distal end of the radial bone (Fig. 4–4).

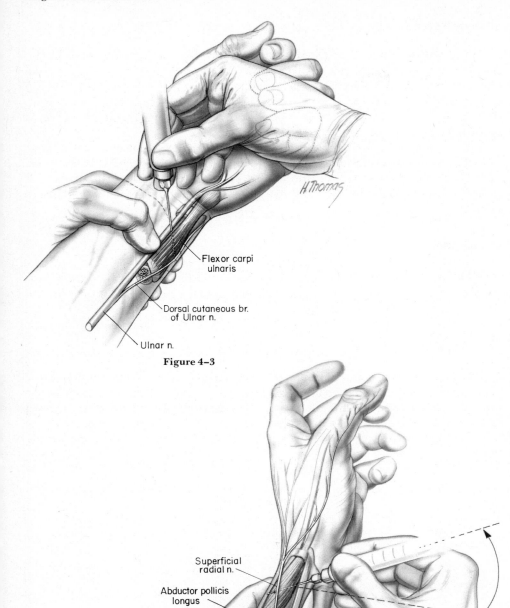

Flexor carpi
ulnaris

Dorsal cutaneous br.
of Ulnar n.

Ulnar n.

Figure 4–3

Superficial
radial n.

Abductor pollicis
longus

Radius

Figure 4–4

Median Nerve Block

One half to three fourths of an inch above the wrist joint, between the tendons of the flexor carpi radialis and the palmaris longus muscles, and one half inch deep to the skin, lies the median nerve (Fig. 4–5). A one inch long, 25 gauge needle is advanced until paresthesia is elicited, then 5 ml of local anesthetic is deposited. Care should be taken not to puncture or damage the nerve, as painful paresthesia may last a few weeks.

Both the median nerve and the radial nerve can also be blocked at or above the elbow, but it is preferable to avoid the ulnar nerve at the elbow. If the ulnar nerve is to be blocked behind the medial epicondyle, a very small amount of local anesthetic should be used and extreme care should be taken not to damage the nerve.

Finger Blocks

The most simple technique is to surround the finger in a ring fashion, for example, with 0.5 per cent xylocaine (without epinephrine). Do not overdistend the tissue, as already mentioned.

Metacarpal Nerve Block

The digital nerve may be blocked at the metacarpal level if 2 ml of a low concentration of anesthetic (for example, 0.5 per cent lidocaine) is injected immediately lateral and adjacent to the flexor tendons of the fingers at the level of the distal palmar crease. This is a safer technique, as the block is proximal to the distal palmar arch where cross anastomosis with other arterial blood supply to the finger occurs.

Lower Extremity

The three most frequently blocked nerves are the femoral, the sciatic and the lateral femoral cutaneous.

Femoral Nerve Block

The femoral artery is palpated. The femoral nerve is located immediately lateral to it. Through a skin wheal, a 22 gauge, 2 inch needle is inserted ½ inch lateral to the artery, ½ to 1½ inches deep, depending on the amount of fat. At this point, 5 to 10 ml of a suitable anesthetic agent is injected.

Sciatic Nerve Block

A line is drawn between the posterior superior iliac spine and the greater trochanter, then at the midpoint of this line, a perpendicular line is dropped 3 to 3½ inches long; at the end of this line a skin wheal is raised, and a needle is insert-

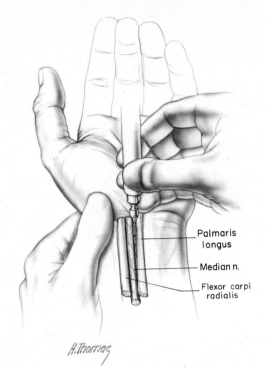

Palmaris
longus

Median n.

Flexor carpi
radialis

H.Thomas

Figure 4–5

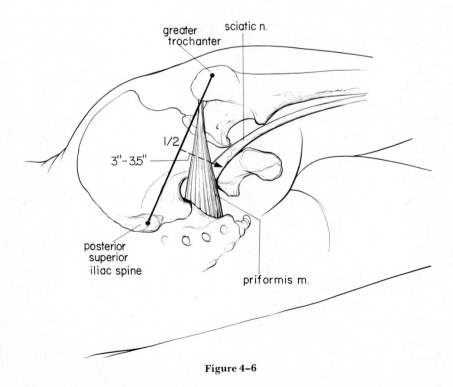

greater
trochanter

sciatic n.

1/2

3"–3.5"

posterior
superior
iliac spine

priformis m.

Figure 4–6

ed perpendicular to the skin (Fig. 4–6). The nerve is usually one to two inches deep depending on the thickness of the buttocks. Paresthesia is then elicited. Inject 10 to 15 cc of 2 per cent lidocaine or a comparable strength of another local anesthetic. If epinephrine is used, anesthesia is usually complete within 15 or 20 minutes.

Lateral Femoral Cutaneous Nerve Block

One inch medial to and one inch inferior to the anterior superior iliac spine, the needle is inserted perpendicularly until it penetrates the fascia lata; 5 to 10 ml of 1 per cent lidocaine, or a comparable dose of some other local anesthetic are injected in a fanlike fashion cephalad and caudad (Fig. 4–7). The procedure is repeated and another 5 ml is injected in a similar fashion.

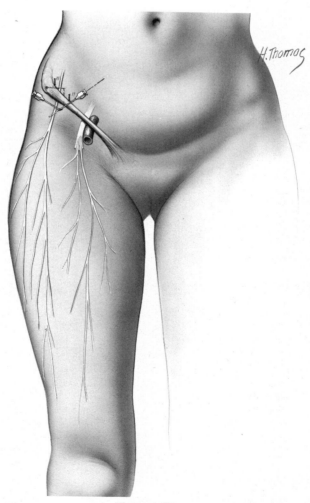

Figure 4–7

Obturator Nerve Block

A wheal is made over the skin ½ inch below and and ½ inch lateral to the pubic tubercle. A 22 gauge, 2 inch needle is advanced perpendicular to the skin through the wheal until it contacts the inferior ramus of the pubic bone. The needle is withdrawn and redirected and readvanced to a depth of ½ inch, at an angle of 60 degrees to the transverse axis, pointing laterally and cephalad (Fig. 4–8). When the needle point is no longer in contact with bone, it is again slightly withdrawn and redirected at an angle of 30 degrees to the transverse axis, pointing more laterally, and then advanced 1½ inches. Paresthesia usually occurs at this point. The usual technique for aspiration is followed, and if blood is obtained the needle should be withdrawn for a few millimeters and re-advanced to elicit paresthesia. A dose of 15 ml of local anesthetic solution is deposited. The needle is withdrawn slowly and another 10 ml is injected.

Figure 4–8

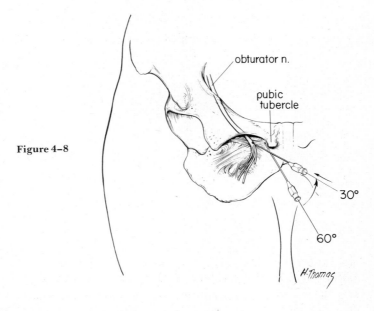

Trunk

Intercostal Nerve Block

The intercostal nerves can be blocked at any point along their course three to four inches from the vertebral spine to the cartilaginous portion of the rib. They run in a neurovascular bundle located in a groove running along the lower border of each rib.

A wheal is raised along the lower border of the rib where the block should be performed. The needle is advanced carefully until the lowermost border of the rib is contacted, then the needle is walked along the lower border of the rib, then readvanced slowly for about one eighth inch (Fig. 4–9). Paresthesia may or may not be elicited at this stage. Careful aspiration for blood or air is made. The

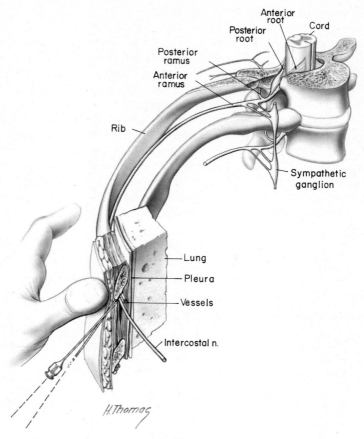

Anterior
root

Posterior
root

Cord

Posterior
ramus

Anterior
ramus

Rib

Sympathetic
ganglion

Lung

Pleura

Vessels

Intercostal n.

H.Thomas

Figure 4–9

needle tip should be always under control and always in contact with the lower border of the rib. A few ml of a weak concentration of the chosen local anesthetic are then injected. Pneumothorax is the most common complication of this procedure. As many ribs as needed can be blocked to effect complete relief of pain. Bilateral blocks are necessary for lesions overlying the sternum or midline. Onset of anesthesia is immediate. High systemic blood levels of the drugs are common in intercostal blocks.

Paravertebral Sympathetic Chain Block

The spine of the second or third lumbar vertebra is palpated and a skin wheal is raised at 2½ to 3 inches lateral to the tip of the spine (Figs. 4–10 and 4–11). A 4 inch 22 gauge needle is inserted through the skin wheal at an angle of 40 to 45 degrees to the perpendicular. The needle is withdrawn a few millimeters and walked off the tip. It is then readvanced at an angle of 40 to 50 degrees so it will contact the ventrolateral aspect of the lumbar vertebral body. It is then withdrawn and redirected until it slides off the lateral surface of the vertebral body.

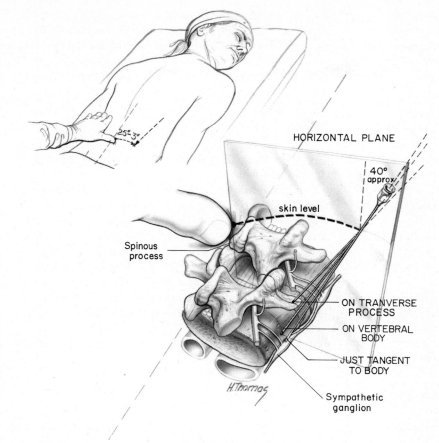

HORIZONTAL PLANE

40° approx.

skin level

Spinous process

ON TRANVERSE PROCESS

ON VERTEBRAL BODY

JUST TANGENT TO BODY

Sympathetic ganglion

H.Thomas

Figure 4–10

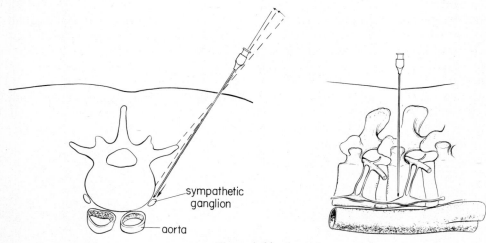

sympathetic ganglion

aorta

Figure 4–11

Advancement is carefully controlled to avoid puncturing any major vessels. The needle is withdrawn ½ cm, and a 5 ml dose of local anesthetic agent is deposited at this point. An image intensifier capable of two-plane visualization and televised x-ray screening can demonstrate the exact location of the tip of the needle in relation to the ventrolateral aspect of the vertebral body (Boas, 1976).

Paravertebral Somatic Nerve Block

In the thoracic region this block is helpful in identifying intercostal neuralgia and cardiac pain, while in the lumbar region it is helpful in localizing the pain in the inguinal region, legs, and lower back.

The same technique is used in both the lumbar and thoracic regions. However, one should note the difference in the anatomical landmarks. The tip of the thoracic vertebral spine corresponds to the body of the vertebra below. In the lumbar region it corresponds to the same vertebral body. Skin wheals are raised over the selected transverse processes. The needle is inserted and advanced perpendicular to the skin until it contacts the transverse process. Then, the needle is withdrawn a few millimeters and redirected, while advanced a few degrees caudad, until it slides off the lower border of the transverse process. Depending on the individual physique, a depth of 4½ to 7 cm is required to contact the appropriate root. Paresthesia should be elicited with utmost care. After careful aspiration for blood and cerebrospinal fluid, a dose of 5 ml of suitable local anesthetic agent is deposited.

Lumbar Plexus Block

The lumbar plexus is sandwiched between the quadratus lumborum and the psoas muscles, hence it is enclosed in fascial envelopes. This block can be accomplished by a single injection using an anterior, inguinal paravascular approach (Winnie, 1975). The technique is a simple modification of the femoral nerve block.

The femoral artery is palpated and retracted medially. Just lateral to the femoral artery, a skin wheal is raised. The needle is inserted into the fascial sheath and advanced until paresthesia of the femoral nerve is elicited. Digital pressure is applied firmly just distal to the needle while a suitable local anesthetic agent is injected. A volume of 30 to 35 ml is necessary. Following the injection, the needle is removed but digital pressure should be maintained for another few minutes.

Classic regional anesthesia texts such as Moore, 1965, Bonica, 1953, and Collins, 1976, should be referred to for further details regarding techniques or other blocks, particularly the commonly used screening blocks; for example, epidural, caudal, and spinal.

REFERENCES

Bietar, R.: Comparison of local anesthetics. J. Pharmacol. 56:221, 1936.

Boas, R. A: Lumbar sympathectomy — a percutaneous chemical technique. In Bonica, J. J. and Albe-Fessard, D.: Advances in Pain Research and Therapy, New York, Raven Press, 1976, Vol. 1.

Bonica, J. J.: The Management of Pain. Philadelphia, Lea and Febiger, 1953.

Bonica, J. J.: Current role of nerve blocks in diagnosis and therapy of pain. In Bonica, J. J.: Advances in Neurology, New York, Raven Press, 1974, Vol. 4.

Bonica, J. J.: Neurophysiologic and pathologic aspects of acute and chronic pain. Arch. Surg. 112:750, 1977.

Bonica, J. J., and Albe-Fessard, D.: Proceedings of the first world congress on pain. In Bonica, J. J., and Albe-Fessard, D., Advances in Pain Research and Therapy, Vol. 1. New York: Raven Press, 1976.

Burgess, P. R.: Patterns of discharge evoked in cutaneous nerves and their significance for sensation. In Bonica, J. J.: Advances in Neurology, New York, Raven Press, 1974, Vol. 4.

Chapman, C. R.: Psychological aspects of pain patient treatment. Arch. Surg. 112:767, 1977.

Collins, V. J.: Principles of Anesthesiology. Philadelphia, Lea and Febiger, 1976.

Condouris, G. A.: Effects of local anesthetics on the refractory periods of peripheral nerves. Pharmacologist 8:187, 1966.

Condouris, G. A.: Local anesthetics as modulators of neural information. In Bonica, J. J., and Albe-Fessard, D.: Advances in Pain Research and Therapy, New York, Raven Press 1976, Vol. 1.

Convino, B. G.: New local anesthetics for pain therapy. In Bonica, J. J.: Advances in Neurology, New York, Raven Press, 1974, Vol. 4.

Doupe, J., et al.: Post traumatic pain and causalgesic syndrome. J. Neurosurg. Psychiatry, 7:33, 1944.

Evans, J. A.: Reflex sympathetic dystrophy. Surg. Clin. N. Am. 26:780, 1946.

Evans, J. A.: Reflex sympathetic dystrophy. Surg. Gynecol. Obstet. 82:36, 1946.

Evans, J. A.: Sympathectomy for reflex sympathetic dystrophy: report of 29 cases. J.A.M.A. 132:620, 1946.

Evans, J. A.: Reflex sympathetic dystrophy; a report on 57 cases. Ann. Intern. Med. 26:417, 1947.

Fetz, E. D.: Pyramidal tract effects on interneurons in the cat lumbar dorsal horn. J. Neurophysiol. 31:69, 1968.

Hallin, R. G., and Torebjork, H. E.: Activity in unmyelinated nerve fibers in man. In Bonica, J. J. Advances in Neurology. New York, Raven Press, 1974, Vol. 4.

Hay, R. C., et al.: Control of intractable pain in advanced cancer by subarachnoid alcohol block. J.A.M.A. 169:1315, 1959.

Iggo, A.: The case for pain receptors. In Payne, J. P., and Burt, R. A. P.: Pain: Basic Principles, Pharmacology Training. London, Churchill Livingston, 1972.

Jefferson, A.: Trigeminal neuralgesia: Trigeminal root and ganglion injections using phenol in glycerine. In Knighton, R. S. and Dumke, P. R., Henry Ford Hospital International Symposium on Pain, Detroit, 1964. Boston, Little Brown and Company, 1966.

Kramer, H. S. and Schmidt, W. H.: Regional Anesthesia of the Maxillofacial Region in Facial Pain, 2nd ed., Philadelphia, Lea and Febiger, 1977.

Maher, R. M.: Relief of pain in incurable cancer. Lancet 1:18, 1955.

Mark, V. H., et al.: Intrathecal use of phenol for the relief of chronic severe pain. N. Engl. J. Med. 267:589, 1962.

McIntyre, A. R., and Sievers, R. F.: Pharmacology of some new local anesthetics. J. Pharmacol. Exper. Ther. 63:369, 1938.

Melzack, R.: Psychological concepts and methods for the control of pain. In Bonica, J. J.: Advances in Neurology. New York, Raven Press, 1974, Vol. 4.

Melzack, R., and Casey, K. L.: Sensory motivational and central control determinants of pain. In Kenshalo, D. R.: The Skin Senses. Springfield, Charles C Thomas, 1968.

Melzack, R., and Wall, P. D.: Pain mechanism: A new theory. Science 150:971, 1965.

Merskey, H., and Spear, F. G.: Pain: Psychological and Psychiatric Aspects. London, Balliere Trindall and Cassell Ltd., 1967.

Moricca, G.: Chemical hypophysectomy for cancer pain. In Bonica, J. J.: Advances in Neurology, New York, Raven Press, 1974, Vol. 4.

Moore, D. C., et al.: Bupivacaine compared with etidocaine for vaginal delivery. Anesthesia and Analgesia; Current Researches, 54:250, 1975.

Moore, D. C.: Regional Anesthesia. Springfield, Charles C Thomas, 1965.

Moore, D. C.: Factors determining blood level and dosage of anilid type local anesthetic agents. Presented to ASA annual meeting, 1976.

Murphy, T.: Current status of diagnostic and therapeutic nerve blocks. In 28th Annual Refresher Course Lectures. American Society of Anesthesiologists, 1977.

Noordenbos, W.: Pathologic aspects of central pain states. In Bonica, J. J.: Advances in Neurology. New York, Raven Press, 1974, Vol. 4.

Pagni, C. A.: Pain due to central nervous system lesions: physiopathological considerations and therapeutical implications. In Bonica. J. J.: Advances in Neurology, New York, Raven Press, 1974, Vol. 4.

Perl, E. R.: Is pain a specific sensation? J. Psychiatr. Res., *8*:272, 1971.

Sessle, B. J., and Greenwood, L. F.: Role of trigeminal nucleus caudalis in the modulation of trigeminal sensory and motor neuronal activities. *In* Bonica, J. J., and Albe-Fessard, D.: Advances in Pain Research and Therapy. New York, Raven Press, 1976, Vol. 1.

Sternback, R. A.: Pain: A Psychophysiologic Analysis. New York, Academic Press, 1968.

Taub, A.: Local, segmental supraspinal interaction with a dorsolateral spinal cutaneous afferent system. Exper. Neurol. *10*:357, 1964.

Ventafridda, V., and Martino, G.: Clinical evaluation of subarachnoid neurolytic blocks in intractable cancer pain. *In* Bonica, J. J., and Albe-Fessard, D.: Advances in Pain Research and Therapy. New York: Raven Press, 1976, Vol. 1.

Wall, P. D.: The laminar organization of dorsal horn and effects of descending impulses. J. Physiol. *188*:403, 1967.

Winnie, A. P.: Regional anesthesia. Surg. Clin. North Am. *55*(4):861–892, 1975.

5

SPECIAL DIAGNOSTIC STUDIES

E. F. SHAW WILGIS

There are many special diagnostic studies that can be utilized in the search for an answer to peripheral nerve problems. Some of these can be performed by the examining surgeon; others need the aid of ancillary personnel, including radiology, physical therapy, and other surgical modalities. It must be emphasized that no one of these studies is in itself diagnostic but should be used only as a diagnostic aid in the complete clinical assessment of any given problem.

MYELOGRAPHY

Myelography is the radiologic visualization of the subarachnoid space in any given part of the spine. It involves the combined disciplines of radiology and neuro- or orthopedic surgery. It is always done secondary to complete physical examination. Its main advantage is in attempting to further define whether a lesion has a spinal origin or is peripheral. Usually, contrast medium is injected into the lumbar subarachnoid space and is visualized throughout the entire spinal canal by tilting the patient. Compressive root defects can be determined as well as defects in the covering surfaces of the spinal cord. Myelography is useful in brachial plexus injuries, in cervical spine as well as lumbar spine compressive defects, and in determining spinal cord tumors. Its main disadvantage is that it is an invasive study and the usual sterile precautions of lumbar puncture must be observed. In rare instances patients can develop spinal headache and have lingering problems as a result of myelography.

VASCULAR TESTS

The function of the peripheral nerves in an extremity can be directly related to the quality of the circulation in that given extremity. Nerves respond quickly to ischemia, and if that ischemia is prolonged, they show a prolonged recovery period. Studies by this author as well as others have shown this to be true (Wilgis, 1971). In 1917, Tinel described the consequences of ischemia from severance of a main artery. This was reconfirmed by Seddon (1972). Ischemia can be produced in several different ways. First, as a result of injury, there is occlusion of a major vessel that includes division, thrombosis, or embolism. Secondly, ischemia can be produced by a compressive force such as hematoma, subfascial edema, or a tumor growing in a closed space. These two methods of producing ischemia have two separate effects. First, there is a local effect on the adjacent nerve. This local effect is an ischemic neuritis or compression defect within a segmental area of the adjacent nerve, or both. This can produce all of the symptoms of a lesion of that given nerve. Secondly, and just as important, is the distal effect of an ischemic event. This can involve the entire physiologic function of the nerve, including the sensory and motor end organs. We see this distal effect more often in the vascular lesions of diabetes, collagen vascular diseases, and severe peripheral arteriosclerosis where the entire circulatory input into the extremity is diminished.

For all of these reasons it is most important to include a thorough vascular examination in any patient with a peripheral nerve lesion. The normal physical examination including blood pressure recordings and the palpation of pulses should be done. Specific maneuvers such as the Adson test, which examines the peripheral radial pulse in varying positions of extension and abduction of the shoulder, can be helpful in pinpointing local compressive forces. There are several special diagnostic studies of varying degrees of complexity which we shall now consider.

Allen Test

The Allen Test is a useful clinical test to determine the patency of one of the arteries in a double arterial supply system. This is particularly useful in the hand, which is supplied by both the radial and ulnar arteries. The Allen test consists of compressing both the radial and ulnar arteries and then emptying the hand of all blood by flexion and extension of the digits. The pressure is then removed from the radial artery, and the hand is allowed to fill. The test is repeated by releasing pressure to the ulnar artery, and again the hand is then allowed to fill. If one of the two arteries is occluded or if the palmar arch is incomplete, the compromised circulation will then become evident. In a study of 70 healthy subjects Mozersky et al. (1973) reported that 1.6 per cent had an incomplete radial dominant palmar arch with no antegrade circulation and that 8.4 per cent had poor antegrade and retrograde collateral circulation, indicating the importance of detecting the adequacy of the entire arterial tree. A variant of this test can also be used in the digit by selectively compressing either digital artery and testing the capillary filling of that particular digit.

Doppler

The ultrasonic flow detector (Fig. 5–1) is a noninvasive monitor of arterial and venous flow (Strandness et al., 1966). Ultrasound waves emitted through

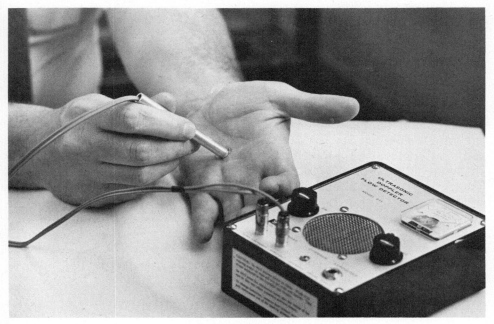

Figure 5–1 Doppler ultrasonic flow detector.

piezoelectric crystals are transmitted through the skin's subcutaneous tissue and superficially located blood vessels. The radial, ulnar, palmar arch, and digital vessels are accessible for monitoring with this instrument. The emitted high frequency sounds of five to ten million cycles per second strike the soft tissues and the blood cells moving through the blood vessels. The blood cells, which are in rapid motion, cause an alteration in the pitch of the sound waves upon impact. These reflected waves, varying in volume and pitch depending upon the velocity and quantity of moving blood cells, are received by the recording part of the probe and are amplified and converted to signals in an audible range. The experienced listener can readily separate arterial and venous flow signals. It is also possible to differentiate arterial flow signals through normally patent versus stenotic vessels and to recognize arterial flow arriving by collateral vessels bypassing a proximal obstruction. This information can be transferred to a recording device so that a pictorial pulse wave can be elicited. Other applications of the ultrasonic detector include the following:

1. Determination of systolic pressures at various levels of the arm that has no pulses at the wrist.
2. Determination of the adequacy of cross circulation to the hand and to each digit prior to any surgical procedure or cannulation of either the radial or ulnar artery.
3. Determination of patency of digital vessels transiently occluded by vasospasm.
4. Determination of prognosis for survival of individual digits based on the presence of demonstrable pulse flow in the digital arteries.
5. Determination of the precise level of digital arterial occlusions.

6. Determination of whether the hand circulation is supported by direct flow by normally patent arteries or whether flow is most likely via collateral vessels.

Arteriography

The contrast angiogram has enjoyed a long history of being a useful diagnostic method in the evaluation of the vascular status of an extremity. It involves the intra-arterial injection of contrast medium and the subsequent visualization of the arterial and venous phases of circulation. This method is invaluable for the location of specific arterial defects. The femoral route is the safest puncture site. Severe complications have been reported from the transaxillary route as well as the brachial injection sites. However, the discomfort of this method, the requirements of special personnel and equipment, the hazards of administration of iodides, and the possible complications at the site of arterial puncture limit its application. It cannot be used routinely nor can it be used repetitively. One of the disadvantages is that the arteriogram is mainly an anatomical study and gives no information as to the dynamic state of the circulation.

Plethysmography

Another noninvasive technique for evaluating peripheral blood flow that we have found helpful is plethysmography (Wilgis, 1974). A plethysmograph is an instrument that measures volume. There are many types of plethysmography: strain gauge, impedance, pneumatic, hydraulic, and inductance. Essentially, all of these methods utilize volume displacement attached to a recording device and amplifying system to obtain not only quantitative but also qualitative recording of a pulse wave. The pulse wave can then be examined. Each normal digital pulse wave reveals a sharp systolic peak and a dicrotic notch on the downslope. Vasospasm is revealed by a decreased amplitude of the wave with normal configuration. Proximal obstruction in the arterial tree, which alters normal pulsatile flow, produces a digital pulse wave with decreasing amplitude, a rounded peak, and absence of the dicrotic notch on the downslope. These pulse waves can then be compared to those of other digits and the contralateral hand to obtain a percentage of normal circulation.

The latest development in plethysmography is the pulse volume recorder. This was developed by Raines (Darling et al., 1972; Raines et al., 1973). It produces a quantitative, reproducible segmental plethysmographic recording of the area studied with a minimum of complexities. This device records volume change within a given segment of a digit. This includes all segments of the arterial system and this limb segment during a specific cardiac cycle. The system consists of one or two digital cuffs, one of which is used to pick up the pressure changes. These cuff pressure changes affect alteration in the cuff volume, which, in turn, reflects changes in limb value. The electronic package then transmits and records the data on hard copy paper for the clinician to read (Fig. 5–2). It can be used in conjunction with the Doppler ultrasonic flow detector.

The second cuff is used to record the digital perfusion pressure. The digital perfusion pressure, measured in millimeters of mercury, represents the circula-

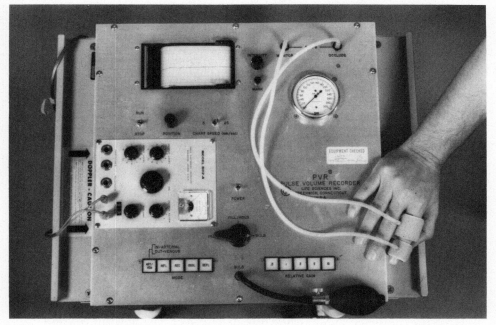

Figure 5–2   Pulse volume recorder with digital cuffs in place.

tory pressure in the digit being studied. We have found this to be the most reproducible and reliable method of recording circulation in a digit. More simply, it is a blood pressure recording of a finger taken with miniature apparatus (Fig. 5–3). This figure can then be correlated, as in the upper extremity, with the other areas of physical examination including the nervous system.

The pulse volume recording and digital perfusion pressures can then be used to study the circulation in various dynamic states: before and after exercise and before and after exposure to cold. It is our routine to examine the patient

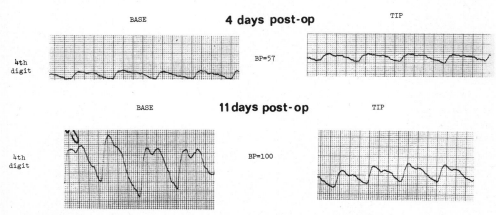

Figure 5–3   Pulse volume recording four and 11 days after digital replantation. The recordings of the pulse waves are from the base and tip of the revascularized digit.

before exercise and then to exercise the involved limb for five minutes. We then examine the patient again and record digital perfusion pressures after exercise. This gives information as to whether the blood supply in the extremity is adequate to sustain prolonged exercise. It is particularly helpful in elucidating claudication symptoms of a vascular nature.

In examining the patient for cold intolerance, the pulse volume recording and digital perfusion pressures are recorded at room temperature. The extremity is then immersed in iced water for three minutes and the patient is again examined. If the recording does not return to near normal after five minutes at room temperature, it is abnormal and could be diagnostic of vasospasm.

Another variety of cold stress testing is the Foster Test. This method studies variation in temperature as the extremity is cold stressed in iced water. The temperature of the hand is measured prior to and after immersion in cold water for three minutes. Temperature is again studied and charted relative to time until it returns to its preimmersion level.

Vasospastic disorders and other abnormalities of the sympathetic nervous system should be so investigated.

Radionuclide Studies

In our experience radionuclide intravenous dynamic flow studies and static perfusion scans of the extremity have been useful (Wagner, 1972). Multiple modifications are possible either with the equipment, or with choice of nuclide or compounds used for tagging, thus improving the quality of the image or increasing the diagnostic accuracy, or both. An image or image series is obtained that provides useful information in a significant number of patients (Wilgis et al., 1974).

This method is as follows:

The scintillation camera (Nuclear of Chicago Pho Gamma III) (Fig. 5–4) is fitted with a 4000 parallel hole high sensitivity low-energy collimator. Technetium 99m as pertechnetate is eluted from a molybdenum 99m generator. The minimum nuclide dose needed to obtain a satisfactory dynamic handflow study is 10 millicuries given intravenously. By studying normal controls (patients referred for brain scanning), it was established that smaller doses gave unsatisfactory handflow studies. However, doses of 10 millicuries were adequate for static hand images. We routinely used 20 millicuries for the dynamic flow study. High specific-activity technetium 99m (8 to 12 millicuries per milliliter) is injected as a bolus in the antecubital fossa. In our experience, basilic vein injections using a 19 gauge needle gave better studies than the cephalic vein injection. A significant factor to be considered in this procedure is the temperature influence on the capillary bed — the examined extremity should be normalized to room temperature.

The hand is placed on the camera detector or directly underneath it. Satisfactory information density for the flow study using Polaroid film is obtained with three to six seconds of exposure time per image (approximately 250 to 600 counts per image). The appearance of the nuclide in the examined segment is monitored on the C.R.T. display screen. If at all possible, the injection should be performed in the opposite extremity, although excellent studies were obtained with careful positioning venipuncture in the ipsilateral antecubital

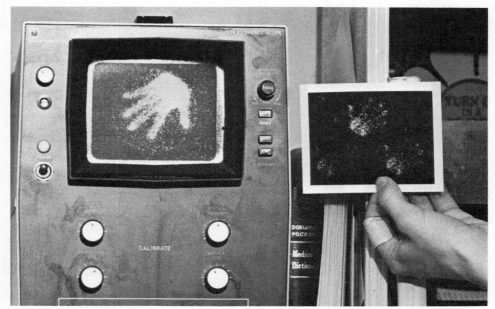

Figure 5–4 Radionuclide angiogram is projected on the x-ray screen, and the collective images are recorded on polaroid film.

fossa. The study is completed with static cumulative imaging: an image or images of 100,000 to 300,000 count exposures are obtained immediately after the dynamic study.

SUMMARY

In conclusion, there are many and varied ways in which the vascular system can be studied.

Each diagnostic test has its own merits. We have used the clinical physical examination, including special pulse tests such as Allen and Adson routinely. More sophisticated testing methods, such as radioactive scanning or pulse volume recording can be used to provide further information in case of a diagnostic dilemma. Recent quantitative studies of circulation after replantation confirm that ultimate nerve function is dependent on circulation. The results of these studies then have to be applied to the relationship of the vascular system to the nervous system. One must be constantly cognizant of vascular lesions or vascular complications that can lead to clinical problems of the peripheral nerves.

REFERENCES

Darling, R. D., Raines, J. K., Brener, B. J., and Austen, W. G.: Quantitative segmental pulse volume recorder: A clinical tool. Surgery 72:873, 1972.

Mozersky, D. J., Buckley, C. J., Hagood, C. O., Jr., Capps, W. F., Jr., and Dannemiller, F. J., Jr.: Ultrasonic evaluation of the palmar circulation—a useful adjunct to radial artery cannulation. Am. J. Surg. 126:810, 1973.

Raines, J. K., Jaffrin, M. Y., and Rao, S.: A non-invasive pressure pulse recorder development and rationale. Med. Instrum. 7:245, 1973.

Seddon, H.: Surgical Disorders of the Peripheral Nerves. Baltimore, The Williams & Wilkins Co., 1972.

Strandness, D. E., Jr., McCutcheon, E. F., and Rushmer, R. F.: Application of a transcutaneous Doppler flowmeter in evaluation of occlusive arterial disease. Surg. Gynecol. Obstet. *122*:1039, 1966.

Tinel, J.: Nerve Wounds. London, Bailliere, Tindall and Cox, 1917.

Wagner, N. H.: Nuclear medicine in cardiovascular disease. Hosp. Pract. 7:108, 1972.

Wilgis, E. F. S., Jezic, D., Stonesifer, G. L., Jr., Classen, J. N., and Sekercan, K.: The evaluation of small vessel flow. J. Bone Joint Surg. *56A*:1199, 1974.

Wilgis, E. F. S.: Observations on the effects of tourniquet ischemia. J. Bone Joint Surg. *53A*:1343, 1971.

6

NORMAL AND ANOMALOUS INNERVATION PATTERNS IN THE UPPER EXTREMITY

EMANUEL B. KAPLAN and
MORTON SPINNER

Anomalies associated with interjoining of neural elements can occur anywhere from the origin of the brachial plexus to the digits. At the brachial plexus level it is usual to find major shifting of neural components, seen easily with the naked eye, while more peripherally, such neural interchange is observed only microscopically.

Knowledge of these neural variations is vital in order to effectively treat patients who present with problems of pain, paralysis, or paresthesias that often differ from the more classic clinical manifestations of specific peripheral neural disorders. This chapter will emphasize the clinical aspects and significance of these variations. It is impossible to list all the neural anomalies of the upper extremities but we shall present the basic patterns of the significant neural anomalies and their clinical importance, focusing attention on representative examples, as seen in the brachial plexus, arm, forearm, and hand.

At all levels there are four basic patterns of neural variations:

1. Inconstancy in the number of branches to muscles or to skin, or both. Additionally, there are significant variations in the level of origin of the major branches from their parent trunk (Brash, 1955).
2. Neural loop formations of the short and long varieties (Hartmann, 1887; Kaplan, 1963; Winkelman and Spinner, 1973).
3. Neural variations within an individual muscle or an individual muscle group; (Figs. 6–1 and 6–2); that is, the flexor digitorum profundus muscle or the thenar muscle group (Brooks, 1886; Roundtree, 1949; Harness and Sekeles, 1971).
4. A significant communicating branch between one major peripheral nerve trunk and another, as seen with the Martin-Gruber anastomosis (neural connection between the median and ulnar nerves, Fig. 6–1) in the forearm; a neural pathway connecting the musculocutaneous and median nerves in the arm (Figs. 6–10*B* and 6–11*E*, and the Riche-Cannieu anastomosis (neural connection between the deep branch of the ulnar nerve and the median nerve, Fig. 6–2) in the hand.

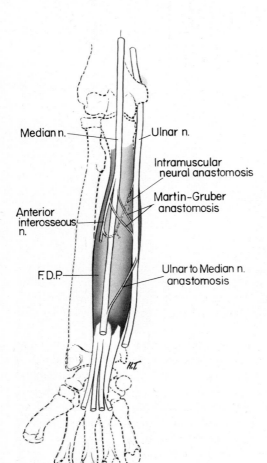

Figure 6–1 An intramuscular neural anastomosis within the flexor digitorum profundus (F.D.P.) between the anterior interosseous branch of the median nerve and the motor branch of the ulnar nerve to this muscle is depicted. It is through this connection that variations in supply to the flexor digitorum profundus between the ulnar and median nerves occur. The Martin-Gruber anastomosis and the ulnar nerve to median nerve anastomosis are also represented.

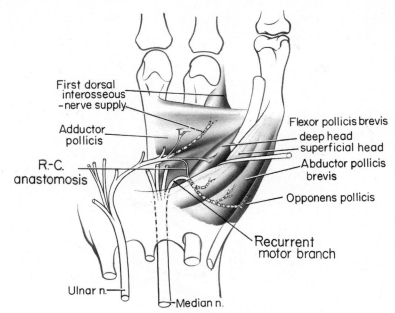

First dorsal
interosseous
-nerve supply

Adductor
pollicis

R.-C.
anastomosis

Flexor pollicis brevis
deep head
superficial head

Abductor pollicis
brevis

Opponens pollicis

Recurrent
motor branch

Ulnar n.

Median n.

Figure 6–2 There are significant variations in the neural supply of the thenar group of muscles. These muscles are usually supplied by the recurrent branch of the median nerve but they can be innervated by the ulnar nerve to varying degrees through the Riche-Cannieu anastomosis (R.–C.).

BRACHIAL PLEXUS

The brachial plexus is usually formed in the following manner: the fifth and sixth cervical nerve roots combine, soon after their origin, to form the upper trunk; the seventh cervical nerve passes on directly to the middle trunk; while the eighth cervical and first thoracic roots combine, soon after their origin, to form the lower trunk. Classically, each of the trunks separates into an anterior and a posterior division.

The basic pattern of a normal brachial plexus at this level thus resembles an inverted letter "Y" placed between two "X"'s (Fig. 6–3).

All of the posterior divisions combine to form the posterior cord. While the anterior divisions of the upper trunk and middle trunk combine to form the lateral cord, it is the anterior division of the lower trunk that continues on as the medial cord. In the axilla, the lateral cord gives rise to the musculocutaneous nerve and the lateral root of the median nerve, while the medial cord gives rise to the ulnar nerve, the medial root of the median nerve, and the medial cutaneous nerves of the arm and forearm. The posterior cord gives rise to the axillary nerve and the radial nerve.

Elements of the brachial plexus which are anterior remain in that plane and there is no communication between the anterior and posterior elements, the

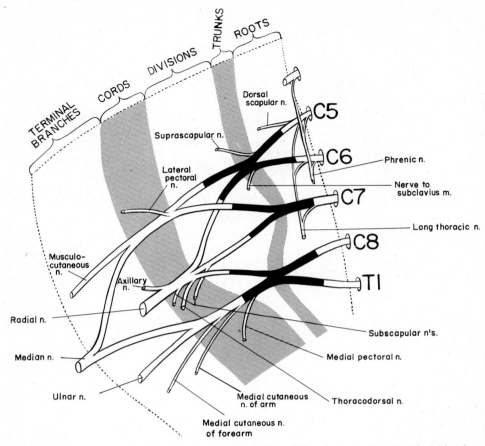

Figure 6–3 The pattern of the proximal formation of the plexus in the supraclavicular fossa of the roots, trunks, and divisions is that of two "X"'s surrounding an inverted "Y."

latter including the posterior divisions and posterior cord. Similarly, there is no communication from the posterior to the anterior neural structures.

Common Variations in the Major Elements of the Supraclavicular Portion of the Brachial Plexus

The most frequent variation of the plexus results from accessory contributions from the fourth cervical level and occurs in 62 per cent of the population (Kerr, 1918).

In addition, the second thoracic nerve frequently participates in the formation of the brachial plexus (Cunningham, 1877; Paterson, 1887). These findings indicate that the plexus frequently has its origin from as high as the fourth cervical nerve to as low as the second thoracic nerve. If the elements from the fourth cervical nerve predominate, the brachial plexus is referred to as being in a *pre-fixed* position; if the lower elements predominate, then the term *post-fixed* is utilized. Bilateral symmetry of the plexus was found to exist in 61.9 per cent of 63 cadavers (Kerr, 1918).

Less Common Variations in the Major Elements of the Supraclavicular Portion of the Brachial Plexus

The upper trunk may occasionally arise from C5, C6, and C7 nerve roots, rather than the more usual C5 and C6 roots. Rarely, this trunk may be formed by C6 and C7 nerve roots only. The posterior cord infrequently arises from C6 and C7, rather than by divisions of all the roots (Turner, 1871). In one subject, the seventh cervical root decussated into three elements, one going to the lower trunk, one to the posterior cord, and one entering the median nerve directly.

According to Herringham (1887), the upper trunk is inconstantly formed, C5 and C6 roots each dividing into an anterior and a posterior branch. In 8 of 10 specimens, Schumacher (1913) observed an anastomosis of the lateral and medial cords which passed anterior to the axillary artery and carried the fibers of C7 to the ulnar nerve; it reached the medial cord at variable levels but above the origin of the ulnar nerve in all 8 specimens. Rarely, the upper trunk is formed by C5, C6, and C7 nerve roots dividing into two planes, an anterior and a posterior division. ·

Kerr noted that in 14 of 175 plexuses studied the upper trunk did not exist; C5 and C6 roots each divided into an anterior and a posterior division, which then united. The middle trunk bifurcated into its usual anterior and posterior elements in the vast majority of instances. In five specimens, the middle trunk was observed to divide into three branches, one posterior and two anterior branches. One of the anterior branches entered the lateral cord and the other entered the medial cord (Fig. 6–4).

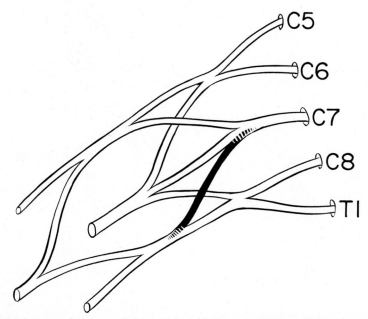

Figure 6–4   An anomalous extra division of the middle trunk which traveled to the medial cord.

With regard to the lower trunk, in Kerr's study it was formed in 166 of 175 dissections by C8 and T1. In 165 of 166 specimens, the lower trunk divided into an anterior and a posterior division. In the remaining specimen it divided into the ulnar nerve and the medial root of the median nerve. In two cases, C8 sent a branch to the lateral cord, in one case C8 united with the lateral root of the median nerve, and in one instance C8 joined with the middle trunk (Fig. 6–5). In six specimens, the C8 root divided into an anterior and a posterior element, the anterior joining T1 to form the medial root of the median nerve and the ulnar nerve (Fig. 6–6). In 45 dissections, Herringham found that the posterior cord received a contribution from T1 in six instances. Cunningham (1877) felt that T1 did not participate in the formation of the posterior cord, but Harris (1904, 1939) found a contribution from T1 to the posterior cord in 9 of 14 specimens.

An extreme variation of the plexus has been described in which all the roots united to form a single cord (Singer, 1933; Hasan and Narayan, 1964).

It is impossible to give the average length of each trunk because of the myriad variations which occur, even comparing one extremity to its mate. Hovalacque (1927) has observed the upper trunk measurement to vary from 12 mm to 4 cm, while the lower trunk varied from 4 to 5 cm in length.

Valentin (1843) and Soulie (1904) concluded that the anterior branch of C6 was almost always larger than the other branches, but there is disagreement with this observation (Kerr, 1918; Hovelacque, 1927).

It is common for the C5 and C6 roots either to pass through the scalenus anticus muscle or to pass between the scalenus anticus and the scalenus medius muscles. The C5 root may occasionally pass anterior to the scalenus anticus muscle. The cords are formed at the level of the summit of the axilla. At this level, the two anterior cords (the lateral and medial) are almost always the same size. The posterior cord is twice the diameter of the anterior cords.

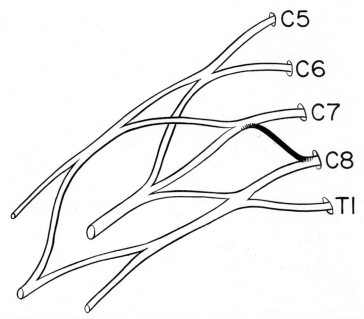

Figure 6–5   An anomalous branch of the C8 root is seen passing to the middle trunk.

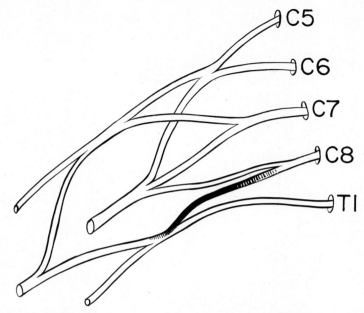

Figure 6-6 Anomalous lower portion of the brachial plexus. There is no inferior trunk. The C8 root has divided into two components, one to the posterior cord and the other, an anterior element, joined T1 distally to form the medial root of the median nerve and the ulnar nerve.

PERIPHERAL NERVES OF THE SUPRACLAVICULAR PORTION OF THE BRACHIAL PLEXUS

Four major branches that arise from elements of the brachial plexus above the clavicle are comparable to peripheral nerves at the termination of the distal plexus; these proximal nerves are the suprascapular, dorsal scapular, long thoracic, and phrenic. The nerve to the subclavius muscle is a less significant branch. All of these branches arise from anterior components of the roots or trunks.

Suprascapular Nerve

The suprascapular nerve arises from the upper trunk in 63 per cent of cases. In 69 of the 172 brachial plexuses dissected (Kerr, 1918), it received a contribution from C4 itself or a separate branch from C6. The nerve can rarely arise from the distal end of C5 root.

Dorsal Scapular Nerve

In the majority of instances the nerve to the levator scapulae and to the rhomboids is a single branch, but occasionally the nerve may be double, with the two branches running close together. Whether single or double, the nerve constantly originates from C5, close to the exit from the intervertebral foramen

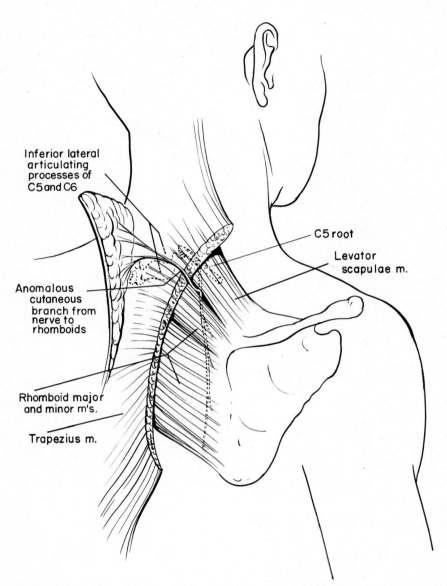

Figure 6–7   An anomalous branch of the dorsal scapular nerve (the nerve to the levator scapulae and rhomboids) can supply the skin on the dorsum of the back. This anomalous branch penetrates the trapezius to reach the skin over the upper dorsal spine. The dorsal scapular nerve is usually motor. A proximal entrapment lesion of this nerve usually does not leave sensory disturbance. However, some lesions of this nerve can present with sensory findings in addition to paralysis of the levator scapulae and the major and minor rhomboids if this neural variation was present.

(Herringham, 1887). On occasion it may receive a branch from the root of C4 and, rarely, it arises only from C4. In one interesting dissection, the nerve to the rhomboids not only supplied the levator scapulae and the rhomboids but sent a branch through the trapezius muscle to supply an area of skin in the region of the fifth and sixth dorsal vertebrae (Fig. 6–7).

Long Thoracic Nerve

The long thoracic nerve (the nerve of Bell) originates from two or three roots. This nerve innervates the serratus anterior muscle. The proximal origin of the nerve originates from C5, frequently in common with the nerve to the levator scapulae and rhomboids. The largest component of the long thoracic nerve usually arises from C6, the inconstant branch emanating from C7. On occasion, there can be contributions from C4. A supernumerary branch may arise from C8. On occasion, two separate branches may supply the serratus anterior, one from C5 supplying several of the digitations of the serratus anterior while another from C5 and C6, or from C6 alone, innervates the adjacent digitations (Curnow, 1873). Herringham found that the upper digitations of the muscle were usually supplied by C5, the middle digitations by C5 and C6, and the inferior digitations by C7.

Phrenic Nerve

The phrenic nerve, which innervates the diaphragm, arises from the roots of C5 and C6 and receives occasional contributions from C4.

The nerve to the subclavius usually arises from the lateral trunk and is formed by C4 and C5, with infrequent twigs arising from C6 or C7. Turner (1872) observed that the nerve to the subclavius on rare occasions gives a branch to the clavicular portion of the sternomastoid muscle.

BRANCHES OF THE MIDPORTION OF THE PLEXUS

These branches usually arise from the medial, lateral, and posterior cords. These include the nerves to the pectoralis major and minor, the subscapular nerves, and the thoracodorsal nerve.

Pectoralis Major

Herringham demonstrated that nerve innervation to the pectoralis major is usually double. The lateral pectoral nerve is usually thinner, arising either from the distal end of the upper trunk, from the anterior division of the upper trunk, or from the lateral cord. The inferior branch arises either from the lower trunk, its anterior division, or from the medial cord (Fig. 6–3). The pectoralis major may also receive twigs from the intercostal nerves.

Pectoralis Minor

The nerve to the pectoralis minor, after penetrating this muscle, may anastomose with the inferior pectoral nerve. After innervating a portion of the pectoralis major, it usually supplies an area of skin at the base of the axilla.

It has been shown that a branch of the pectoralis major nerve may supply the clavicular portion of the deltoid muscle (Luschka, 1850; Turner, 1872; Frohse and Fränkel, 1908). This is common if the cephalic vein is absent and there is partial fusion of the pectoralis major and deltoid muscles. In addition, there are anastomoses between the supraclavicular nerves (sensory) and the perforating branches of the nerves to the pectoralis major in the region of the deltopectoral groove.

Subscapular Nerves

The nerve supply to the subscapularis muscle usually has a superior and an inferior branch. The superior nerve is most frequently derived from the terminal portion of the middle trunk or its posterior division (Fig. 6–3) and is frequently double-branched (40 per cent) or even triple-branched (6 per cent) (Kerr). Almost from its origin, the nerve enters the axilla, running along the lateral side of the posterior cord. It may arise from the union of the posterior divisions of the lateral and lower trunks. In 13 of 157 plexuses, Kerr noted that it arose from the posterior cord. It can arise from C5 root or from two roots. It can rarely arise with the suprascapular nerve from the lateral trunk. It can even originate from the radial nerve so that significant variations in the origin of the superior branch of the nerve to the subscapularis muscle are seen. The subscapularis muscle does not usually receive any fibers from C7, most of them coming from C5 and C6, or from C5 or C6 alone. The inferior nerve to the subscapularis muscle is very inconstant and diverse, and is related to the variations of the branches to the latissimus dorsi and teres major muscles. When these latter branches are reduced or totally absent, the inferior subscapular nerve is well developed and will frequently supply the latissimus dorsi and teres major muscles, in addition to the subscapularis muscle. If, on the other hand, the nerve branches to the latissimus dorsi and the teres major muscles are well developed, then the inferior nerve branch to the subscapularis muscle is reduced or is totally absent. This latter branch most frequently arises in the axilla either directly from the posterior cord or from a common branch, together with the axillary nerve and the nerve to the teres major. It seldom takes origin from the union of the posterior division of the lateral and middle trunks, and may occasionally arise from the radial nerve. The inferior subscapular nerve can receive a branch from the superior subscapular nerve and supply the latissimus dorsi and teres major muscles.

Thoracodorsal Nerve

The thoracodorsal nerve (occasionally referred to as the long or middle subscapular nerve) derives its fibers from C5 through C8 and in 50 per cent of instances from C7 alone (Kerr, 1918). It emanates usually from the posterior cord to innervate the latissimus dorsi muscle.

EXAMPLE OF NEURAL ANOMALY OF THE
BRACHIAL PLEXUS WHICH HAS
CLINICAL SIGNIFICANCE

The flexor carpi ulnaris can be found functioning with a complete lower trunk lesion.

In 5 to 10 per cent of upper extremities the motor funiculi to the flexor carpi ulnaris muscle arise from the C7 root rather than from the C8 and T1 nerve roots. These aberrant funiculi pass down the middle trunk, cross over through at least two distinct pathways in the distal portion of the brachial plexus, and enter the ulnar nerve to innervate the flexor carpi ulnaris muscle (Fig. 6–8). It is therefore not uncommon to observe a functioning flexor carpi ulnaris muscle despite a complete C8–T1 lesion.

THE TERMINAL BRANCHES OF THE
BRACHIAL PLEXUS IN THE ARM

These peripheral nerve branches include the median, musculocutaneous, radial, axillary, ulnar, and medial cutaneous nerves of the arm and forearm.

Median Nerve

The median nerve is formed in the axilla by the union of neural elements of the lateral and medial cords. The lateral and medial roots of the median nerve usually unite anterior to the axillary artery to form the median nerve (Fig. 6–9A).

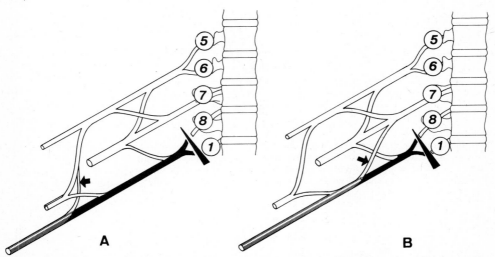

A   **B**

Figure 6–8 The flexor carpi usually receives its motor supply from C8. It can arise from C7, and these neural fibers pass via an anomalous course (arrows) to the ulnar nerve distal to the C8–T1 lesion. This occurs via an anomalous branch of the lateral root of the median nerve (*A*) or through an extra division of the middle trunk (*B*). The ulnar nerve in these instances has a "lateral root" very much as the median nerve characteristically has two roots. In this anomaly, the ulnar nerve also has two roots. It is through this "lateral root" of the ulnar nerve that aberrant functioning neural fibers can reach the flexor carpi ulnaris with a complete lower plexus root lesion.

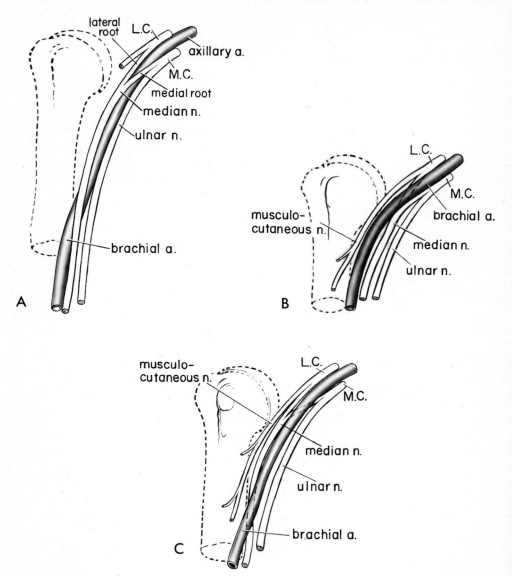

Figure 6–9 *A*, In the axilla the median nerve is formed by the union of the lateral root of the median nerve and the medial root of the median nerve from the lateral and medial cords, respectively. The median nerve and its roots usually pass anterior to the axillary artery. *B*, The lateral root of the median nerve can pass posterior to the axillary artery. *C*, The medial root of the median nerve can pass posterior to this artery.

There are significant anatomical variations in the formation of the median nerve and its relationship to the axillary artery. On occasion, the lateral root of the median nerve passes posterior to the axillary artery, while in other instances the medial root of the median nerve passes posterior to this major artery (Fig. 6–9*B* and *C*). The medial root is usually constant in its size and course. The lateral root is extremely variable. It can be extremely small, and it may be double or triple (Fig. 6–10*A*). The smaller the lateral root of the median nerve, the more

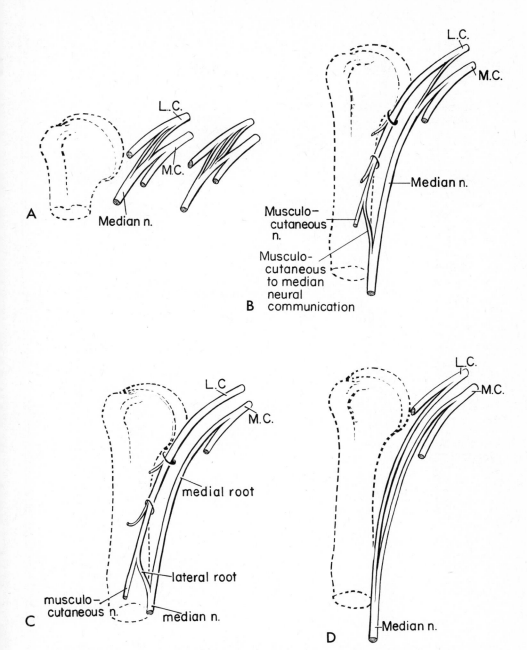

Figure 6–10   There are numerous variations of the lateral root of the median nerve. *A,* It may be double or triple. *B,* It may be thin. When this occurs there is usually a communication between the musculocutaneous nerve and the median nerve in the arm. *C,* The lateral root of the median nerve can have a low take-off. It can pass with the musculocutaneous nerve for a varying distance in the arm before joining the medial root to form the median nerve. *D,* The two roots of the median nerve can arise at their usual axillary level but may unite to form the median nerve at varying levels in the arm. It appears as if the median nerve is "reduplicated" when in reality it had not united or completely formed.

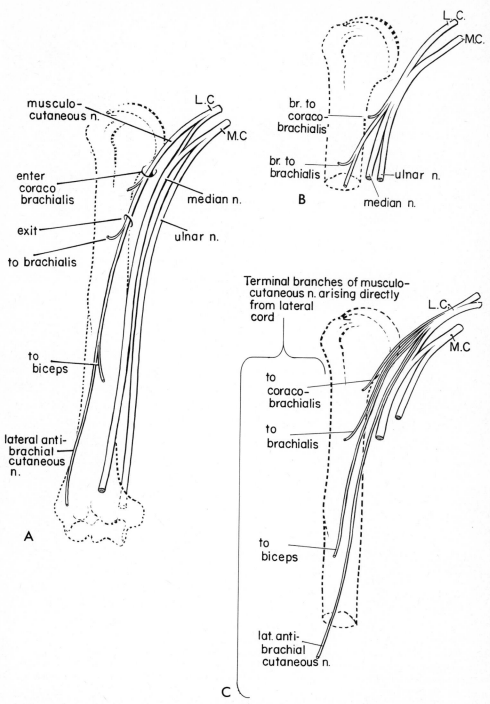

Figure 6–11 *A*, The musculocutaneous nerve usually arises from the lateral cord (L.C.) and penetrates the coracobrachialis muscle in·the proximal region of the arm. *B*, It can arise from a common neural structure which gives origin to the median, ulnar, and musculocutaneous nerves. *C*, It may divide into some or all of its terminal branches in the axilla. All of the branches may then perforate the coracobrachialis muscle at multiple sites.

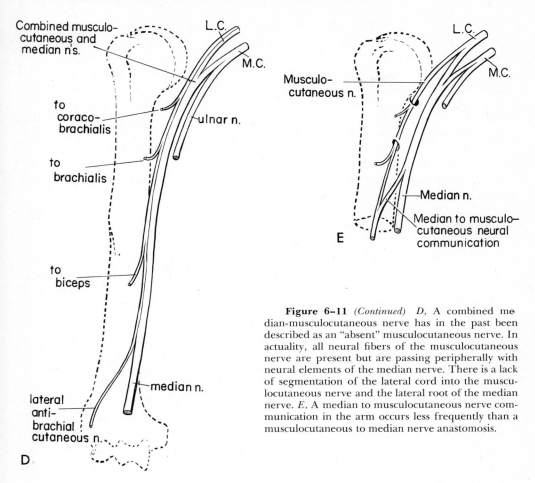

Figure 6–11 *(Continued)* D, A combined median-musculocutaneous nerve has in the past been described as an "absent" musculocutaneous nerve. In actuality, all neural fibers of the musculocutaneous nerve are present but are passing peripherally with neural elements of the median nerve. There is a lack of segmentation of the lateral cord into the musculocutaneous nerve and the lateral root of the median nerve. E, A median to musculocutaneous nerve communication in the arm occurs less frequently than a musculocutaneous to median nerve anastomosis.

likely it is that a communication exists between the musculocutaneous nerve and the median nerve in the arm (Fig. 6–10*B*). This has a 24 per cent occurrence rate (Vallois, 1922). All neural elements of the lateral root of the median nerve may pass with the musculocutaneous nerve to join the medial root of the median nerve at varying levels in the arm (Fig. 6–10*C*). In this instance, no lateral root is found in the axilla. Occasionally, the lateral and medial roots of the median nerve join in the formation of the median nerve at variable levels in the arm (Fig. 6–10*D*). If the union of these roots is distal to the elbow, "two" median nerves in the arm would be found at surgery.

Musculocutaneous Nerve

The musculocutaneous nerve arises from the lateral cord in 88 per cent of the population (Kerr, 1918). It usually penetrates the coracobrachialis muscle in the proximal arm (Fig. 6–11*A*), but it may not do so in 10 to 19 per cent of cases (Testut, 1884; Vallois, 1922). The musculocutaneous nerve can arise from a common neural structure, giving origin to the median, ulnar, and musculocutaneous nerves (Fig. 6–11B). It may divide soon after origin into its terminal branches before perforating the coracobrachialis muscle and, indeed, may perforate this muscle at multiple sites (Fig. 6–11C). It may even appear that this nerve is "reduplicated" or that a "double" musculocutaneous nerve is present. This nerve may penetrate an anomalous muscle in this region rather than the coracobrachialis. In the past, the term "absence" of the musculocutaneous nerve had been utilized. This anomaly is essentially a combined median-musculocutaneous nerve (Fig. 6–11D). The incidence of this neural variation is as high as 2 per cent. There can be gradations of this anomaly from partial to complete. Variations of the musculocutaneous nerve are therefore relatively frequent. It can even arise from the medial root of the median nerve.

The musculocutaneous nerve usually takes origin from C5 and C6. When fibers from C7 enter this nerve, they usually correct their position by passing through a communication from the musculocutaneous nerve to the median nerve (Fig. 6–10B). This anastomosis occurs in approximately 24 per cent of upper extremities. A median nerve to musculocutaneous nerve communication occurs much less frequently — approximately 2 per cent (Fig. 6–11E).

Radial Nerve

The radial nerve, the largest terminal branch of the plexus, is one of the branches of the posterior cord (Fig. 6–3). In 20 per cent of specimens Kerr (1918) observed the posterior cord to be absent, and frequently a common radial-axillary nerve was noted to be formed by the union of the posterior divisions of the upper and middle trunks. More distally the radial nerve received a contribution from the posterior division of the lower trunk. The posterior divisions of the upper and middle trunks have been seen to form the axillary nerve, while the posterior division of the lower trunk was found to form the radial nerve, receiving an anastomosis from the lateral trunk.

Anomalous perforation of the subscapularis muscle by elements of the radial nerve has been noted. A variant muscle of the posterior wall of the axilla, the accessory scapularis-teres-latissimus, has been observed to penetrate variant neural components of the posterior cord, radial, and axillary nerves (Kameda, 1976).

In the arm the radial nerve may communicate with the ulnar nerve.

The branches of the radial nerve to the triceps arise from varying levels in the axilla or proximal arm, usually from the junction of the middle and upper third of the arm. One or two branches to the long head of the triceps often arise from the radial nerve soon after its formation in the axilla. This muscle can also be supplied by motor branches arising more distally. The lateral and medial heads of the triceps are usually innervated by branches of the radial nerve arising in the brachioaxillary region and in the midarm.

Axillary Nerve

The axillary nerve is a terminal branch of the posterior cord. It usually arises high in the axilla on the subscapularis muscle posterior to the pectoralis minor. On occasion it can arise below the inferior border of this latter muscle.

The circumflex nerve can penetrate the subscapular muscle rather than going into the quadrilateral space distal to the subscapularis muscle (Macalister, 1875). The nerve to the teres minor is quite large. It usually is a solitary branch. Frequently, the nerve to the teres minor arises from a common trunk with nerve fibers that supply the posterior part of the deltoid. Herringham and Harris never found fibers of C7 contributing to the axillary nerve; only fibers of C5 and C6 were noted (Harris, 1903; Herringham, 1887).

Ulnar Nerve

The ulnar nerve is a continuation of the medial cord below the origin of the medial cutaneous nerves of the arm and forearm and the medial root of the median nerve. The ulnar nerve may have additional neural elements joining it frequently from the lateral cord or from the middle trunk or its anterior division. These supplemental neural elements of the ulnar nerve have been termed the "lateral root" of the ulnar nerve (Hirschfeld, 1866). This anomalous root usually joins to form the ulnar nerve at the level of the inferior border of the subscapularis muscle but it can do so very much lower (Fig. 6–8B).

Medial Cutaneous Nerve of the Arm

The medial cutaneous nerve of the arm arises from the medial cord more proximally than does the medial cutaneous nerve of the forearm.

It may arise from a common branch with the nerve of the pectoralis minor or together with the medial cutaneous nerve of the forearm or in common with the first or second intercostal nerve. It may even arise from the lower trunk.

The Medial Cutaneous Nerve of the Forearm

The origin of the medial cutaneous nerve of the forearm is quite variable. In the largest group of cases it arises from the medial cord just below the medial cutaneous nerve of the arm (Fig. 6–3). This nerve is usually about 2 mm in diameter; it is rarely larger. Sometimes it is double or triple. On occasion it is absent.

The medial cutaneous nerve of the forearm usually arises from the medial cord, although it can also arise from the lower trunk, the posterior division of the lower trunk, the first thoracic root, the ulnar nerve, or directly from the eighth cervical and first dorsal roots by two connecting branches. Not infrequently, it may arise from a common branch with the medial cutaneous nerve of the arm and the pectoralis minor nerve.

When the medial cutaneous nerve of the forearm is small, the intercostohumeral nerve is larger than usual. When it is larger or has multiple branches, the intercostohumeral nerve is smaller. Finally, it is not uncommon to have an anastomosis in the axilla or proximal humerus between the intercostohumeral nerve and the medial cutaneous nerve of the forearm. Other communications between the medial cutaneous nerve of the forearm and the medial cutaneous nerve of the arm are frequently observed in the arm.

The medial cutaneous nerve of the forearm is most frequently derived from the first thoracic root, less commonly from the eighth cervical, and anomalously from C7 (Walsh, 1877).

AN EXAMPLE OF A NEURAL ANOMALY OF THE ARM WHICH CAN HAVE CLINICAL SIGNIFICANCE

If a complete fusion of the median and musculocutaneous nerves (Fig. 6–11D) existed in an arm, a small puncture wound which was critically placed would produce a complex deformity of the limb. There would be marked motor loss in the arm and hand, as well as vital sensory loss. The hand would characteristically present with paralysis of the high median nerve type, with loss of function of the thenar muscles, radial two lumbricals of the hand, and specific long flexors of the forearm innervated by the median nerve — the flexor carpi radialis, palmaris longus, flexor digitorum superficialis, flexor pollicis longus, and the index and long finger flexor digitorum profundus muscles. The pronator teres and quadratus muscles would be paralyzed. Thus, the forearm would be supinated because of this paralysis.

Furthermore, with the biceps and the brachialis muscles paralyzed, there would be marked weakness of elbow flexion and some weakness of supination of the forearm. Elbow flexion that was present would be achieved by the brachioradialis muscle and supination of the forearm by the supinator muscle — both radial-nerve innervated.

The sensory loss with this anomaly would include the radial 3½ digits, the radial side of the palm (median nerve), and the lateral aspect of the forearm (musculocutaneous nerve).

A puncture wound of the axilla or upper arm could result in devastating motor and sensory loss at multiple levels — elbow, forearm, and hand — of an arm in which a combined median and musculocutaneous nerve existed.

ANOMALOUS NEURAL PATTERNS OF THE FOREARM AND HAND

In the forearm there are four major neural connections between the ulnar and median nerves. There are, in addition, other significant variations of each of the major peripheral nerve trunks and their branches which will be presented.

1. Within the substance of the flexor digitorum profundus muscle an anastomosis exists between the anterior interosseous branch of the median nerve and the motor branch of the ulnar nerve to this muscle (Fig. 6–1). In the classic anatomical description, the flexor digitorum profundus muscles of the index and long fingers are usually innervated by the median nerve, while those of the ring and little fingers are supplied by the ulnar nerve. Extreme variations can occur in this pattern of innervation. The median nerve can supply all of the

flexor digitorum profundus muscle (as in the "all median nerve hand") or, in the opposite extreme, the ulnar nerve can supply almost all of this deep muscle group. Usually, the index finger profundus is median-nerve innervated but on isolated occasions the ulnar nerve may even supply the index profundus as well. From these extremes, all types of variations exist, from dual innervation of the flexor digitorum profundus of the long finger to dual innervation and various degrees of innervation of the deep flexors of all the digits (Sunderland, 1945).

2. The Martin-Gruber connection (Martin, 1763; Gruber, 1870; Mannerfelt, 1964). This neural communication occurs between the median nerve in the proximal forearm or from its anterior interosseous branch and the ulnar nerve. It frequently carries motor fibers from the median nerve to the ulnar nerve to many of the intrinsic muscles of the hand (Mannerfelt, 1966). There is a 15 per cent occurrence of this neural anomaly. This neural communication usually passes adjacent to the ulnar artery in the proximal forearm.

3. There is also a neural connection from the ulnar nerve to the median nerve in the distal forearm. This anomalous communication is far less frequent than the Martin-Gruber communication. In one of the cases in which we had observed this branch, it was rather large. On electrical stimulation, only a small amount of response in the proximal hypothenar musculature was noted. It was interpreted that the major supply of this aberrant branch was anomalously supplying sensation to the long and ring fingers. Peripheral nerve block of the ulnar nerve at the wrist and elbow could confirm this conclusion.

4. In the hand, Riche (1897) and Cannieu (1897) described a neural connection between the recurrent branch of the median nerve in the thenar eminence and the deep branch of the ulnar nerve (Fig. 6–2). This connection is thought by many to be of the motor variety (Brooks, 1886; Foerster, 1929; Mannerfelt, 1966; Harness and Sekeles, 1971). Gehwold (1921) was of the opinion that this aberrant neural pathway was sensory. Harness and Sekeles reported a 77 per cent incidence of this neural communication between the deep branch of the ulnar nerve and the median nerve or its major branches.

These aberrant neural pathways occasionally permit a hand without deformity even though a complete high or low nerve lesion exists. The two radial lumbricals are usually supplied by the median nerve, but the ulnar nerve may do so. When a three-finger ulnar-claw hand is observed following an ulnar nerve lesion, the paralyzed second lumbrical is anomalously supplied by this nerve. In contrast, the third lumbrical has dual innervation from both the median and the ulnar nerves in 50 per cent of limbs. A complete low lesion of the ulnar nerve would produce only a claw-digit of the little finger when the long finger lumbrical is supplied by the median nerve. On extremely rare occasions, the median nerve may even innervate all the lumbricals. In this instance, with a complete low ulnar nerve there would be no clawing of any of the digits. Similarly, the ulnar nerve may, on isolated occasions, supply all the lumbricals (Sunderland, 1945), in which case a complete ulnar nerve lesion would result in a claw deformity of all the digits. Here, the hand would simulate a combined low median and ulnar nerve lesion.

The first dorsal interosseous muscle is usually innervated by the ulnar nerve, but in 10 per cent of hands it is supplied completely or in part by the median nerve. In 1 per cent of hands the first dorsal interosseous muscle and, on occasion, the second and third interosseous muscles may be supplied by the radial nerve either by way of the terminal branches of the posterior interosseous nerve or by the superficial radial nerve (Froment, 1846; Rauber, 1865; Fahrer, 1968).

There are other anomalies of the nerves of the forearm. Funicular elements of the nerve may split off from the main nerve trunk to rejoin it at a more distal site. These gross neural loops may occur over a short or long distance (Kaplan, 1963; Winkelman and Spinner, 1973). They have been observed about the pisiform or the hook of the hamate (Fig. 6–13D). They may even occur the entire length of the forearm (Fig. 6–12). French anatomists have termed these anomalies "petite ellipse" and "grande ellipse," depending on their length (Hartmann, 1887).

The clinical significance of these variant neural elements is clear (Fenning, 1965; Lanz, 1974; Lassa and Shrewsbury, 1975). If the main nerve trunk has been severed distal to the origin of a neural loop, significant function of the particular nerve may still be present because of the intact neural fibers of the loop (Fig. 6–12).

There are many anomalies of the motor branch of the median nerve, including aberrant course, reduplication, and unusual point of take-off from the median nerve (Spinner, 1978). Knowledge of these variations is critical, especially in surgery for the ubiquitous carpal tunnel syndrome.

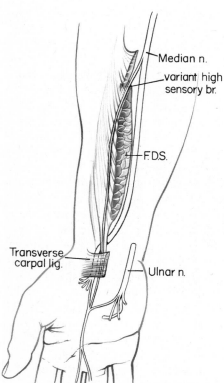

Median n.

variant high
sensory br.

F.D.S.

Transverse
carpal lig.

Ulnar n.

Figure 6–12 A large neural loop formation of the median nerve is shown about the flexor digitorum superficialis (F.D.S.) in the forearm. This has been reported on occasion. In the palm the commonly observed ulnar nerve to median nerve communication is demonstrated.

Sensory variations of the ulnar nerve are frequent. Usually, the ulnar nerve innervates the medial 1½ digits. Furthermore, the dorsoulnar aspect of the hand is usually supplied by its dorsal branch. Nevertheless, we have seen patients in whom the dorsoulnar aspect of the hand was supplied by the superficial radial nerve. This anatomical sensory variation of the superficial radial nerve, described by Learmonth (1919), has important clinical significance because, with normal sensation of the dorsoulnar aspect of the hand, one would suspect a lesion of the ulnar nerve to be low. In actuality, it is high, at the elbow; the superficial radial nerve supply to the dorsoulnar aspect of the hand leads to the false clinical localization. Either by blocking the superficial radial nerve or with the aid of electrical conduction studies across segments of the ulnar nerve, one can avoid this clinical diagnostic error.

It is not uncommon to have an anomalous sensory communication in the palm between the ulnar and median nerves (Fig. 6–12). These sensory connections found in the hand and those found in the distal forearm are the likely pathways for increased ulnar nerve sensory supply to more than the usual medial 1½ digits innervated by the ulnar nerve (Fig. 6–1).

Sensory branches can arise from a more proximal site on a nerve and can travel an anomalous course in the forearm (Turner, 1874). The ulnar digital nerve to the fourth web space has been observed to arise from the ulnar nerve in the midforearm and even pass superficial to Guyon's tunnel rather than deep to it (Fig. 6–13*B*). Similarly, the dorsal cutaneous branch of the ulnar nerve has been observed to arise just distal to the elbow and pass subcutaneously the entire length of the forearm (Fig. 6–13*C*). This nerve usually arises in the distal forearm 6 to 8 cm proximal to the wrist (Fig. 6–13*A*). Lastly, the posterior cutaneous nerve of the forearm, usually a branch of the radial nerve, may arise from the ulnar nerve (Turner, 1874).

AN EXAMPLE OF A NEURAL ANOMALY OF THE FOREARM AND HAND WHICH HAS CLINICAL SIGNIFICANCE

In the classic low ulnar hand with total denervation, one sees clawing of the ring and little fingers. Clawing is characteristically observed with hyperextension of the metacarpophalangeal joint of the ring and little fingers and with subsequent compensatory flexion of the proximal and distal interphalangeal joints.

Clawing does not occur if there is anomalous innervation of the third and fourth lumbricals by the median nerve. In addition, no clawing is observed in a low ulnar nerve lesion if the flexor digitorum profundus tendons to the medial two digits are severed at the time of the low ulnar nerve laceration.

*   *   *   *   *

All the nerves of the extremities can have some degree of deviation from classic anatomical description. These variant sensory and motor innervation patterns are extremely common. It is essential to appreciate these variations in order to effectively manage peripheral nerve lesions.

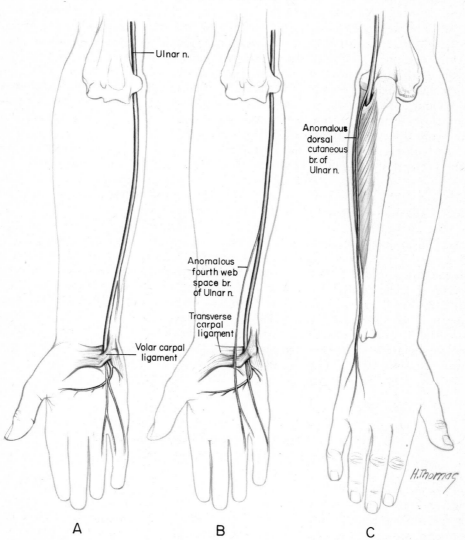

Ulnar n.

Anomalous
dorsal
cutaneous
br. of
Ulnar n.

Anomalous
fourth web
space br.
of Ulnar n.

Transverse
carpal
ligament

Volar carpal
ligament

H. Thomas

A   B   C

Figure 6–13 *A,* The usual branches of the ulnar nerve—the dorsal cutaneous nerve, the deep motor branch, and the sensory branches to the fourth web space and to the medial side of the fifth finger—are depicted in the distal right forearm and hand. *B,* An anomalous branch of the ulnar nerve which arose in the forearm rather than in the palm. This variant branch to the fourth web space passed superficial to Guyon's tunnel rather than deep to the volar carpal ligament. *C,* The dorsal cutaneous branch of the ulnar nerve can arise as far proximal as the elbow and traverse a subcutaneous course superficial to the flexor carpi ulnaris.

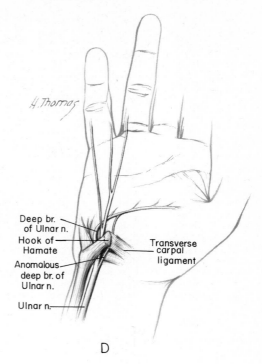

Figure 6–13 (*Continued*) *D,* The motor branch of the ulnar nerve can be split about the hook of the hamate. Part of this nerve can pass in an anomalous course radial to the bony protuberance.

Deep br. of Ulnar n.

Hook of Hamate

Anomalous deep br. of Ulnar n.

Ulnar n.

Transverse carpal ligament

D

REFERENCES

Brachial Plexus

Cunningham, D. J.: Note on a connecting twig between the anterior divisions of the first and second dorsal nerves. J. Anat. Physiol. *11*:539, 1877.

Curnow, J.: Notes of some irregularities of muscles and nerves. J. Anat. Physiol. *8*:304, 1873.

Dixon, A. F.: Abnormal distribution of the nervus dorsalis scapulae and certain of the intercostal nerves. J. Anat. Physiol. *30*:209, 1896.

Frohse, F. and Fränkel, M.: Die Muskeln des menschlichen armes. *In* Handbuch der Anatomie des Menschen. Herausgegeben K. von Bardeleben, Jena. Gustav Fischer, 1908.

Harris, W.: The true form of the brachial plexus and its motor distribution. J. Anat. Physiol. *38*:399, 1904.

Harris, W.: The Morphology of the Brachial Plexus. London, Oxford University Press, 1939.

Hasan, M. and Narayan, D.: A single cord human brachial plexus. J. Anat. Soc. India, *13*:103, 1964.

Herringham, W. P.: The minute anatomy of the brachial plexus. Proc. Roy Soc. Lond. *41*:423, 1887.

Hirschfeld, L.: Traité et iconographie des systèmes nerveux et des organes des sens de l'homme. 2nd ed. Paris, Masson, 1866.

Hovelacque, A.: Anatomie des nerfs craniens et rachidiens et du grand sympathique chez l'homme. Paris, Masson, 1927, Vol. 2.

Kameda, Y.: An anomalous muscle (accessory scapularis-teres-latissimus muscle) in the axilla penetrating the brachial plexus in man. Acta Anat. *96*:513, 1976.

Kerr, A. T.: The brachial plexus of nerves in man, the variations in its formation and branches. Am. J. Anat. *23*:285, 1918.

Luschka, H. von: Die Nerven des menschlicher Wirbelkanales. Türbigen, H. Laupt, 1850.

Macalister, A.: Notes on some anomalies in the course of nerves in man. Proc. Roy. Irish Acad. Dublin *12*:426, 1875–1877.

Paterson, A. M.: The limb plexuses of mammals. J. Anat. Physiol. *21*:611, 1887.

Schumacher, S.: Nochmals die Frage der kollateralen Innervation. Anat. Anzeiger *44*:14, 1913.

Singer, E.: Human brachial plexus united into a single cord. Anat. Rec. *55*:411, 1933.

Soulié, A.: Les nerfs rachidiens. *In* Traité d'anatomie humaine publié par P. Poirier et A. Charpy. 2nd ed., Paris, Masson, 1904.

Sunderland, Sir: Nerves and Nerve Injuries. 2nd ed., Edinburgh, Churchill Livingstone, 1978.

Turner, W.: Some additional variations in the distribution of nerves of the human body. J. Anat. Physiol. *6*:101, 1871.

Turner, W.: Further examples of variations in the arrangement of nerves of the human body. J. Anat. Physiol. *7*:297, 1872.

Valentin, G. G.: Traité de neurologie. Paris, J. B. Baillière, 1843.

Arm

Lang, J., and Spinner, M.: An important variation of the brachial plexus — complete fusion of the median and musculocutaneous nerves. Bull Hosp. Joint Dis. *31*:7, 1970.

Linell, E. A.: The distribution of nerves in the upper limb with reference to variabilities and their clinical significance. J. Anat. *55*:79, 1920–1921.

Mrvaljevi'c, D., and Djordjevi'c-Camba, V.: Anatomic variation of the passage of the musculocutaneous nerve through the caput longum of the biceps muscle. Srp Arh Celok Lek. *99*:303, 1971.

Testut, L.: Mémoire sur la portion brachiale du nerf musculocutané. Internat. Monatschr. f. Anat. u Histol. *1*:305, 1884.

Vallois, H. V.: Recherches sur le trajet et les anastomoses du nerf musculo-cutané au niveau du bras. Arch. Anat. Histol. Embryol. *1*:183, 1922.

Walsh, J. F.: Anatomy of the brachial plexus. Amer. J. Med. Sci. *74*:387, 1877.

Zeuke, W., and Heidrich, R.: Pathogenesis of isolated postoperative paralysis of the musculocutaneous nerve. Schweiz. Arch. Neurol. Neurochir. Psychiatr. *114*:289, 1974.

Forearm and Hand

Brash, J. C.: Neurovascular Hila of Limb Muscles. Edinburgh, E. & S. Livingstone, 1955.

Brooks, H.: Variations in the nerve supply of the flexor pollicis muscle. J. Anat. Physiol. *20*:641, 1886.

Cannieu, J. M. A.: Recherches sur une anastomose entre la branche profunde du cubitale et le médian. Bull. Soc. Anat. Physiol. Bordeau *18*:339, 1897.

Fahrer, M.: Rare variations in a left radial nerve — Case Report. J. Anat. (Lond.) *103*:208, 1968.

Fenning, J. B.: Deep ulnar-nerve paralysis resulting from an anatomical abnormality. J. Bone Joint Surg. *47A*:1381, 1965.

Foerster, C.: Die Symptomatologie der Schussverletzungen der peripheren Nerven. *In* M. Levandorosky (Ed.): Handbuch der Neurologie. Berlin, Springer, 1929.

Froment, J.-B.-F.: Traité d'anatomie humaine. Paris, Méguignon-Marvis, 1846, p. 494.

Gehwolf, S.: Weitere Fälle von Plexus Bildung in der Hohlhand. Anat. Anz. *54*:435, 1921.

Gruber, W.: Ueber die Verbindung des Nervus medianus mit dem Nervus ulnaris am Unterarme des Menschen und der Sängethiete. Arch. Anat. Physiol. *37*:501, 1870.

Harness, D. and Sekeles, E.: The double anastomatic innervation of the thenar muscles. J. Anat. *109*:461, 1971.

Hartmann, H.: Etude de quelques anastomoses elliptiques des nerfs du membre supérieur. Bull. Soc. Anat. Paris *62*:860, 1887.

Kaplan, E. B.: Variation of the ulnar nerve at the wrist. Bull. Hosp. Joint Dis. *24*:85, 1963.

Lanz, U.: Lahmung des tiefen. Hohlhandastes des Nerves ulnaris bedingt durch eine anatomische Variante. Handchirurgie *6*:83, 1974.

Lassa, R., and Shrewsbury, M. M.: A variation in the path of the deep motor branch of the ulnar nerve at the wrist. J. Bone Joint Surg. *57A*:990, 1975.

Learmonth, J. R.: A variation of the radial branch of the musculospiral nerve. J. Anat. *53*:371, 1919.

Mannerfelt, L.: Studies on anastomosis between the median and ulnar nerves in the forearm. Acta Universitatis Lundensis Sectio II, No. 6, 1964.

Mannerfelt, L.: Studies on the hand in ulnar nerve paralysis. A clinical-experimental investigation in normal and anomalous innervation. Acta Orthop. Scand. Suppl. 87, 1966.

Martin, R.: Tal om nervus allmanna egenskaper 1 mannsikans kropp. Stockholm, Lars Salvius, 1763.

Rauber, A.: Vater'sche Köper der Bänder und Periostnerven, Inaug. Diss., Munich, 1865.

Riche, P.: Le nerf cubitale et les muscles de l'éminence thenar. Bull. Mem. Soc. Anat. Paris *5*:251, 1897.

Roundtree, P.: Anomalous innervation of the hand muscles. J. Bone Joint Surg. *31B*:505, 1949.

Spinner, M.: Injuries to the Major Branches of Peripheral Nerves of the Forearm. 2nd ed., Philadelphia, W. B. Saunders, 1978, pp. 203–210.

Sunderland, S.: The innervation of the flexor digitorum profundus and lumbrical muscles. Anat. Rec. *93*:317, 1945.

Turner, W.: Further examples of variations in arrangement of nerves of the human body. J. Anat. Physiol. *8*:297, 1874.

Winkelman, N. Z., and Spinner, M.: A variant high sensory branch of the median nerve to the third web space. Bull. Hosp. Joint Dis. *34*:161, 1973.

7

NORMAL AND ANOMALOUS INNERVATION PATTERNS IN THE LOWER EXTREMITY

LAWRENCE PRUTKIN

GENERAL PATTERN OF PERIPHERAL NERVES TO LOWER EXTREMITY

The peripheral nerve supply to the lower extremity is derived from the lumbosacral plexus, which in itself is composed of the lumbar and sacral plexuses. The lumbar plexus is distributed to the anterior and medial aspects of the thigh except for the saphenous nerve (from the femoral nerve), which is a cutaneous nerve distributed to the medial and somewhat anterior surface of the leg and medial side of the foot. The chief nerves of the lumbar plexus are the femoral nerve (to the flexor muscles) and the obturator nerve (to the adductor muscles).

The sacral plexus has a greater distribution to the lower limb than does the lumbar plexus. Most of the sacral plexus is continued into the thigh as the sciatic nerve, which innervates the skin of most of the leg and all of the foot. It supplies the muscles in the posterior aspect of the thigh, and all the muscles in the leg and foot, and contributes innervation to all the joints in the lower extremity.

LUMBOSACRAL PLEXUS

Composition

The lumbosacral plexus is formed by a combination of all the ventral rami of spinal nerves from the first lumbar nerve, often including the last thoracic nerve down to the sacral nerves. The lumbar plexus is formed in the psoas major muscle lying in the abdomen, while the sacral plexus is formed anterior and lateral to the sacrum (in the pelvis). Although both plexuses supply the inferior extremity, some nerves go to the anterior abdominal wall, while others supply the perineum and coccygeal region.

Variations

The lumbosacral plexus will present many variations, most of them minor. Although the normal collection of nerves usually ranges from the first lumbar down to the third sacral nerve, it is not uncommon to have higher nerves from the last thoracic (T12) enter the plexus or lower nerves from the fourth sacral (S4) contribute to the plexus. This pattern of variation can enlarge the plexus, or the plexus may be contracted by a higher or lower nerve failing to contribute to the plexus. Hollinshead (1968), in discussing this shifting of nerves (enlarging or contracting the plexus), feels it is important when a given spinal nerve instead of contributing its usual complement of fibers to a specific branch of the plexus contributes less to that branch and more to another. He specifically mentions the fourth lumbar nerve, which usually is the major contributor to the femoral nerve of the lumbar plexus but can shift and send most of its fibers to the sciatic nerve of the sacral plexus (Fig. 7–1).

It is most difficult to classify the normal lumbosacral plexus pattern. Bardeen and Elting (1901) designated a lumbosacral plexus as normal if it had either the first or second lumbar nerve as its highest nerve, the third sacral nerve as its lowest nerve, and the fourth lumbar nerve as a major contributor to the lumbar rather than to the sacral plexus. Using this definition, they found 42.3 per cent of 256 specimens examined had normal plexuses.

In defining a normal lumbosacral plexus, Horwitz (1939) stated that the highest nerve entering the plexus is the second lumbar nerve; the nerve that goes to both the lumbar and sacral plexuses (the furcal nerve) is the fourth lumbar; and the sacral plexus is to be supplied by the fourth lumbar nerve through the fourth sacral nerve. Of 114 bodies he examined (228 plexuses), 71.93 per cent were normal according to his definition.

Hollinshead (1968) reported some interesting variations to the furcal nerve. Usually the fourth lumbar nerve will distribute to both the lumbar and sacral plexuses. Occasionally, the third and fourth lumbar nerves will be furcal nerves; or the fourth lumbar nerve will entirely distribute to the femoral nerve, while the fifth lumbar nerve will entirely distribute to the sciatic, a combination yielding no furcal nerve; or the fifth lumbar nerve will be the furcal nerve, giving fibers to both the femoral and sciatic nerves (Fig. 7–1).

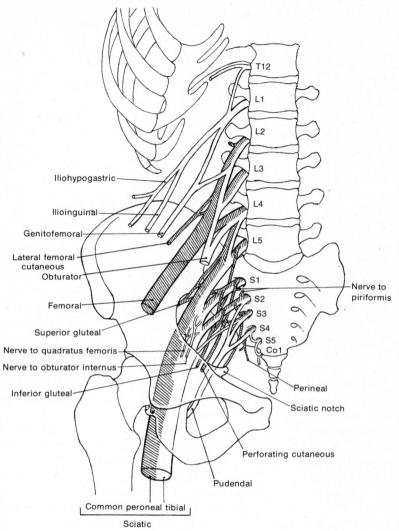

Figure 7–1

LUMBAR PLEXUS

Composition

The lumbar plexus is formed either within the psoas major muscle or posterior to it. The nerves that emerge are the iliohypogastric, the ilioinguinal, the genitofemoral, the lateral femoral cutaneous, the obturator, the accessory obturator, the femoral, and a branch to the lumbosacral trunk. The iliohypogastric, ilioinguinal, lateral femoral cutaneous, and femoral nerves are found at the lateral border of the psoas major muscle. The genitofemoral nerve travels on the anterior aspect of the psoas, while the obturator, accessory obturator, and the branch to the lumbosacral trunk appear medial to the psoas.

The lumbar plexus is formed by the ventral primary divisions of the first, second, and third lumbar nerves and the greater part of the fourth lumbar nerve. In most instances, the twelfth thoracic nerve will send fibers to communicate with the first lumbar nerve. The latter nerve will then split into two branches: the cranial, forming the iliohypogastric and ilioinguinal nerves, and the caudal, joining a branch of the second lumbar to form the genitofemoral nerve. The remainder of the second lumbar nerve along with the third and fourth lumbar nerves divide into a larger, posterior, division and a smaller, anterior, division. The anterior divisions unite to form the obturator nerve, while the posterior divisions give rise to the lateral femoral cutaneous nerve and the femoral nerve. The accessory obturator, present in about 30 per cent of individuals (Goss, 1973), arises from the third and fourth lumbar nerves. Part of the fourth lumbar nerve joins the fifth lumbar to form the lumbosacral trunk.

Variation

The most common composition of the lumbar plexus is from L1 to L4. The highest nerve to enter into the formation of the lumbar plexus is usually, but not always, the twelfth thoracic nerve. Hollinshead (1968) reports that occasionally the eleventh thoracic nerve will enter into the formation of the lumbar plexus. At the other end of the lumbar plexus, Horwitz (1939) reports that in 12 per cent of the plexuses he examined, the fifth lumbar nerve sent a branch to the lumbar plexus.

The Iliohypogastric Nerve

The iliohypogastric nerve arises from the first lumbar nerve and usually from the twelfth thoracic nerve. It leaves the lateral border of the psoas major and runs to the posterior part of the transversus abdominis, near the crest of the ilium. The nerve gives off a lateral cutaneous branch, which is distributed to the posterior and lateral part of the skin of the buttock. The iliohypogastric will also give off an anterior cutaneous branch, which is distributed to the skin above the pubic symphysis (hypogastric region).

The variations in the iliohypogastric nerve that have been reported refer to the origin of this nerve. Bardeen (1907) found that in 34 per cent of cases, the nerve arose from the first lumbar and twelfth thoracic nerves, in 32 per cent, it arose solely from the twelfth thoracic nerve, and in 32 per cent it arose solely from the first lumbar nerve. In 2 per cent of cases, the nerve arose from both the eleventh and twelfth thoracic nerves.

The Ilioinguinal Nerves

The ilioinguinal nerve arises from the first lumbar nerve and leaves the lateral border of the psoas major just inferior to the iliohypogastric nerve. It runs to the crest of the ilium, enters the transversus abdominis, and then penetrates the internal oblique muscle, to which it sends fibers. After leaving the muscle, the nerve goes through the superficial inguinal ring and is distributed to the skin over the medial and proximal part of the thigh, in the male to the skin over the root of the penis and scrotum, and in the female to the mons pubis and labium majus.

Bardeen (1907) reported that in 51.5 per cent of instances studied the ilioinguinal nerve arose from L1, in 38.3 per cent it arose from T12 and L1, in 3.5 per cent it arose from only T12, and in 6.6 per cent the nerve was absent. When the nerve is absent, the genital branch of the genitofemoral nerve may supply its branches (Goss, 1973).

The Genitofemoral Nerve

The genitofemoral nerve arises from the first and second lumbar nerves and emerges on the ventral surface of the psoas major. While on the muscle, or occasionally within it, the nerve divides into a genital (external spermatic) branch and a femoral (lumboinguinal) branch. In the male, the genital branch passes through the inguinal canal, lies adjacent to the spermatic cord, and supplies the cremaster muscle and the skin of the scrotum and adjacent thigh. In the female, the genital branch is distributed to the skin of the labium majus. The femoral branch, accompanied by the external iliac artery, passes under the inguinal ligament. In the thigh, it enters the femoral sheath and lies lateral to the femoral artery. It is distributed to the skin of the proximal part of the anterior surface of the thigh.

The genital branch of the genitofemoral nerve may be absent, the ilioinguinal nerve substituting for it (Goss, 1973). Bardeen (1907) found no femoral branch to be present in 1.2 per cent of cases. Bardeen found the femoral branch in its usual position in the thigh in 81 of 133 instances (60.9 per cent). In 18.8 per cent of instances, it was distributed more internally (medially), and in 20.3 per cent it was distributed more externally (laterally). He also believed that the femoral branch may have a slight, moderate, or extensive distribution (i.e., considerable variation) to the skin.

The Lateral Femoral Cutaneous Nerve

The lateral femoral cutaneous nerve arises from the second and third lumbar nerves and emerges from about the middle of the lateral border of the psoas major. It runs to the anterior superior iliac spine, passes behind the inguinal ligament and anterior to the sartorius muscle, and then into the subcutaneous tissue of the thigh. It divides into an anterior and a posterior branch, to be distributed to the skin of the lateral region of the thigh. The anterior branch supplies the skin of the lateral and anterior aspect of the thigh as far as the knee. The posterior branch supplies the skin from the level of the greater trochanter to the middle of the thigh (on the lateral and posterior surface of the thigh).

Bardeen (1907) found that the lateral femoral cutaneous nerve varies considerably in its origin as well as its distribution. In 39 per cent of 287 cases the nerve arose from T12, L1, and L2. In 43 per cent, the nerve arose from the first three lumbar nerves, and in 18 per cent, the nerve arose from the main trunk of the femoral nerve. Horwitz (1939) found the nerve to arise from the femoral nerve in 65.3 per cent of cases. Paterson (1893) found no origin from T12 in 23 plexuses examined.

Bardeen (1907) found that in 45 of 146 instances (30.8 per cent) the lateral femoral cutaneous nerve extended medially over the anterior portion of the thigh, substituting for the anterior cutaneous branches of the femoral nerve. He claimed that there is no relationship between race, sex, or side of body and variation in the distribution of the lateral femoral cutaneous nerve.

The Obturator Nerve

The obturator nerve arises from the second, third, and fourth lumbar nerves. It emerges from the medial border of the psoas major muscle, above the brim of the pelvis and under the common iliac vessels. It courses between the muscle and the lateral border of the vertebral column, then runs along the lateral wall of the lesser pelvis and enters the obturator foramen accompanied by the obturator vessels. Upon entering the obturator canal, it divides into anterior and posterior branches, named because of their relation to the adductor brevis muscle.

The anterior branch passes anterior to the obturator externus and adductor brevis but posterior to the pectineus. If an accessory obturator nerve is present the anterior branch will communicate with it. It supplies the adductor longus, the gracilis, and the adductor brevis, and ends in the subsartorial plexus by communicating with the anterior cutaneous and saphenous branches of the femoral nerve. The anterior branch of the obturator nerve gives off an articular branch which enters the fibrous capsule of the hip joint through the pubofemoral ligament. Occasionally, a cutaneous branch (derived from L1) from the anterior branch of the obturator nerve is found. It is superficially located between the gracilis and sartorius muscles in the middle third of the thigh, and is distributed to the skin of the medial side of the proximal half of the leg. When this nerve is present, the medial anterior cutaneous branch of the femoral nerve is small (Goss, 1973).

The posterior branch pierces the obturator externus and supplies that muscle, passes posterior to the adductor brevis and anterior to the adductor magnus, supplying the latter muscle.

Bardeen (1907) stated that in most instances the obturator nerve, like the femoral, arises from the second, third, and fourth lumbar nerves. However Horwitz (1938), in examination of 228 plexuses, found the obturator nerve to arise most commonly from the third and fourth lumbar nerves (almost 77 per cent of plexuses examined), while in only 1 per cent did the obturator arise from the second, third, and fourth lumbar nerves.

The Accessory Obturator Nerve

The accessory obturator nerve is present in about 29 per cent of cases (Goss, 1973). When present, it arises from the third and fourth lumbar nerves, emerges from the medial border of the psoas major, descends along the medial aspect of the muscle, and crosses anteriorly, over the superior ramus of the pubis. It does not follow the obturator nerve through the obturator foramen. Entering the thigh, the accessory obturator nerve passes posteriorly to the pectineus muscle, which it supplies, sends a branch to the hip joint, and communicates with the anterior branch of the obturator nerve. In most instances, an anastomotic branch could be traced to the cutaneous branch of the obturator nerve (Goss, 1973).

Bardeen found the accessory obturator nerve to be present in 8.4 per cent of 250 plexuses examined (21 plexuses). Horwitz (1939) found the nerve in 17.1 per cent. Bardeen expressed the belief that the accessory obturator is found more frequently in males (9.3 per cent) than in females (5.4 per cent), and more frequently in caucasians (10.8 per cent) than in blacks (6.4 per cent).

The origin of the nerve appears to be variable. Bardeen and Elting (1901) found the nerve to arise most frequently from the third and fourth lumbar nerves. Lockhart (1969) states that the nerve arises from the second and third lumbar nerves, while Horwitz (1939) found the nerve to arise from either the femoral or the obturator nerve.

The Femoral Nerve

The femoral nerve arises from the second, third, and fourth lumbar nerves. It is the largest branch of the lumbar plexus, and is the major nerve to the anterior aspect of the thigh. The nerve emerges from the substance of the psoas major at its lateral border, passes caudal between the psoas and iliacus muscles and then courses posterior to the inguinal ligament, lateral to the femoral artery. In the femoral triangle, the nerve separates into many cutaneous and muscular branches.

While in the abdomen, the femoral nerve gives off branches to the iliacus muscle. Immediately below the inguinal ligament, a branch is sent to the anterior surface of the pectineus muscle. A branch is also sent to the sartorius, this branch arising in common with the intermediate anterior cutaneous branch. Several muscular branches of the saphenous nerve supply the quadriceps femoris. Those branches to the rectus femoris and the vastus lateralis follow the descending branch of the lateral femoral circumflex artery. The branch to the vastus medialis runs with the saphenous nerve outside the adductor canal. There are usually two or three branches to the vastus intermedius, one branch piercing the muscle to reach the articularis genu and the knee joint. The main nerve supply to the anterior aspect of the knee joint capsule is derived from the articular filaments of the femoral nerve, which are distributed to the three vastus muscles.

The femoral nerve has three large cutaneous terminal branches. The intermediate anterior cutaneous nerve divides into two branches, which descend over the sartorius muscle to supply the skin on the anterior thigh as far distally as the anterior knee. The distribution overlaps superiorly with the skin supplied by the genitofemoral nerve and laterally with the skin supplied by the lateral femoral cutaneous nerve (Goss, 1973). The medial anterior cutaneous nerve passes obliquely in front of the proximal part of the femoral artery, and gives off a few twigs, which pierce the fascia lata and distribute to the skin of the medial side of the thigh near the great saphenous vein. The nerve divides into an anterior branch and a posterior branch. The anterior branch passes caudally on the sartorius muscle, supplies the skin on the medial side of the knee, and communicates with the saphenous nerve (patellar plexus) in front of the knee. The posterior branch runs distally along the medial aspect of the sartorius muscle to the knee, communicates with the saphenous nerve, and continues down to the skin of the medial side of the leg, which it supplies. At the lower border of the adductor longus, the nerve takes part in the formation of the subsartorial plexus by communicating with branches of the saphenous and obturator nerves. The medial anterior cutaneous nerve tends to be small when the obturator nerve has a cutaneous branch (Goss, 1973).

The saphenous nerve is the largest cutaneous branch of the femoral nerve. It is distributed to the integument of the medial side of the leg. The nerve passes with the femoral artery, first lying lateral to the artery and then within the adductor canal, crossing to the medial side of the artery. In the

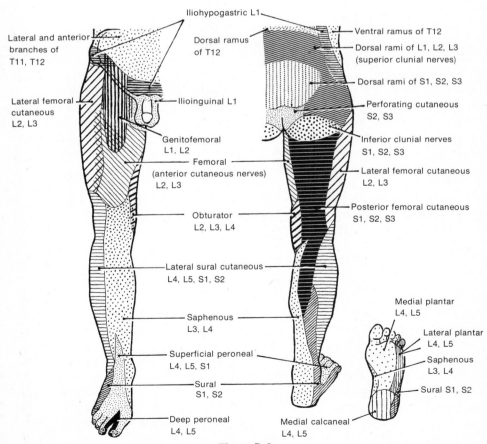

Figure 7–2

canal, the nerve sends a branch to join the medial anterior cutaneous nerve and obturator nerve to form the subsartorial plexus. The saphenous nerve then leaves the canal and, at the hiatus of the adductor magnus, quits company with the artery, runs deep to the sartorius, along the medial side of the knee, where it gives off a large infrapatellar branch. This branch supplies the skin in front of the patella and communicates with branches of the lateral femoral cutaneous nerve, branches of the saphenous nerve, and the anterior cutaneous branches of the femoral nerve to form the patellar plexus. The saphenous nerve becomes superficial between the tendons of the sartorius and gracilis muscles, and passes with the great saphenous vein along the medial side of the leg. It supplies the skin of the anterior and medial aspect of the leg, communicating with the medial anterior cutaneous nerve. The nerve continues to the ankle, where it supplies the skin over the medial malleolus and medial side of the instep and ends at the medial side of the foot as far as the ball of the great toe. It anastomoses with the medial branch of the superficial peroneal nerve (Goss, 1973) (Fig. 7–2).

Although the femoral nerve usually arises from the second, third, and fourth lumbar nerves, Bardeen (1907) stated that the first lumbar nerve usually contributes to the origin of the femoral nerve; occasionally, the twelfth thoracic and fifth lumbar nerves contribute also.

There is great variation in the distribution of the anterior cutaneous nerves of the thigh. In five of 80 cases, Bardeen (1907) found the proximal branches of the medial anterior cutaneous nerve to be distributed in the region of the ilioinguinal nerve. In two of 80 cases, he found that the same nerve sent a branch as far distally as the ankle, accompanied by the saphenous nerve. In the distribution of the nerve supply over the anterior aspect of the thigh, he found the lateral femoral cutaneous nerve to be associated with the anterior cutaneous nerves in 64 per cent of instances. However, in 33 per cent the lateral femoral cutaneous nerve had an extensive distribution over the anterior aspect of the thigh, while there was a limited distribution of the anterior cutaneous nerves.

Bardeen (1907) believed the saphenous nerve to be fairly constant in its general pattern of distribution. When variation is present, it is more likely to be seen in the distal portion of the nerve. In three of 75 cases, the nerve extended all the way to the great toe (Fig. 7–2).

SACRAL PLEXUS

Composition

The sacral plexus is formed by the lumbosacral trunk, from the fourth and fifth lumbar nerves, and by the first three sacral nerves. The plexus is formed posteriorly to the internal iliac vessels and ureter in the posterior wall of the pelvis, where these nerves converge to the inferior border of the greater sciatic foramen. The nerves unite into a large band that is flattened and conveyed into the thigh as the sciatic nerve. The nerves that contribute to the formation of the sacral plexus (L4, L5, S1, S2, S3) split into ventral (anterior) and dorsal (posterior) divisions. The posterior divisions of all the nerves except the third sacral form the common peroneal part of the sciatic nerve, and all the anterior divisions form the tibial part of the sciatic nerve.

Branches from the anterior divisions of S2 and S3 unite with most of S4 to form the pudendal nerve of the perineum.

The following nerves are branches of the sacral plexus:

1. Nerve to the quadratus femoris and gemellus inferior
2. Nerve to the obturator internus and gemellus superior
3. Nerve to the piriformis
4. Superior gluteal nerve
5. Inferior gluteal nerve
6. Posterior femoral cutaneous nerve
7. Perforating cutaneous nerve
8. Sciatic nerve — tibial
                 — common peroneal

Variations

In the most common formation of the sacral plexus, the fourth lumbar nerve is the most superior. However, Horwitz (1939) found that the third lumbar nerve contributed to the plexus in about 5 per cent of cases. Bardeen and Elting (1901) found a branch from the third lumbar nerve to the sacral plexus in six of 256 instances. The third sacral nerve is usually the lowest nerve in the sacral plexus. Both Hollinshead (1968) and Lockhart (1969) found the most caudal contribution to be the fourth sacral nerve. Horwitz (1939) described the pudendal nerve as the caudal border of the sacral plexus.

The Nerve to the Quadratus Femoris and Gemellus Inferior

The nerve to the quadratis femoris and gemellus inferior arises from the fourth and fifth lumbar nerves and the first sacral nerve, and leaves the pelvis through the greater sciatic foramen ventral to the sciatic nerve. It courses deep to the tendon of the obturator internus, gives a branch to the gemellus inferior and to the hip joint, and ends by piercing the deep aspect of the quadratus femoris.

Paterson (1893) pointed out that the nerve may arise either only from the fourth and fifth lumbar nerves with no contribution from the first sacral nerve or only from the fifth lumbar and first sacral nerve. Bardeen (1907), in describing the distribution of the nerve, found branches to both the gemellus inferior and the gemellus superior. The nerve may not end in the quadratus femoris but may continue down to the proximal portion of the adductor magnus or to the obturator externus (Goss, 1973).

The Nerve to the Obturator Internus and Gemellus Superior

The nerve to the obturator internus and gemellus superior arises from the fifth lumbar nerve and the first two sacral nerves. It leaves the pelvis through the greater sciatic foramen, then gives a branch to the gemellus superior and crosses the ischial spine, where it is lateral to the internal pudendal vessels. It re-enters the pelvis via the lesser sciatic foramen, and supplies the obturator internus.

Paterson (1893) found that in some instances the first three sacral nerves were the sole contributors to the origin of the nerve to the obturator internus. Bardeen (1907) found that, occasionally, the third sacral nerve takes part in the origin of the nerve, along with the fifth lumbar and first two sacral nerves.

The Nerve to the Piriformis

The nerve to the piriformis usually arises from the first and second sacral nerves and pierces the anterior surface of the piriformis. Occasionally, the nerve may be double (Goss, 1973). Bardeen (1907) found a twig entering the piriformis from the ascending branch of the superior gluteal nerve.

The Superior Gluteal Nerve

The superior gluteal nerve arises from the fourth and fifth lumbar nerves as well as the first sacral nerve. It leaves the pelvis, anterior to the piriform muscle, via the greater sciatic foramen, runs with the superior gluteal vessels, and divides into a superior and inferior branch. The superior branch supplies the gluteus minimus. The inferior branch distributes to the gluteus medius and gluteus minimus, and ends in the tensor fasciae latae.

Hollinshead (1968) states that if the fifth lumbar is the furcal nerve and the fourth lumbar has no contribution, the superior gluteal nerve can receive some fibers from the second sacral nerve.

The Inferior Gluteal Nerve

The inferior gluteal nerve arises from the fifth lumbar nerve and the first two sacral nerves. It leaves the pelvis through the greater sciatic foramen, and distributes on the deep aspect of the gluteus maximus.

According to Hollinshead (1968), the nerve may receive fibers from the fourth lumbar nerve and can also receive a few fibers from the third sacral nerve. Bardeen (1907) found that the third sacral nerve rarely contributes to the inferior gluteal nerve. In addition, the inferior gluteal nerve may be bound at its origin with the trunks of origin of the posterior femoral cutaneous nerve and, occasionally, with the sciatic nerve.

The Posterior Femoral Cutaneous Nerve

The posterior femoral cutaneous nerve supplies the integument of the perineum, and the posterior aspect of the thigh and leg. It arises from the first three sacral nerves, leaves the pelvis through the greater sciatic foramen, and accompanies the inferior gluteal vessels to the gluteus maximus. Deep to that muscle the nerve gives off three to four inferior cluneal (gluteal) branches, which supply the skin over the lateral and lower part of the gluteus maximus (as far as the greater trochanter). The nerve also gives off perineal branches, running over the hamstring muscles below the ischial tuberosity to supply the skin of the external genitalia and adjacent proximal medial surface of the thigh. One branch, the inferior pudendal, will supply the skin of the scrotum in the male and the labium majus in the female.

The nerve continues down the posterior thigh, anterior to the long head of the biceps femoris, and accompanies the small saphenous vein to the middle of the back of the leg, where it supplies the skin of that region. It will send branches to the popliteal fossa, where it will communicate, via sural branches, with the sural nerve.

Bardeen (1907) found the posterior femoral cutaneous nerve to have considerable variation in its origin and distribution. The nerve may arise from either the fifth lumbar and first sacral nerves, the first two sacral nerves, the second and third sacral nerves, or the third and fourth sacral nerves.

When the tibial and peroneal nerves arise separately, the posterior femoral cutaneous nerve also arises separately. The ventral portion accompanies the tibial nerve and gives off perineal and medial femoral branches; the dorsal portion accompanies the peroneal nerve and gives off gluteal and lateral femoral branches (Goss, 1973). In 81 of 110 cases, Bardeen (1907) found the terminal branches of the posterior femoral cutaneous nerve in the upper third of the back of the leg. Rarely did he find an anastomosis of the nerve with the sural nerves, as is usually described.

The Perforating Cutaneous Nerve

The perforating cutaneous nerve arises from the second and third sacral nerves. It pierces the sacrotuberous ligament, and supplies the skin over the medial and lower part of the gluteus maximus.

In 33 per cent of instances the perforating cutaneous nerve is absent (Goss, 1973). When absent, it may be replaced by a branch of the posterior femoral cutaneous nerve. The nerve may arise in common with the pudendal nerve (Goss, 1973). Bardeen (1907) found the perforating cutaneous nerve in only eight of 94 instances.

The Sciatic Nerve

The sciatic nerve is considered to be the continuation of the major part of the sacral plexus into the lower extremity. It arises from the fourth and fifth lumbar nerves as well as from the first three sacral nerves. It emerges from the pelvis through the greater sciatic foramen, is anterior to the obturator internus, the two gemelli muscles, and the quadratis femoris, and is posterior to the gluteus maximus. It lies upon the adductor magnus and, usually, at the distal third of the thigh near the popliteal fossa will split into its two large terminal divisions, the tibial nerve and the common peroneal nerve. In some instances, the splitting of the sciatic nerve occurs near the origin of the sacral plexus, thus separating the two terminal nerves throughout their course with no true sciatic nerve being present.

In the proximal part of the sciatic nerve, articular branches are given to the hip joint, and muscular branches are distributed to the long head of the biceps femoris, the semitendinosus, the semimembranosus, and the adductor magnus (all from the tibial nerve), and a muscular branch to the short head of the biceps femoris, derived from the common peroneal nerve.

The Tibial Nerve

The tibial nerve arises from the anterior divisions of the fourth and fifth lumbar nerves as well as from the first three sacral nerves. It passes through the popliteal fossa, then between the two heads of the gastrocnemius muscle, and runs deep to the tibialis posterior down to the tendo calcaneus and the flexor retinaculum, where it divides into medial and lateral plantar nerves. In its course, the tibial nerve gives off several branches. Articular branches are distributed to the knee, ankle, and tibiofibular joints. Muscular branches supply the following muscles: the gastrocnemius, plantaris, soleus, popliteus, tibialis posterior, and flexor digitorum longus.

Below the knee, between the two heads of the gastrocnemius, the tibial nerve gives origin to the medial sural cutaneous nerve. This nerve descends to about the middle of the back of the leg, and is joined by a communicating branch of the lateral sural cutaneous nerve off the peroneal nerve to form the sural nerve. The sural nerve passes on the lateral side of the tendo calcaneous, supplying the skin of the back of the leg and communicating with the posterior femoral cutaneous nerve (Goss, 1973). The nerve courses anteriorly below the lateral malleolus, where it is now named the lateral dorsal cutaneous nerve. It supplies the side of the foot and little toe, and communicates with the intermediate dorsal cutaneous nerve, a branch of the superficial peroneal (Goss, 1973).

Of the two terminal branches of the tibial nerve, the medial plantar is the larger. The nerve passes posterior to the abductor hallucis, and appears in the sole of the foot between that muscle and the flexor digitorum brevis. It innervates these two muscles and gives off to the great toe the proper plantar digital nerve, which innervates the flexor hallucis brevis and the skin of the medial side of the great toe. The medial plantar nerve ends at the base of the metatarsal bones in three common digital nerves. The first common digital nerve will supply the first lumbrical muscle.

The three common digital nerves pass between the plantar aponeurosis, where they each split into two proper digital nerves. These supply the adjacent and plantar sides of the first four toes and the distal surface of the terminal phalanges.

The lateral plantar nerve passes diagonally toward the base of the fifth metatarsal bone. It supplies the skin of the fifth toe and the lateral half of the fourth toe. Between the flexor digitorum brevis and the abductor digiti minimi, it innervates the latter muscle and the quadratus plantae and then divides into a superficial and a deep branch. The superficial branch splits into two plantar digital nerves, one to supply the adjacent sides of the fourth and fifth toes and the other to supply the two interossei of the fourth intermetatarsal space, the flexor digiti minimi brevis, and the lateral side of the little toe. The deep branch courses posteriorly to the flexor muscles and distributes to the adductor hallucis, all the interossei except those in the fourth intermetatarsal space, and the second, third, and fourth lumbrical muscles.

In 10 to 15 per cent of cases, the sciatic nerve will separate at its origin into two nerves, the common peroneal and the tibial (Hollinshead, 1968). Paterson (1893) found this condition in three of 23 plexuses he examined.

In the distribution of the tibial nerve, Horwitz (1938) found in 98 of 100 cases that the sural nerve divided 0.5 inch behind and above the tip of the lateral malleolus into a small posterior branch and a large anterior one. The larger branch passed to the dorsum of the foot, anastomosed with the intermediate dorsal cutaneous division of the superficial peroneal nerve, and ended as the lateral digital branch of the fifth toe. An additional lateral calcaneal branch came off the sural nerve two inches above the lateral malleolus.

Bardeen (1907) found that the tibial nerve may occasionally have double branches in its supply to the long head of the biceps femoris and the semitendinosus. Frequently, the muscular branches to each of these muscles are combined into a common trunk for a part of their course. In addition, he found that, compared with the other nerves of the foot, the plantar nerves seem to be unusually constant in their distribution. The quadratus plantae was always innervated by the lateral plantar nerve. The lateral plantar nerve only occasionally gave a branch to the lateral head of the flexor hallucis brevis, and in about one in 10 cases the medial as well as the lateral plantar nerves supplied both the first and second lumbrical muscles.

The Common Peroneal Nerve

The common peroneal nerve arises from the posterior divisions of the fourth and fifth lumbar nerves and the first two sacral nerves. It is the smaller of the two terminal branches of the sciatic nerve. It runs obliquely through the popliteal fossa, close to the biceps femoris, and descends on the lateral border of the fossa anterior to the lateral head of the gastrocnemius. At the knee, the common peroneal gives off articular branches to the knee. It also gives off the lateral sural cutaneous nerve, which supplies the skin of the posterior and lateral aspects of the calf. The lateral sural cutaneous nerve, at the head of the fibula, gives off a peroneal communicating ramus, which passes anterior to the lateral head of the gastrocnemius to join the medial sural cutaneous nerve and form the sural nerve.

The common peroneal nerve winds around the neck of the fibula, where it is superficial and can be palpated, and runs posterior to the peroneus longus to divide into the superficial and deep peroneal nerves.

The superficial peroneal nerve passes between the peroneus longus and peroneus brevis, gives muscular branches to them, and then runs vertically between these two muscles and the extensor digitorum longus. In the lower third of the leg, it becomes superficial, gives branches to the skin of the lower leg, and divides into the medial dorsal cutaneous nerve and the intermediate dorsal cutaneous nerve.

The medial dorsal cutaneous nerve follows a course anterior to the ankle joint, and splits into two dorsal digital nerves, which supply the medial side of the great toe, the adjacent sides of the second and third toes, and the skin of the medial side of the foot and ankle. The medial dorsal cutaneous nerve communicates with the deep peroneal nerve and the saphenous nerve (Goss, 1973).

The intermediate dorsal cutaneous nerve runs along the lateral part of the dorsum of the foot, where it supplies the skin of that region, and splits into two dorsal digital nerves, which supply the adjacent sides of the third, fourth, and fifth toes. It has been found that, frequently, when some of the lateral branches of the superficial peroneal nerve are absent their places are taken by branches of the sural nerve (Goss, 1973).

The deep peroneal nerve courses vertically down, deep to the extensor digitorum longus. It accompanies the anterior tibial artery, passes deep to the extensor retinaculum and divides in front of the ankle into a medial and a lateral branch. It innervates the tibialis anterior, extensor digitorum longus, peroneus tertius and extensor hallucis longus while in the leg.

The medial branch, supplying the first dorsal interosseous muscle, runs with the dorsalis pedis artery and, at the first intermetatarsal space, splits into two dorsal digital nerves to supply the adjacent sides of the great and second toes. It communicates with the medial dorsal cutaneous branch off the superficial peroneal nerve.

The lateral branch passes deep to the extensor digitorum brevis, which it supplies, and becomes enlarged (Goss, 1973). It sends filaments to the tarsal joints, and muscular branches to the second dorsal interosseous muscle and perhaps the third dorsal interosseous muscle (Lockhart, 1969).

Bardeen and Elting (1901) found, in rare instances, that the third lumbar nerve or the third sacral nerve contributed to the origin of the common peroneal. In one case they found the sole contribution to the common peroneal nerve to be derived from the fourth and fifth lumbar nerves.

Horwitz (1938) found the normal course of the deep peroneal nerve in the leg (95 of 100 cases) to first be lateral to the anterior tibial artery, then anterior to the artery four inches above the ankle joint, and then lateral to the artery again. In four cases, he found the nerve lateral, then posterior, and then medial to the artery, and in one case, the nerve was lateral, then anterior, and finally medial to the artery. He described these five cases as infrequent variations.

Horwitz (1938) described the course of the superficial peroneal nerve and found that in 90 of 100 cases the nerve became superficial five inches superior to the lateral malleolus, in the groove between the peroneal muscles and the extensor digitorum longus. In five cases, the nerve became superficial three inches above the malleolus, two inches above the malleolus in two cases, four inches above the malleolus in two cases and six inches above the malleolus in one case.

Usually the extensor digitorum brevis is innervated by the lateral branch of the deep peroneal nerve. However, in 25 to 30 per cent of cases, it will receive its nerve supply from an accessory deep peroneal nerve originating off the superficial peroneal nerve (Lambert, 1969; Infante and Kennedy, 1970; Goodgold and Eberstein, 1972).

REFERENCES

Bardeen, C. R.: Development and variation of the nerves and the musculature of the inferior extremity and of the neighboring regions of the trunk in man. Am. J. Anat. 6:259, 1907.

Bardeen, C. R., and Elting, A.: A statistical study of the variations in the formation and position of the lumbo-sacral plexus in man. Anat. Anz. 19:124, 209, 1901.

Goodgold, J., and Eberstein, A.: Electrodiagnosis of Neuromuscular Diseases. Baltimore, The Williams & Wilkins Co., 1972.

Goss, C. M.: Anatomy of the Human Body by Henry Gray. Philadelphia, Lea and Febiger, 1973.

Hollinshead, W. H.: Anatomy for Surgeons. Hagerstown, Harper and Row, Inc., 1968, Vol. 3.

Horwitz, M. T.: Normal anatomy and variations of the peripheral nerves of the leg and foot: Application in operations for vascular diseases: Study of one hundred specimens. Arch. Surg. 36:626, 1938.

Horwitz, M. T.: The anatomy of the lumbosacral nerve plexus — its relation to variations of vertebral segmentation, and the posterior sacral nerve plexus. Anat. Rec. 74:91, 1939.

Infante, E., and Kennedy, W. R.: Anomalous branch of the peroneal nerve detected by electromyography. Arch. Neurol. 22:162, 1970.

Lambert, E. H.: The accessory deep peroneal nerve: A common variation in innervation of extensor digitorum brevis. Neurology 19:1169, 1969.

Lockhart, R. D., Hamilton, G. F., and Fyfe, F. W.: Anatomy of the Human Body. Philadelphia, J. B. Lippincott Co., 1969.

Paterson, A. M.: The origin and distribution of the nerves to the lower limb. J. Anat. Physiol. 28:84, 169, 1893–94.

Pain

II

8

PAIN: EXTREMITIES AND SPINE— EVALUATION AND DIFFERENTIAL DIAGNOSIS

J. LEONARD GOLDNER

INTRODUCTION

The physiology of pain's reception and the recognition of pain necessitate a brief review of the receptors, the pathways, and the brain centers through which painful stimuli are conducted and recognized. The classic definition of the physiologic processes involved in the recognition of heat, cold, sharp, and dull has been modified by more recent observations in the field of neurophysiology (Horch, 1978).

Free nerve endings of the C–fibers are considered the primary receptors that signal pain. Recent physiologic evidence indicates that these free nerve endings also function as receptors for other kinds of sensation. At the peripheral end, fine cutaneous afferent activity is a necessary condition for individuals to experience pain. Functional localization of pain is important, but spatial and temporal mechanisms involved in the coding of sensory experience within the central nervous system must be considered a part of the entire mechanism. This concept is important in determining methods of relieving pathologic pain conditions (Wall, 1974; Wagman and Price, 1969).

Pain is transmitted in the lateral spinothalamic tracts. Thermal sensation is carried in the same area in the anterior quadrant of the spinal cord. Other pathways for transmission of the pain stimuli are available. The lateral spinothalamic tract, if followed genetically, is a recent pathway with input directly to the sensory thalamus. Rapid transmission of the pain occurs through the spinothalamic route to the thalamus, where higher levels of integration occur through

119

the thalamocortical connections. A definite topographic scheme of the body's sensory image exists within the cord and the thalamus, with input from the facial region being medial to that of the body, and the input from the leg regions being lateral (Melzack, 1975; Miller, 1966).

Pain resulting from electrical stimulation of the spinothalamic tract pathways is usually experienced by the patient as a sharp, well demarcated sensation referred to a localized region of the body. Diffuse pain pathways appear to have multiple routes through the spinal cord, with distribution to the mid brain, thalamus, and hypothalamus in the spinal recticular pathways, and if followed genetically are older than the newer lateral spinothalamic tracts and are designated as the paleothalamic system. These tracts may be crossed or uncrossed and are composed of short chains of neurons that make several synaptic connections at successive rostral levels in the central nervous system. Pain transmitted via these routes appears to be slower in transit to higher levels, and the sensation experienced by alert patients during stimulation is ill defined and unpleasant, being diffusely localized to the regions in the central parts of the body, including the head, chest, and abdomen (Melzack, 1975).

A primary pain syndrome may involve the pain pathways themselves. An example of a primary pain syndrome is the painful dysesthesia occurring from operative cordotomy, tractotomy, or thalamotomy. Other examples are the pain of the thalamic syndrome, with its characteristic severity and hand position, and the painful phantom limb syndrome. Also, central pain syndromes occur after trauma, vascular occlusion, tumor, or other conditions involving the central nervous system such as herpes zoster (Sweet and Wepsic, 1968).

The reader is referred to the chapters in this book on Neurophysiology in order to reinforce the anatomic designation of pathways and the neurophysiologic interpretation of pain syndromes.

PAIN RESULTING FROM EXTERNAL AND INTERNAL FACTORS

Examples of various pain responses and the cause of pain complaints may be described on the basis of clinical observation as well as experimental studies. These examples illustrate pain responses of different intensity and different characteristics. Several examples are listed with descriptions of the pain and explanatory comments concerning the etiologic factors.

1. *Expansion of a hollow viscus* may be associated with an abdominal cramp. The resulting pain is of varying degree and may be mild or severe.
2. *Migraine headache* associated with vascular alteration such as vasodilatation is severe and throbbing, and is frequently associated with nausea, aura, and other unpleasant feelings that aggravate the intensity of pain.
3. *Periodontal tissues* when irritated cause a unique painful sensation. If the dentine layer is exposed after removal of plaque or resorption of gingival tissue, hot or cold fluid causes exquisite pain that is intense and severe. Pressure on a tooth surrounded by inflamed periodontal tissue or a tooth that is covered by sensitive dentine causes a dull ache.
4. *Severe joint pain* may occur when the synovium and capsule are stretched by

fluid under tension or by irritation of the periosteal area at the edge of the articular cartilage. If the tension occurs rapidly and the pressure is high, diffuse severe pain will occur around the involved joint (Kellgren and Samuel, 1950; Clippinger and Goldner, 1973).

5. *Thermal variations* on the skin, including excessive heat or cold, cause a characteristic withdrawal response of the involved part. The stimulus from ice or liquid nitrogen is better tolerated momentarily than the stimulus from an excessively hot object.

6. *A sharp stimulus* on the skin or other sensitive tissue causes a rapid pain response, as does cutting, scraping, pinching, or twisting (Nosik, 1954).

7. Stimulation of *myofascial attachments* to periosteum or bone by sudden stress, constant stretch, or pressure causes a deep dull aching response that is readily tolerated as compared with the acute pain that results from sharper stimuli (Goldner, 1954, 1956).

8. *Muscle claudication due to arterial insufficiency* causes involuntary muscle cramping or aching as the result of hypoxia. The degree of pain varies according to the severity of the ischemia (Hill, 1973; Mavor, 1956).

9. *Increased compartment* pressure of 35 mm Hg from direct trauma results in severe throbbing, gnawing, aching, diffuse deep pain which is relieved almost immediately by fasciotomy throughout the entire length of the compartment.

10. *Ischemia of peripheral nerves* results in paresthesias and periods of painful numbness associated with episodes of diminished peripheral blood flow. Nerve compression causes alteration of axon conduction and relative ischemia. A combination of ischemia and compression results in a persistent, painful paresthesia.

11. *Muscle cramping or painful contractions* occur as a result of peripheral nerve irritation or motor end-plate sensitivity or unexplained muscle contraction with subsequent soreness of the muscle belly after the acute, deep, dull aching sensation associated with the cramping has been alleviated.

12. *Irritation of a posterior sensory root* ganglion causes peripheral cutaneous burning, stinging, throbbing, alterations of skin sensation, and a deep aching pain. These signs are noted in herpes zoster, which affects the posterior root ganglia. The pain may be unrelenting, searing, and burning and may be associated with hypersensitivity of hair in the cutaneous dermatome. A cyst of the nerve root may cause the same complaints.

13. *Nerve root irritation* from mechanical or inflammatory stimuli causes hypesthesia, paresthesia, muscle cramping, vague aching in the deep structures, and dermatome alterations.

14. *The deep aching bone and periosteal pain* caused by increased pressure and vascular alteration of osteoid osteoma has pain characteristics different than those from dermatome and myotome pain stimuli.

15. *Distention of the intervertebral space* recognized during discography causes a deep, diffuse, radiating stimulus not well localized. Radiation may occur to the sacrum, buttocks, deeper areas of the pelvis, or lateral trunk.

16. *Hypertonic saline* injected into the subcutaneous and fascial tissues causes deep, radiating pain which resembles that resulting from mild irritation of fascial attachments, by either calcification, tearing, or pressure (Lewis, 1942).

17. *The exquisite tenderness of a glomus tumor* in the digit is a combination of cutaneous and deep pain and is associated with rapid withdrawal of the part and intolerance of the individual to even the slightest pressure.

18. *Digital nerve irritation due to laceration,* infection, or trauma in the finger pulp is a combination of pressure and direct irritation in closed compartments and is associated with throbbing, burning, and aching.

19. *A lacerated digital nerve* that is untreated will cause a hypersensitive neuroma that is characterized by dysesthesia, paresthesias, cold intolerance, and hypesthesia.

20. *Sensory nerve compression* lesions of the superficial radial, median, or ulnar nerve will cause tingling, burning, and numbness with diffuse altered sensations throughout the involved digits.

PAIN ASSESSMENT

The differential diagnosis and evaluation of pain depend on a description of the intensity of the unpleasant sensation, a comparison by the patient to other known sensations, and an attempted designation of the severity of pain based on a number system. The spectrum of pain awareness and severity varies from a minimal pain response that is tolerated and easily overlooked to an unbearable sensation that interferes with the individual's productive activity. Examples of painful sensations of varying degrees caused by different lesions are clarified by relating specific patient examples.

1. *Separation of the finger pad from the nail plate such as occurs when paper is accidentally forced between the nail plate and the nail bed.* The resulting immediate pain is sharp, burning, lancinating, and well localized with a high level, discrete pain response diminished by firm compression of the part and improved by immobilization and by clipping away the unopposed fingernail in order to avoid repeated stress on the skin (Goldner et al., 1972).

2. *Hematoma under the nail plate from a direct blow* causes a deep, dull aching, diffuse hypersensitivity associated with throbbing which is aggravated when the hand is dependent.

3. *Tight, contracted connective tissue in the hand associated with limited finger flexion* and a *sensation of stiffness* results in a nondescript diffuse aching sensation more obvious after inactivity and aggravated by stressful actions. Scleroderma, rheumatoid arthritis, and osteoarthritis are frequently associated with this kind of pain (Goldner, 1955, 1975).

Patient Examples

Case 1. Upper Extremity Pain Syndrome

DIFFERENTIAL DIAGNOSIS.   A 50-year-old female complained of an aching neck, a painful shoulder, localized tenderness around the elbow, and intermittent paresthesias in the hand. The anatomic structures suggested a cervical root compression syndrome with radiation into the shoulder and the scapular region and dermatome, myotome, and sclerotome distribution of pain in the anatomic region supplied by C6, C7, and C8 nerve roots. Physical examination suggested a lateral epicondylitis with pain over the extensor tendons, a medial epicondylitis with tenderness over the forearm flexor mass, and shoulder pain when the humerus was abducted. The shoulder impingement syndrome was differentiated from the radicular pain usually associated with nerve root irritation. A scapulothoracic syndrome associated with degeneration of fascial and tendon attachments is accentuated by unusual positions of the extremity. Anxiety and tension result in a painful extremity from the neck to the hand. Minimal symptoms can be aggravated by emotional depression, with the patient's ability to tolerate the pain diminished to a low level. Physical examination aids in establishing a diagnosis:

1. Cutaneous sensory impairment is detected if present. Hypesthesia in a dermatome distribution is suggestive of cervical root or cutaneous compression lesions.
2. Diminished tendon reflexes such as deltoid, triceps, biceps, and radial reflexes are significant in localizing and suggesting a cervical root lesion.
3. Diminished muscle tone and moderate atrophy if generalized throughout the extremity suggest disuse, as might be noted with an adhesive capsule of the shoulder. However, localized atrophy or diminished tone indicates a nerve root irritation or motor fiber involvement of the peripheral nerve.
4. Muscle strength, if diminished, suggests nerve root or mixed nerve involvement.
5. Tender muscle motor points are noted when a nerve root is affected.
6. Digital pressure over the nerve root or nerve trunk and stretch of the nerve by separating the head from the tip of the shoulder aggravate local pain or radiating pain.

Accessory studies and clinical and laboratory tests provide additional information:

1. *A positive nerve percussion* test may indicate nerve irritation at the point of percussion, such as a compressed median nerve at the wrist; or palpation along the entire course of the nerve suggests sensory irritation at a higher level.
2. *Physical stress and stretch of the nerve* may aggravate pain; a local anesthetic injection into a cervical root or nerve trunk may diminish pain. This therapeutic test aids in localization of the site and anatomic distribution of pain.
3. *Sensory conduction studies* at the wrist, elbow, and across the thoracic outlet are helpful in determining the site of nerve compression or irritation. There is a special method of determining sensory conduction across the supraclavicular region which requires an integrator for accurate reading.
4. *Thermography* will provide relatively quick information about peripheral blood flow and excess heat being given off by soft tissue or bone lesion (Venters et al., 1972).
5. A *technetium 99* bone scan will provide information concerning increased vascularity of a particular part of the extremity and aid in differentiating nerve pain from bone pain.

This patient's studies were completed and myelography demonstrated a cervical root filling defect. Other studies were suggestive of a root lesion. After discectomy and fusion, the radicular component of pain was relieved but the impingement syndrome of the shoulder and the epicondylitis of the elbow persisted. Two distinct conditions were present but they blended as one diffuse pain syndrome of the upper extremity. Also, a third factor was the patient's desire to retire after 30 years of teaching and this influenced her rate of recovery and the slow elimination of her "pain syndrome."

Nerve root compression results in different pain patterns involving a dermatome, a myotome, or a sclerotome; frequently the pain pattern is a combination of all three of these sensations. The nerve root components related to the myotome and sclerotome are similar to the pain pattern that arises from a pathologic connective tissue stimulus associated with adhesive capsulitis of the shoulder, an impingement syndrome of the shoulder, or a partial tear of the lateral extensor muscle mechanism at the elbow known as "tennis elbow" (Sherman, 1963; Feinstein et al., 1954).

FACTORS AFFECTING THE INTENSITY OF PAIN

There are *physiologic variations* of the pain threshold from one person to another; that is, there is an inherent definable difference in the pain level which varies from congenital insensitivity to pain to a state of hyperreactivity to almost any external stimulus. This spectrum is divided as follows:

1. *Congenital insensitivity* to pain is recognized as a true syndrome in which the person does not respond to epicritic stimuli or fractures of the extremities by other than a descriptive comment concerning the injury. These patients do not complain of pain (Black, 1954; Feindel, 1953; Petrie, 1953).
2. *A high threshold of pain* is recognized by many individuals who tolerate painful stimuli such as heat, cold, sharp, or heavy pressure with recognition of the abnormal sensation and the kind of sensation but who are able to accept the stimulus with minimal response.
3. *A temporary limited awareness* of pain occurs immediately after certain severe injuries, such as a tear of major ligaments about the knee during a football game or a severe inversion injury to the ankle resulting in massive ligamentous tear. The individual experiences sudden, exquisite, severe pain at the time of the injury and may become hypotensive, nauseated, and faint. During the recovery phase the injured part may be manipulated with little or no discomfort in certain instances. Within several minutes after injury, however, the pain pattern associated with periosteal injury, distended synovium and capsule, and pressure from hematoma becomes severe.
4. *An average reaction to pain stimuli* characterizes that which most individuals have to a sudden sharp point, to excessive heat, or to a severe rotary injury to a joint. The individual with average pain tolerance will describe pain in the shoulder as being dull and aching but compatible with moderate limitation of the activities of daily living. If the pain is more severe, the condition will be described as sharp, lancinating, and intermittently severe. The circadian

cycle affects the intensity of the pain. Pain complaints are usually greater at night and also increase as barometric pressure increases. External modalities such as excessive heat or cold, or an unusual degree of compression or forcible rotation cause pain to increase.

5. *The individual's personality* affects this average reaction to pain. Those with hysterical personalities or with a tendency to hypochondriasis or those who are anxious and depressed respond with more frequent and intense complaints concerning pain and overreact to the severity of the stimulus (Welsh and Dahlstram, 1956). Other items that affect the intensity of pain include sleep deprivation, absence of certain habit forming medications, and an unnaturally high anxiety level. Individuals with labile personality who have acute pain may overreact to a painful stimulus. The same individuals may become dependent and passive and accept chronic pain although frequently complaining about the effect of the pain on their personality. For example, they state that pain causes them to be tired, that it decreases their ability to concentrate, that it lessens their sex drive and performance, and that it alters their disposition. The emotional aspects of pain cannot be separated from the physical aspects. A severe toothache that interferes with sleeping, eating, and working is represented by a much higher degree of pain and responds less well to medications and external applications than does the acute form of pain that is present for only a short period of time and does not affect rest and nutrition.

Conditions in Extremity and Environment That Alter Severity of Pain

A painful amputation stump may be temporarily relieved by compression with a temporary socket, by external wrapping, or by firm pressure from the patient's hands. The severity of phantom pain may be increased or decreased by altering the state of a peripheral nerve by nerve block. Peripheral electrical stimulation may temporarily affect the severity of both phantom pain and phantom sensation (Goldner and Hendrix, 1977; Melzack, 1975).

Adherent tight skin over a lacerated peripheral nerve may cause unplesant stimuli when the skin is stretched and the nerve is irritated. External pressure over thin adherent skin covering a peripheral nerve may result in an acute painful response. When a peripheral nerve is adherent to tendon, bone, or skin a forceful stretch of the fingers or hand into an extended position applies traction to the nerve and results in painful sensory stimulation.

Compression of a peripheral nerve within the carpal canal or indirect irritation of the posterior tibial nerve by a proliferative posterior tibial tendon sheath causes local sensory stimulation of the nerve, development of an area of compression or enlargement, interference with the vascular supply to the nerve, and subsequent painful stimuli both at the point of irritation and in the autonomous zone of the nerve (Goldner, 1975).

Direct or indirect ischemia of a peripheral nerve causes paresthesias, dysesthesias, and varying degrees of claudication. Cold intolerance is related to vasoregulatory deficiencies affecting peripheral nerves, the sympathetic nervous system, or the various geographic segments of the peripheral arterial

tree. Vasospasm may result from a high concentration of epinephrine, sero-
tonin, or chemical agents such as ergot. Pain is a factor in all of these conditions, and the degree of pain depends upon the rapidity of the onset of the
pathologic condition and the chronicity of the etiologic factor. An abnormal
increase in compartment pressure compromises the perfusion process or the
capillary closing pressure, which leads to ischemia, the accumulation of metabolites, and pain (Goldner, 1955, 1975).

Classification of Patients with Major Peripheral Pain Syndromes

From 1974 through 1978, we have used a *transcutaneous* nerve stimulator
on approximately 400 patients with chronic pain syndromes (Goldner and
Hendrix, 1977). The selection of the patients to receive the stimulator was
dependent on many factors but the common thread was the existence for
many months of a pain syndrome that had not responded to many different
efforts at relieving or diminishing pain and a patient who was willing to try
the stimulator. About 25 per cent of the 400 patients responded favorably in
that their pain pattern was diminished significantly. The response, however,
was assessed according to the presumed cause of pain and the emotional profile of the patient, and consideration was given to many factors that influence
pain, such as the placebo effect.

A group of patients at Duke have been managed by *microelectrode* peripheral nerve implants (Nashold, Goldner, and Bright, 1975). The patients treated
in this way had severe pain patterns, usually associated with a particular peripheral nerve lesion or a nerve root lesion. These patients frequently responded
satisfactorily to peripheral nerve block and were improved temporarily by the
transcutaneous stimulator. Many other factors in the area of social adjustment, financial gain, and other secondary gain syndromes had to be considered in the final results.

A large group of patients were categorized as *"reflex sympathetic dystrophy"*
types. In these patients the pathologic lesion varied from peripheral neuroma
to cervical root lesion. Symptoms included burning pain in the extremity, dysesthesia, constant pain which was worse at night, a pain pattern partially relieved by sympathetic nerve block or intra-arterial or intravenous reserpine,
and pain complaints that were occasionally relieved by peripheral nerve decompression or by bypass arterial graft or sympathectomy to improve peripheral blood flow (Goldner and Bright, 1979).

Patients with demonstrable *vascular insufficiency* determined by skin temperature readings, cold tolerance tests, thermography, and angiography had
pain syndromes associated with exposure to cold, to exercise, or to emotional
disturbances affecting their vasoregulatory capabilities. A connective tissue
disease such as scleroderma or any of the collagen conditions causing Raynaud's syndrome were included in the group with pain due to vascular insufficiency (Porter, 1977; Stirrat et al., 1978; Urbaniak et al., 1978).

Patients with *peripheral nerve trauma* resulting in a complete nerve lesion
developed chronic pain syndromes associated with inadequate nerve repair or

nonphysiologic nerve regeneration. Other patients, with partial peripheral lesions, were prone to persistent pain caused by partial interruption of conduction and causalgic syndromes that were associated with diminished peripheral blood flow secondary to the nerve injury and persistent painful stimuli from the incomplete nerve lesion (Goldner, 1977).

DESCRIPTIVE TERMINOLOGY ASSOCIATED WITH PERIPHERAL NERVE LESIONS AND COMBINED PERIPHERAL NERVE AND VASCULAR LESIONS (Goldner, 1977)

Anesthesia: no demonstrable recognition of external stimuli except movement of the part or extreme pressure which causes tendon or bone stimulation.

Hypesthesia: diminution of the ability to recognize cutaneous stimulation caused by pressure made with a sharp point or a dull object. This description usually designates alteration of a dermatome.

Dysesthesia: an uncomfortable, unpleasant sensation resulting from stimulation of a cutaneous region, usually affected by peripheral nerve trauma or regeneration. Stimulation of one side of a digit may actually be felt in adjacent digit.

Paresthesia: painful tingling, aching, and burning along the course of a peripheral nerve resulting from percussion of the involved nerve or stimulation of the skin in the autonomous zone of the involved nerve.

Hyperesthesia: unpleasant feelings of excessive sensation resulting from cutaneous stimulation. Hair in the geographic dermatome is excessively sensitive to touch, as are the skin and fingernail which are part of that digit.

Cold intolerance: this is the dull, deep, aching sensation in a segment of the extremity that occurs as the environmental temperature is lowered. The more rapidly the temperature drops the greater is the pain. The pain distribution is not well localized and is not relieved immediately by warming the part. The pain associated with cold intolerance may be minimal if the temperature is dropped slowly but may be severe if warm-up is done too rapidly.

Burning, searing, cutting and **hot** are terms commonly used by individuals with peripheral nerve lesions that result from complete or partial nerve trauma.

PAIN SYNDROMES: EXAMPLES AND DESCRIPTIONS

Pain syndromes vary from those of minimal intensity to those of severe intensity that are not readily relieved by any method of treatment. Patient examples are presented in order to emphasize the spectrum observed, the diagnostic methods, and the selection of treatment used in attempting to solve these complex problems.

Patient Examples

Case 2. Puncture Wound of a Digit

A 38-year-old woman received a puncture wound of the pad over the distal phalanx of the long finger by a piece of glass. On three occasions, the attending physician attempted to remove glass slivers using local anesthesia and radiographic control. As a result of the original trauma and the subsequent alterations of the finger pad, the pulp became atrophic, cutaneous sensation decreased, and hypersensitivity of the entire tip occurred with persistent hypesthesia, dysesthesia, and hyperesthesia. Fibrosis of the pad resulted in tethering of the arborized branches of the digital nerve, causing fixation of nerve endings in periosteum and bone. Whenever the pad was compressed by pinch or grasp, the nerve stimulation was severe. Without protective fat, the sensory end receptors are constantly compressed and irritated, and painful stimuli occurred repetitively. The patient attempted to protect the finger with a Bandaid or a thimble in order to diminish the sensory input. (Inadequate skin and fat and insufficient protection of the end receptors results in persistent pain.)

TREATMENT. Avoidance of stimulation is a method of diminishing the intensity of pain in any of the pain syndromes involving the upper extremity. Compression of the finger pad or counterirritation by stimulation may alter the sensory input. External heat may cause peripheral vasodilatation and alter the blood flow, which in turn may diminish the intensity of pain. Temporary alteration of sensory input by nerve block, by intermittent drip of a local anesthetic through a percutaneous tube, may diminish the cycle of painful afferent impulses and influence the effect on the centers in the spinal cord and brain. Steroid as an anti-inflammatory may be injected locally or given orally in order to change the local membrane potential and to affect adherent fibrous tissue. Local steroid injections are usually done deep to the dermis or the fatty layer and deep to or just around the nerve. Steroid causes fat atrophy and thinning of the skin around the painful area as well as depigmentation. Several patients have been observed who have had steroid injections into or around the fingertips for management of painful digital nerve conditions. In a peripheral neuroma, this treatment will occasionally decrease pain associated with an amputation. But if fat and skin atrophy occur, the digital nerve may ultimately have less protection than before the injection, and pain may become worse.

This patient had a persistently thin fingerpad, a hypersensitive fingertip, and pain with pinch and pressure. This was managed by elevating the entire pad through radial and ulnar incisions, mobilizing the soft pulp with the neurovascular structures intact, and advancing the tip to the edge of the fingernail after the thin skin had been trimmed. A segment of bone was also trimmed so that a new pad was constructed. The procedure was reasonably successful for this patient. Several months after the operation, her sensitivity had diminished over 70 per cent, the protection from the skin pulp had improved, and she was using the digit for typing, writing, and turning pages (Goldner, 1977).

Case 3. Digital Nerve Laceration

A patient with a laceration of both digital nerves developed adhesions of the nerve endings to the dermis. The proximal neuroma and distal fibroma were adherent and tethered. How does one eliminate pain from the neuromata, from adherent nerve endings causing traction of nerves, and still provide continuity of the nerve? The nerve should be mobilized, the neuroma resected, and resuture done without excess tension. Usually an epineurial end-to-end suture is possible. If, after the segments are mobilized, there is a gap of 2 cm or less, measured with the wrist in neutral position and the digit straight (zero degrees at all digital joints), the gap can be eliminated by flexion of the finger to about 40 degrees. If the gap is greater than 2 cm, an intercalated nerve graft is inserted in order to restore protective sensation and to diminish the escape of unmyelinated axons from the proximal end. This procedure usually diminishes or relieves the hypersensitivity after regeneration across the graft occurs, and will diminish pain, provided a biologic tube exists into which axons will advance. Nerve adhesions caused by inadequate skin coverage provide an unfavorable environment for traumatized digital nerves or those that have been repaired by end-to-end suture or nerve graft. In most instances, end-to-end suture of lacerated nerves is possible, and, if done within a year of the original accident, will diminish sensitivity and allow the development of protective sensation. One must inform the patient that progressive improvement will occur up to five years after the repair, provided that the suture is completed in an appropriate way. Our experience has been that, although sensory nerve repair should be done within a year after injury, pain has been diminished and sensation improved after nerve repair even five years after injury (Goldner, 1968–1974).

Case 4. Digital Nerve Injury Resulting in Neuroma Within an Intact Nerve

A 40-year-old female accidentally pushed an oyster knife into the palm of her hand and lacerated the palmar fascia, a common digital nerve, and the adjacent artery. Initial treatment was wound excision and closure of the wound with two large silk sutures. Anesthesia and paresthesias were present within a few days, and hyperesthesia developed. A nerve lesion in continuity may result in a complete block of axon conduction and local dysesthesia. An available human model is the patient with an injured saphenous nerve at the knee affected by either the incision or a suture at the time that an arthrotomy is done. Immediately after the knee operation, the patient complains of a numbness and dullness and may have hypersensitivity as well. Hypesthesia and paresthesia may exist simultaneously, and dysesthesia, the unpleasant sensory response, may be part of this syndrome. Furthermore, if the nerve is attached to the flexor tendon or to the lumbrical muscle of the long finger, pain will occur as the digit is extended because traction is exerted on the nerve. When the wrist is flexed and the finger is extended, radiculopathy is minimal. When the wrist is at neutral and the finger is extended, paresthesias are severe.

TREATMENT. This hypersensitive finger and its digital nerve were operated upon three months after the initial injury. The neuroma was resected and the digital nerve resutured. After the nerve suture, the patient continued to have a burning sensation and dysesthesias. The operative procedure was performed under general anesthesia, and postoperative stellate blocks were used. Our clinical and laboratory studies indicate that vasospasm results in diminished blood flow and that pain persists so long as blood flow is diminished. Postoperative stellate blocks, intra-arterial or intravenous reserpine, and postoperative oral steroid for 10 days are the methods used to reverse vasospasm and improve blood flow in order to decrease pain. Biofeedbacks may be helpful. Prior to the treatment of vasospasm the hand was intermittently cool and dry as a result of the peripheral nerve injury. Sweating was not excessive in the adjacent nonaffected area, suggesting that a true sympathetic dystrophy was not present. The skin supplied by the repaired digital nerve was dry as was expected.

Causalgia (burning pain) usually occurs when there is nerve injury associated with vascular insufficiency and the lesion usually involves part of the nerve but is not associated with complete nerve laceration. This patient had causalgia prior to nerve suture, persistent pain associated with vasospasm, and pain associated with collagen tightness in the adjacent joints (Goldner and Bright, 1979). Also, acute nerve trauma (for example, to the cervical roots, median nerve, sciatic nerve, or ulnar nerve) may result in fiery, lancinating, burning, shooting pain, hypersensitivity—that is, causalgia or St. Anthony's fire, which usually recedes rapidly if due to contusion of the nerve.

The procedures performed were: 1) stellate ganglion block with resulting increase in skin temperature and partial relief of pain. The stellate block would not be expected to eliminate all the pain if the connective tissue was tight and if the nerve was tethered. 2) Median nerve block into the carpal canal resulted in immediate temporary relief. Patients with a swollen hand and a tethered digital nerve have developed secondary median nerve compression due to tenosynovitis and intermittent traction and compression of the nerve. This is noted in patients with finger amputations who have persistent phantom pain in the zone of the median nerve. Release of the median nerve compression frequently has diminished the phantom pain and pain in the autonomous zone of the median nerve, provided that the digital nerves are not adherent to the amputation stumps and the neuromata are not constantly irritated (Grant, 1951).

Additional treatment for this patient's pain problem included steroid injection into the flexor tendon sheaths, constant elevation of the hand and arm to reduce edema, a dorsal plaster splint to limit wrist motion and decrease trauma to the median nerve, and a two week course of oral steroids, with the first dose being 40 mg of prednisone, diminishing 5 mg daily to 10 mg each day. The patient's range of motion improved dramatically within 48 hours, pain was lessened, and improvement occurred gradually during the next three months.

Electrical studies during the postoperative period did show a minimal median nerve conduction time delay. Because of the continued clinical improvement, the decision was made not to operate on the median nerve, since a satisfactory digital repair had been done and the patient was improving by nonoperative methods, whereas an operation on this hand which was affected by a sympathetic dystrophy due to vasospasm could result in recurrence of vasospasm and aggravation of the pain syndrome. If progressive compression of the median and ulnar nerves occurs at the wrist, and if the nonoperative methods of treatment described are insufficient to decrease pain, then decompression of the nerve is essential. The possible benefits derived outweigh the risk of postoperative hand stiffness.

Occasionally patients with this kind of problem have required late median nerve decompression, release of palmar fibrosis, and application of a sheet of silicone between the skin and the nerve. There is a scarcity of fat in the palm and the wrist, and the nerve may need protection during the healing phase. Other substances used are Gelfoam and Surgicel wrapped around the nerve. These provide temporary insulation from the surrounding tissue. Fat grafts are currently popular, although the author's personal past experience with free fat has been with the formation of free fibrous fat, which revascularizes slowly. Even the fat on the undersurface of a full thickness pedicle skin flap with good vascularization becomes fibrous and adherent to the nerve. Our experience has been that Surgicel around the nerve will protect the nerve from the adjacent skin. If the nerve needs protection from surrounding tendons, silicone sheeting is added as a temporary measure. Usually the silicone must be removed, although not always.

Case 5. Digital Nerve Laceration in the Palm

A 4-year-old child was examined four months after a palmar injury which occurred as the result of a fall on a glass bottle. She demonstrated severe hypersensitivity of the hand and had persistent pain in the palm, probably associated with a piece of glass in the deep layers of the palm. Atrophic ulcer was present on the tip of the digit. The initial treatment by the attending physician had been irrigation of the wound under general anesthesia, suture of the flexor digitorum superficialis and flexor digitorum profundus in the palm, and repair of the common digital nerves with a large silk suture. The hand had been immobilized for three weeks, but pain persisted. After the dressing was removed, the child would not move the fingers, but would move the thumb. The child was known to "bite her nails when anxious," and this particular finger showed evidence of loss of part of the finger pulp associated with nail biting and lack of sensitivity of the skin. The child held the digits in acute flexion and would not allow passive efforts at extension because of severe pain. Four months after the initial injury, the digit was dry, sweating was absent, a water wrinkle test was negative, and no fingerprints were noted on the fingerpad. Improvement did not occur as time passed and there was no evidence of peripheral nerve regeneration. Percussion of the healed laceration in the palm resulted in an exquisite pain reaction.

The author has observed this pattern of painful injury syndrome in children on numerous occasions and, therefore, will discuss several basic concepts.

Children with digital nerve injuries develop pain syndromes that will not disappear merely because of their age.

In a child, absent sensation due to common digital nerve injury can persist as an area of hypesthesia only or dysesthesia and anesthesia for months or years. Overlap innervation from adjacent intact digital nerves may not be sufficient to reinnervate the area.

Penetrating injuries in children must be managed under general anesthesia; the traumatic incision usually must be enlarged and a meticulous exploration of the area for foreign body done. At that time, the decision to suture lacerated tendons, nerves, and vessels depends on the degree of wound contamination and the *experience* of the surgeon. A safe physiologic approach if the wound is contaminated and if the surgeon is inexperienced with this kind of injury is to leave the wound open and proceed with early delayed closure and repair of the tendons and nerves five days after the injury.

Once the repair has been done, however, whether immediate or delayed, the repaired digital nerves should show progressive improvement of at least 1 mm a day in the adult and 2 to 3 mm a day in the child. This is determined by a percussion test at regular intervals. If excessive pain persists and an orderly pattern of regeneration is not evident, the nerve should be reoperated upon. This decision is usually possible by four to six weeks after the initial injury.

Digital nerve injuries resulting in tethering or fixation of the nerve to an adjacent tendon frequently result in median nerve compression and irritation at the wrist. Synovitis from inflammation, hemorrhage, trauma, or tendon retraction may irritate or fill the carpal canal and cause nerve compression and abnormal fixation of the median nerve by the digital nerve, which is not gliding distally. The same observations have been made concerning the ulnar nerve in the ulnar canal after common or proper digital nerve trauma to the ring or little finger.

The pathologic lesions described may mimic a reflex sympathetic dystrophy syndrome. Stellate ganglion block will improve blood flow and lessen the symptoms of a sympathetic dystrophy. However, if nerve tethering or compression persists, the stellate block alone diminishes but will not eliminate the pain syndrome. Block of the sympathetic fibers will not eliminate pain associated with nerve tethering, nerve compression, a neuroma in continuity, or wild axons undergoing disorderly growth. Temporary mild improvement occurs after the block as a result of increased blood flow or as a result of the anesthetic solution bathing nonmyelinated sensory fibers in the brachial plexus, or both.

True "causalgia" (Weir Mitchell, 1872) usually includes sudden onset of an incomplete nerve lesion alone, or a severe incomplete nerve injury associated with a prominent element of vascular insufficiency (Goldner and Bright, 1979). Major arterial insufficiency or small vessel compression by a tight compartment or vasospasm results in inadequate capillary perfusion, muscle fibrosis, and pain. The vascular insufficiency may be extensive, involving the entire upper extremity after injury in the axilla, or the pain syndrome may involve the forearm and hand if injury has occurred at the elbow, or, as was the case in the four-year-old child's palmar injury, the pain may result from ischemia of the lumbrical muscle and injury to the digital nerve and flexor tendons.

TREATMENT.   The child's palm was reoperated upon four months after the original injury. The common and proper digital nerves were isolated, freed from the surrounding palmar fascia and scarred flexor tendons, and removed from the ischemic fibers of the lacerated lumbrical muscle. The median nerve was under moderate compression at the wrist, and the digital nerves were compressed as they entered the finger. A piece of glass was removed from the deep muscle layer in the palm. A flexor tendon repair was possible by suturing the tendon distally at the metacarpophalangeal joint level and lengthening the flexor profundus at the base of the palm. A 14 mm defect occurred in the common digital nerve to the long and ring fingers after the nerve had been mobilized and the proximal neuroma and distal fibroma had been cut back so that good fascicles were present. This defect was readily made up by mobilizing the median nerve at the wrist, by mobilizing the digital nerves in the palm, and by flexing the wrist 30 degrees and the fingers 60 degrees. The hand was immobilized for four weeks in a dorsal plaster splint that extended above the elbow. During this period of 28 days, nerve regeneration progressed rapidly, as was indicated by an advancing percussion test through almost 40 mm. At six weeks after the delayed repair, the child had 50 per cent finger flexion and extension and sufficient improvement in sensation to eliminate the trophic stimulus. *Nerve grafting was unnecessary.* Four years after the delayed repair, the child could flex the fingertip to the distal palm crease and she demonstrated normal sweating, normal fingerprints, 4 mm two-point discrimination similar to the adjacent digits, and no atrophy or trophic change. A moderate degree of peritendinous adhesion occurred, limiting hyperextension. Tenolysis may be necessary as rapid growth occurs.

The child's problem indicates that a pain syndrome requires detailed analysis in order to determine if pain is due to persistent foreign body in the hand, tethering or adherence of injured nerves to damaged tendons, vascular insufficiency, or abnormal afferent stimuli coming from one or all of these unphysiologic conditions. If both digital arteries are lacerated and not repaired, axon regeneration will be hindered and pain from any source will be prolonged. Gelberman et al. (1978) demonstrated that when both digital vessels were involved and when both digital nerves were lacerated, the quality of sensory recovery after nerve suture was less satisfactory than when two digital nerves were lacerated and one digital vessel was intact. There is a significant relationship between nerve trauma, vascular damage, and pain.

Case 6. Incomplete Nerve Laceration in the Palm

A 38-year-old woman received a vegetable knife injury of the palm which resulted in flexion deformity of the fingers, tenosynovitis, and adherence of digital nerves to the flexor tendons. Laceration of the common digital nerve supplying the long and ring fingers had occurred at the time of the original injury and necessitated mobilization of the nerves, resection of the fibrotic segments, and suture. After the operation, pain lessened but stiffness persisted. Collagen fibrosis and adhesions caused pain. Part-time elevation, external splinting (both day and night), an active exercise program, desensitization of the hand as described by Curtis and Dellon in Chapter 47, application of paraffin to increase temperature, elimination of nicotine, avoidance of repetitive trauma, and use of salicylates resulted in gradual improvement. Elevation may decrease capillary flow and distal perfusion and should be intermittent, not constant.

Items that affect diminution of pain and improved range of motion are: a) lessening of edema; b) gradual stretch and realignment of collagen, using Velcro straps and night splints; c) active assistive exercise hourly; d) avoidance of excessive heat or cold; e) intermittent elimination of pain by anesthetic blocks; f) anti-inflammatory medications; g) adequate sleep and avoidance of anxiety to lower the level of pain and hasten the speed of recovery; and h) increase in capillary perfusion distally by multiple methods.

The discussion of the *spectrum of pain syndromes* continues with emphasis on variations of the severity of the injury involving certain peripheral nerves frequently damaged during trauma or operative procedures. The superficial radial nerve is particularly affected by incisions and trauma to the dorsum of the wrist and the hand.

Case 7

A 26-year-old woman was treated for stenosing synovitis of the abductor pollicis longus and extensor pollicis brevis by release of the annular ligament. Postoperatively she noted hypesthesia in the region of the superficial radial nerve supply to the thumb and to the index finger. The cause of this was nontraumatic mobilization of the nerve and careful isolation of the nerve by placement of a flexible rubber dam around the nerve with non-contact by a rigid retractor. This minimal handling can cause temporary hypesthesia. As the force of retraction increases, the extent of hypesthesia is intensified and prolonged. When the nerve was tapped at the site of partial interruption of conduction, the test was moderately positive, and profound hypesthesia was not present. Gradual improvement occurred during the next several months, and after a year sensation was normal. This mild temporary sensory change is usually not painful and is noted only when the patient touches or rubs the area of involvement.

This patient demonstrated *moderate involvement of the superficial radial nerve*, caused either by a suture being placed around the nerve during wound closure or by prolonged retraction or compression of the nerve. After the initial operative procedure had been completed, anesthesia existed in the zone innervated by the superficial radial nerve, and the question of whether or not a complete laceration existed was determined by a period of observation of three months. If the nerve had been traumatized but not lacerated or constricted, then sensation would improve. If a painful sensation persisted, nerve block with local anesthetic should be done proximal to the point of trauma. If complete anesthesia occurred with the nerve block, and if partial sensory recovery occurred after the block wore off, then conduction was probably present and the nerve injury was only partial. If the superficial radial nerve continued to be hypersensitive at the site of operation or trauma and if no improvement occurred after several weeks, then exploration of the nerve was indicated. The sensory conduction study of afferent impulses was also helpful in determining whether the nerve was partially or completely lacerated.

Complete laceration of one or more branches of the superficial radial nerve may occur when a tenosynovectomy is being performed or at the time that a direct laceration of the extensor pollicis longus tendon occurs. Anesthesia and dysesthesia persist in the area of nerve trauma, and a percussion test results in dysesthesia. Pain persists without evidence of improvement. Exploration of this nerve usually demonstrates a laceration with minimal nerve gap which allows end-to-end suture rather than resection. Although resection does not diminish the local "hot spot" in many instances, hypesthesia and anesthesia which are unpleasant persist for many months or even years and pain is not always relieved sufficiently to justify the resection. A successful treatment in many instances is to mobilize the nerve, resect the neuroma and fibroma, and attempt an end-to-end suture. A gap of 2 or 3 cm can be made up by dorsiflexing the wrist and extending the thumb. This procedure has been done by the author several times, and as long as a year after the original injury, with elimination of pain and eventual restoration of adequate sensation. If a gap in the nerve measures 3 or 4 cm and if the patient is in an age group where immobilization for more than three weeks is not desired, a nerve graft is performed. An alternative method of treatment is to isolate all of the proximal fibrotic ends of nerves and use a bipolar cautery to obliterate conduction proximally and place the proximal nerve endings in muscle tissue so that tethering will not occur. Epineurium is sutured over the cauterized axonplasm with 9–0 suture (Goldner, 1977).

Case 8

A 50-year-old man had received a *laceration of the superficial radial nerve* in three locations on the wrist and at the base of the thumb. Two prior efforts had been made to resect the nerves, to ligate them, and to eliminate skin hypersensitivity. Because of the failure of prior resections, prior folding back of the ends of the nerves into muscle, and prior coagulation, the nerve endings were identified and a sural nerve graft of 4 cm was done, gathering the proximal major nerves and the distal endings into the graft. A thin sheet of silicone was sutured over the fibrous tissues on which the nerve was placed and Gelfilm was wrapped around the suture lines to protect the nerve from the overlying skin. Eight months later, the hypersensitivity had diminished 70 per cent and sensation had improved about 30 per cent. Pain was diminished significantly. An external plastic covering was used to avoid unnecessary stimulation to the hand (Goldner, 1977).

Case 9. Laceration of the Ulnar Nerve in the Distal Forearm

A 40-year-old male received a laceration of the ulnar aspect of the forearm 4 cm proximal to the pisiform bone. At examination of the patient six weeks after the injury had occurred and after the initial surgeon had ligated the ulnar artery and repaired the ulnar nerve during the primary procedure, the patient continued to have pain, paresthesias, dysesthesias, and anesthesia. Percussion at the site of the laceration demonstrated exquisite tenderness. The digits showed lack of sweating, the entire hand was cool, and vascular compression test of the median and ulnar artery showed no flow in the ulnar artery. Cooling of the hand increased the severity of pain, and warm-up time was extremely slow.

The findings were in keeping with vasospasm, vascular insufficiency on the ulnar side of the hand, and a nonphysiologic nerve repair. The original site of injury was operated upon and the ulnar nerve showed a large neuroma which was not conducting action potentials at any site. The neuroma was hard and the nerve had the appearance of having been repaired through an area of fibrosis rather than through healing axons. The neuroma and fibroma were resected, and a defect of approximately 3 cm resulted. The nerve was mobilized proximally for 9 cm and distally into the hand. Anterior transfer to obtain an end-to-end suture with 7–0 nylon was unnecessary. Anterior transfer would have been done if adequate apposition of the nerve endings had not been possible. The dorsal sensory branch was isolated and sutured separately, as this had not been repaired at the initial primary suture. Nerve graft was unnecessary at either site (Goldner, 1958–1968; Goldner, 1968–1974; Goldner et al., 1975).

The ulnar artery was adherent to a large mass of fibrous tissue both proximally and distally. End-to-end repair would have been possible, but in view of the author's past experience with patients with ulnar artery thrombosis in whom arterial grafts and repairs have not been particularly successful this was not done (Goldner and Eguro, 1973). Radial artery flow was strong when vasospasm did not exist. Mobilization of the ulnar ends of the artery and placement away from the nerve suture was performed, and this may have had some effect on diminishing vasospasm and eliminating local pain. Blood vessels are painful when manipulated, and when irritated or tethered may cause adjacent vasospasm (Goldner, 1975).

Immediately after the operative procedure was completed, the burning pain in the hand was absent, anesthesia persisted, and the entire hand was warmer, indicating that vasospasm was less and that motor power was the same. As nerve regeneration occurred, the dysesthesias increased slightly but were maintained at a minimum by a lightweight plastic covering over the site of suture, an active exercise program, a low blood level of anti-inflammatory medication, avoidance of sleep deprivation, prevention of cooling, elimination of smoking, and diminution of anxiety. Three years later the patient has regained sweating and fingerprints, has two-point discrimination of 7 mm, and the hypothenar and first dorsal interosseous muscles have 40 per cent of normal strength. Clawing has been eliminated, cold tolerance is satisfactory, and pain is not a problem.

This patient demonstrated the pain syndrome that results from trauma, unphysiologic nerve repair, vascular insufficiency, excessive fibrosis, and internal and external vasoregulatory conditions causing vasospasm. A combination of all these factors results in a high level of pain. Elimination of primary nerve irritation, diminution of fibrosis, improvement of vascular flow, and decreased anxiety or depression result in a diminution of pain to a level of tolerance.

Case 10. Pain Oriented Problem Associated with Bilateral Thumb Amputations Aggravated by Social and Financial Problems

A 45-year-old male was examined four years after his right thumb had been amputated at the level of the metacarpophalangeal joint as a result of an avulsion injury. Pain persisted, severe hypersensitivity was present, and the index finger, which had not been involved in the accident, showed diminished sensation and dryness. The long finger was the site of burning and aching and the entire hand became painful.

The volar aspect of the wrist was painful to percussion, the phantom thumb pain was aggravated by tapping the median nerve, and the radiation into the index and long fingers occurred consistently. Volar flexion of the wrist aggravated pain in the thumb, index, and long fingers, and dorsiflexion of the wrist caused pain in the same digits. A tourniquet was applied to the arm and elevated to 60 mm Hg, which resulted in venous congestion and a rapid increase in pain. Without the tourniquet, sensory conduction was prolonged as was motor conduction across the wrist. Abnormal action potentials were present in the opponens and abductor muscles consistent with median nerve compression.

Phantom sensation occurs in every adult who has an amputation. The sensation may persist for weeks or months and changes as time passes. The phantom sensation of the missing part migrates proximally and as it approaches the amputation stump, pain diminishes. This is probably due to conditioning and passage of time. Patients may recall quickly and vividly the position of the amputated part at the time of an accident or prior to amputation for a neoplasm. This image eventually fades, but may not be lost permanently (Goldner, 1972). Phantom pain described as pathologic has been noted in 5 per cent of the patients attending the Duke Orthopaedic Amputation Clinics during the past 25 years. The duration of preamputation pain, the patient's emotional profile, and the persistence of fibrosis around the nerve endings or inadequate skin covering the nerves are factors that may cause or aggravate continuation of the pain. Relief of phantom pain has been accomplished by stump revision, resection of fibrotic and adherent nerve endings, relief of abnormal skin tension, improvement of peripheral blood flow, diminution of vasospasm, and elimination or improvement of emotional depression. A transcutaneous nerve stimulator has diminished pain in certain patients (Goldner and Hendrix, 1977), and microelectrode implants placed directly on peripheral nerves well above the site of the amputation have diminished phantom pain and phantom sensation and improved the patient's capability of wearing one or more prostheses (Goldner, Bright, and Nashold, 1975, Jeans, 1975).

The patient with the thumb amputation being discussed here was operated upon both at the wrist and in the hand. The median nerve was found to be severely compressed, the epineurium was constricting the fascicles, and an hourglass deformity had occurred. Epineurial splitting was necessary, and fascicular dissection was done. Fascicular dissection is performed only if there is profound motor loss and dysesthesias or profound sensory disturbance prior to the procedure. Those patients who have satisfactory motor function who do not have severe hypesthesia but only paresthesias should have the epineurium split but should not have the fascicular dissection. The latter causes profound delay in sensory recovery and delay in motor recovery (Goldner, 1972, 1977).

This patient had moderate relief of pain after the median nerve dissection and significant relief after a transcutaneous stimulator was applied. He has used this stimulator now on a day-to-day basis as many as four hours during the day and at night to aid in maintaining a satisfactory sleep pattern. He works as a heavy equipment operator and does his job without difficulty. Certain pharmacologic agents have been helpful in diminishing his pain and allowing him to maintain emotional stability. These are Dilantin, Prolixin, Elavil, and Sinequan. Occasionally, when the pain pattern becomes severe, either from local trauma or emotional disturbance, a peripheral block of the median nerve using a long-acting anesthetic will provide the patient with several hours of relief and allow him to regain his physical and emotional stability so that he readjusts to his chronic pain problem. *Restoration of sleep pattern is important.*

The patient's opposite thumb, which had been amputated at the level of the proximal interphalangeal joint, was painful because of adherence of the digital nerves to the distal end of the proximal phalanx. This is a frequent finding after traumatic amputation and repair by a surgeon who is unnecessarily concerned that proximal resection of the digital nerve will result in loss of sensation to the amputation stump. Our experience has demonstrated that a digital nerve can be cut back at least 1 cm from the amputation stump without significantly affecting the sensation of the skin flaps over the stump. Proximal transposition of the neuroma and nerve of more than 2 cm affects sensation of the overlying skin. Dissection of both digital nerves was done, the proximal ends were coagulated with bipolar cautery, the epineurium was sutured over the axons, the articular surface and a portion of the condyles were removed from the phalanx, and closure of the skin without tension was performed. The "hot spots" and the unpleasant pain sensations were eliminated, and within six months the amputation stump was completely painless (Goldner and Fisher, 1972).

PAIN PROBLEMS — DIFFERENTIAL DIAGNOSIS

Pain problems can be categorized as: a) pure nerve pain, b) pain associated with nerve and vascular insufficiency, or c) pain related to numerous local alterations, such as inadequate skin coverage, fibrosis, bone pressure, tendon irritation, and collagen fibrosis. Also, the alterations that occur in central pain connections are recognized as a part of the persistent chronic pain syndrome. Patient examples provide a method of investigating the types of pain using the syndromes and relating the onset to history and known events, and provide a way of analyzing the different forms of treatment. This information may result in lessening the severity of or eliminating a pain syndrome. The more complex the problem, the more complex is the treatment. A multifactorial approach is necessary. Patients to be presented make up part of the author's experience with these problems; these cases emphasize the necessity of avoiding a simplistic approach, whether it be psychological, operative, pharmacologic, or that of peripheral nerve blockade with local anesthetic.

Case 11. Forearm Nerve and Artery Laceration with Persistent Pain

A 35-year-old male received a laceration of the forearm that included the radial artery and the median nerve. Primary treatment consisted of ligation of the radial artery and repair of the median nerve. Observations during the next year showed a persistent area of local pain at the site of the laceration, a nonconsistent regeneration pattern, and development of dysesthesia and hypesthesia. Cold tolerance was low and sweating was absent. The attending surgeon performed a second operative procedure approximately six months after the initial injury. Neurolysis was done, and the neuroma in continuity was described as being hard and adherent, and would not conduct gross electrical stimulation. Neurolysis of a previous sutured primary nerve laceration is usually not successful in improving conduction. The nerve that does not show an orderly progression of regeneration after primary repair should be resutured within three to six months. Evoked potential readings at the time of the second operation may be helpful. If evoked potentials are absent, resuture is mandatory. If pain is severe, resuture is indicated.

TREATMENT.   The patient was seen for examination one and one half years after the initial injury and after two operations had been performed. Pain, both day and night, was the major complaint. Cold intolerance was noted, and the pain interfered with the patient's sleep pattern. The percussion test was strongly positive at the site of injury but was not present more than a centimeter distal to the site of injury, indicating that nerve regeneration had not occurred. Sweating was absent, the fingerprints were smooth, and the existing motor power of the intrinsic muscle of the thumb was determined, by blockade of the ulnar nerve at the elbow, to be related to an anomalous innervation pattern (Goldner and Jones, 1966). Vascular insufficiency was evident although the ulnar artery was carrying sufficient blood to nourish the hand even though the radial artery had been ligated.

Sympathetic blockade did diminish cold intolerance moderately, but did not eliminate the pain associated with the nerve lesion. Sympathectomy will not relieve the pain associated with a nonphysiologic nerve suture. A dorsal column stimulator may diminish the pain but will not solve the local problem, nor will a microelectrode implant on the nerve improve nerve regeneration, even though the severity of pain may be diminished moderately (Goldner and Bright, 1979).

A year and a half after the initial injury the site of nerve injury was exposed, and the median nerve was mobilized at the wrist, in the forearm, and at the elbow. The involved area of the nerve was resected and a 4-cm defect was created. The nerve ends were brought together with relative ease by flexing the wrist 30 degrees, flexing the elbow 90 degrees, and bringing the arm to the side. Nerve grafting is not necessary if extension is carried out slowly after four weeks of healing. The inherent elasticity of the nerve allows up to 15 per cent stretch of the total length of the nerve (Goldner, 1978).

Postoperatively, the patient was free of burning pain and dysesthesia, or uncomfortable sensation, in the hand, and the digits were somewhat warmer due to diminution of vasospasm. Motor power to the fingers and in the intrinsic muscles of the thumb was not altered. The goal was relief of pain and recovery of protective sensation, as motor power provided by the anomalous innervation from the ulnar nerve carrying fibers from the median nerve (the Martin-Gruber anastomosis [Goldner and Jones, 1969]) provided adequate intrinsic function for pinch and grasp. Three months after the operation, a percussion test over the site of the suture caused minimal discomfort rather than the excessive pain and paresthesias that had occurred preoperatively. Percussion from distal to proximal showed advancement of regeneration at a rate of 1 mm per day. The postoperative percussion test was not accompanied by apprehension and generalized sweating as was the preoperative test. The patient would smile while the original pain pattern was discussed. and he tolerated manipulation of the forearm and the hand without apprehension. Postoperative diagnostic tests such as the cooling test, measurement of blood flow, and thermogram readings all showed diminished vasospasm, improved peripheral blood flow, improved cold tolerance, and diminished pain.

DIFFERENTIAL DIAGNOSIS. Pain syndrome aggravated by median nerve compression or trauma at the wrist, also pain associated with sympathetic dystrophy or a *causalgic* syndrome.

Case 12. Median Nerve Compression due to Chronic Tenosynovitis, Reactive Fibrosis After Prior Nerve Decompression

The patient was a 45-year-old woman, moderately obese and with thick fingers and tight compartments. She had developed a spontaneous median nerve compression syndrome due to obesity. Her attending surgeon had released the volar retinacular ligament without resecting the hypertrophied synovium around the flexores digitorum profundi. Intrinsic atrophy of the thumb, which had been described preoperatively, persisted as did hypesthesia and dysesthesia. Several months after the initial decompression the patient showed no evidence of motor recovery or sensory recovery and pain was increasing.

TREATMENT. At the time the median nerve was reoperated upon our findings were those of persistent perineural fibrosis, absence of motor fiber conduction (tested by proximal electrical stimulation), and persistent tenosynovitis of the flexor tendons. Treatment included splitting of the epineurium under 4 × magnification, funicular dissection of the major segments of the nerve, and fascicular dissection of the motor segment including release of the fascia around the motor branch of the median nerve. A subtotal tenosynovectomy of the flexor tendons was accomplished and a small piece of Surgicel was placed around the split nerve. Postoperatively, pain and sensation were diminished and sweating was absent. In patients with severe compression or entrapment this kind of dissection usually results in temporary loss of painful sensations, but preoperative sensory and motor deficiencies continue as expected until regeneration occurs. The patient was examined one and a half years after the nerve dissection and decompression and showed recovery of sweating, two-point discrimination of 5 mm, recovery of the intrinsic muscles of the thumb, and no pain.

I have treated several other patients with profound *pain syndromes associated with compression neuropathy* in which the nerve had not been lacerated, but in which the fascicles were not conducting. These nerves will show improved conduction after epineurial splitting and fascicular neurolysis. *This kind of dissection should not be done, however, if motor power is present and the sensory disturbance is minimal.* A median nerve that is treated for compression symptoms only does not require fascicular dissection. Furthermore, a nerve that has been previously lacerated and repaired which is not conducting well will not respond to fascicular dissection in a favorable way. Improvement, if any, after the neurolysis may be diminution of external compression associated with fibrosis around the nerve, rather than from improving conductibility by diminishing intraneural fibrosis (Goldner, 1958–1978).

Case 13. Partial Laceration of Median Nerve at Wrist, Treated by Primary Repair and Subsequent Development of Large, Painful Neuroma

A 35-year-old woman received a laceration of the wrist on a piece of broken glass, which incised the palmaris longus muscle and the sensory components of the median nerve. The attending surgeon attempted primary repair. Several months later, the patient had a large, proliferating, painful neuroma, dysesthesia, and paresthesia over the median nerve distribution and normal thumb intrinsic muscles that were proven by nerve block to be innervated by fibers carried in the median nerve (Goldner and Jones, 1969).

TREATMENT. The choices of treatment were resection of the fibrous neuroma and separation of the motor segments followed by either nerve grafting or resuture. The sensory neuroma was resected using 3.5 × magnification, the motor fibers were identified by electrical stimulation, and fascicular suture was done without nerve grafting. The defect measured approximately 2 cm. The sensory components were brought together as an epineural suture, and the motor segment made a "U" shaped turn at this point. Postoperatively, the painful mass at the wrist was eliminated, hypersensitivity was diminished, and the patient's anxiety and depression lessened. During the following year, the patient's hand showed good evidence of sensory regeneration and a return of sweating, and at the end of the three years 6 mm two-point discrimination was present. Although there was a noticeable difference in sensation between the index and the little fingers, the recovery was excellent. The patient's social situation, her economic problems, and other factors which were also affecting her pain syndrome, such as smoking, caused measurable vasoconstriction. The patient wears a plastic cup held on with a Velcro strap over the neuroma and avoids bumping the wrist (Goldner, 1968–1974).

Case 14. Laceration of the Median Nerve (Fig. 8–1)

A 16-year-old male received a laceration of the volar aspect of the wrist by a metal object. *Primary repair* was done by the attending surgeon but the carpal ligament was not released. Sensory and motor recovery did not occur, and the surgeon attempted a *second repair*. Review of the histologic sections from that operation showed incomplete resection, both proximally and distally. The surgeon was misled as to the success of the initial operative procedure because the abductor pollicis brevis was functioning. However, local injection of the median nerve proximal to the site of laceration resulted in elimination of pain in both the site of laceration and the fingers, but did not eliminate intrinsic motor function of the abductor pollicis brevis. Local anesthetic block of the ulnar nerve at the elbow level did not weaken the abductor pollicis brevis, but when the injection was done at the wrist level, the abductor pollicis was paralyzed (Goldner and Jones, 1969).

TREATMENT.   At a later date, during the course of regeneration, when the median nerve was injected just proximal to the site of laceration the abductor pollicis was not paralyzed, but when the median nerve was injected proximal to the elbow joint, the abductor muscle was paralyzed. This combination of injections indicated that the crossover was from the median nerve in the upper forearm to the ulnar nerve in the mid forearm and to the intrinsics of the thumb distal to the median nerve laceration (median nerve crossover to ulnar nerve and innervate median nerve muscle mass).

At the time of the *third operation*, on the median nerve, the neuroma was isolated and the nerve was mobilized both into the hand and proximally to the level of the pronator. A 3 cm defect was created by resection of the neuroma, and an end-to-end suture was done with 7–0 and 8–0 suture without tension by flexing the wrist 40 degrees (1 cm), flexing the elbow 90 degrees (2 cm), and placing the arm at the side (1 cm). Once the suture was completed, the inherent elasticity of the nerve segments allowed the wrist to be extended to 30 degrees before slight tension occurred on the suture line. A posterior plaster splint was used for four weeks, and gradual extension of the wrist and elbow was allowed during the next two months (Goldner, 1978).

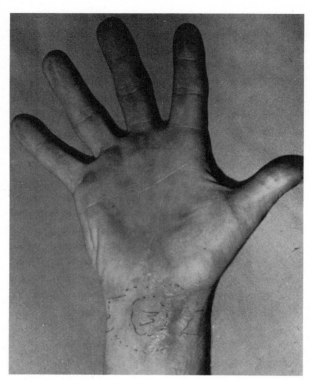

Figure 8–1 This hand of a 16-year-old male received a laceration of the *median* nerve at the wrist two years prior to the initial assessment for a chronic pain syndrome. Two efforts at nerve repair had been done but sensory regeneration had not occurred. The patient had paresthesias, dysesthesia, and hyperesthesia in the hand but no recovery of sweating, fingerprints or light touch. Motor power of the thumb intrinsic muscles was good because of an anomalous innervation pattern (Martin-Gruber crossover) from the adjacent ulnar nerve. A palpable mass on the volar aspect of the wrist was exquisitely tender to touch and interfered with his attempts at work. Diagnostic studies included median and ulnar nerve blocks, electrical testing, cold tolerance tests, and thermogram. Treatment required mobilization of the median nerve from the hand to the upper arm, resection of the proximal neuroma and distal fibroma to good fascicles, and an end-to-end epineurial suture with 6–0 and 7–0 nylon suture. Sensory regeneration was relatively rapid and within 18 months the patient regained sweating, fingerprints, improved nail growth, increased cold tolerance, and relief of the hyperesthesia and paresthesias. The acute pain at the wrist was eliminated. Thus, even after two years, pain from inappropriate axon regeneration can be improved by a physiologic nerve suture. Sympathectomy would not eliminate this burning pain and would not result in improved regeneration. Transcutaneous stimulation diminished the hypersensitivity only about 10 per cent.

Six months after the repair, a positive percussion test and stroking test at the fingertip level were present, indicating that regeneration had occurred at approximately 1 mm a day. The patient could recognize heat and cold and had protective sensation within six months. At the end of two and a half years, he demonstrated two-point discrimination of 8 mm, even though the definitive repair was not done until more than a year after the initial injury. Pain was eliminated immediately after the definitive repair, the painful nodule at the wrist did not recur, and motor function was intact. *A nonphysiologic primary or delayed nerve repair will result in pain at the site of nerve repair and dysesthesias distally.* Nerve repair without adequate axon penetration of the distal segment will result in a painful neuroma in continuity with continued proliferation locally and persistent severe pain. Anomalous innervation patterns of motor segments of the median or ulnar nerve must be recognized, as they can be misleading in determining the proper course of management of a peripheral nerve injury and pain syndrome.

DIFFERENTIAL DIAGNOSIS. Pain syndromes in the hand simulating nerve compression caused by arterial emboli.

Case 15

A 36-year-old male complained of intermittent sensations of tingling, burning, and numbness in the hand. Examination showed that the radial and ulnar pulses were present, and these pulsations were frequently diminished. When the extremity was elevated for a few minutes, the patient complained of paresthesias and dysesthesias. Roentgen examination of the clavicle showed a congenital pseudarthrosis. Arteriography demonstrated alteration of the subclavian artery at the level of the bony change. The intermittent emboli resulting from this damage to the intima caused the tingling and color change in the hand and the coolness and nerve ischemia associated with vascular ischemia. Treatment required resection of the center of the clavicle, resection of the damaged segment of artery, and replacement by a Dacron graft. The patient's pain complaints were eliminated.

ANALYSIS AND COMPARISON OF PAIN TYPES

Analyzing and comparing the pain caused by different conditions will assist in determining the actual diagnosis. Certain examples deserve discussion:

Compression of the sciatic nerve caused by a dislocated femoral head causes contusion or compression of the nerve and partial ischemia of the nerve as a result of compression of the artery within the nerve, but there is no major vascular insufficiency of the extremity. Pain is primarily neural in origin, with secondary vasospasm resulting from pain.

A direct contusion of the ulnar nerve at the elbow results in immediate momentary hyperesthesia and dysesthesia without a major ischemic component other than that which affects the vasoregulatory system.

A muscle compartment syndrome, such as of the anterior compartment of the leg, causes muscle ischemia due to diminished capillary perfusion. The compartment pressure exceeds the capillary closing pressure, and pain results. Nerve function may be affected primarily or secondarily (Porter, 1977).

A tourniquet applied above the elbow and elevated to a pressure of 300 mm Hg causes loss of motor function in the forearm and hand and loss of sensation after motor weakness occurs (30 to 40 minutes). The patient notices moderate paresthesias in the hand and a heavy, tight compressive feeling around the arm and the forearm. Nerve compression over a wide area causes less burning sensation than does localized nerve compression involving a short segment of the nerve.

Stretch injuries of the cervical roots and segments of the brachial plexus causes neck pain, dysesthesia in the proximal segments of the extremity, and anesthesia distally. If the lesion is complete, motor and sensory regeneration will not be evident. Pain may be severe if the roots are avulsed or may be moderate if the cords or peripheral nerves are damaged. If the lesion is irreparable and amputation is done above the elbow, the patient may continue to have phantom pain for years. This sensation may recur intermittently. Certain mechanical manipulations, such as depression of the shoulder and tilting of the head, aggravate the phantom pain and the phantom sensation. Also, percussion of the major nerves in the supraclavicular area has caused phantom paresthesias in the forearm and hand. The affected patient noted that wrapping the stump firmly and applying the artificial limb socket at night improved his sleep and decreased his phantom pain. The phantom forearm and hand are located in the "mid forearm region." The patient has not noted regression of the phantom proximally, and, in my experience, unless the phantom moves up to the end of the stump, the phantom pain will persist along with the phantom sensation.

THE GRADATIONS OF PAIN

The clinical syndrome as it affects a particular patient is described and the gradation of severity is determined. Minimal treatment may improve a mild pain syndrome, whereas maximum treatment may be necessary for a severe syndrome. Varying shades of pain do occur. Individuals tolerate pain in different ways. The patient's physical condition, the environment, and the individual's emotional makeup affect the severity of pain. The assessment must be historical and biographical, must include physical examination, and must utilize certain mechanical modalities for diagnosis. Patients with chronic upper or lower extremity pain may be classified into five categories:

1. *The pain is agonizing and intolerable,* results in severe loss of sleep and loss of appetite, and is unaffected by environmental changes. Examples of this would be kidney colic and the pain associated with pancreatitis, acute gallbladder attack, and interspace infection of the spine.
2. *The patient with chronic pain syndromes* that are partially alleviated by rest but aggravated by physical activity or by emotional stress. These patients obtain reasonable relief with moderate doses of pain and anti-inflammatory medications but do not require opiates. Examples are individuals with chronic low back pain without radiculopathy, cervical intervertebral disc disease with minimal nerve root irritation, median nerve compression at the wrist, and intermittent motor and sensory ulnar neuropathy at the elbow.
3. *Patient with an intermittent pain syndrome* related to environmental changes, emotional stress, or irritation of a sensitive point, such as a digital neuroma. The residual changes from a sympathetic dystrophy, the persistent chronic pain from a resolving compartment syndrome, or the pain resulting from arthrofibrosis of the joint may require anti-inflammatory medications, external splinting or protection, and medications to assist in a good sleep pattern.
4. *Certain patients with chronic, severe,* persistent pain require opiates and/or special medications such as Dilantin, Elavil, Prolixin or other medications that have a central effect on the pain centers. For example, patients with cancer may require Dilaudid, Codeine, Demerol, or morphine, and to this are added the salicylates or other anti-inflammatory medications.
5. *Patients with intermittent nerve root irritation* or vascular insufficiency of the

extremity or a combination of both may have moderate episodes of acute or chronic pain syndromes that may be affected by limitation of activity, a transcutaneous stimulator, and/or certain medications (Goldner and Hendrix, 1977).

PLANNING TREATMENT PROGRAMS FOR PATIENTS WITH CHRONIC PAIN SYNDROMES

The physician should consider the severity of the pain syndrome and the primary diagnosis in prescribing medications and other forms of treatment.

1. Pain medication given primarily for relief of acute pain complaints for a patient who does not have any basic emotional component to his or her pain. Postoperative pain or post-traumatic pain are in this category.
2. Medications prescribed to assist the patient in sleeping.
3. Medications prescribed to diminish pain in order to allow the patient to maintain a reasonable appetite.
4. Medications to assist the patient in performing daily activities that require concentration, reading, writing, and planning.
5. Those patients who have persistent aching and pain associated with bending, twisting, walking, and standing need a rest program and external applications of heat or immobilization and possibly anti-inflammatory medications but do not require pain medication.
6. Many patients with pain syndromes are readily managed by transcutaneous stimulator, protection of sensitive points by plastic covers or caps, and protection of the extremity from excess cold or heat. Physical therapy programs aid the patient in carrying out active joint muscle and tendon stretching, and provide the patient with a self-motivating program as well as the reinforcement and confidence that comes with the presence of another individual who is touching and soothing him.

ANALYSIS OF PAIN COMPLAINTS

The physician must not only assess the severity of the patient's complaints but also attempt to determine the specific tissues involved. *Sensory* and *motor* assessment of the extremity, determination of the presence or absence of sweating, recording the skin temperature, testing two-point discrimination, and recording of the strength of grip and pinch will give important information about the lesions affecting peripheral nerves. A *sensory* nerve is assessed by attempting to localize a specific point of *hypersensitivity* (a trigger area or sensitive spot) where a compression lesion or irritative lesion exists. Tension on the nerve can be applied by flexing or extending a joint proximal or distal to the nerve. Median *nerve compression* at the wrist is affected by wrist flexion or extension. A compression lesion at the elbow involving the ulnar nerve may be affected by acute elbow flexion. Forcible eversion and dorsiflexion of the foot may irritate a compressed posterior tibial nerve where the nerve is affected by the abductor hallucis muscle.

Muscle strength is determined by clinical examination, which includes recording the strength of grip and pinch, and by individual muscle testing. Extreme care may be taken in testing individual muscles that affect the distal, proximal, and metacarpophalangeal joints of the hand and the articulations of the wrist. Substitution patterns must be avoided while muscle testing is performed. The examiner must determine if the patient is withholding strength, or whether the lack of strength is associated with fear, anxiety, or emotional disturbances.

Electrical studies using needle electrodes placed into individual muscles are valuable in determining alterations of the muscle belly. Determination of the speed of *motor and sensory conduction* is also helpful in localizing compressive lesions or in separating myopathy from neuropathy. This is particularly helpful in providing information about the thoracic outlet syndrome (Clippinger, Goldner, and Roberts, 1962).

Vascular assessment of the upper and lower extremities includes such clinical tests as the Allen compression test at the wrist, pulse volume recordings in the hand and foot, Doppler determination of blood flow in small and large peripheral vessels, and recording of skin temperatures. Doppler pressure studies are done by listening to the flow in major arteries, both with and without proximal compression of the blood pressure cuff at determined pressure levels. When major arterial circulation is diminished, the sound will be obliterated at a much lower pressure than that which occurs in an extremity with normal vascular flow. These readings supplement those obtained from plethysmography (Goldner and Bright, 1979).

A patient with subacute or chronic thrombosis of the ulnar artery will show no flow through the ulnar artery at the wrist when the radial and ulnar artery compression test is done. Patients with no flow through the ulnar artery may have an adequate collateral circulation from the deep palmar arch, but in spite of this tend to show cold intolerance and paresthesias in the digits on the ulnar side of the hand when external temperature decreases (Eguro and Goldner, 1972).

Muscle testing will determine weakness that results from vascular ischemia or from nerve injury or compression. A compartment syndrome is accompanied by moderate or severe pain and results from combined tissue injury of muscle and nerve caused by increased compartment pressure as a result of the nonelastic external surrounding fascia confining the soft tissues within the closed space. The muscle is affected by hypoxia and acidosis and the increased capillary closing pressure is greater than that which allows perfusion of tissue to occur. Nerve damage and muscle necrosis result (Goldner, 1975).

Case 16. Mild Compartment Syndrome in Forearm

A 25-year-old male complained of pain in the forearms, painful, tight hands, and tingling of all the fingers after doing heavy work. The symptoms persisted intermittently for a few days after the physical effort and then gradually subsided. This pattern had been present for about three years with no evidence of motor weakness, no persistent peripheral nerve alterations, and no indication of a specific muscle or joint disease.

On palpation the forearm muscles were hard and firm, and repetitive flexion and extension of the fingers combined with repetitive lifting during a short period of time caused pain in the forearms and hands. Rest provided partial relief. Pressure studies with the Wick catheter demonstrated increased pressure in the compartment containing the flexor carpi radialis, the flexor superficialis, and the flexor digitorum profundus muscles. The condition gradually improved as the patient avoided excess physical activity and maintained activities of the hands and forearms on a day-to-day basis.

A similar syndrome is noted in runners with tight anterior compartment fascia of the lower extremities. This same pathologic elevation of compartment pressure accounts for unexplained onset of anterior tibial muscle necrosis and unexplained muscle or nerve alterations associated with trauma and increased compartment pressure (Matsen, 1979; Mavor, 1956).

I have observed certain patients with tight forearm compartments who have had an operation on the hand and wrist. Postoperatively, they evidence hand pain, nerve compression, and limited flexion of the fingers. Release of the forearm fascia to the elbow has resulted in immediate dramatic relief. The acute postoperative pain in these patients results in a differential diagnosis of a) tourniquet palsy, b) direct trauma to the nerve during the operative procedure, c) postoperative hematoma, and d) compartment pressure from intracellular edema and hematoma. The pain is severe and the treatment is exacting (Goldner, 1975).

The same pattern of pathologic events occurs in the patient who, after a high tibial osteotomy or a high tibial fracture, complains of severe pain and burning in the leg and foot and who develops weakness of dorsiflexion within a few hours after the operation or injury. The differential diagnosis is one of peroneal nerve compression or anterior compartment compression. Pain is usually severe for an hour or less and may cease if the compression is primarily causing vascular insufficiency. However, if persistent median or posterior tibial nerve compression occurs, then burning pain and loss of sensation will persist for several hours or even days.

Postoperative Compartment Compression Pain

Case 17

A 22-year-old male demonstrated persistent paralysis of the interosseous and adductor pollicis muscles after a high ulnar nerve laceration. Multiple tendon transfers were performed in order to replace the intrinsic muscles of the fingers and thumb. The tourniquet was released before wound closure. The muscle bellies of the flexor superficialis extended down to the wrist area and into the carpal canal. Postoperatively, the patient complained of dysesthesias in all the fingers and deep aching tightness in the forearm and could not actively extend the fingers because of pain; passive extension of the fingers caused severe pain. The condition did not improve during a 24 hour period of observation during which the dressings were split, and examination showed the large pulses to be palpable and capillary refill to be satisfactory. However, because of the persistent subjective complaints — pain on attempted extension of the fingers and tightness of the lower and mid forearm — he was taken back to the operating room. Local anesthesia was selected so that flexion and extension could be determined readily and so that postoperative assessment of the sensation and range of motion could be determined. Systemic analgesia and nitrous oxide were available to eliminate pain during the procedure. When the incision was reopened the muscle bellies of the flexor superficialis bulged out of the wound, being under high pressure. The incision was extended proximally to the end of the mid forearm, and the superficial fascia was split through the level of the lacertus fibrosus. The fingers could be almost completely extended passively. The transverse retinacular ligament at the wrist was also opened so that the median and ulnar nerves were not under compression. Wound closure was possible after elevation and gentle compression of the arm for several minutes. No further complication occurred (Goldner, 1975).

Case 18

A 23-year-old female received a laceration of both flexor tendons to the little finger through the level of the palmar surface of the metacarpophalangeal joint. Primary repair was attempted in the emergency room by the attending physician. Swelling and pain occurred within 24 hours under the compression dressing and pain was severe. This was described as tense, aching, and burning. Partial splitting of the external dressing provided diminution of pain, but a deep, aching pain persisted. The adjacent ring and long fingers could not be moved without causing deep, sharp, lancinating pain in the wrist and forearm. The wound was opened at five days after the injury and a purulent exudate was released from the ulnar bursa, which extended back to the lower forearm. Streptococci organisms were isolated. An incision was made from the base of the finger to the volar wrist crease and a large amount of exudate removed. Additional tension was noted at the wrist and in the distal forearm, and the superficial fascia was split proximal to the mid forearm, in order to relieve tension of the flexor superficialis, flexor profundi, and median and ulnar nerves. After release of the fluid from the tendon sheath and the carpal canal as well as release of the compartment pressure in the forearm, pain was relieved.

Patients who have trauma to the lower extremity and who experience severe pain that is not relieved by splitting dressings must be managed as if they have persistent direct compression of a peripheral nerve or an expanding hematoma from venous or arterial hemorrhage causing increased compartmental compression with resulting intracellular edema, or a tight compartment from muscle edema. Individuals who inherently have collagen tissue that allows only a minimal amount of expansion are prone to development of compression syndromes.

PAIN SYNDROMES ASSOCIATED WITH COMBINED NERVE AND VASCULAR INSUFFICIENCY

Patients with combined nerve and arterial injury initially require arterial repair or vein graft. Primary nerve repair may fail and leave a painful nonconducting neuroma. Nerve repair should be delayed until blood supply is reestablished.

Case 19

A 32-year-old male received a laceration of the brachial artery and median nerve when he fell through a glass window. Arterial supply was re-established with great difficulty by a vein graft, which thrombosed on three different occasions during a two week period. The median nerve had been sutured with a holding suture but a definitive repair had not been done. The patient developed a cool, painful, and stiff hand, and an aching in the forearm when the environment was cool, and had severe pain when the area of nerve laceration was tapped. Six months after the original injury, and three months after sympathectomy, the median nerve was mobilized proximally in the axilla and distally in the forearm; a fibrous neuroma and fibroma were resected; and 4 cm gap was bridged by end-to-end suture. Postoperatively, the local hyperesthesia and paresthesias were diminished. The radial pulse was intact and finger flexibility improved somewhat.

Nerve regeneration was progressive during the next three months, as determined by the percussion test. About three months after the nerve repair, the patient noted a sudden onset of burning pain in the forearm; the hand was cool, the fingers stiffened rapidly over a four day period, and the radial pulse was not palpable.

An arteriogram demonstrated minimal blood flow into the hand and evidence of a thrombosis proximal to the vein graft in the arm. A bypass graft was done from the axillary artery to the radial artery at the wrist. Blood flow to the hand improved significantly. The acute pain was relieved and the dull aching diminished within the next two weeks. This patient demonstrated the importance of adequate blood flow in order to maintain collagen flexibility in the combined pain syndromes that occur from a nerve laceration in the presence of arterial insufficiency (Goldner and Bright, 1977).

Pain Associated with Index Ray Deletion (Fig. 8–2)

Case 20

A 35-year-old male received a laceration at the base of the index finger which injured the digital nerve, the digital artery, and both flexor tendons. An attempt at repair failed. Because of other complications removal of the index ray was done by the attending surgeon. Postoperatively, the patient showed diminished sensation on the radial side of the long finger, limited flexion of all the digits, a painful phantom sensation of the index finger, and progressive stiffness of the entire hand. The attending surgeon prescribed stellate ganglion blocks, physical therapy, and pain medication. The stellate block improved the pain syndrome temporarily.

Definitive treatment initiated several months after the initial injury and the ray deletion required release of the median and ulnar nerves at the wrist, tenosynovectomy of the flexor tendons, which were surrounded by thickened synovium, microdissection of the adherent digital nerves to the index finger, and isolation of the epineurium, resection and bipolar coagulation of the axonplasm, and suture of the epineurium with 9–0 suture. The nerve was placed in the

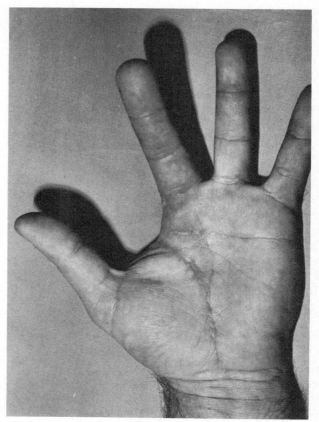

Figure 8–2 This is the hand of a patient who was first seen because of severe pain in the palm at the site of prior index ray deletion. The hand was sweating excessively, had several exquisitely tender hot spots at the base of the long finger and in the palm, and showed limitation of motion of the long finger because of contracture of the intrinsic muscles and tendons. The patient had undergone three prior operative procedures directed toward "neurolysis," "placement of the neuroma in better tissue," and removal of a segment of the second metacarpal which was "pressing on the peripheral nerves." Cold intolerance was demonstrated by thermistor studies; pulse volume recordings and skin temperature readings were diminished with cooling. Pain increased as cooling occurred. Warm up time was exceedingly slow. Stellate ganglion block improved peripheral blood flow and diminished but did not eliminate pain. Several factors were affecting and promoting the pain syndrome: a) smoking; b) tethering of the digital nerves of the amputated index finger to the tendons; c) compression of the median and ulnar nerves at the wrist due to chronic tenosynovitis caused by retraction of the flexor tendons; d) fibrosis and obliteration of the superficial vascular arch; e) fibrosis of the radial digital nerve to the long finger, secondary to prior laceration of this nerve without subsequent repair; f) severe contracture of the intrinsic muscles due to transfer of the first dorsal interosseous to the lateral bands of the long finger with subsequent connective tissue and joint pain, g) vasospasm secondary to all of the points listed. Treatment included repair of the lacerated digital nerve, resection and cauterization with bipolar forceps at a proximal point in keeping with the presence of acceptable surrounding tissue; release of the contracted intrinsics and excision of the first dorsal interosseous, decompression of the median nerve by release of the transverse retinacular ligament and release of the ulnar nerve in Guyon's canal; a postoperative tapering course of steroids, postoperative stellate ganglion block, on three occasions followed by peripheral nerve block, weekly for four weeks, and a protective plastic cap for the hand for several months. The transcutaneous stimulator was used for part of the day and prior to sleep. The patient's pain gradually subsided. Sympathectomy would have been beneficial only to compensate for the vasospasm but would not have eliminated the pain associated with the peripheral nerve lesions. Sympathectomy should be held as an adjunctive last resort procedure rather than as the initial procedure. Intra-arterial or intravenous reserpine injected with an elevated proximal operating tourniquet at 280 mm Hg after a preliminary exsanguination of the limb and utilizing the intravenous Xylocaine technique used in performing regional intravenous anesthesia the frequency of the need for surgical sympathectomy will be reduced.

intrinsic muscle to avoid tethering. The lacerated common nerve to the index and long fingers was repaired. Postoperative stellate blocks were followed by a two-week course of oral steroids and anti-inflammatory medication. The patient was not allowed to smoke, the hand was kept warm, and vasospasm was diminished. The sensitive areas in the palm were covered by a plastic cap to avoid repetitive stimulation. Range of motion improved, pain was diminished, and the phantom pain reverted to a phantom sensation that could be tolerated. Sympathectomy was not necessary to resolve the swelling, stiffness, and burning.

Syndromes such as this are managed by reapposition of lacerated nerves, resection of adherent nerve tissue which is under constant stress, release of compression of major nerves brought on by tenosynovitis resulting from the injury, and diminution of the vasospasm caused by nerve injury, progressive fibrosis, persistent pain, and vasoconstrictors such as nicotine (Goldner, 1977).

Ulnar Nerve Laceration and Compression Associated with Chronic Pain Syndrome

Case 21

A 50-year-old male was treated initially for chronic compression of the ulnar nerve at the elbow. This was associated with dysesthesia and paresthesia in the forearm and hand and minimal motor weakness. According to the records, *the nerve was transferred anteriorly* to the medial condyle, but without relief. Local hypersensitivity of the skin and burning in the little finger persisted. Several months later, because of persistent pain, a *second operation* was done and the nerve was found to be surrounded by a thickened fibrous covering and there was compression proximally at the intermuscular septum and distally where the nerve entered the flexor carpi ulnaris. Additional dissection, removal of the epineurium, and attempted fascicular dissection resulted in diminished motor strength and persistent pain.

A microelectrode was applied proximally, and peripheral nerve stimulation was attempted. Moderate relief was obtained during the procedure, which was performed under local anesthesia, but postoperatively satisfactory relief was not possible. This appeared to be due to an inability to place the electrode directly on the sensory fibers that affected the patient's pain, and to persistent stimuli distal from the nerve in the fibrous scar at the elbow.

At the present time, the solution to this problem is under discussion. One approach is resection of all the affected nerves followed by sural nerve grafting; a second is another attempt at peripheral nerve stimulation; a third is transcutaneous dorsal column stimulation in the cervical region; and a fourth, under consideration, is resection of the substantia gelatinosa (Nashold, 1978; Nashold, Goldner, and Bright, 1975).

Resection of purely sensory nerves such as the superficial radial, the saphenous, or the medial antebrachial cutaneous results in an area of hypesthesia and dysesthesia with partial relief of the persistent pain syndrome. However, incision and resection of major nerves such as the median, the ulnar, or the posterior tibial have resulted in persistent paresthesias, persistent phantom pain, and dysesthesia without improvement of the patient's condition.

Patients with this problem involving the median, ulnar, or posterior tibial nerve continue to present a challenge that requires additional clinical and laboratory investigation. Direct electrical stimulation of peripheral nerves has been beneficial for some and resection and nerve grafting have aided others; proximal surgery with percutaneous dorsal column stimulation or formation of a more proximal lesion in the spinal cord or brain must also be considered (Nashold, Goldner, and Bright, 1975).

Forearm and Hand Pain Syndrome Associated with Combined Nerve Compression, Collagen Fibrosis, Adherent Flexor Tendons, and Secondary Vasospasm

Case 22

This 48-year-old female had an episode of bleeding into the anterior compartment of the forearm after anticoagulation was used for treatment of thrombophlebitis. The attending surgeon had released the forearm fascia but had not extended the incision into the hand or wrist. A second operation included more of the forearm and the proximal wrist. Because of persistent pain and "burning," a sympathectomy was performed. This procedure may diminish the occurrence of vasospasm but will not improve the compression on the median or ulnar nerve in the palm and will not release the adherent flexor tendons, which when stretched cause a deep, dull aching in the arm and hand. The patient described her pain as "burning," "searing," and deep aching. She had received a transcutaneous stimulator which, when the electrodes were placed proximally, provided her with about 25 per cent relief of her pain. She described her major pain as a deep, dull, aching feeling in the hand and the wrist; only when the wrist was elevated and the fingers extended did she feel the burning.

Examination showed the skin to be dry and the hand to be warm as a result of the sympathectomy; no unusual swelling was present. The hand was not hypersensitive to touch. There was no stiffness about the shoulder or the elbow, and the findings were not those of sympathetic dystrophy or causalgia and actually were not consistent with causalgia prior to the sympathectomy. Percussion of the median and ulnar nerves at the elbow was not painful, nor was percussion of the median or ulnar nerve at the wrist uncomfortable. However, when the wrist was forcibly dorsiflexed and the fingers forcibly extended she complained of tightness and burning at the wrist but not into the fingers. Flexion contracture of the flexor superficialis tendons to the long, ring, and little fingers existed; these tendons were adherent to the flexores digitorum profundi, which were affected by the compartment compression syndrome that occurred initially as a result of the bleeding.

Intrinsic contractures involving the lumbrical muscles of the long, ring, and little fingers were evident when the wrist was extended, particularly when the metacarpophalangeal joints were held in maximum extension. Attempts at flexing the interphalangeal joints with the digits fully extended caused significant pain at the level of the interphalangeal joints and in the flexor tendons and the lumbrical muscle bellies. Stretch of the collateral ligaments and the interphalangeal joints, capsule, and synovium caused pain. Arthrofibrosis in the interphalangeal joints was painful when the digits were manipulated.

DIAGNOSTIC STUDIES THAT WERE HELPFUL IN DETERMINING A TREATMENT PROGRAM AND IN DECIDING ABOUT CAUSALGIA AND SYMPATHETIC DYSTROPHY

1. Review of the history with emphasis on the compartmental hemorrhage and damage to the muscle fibers.
2. Absence of relief by sympathectomy. Stellate ganglion block may cause temporary improvement because of flow of the anesthetic agent over the brachial plexus which results in diminished pain in the extremity, thought by some to be due to vasodilatation but actually due to hypalgesia from the anesthetic agent. Skin temperature readings aided in elucidating the cause of the partial pain relief (see 6. *Cold tolerance studies* below).
3. *Superficial nerve block,* median and ulnar proximal to the elbow, diminished her severe aching pain when the fingers were manipulated, but she still noted the deep, dull sensation when the fingers were stretched even after the nerve block. This is in keeping with fibrous adhesions and contracture of tendons.
4. *Local block of the ulnar nerve* at the wrist diminished aching in the hand but did not eliminate hand and forearm pain when the digits were placed under tension in the extended position.
5. A *transcutaneous nerve stimulator* diminished her pain intensity about 25 per cent. However, all of the pain was not eliminated.
6. *Cold tolerance studies* were done. Cooling time was slow, and warmup time was more rapid than in the opposite, nonoperated, nonpainful hand. This observation indicated that persistent vasodilatation had occurred as a result of the sympathectomy.
7. A *thermogram study* showed increased heat from the extremity on which the sympathectomy had been performed.

TREATMENT

Operative treatment included:

1. Release of the intrinsic tendons medial and lateral of the long, ring, and little fingers, with considerable improvement of range of motion when the digits were extended.
2. Incision of the central slip of the extensor mechanism over the middle phalanx, proximal to the distal interphalangeal joint, as this tendon was adherent and contracted, and was affected by the contracture of the retinacular ligaments.
3. Lengthening of the flexor digitorum profundi at the wrist of the long, ring, and little fingers.
4. Neurolysis and decompression of the median and ulnar nerves at the lower forearm, at the base of the palm, and into the hand. The nerves were definitely adherent to the fibrous sheaths of the flexor tendons.
5. Reconstruction of a volar retinacular ligament to avoid bowstringing of nerves and tendons at the level of the carpal canal.

Postoperatively, the patient had dramatic relief of pain, and could tolerate stress on the fingers with minimal discomfort. The observation of findings compatible with a compartment compression ischemia and temporary capillary insufficiency (Volkmann's ischemia) was consistent with the changes in the muscle fibers, the fibrosis of the flexor tendons, the adherence of nerves to tendons, and the deep, aching pain in the forearm and hand (Goldner, 1955, 1975).

The concept must again be emphasized that a muscle belly will undergo ischemic necrosis when the blood supply is inadequate, while the external skin in the same region will remain viable.

CHRONIC PAIN SYNDROMES — RELATIONSHIP
BETWEEN TIME AND REFRACTORINESS

Many conditions lead to chronic pain syndromes. Examples that have been presented include: a) perineural fibrosis with local ischemia; b) neuroma within an intact nerve; c) external compression of a peripheral nerve; d) muscle compartment syndromes; e) fascial syndromes, f) intermittent capillary, arteriolar, or arterial insufficiency; g) systemic disease such as diabetes or scleroderma affecting large or small blood vessels; h) chemical alterations of vessel size, vasoregulatory instability; and i) peritendinous and adhesion pain. Pain stimuli from collateral ligaments, synovium, and periarticular tissues add to the intensity and degree of pain and diminish the likelihood that any single modality of therapy will eliminate all afferent stimuli.

Various forms of therapy already described in the pain problem case studies should be initiated early and simultaneously or at least progressively. The physician must recall the importance of blood supply to the involved part, of vasoregulatory variations, of nerve lesions of varying severity, and of compartment compression syndromes that cause persistence of diffuse pain.

The direction of management depends on an accurate and detailed history, and on an analytical examination that includes assessing various systems such as skin coverage, skin sensitivity, motor and sensory nerve conduction, state of end-organ receptors, adhesions between skin and cutaneous nerves, nerve compression, nerve ischemia, and the effect of ligament adhesions, intra- and extra-articular adhesions, and pain from worn articular cartilage.

Time alone will not cure all chronic pain problems caused by pathologic lesion of peripheral nerves. The patient's emotional situation — the sleep pattern, the occurrence of emotional depression, the degree of anxiety, and the degree of conversion hysteria — also affects the complaints and the actual degree and extent to which pain permeates his or her entire awareness. Other important factors are the patient's family history and the existence of chronic pain models, the family history of emotional problems, and the financial state of the patient as it relates to income, debt, and secondary gain, either recognized or unrecognized. Aggressive, nondestructive treatment must be initiated early or the pain syndrome will become ingrained and less responsive to any form of treatment. *However, the presence of pain for years does not necessarily leave a nonreversible image on the central nervous system.*

Case 23

A 32-year-old woman had complained of an area of exquisite tenderness on the inner side of her knee joint for 16 years. When touched, the lesion was exquisitely painful. She could not sit with one leg against the other because of the severe pain. Many of her daily physical functions were affected by this area of severe lancinating, radiating pain. Psychiatric treatment had been attempted and numerous medications had been used, but not until the area was operated upon and a neurilemoma of the saphenous nerve was removed was her pain relieved. Although she had been affected by the same constant pain for over 10 years, her pain was relieved by the day after the operation.

Case 24

A 62-year-old woman had suffered with hypesthesia, paresthesia, and burning of the thumb and index finger for 14 years. There had been no known trauma. Examination showed atrophy of the opponents and abductor muscles, a positive percussion test at the wrist, aggravation of the dysesthesia by wrist flexion, and lack of recognition of vibration. Diagnosis of median and ulnar nerve compression at the wrist was made, and the transverse retinacular ligament at the wrist was released, the ulnar canal in the hand was opened, and the epineurium of both median and ulnar nerves was split to relieve the severe constriction, after which the pain was eliminated and her sensation gradually improved over a period of several months. Motor power improved also.

Case 25

A 22-year-old male with severe, dull, deep aching pain in the thigh for approximately five years was taking 20 aspirin tablets (0.3 gram) daily in order to get temporary diminution of pain. He had been in the armed forces for four years and stopped going to sick call because he had gained the reputation of being a "gold brick."

X-ray of the thigh showed a giant osteoid osteoma in the mid shaft of the femur. Excision of the lateral cortex and removal of the central aspect of the lesion resulted in immediate relief of pain that had been present for five years.

Case 26

A 26-year-old female had exquisite pain and tenderness in the tip of her left long finger. She had had the pain almost constantly for seven years, had been examined by numerous physicians, and the hand and finger had been investigated by several x-rays. The diagnosis of glomus tumor was made and when the subungual lesion was removed she was relieved of her pain by the following day.

REFERRED PAIN
(Bourdillon, 1957, Goldner, 1954, 1956)

Recognition of pain in one area with actual origin of the pathologic lesion in another is a well recognized concept that must be considered when pain syndromes are being analyzed. For example, the drinking of cold fluid can irritate the fifth cranial nerve, subsequently causing pain in the eye. Shoulder pain may originate from irritation of the diaphragm mediated through C3 and C4. Otitis media may be felt below the angle of the mandible referred through the fifth cranial nerve, and occipital headache may result from irritation of C3 in osteoarthritis of the upper cervical spine.

Shoulder pain in the deltoid insertion usually denotes the presence of a lesion in the subacromial bursa or in the supraspinatus tendon. Pain along the inner border of the scapula may originate from a compression lesion of C5 root. Burning sensation on the dorsum of the index finger may be related to compression of the sensory component of the radial nerve at the elbow, rather than to irritation of the digital nerves in the index finger. A sensation of burning and hyposensitivity in the thumb may be associated with moderate changes from a cerebral thrombosis rather than with irritation of the superficial sensory branch of the radial nerve or with irritation of the main radial nerve. Knee pain, particularly on the inner aspect of the knee, may be referred from a pathologic lesion in or about the hip through the obturator nerve. Pain on the dorsum of the foot may be secondary to a lesion of the proximal fibula affecting the superficial branch of the peroneal nerve. Lesions affecting the cervical nerve roots may cause peripheral sensory alterations and pain that do not follow an expected anatomic pattern. This may be due to the presence of a prefixed or postfixed brachial plexus. The prefixed brachial plexus, which is a developmental anomaly, includes the root of C3 as part of the proximal trunk and cord and includes less of T1 nerve root in the distal peripheral nerves to the upper extremity. The postfixed plexus excludes C3 and possibly C4 and includes more of T1 and T2 roots in the plexus. Thus the localization of a lesion affecting a nerve root or the brachial plexus, or the determination of the exact site of the pathologic lesion several years after trauma, must be interpreted with the realization that these variations in motor nerve distribution may also be accompanied by anomalous innervations of sensory fibers (Goldner and Jones, 1966).

Nerve crossovers do occur in the supra- or infraclavicular region or in the axillary region and may result in the median nerve temporarily or ultimately carrying motor fibers that usually make up part of the ulnar nerve. Thus an interruption of the ulnar nerve at the elbow may not affect the strength of the interosseous muscles if the motor fibers supplying these muscles had crossed over to the median nerve in the mid-arm region and were carried distally by the ulnar nerve. These findings may include motor alone, motor and sensory, or sensory alone (Goldner and Jones, 1966). Electrical stimulation and nerve block studies are important in assessing both motor and sensory components of a nerve that may be involved in a chronic pain syndrome.

CAUSALGIA

Causalgia (burning pain), which was described in 1864 by Weir Mitchell, Morehouse, and Keen, is a syndrome first noted in Civil War soldiers with gunshot wounds of the extremities involving major nerve trunks (Weir Mitchell, 1872). The hand or the foot demonstrated swelling, erythema, excessive sweating, absence of skin creases, glossiness, stiffness, and slow growth of fingernails.

The person afflicted with this kind of hand usually covered it with a cloth, did not allow anyone to touch it, and refused to have the nails trimmed. In severe causalgic states, a sudden or unexpected noise or touch or modest alterations of heat or cold brought on a paroxysm of pain. Our experience with this lesion during World War II and since that time has shown this to be a peripheral nerve injury associated with a vascular insufficiency or a vasoregulatory condition. The spectrum of causalgia ranges from minimal, which results from relatively minor trauma to a digit, with resulting mild swelling and moderate limitation of joint motion and modest pain, to a severe injury to a digital nerve, with resulting hypersensitivity, limited joint motion, and excessive sweating in certain parts of the extremity and dryness in other parts (Goldner, 1955, 1975).

The exact neurophysiologic explanation of causalgia has been discussed by many, but the human model, as the author has observed, occurs after trauma to a large peripheral nerve such as the sciatic or the median, or to the brachial plexus, and is accompanied by injury to major arteries or is associated with increased compartment pressure. Incomplete nerve lesions occur with gunshot wounds such as rifle injuries, with fractures or dislocations associated with trauma to the median nerve at the elbow after supracondylar fracture, and with trauma to the sciatic nerve after a fracture dislocation of the hip. A possible explanation for the burning and dysesthesia is that it is the result of a short-circuiting of the C fiber impulses or the shunting of afferent sympathetic impulses through the injured somatic nerve, which in turn activates pain fibers. The burning pain of causalgia (hyperesthesia–dysesthesia) may involve the hand or the foot. The skin of the extremity becomes smooth; hair is lost; the color becomes erythematous; the surface is glossy; sweating increases; and the limb becomes intermittently cold. Causalgia syndrome is characterized by increased sweating if the peripheral nerve is *incompletely* affected and vascular impairment is present. If the nerve is *totally severed,* sweating ceases, fingerprints disappear, the digits atrophy, the nails become brittle and grow slowly, and the peripheral joints stiffen in varying degrees, somewhat depending on the age of the patient.

In the *causalgic syndrome,* sweating persists and may be excessive, sensitivity to touch and to environmental stimuli increases, the part of the extremity involved becomes cool, and vasoregulatory alterations are evident. Diminished blood flow, which is measurable, is due either to actual injury to large vessels, to multiple injuries to smaller vessels, to secondary vasospasm, or to any or several of the conditions that cause alterations of vascular tone.

A patient with a major causalgia expresses apprehension by withdrawing the extremity quickly when the examiner approaches the involved part. The hand is protected by a warm cloth or by the patient grasping it if the pain becomes severe. These individuals evidence severe sleep deprivation, irritability, fearfulness, anxiety, and loss of confidence. Loud external stimuli are avoided; alterations of environmental temperature extremes are managed by covering the part; and the patient usually becomes withdrawn. Severe pain can be temporarily lessened by using warm water soaks, a heat lamp, or other forms of external temperature elevation. Complete stellate ganglion block, which increases peripheral blood flow, and which diffuses the anesthetic over the roots of the brachial plexus at the time the sympathetic block is given, may relieve pain dramatically for a few hours. Overactivity of the sympathetic system is temporarily neutralized. If the painful condition cannot be successfully reversed by sympathetic block and by altering the sensitive points then sympathectomy will not be useful. However, if pain is diminished significantly after sympathetic block, then sympathectomy is indicated. Frequently, however, sympathetic block, peripheral nerve block, intra-arterial or closed intravenous reserpine, intra-arterial or intravenous steroids, or a combination of stellate block and anti-inflammatory medications may alter the causalgic pattern. *Sympathectomy is indicated* in patients with a severe vasoregulatory problem who have had adequate local therapy, such as neurolysis, nerve repair, isolation of painful neuroma in scar, and other kinds of local therapy, with persistence of the burning pain and diminished peripheral blood flow detected by pulse volume recordings and cold intolerance.

True causalgia is usually improved by sympathetic block and by sympathectomy, if necessary. However, if a peripheral nerve compression lesion, neuroma in continuity, or vascular insufficiency persists, it must be managed even though the burning pain may be temporarily or permanently eliminated by blockade of the sympathetic fibers.

Minor causalgia may occur as a result of trauma to a cutaneous nerve such as the superficial radial nerve at the wrist, the saphenous nerve on the medial aspect of the knee joint, or the dorsal branch of the ulnar nerve on the dorsal or volar aspect of the hand. After nerve injury, these areas become hypersensitive, dysesthetic, and hyperpathic, and require treatment. They are best managed by using plastic caps with Velcro straps over the sensitive zone and also by diminishing excessive motion of the part if joint motion will cause undue stretch on a tethered nerve (Goldner, 1972). Sensory zones usually supplied by these nerves are affected after trauma and become hypersensitive, dysesthetic, and hyperpathic, and may require aggressive treatment. Local nerve blocks, protection from external stimuli by plastic caps, use of the transcutaneous nerve stimulator, and small doses of anti-anxiety or antidepressant medication are helpful.

Patients with Varying Degrees of Causalgia

Case 29

A 35-year-old male received a fracture dislocation of the hip and contusion of the sciatic nerve. Partial motor weakness resulted, and sensory deficit was present, as were hyperpathia and burning of the foot and calf. Peripheral blood flow, determined by skin temperature readings, Doppler, and pulse volume recordings showed no deficiency. The patient stated, however, that cool weather aggravated the pain, and when the part was cooled there was obvious peripheral vasoconstriction.

Lumbar paravertebral nerve block warmed the foot, increased peripheral blood flow, and temporarily diminished pain. Lumbar sympathectomy increased blood flow and diminished pain and burning. The patient noted, however, that when he was anxious, under stress, or fatigued the burning worsened. In spite of the sympathectomy, the foot showed diminished blood flow when exposed to a cool environment; pain was aggravated but to a lesser extent than preoperatively by cooling the foot, but comparative examination showed fewer problems following sympathectomy than before. Medications such as Elavil, Dilantin, and Prolixin also diminished the intensity of pain if the medications were taken regularly but did not completely eliminate the foot complaints.

Psychological testing showed the patient to have no major abnormal emotional characteristics such as hypochondriasis or hysteria or malingering. Financial or emotional secondary gain factors could not be detected.

A transcutaneous stimulator, placed high on the buttock, diminished a small percentage of the burning pain but did not eliminate it completely. Six months after the sympathectomy, transcutaneous stimulation was discarded because of this, and the patient was able to accommodate reasonably well. The foot was protected from excessive dorsal stretching and the patient avoided prolonged sitting, which caused compression of the sciatic nerve and prolonged fatigue. Another form of therapy available to him would have been a percutaneous dorsal column stimulator (Nashold, 1978) but the condition was not severe enough to warrant that treatment. Although the classic description of causalgia is known and recognized, the relationship to vasospasm, insufficient peripheral blood flow, and an incomplete nerve lesion or some other source of abnormal sensory input is less well recognized.

In most patients, the lesser or minor causalgic variations are not aggressively treated. Minor causalgia may occur after injury to a cutaneous nerve such as the superficial radial nerve at the wrist, the saphenous nerve at the knee, or the dorsal branch of the ulnar nerve at the wrist. The areas supplied by these nerves become hypersensitive, dysesthetic, and hyperpathic, and sweating may increase slightly but not excessively. These syndromes are managed by appropriate diagnostic studies, peripheral nerve block, cold tolerance test, thermogram, stellate ganglion block, and anti-inflammatory agents. The hypersensitive dysesthetic or hyperpathic skin areas are managed by being protected from external sources and avoidance of excessive stress and motion. Intravenous reserpine (2.5 mg) and Lidocaine (20 cc 0.4%) using the double tourniquet technique will warm the hand and decrease pain. The effect is usually noted with 24 hours after injection (Goldner and Donahoo, 1960–1978).

Case 30

A 43-year-old female traumatized the palm of her hand when a piece of furniture that she was moving fell on the hand. No fracture occurred. The attending physician wrapped the hand in an elastic bandage; after this, the fingers swelled, the hand became cool, and there was excessive sweating and erythema of the hand. Sweating and joint stiffness increased and the patient noted almost constant burning and aching. Inadequate cold tolerance was proved by cooling tests and by slow warmup tests.

The patient was given three peripheral nerve blocks on three consecutive days with long acting local anesthetic (Marcaine), a dorsal plaster splint to stabilize the metacarpophalangeal joints when active flexion was being done, a plastic molded cap for the palm held in place with a Velcro strap in order to avoid constant contusion of the hand when attempting to work at home, and a two week course of oral prednisone beginning with 40 mg daily and tapering 5 mg per day until a maintenance dose of 5 mg twice a day was reached, for a total of 14 days for all of the anti-inflammatory medication. At the end of that time, the patient showed relatively dramatic relief of pain, diminished sweating, improved range of motion, and improved sleep. An operative procedure was not necessary. The diagnosis was perineurial fibrosis and intraneural fibrosis of the palmar digital nerve. The patient was maintained on anti-inflammatory medications for about six months and her symptoms gradually stabilized to a point where she could return to doing all of her household activities.

Designations of various syndromes involving the upper extremity have confused the concept of the pathologic lesions that result in varying degrees of vasoregulatory conditions. Major causalgia, as described by Weir Mitchell (1872), and minor causalgia are at opposite ends of a spectrum associated with intermittent vasospasm, collagen contracture, and peripheral pain.

The sensitive point ("trigger point") or the area of pathology that stimulates overactivity of the sympathetic nervous system is usually initiated by pain, chronic disease, or a vasoregulatory problem.

The terms reflex sympathetic dystrophy, shoulder–hand syndrome, upper limb dystrophy, and lower limb dystrophy refer to conditions that occur after major or minor trauma to digits or peripheral nerves as a result of vasospasm from any locus of pain. Other systemic conditions that may be associated with dystrophy of a limb are coronary artery disease, chronic pulmonary disease, and retroperitoneal lesions. The common elements in all of these conditions are vasospasm and a locus of pain, whether it be cardiac, shoulder (Johnson, 1959), cervical root, peripheral nerve lesion or nerve compression with secondary diminution of peripheral blood flow. The upper or lower extremity may show erythema or cyanosis, excessive or diminished sweating, collagen tightness, and pain.

Differences in sweating occur in many individuals. Certain persons normally show little or no sweating on the palmar aspects of the hands and feet. These individuals will not sweat even when the sympathetic nerves are stimulated in a totally cold environment. Other persons show excessive sweating without true sympathetic stimulation or without demonstrable pathologic lesions. If excessive sweating occurs and if other aspects of sympathetic dystrophy are present, the diagnosis can be ascertained by performing cold tolerance tests and recording peripheral blood flow as the temperature is lowered and raised.

Pain and joint stiffness are more critical findings than sweating.

Sympathectomy is seldom required for patients with reflex sympathetic dystrophy. Sympathetic nerve block, intra-arterial or intravenous reserpine medications to improve sleep and diminish anxiety, and treatment with an anti-inflammatory such as corticosteroids or other medication is usually sufficient.

LOW BACK AND LOWER EXTREMITY PAIN

Pain syndromes associated with the back, the pelvis, and the lower extremities are constant problems that demand solution. Localization of the lesion is essential and a determination of the specific tissue involved (for example, skin, fascia, nerve, periosteum, bone) is necessary in order to correlate the tissue, the description of pain, and the location and kind of pain receptors (Goldner, 1954, 1956). Alterations of the skin surface by decreased or increased sensation represent a dermatome distribution. Muscle fascia or tendon aching and discomfort are of myotome origin, and the deep, dull, gnawing bone pain follows a sclerotome pattern (Kerr, 1975).

Interpretation of the patient's complaints requires a careful history, a detailed physical examination, appropriate laboratory studies, roentgenographic assessment, and special studies determined by the preliminary diagnosis. The patient's age, occupation, daily activities, physical stress, and emotional makeup must all be carefully considered in determining the probable cause of a backache or a radiating sensation into the extremity (Levine, 1971).

The patient's occupation is reviewed, and if the individual works in a cold storage area or in an excessively hot temperature, or does repetitive motions many times each day, or is required to lift and stretch or move objects from overhead to the floor, then a correlation between the complaints and the physical activities might be made. The individual who is known to have a sensitive nerve around the knee, the foot, the hand, or the elbow may aggravate this point many times a day, by repetitive trauma. Either the area must be protected, or the way the work is done must be changed, or the job must be changed.

Special Studies with Reference to Back and Lower Extremity Pain

Emotional Profile

The patient's affect and personality may give a clue to the pain pattern, to his or her tolerance level to pain, and to whether the complaints are due to a hypochondriacal pattern, a conversion syndrome, or malingering. If the pain pattern is chronic and the problem not solved easily, then a battery of clinical psychological studies and a psychiatric assessment are necessary. Pain tolerance is affected by anxiety, sleep deprivation, and alterations in the internal and external environment. In patients with pain syndromes related to discrete tumors lessening of pain intensity has been accomplished by minor medications, by alteration of body position, by increasing the sleep period, and by the avoidance of anxiety (Gentry et al., 1977; Goldner, 1976).

Roentgenographic Studies

Roentgenographic studies of the spine, pelvis, and extremities aid in detecting primary bone lesions, alterations of bone density, or changes in the joints associated with trauma or aging.

Special roentgenographic studies include the following:
1. *Tomography* in the anterior, posterior, and lateral planes will provide information about the appearance of bone, articular surface, or soft tissue that might not be evident in the plain projections.
2. *Transaxial tomography* gives information about the spinal canal, the contour of bone around nerve roots, and the anterior, posterior, medial, and lateral size of the canal. Spinal stenosis, unilateral exostoses, or impingement from acute or chronic trauma may become evident whereas the plain roentgenograms or even the myelogram may not show this.
3. *Computerized axial tomography (CAT)* with small amounts of contrast will outline the skeleton, the nerve roots, and the cauda equina at multiple levels to aid in

defining the presence of a lesion. The cross section of the hip joint region, the thigh, or the knee joint will supply information about a benign or malignant neoplasm that is not obtainable by arteriography alone.

4. *Spinal contrast* (Pantopaque or water-soluble contrast Metrizamide) is an aid in determining nerve root lesions or an extrinsic lesion that causes compression. Special techniques are required, such as having the patient supine, prone, or vertical, and performing flexion extension movements of the spine while the contrast is in place.

5. *Bone scan* with technetium 99 provides special information about cellular activity and the presence or absence of information. Gallium scan is also used to give additional data about osteomyelitis.

6. *Epidural venography* has been helpful in defining compression lesions about nerve roots, in determining the limits of a lesion that is blocking the epidural space, and in recognizing lateral compressive root lesions that might not be detected by other contrast studies.

Thermography

This special test detects the infrared light from the body. Increased heat is caused by thrombosis, inflammatory reaction, increased blood flow associated with a vascular lesion, and numerous other pathologic lesions. Also, diminished heat, as detected by the thermogram, is significant in localizing ischemic areas in the skin or vasospasm in a digit.

Electromyography

This will provide information about the peripheral nerve muscle complex. It is helpful in determining alterations of motor action potentials which can be correlated with the sensory dermatome. Motor and sensory nerve conduction studies are valuable in determining whether a conduction delay exists and in localizing the site of a compressive or ischemic nerve lesion (Clippinger, Goldner, and Roberts, 1962).

Differential Spinal Anesthesia

Differential spinal anesthesia (Goldner, 1956; McCollum and Stephens, 1964; Gentry, Newman, and Goldner, 1977) is useful in assessing the patient's pain complaints. The test must be done while the patient is actually suffering the back and lower extremity pain and, if possible, certain manipulations such as straight leg raising are documented as aggravating or lessening the pain. The patient's response to each step of the procedure is important in determining pain tolerance and in determining the effect on pain of needle injection (the placebo effect) and of varying concentrations of local anesthetic such as procaine, varying from normal saline to 1 per cent procaine. The initial injection of saline may cause an alteration of pain that may be significant (Urban and McKain, 1978). The sympathetic dose of 0.2 per cent causes the foot to warm up, but motor power is not affected. If there is an element of sympathetic dystrophy involved, the patient may state that pain has been partially eliminated by that concentration of medication. Occasionally, even after motor block is obtained and extremities are totally anesthetized, the patient complains of persistent pain in the extremity. This is interpreted as being of psychogenic origin and not related to a specific tissue lesion.

Nerve Root Block

Done under control with the image intensifier, nerve root block allows the physician to place the needle in the nerve root foramen and to inject an anesthetic that will provide motor and sensory blockade to a specific root. If this relieves all of the pain, the examiner has positive information concerning the source of the pathology and the probable success of treatment. Anatomic variations do exist and two roots may require blockade, since variations in the lumbosacral plexus may result in overlap from one root to another. The same technique is possible in the cervical region. Before a nerve root block is done, the extremity should be manipulated and the patient put through sufficient physical activity to cause pain to occur.

Peripheral Nerve Block

This is helpful in both diagnosis and treatment. Nerve block will provide information concerning anomalous sensory or motor innervation and will provide specific information about the localization of a dermatome, myotome, or sclerotome. Also, if a peripheral nerve is blocked at a high level and eliminates all of the pain distal to this, then procedures such as placement of a microelectrode may have a reasonable chance of success. For example, if the patient has pain in the ulnar nerve distribution and injection of the ulnar nerve at the elbow level does not relieve pain but injection of the nerve 5 cm higher does, then placement of the microelectrode will be more accurate and the chances of success will be greater. Nerve block will provide a temporary partial sympathectomy and give information about vasospasm and peripheral blood flow (Wall and Gutnick, 1974, Wall and Sweet, 1967, Wagman and Price, 1969; Torebjork and Hallin, 1974).

Discography

Discography is performed by inserting a small-bore needle into the nucleus pulposus and injecting Renografin. If the patient is awake, he or she will give information about any pain that may occur from the injection. This has been very helpful in defining sites of referred pain and determining aberrant pain complaints in certain patients. Injection into the L4 interspace may cause severe pain in the groin or testicle. This is not the standard distribution from the L4 root, but in certain patients will explain the variations of their pain complaints. Injection into the L5 interspace may cause pain in the sacrum or coccyx rather than in the extremity. The patient's chronic pain problem is arising from that interspace and not from the tip of the coccyx itself. The referred pain can be relieved by injecting a local anesthetic into the interspace. Alleviation of the pain is additional information about the localization of the interspace and the adjacent roots as they relate to the pain syndrome. Another method of using discography in pain syndromes — for example, in a cervical syndrome — is to cause the patient's pain to occur by movement of the head, heavy lifting, twisting, and turning, and when the neck and arm pain is present a small quantity of local anesthetic mixed with absorbable contrast is injected into the interspace to determine if the pain is relieved and if the contrast runs out of the interspace. Discography is valuable if these various ancillary studies are done rather than just depending on whether the contrast does or does not run out of the interspace. If the contrast remains in the interspace in a uniform contour, it is unlikely that the source of pain is coming from within the interspace. If the contrast runs out of the interspace, which does happen in many asymptomatic individuals, the proper interpretation must be given after coordinating this information with other data.

Vascular Studies

Information concerning pain complaints can be obtained by determining the effects of diminishing the arterial blood supply, by observing the effects of capillary constriction in cold tolerance tests, by noting the changes that occur with increased venous congestion after a tourniquet is applied, and by measuring compartment compression and observing the effects of exercise on peripheral blood flow (Hill et al., 1973; Silver, 1977).

These studies require use of arteriography to determine if a segmental block exists in a large vessel or if the peripheral arterial bed will not fill because of vasospasm or vasculitis. *Venography* gives information about the flow of blood in the venous system. *Plethysmography* gives information about blood flow at varying pressure levels. The *thermogram* will give indirect information about arterial flow or venous congestion, depending upon the heat given off and the infrared rays detected by the thermograph. *Doppler* studies give information about blood flow in small and large arteries by detecting a sound that correlates with vibration of fluid in the vessel. A *pulse volume recorder* depends on a piezoelectric contact with the digit pulp and a pulse wave recorded on an oscilloscope as a digital indicator.

1. The *Allen test* is done by manual arterial block at the wrist or at the base of the fingers. Pain may result from temporary ischemia or from local compression of the ulnar artery by the examiner's fingers.
2. The result of increasing venous compression can be determined by applying a tourniquet at 60 mm Hg and causing engorgement distal to the tourniquet, which may increase compartment pressure and cause pain or increase compression on a sensitive nerve and cause pain.
3. Compartment pressure increases during exercise or following application of a proximal tourniquet. The *Wick catheter pressure studies* give helpful information about the effect of trauma on compartment pressure, and allow a compartment to be monitored on a digital write-out transducer in order to determine if its pressure is increasing after trauma. Also, individuals with

tight compartments or large muscles are benefited by monitoring their compartmental pressure after exercise in order to determine the rate of recovery of normal pressure. If the absolute reading of the compartmental pressure is 35 mm of Hg or higher or if the length of time for the pressure to return to normal is prolonged when compared with the average (5–15 minutes) then the compartment should be released (Matsen, 1979; Goldner, 1975).

LESIONS SIMULATING INTERVERTEBRAL DISEASE IN BACK AND LOWER EXTREMITIES
(Goldner, 1954; 1956)

Figures 8–3 to 8–10 are diagrammatic representations of pathologic lesions that cause pain which simulates the pain caused by nerve root compression or

Text continued on page 169.

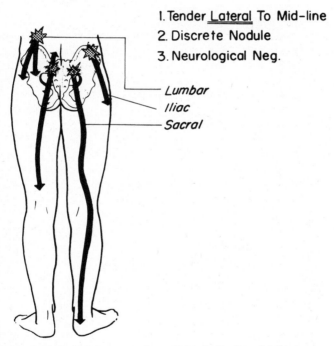

1. Tender <u>Lateral</u> To Mid-line
2. Discrete Nodule
3. Neurological Neg.

Lumbar
Iliac
Sacral

Figure 8–3   Painful fat nodules. Deep fat nodules, located on the fascia over muscle or bone, may be painful to direct pressure or trunk bending. The aching and radicular sensation occurring when the nodule is palpated are readily identified with the painful mass, and all pain is temporarily relieved by local injection of an anesthetic. The radicular component is referred pain similar to that associated with the painful tendon attachment, or periosteal pain or the deep aching associated with compression of the small blood vessels, and the irritation of a sensory nerve penetrating the fascia. This diagram represents the usual locations of painful fat nodules. Straight leg raising may be uncomfortable but is not truly radicular. All peripheral examinations are otherwise normal and there are no x-ray changes. The findings are different from but easy to confuse with nerve root radiculopathy. All tender areas in the buttock are not fat nodules, and many tender areas may represent pain referral from an irritated nerve root. A nerve root ganglion or cyst, for example, may cause pain in the buttock similar to that which occurs with a painful fat nodule that is more proximal. The arrows represent the zones of radiation in a large number of patients who have been treated for painful fat nodules. The patient's subjective localization of pain has been designated by the heavy black arrow.

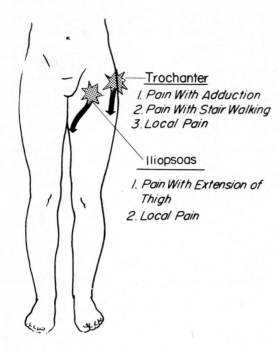

Trochanter
1. Pain With Adduction
2. Pain With Stair Walking
3. Local Pain

Iliopsoas

1. Pain With Extension of
   Thigh
2. Local Pain

Figure 8-4 Patients with complaints of trochanteric tendinitis or bursitis do occasionally have thigh radiation, pain on adduction of the extremity which is aggravated by resting on the involved side; early morning stiffness occurs as a result of limited activity during the night. Local palpation is also painful. The differential diagnosis requires consideration of buttock pain associated with nerve root irritation. Injection with a local anesthetic will eliminate all of the pain if the material is placed in the proper location. Complete relief is usually not the response if there is nerve root involvement. An iliopsoas bursitis resembles an L4 or L3 root lesion or a painful hip. Aspiration of the bursa may result in recovery of fluid from the bursa. Also, a snapping iliopsoas tendon may result in a tendinitis or bursitis.

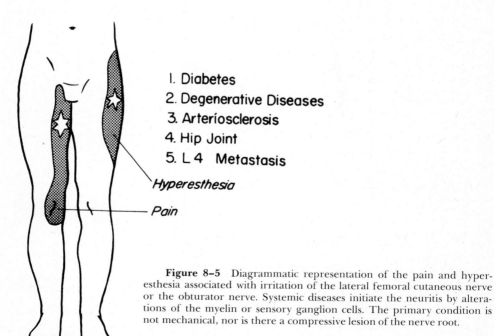

1. Diabetes
2. Degenerative Diseases
3. Arteriosclerosis
4. Hip Joint
5. L 4 Metastasis

Hyperesthesia

Pain

Figure 8-5 Diagrammatic representation of the pain and hyperesthesia associated with irritation of the lateral femoral cutaneous nerve or the obturator nerve. Systemic diseases initiate the neuritis by alterations of the myelin or sensory ganglion cells. The primary condition is not mechanical, nor is there a compressive lesion of the nerve root.

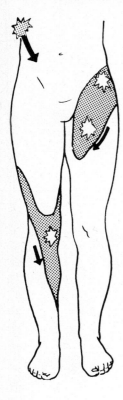

I. Herpes Zoster

2. Other Virus Infections

Figure 8-6 This diagram represents the zone of hyperesthesia or hypesthesia associated with inflammatory involvement of the sensory ganglion with secondary changes in the cutaneous zone of innervation. The development of cutaneous bullae and systemic symptoms is suggestive of a viral cause of nerve inflammation accompanied by peripheral pain.

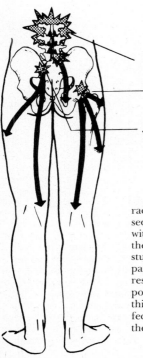

I. Fever—Chills
2. Previous Surgery

Local Pain

— *Hip Joint*

— *Sacro-iliac*

Figure 8-7 The onset of sudden severe back pain, associated with radiation into both thighs, accompanied by fever, chills, elevation of the sedimentation rate, and findings suggestive of septicemia are compatible with an inflammatory lesion of the vertebra with secondary irritation of the adjacent nerve roots. Bone scan, roentgenogram, and serologic studies will aid in the diagnosis, and aspiration may yield bacteria. The pain is severe, aggravated by minimal motion and improved by absolute rest. If the principal site of infection is the hip joint, then pain radiates posteriorly or laterally and may be present along the inner side of the thigh and the knee, secondary to a referred pattern. Sacroiliac joint infection is the cause of severe generalized pain in the posterior aspect of the pelvis and the thigh.

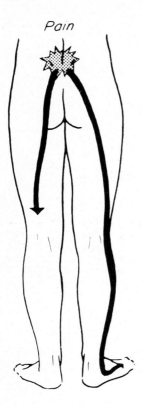

Pain

1. Pain With Extension
2. Mid-line Pain With Pressure
3. Thigh Radiation
4. Sciatic Radiation
5. Oblique X-ray Positive

Figure 8-8 The pain pattern in nerve root irritation due to a movable laminal arch or neural arch resembles that caused by compression of a nerve root by an intervertebral disc or by compression of a nerve root by other mechanical means. Pain usually occurs when the spine is extended or when the spinous process is compressed or manipulated, causing secondary irritation of the dura. Radiation may be along the course of the femoral or sciatic nerve, but this depends on the site of the bone abnormality. Special x-ray studies elicit the skeletal defect that usually accounts for the pattern of pain radiation.

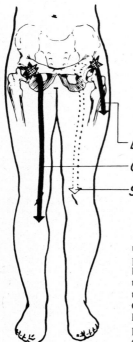

1. Rotation Of Thigh
   Limited
2. "Hip Limp"
3. Neurological Neg.
4. X-ray— Positive

Lat. Femoral Cut.
Obturator N.
Sciatic N.

Figure 8-9 Degenerative arthritis about the hip joint, alteration of the hip joint capsule, or of the surrounding osseous structures may cause pain in the groin anteriorly, laterally, or posteriorly. Pain radiation may be associated with this through the lateral femoral cutaneous nerve distribution, through the obturator nerve along the medial aspect of the thigh, or through branches of the sciatic nerve along the posterior thigh. Clinical examination will allow detection of intra-articular or extra-articular lesions because pain is associated with manipulation. The radicular pattern must be differentiated from other causes of pain in the thigh or extremity.

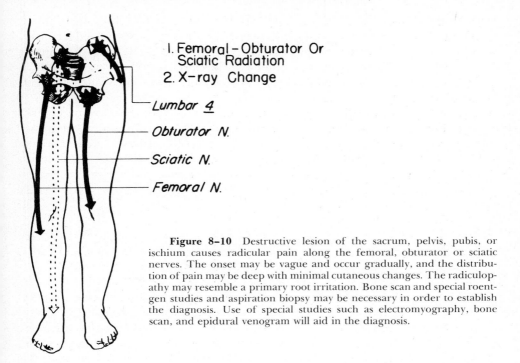

I. Femoral–Obturator Or
  Sciatic Radiation
2. X–ray Change

Lumbar 4

Obturator N.

Sciatic N.

Femoral N.

Figure 8–10 Destructive lesion of the sacrum, pelvis, pubis, or ischium causes radicular pain along the femoral, obturator or sciatic nerves. The onset may be vague and occur gradually, and the distribution of pain may be deep with minimal cutaneous changes. The radiculopathy may resemble a primary root irritation. Bone scan and special roentgen studies and aspiration biopsy may be necessary in order to establish the diagnosis. Use of special studies such as electromyography, bone scan, and epidural venogram will aid in the diagnosis.

irritation. These lesions may be cutaneous or may follow a dermatome pattern; they may be in the fascia, muscle, blood vessels, or peripheral nerves and follow a myotome pattern; or they may be in the bone, joint, periosteum, or deep fascial compartment layers and have a sclerotome distribution (Goldner, 1954, 1956; Schurr, 1955; Sinclair et al., 1948; Toumey, Roppen, and Hurley, 1950).

In order to emphasize the importance of differential diagnosis and the spectrum of lesions, the clinical syndromes that the author has observed and documented are listed. All of these patients were subjected to myelography prior to the author's examination because of the radicular nature of their pain.

1. *Ankylosing spondylitis* may mimic back and lower extremity pain from many causes. Limited chest expansion, sclerosis in the sacroiliac joint, a history of back pain at two to three o'clock AM, and HLA B27 serologic tests are helpful in establishing the diagnosis.
2. *Sciatic nerve* compression by neurofibroma, neurilemoma, ischial bursitis, or endometrial implant on the sciatic nerve has been recognized as a cause of peripheral pain mimicking nerve root compression.
3. *Lateral femoral* cutaneous nerve irritation causing hyperesthesia or hypesthesia may be spontaneous in onset in obese patients. As the nerve leaves the pelvis and crosses over the ilioinguinal ligament, compression caused by adipose tissue, a tight pants belt, prolonged seat belt compression, or pro-

longed flexion of the hip associated with sitting or driving has been noted. Systemic conditions associated with obesity, such as diabetes, must be considered. The postoperative paresthesia is noted frequently after iliac bone grafts are removed as a result of local edema or nerve retraction. Nerves should be carefully retracted or isolated, the fascia sheath split, and stretch by rigid retractors avoided (Fig. 8–5).

4. *Peroneal nerve compression* is evidenced by pain along the course of the superficial peroneal nerve in both the leg and the foot. A traction pin in the upper tibia, an external device for fixation of a fracture, a flexed knee and leg during a cross-leg flap, constant knee crossing by an individual who has lost weight, and postoperative compression of the nerve by plaster cast, compression dressings, or a suspension sling can cause pain that may be severe for 24 to 48 hours and then abate when conduction ceases. Early recognition of the cause of compression or traction is essential.

5. *Posterior tibial nerve* compression lesions associated with a fractured calcaneus, tenosynovitis of the posterior tibial tendon, rupture of the posterior tibial tendon with associated peripheral edema, and a large abductor hallucis muscle that compresses the posterior tibial nerve must be considered when the patient complains of burning, hyperesthesia, paresthesias or hypesthesia on the plantar surface of the foot. Other systemic conditions such as peripheral neuropathy from diabetes, neuropathy from ethanol, heavy metals, or other systemic conditions may cause severe paresthesias. Progressive changes in the joints and bones of the foot noted in rheumatoid or degenerative arthritis may cause a similar pain. The diagnosis depends on history, a local percussion test, electromyographic and nerve conduction studies, appropriate roentgenographic studies and review of the areas proximal to the foot that might involve sciatic radiation (Clippinger, Goldner, and Roberts, 1962, Edwards, Lincoln, Bassett, and Goldner, 1969).

6. *Saphenous nerve lesions* cause hyperesthesia, dysesthesia, or hypesthesia on the medial aspect of the knee and leg. Oppenheimer described this as gonalgia paresthetica. This may be due to direct trauma, to compression by a fascia tunnel where the nerve exits from Hunter's canal, or to postoperative edema, fibrosis, or laceration associated with an arthrotomy of the knee.

7. *Peripheral nerve trauma*, with or without a primary vascular injury, and a resulting sympathetic dystrophy with the spectrum of pain varying from minimal to severe has been discussed under causalgia and includes consideration of primary vascular insufficiency or secondary vasospasm due to nerve injury.

8. *Spillane–Parsonage–Turner syndrome* presents initially with severe pain followed by dermatome and myotome deficiencies and may involve the cervical plexus or the lumbosacral plexus. The initial pain is suggestive of herpes zoster involving a posterior ganglion or an acute compression of a sensory component of a nerve root or peripheral nerve. Dermatome and myotome distributions are irregular. The condition resolves spontaneously but may leave permanent sensory and/or motor deficits (Fig. 8–6).

9. *Segmental ischemia* of peripheral nerve due to vasculitis, an inflammatory process, or idiopathy may cause pain, sensory deficiency, and irregular motor weakness (Spinner, 1976). Arteriography may be helpful in establishing the diagnosis (Silver, 1977; Porter, 1977).

THE MUSCULOSKELETAL ASPECTS OF EMOTIONAL PROBLEMS AS RELATED TO PAIN IN SPINE AND EXTREMITIES
(Goldner, 1976)

The patient with a chronic pain syndrome has complex problems that in many instances can only be defined by a psychiatrist or a clinical psychologist. The assessment of an individual with chronic pain requires more than a brief interview and a cursory examination. The management of this individual necessitates an understanding of his or her past experience, education, basic intellect, prior occupations, relationship to family and employers, understanding of self, and motivation for recovery or desire to retire. I have classified several hundred patients that I have assessed, studied, and treated into five categories.

Category I

Patients who complain of severe pain that affects their daily life but who have no demonstrable organic lesion. This patient is considered to have a "depressive equivalent" (Hohman, personal communication, 1953) and are using pain as an expression of underlying depression. This is not malingering; it is involuntary, serving as a way to sublimate a stressful problem. Biofeedback programs (Ziezat, 1978) may be helpful and psychiatric treatment may be beneficial if the patient is willing to accept this and understands the basis of the pain. Patients with headache, painful feet of a certain characteristic, and intermittent chronic back pain may be in this category.

Category II

Individuals with a documented injury whose complaints persist although the injury was not severe and the objective findings are minimal. These patients are seeking secondary financial or personal gain. Financial recovery is not always the most important aspect of secondary gain. Individuals may seek more attention from other members of the family, or may use the injury as a way of avoiding return to an unpleasant work situation or as a way of rejecting an unpleasant supervisor. A particular patient in this category continued to have extremity pain after a mild back injury. She was comfortable so long as her supervisor did not demand that she increase her work load and did not question her extensively whenever she stayed home from work because of "pain." Her request for a different chair and a different desk were ignored. Her anxiety and hostility levels increased. Once these aspects of her work environment were settled, the patient's pain complaints disappeared. The physician must document the absence of an organic lesion by appropriate clinical examination, careful history, and accessory studies as indicated (Goldner, 1956).

Category III

These patients have a documented pain syndrome. In one example, the cause was a large neuroma of the median nerve at the wrist resulting from a partial laceration of the median nerve a year prior to assessment for chronic pain syndrome. This patient had a hypersensitive mass on the volar aspect of the wrist, extreme anxiety, alterations of blood pressure, and other evidence of sympathetic nerve stimulation when the area was manipulated or touched. She could not concentrate, could not perform her usual job and had an irregular sleep pattern. Dilantin and Elavil diminished her pain awareness but interfered with her ability to drive an automobile and to stay awake during the day. Patients such as this who have a real cause for pain may, however, resort to their pain syndrome as a way of obtaining disability benefits, temporary sick leave, or a change in job location. The physician must be fully informed of the home and job conditions in order to assist the patient in making a reasonable adjustment. This patient was managed by resection of the partially lacerated nerve and resuture by an end-to-end epineural suture of the fibrous area. Pain was diminished and the patient was making gradual improvement. Several months after the operation, however, social and financial alterations occurred that caused the patient to become "worse." Psychiatric and psychological assessments were helpful in determining the cause of the patient's problems and in correcting these deficiencies. When that aspect of her life was improved, her pain diminished. A transcutaneous stimulator was used temporarily but was not helpful; however, certain patients in this category are aided by transcutaneous stimulation (Goldner and Hendrix, 1977).

Category IV

These patients have a distinct lesion, such as the man in this example, who had a nerve injury with regenerating axons but with vascular insufficiency because of a previously placed vein graft that was gradually narrowing and becoming fibrotic. As the graft fibrosed, peripheral blood flow diminished and the pain syndrome increased. Replacement of the vein graft was necessary in order to increase the blood flow. Also, the patient was taken off of a job that requred constant repetitive trauma to the nerves and vessels of the extremity and was taken out of the cool environment in which he was trying to work. Hand pain was diminished and his overall condition improved (Goldner, 1956).

Category V

These patients have had a known pathologic lesion and were given adequate treatment. Observation of their improvement shows that they have steadily been getting better. Suddenly, however, they seem to be at a standstill or complain of being worse. This frequently coincides with impending negotiations for settlement of litigation at which time the patient will be benefited by consciously or unconsciously "getting worse." Unfortunately, the physician may become impatient and suspicious rather than empathetic and understanding. Yochelson (1972) emphasized the importance of the physician's accepting the patient's complaint of pain rather than expending great energy in attempting to convince the patient that the pain syndrome may not be as severe as the patient thinks it is. The physician should remember that pain may be equated with depression or may cause a secondary reactive depression. Certain patients respond to psychiatric treatment by a diminishing of their pain complaints. Others do not accept the fact that there is an emotional component to their pain syndrome and are not willing to undergo any form of psychiatric treatment.

A study of patients with chronic low back pain (Gentry, 1974) emphasized several factors characteristic of patients with chronic low back pain (Silverman, 1968).

1. Patients experienced unmet dependency needs early in life. They had postponed the gratification of such needs until a minor injury provided a rational and socially acceptable means of depending on others for emotional and economic support.
2. Most males had financial compensation available that would cover the cost of an extended disability and medical and surgical treatment, and spouses who were either already working or who quickly returned to work to provide for the family. Other members of the family would take over domestic responsibility such as housework or yard work until the patient could again perform them without pain.
3. Family models of chronic pain or other types of debilitating physical disorders existed during early life in many of these patients. These models predisposed them toward responding with somatic symptomatology under conditions of life's stress.

This kind of study suggests a way of determining the most relevant factors, either biographical or psychometric, that should be incorporated into a prospective assessment of each patient, the goal of which would be the identification of individuals who will and will not profit from medical and surgical management of pain.

Indications for an operative procedure on the spine or extremities should be well defined, and the available evidence indicating an existing lesion should be considerable. Exploratory operation of nerve roots in the face of negative electromyography, normal venography, a questionable myelogram, and a normal x-ray may lead to increasingly severe depression and reinforce the patient's pronounced tendency to somatize. Reoperation at a later time may become necessary because of complications that occur from the laminectomy or the infection that might ensue.

In many instances, we, as physicians who are attempting to manage patients with chronic pain, are interested in diminishing the patient's use of addicting medications to improve the patient's quality of life, but should not necessarily be directed toward getting the patient back to work. In many instances, the final solution may be that the male patient stays home and looks after the children and maintains the home. The female member of the family may readily accept the role of the family provider and perform well with a regular job. The alleged goal of "getting the person back to work" is not always the basis of success in managing a patient with a chronic pain syndrome (Goldner, 1976; Sternback, 1974).

REFERENCES

Black, J. R.: Congenital indifference to pain. J. Bone Joint Surg. *36*(A): 197, 1954.

Bourdillon, M. J.: Some aspects of referred pain. Proceedings of Southwest Orthopaedic Club Meeting. J. Bone Joint Surg. *39*(B):790, 1957.

Clippinger, F. W., Goldner, J. L., and Roberts, J. M.: Use of the electromyogram in evaluating upper extremity peripheral nerve lesions. J. Bone Joint Surg. *44*(A)1047, 1962.

Edwards, W. G., Lincoln, C. R., Bassett, F. H., and Goldner, J. L.: The tarsal tunnel syndrome: Diagnosis and treatment. J.A.M.A. *207*:716, 1969.

Eguro, H., and Goldner, J. L.: Bilateral thrombosis of the ulnar arteries in the hands. Case Report. Plast. Reconstr. Surg. *53*:573, 1972.

Feindel, W.: Note on the nerve endings in a subject with arthroplasty and congenital absence of pain. J. Bone Joint Surg. *35*(B):402, 1953.

Feinstein, B., Langston, J. N. K., Jameson, R. N., and Schiller, F.: Experiments on pain referred from deep somatic tissues. J. Bone Joint Surg. *36*(A):981, 1954.

Gelberman, R. H., Urbaniak, J. R., Bright, D. S., and Levin, L. S.: Digital sensibility following replantation. J. Hand Surg. *2*(4):313, 1978.

Gentry, W. D.: Factors noted in a chronic pain syndrome. Personal communication. Duke Medical Center Course on Low Back Pain, 1974.

Gentry, W. D., Newman, M. C., Goldner, J. L., and Baeyer, C. V.: Relation between graduated spinal block technique and MMPI for diagnosis and prognosis of chronic low back pain. Spine *2*(3):1977.

Goldner, J. L.: Lesions of the spine resembling ruptured disc. Proceedings Virginia Orthopaedic Society Meeting, March, 1954. J. Bone Joint Surg. *36*(A):1093, 1954.

Goldner, J. L.: Volkmann's contracture. J. Bone Joint Surg. *37*(A):621, 1955.

Goldner, J. L.: Lesions of the low back and lower extremities simulating ruptured discs. North Carolina Med. J. *17* #6, 1956.

Goldner, J. L.: Peripheral nerve mapping, motor fibers. 1958–1978. Unpublished.

Goldner, J. L., and Jones, W. B.: Anomalous innervation of the forearm and hand. J. Bone Joint Surg. *48*(A):604, 1966.

Goldner, J. L., and Eguro, H.: Distribution of superficial radial nerve in fifty normal patients — observation, variations, pattern of sensation in the index and thumb. Unpublished observations, 1971.

Goldner, J. L., and Fisher, G.: Index ray deletion — complication and sequelae. J. Bone Joint Surg. *54*(A):898, 1972.

Goldner, J. L., and Bright, D. S.: Peripheral nerve gaps managed by mobilization of proximal and distal segments and epineural suture. Presented at Course on Peripheral Nerve Injuries — Diagnosis and Treatment. Duke University Medical Center, Durham, North Carolina, 1979.

Goldner, J. L., Yochelson, D., Nashold, B. S., Brown, H., Hunter, J., Omer, G., Kleinert, H., and Green, D.: Upper limb pain. Proceedings ASSH. J. Bone Joint Surg. *54*(A):899, 1972.

Goldner, J. L., and Clippinger, F. W.: Arthrosis of the first metacarpal trapezium joint. J. Bone Joint Surg. *55*(A), 1769, 1973.

Goldner, J. L.: Sensory mapping of peripheral nerves in conjunction with geographic repair of lacerated nerves under local anesthesia. 1968–1974, Unpublished observations.

Goldner, J. L.: Volkman's ischemia contracture. *In* Flynn, J. E.(ed.): Hand Surgery. 2nd ed. Baltimore, Williams & Wilkins, 1975.

Goldner, J. L., Bright, D. S., and Nashold, B. S.: Direct electrical stimulation of the peripheral nerves for relief of intractable pain. J. Bone Joint Surg. *57*(A):729, 1975.

Goldner, J. L.: Musculoskeletal aspects of emotional problems. Editorial. South. Med. J. *69*: #1, 1976.

Goldner, J. L.: Moderator: Panel on Pain Syndromes Involving the Upper Extremity. ASSH, Las Vegas, 1977.

Goldner, J. L., and Hendrix, P. C.: Use of transcutaneous electrical stimulation in the management of chronic pain syndromes. Current Concepts in the Management of Pain, 1977.

Goldner, J. L., and Donahoo, S.: The effect of the tourniquet and intravenous Lidocaine. Clinical Observations, 400 Patients 1960–1970. Unpublished data.

Goldner, J. L., and Bright, D. S.: The effect of extremity blood flow on pain and cold tolerance. *In* Omer, G., Jr., and Spinner, M.: Peripheral Nerve Injuries. Philadelphia, W. B. Saunders Co., 1979, Chap. 9.

Grant, G. H.: Methods of treatment of neuromata of the hand. J. Bone Joint Surg. *33*(A):841, 1951.

Hill, G., Moeliono, J., Tumewu, F., Brataamadjan, D., and Tohardi, A.: The Buerger syndrome in Java. Br. J. Surg. *60*:606, 1973.

Hohman, L.: Depressive equivalents of pain. Personal communication, Duke University, Durham, North Carolina, 1953.

Horch, K. W.: Physiological response to cutaneous nerve lesions. Paper Presentation, Hand Surgery Course, Duke University, September, 1977.

Jeans, M. E.: Effects of brief, intense transcutaneous electrical stimulation on chronic pain. Ph.D. dissertation, McGill University. (Quoted by Melzack, 1975.)

Johnson, J. T. H.: Frozen-shoulder syndrome in patients with pulmonary tuberculosis. J. Bone Joint Surg. 41(A):877, 1959.

Kellgren, J. H., and Samuel, E. P.: Sensitivity and innervation of the articular capsule. J. Bone Joint Surg. 32(B):84, 1950.

Kerr, F. W. L.: Neuro-anatomical substrates of nociception in the spinal cord. Pain 1:325, Elsevier, North Holland, Amsterdam, 1975.

Levine, M.: Depression, back pain and disc protrusion. Dis. Nerv. Syst. 32:41, 1971.

Lewis, T.: Pain. New York, Macmillan, 1942, p. 181.

Matsen, F.: Measurement of intra-compartmental pressure using infusion technique. Personal communication, University of Washington, January, 1979.

McCollum, D. E., and Stephen, C. R.: The use of graduated spinal anesthesia in the differential diagnosis of pain of the back and lower extremities. South. Med. Assoc. J. 57(4) 410, 1964.

Mavor, G. E.: The anterior tibial syndrome. J. Bone Joint Surg. 38(B):513, 1956.

Melzack, R., and Wall, B. D.: Pain mechanism: A new theory. Science 150:971, 1965.

Melzack, R.: Prolonged relief of pain by brief, intense transcutaneous somatic stimulation. Pain 1:365, Elsevier, North Holland, Amsterdam, 1975.

Miller, N. E.: Learning of visceral and glandular responses. Science 163:434, 1966.

Mitchell, S. Weir: Injuries of the Nerves and Their Consequences. Philadelphia, J. B. Lippincott, 1872.

Nashold, B. S.: Pain in the back and lower extremities treated by percutaneous dorsal column stimulator. Personal communication, 1970–1979, Duke University Medical Center, Durham, North Carolina.

Nosik, W. A.: Pain discussion, Current concepts of physiology of the peripheral nerves. Proceedings ASSH. J. Bone Joint Surg. 36(A):644, 1954.

Petrie, J. G.: A case of progressive joint disorders caused by insensitivity to pain. J. Bone Joint Surg. 35(B):399, 1953.

Porter, J. N.: Raynaud's syndrome. In: Sabiston, D. C. (ed.): Davis–Christopher Textbook of Surgery. Philadelphia, W. B. Saunders Co., 1976, p. 1982.

Schurr, P. H.: Extradural sacral cysts: An uncommon cause of low back pain. J. Bone Joint Surg. 47(B):601, 1955.

Sherman, M. S.: The nerves of bone. J. Bone Joint Surg. 45(A):522, 1963.

Silver, D.: Circulatory problems of the upper extremity. In Sabiston, D. C. (ed.): Davis-Christopher Textbook of Surgery. Philadelphia, W. B. Saunders Co., 1977, p. 198.

Silverman, S.: Psychological Aspects of Physical Symptoms. New York, Appleton-Century-Crofts, 1968.

Sinclair, D. C., Feindel, W. H., Waddell, G., and Faulconer, M. A.: The intervertebral ligaments as a source of segmental pain, J. Bone Joint Surg. 30(B):515, 1948.

Spinner, M.: Cryptogenic infraclavicular brachial plexus neuritis. (Preliminary Report.) Bull. Hosp. Joint Dis. 37:98, 1976.

Sternbach, R.: Hidden meanings of pain. Panel, American Association of Orthopaedic Surgeons, 1974.

Stirrat, C. R., Seaber, A. V., Urbaniak, J. R., and Bright, D. S.: Temperature monitoring in digital replantation. J. Hand Surg. 3(4):342, 1978.

Sweet, W. H., and Wepsic, J.: Treatment of chronic pain by stimulation of fibers of primary afferent neurons. Trans. Am. Neurol. Assoc. 93:103, 1968.

Torebjork, H. E., and Hallin, R. G.: Responses in human AC fibers to repeated electrical intradermal stimulation. J. Neurol. Neurosurg. Psychiatry 37:653, 1974.

Toumey, J. W., Poppen, J. L., and Hurley, M. T.: Cauda equina tumors as cause of low back syndromes. J. Bone Joint Surg. 32(A):249, 1950.

Urban, B., and McKain, C.: Local anesthesia: Effect of intrathecal normal saline. Pain 5:43, 1978.

Urbaniak, J. L., Seaber, A. V., and Bright, D. S.: Mercury-in-rubber strain gauge system for cold stress studies. Personal communication. Duke Hand Examination Laboratory. Durham, North Carolina, 1978.

Venters, W. B. Clippinger, F. W., Goodrich, J., Green, N., Ogden, W., and Goldner, J. L.: Thermography: Its uses in orthopaedics. Duke University and Affiliated Institutions Orthopaedic Training Papers, 1972.

Wagman, I., and Price, D.: Responses of dorsal horn cells of M. mulatta to cutaneous and sural nerve A and C fiber stimuli. J. Neurophysiol. 32:803, 1969.

Wall, P., and Gutnick, M.: Properties of afferent nerve impulses originating from neurons. Nature (Lond.), 248:740, 1974.

Wall, P., and Sweet, W. H.: Temporary abolition of pain in man. Science 155:108, 1967.

Welsh, G. S., and Dahlstram, W. G.: Basic Readings on MMPI and Psychology in Medicine. University of Minnesota Press, 1956.

Ziezat, H.: Personal communication, Duke University, Durham, North Carolina, October, 1978.

9

THE EFFECT OF EXTREMITY BLOOD FLOW ON PAIN AND COLD TOLERANCE

J. LEONARD GOLDNER
and DONALD S. BRIGHT

INTRODUCTION

Significant diminution of blood flow to individual digits or to an entire hand or foot results in pale nail beds, slow capillary recovery after skin compression, diminished bleeding after skin puncture, lowering of the skin temperature, and pain of varying intensity. Symptoms and signs of pain, pulselessness, pallor, paresthesias, and paralysis are indicative of arterial insufficiency or inadequate capillary perfusion (Goldner and Eguro, 1973). The coexistence of pallor with cyanosis and rubor is consistent with vasoconstriction and subsequent vasodilatation (Porter, 1977).

The spectrum of causes of diminished blood flow is apparent when one notes the alterations that occur in the healthy extremity affected temporarily by decreased blood flow due to environmental alterations such as cooling of the hands, neck, or feet, contact of a digit with ice, reaction of a vasoconstricting pharmacologic agent such as epinephrine or ergot (Bancroft, Konzett, and Swan, 1951), or sympathetic nervous system stimulation from anxiety or fear.

In each instance, the occurrence of pallor and a significant drop in skin temperature will cause pain which is moderately severe and described as a deep, dull aching sensation. As the ischemic state persists, pain becomes more intense (Goldner and Eguro, 1973).

The term Raynaud's disease is used to describe the occurrence of vasospasm in the absence of an underlying primary disease. If vasospasm is associated with a known connective tissue disease, then Raynaud's phenomenon is implied. Recognition of a Raynaud's syndrome and the patient's response to this condition is important in explaining pain and cold tolerance associated with known pathologic conditions. When the symptoms of pain occur in a digit of the hand or in the entire extremity, the existence of adequate blood flow in the large and small vessels must be determined.

PATHOPHYSIOLOGY

The individual with no discernible lesion may demonstrate arterial spasm with pallor and pain. The pallor persists so long as there is an external or internal stimulus. Once the stimulus ceases, pallor lessens and the digit warms. Pain increases as long as there is spasm and decreases as vasodilatation occurs. An episode of Raynaud's phenomenon involving arterioles and arteries results in diminished or absent capillary perfusion. After several minutes of hypoxia, lactic acid accumulates, and the capillaries and venules dilate. A small amount of arterial blood enters the capillary bed as spasm diminishes, this blood is deoxygenated, and cyanosis occurs. Rubor depends on entrance of a small amount of blood into dilated capillaries. Other factors affecting blood flow are an abnormal response of the intrinsic vascular wall to cold, or increased activity of the sympathetic nervous system. Either or both may exist in addition to the possibility of certain patients having serum immunologic abnormalities which, through chemical mediators, influence vasoconstriction. This must occur through the sympathetic neuromuscular end-plate, since total pharmacologic blockade at this site with reserpine eliminates Raynaud's symptoms. The normal vasoconstrictive response to cold may be additive with underlying chronic vasoconstriction resulting in vascular wall tension exceeding intravascular pressure, the so-called critical closing pressure (Porter, 1977).

Isolated nerve compression lesions of the median or ulnar nerves at the wrist by the transverse retinacular ligament cause paresthesia and hypesthesia, with varying degrees of pain, and cold tolerance is usually affected, but the capillary closing pressure in the digit is usually not altered. Once pressure on the nerve is relieved, sensation improves, cold tolerance increases, the effect of cold on capillary constriction and dilatation is more consistent, and pain is diminished. Compression of the nerve affects the sympathetic fibers as well as the intrinsic vessels. If external compression does not exist but the blood supply to the nerve is affected by proximal spasm in the brachial artery (Bertho et al., 1969), the hand is cool and partially ischemic. The blood supply to both the nerve and to the digit is affected and cold tolerance is diminished.

Ulnar artery compression at the wrist may alter the lumen of the ulnar artery, causing diminished cold tolerance, slow capillary filling, cool digits, di-

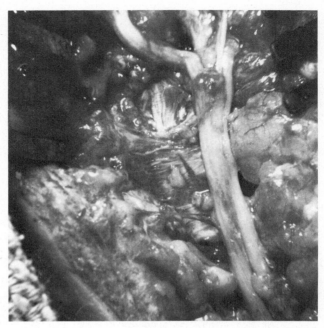

Figure 9–1   This patient had pain in the ulnar aspect of the hand due to ulnar artery thrombosis. The artery has been resected and the ulnar nerve is evident. Pain was due not only to occlusion of the artery but also to compression of the nerve in Guyon's canal. Combined vascular and neural involvement frequently account for pain syndromes not readily explained by involvement of either vessel or nerve alone.

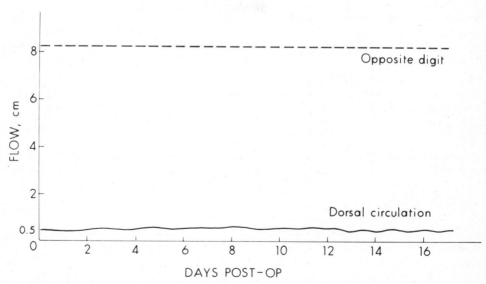

Figure 9–2   These data were obtained after examining the patient several months after laceration of both digital arteries, neither of which was repaired. Low flowmeter recordings indicated the minimal blood supply to the digit through the dorsal circulation in the intact skin flap. Cold tolerance was low, pain was intermittent and severe. Flowmeter studies and skin temperature readings were low and correlate with the occurrence of pain.

minished sensation, and a dull aching pain. Activity aggravates the pain. The cool digit warms up slowly and vasodilatation is slow (Goldner and Eguro, 1973) (Fig. 9–1).

Peripheral nerve trauma without associated extrinsic vascular injury causes sensory diminution and lessened cold tolerance in spite of the absence of trauma to the major vessels of the part. This implies that the influence of vascular tone by the peripheral nerve is altered after nerve trauma. This is clearly evident by observing the rapid onset of pain while the part is cooling and slow warmup time after cooling has occurred. Thus, pain includes at least two demonstrable factors: 1) that which occurs because of vasoconstriction and venous congestion, and 2) neural trauma causing dysesthesia, paresthesia, and hypesthesia (Fig. 9–1).

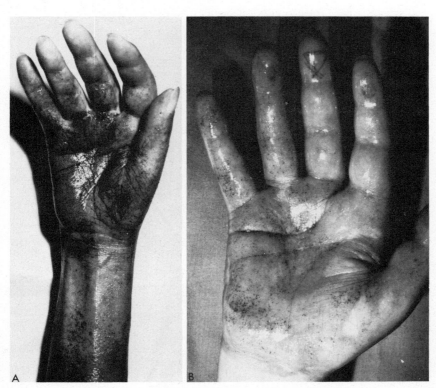

Figure 9–3 *A*, This patient's hand is being assessed by starch-oil-iodine sweat test several months after gunshot injury in the axilla. Severe impairment of blood flow occurred, the median nerve was lacerated, and the ulnar nerve was contused. At that time, the fingertips were dry, blanching was slow, and the hand was cool. All fingers and joints were fibrotic. The combination of vascular and nerve trauma affect the prognosis. Treatment required sympathectomy, bypass vein graft from axilla to elbow, median nerve repair, and ulnar neurolysis. *B*, Repeat starch-oil-iodine sweat test several months after blood supply had been improved by sympathectomy and vein graft, and median nerve and ulnar nerves were showing evidence of regeneration. The sweat test now shows improvement over the thumb, palm, and ring and little fingers, with absent sweating on the palmar surface of the index and long fingers. Improved circulation had resulted in less fibrosis, greater range of joint motion, and improved function of the hand. Thermogram test showed increased heat, pulse volume recording showed increased amplitude, skin temperature had increased comparatively, and Doppler flow studies showed improvement. Cold tolerance increased and pain had diminished.

A digit with known nerve and artery laceration has less cold tolerance than a digit affected by isolated nerve injury without vascular damage (Fig. 9–2). A digit with both nerves and both arteries lacerated is painful while cooling occurs, shows a rapid onset of pallor and cyanosis early in the cooling stage, and demonstrates a slow warmup time (Urbaniak, Seaber, and Bright, personal communication). Also, connective tissue thickens rapidly and fibrosis occurs relatively soon after the injury, particularly if vascular insufficiency is profound, even though the digit may be clinically viable (Fig. 9–3A and B).

Claudication of the extremity occurs after a major vessel is partially or completely obliterated and adds another dimension to the pain spectrum. Fig-

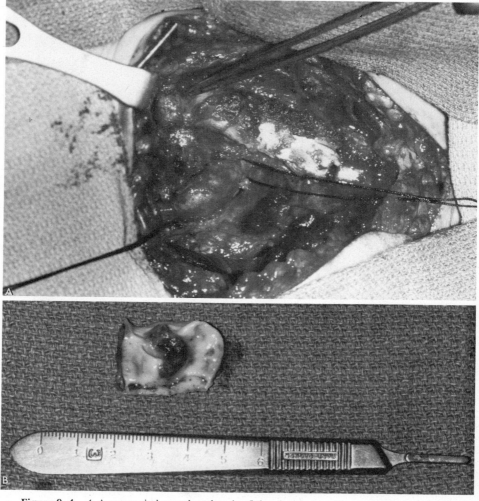

Figure 9–4 *A*, A congenital pseudoarthrosis of the clavicle in a 35-year-old male. The clavicle had been contusing the subclavian artery for many years and an aneurysm formed. *B*, The aneurysm, showing irregularity of the intima and media and expansion of the entire vessel. Emboli formed at this point and caused intermittent pain, pallor, and blanching of the hand. The vascular defect was excised and a Dacron graft was substituted.

ure 9–4*A* and *B* shows compression of the subclavian artery under a congenital pseudarthrosis of the clavicle. The patient was 35 years old. Claudication of the extremity necessitated resection and Dacron grafting in order to relieve pain (Young, 1978). The upper extremities usually tolerate diminished arterial blood flow better than do the lower because of the comparatively greater muscle mass in the lower limbs and the lesser work requirements of the upper limbs.

CLINICAL PAIN SYNDROMES RELATED TO ALTERED EXTREMITY ARTERIAL BLOOD FLOW

Tourniquet Test Model

Application of a pneumatic tourniquet to a normal extremity with pressure elevated to 300 mm. mercury will obliterate arterial inflow and venous outflow, slow motor nerve conduction, decrease sensory conduction, and cause severe pain in the hand and forearm, and at the site of tourniquet compression. Anoxia and nerve compression occur simultaneously, and muscle weakness is evident within three to five minutes. Digital paresthesias occur at the same time and sensation diminishes gradually to anesthesia in about 30 minutes. These painful sensations are a combination of muscle and nerve ischemia as well as nerve compression (Goldner, 1975, Goldner and Donahoo, 1960–78, unpublished data).

In patients known to have a pure nerve compression lesion, such as ulnar nerve compression at the elbow, posterior interosseous nerve compression in the supinator muscle, or median nerve compression at the wrist, diminished blood flow will cause abnormal sensory changes to occur earlier than would happen in the normal patient, and motor weakness occurs more quickly when partial or complete ischemia occurs.

Various conditions such as atherosclerotic stenosis, thromboembolism, or compression of major arteries in the thoracic outlet cause pain, claudication, paresthesias, and intermittent episodes of pallor. The lesions may be partial or complete, and the clinical symptoms vary according to the degree of ischemia. Examples are:

1. *Acute occlusion of the ulnar artery* is associated with unrelenting pain, pallor, and subsequent rubor and cyanosis. Cold tolerance is diminished, and intrinsic muscle weakness occurs (Silver, 1977) (see Fig. 9–1).

2. *Obliteration of the brachial artery* due to trauma and the occurrence of an anterior compartment compression of the forearm muscles, vessels, and nerves causes pallor of the hand, diminished pulse volume, and severe pain. The effect of diminished arterial inflow and lessened venous outflow on pain has been reasonably well calibrated by analyzing effects of traumatic lesions at various levels in the extremity. For example, decompression of a tight compartment anterior to the elbow and in the forearm will diminish pain almost immediately; elimination of nerve compression syndromes at the wrist and elbow will provide measurable relief of pain (Goldner and Eguro, 1973).

3. *Causalgia,* considered by this author to be a mixed nerve lesion

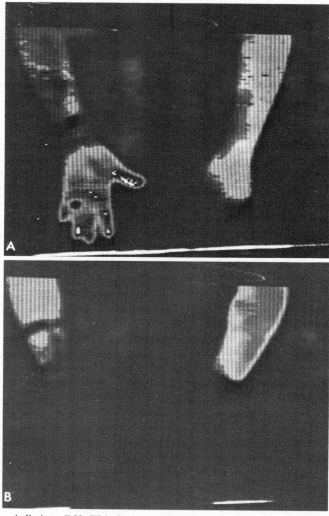

Figure 9–5 *A*, Patient C.H. This figure shows the thermograph recording after both hands were cooled for several minutes. The right hand, which had been injured, showed more rapid cooling than the left, the intensity of pain increased on the right, and pain persisted after the hands were warmed. Warm-up time was much slower on the injured right extremity and pain persisted for over an hour on the right after the cooling episode. *B*, Patient L. G. Thermogram recording showing comparative findings on the left (noninvolved) and right (injury resulted in median nerve laceration and radial artery laceration, mid forearm). Note the decreased emission of infrared from the hand. Other tests showed low pulse volume recordings, diminished Doppler recordings, and lowered skin temperature. After nerve repair and decompression, pain was diminished but vascular insufficiency persists. A bypass graft may be necessary; sympathectomy has increased blood flow and diminished the pain, at least temporarily.

with *accompanying or secondary vascular insufficiency,* is usually relieved by sympathectomy which affects peripheral blood flow. The residual pain may require direct treatment of the peripheral nerve (Mitchell, 1872; Goldner and Eguro, 1973; Silver, 1977) (Fig. 9–5*A* and *B*).

4. *Sympathetic dystrophy* is a part of the spectrum that may occur even though there is no particular nerve injury demonstrated. There is, however, a vasospastic element which occurs secondary to a major or minor insult of the

extremity or an adjacent organ. This improves with sympathetic blockade, although other forms of therapy may be necessary (Goldner et al., 1977). Such measures as intravenous reserpine (Porter, 1977), large doses of corticosteroids, and repetitive peripheral nerve block all cause diminution of pain, lessening of collagen tightness, and improved peripheral blood flow in addition to decreasing pain of neural origin because blood flow to the intrinsic vasa vasorum of the nerves is increased.

EXAMINATIONS FOR DETERMINING BLOOD FLOW AND ITS RELATIONSHIP TO COLD TOLERANCE

Clinical assessment of the hand requires detailed examination of the nail beds as to rapidity of recovery of color after pressure; the amount and color of blood that appears after puncturing the digit pulp; determination of flow through major arteries before and after exercise by the Allen test; assessment of the alterations that occur with arterial and venous tourniquet tests; and cold tolerance tests which affect blood flow as measured through a flowmeter as the skin temperature is lowered and then warmup time is observed. Techniques of determining diminished blood flow, whether mechanical or vasospastic, including the Piezo electric flowmeter (Fig. 9–6), skin thermometer read-

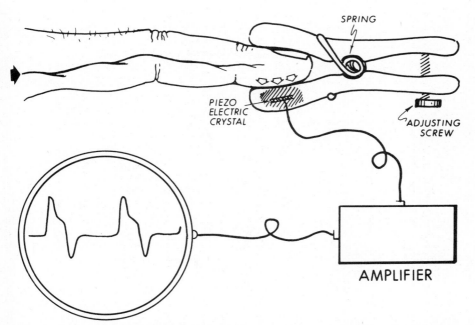

Figure 9–6 Diagram of pulse flow indicator. This apparatus is used to determine increase or decrease of blood flow. The piezoelectric crystal touches the pulp of the digit. Careful adjustment is necessary in order to obtain consistent and accurate readings. This apparatus, which is noninvasive, gives rapid information about blood flow and gives much information quickly in comparison to magnification angiography which requires more time, is a greater risk, and may not provide as much information. The flowmeter provided information about each patient with vascular impairment noted in Table 9–2.

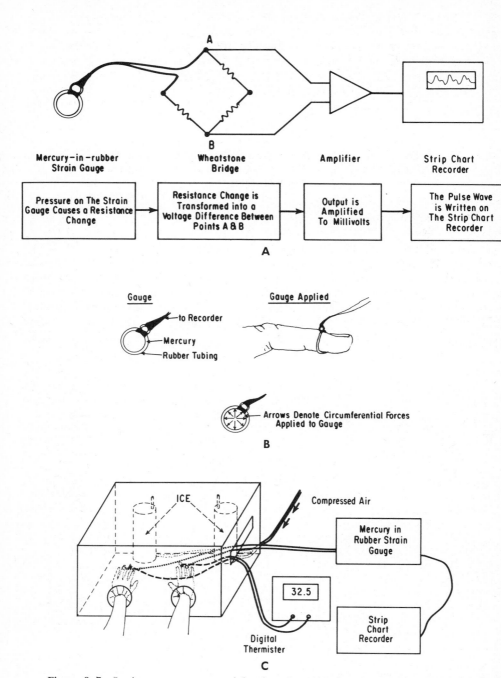

Figure 9–7 Strain gauge system used for detecting alterations in skin temperature in a digit during cooling and warmup. *A* shows the strain gauge, the voltage differences, the amplifier, and the strip recorder. *B* is a detailed diagram of the finger gauges. *C* shows the subject's hands in the cooling box with the strain gauges in place, the skin temperature readings, and the strip chart recorder.

Legend continued on the opposite page

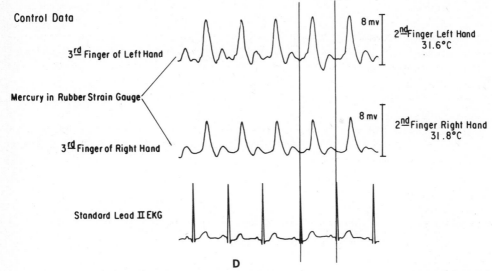

Figure 9–7 *(Continued)*   D, Data obtained prior to placing the hands in the cooling box, alternating from the third digit to the second digit, temperatures as indicated. These are ambient temperatures which are average for this patient. This temperature reading can be a baseline in determining diminished blood flow. If the temperature is less than 29° C, the blood flow is diminished critically.

ings, compartment pressure measurements with the wick catheter (a catheter with a Dexon wick read through a pressure transducer), and thermography (Fig. 9–5), all will provide direct or indirect information about blood flow. Magnification angiography with contrast and the use of intra-arterial vasodilators will also give information about the competence of major and minor blood vessels and data about the collateral circulation. If these studies are used both individually and as a group, important information will be derived that will document normal blood flow and the absence of pain originating from the vascular system as compared with inadequate blood flow associated with varying degrees of pain relieved partially by rest and aggravated by activity. It is possible to separate pain primarily due to nerve injury from pain originating within the vascular system. Combinations of the two are more difficult to differentiate.

Duke Diagnostic Hand Laboratory personnel have developed a technique using an environmental box for cooling (Fig. 9–7A to D) (Urbaniak, Seaber, and Bright). Temperature within the box is 10° C while the cold stress test is in progress. Eleven skin thermometers are used, one for each digit and one to measure the ambient temperature. Initially, mercury in rubber strain gauges are placed on the right and left long fingers and controlled readings are taken at room temperature. The subject's hands are then placed into the test box and remain there at 10° C for 20 minutes. Temperature readings are recorded, and strip chart recordings are made from the strain gauges. Finger pulp pressure is used to determine alterations in arterial blood flow. The data from this test will give information about the direct effect of external temperature on blood flow to the digits and the indirect effect of cooling elsewhere in the body (i.e., the neck or the trunk) as it might affect blood flow when the temperature in the box is ambient (Urbaniak, Seaber, and Bright, 1978).

Doppler Readings

As blood flows within blood vessels, sound waves occur and can be amplified (Fig. 9–8). The Doppler apparatus gives readings that can be qualitated and quantitated, both before and after vasodilation occurs. Subjective pain complaints may then be correlated with the alterations in blood flow. The Doppler flowmeter will provide information about the presence or absence of blood flow within arteries and veins. A blood pressure cuff is used as a tourniquet in both the upper and lower extremities for quantitation of flow at different pressures. Certain critical pressures causing ischemia will be associated with pain.

Pulse Volume Recorder

The pulse volume flowmeter measures the height of the pulse wave and is affected by blood flow (Urbaniak, Seaber, and Bright, 1978).

Skin Thermometer

A surface temperature gauge is used to measure skin temperature, to compare it with ambient temperature and to correlate these with peripheral blood flow. Pain may or may not be a subjective symptom as skin temperature diminishes. The sympathetic nervous system does affect blood flow. Patients who have undergone replantation of a digit or hand show peripheral blood flow to be affected by nicotine, anxiety, thorazine, or physical and emotional changes associated with removal of the dressings. Alterations of blood flow are measured by the flowmeter or skin thermometer. Sympathetic blockade (Fig. 9–9) once or twice each 24 hours with a long-acting anesthetic causes increased blood flow through a patent digital vessel and improves arterial input

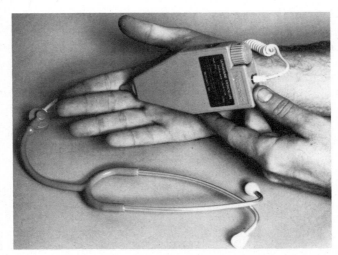

Figure 9–8 Doppler flow studies aid in determining blood flow in an artery or vein. An ultrasound beam is emitted from the ceramic crystal coupled to the skin with a gel with the beam passing through the underlying blood vessel. Ultrasound is reflected from red cells in the blood vessel and is shifted in frequency by an amount proportional to the flow velocity of the red cells.

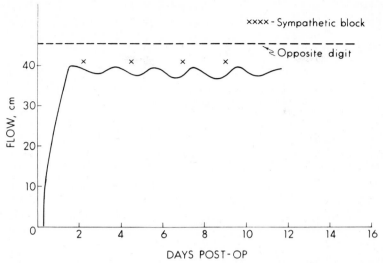

Figure 9–9   Chart showing summary of blood flow measurements after repair of both arteries and improvement in blood flow associated with sympathetic block. Information such as this has correlated with viability of the digit after trauma. In the patient with vascular insufficiency from other causes, pain may be related to lessened blood flow and the information is determined in the same way.

sufficiently to improve viability of the digit. Pain is usually not a problem (Urbaniak, Seaber, and Bright). However, patients who have had arterial injury not repaired, and diminished blood flow as documented by flowmeter readings, will have persistent pain associated with cold and will usually not show improved peripheral flow even after several years (Fig. 9–2). If both digital arteries have been lacerated and neither repaired, time alone will result in somewhat better nutrition to the digit, but the measurable circulation by flowmeter, Doppler, and cold tolerance test will not change (Gelberman et al., 1978). If a large dorsal skin flap is present and both arteries are lacerated, the digit will remain viable but years later, blood flow will be diminished significantly and cold tolerance will be less (Goldner and Eguro, 1973). Those digits which have had both arteries and veins repaired show peripheral flow to normal levels, high cold tolerance, and minimal if any pain with cold exposure (Gelberman et al., 1978).

Table 9–1 gives a pattern showing the relationship between blood flow in the digit, cold tolerance, and the occurrence of pain.

Table 9–1

BLOOD FLOW	COLD TOLERANCE
Blood flow normal Pain, none	⟷ Cold tolerance normal
Blood flow diminished Pain increased	⟷ Cold tolerance down
Nerve laceration Pain increased	⟷ Cold tolerance down
Nerve intact Pain, none	⟷ Cold tolerance normal

Various combinations of blood vessel and nerve injury will show alterations of cold tolerance consistent with the observations made when each individual structure is affected by trauma.

PAIN SYNDROMES RELATED TO UPPER EXTREMITY BLOOD FLOW

Eighty-two patients with chronic pain syndromes after neurovascular injuries were tested for extremity blood flow. Sympathetic nerve block and peripheral nerve block increased blood flow and decreased pain. After the nerve block had worn off, the intensity of the remaining pain was less if increase in blood flow persisted. If the blood flow progressed to the original post-injury condition, pain reappeared. Also, patients who had evidence of chronic vasospasm associated with a chronic pain syndrome, as in reflex sympathetic dystrophy, usually showed decreased blood flow affected by nicotine and anxiety and increased pain.

Data obtained by use of the pulse volume flowmeter indicated that 63 of the 82 patients showed diminished peripheral blood flow of at least 30 per cent and the majority of these patients showed diminution over 50 per cent, while a small number showed diminution of blood flow at 90 per cent. Eighteen of the 63 patients received sympathetic nerve blocks, and 14 of the 18 showed significant increase in blood flow to the involved digits, which approximated that to the uninvolved digits. Pain was consistently decreased while the blockade was effective. This was interpreted as being associated not only with improved blood flow but also an indirect effect of the anesthetic on the pain fibers in the brachial plexus. However, paravertebral blocks in the lower extremity showed vasodilation and warming of the extremity with diminution of pain when the anesthetic was placed around the lumbar sympathetics and not around the lumbosacral plexus.

PATIENT EXAMPLES

1. A 42-year-old mechanic experienced severe chronic pain along the ulnar aspect of the hand. In his occupation, he frequently used the hand as a "hammer." The Allen compression test showed absent blood flow in the ulnar artery and compression tenderness along the course of the artery. Doppler readings showed no flow in the ulnar artery at the wrist (see Fig. 9–1). Flowmeter studies of the little finger showed 50 per cent diminished blood flow as compared with the opposite normal digit. At operation, the artery was thrombosed and enlarged. The ulnar canal was full. The ulnar artery was decompressed and the thrombosed segment of the vessel was excised; no vein graft was used, as in our experience vein grafts in this setting have not been successful. Collateral circulation was increased significantly after segmental resection.

2. A 60-year-old male was examined initially because of pain and bluish discoloration of the ring and little fingers of one hand. The pain pattern

extended from the mid forearm to the fingertips. Viability of the digits was questionable. After a stellate ganglion block was done, pain diminished considerably and the entire hand became pink. Diagnosis was thrombosis of the ulnar artery. At operation, the artery was found to be sclerotic and clotted, and was resected. A vein graft was attempted, but clotting occurred during the procedure and it was removed. Postoperatively, the hand was pink and warm, and pain had been eliminated. A year later, the hand showed a full range of motion, satisfactory peripheral blood flow, and no claudication. This patient demonstrated the same findings made in others when angiography was done, and showed adequate collateral circulation in spite of thrombosis of the ulnar artery. There is a wide individual variation in collateral circulation. Flowmeter studies in this instance improved to about 80 per cent of normal and all pain was relieved.

3. A 47-year-old female fell and fractured the distal end of the radius. The fracture was manipulated and a cast applied prior to our examination. When first seen, she complained of hand pain, numbness along the usual course of the median nerve, coolness of the hand, and limited finger motion. Nerve conduction studies showed conduction over the median nerve to be slow. The radial and ulnar pulses were palpable and were not affected by the compression test. Flowmeter studies, however, showed blood flow in the injured hand to be decreased by about 30 per cent as compared with the uninjured hand. Pain increased when the extremity was elevated and when it was cooled. A Xylocaine injection into the confines of the carpal canal was done and in 20 minutes the flowmeter studies were repeated. During this time, pain was relieved, partial loss of sensation occurred, the skin temperature increased 2° C. as compared to the opposite hand, and blood flow as measured by the pulse volume recorder was 150 per cent greater than prior to the injection. We interpret this as an effect on sympathetic nerve fibers, as the injection was done in the canal near the median nerve and only 1 cc of anesthetic agent was used. We believe that there is a direct relationship between median nerve compression, diminished blood flow, and the occurrence of sympathetic dystrophy and the associated fibrosis. Several patients have shown diminished blood flow associated with progressive fibrosis.

Decompression of the median nerve was done shortly after the initial examination, and the patient continues to show improved peripheral blood flow, improved motor and sensory nerve conduction, and diminished pain.

4. A 16-year-old male received a laceration anterior to the elbow joint with interruption of the brachial artery and partial laceration of the median nerve. The attending physician ligated the artery and repaired the nerve. The patient's major complaint several weeks after the initial injury was pain in the forearm and hand. Flowmeter studies showed low amplitude, with the recording measuring 0.5 cm in height. A sympathetic block resulted in dramatic improvement in flowmeter readings up to 12 cm. Pain was relieved after the block and repeat blocks showed the same pre- and post-block readings. A sympathectomy was done and pain was relieved. The differential diagnosis includes consideration of (a) diminished blood flow associated with interruption of a major artery and inadequate collateral circulation; (b) diminished blood flow associated with excessive vasospasm due to sympathetic nervous system overactivity; (c) diminished blood flow due to increased compartment

pressure associated with trauma or a large muscle mass. In this instance, (a) and (b) accounted for the diminished blood flow and pain.

5. A 36-year-old male received a 12 gauge shotgun wound to the right axilla. A segmental loss of the axillary artery occurred and the median nerve was interrupted in the upper third of the arm. The surgeons who attended the patient initially inserted a saphenous vein graft about 8 cm long and restored a palpable radial pulse. We saw the patient two weeks after the injury, at which time he demonstrated anesthesia in the autonomous zone of the median nerve, a fair radial pulse, and a moderate amount of deep, dull, aching pain in the extremity. Cooling was unpleasant. The hand showed minimal tightness of the joints. During the next six weeks, the volume of the radial pulse diminished and eventually was absent, skin temperature dropped, the hand became cooler, and dysesthesias and paresthesias along the course of the separated median nerve persisted. The pain pattern was one of *causalgia* and was associated with a nerve injury, with the ends of the nerve being fibrosed severely, and a gradual diminution of blood flow. As the pulse diminished and time passed, the hand became more fibrotic (see Fig. 9–3*A*). A median nerve repair was done and a gap of 6 cm was bridged by adducting the humerus, flexing the elbow, and mobilizing the nerve. The vein graft was carrying a minimal amount of blood and had almost stopped functioning. The incision extended down to the wrist so that the anterior compartment of the forearm could be decompressed. After the nerve repair, pain was diminished, anesthesia persisted as expected, but there was less paresthesia and dysesthesia. Blood flow was not altered. About three months after the nerve repair, there was a sudden increase in severe pain, radial pulse was completely gone, and pulse volume recorder readings showed loss of amplitude. Arteriogram was done and showed the vein graft to be completely obliterated with only minimal collateral circulation distally. A bypass graft was done from the mid-arm to the wrist across the elbow joint. Postoperatively the hand was warm, the pain diminished, and the stiffness lessened over a period of eight weeks. Currently, two years later, the patient has recognition of heat and cold, touch, sharp and dull, showing adequate protective sensation. Stereognosis and two point discrimination were not yet recovered, although sweating was returning (see Fig. 9–3*B*). Motor power in the flexor digitorum profundi was good, cold tolerance was improved, and hand function had improved.

Other methods of diminishing the patient's pain during this two and a half year period included use of a stretch nylon glove at night and during exposure to air conditioning or cool weather, oral isoxsuprine HCl (Vasodilan) occasionally when episodes of pain became quite severe, and use of a bias-cut stockinette wrap at night in order to flex the fingers, place the thumb opposite the long finger and keep the fingers in a relatively flexed position. Ethyl chloride spray to the hypersensitive area of the nerve repair or to the sensitive areas along the medial antebrachial cutaneous distribution decreased pain temporarily for a few hours and allowed the patient to accept the syndrome with less anxiety. The patient was provided with a can of plastic spray and if hypersensitive skin areas occurred he was to spray the skin with the resin and thereby diminish external stimuli. He was also given chloral hydrate at night and doxepin HCl (Sinequan) for his intermittent reactive depression. This patient with *causalgia* responded to mobilization and suture of the median nerve and improvement in peripheral blood flow by bypass vein graft. A sympathectomy had been done prior to repair of the median nerve, with improvement for several weeks but with gradual return of pain as blood flow diminished. The vein graft provided sufficient improvement in blood flow during a period of several months that severity of pain was diminished, stiffness of the fingers was decreased, and nerve regeneration proceeded in a satisfactory way. We believe that this *causalgic* syndrome was directly related to both nerve damage and diminished blood flow.

6. A 38-year-old woman complained of bilateral foot pain. She had noted burning and tingling and uncomfortable feelings while walking. In addition to the paresthesias and dysesthesias, she could not tolerate air conditioning or cool weather without extra clothing on the feet. She had been operated upon on two occasions for posterior tibial nerve decompression, although preoperative nerve conduction studies were normal and no evidence of tenosynovitis existed. Our clinical examination showed cool feet, there was increased pain with walking and tiptoeing, and flowmeter studies showed a significant diminution in digital pulse volume in both feet. External cooling diminished the blood flow. A sympathetic nerve block was done and the feet became palpably warmer almost immediately and this was accompanied by increased flowmeter

Table 9–2   Pain Syndromes Related to Diminished Blood Flow With or Without Peripheral Nerve Injury

NAME	CLINICAL HISTORY	FLOWMETER STUDIES	RESULT
T.S.	GSW brachial artery median and ulnar nerve trauma	Normal side 32 cm Injured side 0.5 cm	Sympathectomy with noticeable increase in blood flow; pain diminished 70%
A.S.	Fractured thumb, subsequent development of "dystrophy"	Prior to sympathetic block 3.0 cm After block 10.0 cm	Relief of symptoms after each block; total of three blocks
A.H.	GSW brachial area vascular injury and brachial plexus trauma	Injured side 0.5 cm Normal side 3.5 cm	After sympathectomy, flow increased to 10 cm, major symptoms relieved for prolonged period of time (Fig. 9–10)
C.C.	Trauma to left index finger, "dystrophic" hand	Injured side — left 1 cm Normal side — right 10 cm	Improved by sympathetic blocks; continued to have moderate cold intolerance and a palpably cool digit
P.B.	Crush injury to left hand; injury to radial and ulnar arches	Left 0.2 cm Right 2.0 cm (ten times different)	Clinical findings of insufficient arterial circulation; flow studies showed severe decrease in peripheral flow, left hand. Patient not ready for operative reconstruction. Arteriography — occlusion of both major vessels. Proposed plan: reanastomosis or graft of one major vessel.
G.S.	Incomplete amputation, upper extremity; ulnar artery ligated, radial artery repaired	70% of noninjured side; Radial artery palpable	Cold tolerance good; minimal pain; ulnar nerve intact
K.N.	Punch press injury; digital vessels not repaired	No flow in index No flow in long 40% normal flow in ring	Dry gangrene of index finger distal to PIP joint, and long finger distal to PIP joint. Ring finger survived.
T.P.	Claudication lower extremities	Baseline 2.0 cm. in involved extremity at rest; exercise resulted in decreased flow to 0.25 cm.	Pain associated with diminished flow which occurred within 10 minutes after onset of exercise pain
M.L.	Lumbosacral discectomy; postoperative sympathetic dystrophy, right lower extremity, cool, burning, and painful	Normal 16 cm Affected 4 cm	Paravertebral blocks improved pain

recordings. After the sympathetic block, her pain was relieved completely and the burning was much less noticeable. She was give a course of decreasing doses of corticosteroids to supplement the sympathetic nerve blocks. Over a period of three months, her pain was relieved sufficiently to allow her to return to work. One year later, her feet were painless, she was working full time and, although her feet still got cold when the environment cooled, they were not painful.

We consider this patient's problem to be one of vasospasm of sufficient intensity to involve the peripheral vessels and the peripheral nerves. As blood flow improved, pain decreased.

Table 9–2 provides a brief history of patients with pain syndromes, of flowmeter studies providing data related to diminished blood flow, and of the results of treatment directed toward improving peripheral circulation. The findings of diminished blood flow are consistently related to varying degrees of pain syndromes.

HELPFUL TREATMENT METHODS IN PAIN SYNDROMES RELATED TO DECREASED BLOOD FLOW

1. Warm environment; eliminate nicotine; diminish caffeine; alleviate anxiety as much as possible.

2. Peripheral nerve block for immediate relief of pain and for vasodilation. Peripheral perfusion with a long-acting anesthetic agent through a polyethylene tube or silicone tube (Chapter 15).

3. Stellate ganglion blocks, repeated three to five times; lumbar sympathetic blocks, three to five times; differential spinal block using the appropriate dosage to obtain sympathetic blockade (Figs. 9–10 and 9–11); epidural anesthetic block.

4. Graduated, decreasing doses of oral steroids for one week, beginning with 40 mg daily and diminishing the dose to 5 mg on the last day. Follow this by anti-inflammatory medication; supplement with intravenous reserpine.

5. Graduated exercise activity for both the upper and lower extremities as a permanent program.

6. Decompression of peripheral nerve; or decompression of tight compartments after testing with the wick catheter or with exercise, or both.

Occasionally, compartmental pain is due to intimal damage which requires resection of the blood vessels.

7. Segmental arterial resection and resuture or vein grafting or replacement with Dacron graft (see Fig. 9–4A and B) (Young, 1978).

8. Sympathectomy; cervicodorsal or lumbar.

9. Peripheral nerve block or intra-articular xylocaine. Pain within or around the shoulder, or another joint, may be caused by intra-articular or extra-articular pathology, or a combination of both. A xylocaine anesthetic block of the suprascapular nerve will diminish pain originating from within the joint and to a lesser degree pain that comes from a fibrous capsule outside the joint; and intra-articular injection of steroid and xylocaine will give infor-

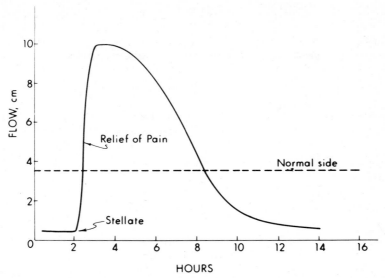

Figure 9-10   This graph shows the low blood flow in a patient who has a chronic pain syndrome after a brachial plexus injury in which the axillary artery was damaged. After the stellate block was done, the measurable improvement in blood flow was almost immediate. Relief of pain occurred as the flow increased significantly. The patient had relief for several hours with a long-acting local anesthetic. Pain recurred in about the same intensity at 14 hours and persisted until vascular insufficiency was improved.

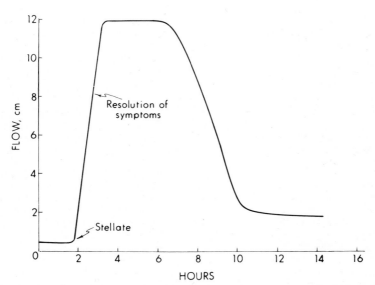

Figure 9-11   This graph demonstrates arterial insufficiency. The diminished blood flow was directly related to activity pain. As the patient performed muscle action, claudication occurred. A stellate block increased blood flow significantly and claudication symptoms were temporarily absent within 30 minutes after the blockade. Pain was completely relieved for two to three hours while the hand was warm. As blood flow diminished, the claudication symptoms gradually recurred. Sympathectomy may give partial relief and a by-pass graft should be considered.

mation about joint pain due to articular change and synovitis, as it will not affect capsular contracture as readily as will the nerve block.

10. Cover painful areas of prior nerve injury with protective plastic caps or protective external covers to prevent repetitive trauma to the suture site of the nerve in the involved hand.

11. Transcutaneous nerve stimulation may improve peripheral blood flow.

12. Electrical stimulation by a microimplant on the peripheral nerve may diminish peripheral vascular spasm and may increase blood flow.

13. Pharmacological agents given orally or intra-arterially or intravenously with double tourniquet technique. Reserpine 3 to 5 mg is helpful for two to three months.

14. Biofeedback techniques may diminish vasospasm in patients who have nonspecific labile syndromes (Wilgis, 1977).

REFERENCES

Bancroft, H., Konzett, H., and Swan, H. J. C.: Observations on the action of the hydrogenated alkaloids of the ergotoxin group on the circulation in man. J. Physiol. *112*:273, 1951.

Bertho, E., Rattle, J., Jean-De-Dieu, J., and Gagnon, J. C.: Iatrogenic ergotism. Report of a case. Angiology *20*:455, 1969.

Gelberman, R. H., Urbaniak, J. R., Bright, D. S., and Levin, L. S.: Digital sensibility following replantation. J. Hand Surg. *3(4)*:313, 1978.

Goldner, J. L.: Volkmann's ischemic contracture. *In* Flynn, J. E. (ed.): Hand Surgery. 2nd ed., Baltimore, Williams & Wilkins, 1975.

Goldner, J. L., and Donahoo, S.: The effect of the tourniquet and intravenous lidocaine, clinical observations, 400 patients, 1960–1978. (Unpublished data.)

Goldner, J. L., and Eguro, H.: Bilateral thrombosis of the ulnar arteries in the hands, Case Reports. Plast. & Reconstr. Surg. *52*:573, 1973.

Goldner, J. L., Gould, J. S., Urbaniak, J. R., and McCollum, D. E.: Metacarpophalangeal joint arthroplasty with silicone-Dacron prostheses, Niebauer type, six and a half years experience. J. Hand Surg. *2(3)*:200, 1977.

Hill, G., Moeliono, J., Tumewu, F., Brataamadja, D., and Tohardi, A.: The Buerger syndrome in Java. Br. J. Surg. *60*:606, 1973.

Mitchell, S. W.: Injuries of the Nerves and Their Consequences. Philadelphia, J. B. Lippincott Co., 1872.

Porter, J. N.: Raynaud's syndrome. *In*: Sabiston, D. C., Jr. (ed.): Davis-Christopher Textbook of Surgery. Philadelphia, W. B. Saunders Co., 1977, p. 1982.

Silver, D.: Circulatory problems of the upper extremity. *In* Sabiston, D. C., Jr. (ed): Davis–Christopher Textbook of Surgery. Philadelphia, W. B. Saunders Co., 1977, p. 1985.

Stirrat, C. R., Seaber, A. V., Urbaniak, J. R., and Bright, D. S.: Temperature monitoring in digital replantation. J. Hand Surg. *3(4)*:342, 1978.

Urbaniak, J. R., Seaber, A. V., and Bright, D. S.: Mercury-in-rubber, strain gauge system for cold stress studies. Personal communication, Duke Hand Examination Laboratory, 1978.

Venters, W. B., Clippinger, F. W., Goodrich, J., Green, N., Ogden, W. S., and Goldner, J. L.: Thermography: Its uses in orthopaedics. Duke University and Affiliated Institutions Orthopaedic Training Program Papers, June 1972.

Wilgis, S.: Personal communication, 1977.

Young, W. G.: Personal communication, 1978.

10

PAINFUL NEUROMAS

RICHARD G. EATON

Symptomatic neuromas are a frequent cause of major hand disability. Of the sequelae of nerve division, the development of a painful neuroma is frequently more disabling than the resulting sensory deficit. This is increasingly true the more distal the lesion. A single digital neuroma on the volar pressure surface of the finger or palm, or a neuroma of the superficial sensory branch of either the median, ulnar, or radial nerves, undergoing tension with wrist or finger motion, is capable of completely disabling an otherwise normal hand or arm. In 1874 Weir Mitchell observed in a patient with a longstanding irreparable median nerve injury that the relief of pain was so gratifying following neuroma resection and transposition that the sensory deficit was readily accepted. (Mitchell, 1874).

Formation of a neuroma is actually a physiologic but usually abortive attempt at spontaneous axon repair. Immediately following axon interruption there is a latent or shock period during which time the nerve cell body adjusts to the loss of a remote portion of its axioplasm. The level of interruption (the more proximal, the greater the loss of axioplasm) and the nature of the trauma (crush, avulsion or sharp laceration), influence the duration of this latent period. The central limb of the divided axon trunk undergoes wallerian degeneration to the level of the next proximal node of Ranvier. As the cell body recovers, the axon stumps begin to elongate distally in a random, primitive attempt to restore continuity to the nerve trunk. In order to compensate for the detached distal segment a large number of Schwann cells appear, serving to provide supernumerary Schwann cell ensheathment in an attempt to conduct budding axon fibers through the disorganized scar. A few such axons may penetrate beyond the capsule. Once through the capsule these branch in many directions in an effort to find a distal Schwann tube (Spencer 1974).

Fortunately, relatively few neuromas become symptomatic. The vagaries of neuroma formation are such that similar nerve trunks sectioned at the same level in the same patient will develop neuromas of varying sizes and symptomatology (Fig. 10–1). Apparently, local tissue factors, anoxia, foreign material, or infected or necrotic tissue at each specific neuroma site play an important role in formation and symptomatology.

195

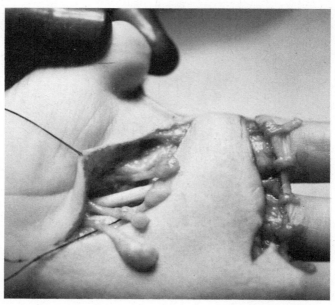

Figure 10–1   Multiple neuromas in the same patient. The varied reaction of each individually transected branch of the median nerve at the same level is not well understood.

CLASSIFICATION OF NEUROMAS

Neuromas can be classified into three distinct anatomic types*

I *Amputation neuromas:* These result from section through a nerve trunk and all adjacent tissue at a single level, the nerve stump lying in an injured composite tissue bed. Such form a terminal bulb neuroma.

II *Terminal branch neuromas:* These result from isolated section of one of the distal ramifications of a peripheral nerve trunk. Since these involve terminal arborizing sensory branches, the injury may intially be unrecognized or considered too small or too difficult to mobilize for repair. Such nerves also form terminal bulb neuromas.

III *Neuroma-in-continuity.* These result from partial division of a nerve trunk. With these lesions, the involved cross-sectional area will contain normal axons as well as intertwining regenerated axons and glial tissue. Grossly, this forms a fusiform or nodular enlargement of the intact nerve trunk.

Treatment of these neuroma types will be considered separately.

TREATMENT

Primary Care

Since the formation of a neuroma is a physiologic consequence of nerve injury, it is inevitable that, unless an accurate primary repair of the nerve is

*Only mixed and sensory neuromas will be considered, since it is these which become symptomatic.

performed, some degree of hypertrophy and scar encapsulation will develop at the site of injury. Though complete elimination of neuroma formation is not yet possible, it is possible to mechanically modify neuroma formation by controlling the environment in which the neuroma forms. Neuromas forming in the primary wound cicatrix are much more likely to become symptomatic than those forming in minimally scarred, well vascularized tissue. Bunnell observed that symptomatic neuromas were relatively rare during World War II because of the widespread practice of staged amputations (Bunnell, 1956). Primary guillotine amputations were performed, with subsequent revisions that permitted the revised nerve stump to retract into a minimally scarred tissue bed. He felt that infection during healing and excessive wound cicatrix were the major causes of painful neuroma (Bunnell 1956).

Optimum primary care of an amputation stump or of an irreparable nerve laceration will markedly decrease the incidence of symptomatic neuromas. The goal of primary care therefore is to provide the best possible tissue bed for the sectioned nerve end to rest as the obligatory neuroma forms. Extensive published reports of elaborate chemical and mechanical treatment modalities have shown them to be unpredictable or to have little documented value in management of freshly divided nerves (Snyder, 1961).

Technique

Type 1 — Amputation Neuroma

The amputation stump is carefully debrided and the involved nerves identified. Just prior to closure or resurfacing, the nerve is dissected free, and, with gentle traction applied, a sharp atraumatic re-section is performed as proximally as possible, permitting the nerve to retract into clean, well vascularized soft tissue. Small adjacent vessels, such as digital arteries, should be left undisturbed. To further ensure a pain-free stump there should be no tension in the final closure or resurfacing. Tension produces anoxia with increased wound induration and subsequent fibrosis.

Type 2 — Terminal Branch Neuroma

The key factor in treatment of an isolated irreparable nerve laceration is early recognition of the anatomic disruption. In any laceration that overlies a known superficial nerve trunk, a sensory deficit *must* be ruled out before local anesthesia is administered for wound closure. Sharply divided sensory nerve trunks greater than 3 millimeters in diameter can be satisfactorily repaired using gross or loupe-assisted visualization, and are the least likely to develop painful symptoms. Primary repair is indicated for those nerves that are particularly difficult to mobilize and approximate once they have healed in a retracted position. Most noteworthy are the dorsal branch of the ulnar nerve, the superficial radial sensory nerve in the wrist, and the sural nerve in the foot. Repair of these intermediate sized nerves is intended to prevent or reduce painful sequelae more than to restore sensibility.

Divided sensory nerves *less* than 3 millimeters in diameter may be more difficult to diagnose because of the smaller sensory deficit. In clean, sharp wounds they may spontaneously retract from the area of wound cicatrix and form asymptomatic neuroma. Prior to closure of the skin, a limited search for the proximal stump is justified, and if the suspected branch can be identified it should be drawn distally, sharply resected, and allowed to retract. The same retraction technique should be used for small sensory branches that must be sacrificed during surgical exposure. Excessive traction on the nerve should be avoided, since intraneural axon ruptures can produce linear microneuromas, which are particularly difficult to treat.

The proximal retraction technique is also applicable to intermediate sized sensory or mixed nerves that have suffered severe crush lacerations, or those that are badly frayed and likewise considered irreparable.

Type 3 — Neuroma-in-Continuity

Partial division of a peripheral nerve is particularly difficult to diagnose. Fortunately, in the larger mixed nerves, owing to neuropraxia, the acute deficit is usually proportionately greater than that which would be expected for the actual number of axons interrupted. Local anoxia, hemorrhage, or compression may contribute to this phenomenon. Such partial lacerations therefore are usually recognized, and exploration and appropriate repair carried out.

In intermediate or smaller trunks, the deficit is smaller and may be overlooked. *There is no other situation in the management of peripheral nerve injuries in which an accurate anatomic diagnosis is more crucial than in partial nerve division.* Proper treatment requires exploration and repair within 3 to 4 days, before axonal architecture and orientation have become obscured by the fibrin, clot, and granulation tissue that rapidly fill the defect in the trunk. Subsequent repair, even assisted by the operating microscope, is less satisfactory in such an edematous, distorted segment, and the risk of injury to the intact fascicles is considerable.

Secondary Care

The treatment of established painful neuromas requires patient and skillful exercise of the art of medicine. Early recognition and treatment are essential, since establishment of a fixed reflex pain pattern triggered by painful neuromas may be extremely difficult to reverse. Once established, the reflex pattern may persist even when the neuroma has been anesthetized or otherwise rendered asymptomatic.

Historically, well over 100 physical or chemical modalities have been proposed for treatment of painful neuroma (Snyder, 1961). Such multiplicity should suggest the obvious lack of a satisfactory treatment method. Since 1880, when Gluck first embedded the transected nerve stump in decalcified bone (Gluck, 1880), all procedures invariably include initial *resection* of the symptomatic neuroma, followed by specific mechanical or chemical modification of the remaining stump in an effort to alter inevitable neuroma reformation. All such techniques, therefore, are subject to much the same intrinsic vagaries in healing as those that resulted in development of symptoms in the initial neuroma. Though techniques produce initial immediate relief in symptoms, within 4 to 10 weeks a significant number of these patients will experience recurrence of symptoms as the second neuroma forms. Tupper, in a recent comparison of surgical treatments of painful neuromas from all causes, found only 34 per cent painless or minimally tender operative sites following the first neurectomy. Those undergoing a second neurectomy achieved only 38 per cent painless or minimally tender operative sites. Those undergoing second neurectomy plus silicone capping following unsatisfactory initial simple neurectomy achieved only 25 per cent painless or minimally tender operative sites (Tupper and Booth, 1976).

A completely different surgical approach to the painful neuroma has been successful for the author. This technique is based upon making every effort to keep the primary neuroma *intact* within its mature encapsulating scar, and atraumatically transposing it en bloc to an adjacent proximal area that is free of scar and less exposed to trauma. By this technique four out of five painful amputation neuromas and two out of three terminal branch neuromas were rendered symptom free in a series of predominantly Workmen's Compensation patients. Seventy-two per cent had absent to mild sensitivity at the point of relocation and 28 per cent had no sensitivity (Herndon, Eaton, and Littler, 1976).

Technique

Type 1 — Amputation Neuroma

Under tourniquet hemostasis the neuroma with its fibrous capsule is atraumatically isolated and mobilized on its proximal trunk. A proximal adjacent area that is free of scar and away from local pressure or trauma is selected. Optimal sites are the dorsal web space within or deep to muscle, and between metacarpal shafts. A dorsal site is preferable to a volar, where the neuroma may be subjected to direct trauma by manual activity such as gripping tools.

The neuroma, in continuity with its nerve stalk, is carefully dissected proximally until the neuroma bulb can be transferred to this optimal relocation site without tension. When a bifurcation is encountered, such as the dorsal sensory branch of a digital nerve, careful teasing of this filament from the main branch using optical loupe assistance, will permit full mobilization. Care must be taken to leave the adjacent digital vessels undisturbed. A 5-0 catgut suture is placed through the capsule (not the neuroma) and tied. The free ends of the suture are passed through a subcutaneous tunnel to the relocation site and then out through the skin proximal to this site. The neuroma is then drawn proximally into this location by traction on these sutures. The free ends are sutured loosely to the skin, leaving subcutaneous fat between the neuroma capsule and the skin (Fig. 10–2). Superficial positioning of the neuroma or fixation to the skin are complications that have an unfavorable influence on the final result. Before closure the nerve trunk is inspected to be certain that it is completely free of tension. The most common cause of failure in this procedure is displacement of the relocated neuroma from rebound due to residual tension in the proximal stalk as the catgut suture resorbs.

It is important to recognize that hypersensitive neuroma is but *one* of the causes of amputation stump pain. Following acute amputation there is a silent

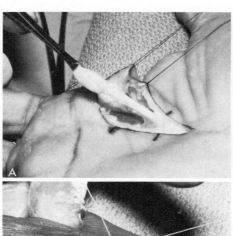

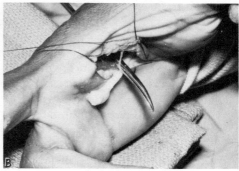

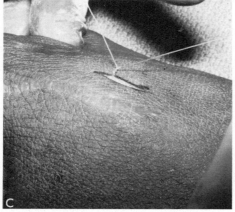

Figure 10–2 Technique for transposing a painful neuroma. *A*, Atraumatic dissection of the encapsulated mature neuroma. There must be adequate proximal mobilization of the stalk so that relocation within or dorsal to the interosseous muscle can be accomplished without tension. *B*, A tract is created through which the neuroma can be passed to the selected site. *C*, A fine, absorbable suture is used to pass the neuroma. When satisfactorily positioned, this traction suture is fixed to the skin, allowing a layer of muscle or subcutaneous tissue to be interposed between the neuroma capsule and the skin.

period of 3 to 6 weeks before the neuroma forms. Immediate and early diffuse stump pain is more likely due to ischemia, flap tension, low grade infection, or traumatic edema in the stump. With resolution of the wound induration, much or all of this pain and sensitivity will subside. At this point, however, patients developing symptomatic neuroma will experience a change in the character of the pain. The new pain has a burning characteristic and becomes more localized. In a small area, such as a finger amputation stump, localization of a radial or ulnar digital neuroma is not always possible. However, unless one is completely certain that only a single proper digital nerve is involved, both neuromas should be transplanted. In digits with diffuse dysesthesia yet having one obviously palpable and sensitive neuroma, experience has shown that following transfer of this obvious neuroma, the remaining neuroma produces equally disabling hypersensitivity. A differential diagnosis can often be made following careful anesthetic infiltration of the proximal trunk of one or both of these proper digital nerves.

Type 2 — Terminal Branch Neuroma

A symptomatic neuroma of one of the branches of an otherwise intact nerve presents a more difficult problem. The superficial branch of the radial nerve, because of its multiple terminal branches and difficulty in mobilization, presents a particularly difficult problem. In symptomatic terminal branch neuroma, the prognosis is dependent on the available length of the proximal trunk: the longer the stalk, the more flexibility in selection of the optimal translocation site. Proximal teasing of the neuroma segment from its parent trunk is helpful but carries a risk of creating multiple microneuromas of the internally spiraling axons, which branch into the mobilized segment.

The surgical technique is basically simlar to that used for amputation neuroma. The atraumatically isolated end neuroma is translocated on a relaxed proximal stalk to a scar-free, well protected area, optimally in proximal muscle substance. Distal neuroma of the radial sensory nerve can be inserted into the fleshy portion of the flexor pollicis longus or flexor carpiradialis muscle; more proximal neuromas can be inserted into the brachioradialis.

In the author's series two thirds of terminal branch neuromas treated by this technique were relieved, including five of seven superficial radial sensory neuromas (Herndon, Eaton, and Littler, 1976).

Type 3 — Neuroma-in-Continuity

The optimal treatment for neuroma-in-continuity is primary repair of the partially divided nerve trunk. Late repair of partially divided mixed nerves, which involves careful microsurgical dissection, is discussed elsewhere. Intermediate- or small-size nerves with painful neuroma-in-continuity may be treated by mobilization of the proximal and distal nerve trunk and a limited transposition of the fusiform mass to a less scarred, less traumatized area. A local fascial or retinacular sling can be improvised and sutured to the dermis to block the return of the thickened nerve trunk to its original location. Such repositioning is effective not only in neuroma following partial nerve division but also for the unique traumatic perineural swellings that develop in bowlers (Dobyns, 1972), tennis players, and even professional drummers, at the site of repeated localized trauma.*

Intermediate or small neuromata-in-continuity in which mobilization of the proximal and distal segment is still not sufficient to ensure *relaxed* repositioning in an untraumatized location may require sectioning of the nerve distal to the neuroma followed by relocation using the same technique as with end neuroma. The sensory deficit produced is rarely increased, whereas the symptomatic relief may be quite dramatic.

Certain intermediate or small neuroma-in-continuity contain predominantly divided axons. In these the neurologic deficit is more pronounced distally. When present in a nerve trunk which can be satisfactorily mobilized, such neuromas can be resected and microsurgically repaired end-to-end. It is important to be certain that the intact axons in such a segment are relatively few.

Neurectomy plus silicone capping as a primary treatment has been recently advocated (Frackelton et al., 1971, Snyder and Knowles, 1965, Swanson et al., 1977). Frackelton noted that his best results were those in which the *transected* nerve and its silicone cap were definitively transposed and transfixed to a separate soft tissue site (Frackelton et al., 1971). All authors stress the critical

---

*Such fusiform thickenings are composed predominantly of hyperplastic perineural elements, and rarely contain divided axons. They are not true neuromas.

nature of the length and fit of the silicone cap. Improper fit may lead to necrosis if the cap is too long or too tight, or proximal and distal axon escape if the cap is short or loose (Biddulph, 1972, Frackelton et al., 1971, Swanson et al., 1977, Tupper and Booth, 1976). These potential problems do not occur with relocation of the *intact* neuroma (Herndon, Eaton, and Littler, 1976).

REFERENCES

Biddulph, S. L.: The prevention and treatment of painful neuroma. J. Bone Joint Surg. *54B*:379, 1972.

Boyes, J. H. (ed.): Bunnell's Surgery of the Hand. 3rd ed., Philadelphia, J. B. Lippincott Co., 1956, p. 426.

Dobyns, J. H., O'Brien, E. T., Linschield, R. L., Farrow, G. M.: Bowlers thumb. J. Bone Joint Surg. *54A*:751, 1972.

Frackelton, W. F., Teasley, J. L., Tauras, A.: Neuromas of the hand treated by transplantation and silicone capping. J. Bone Joint Surg. *53A*:813, 1971.

Gluck, T.: Ueber Neuroplastik auf dem wege der Transplantation. Arch. Klin. Chir. *25*:606, 1880.

Herndon, J. H., Eaton, R. G., Littler, J. W.: Management of painful neuromas in the hand. J. Bone Joint Surg. *58A*:369, 1976.

Mitchell, S. W.: Traumatic neuralgia: Section of the median nerve. Am. J. Med. Sci. *67*:2, 1874.

Spencer, P. S.: The traumatic neuroma and proximal stump. Bull. Hosp. Joint Dis. *35*:85, 1974.

Snyder, C. C.: The surgical handling of tissue. Proc. Seventh Annual Convention, Am. Assoc. Equine Prac., Fort Worth, Tex., Dec. 1961.

Snyder, C. C., Knowles, R. P.: Traumatic neuromas. J. Bone Joint Surg. *47A*:641, 1965.

Swanson, A. B., Boeve, N. R., Lumsden, R. M.: The prevention and treatment of amputation neuromas by silicone capping. J. Hand Surg. *2*:70, 1977.

Tupper, J. W., Booth, N. M.: Treatment of painful neuromas of sensory nerves in the hand: a comparison of traditional and newer methods. J. Hand Surg., *1*:144, 1976.

11

MORTON'S NEURITIS AND MANAGEMENT OF POST-NEURECTOMY PAIN

JOSEPH E. MILGRAM

The patient suffering from Morton's neuritis is usually an adult female who presents with paroxyms of pain in one forefoot on walking, often extending into the central toes and who hastens to remove her shoe for temporary relief. The condition typically involves the third intermetatarsal space (but sometimes the second) radiating to the two adjacent toes. In advanced cases, the pain may be constant and the toes numb. With further evolution, episodes occur at shorter and shorter intervals.

The condition was first recorded in England in 1845 by Durlacher, who throught it was an affliction of the plantar nerves. In 1876, Thomas George Morton, of the Pennsylvania Hospital in Philadelphia, for whom the disease is named, attributed the digital nerve irritation to compression from abnormal mobility of the metatarsophalangeal joint and advised excision of the joint, together with surrounding soft parts.

In 1893, another Morton, Thomas S. K., also advised that resection of the fourth metatarsophalangeal joint would relieve the painful nerve. Robert Jones (1897, 1898, 1929) reported that relief had been obtained by excision of the joint or the metatarsal head; by amputation of the toe and metatarsal head; by inserting a heated needle into the nerve; by injection of carbolic acid; and by partial excision of the digital plantar nerve.

Hoadley (1893) mentioned neuroma as the causal pathology. In Australia, Betts, (1940) reported neuritis of the digital nerve with a pronounced neuroma in all cases. He urged that the surgical treatment for Morton's neuroma be excision of the benign involved area of nerve (Fig. 11–1).

Observers have remarked on a number of anatomic functional factors that may contribute to digital nerve trauma, namely, at the third interspace the

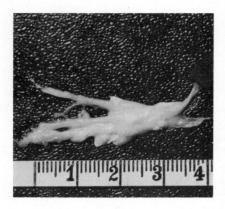

Figure 11–1 *Case 1.* Typical neurectomy specimen of one side of a bilateral case. Unfortunately, excision was followed by bilateral recurrence. The recurrent symptomatology was relieved conservatively by pad separation of metatarsals 3 and 4.

medial longitudinal arch elements (talus, scaphoid, and metatarsals first, second, and third) move on the lateral elements of the foot (os calcis, cuboid, and metatarsals fourth and fifth).

Furthermore, active hyperextension of the digits during gait, which occurs not only in hammer toes and cavus but also often in feet with short heel cords, serves to increase tension forces on the nerves as they pass across the transverse metatarsal ligament.

The partial restriction of motion of the medial plantar nerve by a communicating branch from the lateral plantar nerve possibly contributes to anchorage of the third interspace nerve.

Even the tarsal — metatarsal special mobility of metatarsals third and fourth may add to the handicaps that the nerve and the digtial vessels must experience.

During running, the metatarsal joints, fat pads, bursae, and vessels are subjected to local pounding by forces of several times the body weight.

A short first metatarsal may possibly help to bring on this lesion. In the 1893 paper of T. G. Morton this appears on the early x-ray he reproduced of one of the cases. It also was associated in several of our cases. Metatarsus primus varus did not seem to be often associated with this metatarsalgic pathology.

Wide separation of all the spread toes when standing is often observed in childhood. In adults with hypermobile metatarsus varus primus there is spreading of the first and second toes associated with separation of the first and second metatarsals and increased separation of the medial and middle cuneiform bones on erect x-ray films.

Wide and progressive bilateral separation of the second toe from the third toe develops in the later decades in female patients with metatarsal pain, and is not frequently associated with short heel cords. A number of these "split toes" patients have presented with severe Morton's pain syndrome. On x-ray studies, no metatarsal shaft spreading accompanied the toe divergence.

HISTOPATHOLOGY

Early degenerative repair lesions are revealed on section of even so-called normal metatarsal blood vessels. That in specially vulnerable areas such as interspace 3–4 not only these vessels but also the digital nerves should experience and manifest response to excessive trauma should not occasion surprise. One might expect it to develop more frequently.

Lassman et al. (1976) found in 76 of the 105 cases operated for atypical symtoms histopathology indicating that early stages of Morton's disease were dominated by characteristic findings.

Perineural thickening with endoneural edema and sclerosis, vascular wall thickening and hyalinization, and nerve fiber demyelination and degeneration were present. Wallerian degeneration was absent.

The hyalinized material around endoneurial vessels was amorphous and eosinophilic, and often formed concentric layered inner rings on PAS stain, with negative reactions for amyloid, acid mucopolysaccharides, collagen, and elastin. Electron-dense amorphous or granular material was present between layers, and, in more advanced stages, hyperplastic endoneurial vessels formed loops.

The endoneurium around nerves became filled with similar hyalinized materal arranged in cylindrical structures in the long axis of the nerves. On cross section Lassman described discs made up of tubular filaments 100 to 110 angstroms in diameter.

The perineurium now thickened.

With advancing disease the nerve is transformed into a cord of connective tissue surrounded by thick perineurium and filled with collagenous microfibrillary material. Later, surrounding connective tissue and bursa are involved, so that the proximal part of the nerve terminates in a nodule of connective tissue.

Why endoneurial edema and sclerosis should develop is a matter for speculation. The finding of analogous changes in peripheral vessels of the elderly is of interest. No inflammatory neoplastic (McElvenny) or metabolic process was discerned by Lassman.

The nature of the microfibrillar material is the subject of varied interpretations.

Reed and Bliss in 1973 had directed special attention to the elastogenesis in the fibroadipose tissue adjacent to the so-called neuroma, with the deposition of fibrinoid. They interpreted the condition to be primarily an inflammatory process with deposition of elastic fibers, many of which are abnormal. They suggested the term "regressive and productive intermetatarsal elastic fibrositis" to describe the lesion. They proposed that inflammatory processes adjacent to bursae may convert collagen connective tissue to elastic fibers.

RESULTS OF OPERATIVE TREATMENT

The literature on follow-ups is short, and no detailed data of recurrences after surgery could be accumulated. Recurrences are relatively seldom experienced and seldom reported. Studies are now in progress, but follow-up observations are difficult to interpret.

In 1967, Lelièvre reported 350 excisions with only three failures. New York City colleagues with extensive operative experience (comparable to that of Lelièvre) were asked to estimate their recurrences. Reports varied between 3 per cent and 7 per cent. Others denied personal experience other than with recurrences arising from the surgery of other colleagues.

Recurrences are difficult to evaluate.

Lapidus (1961) related that over recent years he encountered several cases in which there was recurrence of symptoms following neurectomy.

On re-exploration of one case a neuroma of the second common plantar nerve was found. When this was excised all symptoms disappeared.

In another case, reoperation for recurrent symptoms revealed that the stump of the previously removed third common plantar digital nerve was bound down in thick scar tissue. The scar tissue and the proximal portion of the nerve were excised proximal to the original site; the second and fourth digital nerves were also removed, although grossly and macroscopically they appeared to be normal. Symptoms abated permanently.

A third patient (Fig. 11–2), who had bilateral recurrence of symptoms 1½ years after neuroma excision (one side operated by Lapidus, one side by myself), was supplied with small, appropriately shaped and placed metatarsal pads. With these supports the pain was promptly relieved. She has worn supports for the past five years with no return of pain.

In none of Lassman's confirmed cases did amputation neuroma or recurrence appear in follow-up during the last 10 years.

Nissen (1948) relates three recurrences in a series of 26 cases; one was reoperated and relief was obtained by nerve excision in the second to third metatarsal interspace.

Mulder (1951) reported re-formation of neuroma in one of 12 cases reoperated. The neuroma was again operated on but the result was not stated.

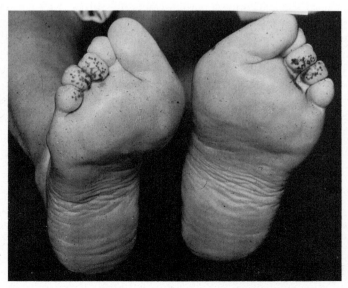

Figure 11–2 *Case 1.* A bilateral bunion with Morton's syndrome both sides recurring 1½ years after bilateral neurectomy. The ink spots localize the area of sensory disturbance at the time of recurrence.

Bartolini (1968) reported on changing weight bearing by surgery. He shortened two or three of the central metatarsals in the mid-diaphyseal region to "invert the arch." Amelioration of subjective symptoms was obtained in 18 cases so treated.

Kite (1964) reported on 105 excisions with but one recurence of pain, which was relieved by reoperation 12 months later. He relates his great satisfaction with neural excision, and provides fine clinical descriptions of the syndrome.

Nora et al. (1965) reported recurrence of burning in five of 42 patients operated, with no improvement in two others (16 per cent). Of particular interest is their report on "controls." They reported that histologic examination of the digital nerves of 10 controls of the same ages revealed changes in varying degrees which were nearly identical to those found in the so-called neuromas; and, in some cases, controls resembled true neuromas more than excised Morton's neuromas from symptomatic cases. They do not believe that Morton's disease is a histologic entity, although they concede it to be a clinical entity. Lassman (1967) also objected to the designation of "neuroma" or "neuromatous pain."

REPORTS OF CONSERVATIVE TREATMENT

Silverman (1976) reports that in the previous three years he saw 110 cases of presumable Morton's neuralgia of mild to severe form, and that conservative treatment by balancing appliances and weekly local injection of corticosteroid provided gratifying and sometimes dramatic relief in 80 per cent of the cases seen in the 12 months prior to publication. Attempts were made to separate the heads of metatarsals three and four by using a felt plug and wearing roomy shoes.

Of interest are the experience of G. Hohmann, the author of "Fuss und Bein" (Foot and Leg), who in 1966 reiterated his opinion that Morton's syndrome arises as a consequence of metatarsal joint ligamentous instability. He reported that when he transferred weight bearing by use of a torsion insole onto the lateral border of the foot, the Morton's pain ceased and did not reappear. He "experienced this in many cases." He once again reports this "to spare patients unnecessary surgery." He does no nerve resections. Incidentally, he reports on two patients who had difficultly after joint excision elsewhere.

PAD TREATMENT IN RECURRENT CASES

In 1964 this author included, in a paper entitled "Office measures for relief of the painful foot," a brief section of the use of small spread pads for Morton's neuritis patients. As a result of that brief note there have been directed to me 20 problem cases from colleagues. These patients all had "neuromas" excised in classic fashion. The pain, initially relieved by surgery, had recurred without known reason three months to five years after surgery. The pain was described as having gradually increased with time, and in each instance to have become disabling. In some burning and radiation were present following operation, and localized pain on weight bearing was similar to, but often more severe than, their preoperative pain. In all cases the pain was worse and was reported to be still elicited by walking or standing, and subsided promptly or gradually on resting the foot. The severity of foot pain in most cases was almost overwhelming.

Irregularly disturbed sensation was found on testing. In six patients on whom excision had been done, examination demonstrated increased apprehension, despite gentleness and reassurance; and there were localized plantar areas of exceptional skin hypersensitivity to fingertip brushing or pressure in the intermetatarsal area. Yet, plantar incisional scars were seldom sensitive, and dorsal scars were quite insensitive.

Attempts to elicit proximal Tinel's signs were usually inconclusive. Compression of metatarsals in less severe cases was not painful; however, in more severe cases the gentlest compression could not be tolerated. Common preoperative painful pressure sites "deep in the fat pad" in the intermetatarsal spaces were not regularly found. Pain was not brought on by motion of the proximal joint or toe. No regular effort was made to click a displaced metatarsal head during compression testing. In general, in postoperative painful feet the most tender area was more accessible and more proximal than in unoperated cases of Morton's disease, although the level of pain on digital manipulation did not correspond to the precise level of nerve division, as described in accompanying operative reports.

TECHNIQUE OF APPLYING METATARSAL PADS FOR MORTON'S NEURITIS

The application of pads is very simple. The physician seeks to spread the metatarsals at the affected interspace and to keep them spread while bearing weight.

One locates and outlines with the fingertip a precise small area where fingertip pressure will cause the two toes to visibly separate.

The foot is supported comfortably at the physician's eye level. The patient is asked to relax his foot and look elsewhere. The area is painted or sprayed with a skin adhesive such as compound tincture of benzoin.

The tip of the index finger explores just behind the palpable metartarsal heads, and presses. Sometimes the resultant toe spread is marked. In the severe pain following operation the toe spread seems less (I have not been able to demonstrate a contracture on erect weight bearing x-ray study).

The other hand outlines the tip of the finger at the "spread site" precisely with a pen.

A foam rubber pad roughly ¼ inch thick, ⅜ to ½ inch wide, and ¾ inch long is cut in advance from adhesive-backed rubber stock of firm resilience.

The pad is now applied at the pressure site; pressure on it must demonstrably separate the toes, or it is shifted to where it will do so (Figs. 11–3 and 11–4).

It is my current practice to provide an additional L-shaped pad outlining the first metatarsal head, separate from the spread pad. The vertical limb is ½ or ¾ inch wide and 2¼ inch long. The horizontal limb is about 1¼ to 1½ inch wide. The vertical limb is placed along the shaft of metatarsal II snugly up to the metatarsal head, and the horizontal limb of the pad is wrapped under the metatarsal I shaft snugly up to but not under the head. This L-shaped pad will hereafter bear

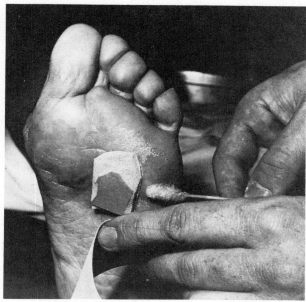

Figure 11–3 *Case 2.* Use of a single spread pad. A small rubber spread pad with beveled edges is glued into place.

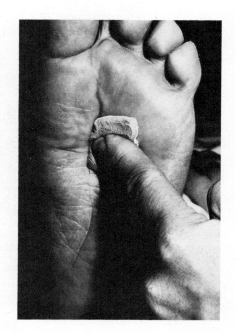

Figure 11–4 *Case 2.* Acute Morton's neuritis, toes 3–4. Evidence of correct placement of spread pad. The toes 3 and 4 are now visibly separated by pressure on the pad. Relief was obtained without surgery.

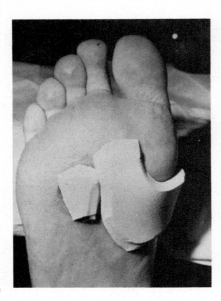

Figure 11–5 *Case 3.* Use of double pads. Pad application for conservative management when Morton's syndrome of toes 3 and 4 accompanies additional anterior metatarsal pad. Small pad spreads metatarsals 3 and 4. A larger, L-shaped pad, in addition, shifts stresses to the necks of metatarsals 1 and 2.

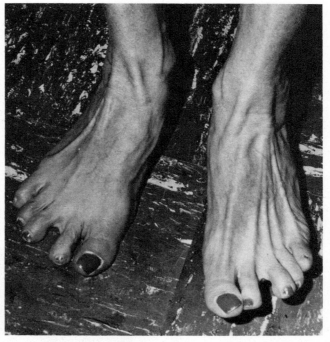

Figure 11–6 *Case 4.* Bilateral "split-toes" feet (2–3) suffering with 3–4 Morton's syndrome which recurred after bilateral neurectomy of the third plantar nerves. (See Figures 11–7 through 11–9 for management.)

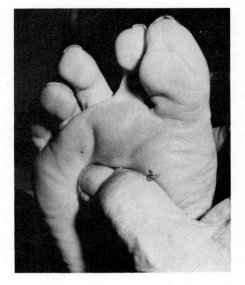

Figure 11–7 *Case 4 (Continued).* "Split-toes" foot. Inability to separate toes 3 and 4 by plantar test point pressure while toes 2 and 3 are left free. If toes 2 and 3 are fastened together, test will locate the proper site to separate toes 3 and 4 by local spread. (See Figure 11–8.)

most of the stress of weight bearing (Fig. 11–5). The edges of the pads are beveled with bandage scissors. Then both pads are loosely encircled with a 2 inch adhesive band, applied while the foot is maximally spread by application of finger pressure.

In Morton patients who have "split toes" (Fig. 11–6), where the second and third toes widely diverge, pressure over the 3–4 interspace fails to produce spreading until the second and third toes are first approximated by an adhesive loop (Figs. 11–7 and 11–8). The foot is again manually explored for a "plantar spread spot" over the metatarsal 3–4 interspace. Now, increased spread of the second and third toes does take place, and the spread spot can be more clearly marked (Fig. 11–9).

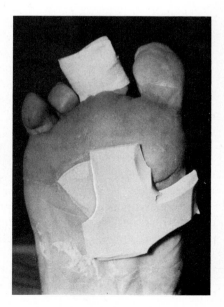

Figure 11–8 *Case 4 (Continued).* Treatment of "split-toes" foot. First, control toes 2 and 3 by the toe loop. Next double pads are applied (the small spread pad is on the left; the L-pad is on the right). Recurrent Morton's syndrome of toes 3 and 4 was controlled conservatively.

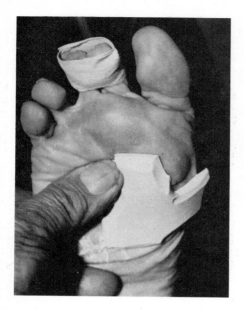

Figure 11–9 *Case 4 (Conclusion).* "Split-toes" foot. The small spread pad is being pressed by the examiner's thumb. Toes 3 and 4 are now visibly separated by the plantar pressure. Later, the treatment consists of removal of the loop about toes 2 and 3 and use of an insole with replicas of the pads on the insole. However, some patients require the constant use of a removable fabric loop in addition to the insole.

Several of the operated patients manifested, in addition to recurrence of preoperative pain, the most severe localized agonizingly painful hyperaesthesia in small plantar skin areas in the intermetatarsal zone, slightly proximal to the metatarsal heads. Brushing this skin very lightly brought on instant paroxysms of pain. Peripheral protective pads and small spread rubber pads glued to the skin proximal to their skin lesions enabled walking and were immediately appreciated. In these patients, padding had to be constant, and in three patients was renewed at 7 to 12 day intervals for several months before insoles were fabricated that would mimic the pad support.

In difficult cases, in addition to spread pads and L pads, special efforts were made to distribute forefoot weight-bearing (by padding) to still other painless areas of the forefoot; namely, the necks of metatarsals I and II and often temporarily the "toe crest areas" under the proximal and middle phalanges of the second, third, fourth, and even fifth toes.

A narrow transverse adherent rubber pad ½ inch wide, and approximately 2 inches long is shaped convex distally to fit the curved hollow under the toes. The convex edge of the pad may be scalloped with a bandage scissors to fit under each toe above. It is covered with a ½ inch wide strip of adhesive tape. Commercial toe crests are available also.

Special reliance was placed on a proximal small spread pad which served to visibly spread the toes of the affected interspace. In two almost intolerably sensitive causalgic cases, an effort was made to provide a rocker sole across the whole width of the foot in addition to the spread pad.

We proximally located a ¾ inch wide transverse pad designed to be the equivalent of a proximal metatarsal bar. This total pad glued to the skin. When it provided immediate standing relief and three weeks subsequent relief it was removed. Contact stresses were now tolerable. The original pad was transmitted to the insole maker to build a replica onto a molded removable insole.

A plaster mold for the insole was at times also made over powdered skin pads in place, with the aid of a two layer plaster of Paris splint. One cannot hope to ask a technician or insole maker to take ordinary molds successfully for such patients. In a real sense these are problems of modest desperation for some pain-worn patients who have refused reoperation after the original operation had failed, and are a challenge to our ingenuity.

Plastic bag protection facilitates bathing while the pads are in place.

Of the previously operated 20 patients treated conservatively since 1962, three left to seek relief elsewhere, and 17 have achieved comfort and have regained the ability to walk freely, provided that they continue to use shoes of adequate width with insoles specially corrected for them. Even bedroom slippers and bath and beach wear are built up, and their fit checked by the physician. I have seen two operated patients so treated prior to 1962 who have persisted with comfort, and experience "only a rare twinge and then only on walking without my corrected shoe," and who have all refused a second neurectomy.

During the initial office visit the patient can usually almost immediately judge wherher the fitted pads will provide pain relief on standing and walking in his shoes. The pad is then fastened in place with glue, and covered by an adhesive circlet applied without constriction.

Shoes of adequate width and depth are essential in every instance, and must be checked by the physician.

Changes at the office are painstaking, and adequate time must be provided for often prolonged trials. These patients are therefore scheduled at the end of the office day.

In the past ten years, 25 other (not operated) "classic Morton's neuritis" patients were offered the choice of such a prolonged program of care, and we have seen complaints of foot pain cease in 21 cases. They continue to wear individually designed molded insoles. It is strange that the nerve mass should presumably persist and the pain so often vanish. We can no longer elicit pain on deep palpation in these old, unoperated cases. Four of these patients did not continue with the conservative effort and were lost to follow-up.

CHOICE OF TREATMENT FOR THE MORTON LESION

In our opinion, surgical excision is still the best method of providing prompt and lasting relief to most patients who present, on detailed examination, strong and presumptive evidence of this disturbing pathologic lesion.

However, we are obliged to offer the alternative of prolonged (and troublesome) conservative care. The non-operative program should be described clearly to the patient, together with the information that only a decidedly small percentage of operated cases of the operatively confirmed lesion will unpredictably persist or recur despite the most careful attention.

Moreover, it must be urged that following operation, balancing of the foot and prolonged careful redistribution of metatarsal stresses by insole and proper nonconstricting footwear should be insistently recommended and provided, in order to diminish the likelihood of late recurrence in the same or an adjacent interspace.

Today, thoroughly informed consent alone can enable a prospective patient to obtain excisional surgery for this painful disability without exposing the surgeon to legal hazards and recrimination if the neuroma excision chances to be in the relatively very small group of excisional failures. Conservative treatment still is very likely to relieve even the unlucky operated foot, for, while the true cause of the Morton's lesion is in a sense a mystery, relief is available for a high percentage of patients afflicted with this complaint.

CAUSALGIA AND MORTON'S LESION

Burning pain is not frequently complained of in Morton's lesions. However, when recurrence of pain develops following neurectomy, causalgic burning pain and osteoporosis are often observed.

Mayfield, who studied causalgia as a consequence of peripheral nerve injuries in World War II, remarked on the incidence (2 to 5 per cent), and conjectured that incomplete rather than complete nerve injuries were responsible. He resorted to interrupting the sympathetic chain by surgical removal of the lower neural components. However, we have not encountered a Morton's lesion requiring such measures for relief.

TRAUMA AND MORTON'S LESION

There appears to be no convincing evidence to indicate that a single traumatic insult to toes or forefoot has incited the lesion. Yet one cannot be sure that repetitive microtraumata arising from abnormal anatomic stresses do not play a part in the development of the lesion in connective tissue of vessel, nerve, and capsule in susceptible patients.

Ulceration of the tip of a partially deinnervated hammer toe analogous to those seen in diabetic neuropathy has not been observed in Morton's neuritis after nerve excision. Local skin thickening does occur, however, and is benefited by toe crest pad protection designed to spread the area of weight-bearing impact over the phalangeal shafts of adjacent toes. Commercial toe crests are available in the form of small sausages which are retained beneath the toes by passing an elastic loop through the toe interspaces. They can be tried to supplement insoles without toe crests. They are seldom as well fitting as crests constructed as an integral part of an insole made on a plaster model. These are worn in shoes checked for adequate width and room for the foot and the appliance.

REFERENCES

Bartolini, G.: La metatarsalgia da inversione della volt a transversa. Archiv. Putti. Chir. Organi. Mov. 23:181, 1968.
Betts, L. O.: Morton's metatarsalgia: Neuritis of the fourth digital nerve. Med. J. Aust. 1:514, 1940.
Durlacher, L.: Treatise on Corns, Bunions, the Diseases of Nails and the General Management of the Feet. London, Simpkin, Marshall, 1845, p. 52.
Hoadley, A. E.: Six cases of metatarsalgia. Chicago Med. Rec. 5:32, 1893.
Hohmann, G.: Über die Mortonsche Neuralgie am Fuss Beitr. Orthop. 13:649, 1966.
Jones, R.: Plantar neuralgia. Liverpool Medico-Chirurgical Jour. 17:1, 1897.
Jones, R., and Tubby, A. H.: Metatarsalgia or Morton's disease. Ann. Surg. 228:297, 1898.
Jones, R., and Lovett, R. W.: Orthopaedic Surgery. London, Oxford Press, 1929, p. 660.
Lapidus, P. W.: In Rothenberg, R. E. (ed.): Reoperative Surgery. New York, McGraw-Hill-Blakiston, 1964, p. 543.

Lassman, G., Lassman, H., and Stockinger, L.: Morton's metatarsalgia. Light and electron microscopic observations and their relation to entrapment neuropathies. Virchows Arch. (Pathol. Anat.) *370*:307, 1976.

Lelièvre, J.: Pathologie du Pied. Paris, Masson, 1967.

Mayfield, F. H.: Causalgia. Springfield, Ill., C. C Thomas, 1951, p. 65.

Milgram, J. E.: Office measures for relief of the painful foot. J. Bone Joint Surg. *56A*:1095, 1964.

Morton, D. J.: The Human Foot. New York, Columbia University Press, 1935.

Morton, T. G.: A peculiar and painful affliction of the fourth metatarsophalangeal articulation. Am. J. Med. Sci., *71*:37, 1876.

Morton, T. G.: The application of x-rays to the diagnosis of Morton's painful affection of the foot, or metatarsalgia. Int. Med. Mag. *5*:322, 1897.

Morton, T. G.: International Medical Magazine and roentgenogram reproduced as Fig. 98, p. 211. Cited by Morton, D. J.: *In* The Human Foot. New York, Columbia Press, 1935.

Morton, T. S. K.: Metatarsalgia (Morton's painful affection of the foot) — with an account of six cases cured by operation. Ann. Surg. *17*:680, 1893.

Mulder, J. D.: The causative mechanism in Morton's metatarsalgia. J. Bone Joint Surg., *33B*:44, 1951.

Nora, P. F., Nora, E. D., and Ghislandi, E.: Morton's metatarsalgia — a misconception. Illinois Med. J. *6*:1665, 1965.

Nissen, K. I.: Plantar digital neuritis. Morton's metatarsalgia. J. Bone Surg. *30B*:84, 1948.

Reed, R. J., and Bliss, B. O.: Morton's neuroma. Arch. Pathol. *95*:123, 1973.

Silverman, L. G.: Morton's toe or Morton's neuralgia: Its recognition and treatment. J. Am. Podiatry Assoc. *66*:749, 1976.

12

REFLEX SYMPATHETIC DYSTROPHY

L. LEE LANKFORD

Reflex sympathetic dystrophy (RSD) is a most distressing and disheartening experience for the patient, the doctor, and almost everyone who comes in contact with the patient. It is distressing to the patient because of the pain, swelling, stiffness, and dysfunction experienced in the affected extremity. It is distressing to the doctor because he is unexpectedly confronted with a severe problem in a patient who has received the proper management. It is distressing to everyone who comes in contact with the patient, because the patient often is difficult and finds it hard to cooperate with those who try to help, and is unable to understand how or why such a calamity should befall him. The doctor is puzzled by this unexpected poor result from a treatment which may well have been identical to that given many others in the past with quite happy results. Reflex sympathetic dystrophy is truly an enigma.

Reflex sympathetic dystrophy is not the only cause of increased pain, swelling, stiffness, and dysfunction. Following the treatment of extremity traumas or extensile surgeries, it is not surprising to find these untoward results occurring in patients with abnormal conditions such as hypertrophic arthritis and Dupuytren's contractures, in those who have a history of collagen problems such as trigger finger, DeQuervain's disease, or "knuckle pads," in patients with severely crushed, infected, or burned hands, and in patients with primary carpal tunnel syndrome (thickening of the transverse carpal ligament). A poor result may also be expected in extremities with less than normal vascularity. Reflex sympathetic dystrophy, however, is known to produce these disastrous symptoms following trauma, disease, or surgery in what may otherwise appear to be a normal hand. It is a separate entity with its own identity, pathogenesis, and diagnosis, and in order to provide the proper treatment we must not be misled by all the other problems which may on the surface appear to mimic reflex sympathetic dystrophy.

216

NOMENCLATURE

In the past, there have been many names given to the condition now universally known as reflex sympathetic dystrophy. Because this condition may follow trauma, it has sometimes been referred to as post-traumatic pain syndrome. Also, because it has been recognized that this condition is connected with the neurovascular system, names such as post-traumatic vasomotor disorders, traumatic angiospasm, reflex nervous dystrophy, post-traumatic spreading neuralgia, and post-traumatic painful osteoporosis have gained favor in the past (Patman and Thompson, 1973).

The most significant contribution to the understanding of this problem was made in 1864 by Silas Weir Mitchell, who reported his findings of gunshot wounds involving nerves during the Civil War (Mitchell, 1864). In 1867, he coined the word "causalgia" from the combination of Greek words meaning "burning pain" (Mitchell, 1867). His description of causalgia (one of the clinical forms of RSD) is so accurate that it remains one of the classical descriptions today. Although Mitchell was unaware of the relationship of this condition to the sympathetic nervous system, he did conclude that a partial nerve injury of a major mixed nerve in the proximal portion of the extremity was likely to cause the very disabling condition, which he called causalgia. It was only natural that John Homans borrowed the term "causalgia" to bring to our attention other conditions which produced a causalgia-like picture, but which unlike Mitchell's cases were not caused by nerve injury (Homans, 1940). These non-nerve injury problems were called "minor causalgia." Mitchell's influence also prompted the use of the words "causalgic state" (deTakats, 1945). At the turn of the century, an "acute bone atrophy" was described in patients with minor traumas to the wrist or ankle but which produced a devastating amount of swelling, stiffness, and pain, which we now recognize as reflex sympathetic dystrophy (Sudeck, 1900).

Inasmuch as RSD occurs with many conditions other than trauma, it is inaccurate to refer to these pathological states as post-traumatic pain syndromes or post-traumatic dystrophy. The role of the sympathetic nervous system in the production of RSD is now universally accepted (Bonica, 1973); and, therefore, the term reflex sympathetic dystrophy is more properly used.

CLINICAL MANIFESTATIONS

Pain

The most important clinical finding in reflex sympathetic dystrophy is pain. However, the distinguishing feature of the pain in RSD is its severity; the degree of pain is completely out of proportion to the inciting trauma. The nature of the pain varies widely, but early in the condition the pain is usually described as a burning or stinging. Later on, it is often referred to as a pressure or cutting pain and becomes constant and unrelenting. Attempted motion severely aggravates the pain; therefore, there is almost a complete cessation of voluntary movement of the extremity. Although the pain may start in one area, it rapidly spreads to adjacent sites and eventually may involve the entire extremity. In untreated severe cases, the pain progresses to the point that the patient may request amputation or even consider suicide. The pain is made markedly worse by attempted active or passive movements of joints, and severe and excruciating paresthesias may be produced by lightly stroking the skin even in uninjured areas. Tenderness is almost always present and is much more severe than one would normally expect. The tenderness is most severe around the joints.

Swelling

Although pain is the most prominent symptom, swelling is the most common physical finding. The swelling usually starts in the area of greatest involvement but soon spreads to the immediate adjacent areas of the extremity proximally and distally (Fig. 12–1). The swelling is soft initially but turns into brawny edema if the condition persists. The brawny edema often gets so severe that it acts as a mechanical block to motion. This "fixed" edema eventually gives way to periarticular thickening and to fibrous tendon adhesions. Elevation of the extremity is more effective in reducing the swelling early in the disease, and it is beneficial at any time.

Stiffness

In RSD, the stiffness is progressive and, unless proper treatment is instigated early, joint stiffness may be permanent. Early, the stiffness is due to the exquisite pain with motion and to the brawny edema. Later, the stiffness is due to increased fibrosis about the joints, along with inelasticity of the ligamentous structures. Flexion contractures are also caused by thickening of the palmar fascia or by adhesion formation in the flexor tendons. All of the tissues of the distal portion of the extremities appear to be infiltrated with fibrous tissue, and

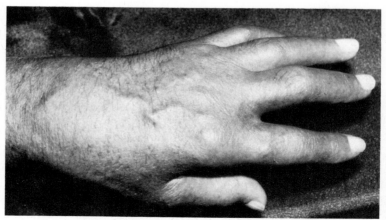

Figure 12–1 Most characteristic findings are swelling, redness, and tight, shiny skin. (From Lankford, L. L., and Thompson, J. E.: Reflex sympathetic dystrophy, upper and lower extremity: Diagnosis and management. *In* The American Academy of Orthopaedic Surgeons Instructional Course Lectures. St. Louis, C. V. Mosby Co., 1977, Vol. 26.

this results in the loss of the normal flexor and extensor skin wrinkles over the joints. It is not uncommon to see shoulder stiffness and loss of forearm rotation, but only rarely is there lack of elbow motion, In many cases, the stiffness and the contractures are permanent.

Discoloration

The outset of RSD is usually manifested by some type of increased coloration, such as redness or blueness. As time goes on, this usually gives way to pallor. Commonly, the first deeper coloration is redness which may be homogeneous, or in the earlier stages it may be located solely over the dorsum of the metacarpophalangeal joints and over the metatarsophalangeal joints. In addition, it may be seen over the dorsum of the interphalangeal joints and in the area of the collateral ligaments. The presence of redness at some stage of RDS has prompted the nickname "red hand disease." It is not unusual to see redness or deeper blueness over the flexor creases of the palm and fingers. If the sympathetic vasoconstrictor stimulation is present primarily in the venous system, the color will be blue or cyanotic; if it is more prominent in the arterial system, the color will be pale. When the sympathetic vasodilator stimulation is greatest, then redness is characteristic.

Sudomotor

Hyperhidrosis, or increased sweating, is commonly seen early but, on occasion, there may well be dryness instead. At times, the increased sweating is profound and may give rise to various dermatological conditions which thrive on increased perspiration.

Temperature

When there is diffuse redness in the hand the temperature of the skin is usually increased; this is more commonly present early than late. When there is cyanosis, or when there is pallor or sweating, the hand is usually cooler. However, the temperature may be increased only around the joints, with a detectable decrease in temperature between the joints.

Osteoporosis

Some demineralization of bone is present in almost any acquired affliction of the extremities and certainly is present with trauma and the immobilization of the part by reflex splinting or cast. However, the degree of osteoporosis present in RSD is so much greater than in any other type of demineralization that it is quite dramatic (Fig. 12–2). The demineralization may first start in the carpal or tarsal bones and give the punched-out appearance seen in "Sudeck's atrophy," but if allowed to continue it will become diffuse. Also, it is much more prominent in the polar regions of the long bones of the hand and foot. In the very late stages, the demineralization becomes very extensive and homogeneous.

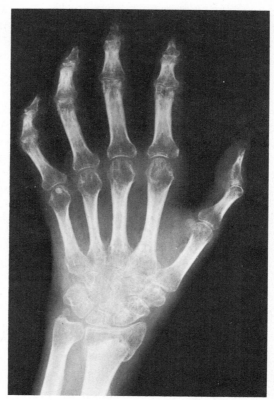

Figure 12–2 Osteoporosis when seen early may be spotty and present only in the ends of long bones. (From Lankford, L. L., and Thompson, J. E.: Reflex sympathetic dystrophy, upper and lower extremity: Diagnosis and management. *In* The American Academy of Orthopaedic Surgeons Instructional Course Lectures, St. Louis, C. V. Mosby Co., 1977, Vol. 26.)

Trophic Changes

The skin becomes thin, tight and shiny. The hairs become sparse and less coarse. The fat pads become atrophic and pull away from the fingernails, and both the tranverse and longitudinal arches of the fingernail increase, producing a tapering point which is referred to as "pencil-pointing." The trophic changes increase with the duration and severity of the condition.

Palmar Fasciitis

In many of the clinical forms of reflex sympathetic dystrophy there is thickening of the longitudinal bands of palmar fascia, and palmar fasciitis nodules make their appearance. This more commonly occurs in the ulnar three fingers than on the radial half of the hand. These nodules may become quite tender. Because these bands contract and produce flexion contractures of the fingers, one might be tempted to excise the nodules and bands. This, however, is ill advised and usually only aggravates the condition.

STAGES

While the symptoms and progress of this disease can be divided into three separate stages, there is considerable overlapping and variation in the stages of each clinical form of RSD.

Stage One

The first pain is. often described as burning, stinging, or cutting and is usually severe and constant. It is aggravated by attempted motion. In stage one, swelling is greatest and usually of the soft or pitting edema type (Fig. 12–3). Lack of active motion is pronounced, and the patient usually finds the part much too painful to attempt exercise or function. Although redness and increased warmth are characteristic of the first part of stage one, cyanosis with coolness and increased sweating may also be present in the latter part of this stage. Demineralization of the bone begins near the end of stage one.

Stage Two

The pain is still constant, and is described more often as a pressure type or tearing type rather than a burning pain. It is still aggravated considerably by attempts at active or passive motion. The swelling becomes a brawny edema and is quite hard and restricts motion (Fig 12–4). Periarticular thickening begins to appear. The hand is more likely to be blue or pale than red during the second

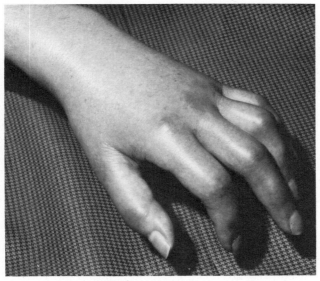

Figure 12–3 Soft swelling and redness over joints is usually seen in first stage. (From Lankford, L. L., and Thompson, J. E.: Reflex sympathetic dystrophy, upper and lower extremity: Diagnosis and management. *In* The American Academy of Orthopaedic Surgeons Instructional Course Lectures, St. Louis, C. V. Mosby Co., 1977, Vol. 26.)

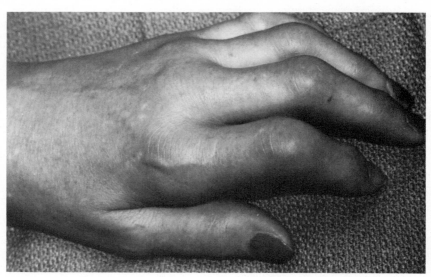

Figure 12–4 In second stage, swelling becomes hard and fixed. Extensor and flexor creases are lost. (From Lankford, L. L., and Thompson, J. E.: Reflex sympathetic dystrophy, upper and lower extremity: Diagnosis and management. *In* The American Academy of Orthopaedic Surgeons Instructional Course Lectures, St. Louis, C. V. Mosby Co., 1977, Vol. 26.)

stage. In the early part of stage two, hyperhidrosis is more likely present. Near the end of this stage, however, the hand begins to get dry and pale, and coolness begins. Subcutaneous atrophy is noted, the flexion and extension creases ("skin joints") are lost, and the skin is flat, smooth, and shiny.

Stage Three

The pain may last for many years, after many months it may become completely quiescent except during attempted motion of the fingers. The swelling has subsided to the point that there is only periarticular thickening remaining. The hand or foot is usually pale, dry, and cool, with atrophic skin and subcutaneous tissues, and the fingers present a shiny, smooth appearance. In many cases, the extremity is completely nonfunctional in the final stage (Fig. 12–5). The degree of osteoporosis is very extensive and becomes diffuse or homogeneous (Fig. 12–6).

ETIOLOGY

There is a great deal that is not known about the etiology and the pathogenicity of reflex sympathetic dystrophy. It is our opinion, however, that these three conditions must be present before a patient can develop RSD:
1. Persistent painful lesion (traumatic or acquired)
2. Diathesis (predisposition, susceptibility)
3. Abnormal sympathetic reflex

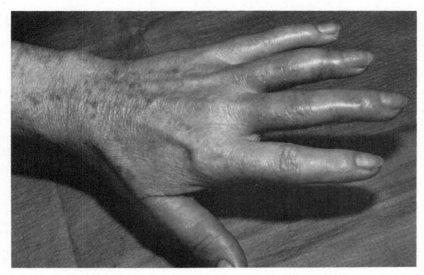

Figure 12–5 Third stage is indicated by decreased digital swelling, pallor, and coolness. The skin is shiny and atrophic. (From Lankford, L. L., and Thompson, J. E.: Reflex sympathetic dystrophy, upper and lower extremity: Diagnosis and management. *In* The American Academy of Orthopaedic Surgeons Instructional Course Lectures, St. Louis, C. V. Mosby Co., 1977, Vol. 26.)

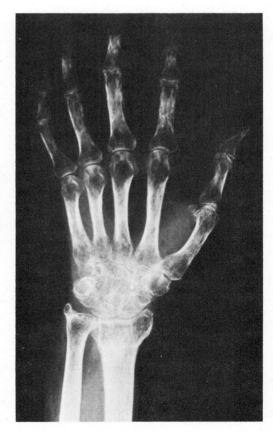

Figure 12–6 In the last stage, osteoporosis is profound and diffuse. (From Lankford, L. L., and Thompson, J. E.: Reflex sympathetic dystrophy, upper and lower extremity: Diagnosis and management. *In* The American Academy of Orthopaedic Surgeons Instructional Course Lectures, St. Louis, C. V. Mosby Co., 1977, Vol. 26.)

Persistent Painful Lesion

Most often, we think of a severe crush injury as causing reflex sympathetic dystrophy, but the degree of trauma need not be extensive. It can be as trivial as the injury caused by a small weight dropping on the extremity, a small laceration, or a digit being mashed in a door. Also, the persistent, painful lesion need not be traumatic in origin, but may be from such acquired disorders as ischemia of tissue, arthritis, stenosing tenosynovitis, or nerve entrapment. In one type of reflex sympathetic dystrophy known as shoulder-hand syndrome, the painful lesion may be caused by a proximal trauma, such as an injury to the shoulder or neck, or it could conceivably be nontraumatic and visceral in origin, resulting from a heart attack, stomach ulcer, or pulmonary lesion (Pancoast tumor).

Diathesis

Diathesis means a predisposition or a natural tendency or susceptibility to certain diseases, in this instance to reflex sympathetic dystrophy. This diathesis is divided into two types. The first relates to increased sympathetic activity on the part of the patient. These "hyper-sympathetic reactors" are patients who generally have a previous history of increased sympathetic action, such as some degree of hyperhidrosis and some evidence of vasoconstriction such as pallor or slight cyanosis and coolness of the fingertips or toes. The capillary filling time is usually somewhat prolonged. These patients frequently have a history of a labile sympathetic nervous system, demonstrated by blushing or fainting. There is a greater incidence of migraine headaches among these patients.

The second type of diathesis refers to the personality and psychological makeup of the individual. While this is not apparent in every patient with reflex sympathetic dystrophy, the majority of the patients seem to fit a pattern often described by psychiatrists in terms such as: "fearful, suspicious, emotionally labile, inadequate personality, chronic complainers, dependent personality, insecure, and unstable personality." These people seek to place the blame for their condition on others. Characteristically, they are not usually cooperative and do not follow the doctor's orders well. They are very good at thinking up excuses for not doing what they are told and often try to control their own treatment. Others give the impression that they enjoy a state of poor health and are looking for something on which to blame their inadequacies. All these conditions, of course, need not be present before a diagnosis of reflex sympathetic dystrophy can be made, but in most instances this diathesis is readily apparent to the skilled observer.

However, these patients are not malingerers. They cannot help what is happening to their extremities and they cannot prevent themselves from developing this condition which produces such devastation in the involved extremity.

Abnormal Sympathetic Reflex

The third condition that must be present before a patient can develop reflex sympathetic dystrophy is an abnormal sympathetic reflex. In the normal state

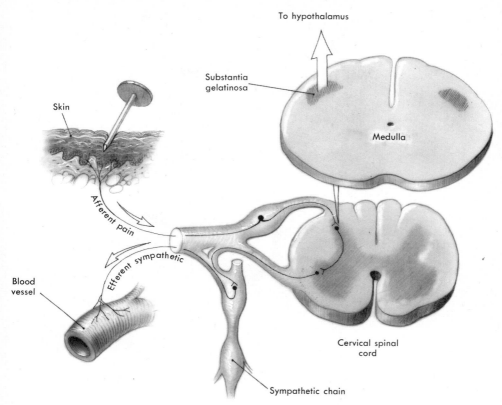

Figure 12-7 Normal reflex arc includes temporary increased sympathetic activity from painful injury, but RSD may develop if this reflex does not shut down at appropriate time. (From Lankford, L. L., and Thompson, J. E.: Reflex sympathetic dystrophy, upper and lower extremity: Diagnosis and management. *In* The American Academy of Orthopaedic Surgeons Instructional Course Lectures, St. Louis, C. V. Mosby Co., 1977, Vol. 26.)

there is a sympathetic reflex that produces vasoconstriction as a response to trauma or to threats to the body's tissues (Fig. 12–7). Certainly, this vasoconstriction reflex is necessary to stop bleeding and to prevent excessive swelling. Soon, however, the vasoconstrictive reflex gives way to vasodilation in order for the body to speed up the repair process, and the orderly mechanism of healing takes place to restore the damaged tissue and to regain function of the part. However, this normal physiological procedure may not take place and instead the initial normal vasoconstrictive reflex may fail to shut down, continuing in an accelerated fashion to the detriment of the tissues. Painful localized ischemia is produced, and thus the "pain reflex" of RSD is set into motion. Livingston (1943) suggested that an abnormal feedback mechanism occurs when afferent pain fiber stimulation persists, causing an abnormal activity in the "internuncial pool" in the spinal cord, resulting in increased sympathetic activity. With increased sympathetic activity, further vasoconstriction occurs, causing more ischemia, and increased pain is produced, which, in turn, causes the sympathetic reflex to further accelerate the vicious cycle (Fig. 12–8).

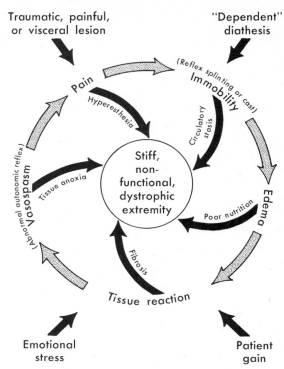

Figure 12–8 Various etiological factors creating the vicious cycle of RSD. (From Lankford, L. L., and Thompson, J. E.: Reflex sympathetic dystrophy, upper and lower extremity: Diagnosis and management. *In* The American Academy of Orthopaedic Surgeons Instructional Course Lectures, St. Louis, C. V. Mosby Co., 1977, Vol. 26.

Melzack and Wall (1965) proposed a theory about the transmission of pain which has been most helpful in understanding the very complicated transmission mechanism of pain. While their "gate control theory" has not been completely supported by experimental evidence and has its share of critics, it has gone a long way to provide us with many answers to this very perplexing subject and remains as the best model yet proposed. This theory suggests that cells in the substantia gelatinosa of the dorsal horn have the capacity to modulate pain fibers coming from the lateral spinothalamic tract. They postulate that the large diameter fibers of pressure, light touch, and joint motion proprioception have the capacity to "close the gate" so that the small diameter pain fibers cannot be transmitted through the transmission cells to be perceived in the cortex as pain. In this manner, a minimum stimulus of pain can be prevented from being interpreted by the cortex as a maximum degree of pain. On the other hand, if the large fiber stimulation (pressure, light touch, and joint motion proprioception) is of sufficient volume, the substantia gelatinosa cells can effectively block or "close the gate" altogether to the small fiber pain stimulation. In other words, if the pressure, light touch, and joint motion stimulation can "outshout" the smaller and slower transmitting pain fibers, the cortex will not perceive pain. The therapeutic implications of this will be discussed under the subdivision of treatment. This system also allows for a central control mechanism of pain perception and explains how psychological and emotional factors can influence the amount and quality of pain.

DIAGNOSIS

Since reflex sympathetic dystrophy is a distinct and definite entity, it has distinct and definite criteria for diagnosis. The diagnosis is not made by exclusion, although, of course, as in any procedure of diagnosis it is important to rule out other conditions having similar symptoms. The diagnosis, however, is made on the basis of distinctive symptoms of RSD.

There are three stages; therefore, the symptoms are somewhat different in each stage. It is necessary to become familiar with each stage so that the symptom picture can be recognized for any of the three stages. The four cardinal symptoms are:
1. Pain
2. Swelling
3. Stiffness
4. Discoloration

The *secondary symptoms* which are most often present, but not necessarily inevitable, are:
1. Osseous demineralization
2. Sudomotor changes
3. Temperature changes
4. Trophic changes
5. Vasomotor instability
6. Palmar fibromatosis

The overriding condition which is paramount in the diagnosis of RSD is the consideration that all of these symptoms are much greater than would be expected for any other traumatic or diseased state. In other words, if the symptoms are markedly out of proportion to the pain-inciting lesion and if the cardinal signs are present with at least some of the secondary signs, then a presumptive diagnosis of reflex sympathetic dystrophy can be made. A confirmed diagnosis, however, can only be made after a temporary or permanent interruption of the sympathetic reflex has produced beneficial results. When this occurs, there can be no doubt that the case at hand is, in fact, reflex sympathetic dystrophy. This is the main distinguishing factor that separates this condition from all other problems of the extremity that are confused with RSD. It must be stated, however, that reflex sympathetic dystrophy cannot be ruled out when the condition fails to show improvement following a sympathetic block that is not truly successful. To be sure that the block has produced ablation of the sympathetic impulses, the extremity must show warmth, dryness, improved coloration, increased capillary flow, and, in the case of the upper extremity, a Horner's syndrome must be present.

SYMPATHETIC NERVOUS SYSTEM

The sympathetic nervous system of the extremities arises principally in the thoracic and lumbar portion of the spinal cord and is composed of sympathetic preganglionic fibers or axons whose cell bodies are located in the lateral horns of the thoracic and lumbar cord. These myelinated sympathetic fibers exit from the spinal cord via the anterior nerve root, from which they separate and form white rami which enter the thoracic and lumbar sympathetic ganglia. A synapse occurs and the postganglionic sympathetic fibers, which are nonmyelinated, exit from the ganglia through the gray rami and enter the peripheral nerve where they eventually reach their target structures such as blood vessels, sweat glands, or hair follicles. This junction of the postganglionic sympathetic nerve fiber with its effector organ is called the neuroeffector junction. Since sympathetic pregangli- onic fibers divide and form plexuses and synapse with many different post- ganglionic cell bodies, a sympathetic discharge may affect several different target organs represented in more than one dermatome. Impulses are transmit- ted from nerve to nerve and from nerve to effector organ by a process called neurohumeral transmission, which involves the release of a neurotransmitter substance from a nerve terminal. The neurotransmitter at most peripheral sympathetic neuroeffector junctions is the catecholamine norepinephrine, which is stored in inactive form within granular structures in the adrenergic nerve ter- minal.

Most sympathetic activity in the postganglionic axons is produced at the neuroeffector junctions by the release of norepinephrine (the sympathetic neurotransmittter) and these nerve fibers are referred to as adrenergic nerves. The sympathetic neurotransmitter for sweat glands, however, is acetylcholine; therefore, these particular fibers are cholinergic fibers. Adrenergic receptors present in a particular tissue may be alpha (α) and beta (β). In skin and subcuta- neous tissue the alpha receptor is vasoconstrictor, while in skeletal muscle the beta receptor produces vasodilation. There is, however, also in skeletal muscle an alpha receptor which produces constriction, but this is not as sensitive as the beta receptor; therefore, vasodilation occurs in muscle at low doses of epineph- rine and vasoconstriction occurs with high doses of epinephrine.

In most tissues, α-receptor activation elicits an excitatory response, and β- receptors mediate an inhibitory response. Activation of an adrenergic receptor may elicit either an excitatory or an inhibitory response in different sympathetic- ally innervated structures, based on the relative potencies of the various cate- cholamines released at the neuroeffector junction.

This may well explain why there can be such great variations in the extremi- ty affected with RSD depending on the severity or the stage of involvement — vasoconstriction or vasodilatation, pallor or increased coloration, sweating or drying, coolness or heat.

CLINICAL FORMS

Much better results can be obtained by starting the treatment of reflex sympathetic dystrophy early. This may best be facilitated by understanding that there are several clinical types of RSD. In the past it was generally thought that only very severe traumas which involved partial nerve injuries could be classified as reflex sympathetic dystrophy. Now, however, it is known that RSD can be produced by many different types of traumas or even nontraumatic painful lesions which may not directly involve a nerve. The wide range of severity of the painful lesion, as well as the many gradations of involvement, have contributed to the misunderstanding of reflex sympathetic dystrophy.

It is for this reason that this author has classified the various clinical types (Lankford, 1977). Since the cases that Mitchell described were all extremely serious and were all produced by a partial injury to a major mixed nerve in the proximal portion of the extremity, we have designated this type as major causalgia. There is, however, a much more common form of RSD produced by an injury to the distal part of the extremity involving a purely sensory branch of a nerve. This has been designated as minor causalgia because, indeed, the trauma and severity of the condition are minor compared to the type described by Mitchell. The term causalgia has also been used in this type, since the causative painful lesion does involve an injury to a nerve.

Most cases of reflex sympathetic dystrophy, however, do not involve trauma to a nerve, whether it be major or minor; therefore, designations of major and minor traumatic dystrophies were felt necessary. In addition to this, the designation of shoulder-hand syndrome was given to those cases that involved either a proximal trauma or that resulted from a painful lesion of the body (rather than the extremity) which was not of traumatic origin.

The various clinical types of RSD are classified in ascending order of severity as follows:
1. Minor causalgia
2. Minor traumatic dystrophy
3. Shoulder-hand syndrome
4. Major traumatic dystrophy
5. Major causalgia

Minor Causalgia

This clinical type includes only those cases that are indeed minor and that are caused by minor traumas to a sensory nerve in the distal part of the extremity. As expected, this type is much more common than the cases described by Mitchell. The painful initiating lesion is most commonly an injury to the dorsal sensory branch of the radial nerve in the hand or the sensory branches of the peroneal nerve in the foot. Since the radial nerve comes out from underneath the protection of the brachioradialis in the vicinity of the distal one inch of the radius and becomes subcutaneous, the sensory branches of the radial nerves are prone to injury from either contusion or laceration. Injury to the palmar branch of the median nerve is the next most frequent cause of minor causalgia. This nerve is easily injured by lacerations and surgical procedures in the volar wrist because it is so superficial. Traumas to any digit or to the digital nerve in the hands or feet may also cause this type of RSD. As is the case in major causalgia, the symptom is primarily of burning pain; there is also dysesthesia to light touch, and this may be so profound that the examiner may find it difficult to examine the patient because of withdrawal of the part when it is touched. There is frequently a Tinel's sign present at the site of the injury. A neuroma may or may not be palpated. Because of the danger of a neurodesis being formed at the site of a repaired lacerated dorsal superficial branch of the radial nerve or the palmar branch of the median nerve, it is hazardous to repair these nerves; and since their function is not absolutely necessary, it is probably wise to simply excise these nerves proximal to the wrist joint where they are well protected beneath surrounding muscles.

All of the cardinal signs of RSD are usually present, but the symptoms are confined to two or three digits and are not as severe as in the other types of RSD. Although the initial involvement seems to be in the area supplied by the damaged nerve, the involvement spreads to adjacent areas if the condition is left untreated.

Minor Traumatic Dystrophy

Unquestionably, this is the most common clinical type of reflex sympathetic dystrophy but, unfortunately, it is also the most commonly overlooked. Since it involves only a few of the fingers and is rarely associated with entire hand involvement, and since it is not induced by a nerve injury, most clinicians in the past have failed to recognize that this is indeed a form of reflex sympathetic dystrophy. However, like all types of RSD, unless its true nature is recognized and the proper early treatment begun, there will most likely be a permanent deformity and dysfunciton.

The causative trauma is usually of minor nature and may be nothing more than a mashing of the finger, a stubbing of the toe, a direct blow over the hand or foot, a partial ligamentous tear, or a fracture. The initial involvement may be limited to the involved digit, but if left untreated, more extensive areas of the hand or foot may become involved. The ulnar three fingers are more commonly involved than the radial two, with the thumb being the least involved. It is in this type of RSD that we more commonly see the redness over the dorsum of the MP and PIP joints and over the collateral ligaments. The swelling is usually fusiform, and pain is present on motion. The eventual loss of motion produces flexion contractures in the PIP joints rather than stiffness in extension. Palmar fasciitis with tender and sometimes red nodules is not infrequent in this type.

Shoulder-Hand Syndrome

This clinical type includes those cases of RSD that are caused by a proximal trauma, such as a shoulder or neck injury, or a painful visceral lesion of the body, such as a heart attack, stomach ulcer, pulmonary lesion or a stroke. The entire extremity is usually involved, with the shoulder joint being the first to produce symptoms of pain, swelling, and stiffness. Although the elbow is involved only to a minor degree, rotary motion of the forearm may become quite limited. There is more swelling in the wrist and over the dorsum of the hand in this form of RSD than in the other types. The residual stiffness of the wrist and fingers is more likely to be in extension than in flexion (Fig. 12–9). Early, there is more pain in the shoulder, but eventually all of the joints in the upper extremity become painful. There is fusiform swelling in the fingers, and the patient makes very little effort to move the fingers because of the pain. The hand is usually dry, and there is less redness present than in most other forms of reflex sympathetic dystrophy. Palmar fasciitis with acute nodules, which may be red and tender, is

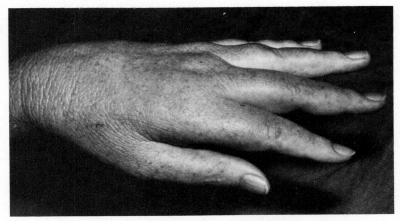

Figure 12–9 Fingers and wrist are characteristically stiff in extension in shoulder-hand type of RSD. (From Lankford, L. L., and Thompson, J. E.: Reflex sympathetic dystrophy, upper and lower extremity: Diagnosis and management. *In* The American Academy of Orthopaedic Surgeons Instructional Course Lectures, St. Louis, C. V. Mosby Co., 1977, Vol. 26.)

more common in this type than in others. The age distribution of shoulder-hand syndrome is usually from age fifty to seventy. While there is a slightly higher incidence in females in all forms of RSD, this is much more evident in shoulder-hand syndrome.

Although this condition has been alluded to in earlier times, the credit for bringing it to our attention should go to Otto Steinbrocker (1947). Following his description of shoulder-hand syndrome and the pronouncement that heart attacks and strokes were the most common cause, there was a rush to include all stiff shoulders following heart attacks, strokes, tendinitis, and capsulitis of the shoulder in this entity. All of these latter conditions can be prevented from producing pain, swelling, and stiffness by the early institution of elevation and gentle motion of the part, and it is a mistake to think of these cases as reflex sympathetic dystrophy. It should be emphasized that all cases of pain, swelling, and stiffness of the shoulder and hand are not reflex sympathetic dystrophy; the diagnosis can be confirmed by the severity of the condition, the presence of the cardinal and secondary signs, and the response to sympathetic interruption.

Major Traumatic Dystrophy

This clinical type usually comes to mind when most people think of reflex sympathetic dystrophy. Certainly, it is the most commonly recognized clinical type of RSD. Not only is it caused by a major type of trauma involving the whole hand and wrist but also it is usually the most severe type seen in a civilian practice. As the name implies, the causative traumatic lesion is usually severe. Colles' fracture and crush injuries lead the list of the types of trauma, but it is felt by this author that, regardless of the initial cause of injury, it is usually a traumatic carpal tunnel syndrome which actually produces the persistent painful lesion that precipitates the reflex sympathetic dystrophy. This is demonstrated in

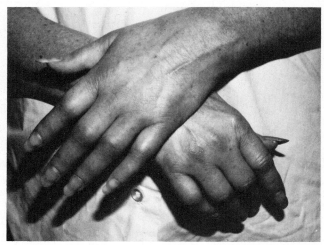

Figure 12–10   Case of bilateral major traumatic dystrophy caused by bilateral traumatic carpal tunnel syndrome secondary to bilateral Colles' fracture. (From Lankford, L. L., and Thompson, J. E.: Reflex sympathetic dystrophy, upper and lower extremity: Diagnosis and management. *In* The American Academy of Orthopaedic Surgeons Instructional Course Lectures, St. Louis, C. V. Mosby Co., 1977, Vol. 26.)

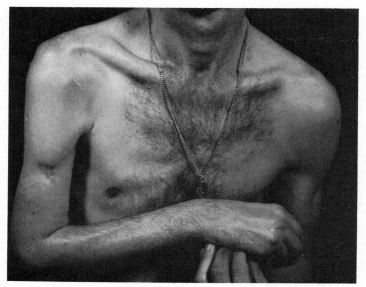

Figure 12–11   Major causalgia resulting from partial injury to median nerve in upper arm secondary to gunshot wound. (From Lankford, L. L., and Thompson, J. E.: Reflex sympathetic dystrophy, upper and lower extremity: Diagnosis and management. *In* The American Academy of Orthopaedic Surgeons Instructional Course Lectures, St. Louis, C. V. Mosby Co., 1977, Vol. 26.)

severe bilateral reflex sympathetic dystrophy (Fig. 12–10) precipitated by bilateral Colles' fractures, neither of which was significantly displaced but which caused a bilateral carpal tunnel syndrome because of the swelling.

The severity of this type of reflex sympathetic dystrophy is so profound that the pain, deformity, and dysfunction may completely change the patient's entire outlook on life.

A much greater degree of osteoporosis is visualized in this clinical type of RSD than in any other. The stiffness which this type produces causes flexion deformities of the interphalangeal joints rather than stiffness in extension.

Major Causalgia

While there is no doubt that this type of reflex sympathetic dystrophy, which was described by Mitchell (1864), causes the greatest devastation of any of the types, it fortunately does not occur very often in a civilian population (Fig. 12–11). It was Mitchell's contention that causalgia was produced by an injury to a part of a major mixed nerve in the proximal portion of the extremity. Usually this is true, but we have seen a severe case of causalgia occur in a nerve that was completely divided. In the lower extremity, trauma to the sciatic nerve produces most cases of causalgia, as does trauma to the median nerve in the upper extremity. In some cases of major causalgia, the symptoms occur quite promptly, but in others there is a delay of several days or weeks. The paramount symptom appears to be an intense burning pain which generally is constant. As in the case of minor causalgia, the pain and painful paresthesias usually occur in the distribution of the nerve that has been injured initially, but with the passage of time the symptoms spread to adjacent areas up and down the involved extremity.

There is usually less redness, swelling, and increased temperature present in the first stages than in other forms of RSD. Pallor or cyanosis, coolness, and sweating are more likely in the second stage, and extreme trophic changes, with stiffness, are present in the third stage.

In severe cases of major causalgia, the pain is aggravated by many types of stimuli such as lightly stroking the skin, wind blowing over the skin, and active or passive movement. Even auditory stimuli such as loud or high-pitched sounds or even certain words may trigger an exacerbation of pain. The pain, swelling, stiffness, and dysfunction may be so profound that severe mental and emotional changes may occur.

Doupe (1944) presented an explanation of how a partial injury to a major mixed nerve can cause this very disabling symptom complex. He proposed that the partial nerve injury caused the loss of the normal myelin sheath with its insulation, and this produced an "artificial synapse" which allowed a "short circuiting" of the impulses being transmitted between the efferent sympathetic fibers and the afferent sensory fibers. He called this abnormal "fiber interaction" a pathological reflex arc because the efferent sympathetic fibers were shunted across at the injury site to the afferent somatic pain fibers, which were then interpreted by the cortex as pain. In the distal reflex arc, the afferent pain impulses were short circuited at the nerve injury site to the efferent sympathetic fibers, which produced antidromic sympathetic activity and increased pain (Fig. 12–12).

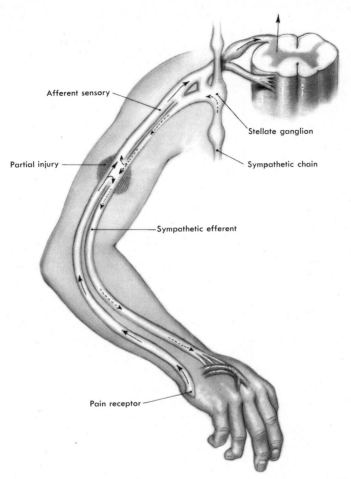

Afferent sensory

Stellate ganglion

Partial injury

Sympathetic chain

Sympathetic efferent

Pain receptor

Figure 12–12   Doupe suggests that partial nerve injury creates "short circuiting" of afferent pain stimuli to efferent sympathetic fibers. (From Lankford, L. L., and Thompson, J. E.: Reflex sympathetic dystrophy, upper and lower extremity: Diagnosis and management. *In* The American Academy of Orthopaedic Surgeons Instructional Course Lectures, St. Louis, C. V. Mosby Co., 1977, Vol. 26.)

TREATMENT

The fibrotic changes produced by reflex sympathetic dystrophy in the gliding tissues and in the joints of the extremities may well become permanent if treatment is not promptly administered. Good results, therefore, require a prompt diagnosis so that treatment may be undertaken before permanent changes have ensued. Awareness of the various clinical types of RSD is, therefore, essential. One must remember that along with the major forms there are also the minor forms of RSD and that the inciting traumas need not be severe.

When the pain, swelling, stiffness, color changes, and osteoporosis are much greater than should be expected for any given condition, then reflex sympathetic dystrophy should be suspected.

It is important to remember that reflex sympathetic dystrophy can develop from an injury, an acquired disease, or after a surgical procedure even in spite of the proper treatment for that condition. Since it can happen in any patient in whom the three etiological factors are present, the occurrence of RDS is not a reflection on the patient's doctor — rather, it is an unfortunate combination of three factors.

The treatment is to eliminate one or more of these predisposing causes and the "pain reflex" chain will then be broken. The most immediate way of eliminating one of the three etiological factors, of course, is to stop the increased sympathetic activity (Spurling, 1930). This may be done by:

1. Local anesthetic block of the sympathetic nerve fibers
2. Use of a sympatholytic drug
3. Surgical sympathectomy

Sympathetic Block

In the upper extremity, the classical way of interrupting the sympathetic arc is to do a stellate ganglion block using a local anesthetic agent to produce a temporary break in the sympathetic stimulation to the extremity. In the lower extremity, this is accomplished with a paravertebral block done in the same manner. If a satisfactory interruption in the sympathetic arc has taken place, the extremity will become warm and dry, and the color will return to a more normal hue or even at times a pink tinge will make its appearance. In the case of the upper extremity, a Horner's sign will be noted. By the time it has been determined that there has been a satisfactory block and that the sympathetic impulses have been stopped, the patient will note a profound relief of pain. Subsequently, there is usually an improvement of motion and some relief of swelling. If there was coldness of the part, hyperhidrosis, and cyanosis, the relief will be even more dramatic because of the complete reversal of these symptoms. The stellate ganglion block and the paravertebral block are, therefore, diagnostic as well as therapeutic. If the pain has been relieved and the burning sensation stopped by the sole means of blocking the sympathetic chain and leaving unaltered the somatic nervous system, then there can be no doubt that the patient's affliction is mediated through an increased sympathetic nerve activity, and RSD has been confirmed.

The pharmacological block of the nerve will last only about one and a half hours if lidocaine (Xylocaine) is used without adrenalin, and possibly twice that long if adrenalin is used. If 0.25 per cent bupivacaine (Marcaine) is used, the block may well last for as long as nine hours. The therapeutic effect of this block, however, will last a great deal longer than the pharmacological interruption of the nerve. On rare occasions, one block might be enough to permanently interrupt the "vicious cycle," but this would only be true if the condition were treated extremely early. Usually, it is necessary to give three to four or more blocks at weekly intervals. This may be sufficient to stop the pain, and more importantly to stop the pain on active and passive motion of the joints of the affected limb. While it is true that decreased swelling and improved motion is commonly noted after a series of blocks, the more important therapeutic effect is the relief of pain. If this can be achieved, then other modalities of treatment can be used to decrease the swelling and improve motion. In some cases, the series of blocks is not sufficient and other modes of sympathetic interruption become necessary.

The technique for *stellate ganglion block* is described in Chapter 17, by Kleinert et al. A block cannot be called successful unless the extremity becomes warmer and dry, and unless the pallor or cyanosis has been replaced with a pink coloration. In addition to this, when the stellate ganglion has been blocked a Horner's sign will be present. Within five to 30 minutes, there should be relief of pain and, more importantly, reduction of pain on motion. In many cases, reduction of swelling and an actual improvement of motion is noted. These beneficial results may last only a few hours or may last from one to two days, depending upon the severity of the condition. The abnormal sympathetic reflex, however, may again be generated and the symptoms can recur. A repeat block should then be done within a few days to one week.

The technique for *paravertebral block* is described in Chapter 17 by Kleinert et al. A successful paravertebral sympathetic block is obtained only if the lower extremity is made warm and dry within 30 minutes after the installation of the local anesthesia. The beneficial results far outlast the actual period of time that the sympathetic nerve has been anesthetized. Several blocks may be necessary at weekly intervals.

Continuous sympathetic blocks using a flexible catheter or tubing directed at the appropriate sympathetic ganglion have been described by Betcher (1953).

Somatic nerve block can also be used to produce an interruption of the sympathetic impulses, since the sympathetic nerve fibers and the somatic nerve fibers are both contained in the peripheral nerves. Radial, median, and ulnar nerve blocks at the wrist serve very well to produce a localized sympathetic interruption to the hand and digits. Median, ulnar, and radial nerve blocks at the elbow will produce a temporary interruption of increased sympathetic activity in the forearm and wrist. Any local anesthetic agent will not only produce a complete sympathetic block but also will relieve the pain by interrupting afferent impulses in the involved extremity. Lidocaine (Xylocaine) is used for short action, and bupivacaine (Marcaine) is used for anesthesia lasting nine hours or longer. The beneficial results of blocking the sympathetics do not last as long when the block is given peripherally rather than at the level of the sympathetic ganglia. They have to be repeated at least two or three times a week to be as beneficial as one stellate ganglion block. This technique is useful when the patient declines to have a sympathetic ganglion block. It is more useful for minor causalgia and minor traumatic dystrophy than for the other clinical forms of RSD.

Periodic perineural infusion (Omer, 1971) has been described as a technique for continuous blocking of somatic nerves and trigger points and produces both afferent pain fiber interruption and sympathetic block by the injection of a local anesthetic serially into an indwelling tube implanted at the site of the offending nerve or trigger point (see Chapter 15).

Sympatholytic Drugs

Unfortunately, there is no perfect pharmacological way to completely inter-rupt the sympathetic activity to the extremities through the use of systemic medication. The most universal effect of sympathetic stimulation is the alpha-adrenergic action, which is the most important vasoconstrictor in the extremity. Phenoxybenzamine (Dibenzyline) undoubtedly is the best alpha blocking agent with the least undesirable effects. Phentolamine (Regitine) also is a good alpha blocking agent, but its use requires careful evaluation of its effect on certain cardiac conditions. Tolazoline (Priscoline) is a good smooth muscle relaxant but has only slight sympatholytic effect and, therefore, requires very large doses for clinical application.

Therefore, the only practical alpha-adrenergic blocking agent (sympatholy-tic drug) is Dibenzyline. The dose is 10 mg orally, one to four times a day. Since the sympatholytic activity causes vasodilation in the entire peripheral circulatory system, it will produce some hypotension with rapid changes in position. The patient must therefore be advised to move from recumbency to a sitting position, and then from a sitting position to the erect position, with a few seconds rest in between. Also, it is necessary to start out with one 10 mg capsule of Dibenzyline a day until the patient has adjusted to its hypotensive effect and then, after four to five days, it may be increased to two capsules daily if the patient has been able to adjust to the medication without symptoms of dizziness or "fuzzy vision." In this careful manner, Dibenzyline may be increased to either three or four times aa day until the desired sympatholytic effect is obtained or until hypotensive symp-toms require that the medication be cut back. Propranolol (Inderal) should not be given in conjunction with Dibenzyline because the former drug is a beta-adrenergic blocking agent and would, therefore, produce a profound hypoten-sion. Dibenzyline, however, can be used with such beta-adrenergic stimulants as nylidrin (Arlidin), which is a peripheral vasodilating agent of muscle more than skin. Dibenzyline may be used in conjunction with a sympathetic ganglion block or a somatic nerve block of the sympathetics in the peripheral nerves. Although it is not effective enough to replace the sympathetic block with an anesthestic agent, it helps to prolong the effect of the sympathetic interruption. It is also given to patients who have had surgery or extremity trauma and who, it is felt, may have the diathesis for reflex sympathetic dystrophy, with the hope that this will prevent the generation of the abnormal sympathetic reflex.

Sympathectomy

If stellate ganglion blocks or peripheral nerve blocks have been beneficial but have not produced lasting results, or if the reflex sympathetic dystrophy has been in progress over a period of many months, it may be necessary to use a surgical sympathectomy to produce a permanent interruption of the abnormal sympathetic reflex. While it is more logical for the extremity surgeon to do the somatic nerve block, it is preferable for the surgeon who will be doing the sympathectomy to give the stellate and the paravertebral blocks so that he may better decide when it is advisable to give up on the sympathetic ganglion blocks and resort to the permanent ablation of the increased sympathetic activity by doing a surgical excision of the sympathetic ganglia.

SYMPATHECTOMY FOR THE UPPER EXTREMITY. The most commonly employed surgical sympathectomy approaches are the posterior approach, as recommended by Smithwick (1940), and the transaxillary approach (Kleinert, 1965). The anterior approach to the lower cervical and upper thoracic sympathetic chain is only rarely used at the present time because of the danger of producing a Horner's syndrome and also because of the difficulty in producing a denervation of the third and fourth dorsal sympathetic ganglia.

In most cases, it is only necessary to obliterate the second, third, and fourth upper thoracic ganglia, but if the stellate ganglion is well segmented, it may be possible to remove the lower segment of this ganglion without producing a Horner's syndrome. When the operation removes these ganglia, it rarely fails to produce a complete cessation of sympathetic stimulation in the upper extremity. This results in an extremely high rate of *relief of pain* in reflex sympathetic dystrophy. The relief is often immediate and dramatic. More significant, however, is the relief of pain on motion, and it is because of this that other modalities of treatment such as exercise and splinting can be instituted with beneficial results. In addition to the relief of pain, resolution of swelling and improved motion are often noted. The sooner the sympathectomy is done, the more profound is the relief of pain and the greater the improvement of motion. The technique for sympathectomy is described in Chapter 17.

SYMPATHECTOMY FOR THE LOWER EXTREMITY. Lumbar sympathectomy is indicated when there has been improvement following the paravertebral blocks, but this improvement has not been of sufficient quality or duration to make more than three or four blocks worthwhile. As in the upper extremity, another indication for the sympathectomy rather than the blocks is prolonged duration of symptoms for more than three or four months. The relief of pain and swelling in the lower extremity is equally as profound as that seen in the upper extremity.

The most commonly used surgical approach is the lateral flank–extraperitoneal section of the sympathetic ganglia. Most commonly, the second, third, and fourth lumbar ganglia are removed, but if the problem involves the thigh or knee it is necessary to excise the first lumbar sympathetic ganglion as well. The technique for sympathectomy is described in Chapter 17.

Other Forms of Treatment

While the main treatment of reflex sympathetic dystrophy is unquestionably the interruption of the increased sympathetic activity (White, 1974), other forms of treatment are helpful. As pointed out in the discussion of etiology, the three necessary ingredients for the formation of reflex sympathetic dystrophy are:
1. Persistent painful lesion
2. Diathesis
3. Abnormal sympathetic reflex

It therefore follows that if any of these three necessary causes can be eliminated or diminished, then this pernicious reflex cycle can be either broken up or decelerated. Elimination of the increased sympathetic activity has been discussed. Relief or elimination of pain can be a productive means of treating RSD.

Diathesis, the second etiological ingredient, cannot be changed significantly, since this is an inherent characteristic or bodily susceptibility which cannot be altered but which may be ameliorated slightly with such mood modifying drugs as diazepam (Valium), trifluoperazine (Stelazine), chlorpromazine (Thorazine), chlordiazepoxide (Librium), amitriptyline (Elavil) or fluphenazine hydrochloride (Prolixin). These medications, while they cannot change the patient's susceptibility to RSD, may slow the vicious cycle down somewhat, but must not be used to replace the need for sympathetic interruption.

Eliminating the painful lesion is an important part of treatment of RSD. If it is suspected that reflex sympathetic dystrophy is occurring after an injury and while the extremity is still immobilized, it is important to make sure that the immobilizing device is not too tight. The cast may need to be split or changed or bony prominences checked to see if the source of pain is from pressure. In the case of injury or surgery around the radial aspect of the wrist or the basal joint of the thumb, a local anesthetic block of the dorsal sensory branches of the radial nerve will not only relieve the pain but will also stop the sympathetic feedback for a period of time. Other trigger points may be injected either by the interrupted technique or by the periodic perineural infusion technique of Omer (1971).

Elevation is an extremely important treatment for reflex sympathetic dystrophy, as it is for any type of extremity affliction that causes swelling. The patient should be sufficiently instructed by the treating physician in regard to the necessity of keeping the part elevated so that it will not become necessary to use other devices to insure elevation that might interfere with the mobility of the patient. A few pillows and a few minutes of explanation are more beneficial to the physiology of the damaged extremity than are the methods requiring the extremity to be tied up or suspended.

One of the most common causes of the painful lesion in the major traumatic dystrophy is the occurrence of a *traumatic carpal tunnel syndrome* along with such other injuries as a crushed hand or a Colles' fracture. Great care must be exercised in evaluating such an injury to make sure that the patient does not have the signs and symptoms of a carpal tunnel syndrome. If this is suspected, then a release of the median or ulnar nerves, or both, in the forearm or wrist may well prevent the occurrence of RSD. To ignore the symptoms of numbness or "dead feeling" is a sure invitation to future trouble. In the case of a comminuted Colles' fracture which must be decompressed in the carpal tunnel area, maintenance of fracture reduction and cast immobilization can be carried out through the use of the .064 in. diameter Kirschner wire drilled through the base of the second and third metacarpals and a small Steinmann pin drilled through both cortices of the radius in the triangular interval between the brachioradialis, the radial wrist extensor, and the abductor pollicis longus tendon. This pin does not penetrate the skin on the other side and therefore is only a "half pin." Another half pin can be used in the proximal ulna, drilling it from the lateral side through both cortices of the bone but not through the skin on the medial side. Care should be exercised not to impale the ulnar nerve. These pins may then be incorporated in plaster, and subsequently the entire palmar aspect of the cast can be removed to dress and inspect the carpal tunnel release wound.

Another way to eliminate or decrease the painful lesion is through the use of *transcutaneous large fiber stimulation* of the peripheral nerve (Wall, 1967). Small, battery operated nerve stimulators using conductive pads as electrodes can be adjusted to a voltage and frequency that will produce a pleasant tingling sensation but not motor activity. In most cases, this will effectively relieve pain while the transcutaneous stimulation is taking place. This will enable the patient to have periods of relief from pain which will not only help him to exercise his previously painful hand but also will temporarily eliminate the pain feedback that keeps the vicious cycle moving. This can effectively be used while the patient receives physical therapy and performs functional activities. The device is customarily used several hours each day with rest periods in between. Most medical supply houses have these units for rent. Although the transcutaneous nerve stimulator cannot take the place of a sympathetic block or a sympathectomy, it is a useful adjunct to the patient's combined treatment. Its effectiveness, however, is limited to early cases.

Another way of relieving pain to break up the etiology triad is through the use of *steroids* (Glick, 1973). There is no interruption of the overactivity of the sympathetic nervous system with the use of steroids, but diminishing pain, swelling, and the fibrotic reaction can be of some value in early cases of RSD. We do not attempt their use in well-established cases, feeling that their only role is in mild and very early dystrophy; therefore, its use does not eliminate the need for sympathetic interruption.

HAND THERAPY

It is not uncommon for the patient's history to reveal that he has received physical therapy elsewhere which has been so vigorous that it has been a very painful experience. Since pain is one of the ingredients of RSD, it is extremely important that the patient not be exposed to any painful stimuli. Any physical therapy that is done vigorously enough to produce pain is definitely contraindicated.

Realistically, it is not possible to carry out any significant degree of hand therapy until the abnormal sympathetic reflex has been interrupted (block or sympathectomy); only then is the patient's pain relieved enough that he can productively do active exercises.

Gentle active exercise of each involved joint of the dystrophic extremity should be started as soon as it is easily tolerated. After the patient has been able to accomplish gentle active exercise without pain, gentle passive exercise may be allowed. No one but the patient, however, should ever do passive exercise, because no one but the patient can tell when the passive force is going to reach the point of pain. Each passive exercise should be just short of the point where it would produce pain. Use of the transcutaneous nerve stimulator helps the patient accomplish exercises without pain.

Gentle rubbing and massaging of the involved extremity by the patient helps to relieve pain, decrease swelling, and improve motion. Although this does not sound like a very sophisticated modality of treatment, it is very effective. Just as one rubs his bumped elbow to relieve pain, rubbing and massaging of the RSD extremity helps to relieve pain. The explanation of this can be found in the "gate

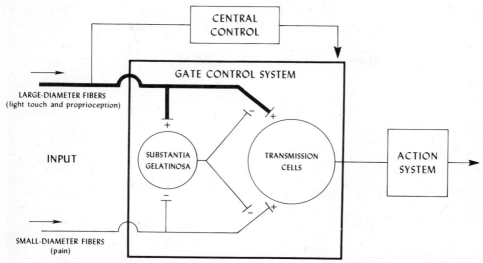

Figure 12–13 Diagramatic visualization of "gate control" theory of pain proposed by Melzack and Wall. (From Melzack, R., and Wall, P. D.: Pain mechanisms: New theory. Science *150*:971, Diagram, 1965. Copyright 1965 by American Association for the Advancement of Science.)

control" theory of pain (Melzack and Wall, 1965), as diagramatically shown in Figure 12–13. Exercising and massaging the extremity (proprioceptive and light touch large fiber impulses) "drown out" or "close the gate" to the small unmyelinated C-fibers of pain, thus dampening or modulating the pain impulses so that very few impulses get through the central transmission system to higher cortical levels.

Heat may be used to help relieve pain and improve motion. This should be done, however, with the extremity elevated. Dependent heat increases swelling and fibrosis and is of questionable value. The two forms of heat treatment that can be used most effectively with elevation are the "paraffin glove" and hot packs.

Splinting is often necessary because of the deformities which are produced by reflex sympathetic dystrophy. For patients having the wrist in flexion, the MP joints in extension, and the PIP joints in flexion, it is very helpful to use dynamic splinting to reverse these deformities. The wrist is the "keystone" in the positioning of the hand. The "resting hand" or "balanced hand" position is with the wrist in extension, the MP joints flexed approximately 60 to 70 degrees, and the interphalangeal joints flexed about 35 degrees. Greatest flexion is present in the small finger, with progressively less flexion in the digits closer to the thumb. In order to regain the "resting hand" position, the wrist must first be brought into extension. Commercially available splints or custom-built splints made in the Hand Therapy Department can be used to accomplish wrist extension but should never be worn so tightly that they cause discomfort. The splints must be removed at least every hour for five to 10 minutes of exercise and massage of the hand. As the patient progresses, the hand therapist should teach the patient how to use the hand again. In many cases, the patient has psychologically completely

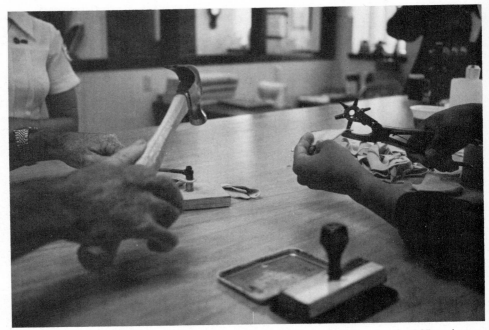

Figure 12–14 Functional activities program in Hand Therapy Unit assists the RSD patients to regain use of their hands.

disassociated himself from his painful, stiff, and deformed extremity. It takes a great deal of patience and effort on the part of the therapist to teach the patient how to use his hand again.

Graduated *functional activities* are planned by the therapist to take advantage of each step the patient gains (Fig. 12–14). The ultimate functional capacity of the extremity is often determined by how well the patient cooperates with the therapy program; obtaining this cooperation sometimes taxes the therapist's ingenuity.

ADJUNCTIVE TREATMENT

Psychotherapeutics may occasionally be indicated in the treatment of RSD, because there is without question a psychiatric problem present in some cases. It is usually difficult, however, to persuade the patient to seek the help of a psychiatrist. This type of treatment usually is time consuming, and therefore, must be done concurrently with the other recognized modalities of treatment.

RECONSTRUCTIVE THERAPY

No elective reconstructive surgery should be done as long as there is any sympathetic reflex activity left. Obviously, the part must be completely pain free before any consideration is given to elective surgery. One very definite indication for a sympathectomy rather than multiple sympathetic blocks is the necessity for some type of reconstructive surgery before full rehabilitation of the patient can be complete. Blocks may be used, however, to control excessive sympathetic stimulation if urgent surgery is required, such as carpal tunnel release or reamputation of a part because of the presence of a painful neuroma or tight skin over the end of the stump. The urgency of this surgery would likely preclude a sympathectomy and instead require the "protective umbrella" of several sympathetic blocks before and after the necessary surgery.

If a sympathectomy has been done, and all reflex sympathetic dystrophy activity has subsided, and if the pain has long since been relieved, such elective surgery as tenolysis and joint release may be judiciously undertaken in order to regain motion if an exhaustive physical therapy program has been faithfully undertaken by the patient. Surgery performed without these specifications and safeguards is ill advised.

CONCLUSION

1. Reflex sympathetic dystrophy should be the all-inclusive term to encompass the various forms of vasomotor and trophic changes produced by painful stimuli, either traumatic or acquired, and mediated through the "sympathetic-pain reflex."
2. Reflex sympathetic dystrophy occurs only when all three of the etiological factors are present:
   a. Persistent painful lesion
   b. Diathesis (patient's susceptibility)
   c. Abnormal sympathetic reflex
3. Clinical forms of RSD are:
   a. Minor causalgia
   b. Minor traumatic dystrophy
   c. Shoulder-hand syndrome
   d. Major traumatic dystrophy
   e. Major causalgia.
4. Reflex sympathetic dystrophy should be suspected when there is more pain, swelling, stiffness, discoloration and osteoporosis than would ordinarily be anticipated for that particular trauma or acquired disease.
5. Early diagnosis and treatment are essential for the best results.
6. Some form of sympathetic activity interruption should be instituted early (sympathetic block or sympathectomy).
7. Be alert to the presence of an acute traumatic carpal tunnel syndrome, and provide adequate surgical decompression of the involved nerves.
8. After interruption of the increased sympathetic activity (resulting in the relief of pain), an intensive rehabilitative program should be initiated.
9. Make sure that physical therapy and splinting do not cause pain, for this will only add to the joint reaction, swelling, and stiffness.
10. Reconstructive surgical procedures to gain motion are only occasionally advisable and should not be done without the "protection" of sympathetic blocks or sympathectomy.

REFERENCES

Betcher, A. M., Bean, G., and Casten, D. F.: Continuous procaine block of paravertebral sympathetic ganglions. J.A.M.A. *151*:288, 1953.

Bonica, J. J.: Causalgia and other reflex sympathetic dystrophies. Postgrad. Med. *53*:143, May, 1973.

de Takats, G.: Causalgia states in peace and war. J.A.M.A. *128*:699, 1945.

Doupe, J., Cullen, C. H., and Chance, G. Q.: Post-traumatic pain and causalgia syndrome. J. Neurol. Neurosurg. Psychiatry 7:33, 1944.

Glick, E. N.: Reflex dystrophy (algoneurodystrophy): Results of treatment by corticosteroids. Reumatol. Rehab. *12*:84–88, 1973.

Homans, J.: Minor causalgia: A hyperesthetic neurovascular syndrome. N. Engl. J. Med. *222*:870, 1940.

Kleinert, H. E., Cook, F. W., and Kutz, J. E.: Neurovascular disorders of the upper extremity treated by transaxillary sympathectomy. Arch. Surg. *90*:612, 1965.

Lankford, L. L., and Thompson, J. E.: Reflex sympathetic dystrophy, upper and lower extremity: Diagnosis and management. *In* AAOS Instructional Course Lectures, St. Louis, C. V. Mosby Co., 1977, Vol. 26.

Livingston, W. K.: Pain Mechanisms: A Physiological Interpretation of Causalgia and Its Related States. New York, Macmillan, 1943.

Melzack, R., and Wall, P. D.: Pain mechanisms: New theory. Science *150*:971, 1965.

Mitchell, S. W.: On the diseases of nerves resulting from injuries in contributions relating to the causation and prevention of disease, and to camp diseases. *In* Flint, A.: United States Sanitary Commission Memoirs. New York, 1867.

Mitchell, S. W., Morehouse, G. R., and Keen, W. W.: Gunshot Wounds and Other Injuries of Nerves. Philadelphia, J. B. Lippincott Co., 1864.

Moore, D. C.: Regional Block. Springfield, Charles C Thomas, 1967.

Omer, G. E., Jr., and Thomas, S. R.: Treatment of causalgia. Texas Med. J. *67*:93, 1971.

Patman, R. D., Thompson, J. E., and Persson, A. V.: Management of post-traumatic pain syndromes. Ann. Surg. *177*:780, 1973.

Smithwick, R. H.: The Rationale and Technique of Sympathectomy for the Relief of Vascular Spasm of the Extremity. N. Engl. J. Med. *222*:699, 1940.

Spurling, R. G.: Causalgia of the upper extremity: Treatment by dorsal sympathetic ganglionectomy. Arch. Neurol. Psychiatry *23*:784, 1930.

Steinbrocker, O.: The shoulder-hand syndrome. Am. J. Med. *3*:402, 1947.

Sudeck, P. H. M.: Ueber die acute entzundliche knockenatrophic. Arch. Klin. Chir. *62*:147, 1900.

Wall, P. D., and Sweet, W. H.: Temporary abolition of pain in man. Science, *155*:108, 1967.

White, J. C.: Sympathectomy for relief of pain. *In* Bonica, J. J.: Advances in Neurology, International Symposium on Pain. New York, Raven Press, 1974. Vol. 4.

13

ACUPUNCTURE

ROBERT J. SCHULTZ

Acupuncture works! That's a strong statement in view of the poor reception the modality has received; however, one cannot deny the numerous reports of success. In writing this section, I am not going to add my endorsement, but will relate my personal experience with acupuncture, both in treating patients and observing the treatment of those patients under the skilled care of master acupuncturists.

New procedures and concepts are difficult to accept. This is especially true when there is little scientific theory or background, and even more so when the concepts are in direct conflict with previously accepted views as determined by the experts. At the meeting of the American Orthopaedic Association in 1977, Dr. Albert B. Sabin related the hardships he encountered in the development of his vaccine and how previous theories accepted by experts who refused to yield set his investigations back for extended periods of time.

In order to properly present a modality, the procedure must first be defined and its variations recognized and categorized separately. The ancient art of acupuncture represents the insertion of needles through the skin at various preselected areas or body parts in order to produce a specific effect and relieve pain and cure disease.

Procedures that are noninvasive, such as massage of acupuncture points, should not be considered acupuncture. Clearly, one must differentiate acupuncture for anesthesia from acupuncture for the management of disease or pain; in addition, the newer variations in technique used in acupuncture analgesia must be differentiated, such as electro-acupuncture.

Acupuncture Anesthesia

Acupuncture anesthesia had as its base the theory that "classical acupuncture" can ease pain and regulate the physiologic functions of the body. As an extension of this concept, Chinese physicians began to question whether acupuncture, which had been long used to treat pain, could be used to prevent pain during surgical procedures. It was felt that following the insertion of needles into specific points of the patient's body, the patient would be able to tolerate surgery while fully conscious. The first reported case, in 1958, was of a dental extraction. Thus acupuncture anesthesia is a modern outgrowth of the classical practice of acupuncture treatment.

Acupuncture Analgesia

The terms acupuncture anesthesia and acupuncture analgesia are not exactly correct and have led to much controversy over the terminology; however, the literature utilizes these terms and, for convenience, I will continue to do the same.

Acupuncture for the management of pain (acupuncture analgesia) is a treatment technique that evolved over thousands of years of vast clinical experience. During this time, it has been performed by a variety of methods, many of which, like acupuncture anesthesia, are modifications or modernizations of traditional acupuncture. Surely, to place an electric charge in contact with a needle could not have been accomplished 5000 years ago. It is possible that these multiple techniques have led to the conflicting reports on the success of acupuncture, since the many methods are lumped together under the common term.

Pain is a subjective complaint. It produces different responses in different people, and, depending on its location and nature, will produce different responses in the same patient. We have been conditioned to accept certain types of pain, such as "arthritic pain," whereas we may refuse to accept pain produced by other etiologies. By the same token, we have also learned to accept or reject the successes and failures of known treatment modalities.

In evaluating the results of acupuncture, one must strongly consider: (1) the expectations, (2) the publicity that has been generated about the modality, (3) the skill of the acupuncturist, and (4) the acupuncture method performed.

EXPECTATION.   A severe problem with acupuncture is the expectation that it is a cure-all with long-lasting results and that failure is unacceptable. This goal is difficult to achieve even with the sophisticated modalities utilized in Western medicine. We accept failure in the medical management of illness, in reconstructive surgical procedures, and certainly in the management of pain. Thus, with acupuncture, as with other treatment modalities, the all or none concept must be put aside and partial success accepted. Acupuncture must not be considered an end-all in itself but a modality to be utilized in concert with other forms of treatment.

PUBLICITY.   Another drawback is the publicity generated about acupuncture. Because the initial practice of acupuncture in the United States began in back alleys and other less favorable locations by unaccredited personnel, an element of suspicion about the technique has developed. As a result, special state licensing procedures were adopted to restrict its use. These restrictions were superimposed upon licensed physicians, which further enhanced the atmosphere of doubt already generated.

SKILL OF THE ACUPUNCTURIST.   In the assessment of results, the skill and expertise of the artist must be strongly considered. Certainly, if total hip replacement, designed and perfected by sophisticated surgeons, were performed by first year medical students or inexperienced surgeons following an introductory course, a high level of sophistication may never have been reached, with the possibility that the procedure would have been considered a failure.

POINTS FOR CHRONIC ARTHRITIS

NECK PAIN	
Feng-Chih	GB-20
Chien-Ching	GB-21
Hou-Hsi	SI-3
SHOULDER PAIN	
Chu-Ku	CO-16
Chien-Chen	SI-9
Chien-Ching	GB-21
Chien-Liao	TH-14
Chien-Yu	CO-15
ELBOW PAIN	
Chu-Chih	CO-11
Tien-Ching	TH-10
Shao-Hai	H-3
WRIST PAIN	
Hou-Hsi	SI-3
Ho-Ku	CO-4
Yang-Chih	TH-4
Pa-Ya	EM-4
HIP PAIN	
Chu-Liao	GB-29
Huan-Tiao	GB-30
Feng-Shih	GB-31
KNEE PAIN	
Tu-Pi	ST-35
Yang-Ling-Chuan	GB-34
Yin-Ling-Chuan	SP-9
Liang-Chiu	ST-34
ANKLE PAIN	
Hsuan-Chung	GB-39
Chiu-Hsu	GB-40
Chung-Feng	GI-4
Chieh-Hsi	ST-4

Figure 13–1 An example of a typical recipe indicating the acupuncture skin points to be needled for the management of regional pain. However, this technique does not permit individualization of treatment, which is so often necessary.

THE METHOD PERFORMED.   In many instances, acupuncture has been performed by persons who were inexperienced or who did not perceive the scope of the field. Because of the great demand on the part of some to perform acupuncture, it began to be taught in rapid group courses. To accomplish this rapid training technique, frequently acupuncture was taught utilizing point recipes. This technique utilizes a given series of acupuncture points to be needled for a particular problem. Thus, if a patient presents with shoulder pain, the acupuncture needles are introduced into a given series of points. If the presentation is knee pain, however, other points are stuck, and so forth. Lists of prescribed points are available for reference (Fig. 13–1).

Many physicians educated in this fashion and utilizing these techniques soon give up in frustration.

Perhaps the greatest stumbling block in the path to acceptance of acupuncture is the lack of a satisfactory explanation of the mechanism of action. To solve this, numerous theories, both Western and Oriental, have evolved. Among the more important are the (1) Meridian Theory, (2) Hypnosis and Conditioning, (3) Gate Control Theory, and (4) Humoral Factors. As yet, none have satisfactorily answered the question.

CLASSICAL ACUPUNCTURE

If acupuncture anesthesia and the newer variations of acupuncture analgesia are developments of traditional acupuncture, then what is traditional acupuncture? The exact beginnings of Chinese medicine are shrouded in legend. Traditional acupuncture is the technique practiced by the early Chinese, dating back to the Stone Age. The first needles were made of sharp pieces of stone; later needles were made of sharpened bone or bamboo and finally of metal.

The initial discovery of acupuncture is believed to have been related to the observations that piercing injuries in warriors produced healing of long-standing pain in entirely different parts of the body. Thus the early primitive experience encompassed the use of only a few skin points. With the passing of time and the gaining of more experience, the acupuncturist looked for and catalogued new body points which, when stimulated, provided therapeutic results. The number of skin acupuncture points consequently increased, and the classic Chinese texts identify 365; however, there have been described throughout the years numbers of acupuncture points ranging from 150 to as many as 1000.

As the new points were added, they were noted to form distinct lines called meridians (Fig. 13–2A). These meridians are believed to connect all the internal organs and other body parts, with the acupuncture points indicating locations on the surface of the body where the meridians emerge. Through the meridians the energy of the body, called Ch'i, circulated, passing from one meridian to another through points of exit and entrance in a constant pattern (Fig. 13–2B). In addition to the points of entrance and exit, there are other pathways or connections between the meridians producing an intricate network.

In the concept of Chinese medicine, there is a constant circulation of Ch'i. This energy flow is felt to contain a harmonious mixture of Yin and Yang, the ever-present opposing forces of nature. Pathology results when either external factors (those outside the body) or internal factors cause an imbalance of Yin and Yang by an interruption or damming of the energy flow. The result is a collection of energy in one or more meridians and deficiencies in others. This alteration in energy balance is then manifested by the presence of pain or other symptomatic complaints. Theoretically, the location of the symptoms, therefore, may not indicate the site of the pathology or interruption of energy. Consequently, treatment may not be performed at the location or site of the pain but directed toward the meridian where the block to energy is occurring, in order to equalize the energy flow by opening the block. Thus, in classical acupuncture different patients with similar symptoms may have the needles placed at different sites, and classical acupuncture be considered a form of systemic acupuncture.

To envision this, we must attempt to block out our concepts of Western medicine and begin to conceive of illness and treatment as presented so many thousands of years ago. There were no diagnoses as to the various forms of arthritides, infections, or metabolic diseases with sophisticated names, nor was

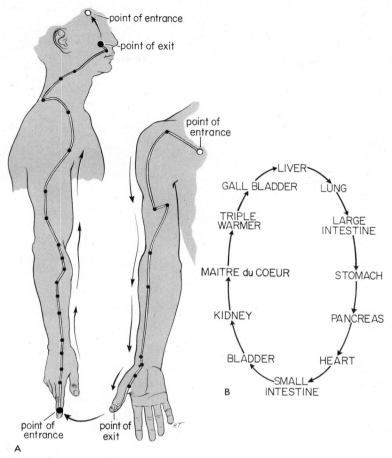

Figure 13–2 *A,* Acupuncture skin points forming meridians. Note the cyclic pattern of energy flow projecting down the arm on the volar surface, and up on the dorsum being connected through points of exit on the thumb and entrance on the index finger. (Adapted from Niboyet, 1970.) *B,* Schematic of circulation of energy flow from one meridian to another.

there instrumentation to conduct x-ray or laboratory studies. For the traditional acupuncturist, diagnosis was made by several methods; namely, inspecting, listening, smelling, inquiring, and, perhaps the most important, palpating the radial pulse (pulse diagnosis), which is supposedly the indicator of the internal flow of energy. In ancient cultures, patients frequently did not undress in front of the physician, and only the wrists and hands were presented to the acupuncturist. In the radial pulse, the master acupuncturist could perceive by palpation multiple sensations. These sensations represent normality or a disturbance in the general flow of energy through the body and are palpated by the examiner, who utilizes both hands simultaneously at the patient's wrist (Fig. 13–3). There are three designated levels along the radial pulse: proximal to, at the level of, and distal to the radial styloids. Comparison is made in palpation of the pulse be-

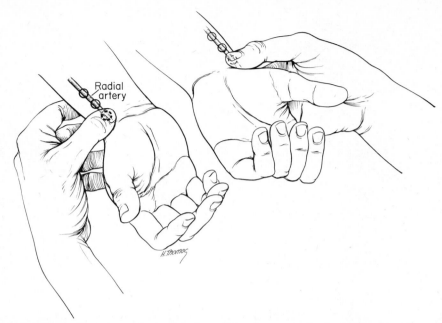

Figure 13–3   Technique of palpating the radial pulse, comparing both sides. Liver, lung, large intestine, etc. are the names of meridians. (Adapted from Niboyet, 1970).

tween the right and the left hand at both a superficial and a deep level at these three positions, producing 12 sites, each of which supposedly represents an organ system whose energy runs in a particular meridian. The difficulty, of course, is that unless we are taught to feel these sensations by a master, we can feel nothing other than the rate and rhythm that we have been taught to feel in Western training, and which is totally unrelated to what the acupuncturist needs to plan his treatment program. The sensations are felt at both a qualitative and quantitative level.

For the traditional acupuncturist, localization of the site of the interruption of energy by utilizing the radial pulse requires serious study, practice, and experience. These pulse sensations are difficult to define, but can be, for simplicity, described as strength, quality, borders, position, and many more. Based on these sensations, the imbalances in energy flow are determined and, subsequently, the acupuncture points selected for needle placement. The pulse, depending on its variations, will record problems of the entire body, of organ systems, or of localized regions. Traditionally, these sensations are said to appear in the pulse prior to the manifestation of symptoms, and a skilled acupuncturist endeavors to keep the pulse regulated so that symptoms will not occur (the so-called balance of Yin and Yang). However, if the block in energy flow is left unchecked, there is an increase in the seriousness of the pathology, with symptoms first localized to a region, and later manifesting as generalized systemic illness.

Once the diagnosis is made, the choice of acupuncture points is determined. The role of the acupuncture point is to restore the flow of energy, or in other words, open the dam when a block to energy flow exists. To do this, a single acupuncture point may have several properties. It may produce a generalized effect, an effect on a specific meridian, a local effect at the site of skin puncture, or a specific visceral or humoral action. In order to gain the desired response, a sophisticated acupuncturist will attempt to find the acupuncture point that will combine many of these effects; and therefore, utilize the least number of needles possible. Thus the key to treatment is to understand the pulse, to be able to palpate it, and then to interpret the sensations and subsequently choose the appropriate acupuncture point. These palpable sensations can only be mastered by dedicated and experienced personnnel with extensive training.

Once the site of needle placement is determined, which can be at one acupuncture point, but more commonly is at several, the needles are placed at varying angles to the skin, and turned briefly in one direction or another, depending on the desired effect. The needles are then left in place without twisting for varying periods of time.

At the time of the needle insertion, the acupuncturist attempts to have the patient experience the phenomenon of Te-ch'i. Te-ch'i is supposed to consist of four sensations: soreness, swelling, numbness, and heaviness. Patients who experience this sensation can be expected to have better results.

Needles of different metals were thought to produce different effects, but now needles of stainless steel are most often used.

With this brief background, how can we then apply acupuncture to patient management? Acupuncture should not be considered an entity in itself but as an adjunct in patient management. In addition, the acupuncture technique should be performed by a skilled person, not one who does it as a sideline. Thus, acupuncture should be utilized in the same fashion that we combine the various specialties, consultations, and modalities to gain a result in Western medicine. It should go without saying that diagnosis should be made prior to acupuncture therapy.

Where, then, does acupuncture work? Where does it produce partial success and where does it fail?

The lists of conditions recommended to be treated by acupuncture are exceedingly long and encompass nearly every pathologic state, whether painful or not, including infections, arthritis, headaches, impotence, paraplegia, metabolic disorders, and others. In my experience, acupuncture works best in cases of nonspecific inflammatory pain. It produces the most gratifying results in low back pain with unilateral radiculopathy and no neurological changes. Results are also satisfactory in nonspecific elbow and shoulder pain. Acupuncture has limited success where there are distinct anatomic pathologic changes. In causalgia with trophic changes, degenerative arthritic changes, and extruded discs the results are poor. However, causalgia-type symptoms without trophic changes can respond to acupuncture therapy. Postoperative pain can be significantly reduced by acupuncture; this in turn will reduce the amount of postoperative medication and permit the patient to begin motion more easily.

Poor response is encountered in patients who need their pain for secondary gain. In most instances, if pain is real, the response will be favorable, as opposed to the general premise that acupuncture only works on an emotional psychic level. There is no doubt that personality has an effect on the results, but this is true for any modality. Similar treatment programs for different patients can produce different results.

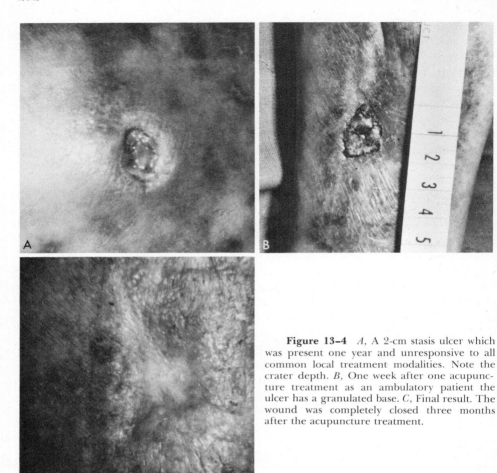

Figure 13–4 *A*, A 2-cm stasis ulcer which was present one year and unresponsive to all common local treatment modalities. Note the crater depth. *B*, One week after one acupuncture treatment as an ambulatory patient the ulcer has a granulated base. *C*, Final result. The wound was completely closed three months after the acupuncture treatment.

Aside from subjective responses, physical changes have been produced by acupuncture. In the management of low back pain, paralumbar muscle spasm has been noted to subside spontaneously with the insertion of the needles. Perhaps one of the most dramatic unsubjective responses is the physical change produced in the healing of vascular ulcers. Stasis ulcers which had been present for extended periods of time and, which were refractory to the usual treatment modalities, responded to treatment by acupuncture in relatively short periods of time. Wounds closed or healthy granulation tissue formed on which skin grafts were placed (Figs. 13–4 and 13–5).

Thus, acupuncture can be called upon to produce desired effects but it must be performed by experienced physicians. Once this occurs, and the experts of the world become the teachers of the future experts, as is presently accomplished in specialty residency programs (certainly extensive surgical procedures are not totally learned while sitting in a classroom for a short few hours), I think we will find that acupuncture works.

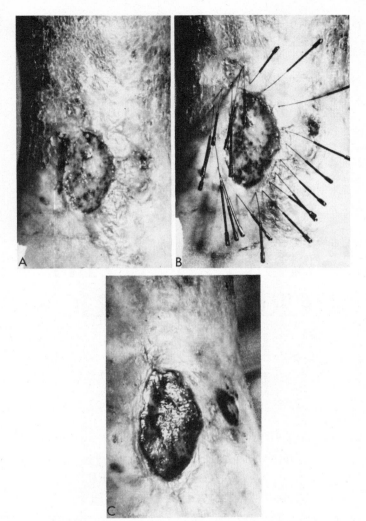

Figure 13–5 *A,* Stasis ulcer of five years' duration with a necrotic base, again unresponsive to conventional modes of treatment. *B,* One hour later, with multiple acupuncture needles inserted in a particular sequence, there is hyperemia of the peripheral margin of the ulcer. *C,* Twenty-five days later the wound is completely filled with healthy granulation tissue. A split thickness skin graft was applied with closure of the ulcer.

RECOMMENDED READING LIST

Casez, R.: Personal communication, 1973.

DeMorant, G. S.: *L'Acuponcture Chinoise.* Paris, Maloine, 1972.

Lu, H. C. (Trans.): *The Yellow Emperor's Book of Acupuncture.* Vancouver, B.C., Academy of Oriental Heritage, 1973.

Mann, F.: *Acupuncture — The Ancient Chinese Art of Healing and How it Works Scientifically.* New York, Random House, 1971.

Melzack, R., and Wall, P. D.: *Gate Control Theory of Pain.* New York, Academic Press, 1968.

Niboyet, J. E. H.: *Traité d' Acuponcture.* Paris, Maisonneuve, 1970, 3 vols.

Niboyet, J. E. H.: *L'Anesthésie par L'Acuponcture.* Paris, Maisonneuve, 1973.

14

ELECTRICAL STIMULATION OF PERIPHERAL NERVES WITH MICRO-ELECTRICAL IMPLANTS FOR PAIN RELIEF

BLAINE S. NASHOLD, JR.,
J. LEONARD GOLDNER,
and DONALD S. BRIGHT

INTRODUCTION

In 1967, Wall and Sweet reported relief of pain by direct electrical stimulation of the ulnar and median nerves for a woman with intractable pain in the left hand. Since that time, electrical stimulation applied to neural tissue at several different levels usually has resulted in partial relief of certain pain syndromes. The exact neurophysiologic mechanism producing pain relief still eludes us, but there appears to be a relationship between large non-nociceptive fibers exerting presynaptic inhibitory effects on the endings of small nociceptive fibers in the

254

dorsal horn (Sweet and Wepsic, 1968; Wagman and Price, 1969; Melzack and Wall, 1973; Melzack, 1975).

Stimulation of a peripheral nerve resulted in reduction of pain sensation over the autonomous zone of the stimulated nerve (Wall and Sweet, 1967). These authors propose that the electrical activity of A fibers of the peripheral nerve in some way interfered with perception of the painful stimulus, probably at the spinal cord level. Wall had shown in animals that when activity of the large A fibers in peripheral nerves was increased by electrical stimulation, there occurred a concomitant inhibition of the activity of the smaller pain fiber within the spinal cord (Wall and Gutnick, 1974a, 1974b; Torebjork and Hallin, 1974).

Other experiments showed that stimulation of the dorsal column of the cat, which is made up entirely of large A fibers, reduced the animal's reaction to noxious stimuli (Wagman and Price, 1969; Kerr, 1975).

In contradistinction to the antidromic inhibitory theory attempting to explain electrical stimulation and how it acts is another more plausible mechanism concerned with the periventricular gray areas known to be capable of inhibiting pain. Electrical stimulation of these areas can dramatically diminish or abolish pain (Melzack, 1975) and inhibit the transmission of impulses at the dorsal horn level. Cells in these areas are known to have large receptive fields, to receive inputs from widespread areas of the body, and to project to all levels of the spinal cord and brain. Intense stimulation would produce a predominantly small fiber input which would give rise to pain but would also activate the central biasing mechanism that would inhibit pain signals from other areas such as the source of pathologic pain (Melzack, 1975).

The complex definition of pain includes many factors, such as the mechanism of the original injury, the location of the pathologic lesion, the patient's personality, the length of time that the pain has been present, the circadian cycle, the patient's fatigue, secondary gain, and determination of whether the pain is primarily central or peripheral and whether it is associated with trauma, soft tissue damage, joint injury, or vascular insufficiency. Definition of the primary pathologic lesion is important if, in fact, this is possible (Goldner and Hendrix, 1977).

Certain pain syndromes have not responded to standard modalities of treatment. Several examples are described (Goldner, 1977).

PAIN SYNDROMES THAT HAVE FAILED TO RESPOND TO DIFFERENT KINDS OF TREATMENT — CLINICAL EXAMPLES

Ulnar Nerve Compression at the Elbow

A patient developed symptoms referable to compression of the ulnar nerve at the elbow. Initial treatment was operative transfer of the ulnar nerve to a location under the origin of the forearm flexor muscles. Pain persisted both locally and in the hand, and, several months later, a second procedure was done in order to place the nerve superficial to the muscle mass and in subcutaneous fat. Pain persisted, and epineural neurolysis was done which was not successful. In addition to the persistent pain, motor atrophy developed and was accompanied by paresthesias about the elbow and dysesthesias of the painful scar and peripheral skin. Pharmacologic agents, local injections with anesthetic agents, sympathetic nerve blocks, and biofeedback were attempted, but the persistent burning pain was not relieved. A transcutaneous nerve stimulator aggravated the pain, but a nerve block done in the axilla did relieve the pain temporarily. Microelectrodes implanted on the peripheral nerve brought temporary partial relief of pain (Fig. 14–6). This case exemplifies just one of many which cannot be managed by local operative treatment alone, and which do not respond to medications. A different approach to relief of pain was attempted by using electroanalgesia, which, in certain patients, has been relatively successful. In this instance, partial relief occurred. (Accornero, Bini, and Manfreidi, 1975; Campbell and Long, 1976; Campbell and Taub, 1973; Goldner and Nashold, 1975; Long, 1973; Torebjork and Hallin, 1974).

Laceration of the Median Nerve in the Mid Arm Associated with Fracture and Arterial Injury

This patient received severe trauma to the mid arm which resulted in a deep laceration, avulsion injury to the brachial artery, laceration of the median nerve, contusion of the ulnar nerve, and fracture of the humerus. Initially, a vein graft was used to re-establish peripheral circulation. This clotted within 12 hours and was replaced. A "causalgia syndrome" occurred as a result of injury to the median nerve and vascular insufficiency. Stiffness of the joints of the hand resulted, contractures of the flexor tendons occurred, and pain persisted. During the subsequent week, the vein graft showed gradual obliteration; as this occurred, pain in the forearm and hand increased noticeably. After sympathectomy was done, blood flow improved moderately and pain diminished moderately. The median nerve was then mobilized and repaired by end to end suture, and the paresthesias and dysesthesias diminished in intensity. However, as time passed, the pain related to vascular insufficiency increased, cold tolerance diminished, nail bed blanching was slow, and hand stiffness increased. Accordingly, after a bypass vein graft from the upper arm to the wrist was done, blood flow was increased and pain was diminished. Over a period of several months pain diminished even more, hand motion improved, and protective sensation developed in the hand. Three to five years must pass before maximum improvement occurs. Release of contractures and tendon transfers to the thumb will improve function once the pain syndrome has been controlled.

Traumatic Arthrosis of the Carpometacarpal Joint of the Hand — Superficial Radial Nerve Trauma

A patient with traumatic arthrosis of the metacarpotrapezium joint was treated by attempted arthrodesis between the first metacarpal and the trapezium. The superficial radial nerve was involved in the surgical scar, and there was evidence that at least two major branches of the nerve had either been severed or were involved by scar compression. Hyperesthesia and dysesthesia were severe, and when the patient attempted to use the thumb or the wrist the pain intensity was aggravated. Treatment included use of a transcutaneous nerve stimulator, with 25 per cent relief, local injection with an anesthetic agent, percussion, use of pharmacologic agents, and application of an external plastic cap protector to avoid stimulation of the area. Isolation of the nerve endings from fibrous tissue and bridging of the fibrous defect with a sural nerve graft diminished the burning pain but did not change cutaneous sensation appreciably; however, it did eliminate a major aspect of the dysesthesia. A peripheral nerve microelectrode implant was not used, although the improvement with transcutaneous stimulation indicates that an implant would have been beneficial. The decision to do the nerve graft rather than the implant was based on the patient's desire to eliminate the power pack and aerial.

The patient who has a peripheral nerve pain syndrome should be managed by multiple diagnostic procedures in an effort to determine the site of the pathologic lesion and the reasons for persistent pain. Several modalities of treatment should be attempted before a peripheral nerve implant is considered. Microelectrode implant is not the initial procedure when peripheral nerve pain persists.

The procedures listed and discussed briefly are the various *modalities* that have been used and should be considered or tried before a microelectrode implant is placed on the peripheral nerve.

1. *Repair of a cutaneous or major peripheral nerve* is done by adequate mobilization, resection of peripheral fibrous tissue, and a careful end to end suture without excessive tension. Gaps of 4 to 5 cm can be bridged by end to end suture if restoration of anatomic position is done slowly after nerve repair occurs. The suture material must be 5-0 or 6-0 for the major holding sutures and 7-0 for interval sutures. Bone shortening may be necessary, particularly of the humerus; this has allowed end to end suture when large gaps are present (Goldner, 1977).

2. *A previously lacerated nerve* that is not appropriate for repair or a nerve associated with an amputation stump should be dissected free from surrounding fibrous tissue and either reamputated and cauterized with a bipolar cautery or transferred proximally into muscle or fat so that a nonconstricting nontethering tissue covering is obtained (Goldner, 1977).

3. *Compression on a peripheral nerve* is released by freeing the retinacular ligament or opening a fascial covering in order to diminish compartment compression and relieve paresthesia and hypesthesia (Goldner, 1977).

4. *Nerve grafting may be done* in order to bridge a large defect after appropriate mobilization and proximal and distal end resection are done. Nerve grafting is preferable to transection of the nerve only if end to end suture cannot be done. However, in certain patients, the donor site of the nerve graft may become painful if an unsatisfied proximal nerve remains (Goldner, 1977).

5. *Silicone capping of lacerated nerves* has been reported. Our experience with capping has not been successful. Either the end should be cauterized and relocated proximally or the gap should be bridged by a nerve graft (Goldner, 1977).

6. *Sympathectomy may be helpful* in diminishing pain associated with nerve and vascular trauma. This is particularly true if vasospasm exists, as noted by readings on the pulse volume recorder, by cold tolerance tests, by skin temperature determinations, and by thermogram. Sympathectomy lessens vasospasm that occurs as a result of alterations by both internal and external stimuli.

Preganglionic as compared with postganglionic sympathectomy will result in a different response in that preganglionic sympathectomy is more permanent (Wall and Gutnick, 1974*b*).

7. *Pharmacologic agents* such as phenytoin sodium (Dilantin), amitriptylene HCl, (Elavil), or fluphenazine HCl (Prolixin) may affect central pain awareness, alter the patient's mood, affect the sleep pattern, and result in temporary diminution of the intensity of pain or partially eliminate the painful sensations. For example, a physician who required an amputation of the arm for treatment of a malignant tumor noted about three months after his amputation that his pain symptoms were less intense when he took Prolixin. However, while busy working with patients, the pain intensity was also less noticeable, and when he awakened in the morning he momentarily would have *no* pain. As soon as he confronted his environment and began his daily activities, the pain recurred (Wall and Gutnick, 1974*a*, 1974*b*; Wall and Sweet, 1967).

8. *Local anesthetic injections with long acting medication* (10 to 12 hours) diminishes the intensity of pain temporarily and provides relief for several hours. If this "block" is repeated at regular intervals, the anxiety and fear related to a persistent unrelenting pain complex is lessened. External trauma to an extremity during the period of nerve regeneration may cause severe pain and require local or peripheral nerve block from time to time in order to decrease the stimuli from regenerating neural elements. If the patient knows that the nerve block can be done after a reasonable waiting period, then anxiety and fear related to a persistent pain complex seem to be less. The summation of regenerating neural elements is frequently more than the patient can tolerate comfortably.

9. *Absolute alcohol injected* into the nerve a few centimeters proximal to the nerve end provides temporary interruption of conduction and diminished hypersensitivity for several weeks. Electrocoagulation may do the same thing (Goldner, 1977).

10. *Epineurolysis that results in freeing the nerve* from constricting fibrous tissue, or surgical splitting of the epineurium that allows release of tension on the fascicles, or, in certain rare instances, fascicular neurolysis may prove beneficial to those patients who have persistent burning pain or dysesthesias. The nerve is placed in soft tissues not under stretch and not subject to repeated external stimulation so that local afferent impulses are not stimulated. Fascicular neurolysis may occasionally decrease the burning and provide improvement in those patients who have had dysesthesia. This treatment has not been helpful after a laceration of the nerve has occurred, it is more likely to succeed when there is prolonged spontaneous compression. Neurolysis may diminish paresthesia and dysesthesia even though sensation may not return completely.

If any or all of these efforts fail, and that has usually been the situation in the patients who were treated by microelectrode implantation, then electrical stimulation should be considered.

DIRECT ELECTRICAL STIMULATION OF PERIPHERAL NERVES

We have used direct electrical stimulation of peripheral nerves with an implantable microelectrode system at Duke since 1969. Pain syndromes have

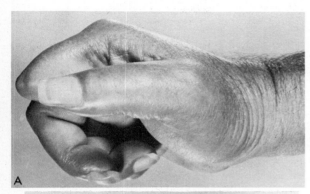

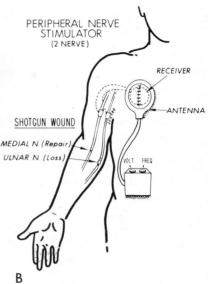

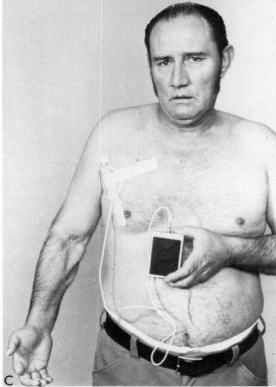

Figure 14–1 *A,* The patient's hand demonstrated absence of the muscles supplied by the ulnar nerve, moderate atrophy of the muscles supplied by the median nerve, smooth, dystrophic skin, and contractures of the fingers. Vascular insufficiency initially, neuromata in continuity, and prolonged fibrosis of the nerve obviated satisfactory local treatment of the nerve. The peripheral nerve stimulator diminished pain and improved overall use of the extremity. *B,* median and ulnar nerve lesions occurred at the elbow as a result of a shotgun injury. The microelectrodes were placed on the median and ulnar nerves at the level of the axillary crease. The wires were placed subcutaneously and were connected to the receiver, which was placed over the pectoral muscle and sutured in place. The antenna is located on the skin, held in place by paper tape, and can be removed by the patient. The power pack, with a separate wire for each nerve, is carried externally by the patient. Injury occurred five years before the stimulators were applied. The patient had persistent pain. He was relieved about 30 to 40 per cent, was able to work, and diminished his intake of medications. *C,* Gunshot wound of the elbow injuring median and ulnar nerves. Prior local treatment of the nerves—sympathectomy, local injections, and pharmacologic agents—was insufficient to relieve the pain. Emotional and social profiles were done, and the patient was considered a satisfactory candidate for the implant. He is holding the power pack in his left hand, the antenna is taped over the receiver.

been managed by placing the electrode or electrodes on either the median or ulnar nerves alone or as a double system in which electrodes are placed on the median and ulnar nerves with separate adjustments for each nerve and a double or single power pack (Fig. 14–1*A*, *B* and *C*) (Goldner and Nashold, 1975).

Etiology of Nerve Lesions Selected for Treatment by Electrical Stimulation

Upper extremity lesions usually involve either the median or the ulnar nerves or both, and lower extremity pain usually results from damage to the sciatic nerve. Causes of nerve lesions include the following:

1. Direct trauma to a nerve with a resulting incomplete nerve lesion.
2. Chemical injections into or around the nerve.
3. Amputation neuromata not improved by reamputation of the neuroma at a higher level.
4. Phantom pain associated with chronic ischemia.
5. Perineural and intraneural fibrosis associated with trauma and ischemia.
6. Isolated injury to the median nerve.
7. Isolated injury to the ulnar nerve.
8. Combined median and ulnar nerve lesions.
9. Isolated injury to the sciatic nerve.

Considerations in Preliminary Preoperative Assessment of Patient Prior to Placement of a Peripheral Nerve Implant

1. Detailed history relative to onset of pain, aggravation of pain, the mechanism of injury, and the presence or absence of vascular pathology.
2. Social, personal, and occupational history including muscle testing, and assessment for anomalous innervation (Goldner, 1969).
3. *Sensory assessment* of the extremity including sweat testing, cutaneous perception test, proprioception determination, alterations of sensory recognition, and the existence of hyperpathia and dysesthesis (Goldner, 1972 [unpublished]; Goldner and Eguro, 1971 [unpublished]).
4. *Pulse volume* recorder readings, skin temperature recording, thermography, cold tolerance tests, and the relationship of all of these tests to pain are essential in defining the cause of pain.
5. *Electrical studies* such as electromyography and nerve conduction determinations aid in defining the degree of motor and sensory alteration of the nerve (Goldner, 1977 [unpublished]).
6. *Nerve block procedures* give information about alterations in blood flow after blockade of the sympathetic ganglia or the peripheral nerve. The nerve block determines if the patient has temporary total relief of pain while afferent stimuli are not perceived. This is helpful in the prognosis regarding placement of the microelectrode on the nerve (Goldner et al., 1972; Goldner, 1977).

7. *Transcutaneous nerve stimulation* provides information about the effect of electrical stimulation on the extremity. The electrodes are placed by trial and error, and the degree of pain relief is noted by the patient. A few days of trial are necessary before an accurate impression concerning the effect of the transcutaneous stimulator can be determined (Goldner and Nashold, 1975; Goldner and Hendrix, 1977; Jeans, 1975; Melzack, 1975).

8. *Clinical psychological* studies and psychiatric assessment provide information about the emotional profile of the patient, the presence of an hysterical pattern, one of hypochondriasis, or one of depression.

Information for Patients Who Are to Have Peripheral Nerve Micro-electrode Implant

These patients are provided information about the possibility of fibrosis occurring around the nerve because of irritation from the implant (Fig. 14–2). They are also informed that the implant will not necessarily relieve all of their pain but may diminish the intensity. Relief may be intermittent and the amount of time that they are required to use the stimulator varies from person to person. Adjustment by reoperation, or even removal, may be necessary.

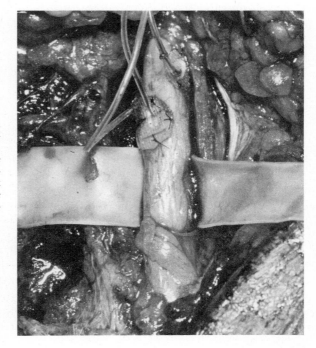

Figure 14–2 Nerve dissection done under local anesthesia. Peripheral nerve isolated on rubber dam. Microelectrodes sutured to the epineurium at two different locations. The site of suture is dependent on electrical stimulation during the procedure and formation of a sensory map.

Operative Technique

The operative procedure includes use of a local anesthetic with an anesthetist "standing by" to provide analgesia and to alleviate the patient's anxiety.

The patient is placed in a comfortable position on the operating table and the procedure is explained. The necessity for accurate responses to questions about the electrical stimulation and its effect on sensation in certain parts of the extremity is emphasized. The patient's participation in preparing a motor-sensory nerve map while low voltage electrical stimulation is performed under local anesthesia is the most important aspect of the procedure. Proper placement of the electrode depends on the patient's responses that pain is partially alleviated or aggravated by low or high voltage stimulation, respectively. If a motor-sensory map is not used, proper placement of the electrode is not ensured, and excessive motor activity may result (Nashold et al., 1977; Goldner, 1968–1974, unpublished).

Pain relief during the assessment stage may be insufficient to warrant placement of an electrode on the nerve, and the patient is advised accordingly. The actual site of electrode placement, if done, is predetermined preoperatively so that the electrode is located far enough proximally in the extremity to avoid crossover sensory branches that might interfere with electrical impulses from the apparatus.

Instrumentation

Magnification of 2.0 to 3.5 times is sufficient for implanting the electrode in an adult. An operating microscope has not been necessary.

Microsurgical instruments should include forceps, scissors, dissectors, and needle holders and clamps for isolating the nerve and for suturing the electrode to the epineurium in the determined location. Microsurgical needles attached to 7-0 nylon suture are adequate.

Procedure

1 per cent lidocaine (Xylocaine) with epinephrine is injected into the skin and subcutaneous tissue at a point far proximal to the pathologic lesion in the nerve. For example, if the ulnar nerve lesion is at the elbow, the electrodes are placed on the ulnar nerve in the upper third of the arm at a point determined by trial electrical stimulation that results in reasonable relief of pain (Goldner and Nashold, 1975; Goldner, 1977).

If the median nerve is affected in the forearm, the electrode is placed on the median nerve in the mid-arm region, proximal to the elbow. A painful phantom in a patient with a below-knee amputation would require placement of the microelectrode on the sciatic nerve in the mid-thigh region below the level where the upper end of the prosthesis would rest (Goldner and Nashold, 1975).

The peripheral nerve is isolated by minimal stripping, the epineurium is not invaded and the blood supply is not altered. Orientation and preparation of the nerve map is obtained by having the surgeon face cephalad and plan the nerve map by looking at a hypothetical cross section of the nerve in that direction. Twelve o'clock on the nerve corresponds to anterior, three o'clock is in the clockwise direction (medial), looking toward the axilla, six o'clock is 180 degrees opposite twelve o'clock (posterior), and nine o'click is opposite the three o'clock point (lateral). Thus, a 360 degree circle is completed (Fig. 14–2) (Goldner and Nashold, 1975).

A complex electrical system has been constructed so that low threshold stimulation of the motor and sensory segments of the nerve is possible (Fig. 14–3A and B). The nerve map is prepared by stimulating the nerve through an arc of 360 degrees and recording points that relate to the location of the patient's recognizable pain. The direction of the electrical stimulation is determined by mapping out appropriate quadrants on the nerve so that proper placement of the electrodes can be done (Nashold and Goldner, 1977).

A subcutaneous dissection is performed which extends from the medial aspect of the upper arm to the anterior pectoral region where the receiver is implanted (see Fig. 14–1C). The subcutaneous dissection is completed from the upper arm incision to the anterior pectoral incision with a blunt hemostat. A hollow polyethylene tube is passed subcutaneously from the site where the electrode will be implanted on the ulnar nerve to the receiver site over the pectoralis major muscles. The electrodes and wire are passed through the hollow tube from the pectoral region to the arm wound, and loops of wire are formed in both the proximal and distal subcutaneous tissues in order to avoid tension on the distal electrodes. The microelectrodes are sutured in place on predetermined sites on the peripheral nerve using 7-0 nylon suture in such a way that tethering and torsion of the wire and nerve are avoided (Figs. 14–2 and 14–4). Recent improvements in design and construction of the electrodes have diminished the occurrence of electrode displacement, lessened the amount of peripheral fibrosis, and provided a sufficient surface for stimulation of the peripheral nerve in order to conduct a current of adequate intensity for maximum pain relief (Fig. 14–5).

The electrode placement is tested by stimulating the nerve with an electrical stimulator. Once the placement of the electrode is satisfactory insofar as pain relief is concerned, the microelectrode is sutured to the nerve and the receiver is anchored subcutaneously in the pectoral region with several sutures. A power source is selected to stimulate the receiver, and this source is adjusted so that the voltage and frequency most comfortable to the patient and most effective in diminishing peripheral pain are selected. The cutaneous contact and the frequency in duration of daily use of the unit are adjusted for each patient (Goldner and Nashold, 1975).

Special instructions about the use of the stimulator are given to the patient, and a period of one to several weeks must elapse before an opinion is given concerning the degree of improvement that might have occurred. Those patients who benefit most by the stimulator implant usually recognize diminution in the intensity of pain while the electrode is being adjusted in the operating room. These patients note the same pattern of improvement early in the course of voltage adjustment in the postoperative period.

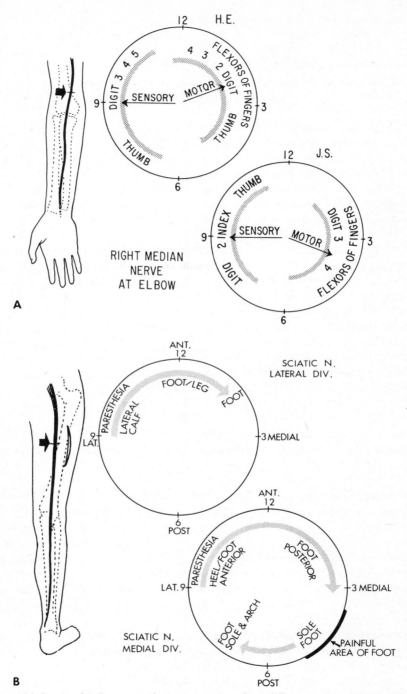

Figure 14–3   *A* and *B*, Sensory and motor mapping of two different patients, showing variations in the nerve at different sites at the elbow and the variation of nerve pathways in different patients. Any selected point along the course of the nerve, the geographic location of motor fibers to a particular muscle or sensory fibers to a particular anatomic area will vary considerably.

Mapping of the right sciatic nerve, both lateral and medial divisions, demonstrates differences in sensory location, depending on the site of electrical stimulation of the nerve at a particular point. The medial division corresponds to the posterior tibial nerve and the lateral to the peroneal nerve.

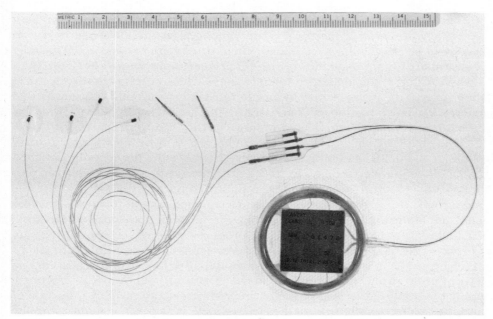

Figure 14–4 Current model, demonstrating receiver, connections between electrodes and wire to the receiver, and four electrodes for placement on a single nerve at different locations.

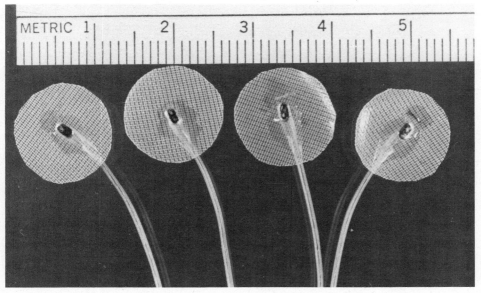

Figure 14–5 Enlargement of microelectrodes for placement on a single nerve. Electrodes as they are placed in contact with the nerve are synchronized with each other, so that current is properly localized as the nerve map is developed.

Descriptions of Electrical Implant Systems

The implant systems (Avery Laboratories, Inc.) are of two types and both depend on the kind of electrical pulse generated at the electrode nerve interspace. The electronic system is made up of three components, which include: 1) electrodes for stimulation (Fig. 14–6), 2) interconnecting wires (Figs. 14–4 and 14–6), and 3) the implanted radio frequency receiver (Fig. 14–6). Electrical stimulation of the nerve is done by an external battery operated transmitter that generates a pulse modulated radio signal fed through an antenna which is placed directly over the implanted radio frequency receiver (Fig. 14–7).

The pulse signal is picked up through the skin by means of inductive coupling, and delivered to the desired nerve site through the specially designed bipolar platinum electrodes. Electrodes are encased in silicone, which is perforated and to which sutures can be applied to anchor the electrode to the epineurium. We currently implant a radio frequency generator whose signal has equal amplitude and duration but an opposite polarity (Goldner and Hendrix, 1977). This alternate pulse stimulator produces negative pulses (B) that are capable of reaching the action potential necessary to neutralize any electrochemical changes brought about by the positive impulses (A). The practical importance of using an alternate pulse system is a lower threshold for peripheral nerve stimulation, reduced fatigue of the peripheral nerve, and possibly reduction of fibrous tissue formation beneath the electrode site at its point of contact with the peripheral nerve. The width of the square wave pulse is set at three microseconds' duration, and the average threshold of stimulation paresthesia varies from 1.5 to 2.0 volts. The patient is able to vary the frequency of the stimulation rate from 15 to 50 Hz.

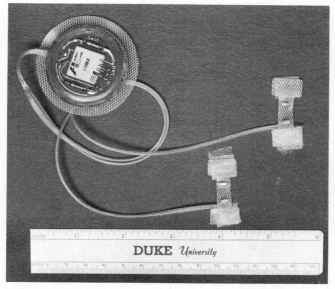

Figure 14–6 Receiver (Avery Laboratories), coated wire, and microelectrode mounted in silicone. One electrode was placed on the median nerve and one on the ulnar nerve. This is an older model and is larger than the present electrodes being used. Electrodes are sutured in place with nylon.

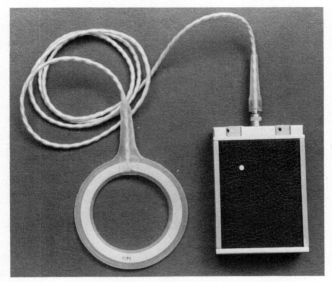

Figure 14–7   The external antenna, which is taped to the skin by the patient. The antenna is placed over the subcutaneous area. The wire is of sufficient length and is protected by a casing that prevents breakage. The power pack can be adjusted to alter the intensity and frequency of the current.

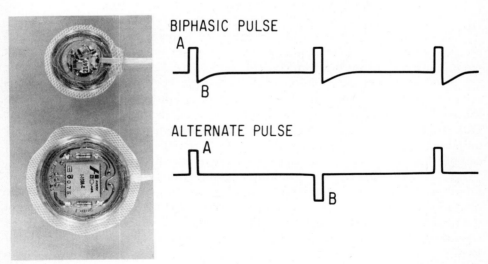

Figure 14–8   Microreceivers with diagram of biphasic pulse from one unit and alternate pulse from another.

Complications of Peripheral Nerve Implant System

Equipment failure has occurred infrequently. The most common problem has been rotation of the electrode on the peripheral nerve. This has resulted in incomplete stimulation paresthesia to a particular area of pain, and occurred when a single large electrode was used and when fixation was being done with large caliber suture.

These earlier electrode implants consisted of a cuff which was wrapped around the peripheral nerve to be stimulated. This cuff can cause serious constriction to the peripheral nerve, and in several patients had to be removed because of the immediate complaint after implantation of pain in and around the site of implantation. At present, we use the small single electrodes which are sutured to the peripheral nerve, thereby eliminating the problem of compression.

Currently, the electrodes are prepared as four separate units and are held in place with 7-0 nylon suture. Abnormal movement occurs less frequently (Fig. 14–2).

There have been no bacterial infections in the group, which included 40 patients One patient of the 40 developed a serosanguineous exudate after removal of the initial electrode and replacement by a second electrode system. Drainage continued, cultures were negative, electrode was removed, and the wound healed primarily. A few months later, a third electrode system was inserted, pain was diminished, mechanical failure did not occur, and drainage did not recur (Goldner and Nashold, 1975).

Results After Implant Placement for Relief of Pain

At the time this manuscript was prepared approximately 40 patients had received peripheral nerve implants in either upper or lower extremities. Each patient has been his or her own control. Placebo implants or false currents have not been used, and a double blind study has not been initiated. The patients selected represent a random sampling of several hundred patients seen during the past 10 years with extremity pain associated with peripheral nerve injury. Our current impression is that if the patient meets the requirements already mentioned in the earlier part of this chapter, a reasonable amount of pain relief can be obtained by use of the peripheral nerve implant system.

Several failures did occur, and these seemed to result from many factors: 1) failure to locate an area on the nerve that resulted in alteration of severity of the pain by the electrical stimulation in the operating room; 2) peripheral fibrosis of the nerve, inflammatory reaction of adjacent tendons, and tethering of the nerve caused pain stimuli greater than the electrical system could relieve; 3) a combination of 1) and 2) that responded to other forms of therapy, such as amputation, which in itself did not eliminate phantom pain or paresthesias but did act to eliminate the afferent stimuli that resulted from chronic irritation of the part. For example, a painful foot or ankle with chronic fibrosis of the peripheral nerve and vascular insufficiency resulted in persistent stimulation of the nerve with weight bearing; amputation eliminated that part of the problem, although the paresthesias and the burning pain may have been improved by continued use of the electrode.

Table 14-1

PATIENT	NERVE INJURY	PRIMARY TRAUMA	PAIN SITE	N. STIMULATOR PLACEMENT	DEGREE OF RELIEF	FOLLOW-UP YRS.
M.M.	Median	Crushed finger six prior operations	Palm, index amputation site	Median	(5 max. 1 min.) 4(70%)	5
H.H.	Median	Laceration, digit, 11 operations phantom	Hand, index, phantom amputation site	Median	5 (80%)	6
McC	Ulnar	Partial laceration, ulnar nerve, tendon	Hand — 4,5 digits	Ulnar	5 (90%)	5
J.M.	Ulnar	Laceration, nerve, tendon, little finger	Palm, 5th digit	Ulnar	1 (20%)	2 Original placement not helpful after 2 yr. follow-up
C.L.	Median and Ulnar	Gunshot wound, elbow several operations	Hand, fingers	Median, ulnar double unit	3 (60%)	3
M.C.	Sciatic	Bilateral, below knee amputation	Amputation stumps phantom, legs	Sciatic, bilateral	5 (90%) wearing prosthesis comfortably	5
K.A.	Sciatic	Fracture dislocation, knee	Leg, foot	Sciatic	3 (60%)	4
TEN	Posterior tibial	Tibia — ankle	Ankle, foot	Sciatic	1 (20%) (amputation) necessary	1 tendon, joint, and vascular problems too great
AB	Posterior tibial	Foot, ankle	Foot	Sciatic	2 (40%)	4

Other factors that may affect the end result and may cause persistent pain of varying degrees include peripheral blood flow deficiency, emotional factors, and secondary gain considerations.

ANALYSIS AND DISCUSSION

Table 14–1 gives a sampling of patients who were referred for management of intractable pain. Most patients had prior nerve and soft tissue procedures, some had prior amputations, and all had more than one operation. The number of operative procedures in itself did not necessarily affect the prognosis.

Several patients had peripheral nerve lesions in continuity, others had nerves that were adherent to bone and tendon and were constantly irritated with motion of the extremity, and certain patients showed diminished peripheral blood flow and severe cold intolerance.

Several patients were benefitted partially by a combination of a thorough dissection of the peripheral nerves, excision of fibrous tissue, and placement of digital or mixed nerves in areas where muscle or fat provided moderate nerve protection. Cauterization of the nerve endings was of some help in certain instances. Improvement of peripheral blood flow by sympathectomy was helpful in certain patients and obviated the need for a stimulator, particularly if a dystrophic syndrome existed. Patients with severe compression of the median and ulnar nerves treated by reoperation, neurolysis, and use of the peripheral implant obtained satisfactory relief and eventually were able to eliminate the microelectrode implant.

One patient with median nerve injury in the forearm with neuroma persisting and without satisfactory regeneration was temporarily improved by nerve block, only slightly improved by the peripheral nerve implant proximal to the elbow, and greatly improved after resection of the neuroma, resuture of the nerve, and release of all peripheral constriction. However, as regeneration occurred, certain components of pain recurred; but with the stimulator in place and used daily during the period of median nerve regeneration, his pain syndrome diminished considerably. Other factors such as avoidance of local trauma were essential for comfort. *This patient demonstrates the important concept that pain is seldom due to one isolated factor. The cause of the pain is usually multifactorial, and relief of pain is dependent on a summation of many of the factors that have been mentioned.*

Several of the patients who were dependent on large amounts of medication were able to eliminate medication once the microelectrode stimulator was functioning properly. Improved sleep, better concentration, and improved daily performance were possible with a successful implant.

The information presented here represents an improvement in our capability of managing patients who have intractable peripheral nerve pain. As more information is gathered concerning the causes of pain and the methods of altering pain by affecting peripheral tissue systems and the patient's emotional response, the pattern of peripheral stimulation will change. Electrical stimulation of the sympathetic nervous system, peripheral blood vessels, peripheral nerves, and other tissues requires more investigation and research.

REFERENCES

Accornero, N., Bini, G., and Manfreidi, M.: Differential block of cutaneous nerve fibers with triangularly shaped electrical impulses. Presented at First World Congress of International Association for the Study of Pain. Florence, Italy, September, 1975.

Campbell, J. N., and Long, D. M.: Peripheral nerve stimulation in the treatment of intractable pain. J. Neurosurg. *45*:629, 1976.

Campbell, J. N., and Taub, A.: Local analgesia from percutaneous electrical stimulation. A peripheral mechanism. Arch. Neurol. *28*:347, 1973.

Goldner, J. L.: Anomalous innervation pattern of the hand and upper extremity. Proceedings of American Society for Surgery of the Hand. J. Bone Joint Surg. *48*:604, 1966.

Goldner, J. L., Yochelson, D., Nashold, B., Brown, H., Hunter, J., Omer, G., Kleinert, H., and Green, D.: Upper limb pain. Proceedings of the American Society for Surgery of the Hand. J. Bone Joint Surg. *54A*:899, 1972.

Goldner, J. L., and Nashold, B. S.: Electrical stimulation of peripheral nerves for relief of pain. American Orthopaedic Association Meeting, San Francisco. J. Bone Joint Surg. *57A*:729, 1975.

Goldner, J. L.: Moderator, Panel on Pain Syndromes Involving the Upper Extremity. Las Vegas, American Society for Surgery of the Hand, February, 1977.

Goldner, J. L., and Hendrix, P.: Use of transcutaneous electrical stimulation in the management of chronic pain syndromes. Current Concepts in the Management of Chronic Pain, 1977.

Goldner, J. L., and Eguro, H.: Distribution of superficial radial nerve in 50 normal patients — observation, variation, pattern of sensation in the index and thumb. (Unpublished, 1971).

Goldner, J. L.: Sensory mapping of peripheral nerves in conjunction with geographic repair of lacerated nerves under local anesthesia, 1968–1974 (Unpublished).

Goldner, J. L: Peripheral nerve mapping, motor fibers, 1958–1978 (Unpublished).

Jeans, M. E.: Effects of brief, intense transcutaneous electrical stimulation on chronic pain. Ph.D. Dissertation, McGill University, 1975. (Quoted by Melzack).

Kerr, F. W. L.: Neuroanatomical substrates of nocioception in the spinal cord. *In:* Pain. Amsterdam, Elsevier/North Holland, 1975, Vol. 1, p. 325.

Long, M.: Electrical stimulation for relief of pain from chronic nerve injury. J. Neurosurg. *39*:718, 1973.

Melzack, R., and Wall, P. D.: Pain mechanisms: A new theory. Science *150*:971, 1965.

Melzack, R.: The Puzzle of Pain. New York, Basic Books, 1973.

Melzack, R.: Prolonged relief of pain by brief, intense transcutaneous somatic stimulation. *In:* Pain. Amsterdam, Elsevier/North Holland, 1975, Vol 1, p. 357.

Nashold, B. S., Goldner, J. L., Bright, D. S., Mullen, J., and Meyer, P.:Topography of sensory and motor fasciculi in human median and sciatic nerves determined by electrical stimulation. (Unpublished; presented at American Association of Neurological Surgeons Meeting, Toronto, Canada, April 24–28, 1977.)

Sweet, W. H., and Wepsic, J. G.: Treatment of chronic pain by stimulation of fibers of primary afferent neurons. Trans. Am. Neurol. Assoc. *93*:103, 1968.

Torebjork, H. E., and Hallin, R. G.: Responses in human AC fibers to repeated electrical intradermal stimulation. J. Neurol. Neurosurg. Psychiatry *37*:653, 1974.

Wagman, I. H., and Price, D. D.: Responses of dorsal horn cells of M. mulatta to cutaneous and sural nerves. A and C fiber stimuli. J. Neurophysiol. *32*:803, 1969.

Wall, P D., and Gutnick, M.: Properties of afferent nerve impulses originating from the neuroma. Nature (Lond.) *248*:740, 1974.

Wall, P. D., and Gutnick, M.: Ongoing activity in peripheral nerves: The physiology and pharmacology of impulses originating from the neuron. Exper. Neurol. *43*:580, 1974.

Wall, P. D., and Sweet, W. H.: Temporary abolition of pain in man. Science *155*:108, 1967.

15

CONTINUOUS PERIPHERAL EPINEURAL INFUSION FOR THE TREATMENT OF ACUTE PAIN

GEORGE E. OMER, JR.

There are only two principles in a treatment program for extremity pain: (1) relieve the pain, and (2) institute active use of the involved extremity. In those patients with an established pain pattern, it is very useful to differentiate localized pain along the course of major peripheral nerves, such as a painful neuroma, from generalized pain that may be stocking-level in distribution or that may follow the watershed, delta-shaped area of major blood vessels. The continuous peripheral epineural infusion technique will identify localized pain and can be an effective treatment modality.

When the patient is first examined, the involved extremity should be palpated and tapped very gently from distal to proximal to demonstrate any "trigger points" of extreme irritation. If a trigger point is obvious, it is marked with a sterile marking pen, and the area is surgically prepared and draped. After local cutaneous anesthesia, a 16 gauge needle is inserted into the trigger point area (Fig. 15–1). The needle is aspirated to avoid blood vessel penetration, and a flexible 18 gauge polyethylene intravenous catheter is inserted through the 16 gauge needle (Fig. 15–2). If performed in this manner, the intravenous catheter should

273

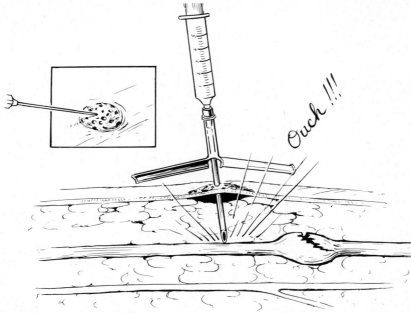

Figure 15–1 Introduction of a 16 gauge needle into the "trigger point" of pain after local cutaneous anesthetic block. (From Omer, G. E.: Complications of treatment of peripheral nerve injuries. *In:* Epps, C., Jr. (ed.): Complications of Orthopaedic Surgery. Philadelphia, J. B. Lippincott, 1978, Chapter 25. By permission of the publisher.)

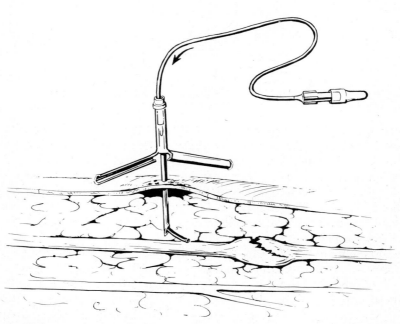

Figure 15–2 Introduction of an 18 gauge intravenous catheter into the "trigger point" of pain. (From Omer, G. E.: Complications of treatment of peripheral nerve injuries. *In:* Epps, C., Jr. (ed.): Complications of Orthopaedic Surgery. Philadelphia, J. B. Lippincott, 1978, Chapter 25. By permission of the publisher.)

not penetrate a nerve or blood vessel. The large-bore 16 gauge needle is then removed, leaving the 18 gauge intravenous catheter in place (Fig. 15–3). One-half milliliter of 0.5 percent lidocaine hydrochloride (Xylocaine) is then injected through the intravenous catheter for local anesthetic effect (Fig. 15–4). If the trigger point pain is relieved, the intravenous catheter is capped and taped in place (Fig. 15–5). The anesthetic block usually is insufficient for complete motor and sensory paralysis, and the pain-free patient is asked to exercise the extremity, to walk, and to perform assigned physical therapy. If the anesthetic block is not effective to relieve the trigger point pain, an additional milliliter of lidocaine hydrochloride is injected, and if the additional amount also is not effective, the intravenous catheter is withdrawn. The peripheral epineural infusion block may be repeated once if the first attempt is unsuccessful.

If the peripheral epineural infusion block is effective, it should be used for treatment. Additional periodic injections of anesthetic solutions such as lidocaine hydrochloride (Xylocaine), mepivacaine hydrochloride (Carbocaine), bupivacaine hydrochloride (Marcaine), or prilocaine hydrochloride (Citanest) may be utilized. The patient decides the frequency of injection, depending upon the time of pain free activity. Our usual regimen has been one-half millimeter of 2 percent lidocaine hydrochloride (Xylocaine) solution with 1/100,000 epinephrine or mepivacaine hydrochloride (Carbocaine) every four hours. The volume for each injection has ranged from 0.5 to 1 milliliter, and the time range between injections has been 1 to 10 hours. The average time range between injections was

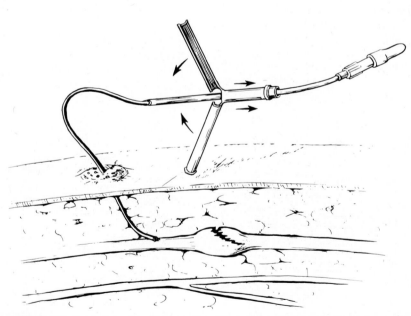

Figure 15–3 Removal of the 16 gauge needle with the 18 gauge intravenous cathether in place near the epineurium. (From Omer, G. E.: Complications of treatment of peripheral nerve injuries. *In:* Epps, C., Jr. (ed.): Complications of Orthopaedic Surgery. Philadelphia, J. B. Lippincott, 1978, Chapter 25. By permission of the publisher.)

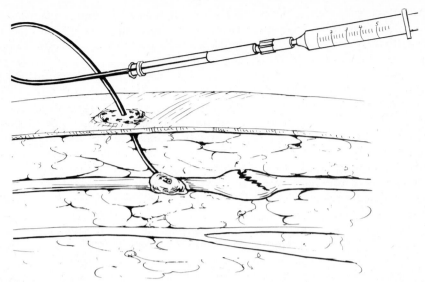

Figure 15–4 Injection of local anesthetic agent to obtain a peripheral perineural infusion block. (From Omer, G. E.: Complications of treatment of peripheral nerve injuries. *In:* Epps, C., Jr. (ed.): Complications of Orthopaedic Surgery. Philadelphia, J. B. Lippincott, 1978, Chapter 25. By permission of the publisher.)

2.2 hours during the acute stage lengthening to 3.4 hours as the cumulative effect of the periodic peripheral epineural infusion and extremity activity decreased pain and improved muscle function (Omer and Thomas, 1972). The periodic infusion is injected through the intravenous catheter without need for further skin puncture, and has been continued for two weeks in only a few cases (Omer and Thomas, 1974). If there is more than one area of localized irritation,

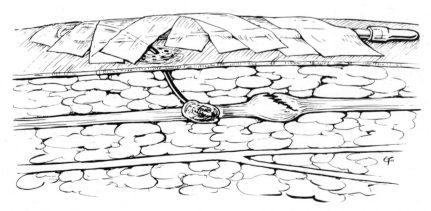

Figure 15–5 The intravenous catheter is capped and taped in place for continuous (periodic) peripheral perineural infusion blocks. (From Omer, G. E.: Complications of treatment of peripheral nerve injuries. *In:* Epps, C., Jr. (ed.): Complications of Orthopaedic Surgery. Philadelphia, J. B. Lippincott, 1978, Chapter 25. By permission of the publisher.)

separate intravenous catheters should be used for each trigger point. In contrast to a central chemical sympathetic block, the peripheral epineural infusion is a ward procedure that can be performed simultaneously with other modes of treatment.

The indications for the periodic peripheral epineural infusion include a trigger point of pain, and for the infusion in combination with a central chemical sympathetic block (stellate ganglion) when the central block had an initial effective duration but subsequent central blocks have given progressive shorter pain free periods and there is a peripheral "trigger point" of pain. The contraindications for the periodic peripheral epineural infusion include established pain syndromes that have been unrelieved for three months or longer and brachial plexus or lumbar plexus level pain, particularly when pain has occurred in the unaffected contralateral extremity. In addition, there is potential for necrosis at the injection site in a severely injured extremity with marginal vascularity. One should expect the periodic peripheral infusion to relieve painful symptoms for a variable period of time, but the technique will not produce permanent relief of pain without associated active use of the extremity by the patient. The technique is much less effective in those cases in which the pain has been untreated and unrelieved for three or more months.

REFERENCES

Omer, G. E., Jr., and Thomas, S. R.: Peripheral periodic infusion sympathectomy for the treatment of causalgia. *In*: Proceedings of the American Society for Surgery of the Hand. J. Bone Joint Surg. *54A*:898, 1972.

Omer, G. E., Jr., and Thomas, S. R.: The management of chronic pain syndromes in the upper extremity. Clin. Orthop. *104*:37, 1974.

16

THERAPEUTIC NERVE BLOCKS FOR THE RELIEF OF CHRONIC PAIN

ADEL R. ABADIR

Therapeutic nerve blocks are utilized mostly to alleviate chronic pain. For optimum results, the following important criteria should be fulfilled:

1. Prior evaluation with diagnostic nerve blocks. Therapeutic blocks should be performed only after evaluation with repeated diagnostic blocks of long duration that have been successful in eliminating or considerably reducing the degree of pain. Diagnostic or prognostic blocks with an indwelling catheter are recommended for this purpose.

2. Patient acceptability. Only after repeated long duration diagnostic blocks by an indwelling catheter, can it be ascertained if the patient finds denervation unacceptable. Permanent anesthesia may not be tolerated by some patients. Unfortunately, long duration reversible blocks will not predict the possibility of painful paresthesias or dysesthesias, which on occasion are a complication, as these occur only with the actual nerve injury of the therapeutic block.

3. Denervation should not be attempted or should be resorted to only if pain is extremely severe in areas exposed to constant pressure, as decubitus ulcerations might develop. The buttocks and the back are particularly prone to this complication.

4. Motor disability should be minimal. Differential nerve blocks that would only denervate sensory fibers with minimal involvement of motor function are

278

certainly of great value. However, there can be no guarantee that some motor power would not be lost.

5. Bladder and rectal function should be preserved. Only in terminal cancer patients should injection of alcohol and phenol into the spinal cord be attempted, gradually increasing the concentrations and volumes of the drugs to achieve maximum relief with minimal disability.

6. Only physicians with experience in this form of therapy should ever attempt permanent blocks.

Other forms of therapy that have been included under therapeutic nerve blocks are: 1) subarachnoid saline injections; and 2) steroid injections peridurally or perineurally; and 3) pituitary ablation by alcohol injection (Moricca, 1976).

Steroids are considered to have the ability to soften scar tissue, producing chemical neurolysis. They are also potent anti-inflammatory agents.

It has been suggested that pain relief from pituitary ablation by the injection of alcohol is due to the interruption of some of the hypothalamic-thalamic pathway by the alcohol rather than to destruction of the pituitary gland itself (Miles and Sampson, 1976).

AGENTS USED IN NERVE BLOCKING PROCEDURES

This group of drugs owes its anesthetic properties to its neurolytic action (McIntyre, 1938; Moore, 1965). The drugs should not be considered for use in a reversible block; although regeneration of nerve fibers may occur from three months to one year later when lower concentrations are used.

Ethyl alcohol

Ethyl alcohol may be used in concentrations from 50 per cent for sympathetic and unmyelinated nerves, to 95 per cent or absolute alcohol (Bieter, 1936; McIntyre, 1938) for large myelinated nerve trunks. It is hypobaric; that is, in any concentration its specific gravity is less than that of the cerebrospinal fluid. In higher concentrations, it produces necrosis of surrounding tissues with extensive scarring (McIntyre, 1938). The onset of action is immediate, allowing a single injection to be tailored to the desired degree and extent of anesthesia required. Although it is quite painful on injection, the pain is tolerated well by most patients. Small amounts of local anesthetics may be used prior to alcohol injection, if desired, to reduce the degree of pain experienced, particularly when it is used in higher concentrations.

Phenol

The usual solution is 5 to 10 per cent aqueous (Moore, 1965; Murphy, 1977), although occasionally up to 15 per cent may be used. This solution is useful for denervation of the trigeminal ganglion. When used in the subarachnoid space, phenol is mixed with glycerine to form a hyperbaric solution (Jefferson, 1966). This heavier solution is useful for limiting denervation to a small area or to one side in the spinal cord. Anesthesia is established slowly and it recedes over the following 24 hours. The reason for this is that phenol possesses a local anesthetic action as well as a neurolytic action.

The extent of denervation can only be evaluated 24 hours after the injection, and sometimes repeated injections with smaller doses are necessary. Fortunately, it is almost painless and is accepted more readily than alcohol by the patient. Far less scarring is produced with phenol than with alcohol. Neuroma formation by regeneration of the nerve is not common. Although phenol is the preferred neurolytic agent for localized denervation, alcohol is still used for intrathecal injection (Bonica, 1953; Hay, 1959; Maher, 1955; Mark, 1962; Ventafridda and Martino, 1976) and chemical hypophysectomy (Moricca, 1974) in terminal patients with malignant tumors.

Alcohol and phenol should be used with care, as erosion of large vessels may produce bleeding and hematomas, and this is particularly hazardous in the brain and spinal cord.

CONDITIONS WARRANTING NERVE BLOCKS

Some of the conditions that can benefit the most from therapeutic nerve blocks are described briefly below.

Trigeminal Neuralgia

In many cases of true trigeminal neuralgia, denervation of the trigger area will relieve pain. In neuralgia whose pain is due to local pathology involving a branch of the trigeminal nerve, denervation of that branch will also render relief.

Destruction of the gasserian ganglion itself may be necessary whenever interruption of the neuropathway of the trigger zone fails to provide relief. The main consideration is to spare the ophthalmic division, which fortunately is rarely involved. Controlled thermocoagulation or chemical ablation of ganglia are currently used. Regardless of the technique used, it is desirable that preservation of some touch sensation be attempted, because when touch was not completely lost paresthesia was less frequent and patient acceptability was high.

The chemical means of denervation include hyperbaric phenol 5 percent in glycerine (Jefferson, 1964), and hypobaric alcohol solution (Ecker, 1974). Phenol may be easier to control, and corneal anesthesia can be avoided in almost 25 per cent of patients.

Differential thermocoagulation of ganglia is accomplished by a radio frequency current heated probe inserted percutaneously (Sweet and Wepsic, 1974). The degree of anesthesia produced can be controlled during the procedure by increasing both the temperature of the probe and the duration of thermocoagulation while testing for the amount of superficial pressure sensations preserved. In this procedure, first division is usually spared.

Surgical interruption of the mandibular and maxillary divisions of the trigeminal ganglia is less frequently performed except where pain persists in spite of the blocks mentioned. Resection of the portio major of the involved nerve by microsurgical techniques, sparing the intermediate nerves and the portio minor, which are considered to be responsible for touch sensations and motor activity, has certainly improved the results of surgical resections and has reduced the sensory deficit and motor loss (Pagni and Maspes, 1976). Only in healthy or younger patients should surgery be considered, as the results of transcutaneous blocks are almost the same without the added surgical risk.

Surgical decompression around the foramen ovale has been credited with good results. However, with this technique, the success rate seems to be related to the amount of trauma to the ganglion during the performance of the procedure. Vigorous rubbing of the ganglia to the degree that sensory loss has been produced has increased the success rate. This technique can really be considered a means of physical denervation rather than simple decompression of the neurological structure (Pudenz, 1952; Taarnhoj, 1952).

In postherpetic neuralgia, relief by permanent blocks is infrequent and recurrence of pain is high.

Occipital Neuralgia

A syndrome generally believed to be secondary to entrapment of occipital nerves as they enter the scalp will respond well to denervation when other methods fail. Chemical denervation or denervation with a heated electrode will also produce acceptable results (Blume, 1976).

Intercostal Neuralgia

These nerves, because of their anatomical location, can be denervated precisely by chemical means or radio frequency current. These blocks are particularly useful for chronic pain of the chest wall and in cases of nonresectible malignant tumor involving the chest wall or breast with intractable pain. In denervation of the breast in terminal cases, ulcers can develop in the inflammatory fold, particularly in obese patients with large breasts, unless excellent hygiene is maintained. Routine denervation following chest procedures should never be performed, particularly in females.

Subarachnoid Differential Nerve Blocks

Differential nerve block with results lasting up to one year is still the most useful technique available for control of pain for patients with terminal metastatic cancer (Bonica, 1953; Hay, Yonezova and Derrick, 1959; Maher, 1955; Mark, White, Zervas et al., 1962). Unfortunately, it is of limited value in relieving visceral pain caused by metastatic cancer in the peritoneal cavity (Ventafridda and Martino, 1976). Results are good if non-visceral structures such as the breast, chest, and abdominal wall are involved.

Hypobaric alcohol solution 50 to 90 per cent and hyperbaric phenol 5 to 15 per cent in glycerine are the two agents most frequently used. The primary objective of this procedure is to reduce pain without producing excessive weakness in the extremities or loss of sphincter control. After careful positioning of the patient, and with the use of phenol in glycerine, it is probably easier to limit the site of action to the affected segments. Denervation is not immediate and 24 to 48 hours will elapse before permanent results are achieved.

The blocks can be repeated with increasing doses to achieve optimal results. The volumes involved are 1 to 4 cc of 50 to 90 per cent alcohol or 5 to 15 per cent phenol, depending on the size of the area involved and the degree of denervation required. As mentioned before, repeated differential block with an epidural indwelling catheter with bupivacaine (Marcaine) 0.25 per cent without epinephrine should be attempted prior to alcohol and phenol injections.

Sympathectomy

The common sympathectomy procedures are stellate ganglion blocks and lumbar sympathectomy.

Therapeutic Stellate Ganglion Blocks

In causalgia of the upper arm, frequently repeated stellate ganglion blocks at 24 to 48 hour intervals with bupivacaine will provide relief that exceeds the duration of the block, and sometimes even affords permanent relief. It is important not to perform surgical sympathectomy until previous symptoms recur. In patients with partial relief lasting from several days to a few weeks, the blocks should be repeated and the patient re-evaluated prior to surgery.

Injection of alcohol or phenol into the stellate area is not recommended, as the area is surrounded by vital structures, and the dose required to produce permanent block may produce damage to some of these, particularly the carotid artery, vertebral artery, phrenic nerve, and recurrent laryngeal nerve. Moreover, the block is usually not complete, and recurrence rate is high. We think that surgical sympathectomy with careful interruption of the thoracic component by the transaxillary exposure is safer and the results are superior.

Lumbar Sympathectomy

The lumbar sympathetic chain can be interrupted by phenol in contrast media, with the aid of a televised x-ray screening with biplane visualization capability (Boas, Hatangdi, and Richards, 1976). The ventrolateral aspects of the bodies of the third and fourth lumbar vertebrae are contacted with 13.5 cm needles, with careful aspiration, and, after injection of a small test dose (0.3 to 0.5 cc) of phenol crystal in Conray 420 to give 70 per cent phenol, sterilized through Cay V-2 mm filter.

To assess the location and insure that there is no intravascular injection, 3 to 5 cc of a local anesthetic solution is injected prior to the administration of the phenol or alcohol. A rise in skin temperature is noted after 30 to 40 minutes, and the prognosis in longterm follow-up is favorable. The only complication reported is dysesthesia in the groin region for two to three months; however, the incidence was less than that following surgical sympathectomy.

Celiac axis block with 50 per cent alcohol or 5 to 10 per cent phenol is used in terminal cancer patients with abdominal metastasis in whom pain is so severe as to be totally incapacitating. The percutaneous techniques described by Bonica (1953) are utilized.

COMPLICATIONS OF ALCOHOL AND PHENOL BLOCK

A condition described as analgesia dolorosa is produced frequently following injections of high concentrations of alcohol; it occurs less frequently following injections of phenol. It also follows partial injury to a nerve, even though no neuromata are apparent, and on microscopic examination a large number of regenerating axons enveloped in scar tissue are seen. Any injury that destroys the neurilemmal sheath is liable to produce this complication.

A similar condition is produced in cases of partial or complete injury to a nerve by physical means. Treatment has been very difficult. In the acute stage, very good results have been obtained by inserting the catheter adjacent to the injured nerve and injecting local anesthetics. (This procedure is described in Chapter 15. A structured program for increasing stimulation in areas where dysesthesias have developed, starting by very light touch and proceeding to deep pressure over a period of several weeks will reduce painful touch sensation (see Chapter 47).

REFERENCES

Bieter, R.: Comparison of local anesthetics. J. Pharmacol. 56:221, 1936.

Blume, H. G.: Radio frequency denaturation in occipital pain: A new approach in 14 cases. *In* Bonica, J. J., and Albe-Fessard, D. (eds.): Advances in Pain Research and Therapy. New York, Raven Press, 1967, Vol 1, p. 691.

Boas, R. A., Hatangdi, V. S., and Richards, E. G.: Lumbar sympathectomy — a percutaneous chemical technique. *In* Bonica J. J., and Albe-Fessard, D. (eds.): Advances in Pain Research and Therapy. New York, Raven Press, 1976, Vol 1, p. 685.

Bonica, J. J.: The Management of Pain. Philadelphia, Lea and Febiger, 1953.

Ecker, A.: Tic douloureux: Eight years after alcoholic Gasserian injection. N.Y. State J. Med. 74: 1586, 1974.

Hay, R. C., Yonezowa, T., and Derrick, W. S.: Control of intractable pain in advanced cancer by subarachnoid alcohol block. J.A.M.A. 169:1315, 1959.

Jefferson, A.: Trigeminal neuralgia: Trigeminal root and ganglion injection using phenol in glycerine. *In* Knighton, R. S., and Dumke, P. R. (eds.): Henry Ford Int. Symposium on Pain, Detroit. Boston, Little, Brown and Co. 1966, pp. 365–371.

Maher, R. M.: Relief of pain in incurable cancer. Lancet 1:18, 1955.

Mark, V. H., White, J. C., Zervas, N. T., et al: Intrathecal use of phenol for the relief of chronic severe pain. N. Engl. J. Med. 267:589, 1962.

McIntyre, A. R.: Pharmacology of some new local anesthetics; J. Pharm. Exper. Ther. 63:369, 1938.

Miles, J., and Sampson, L.: Mode of action by which pituitary alcohol injection relieves pain. *In* Bonica J. J., and Albe-Fessard, D. (eds.): Advances in Pain Research and Therapy. New York, Raven Press, 1976, Vol 1, pp. 691.

Moore, D. C.: Regional Anesthesia. Springfield, Ill., Charles C Thomas, 1965.

Moricca, G.: Advances in Neurology, New York, Raven Press, 1974, Vol 4 p. 707.

Moricca, G.: Neuroadenolysis for diffuse unbearable cancer pain. *In* Bonica J. J., and Albe-Fessard, D. (eds.): Advances in Pain Research and Therapy. New York, Raven Press, 1976, Vol 1, p. 683.

Murphy, T. (1977): 28th annual refresher course lectures, presented 10/16/77 at the New Orleans, ASA meeting.

Pagni, C. A., and Maspes, P. E.: Microneurosurgical treatment and trigeminal neuralgia by selective juxtapontine rhizotomy of the portio major sparing the intermediate fibers. *In* Bonica J. J., and Albe-Fessard, D. (eds.): Advances in Pain Research and Therapy. New York, Raven Press, 1976, Vol. 1, p. 849.

Pudenz, R. H., and Sheldon, C. H.: Experiences with foraminal decompression in the surgical treatment of tic douloureux. Presented at American Academy of Neurological Surgery, New York, 1952.

Sweet, W. H., and Wepsic, J. G.: Controlled thermocoagulation of trigeminal ganglion and rootlets for differential destruction of pain fibers: 1. Trigeminal neuralgia. *In* Moricca, G. (ed.): Advances in Neurology, New York, Raven Press, 1974, Vol. 4.

Taarnhoj, P.: Decompression of the trigeminal root and the posterior part of the ganglion as treatment in trigeminal neuralgia, J. Neurosurg. *9*, 228, 1952.

Ventafridda, V., and Martino, G.: Clinical evaluation of subarachnoid neurolytic blocks in intractable cancer pain. *In* Bonica J. J., and Albe-Fessard, D. (eds.): Advances in Pain Research and Therapy. New York, Raven Press, 1976, Vol. 1, p. 699.

17

SURGICAL SYMPATHECTOMY— UPPER AND LOWER EXTREMITY

HAROLD E. KLEINERT
HANS NORBERG
JOHN J. McDONOUGH

INTRODUCTION

Neurovascular disorders of the extremities face the clinician with both diagnostic and treatment quandaries. The plethora of names given to what most clinicians call sympathetic dystrophy (SD) mirrors these difficulties. The classic signs and symptoms of sympathetic dystrophy, first clearly described by Mitchell, Morehouse, and Keen (1864), were based on their observations of nerve injuries on the wounded in the Civil War. They first called attention to the intense burning pain that is the hallmark of the disease. Following their description, similar, non-military clinical entities were described involving both open and closed injuries. A multitude of names has been given to these entities, the more commonly used term causalgia being coined in 1867. DeTakats (1943) masterfully noted that a wide spectrum of severity of involvement of a single disease process is present rather than a multitude of distinct diseases, which had accounted for the many names formerly applied to the disease. He further resolved some of the controversies by pointing out that the disease, depending on the severity and the treatment rendered, can progress through three different stages.

STAGES OF DISEASE

The first stage is characterized by vasodilatation (Fig. 17–1). The extremity is erythematous and swollen, the skin is dry, the joints are stiff, and there may be an overgrowth of hair and nails (Fig. 17–2). Pain is almost always intense,

285

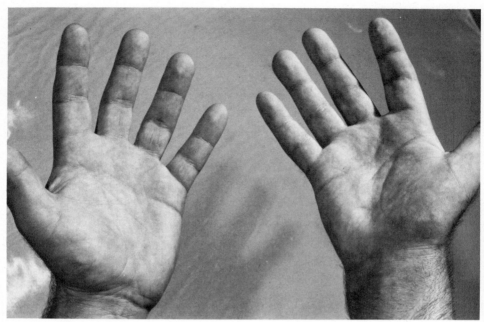

Figure 17–1 This man, referred six weeks after a secondary extensor tendon repair, demonstrates the vasodilatation and rubor of early dystrophy.

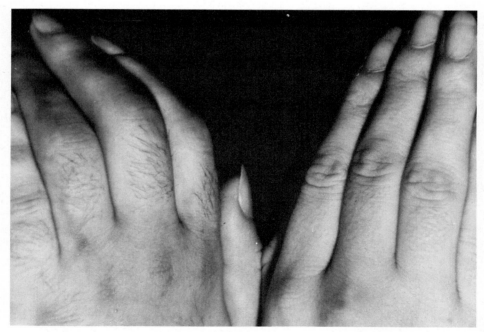

Figure 17–2 Hair overgrowth—one of the early signs of sympathetic dystrophy.

continuous, and burning in nature; however, it may vary in intensity and description. Emotional and environmental stress trigger paroxysms of pain. Hyperesthesia and trophic changes often begin shortly after the injury and initially are limited to the distribution of the involved nerve. With time, these disorders spread to involve the entire extremity. Ideally, cases are recognized in this stage of hyperemia and are arrested and cured by conservative therapy.

The second stage, characterized by vasoconstriction, gradually evolves from the first. In this stage the skin is thin and soft, and sweating is excessive. Pain, undiminished in intensity, has extended to involve the entire extremity. The patient has learned to protect the involved extremity and assumes a characteristic protective posture while awake (Fig. 17–3). Malnourishment and severe psychologic disturbances are common associated problems, but may simply reflect the patient's attempts to protect the involved extremity. More involved and aggressive therapy is required to control symptoms during this stage.

The third and last stage, as outlined by deTakats, is one of atrophy resulting from both protective disuse and chronic vasoconstriction. The extremity is held fixed in a protective position.

Radiographic bony changes of Sudeck's-type atrophy are present (Fig. 17–4A and B). This advanced stage of atrophy is the most difficult to treat because all therapeutic modalities may be ineffective. Some have described this stage as a relative contraindication to operative intervention except amputation. Amputation, however, does not control the pain and adds to, rather than reduces, the patient's physical and psychological disabilities. Conservative or indicated operative therapy, or both, will produce some degree of functional return and pain control even at this stage.

Any patient with pain and/or swelling out of proportion to the extent of injury must be suspected of having sympathetic dystrophy. Damage to any nerve carrying sympathetic fibers may produce a sympathetic dystrophy. It can occur following what appears to be insignificant trauma. In the upper extremity the median nerve is the one most commonly involved. However, injury to a major nerve of the extremity need not be present, for the disease may occur with minor injuries, such as a finger tip crush followed by involvement of the hand and extremity (Fig. 17–5). Sympathetic dystrophy is frequently seen with carpal tunnel compression of the median nerve both prior to and after operative release of the carpal tunnel, and following palmar fasciectomy for Dupuytren's contractures. It can occur from either the trauma of fracture or the corrective manipulation of a Colles' fracture.

Differential Diagnosis

Table 17–1 contains only a partial listing of the chronic pain syndromes that may be confused with sympathetic dystrophy. A difficult differentiation is between sympathetic dystropy and the psychogenic pain syndromes, particularly factitious lymphedema. The onset of sympathetic dystrophy occurs soon after injury, whereas there may be a significant interval between injury and the onset of psychogenic disorders. Psychiatric evaluation aids in the differentia-

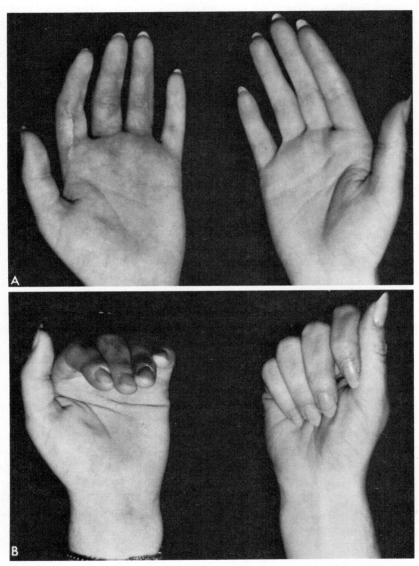

Figure 17–3 *A* and *B*, This patient, whose hand received a crushing type injury, has an unusual amount of burning pain associated with swelling and stiffness in both flexion and extension.

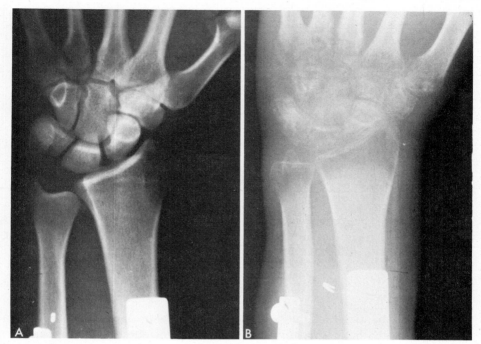

Figure 17–4   *A* and *B*, These marked radiographic changes occurred over a three month period in a patient with a forearm fracture and severe dystrophy.

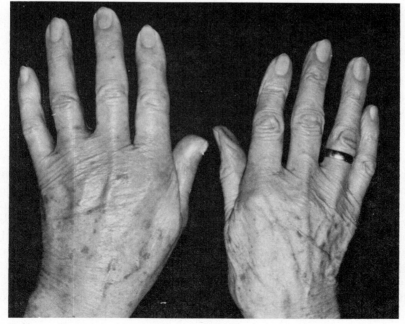

Figure 17–5   Advanced sympathetic dystrophy four months following a crush injury to the left thumb tip. Radiographic changes of osteoporosis were also present.

Table 17–1   **Differential Diagnosis**

Nerve compression (more common)	Vascular insufficiency
Thoracic outlet syndrome	Secondary to trauma
Carpal tunnel	—Chronic Volkmann's contracture
Cubital tunnel	—Ulnar artery thrombosis
Cervical radiculitis	—Axillary vein thrombosis
Cervical disc	Secondary to disease
Radial tunnel	—Raynaud's phenomenon
	—Raynaud's disease
Chronic inflammatory disease	—Early scleroderma
Tenosynovitis	
Synovitis of joints	Psychogenic diseases
Chronic infectious diseases	

tion. The initial anatomic localization of sympathetic dystrophy is rarely observed in psychologic disorders. A diagnostic sympathetic block can help differentiate these disorders.

Conservative Therapy

One must be aware of the potential for drug abuse and addiction in patients with sympathetic dystrophy. Initial treatment should be conservative. This includes intermittent splinting, physical therapy, medications, and temporary interruption of the sympathetic nervous system. Light, comfortable splints in a neutral position are worn at night and can be easily removed during the day for physical therapy. A program is outlined to gradually increase range of motion in the affected part. Gradual desensitization procedures are initiated and have proved to be beneficial.

Desensitization Procedures*

The first stage of desensitization consists of the application of local heat or transcutaneous nerve stimulation, or both. Transcutaneous nerve stimulation (TNS) is the treatment of choice, since it allows more mobility as desensitization is carried out. Transcutaneous nerve stimulation is normally applied to the affected nerves for durations of one hour or greater, depending on individual comfort. Applications of heat may provide relief from discomfort for up to 30 minutes following treatment. Active exercise is performed to increase joint mobility. Although joint capsules are tight from swelling, they usually have not shortened significantly in this first stage. It is not unusual to see an individual regain full range of motion in the hand while exercising on TNS. Resistance to muscular efforts is gradually increased to maximize the muscular pumping mechanism. Compressible materials that allow the hand to progress through full range of motion are utilized. These materials may be used interchangeably to graduate the amount of resistance.

In the second and third stages, the involved nerves may become too irritable to utilize TNS. In the most hyperirritable conditions of the nerves, the

---

*Mark Lindsay, L.P.T.

muscle of the hand and forearm may fasciculate as soon as the TNS apparatus is activated. Under these circumstances, local heat becomes the treatment of choice until the nerve irritability is reduced to the extent that the patient will accept TNS. Exercise begins with active movement through the available range of motion. Edema control procedures may be necessary. Since, by the second and third stages the dystrophy has progressed for some time, joint capsule contracture is present. Specific joint mobilization exercises and active assistive exercises are performed to prevent further capsule tightening and increase the available range of motion.

Chlorpromazine hydrochloride (Thorazine) is an excellent drug for treatment of sympathetic dystrophy. In doses of 10 to 25 mg b.i.d. to q.i.d. it has proved quite effective. In patients over 40 years of age, we prefer trifluoperazine hydrochloride (Stelazine) (2 mg b.i.d.) because of possible Thorazine side effects in the older age group. High dose steroid therapy may also be beneficial.

A trial period of two to three weeks on this regimen is recommended. If favorable response is obtained, the regimen is varied to achieve the best possible results. According to the reponse obtained, physical therapy may be increased or decreased as well as splinting time and drug dosages. In an original investigation of over 500 patients with post-traumatic sympathetic dystrophy, we found that 64 per cent required no further treatment (Kleinert et al., 1973). Of these patients, 46 per cent had complete remission of symptoms, and the remainder indicated that their residual symptoms were minor and that additional treatment was not indicated. Occasionally, cases may regress without continued treatment.

Stellate Block

If there has been no response or an incomplete response to medication as outlined above, temporary interruption of the sympathetic dystrophy in the form of a stellate or paravertebral block is used. The anterior approach for stellate ganglion block is preferred because of its ease and safety. The patient is informed of the symptoms and signs of a satisfactory block and warned that rarely a transient partial brachial plexus block may occur (Table 17–2). All blocks are performed in the hospital outpatient facility as a precaution against infrequent complications, such as pneumothorax, which could require resuscitative measures not readily available in the non-hospital setting.

The block is performed with the patient resting supine and the neck mildly hyperextended. This is managed by placing a pillow or roll under the patient's scapulae and resting the head on the treatment table. The finger tips

**Table 17–2   Symptoms and Signs Associated
with Stellate Block**

Hoarseness
Difficulty in swallowing
Rarely, partial brachial plexus block
Cessation of sweating
Corneal irritation

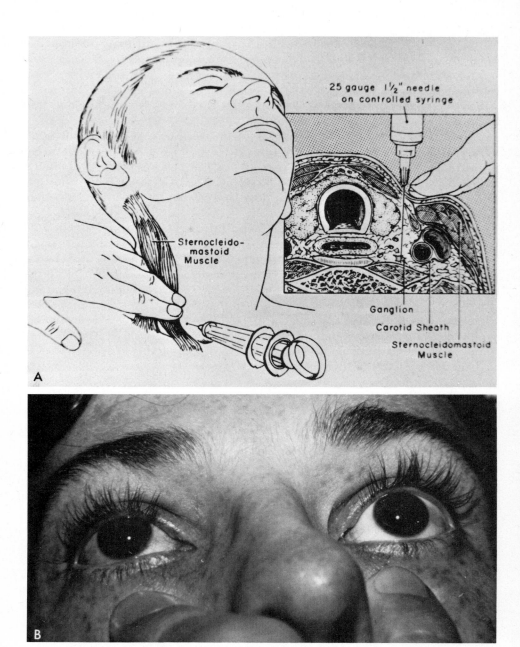

Figure 17–6 *A*, Anterior approach to stellate block. The carotid sheath is retracted with the fingertips and the needle inserted to the transverse process of the sixth cervical vertebra. (From Kleinert, H. E., et al.: Post traumatic sympathetic dystrophy. Ortho. Clin. North Am. *4*(4):917, 1973.) *B*, After injection of properly placed anesthetic solution, an almost immediate Horner's syndrome is noted.

of one hand retract the sternocleidomastoid muscle and the contents of the carotid sheath laterally (Fig. 17–6A). With a 4 cm, 25 gauge needle on a 10 cc control syringe, a skin wheal is raised 2.5 cm above the sternal notch, between the trachea and the sternocleidomastoid. The needle is advanced to the readily palpable transverse process of the sixth cervical vertebra. The needle is withdrawn slightly and, after taking the usual precautions against intravascular injection, 10 to 20 cc's of 0.5 per cent bupivacaine hydrochloride (Marcaine) are injected. The patient is immediately placed with his head and neck elevated to facilitate gravitational flow of the anesthetic toward the stellate ganglion. The patient is held in the hospital for a few hours to (1) observe the adequacy of the block, (2) preclude any untoward reactions and, (3) note changes in the signs and symptoms of the sympathetic dystrophy after the block (Table 17–3).

A successful block has been achieved if a Horner's sign is noted, if vasodilation of the hand and forearm occurs, and if extremity symptoms improve, provided the diagnosis is correct (Fig. 6B). The average block employing Marcaine is of 12 to 18 hours' duration. Blocks are usually given on alternate days. In more refractory cases, a series of blocks is carried out. Hospitalization is recommended to minimize external emotional stress and to permit intensive physical therapy during the pain-free periods following effective blocks. If, after a series of six to eight successful blocks, the patient continues to experience severe symptoms, surgical sympathectomy must be considered.

No response to an objectively successful stellate block indicates that the diagnosis of sympathetic dystrophy should be re-evaluated.

In our series, 84 per cent of the patients who received a series of stellate blocks achieved permanent cessation of pain and required no further treatment. The remaining patients (16 per cent), who received only transient improvement, were treated with transaxillary sympathectomies.

Re-exploration of the wound for entrapped or lacerated nerve is indicated prior to sympathectomy, particularly if a "trigger point" which initiates or exacerbates the pain is present or suspected.

Thoracic Sympathectomy

The importance of patient selection cannot be overemphasized. An adequate response with relief of symptoms must occur with stellate blocks (a medical sympathectomy) before a patient can be considered for surgical sympathectomy. Many surgical misadventures can be avoided if this rule is followed. Not only patients with sympathetic dystrophy but also those with Raynaud's disease, scleroderma, or other collagen diseases, such as Raynaud's

Table 17–3 Signs of Satisfactory Stellate Block

Horner's
Unilateral ptosis
Unilateral scleral injection
Vasodilatation — veins and arteries
Increased R.O.M. of involved extremity ⎱ if patient has
Complete or partial pain relief ⎰ sympathetic dystrophy

phenomenon, thromboangiitis obliterans (Buerger's disease), vascular insufficiency secondary to trauma, arteriosclerosis with thrombosis, painful cold injury, and hyperhidrosis, may be considered candidates for sympathectomy (Homans, 1942). As in sympathetic dystrophy an adequate response to medical sympathectomy is a prerequisite for surgery.

Contraindications to sympathectomy are absence of pulmonary reserve and factitious lymphedema. Other contraindications where only temporary relief might be obtained are metastatic carcinoma and Pancoast tumors. Shoulder disease, apical pulmonary disease, cardiac insufficiency, and poor pulmonary reserve are relative contraindications and require thorough evaluation before surgery is considered. These associated problems plus body type may dictate the type of surgical approach chosen.

In addition to the routine laboratory studies, such as roentgenograms and electrocardiograms, pulmonary function tests and apical lordotic views are obtained. Any abnormality detected requires thorough evaluation before proceeding.

There are a number of surgical approaches to upper extremity sympathectomy, each with advantages and disadvantages. Our preference for most patients is the transaxillary transthoracic approach (Kleinert, 1965), which provides excellent exposure of the stellate ganglion as well as the first four dorsal ganglia with minimal dissection. However, if bilateral sympathectomies are planned, a second procedure one week after the first is required. The transcervical approach, which has the advantage of being relatively simple, causes minimal disruption of normal anatomy but fails to expose the third and fourth ganglia, and should bleeding from an intercostal vessel occur, it would be difficult to control. This approach is indicated in patients with pulmonary disease that militates against thoracotomy. The anterior transthoracic approach of Palumbo (1966) provides excellent exposure of the sympathetic trunk but requires splitting the pectoralis major. The resultant cosmetic deformity is considerable and is of significance, since many of these patients are women. The posterior transthoracic approach, as first described by Adson and Brown (1929) and recently well illustrated by Urschel and Razzuk (1977), facilitates bilateral sympathectomies and simultaneous correction of thoracic outlet syndrome. It is technically the most difficult and time-consuming, requiring major tissue resection. Furthermore, it fails to provide exposure of the lower sympathetic chain and frequently results in an unsightly scar and prolonged postoperative pain.

When obtaining consent for operation, not only is the procedure explained but also the patient is warned of the possibility of a permanent Horner's syndrome — less than 10 per cent in our series. In addition, absence of sweating and the possibility of postoperative intercostal pain are discussed. The patient may be reassured that this intercostal pain from traumatic neuritis is temporary and usually responds to heat, analgesics and intercostal blocks.

Operative Technique

Following the induction of general anesthesia, the patient is placed in the lateral position with padding under the shoulder and between the flexed

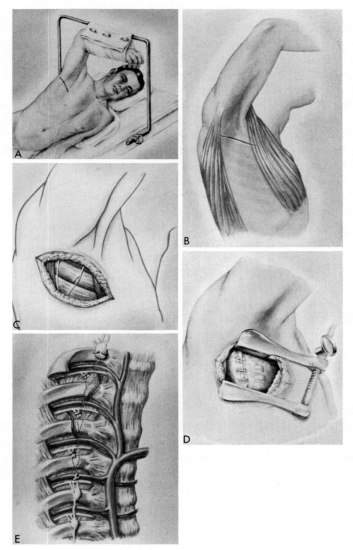

Figure 17–7   Technique of transaxillary sympathectomy. (From Kleinert, H. E., et al.: Neurovascular disorders of the upper extremity. Arch. Surg. *90*·612, 1965.)

knees. Adhesive tape and padded kidney rests are used to maintain the position. The arm may be held abducted 90 degrees by an assistant or may be held suspended by the hand and forearm from a padded ether screen or Mayo stand (Fig. 17–7*A*). Care must be taken not to exceed 120 degrees of abduction to avoid stretch damage to the brachial plexus. The incision is made overlying the second intercostal space from the lateral border of the pectoralis major to the anterior border of the latissimus dorsi, just below the axillary hair line (Fig. 17–7*B*). The axillary fat is swept cephalad by blunt dissection, revealing the serratus anterior muscle (Fig. 17–7*C*). The long thoracic nerve and the intercostobrachial nerve are found in the posterior portion of the wound and preserved. The long thoracic nerve is found in the posterior part of the wound, running parallel and next to the latissimus dorsi. The intercostobrachial nerve, the sensory nerve to the medial aspect of the arm, is found in the superior portion of the wound, arising primarily from the second intercostal space and running in an anteroposterior direction. The pectoralis muscles are bluntly elevated off the chest wall in the area of the second intercostal space by finger dissection. The serratus anterior is divided in the direction of its fibers over the second intercostal space. After hemostasis is achieved, the chest cavity may be entered through the second intercostal space, opening the intercostal musculature and parietal pleura for the entire length of the wound. An extrapleural approach can be used but we prefer the transpleural approach for its technical ease and its speed, and to avoid retropleural hematoma. A self-retaining rib retractor is inserted and slowly opened until sufficient exposure is obtained. Slow opening of the rib retractor will allow excellent exposure without fracturing ribs. Adhesions, when present, are sharply dissected, and the lung is packed away inferiorly and anteriorly.

The sympathetic chain is readily visualized in the posterior mediastinum, lying on the heads of the ribs beneath the parietal pleura (Fig. 17–7D). On the right side, the sympathetic chain is lateral to the azygos vein and vagus nerve. On the left it may be found lateral to the vagus and phrenic nerves as well as the origin of the subclavian artery. The first intercostal vein may cross on top of the sympathetic chain if it joins the innominate vein. The stellate ganglion, formed by fusion of the inferior cervical and first thoracic ganglia, is identified as dumbbell shaped, with its upper pole overlying the head of the first rib. Occasionally, the second thoracic ganglion may be incorporated with the stellate ganglion.

The pleura overlying the sympathetic chain is incised to the level of the fourth thoracic ganglion. The chain is bluntly elevated and exposed with a peanut dissector. Using a nerve hook, the fourth thoracic ganglion is isolated and divided between hemoclips. The dissection is carried cephalad, clipping and dividing the rami. The stellate ganglion is divided by placing clips so as to divide it into halves and excising the caudal portion (Fig. 17–7E). A chest tube of 24 French caliber is placed in the apical posterior region and brought out through a stab-wound incision in the skin of the mid-axillary line. The chest cavity is copiously irrigated with Ringer's or saline solution. Three or four 2-0 chromic pericostal sutures are inserted over the upper rib and through holes drilled in the lower rib to avoid damage to the intercostal artery and nerve. A rib approximator is used to facilitate closure. The serratus anterior is reapproximated with running 4-0 polyglycolic acid sutures (Dexon), as are the subcutaneous tissues. The skin is closed with a subcuticular running 5-0 nylon. The chest tube is sutured into place and placed on water seal suction. A padded dressing is applied.

Postoperative pain may be minimized by intercostal nerve blocks — two interspaces above and below the incision site — using 0.5 per cent Marcaine. These blocks may be performed after closing or under direct vision at the termination of the resection of the sympathetic chain.

Chest x-ray is obtained to verify complete lung expansion. Rigorous chest toilet, deep breathing and coughing exercises, and intermittent positive pressure breathing are begun immediately. Early mobilization is started on the evening of surgery. The chest tube is usually removed on the second postoperative day and complete lung expansion verified by followup x-ray. The majority of patients have been discharged by the sixth postoperative day. The subcuticular pullout suture is removed two weeks postoperatively.

Postoperative Complications

Our most common postoperative complication is intercostal neuritis. This may be minimized at the time of surgery by intercostal blocks. Local heat and analgesics are usually sufficient to control postoperative pain but further intercostal blocks may be required. The potential for pneumothorax is present but is avoided by careful maintenance of the chest tube and followup x-rays. In our series less than 10 per cent experienced a permanent Horner's syndrome.

Recurrent upper extremity pain following thoracic sympathectomy presents a special problem. First, it must be differentiated from intercostal neuritis and other nonrelated diseases. If the recurrent pain seems to be secondary to sympathetic dystrophy, then completeness of the sympathectomy can be checked by the simply performed starch test. If this indicates that the sympathectomy is complete, one can only conclude that problems other than sympathetic dystrophy exist. If the test indicates that an incomplete sympathectomy was performed, reoperation can be considered.

Failure to remove the third and fourth thoracic ganglia is often the cause of incomplete sympathectomy. Cases have been reported in which after reoperation with additional removal of the third and fourth ganglia there was complete cessation of symptoms. Skoog (1947) pointed out that in some patients a significant number of sympathetic ganglia may lie within the spinal nerves, primarily in the second thoracic nerve. Section of this nerve may be considered at reoperation.

Lower Extremity Neurovascular Disorders

Sympathetic dystrophy may occur in the lower extremity as well. We have found it to be less common here, but it responds equally well to the regimen previously outlined. Initial treatment is always conservative and consists of physical therapy, intermittent splinting, and medication. If there is a positive response, the regimen is modified accordingly to produce the maximum benefit. Accurate diagnosis is important. Sympathetic dystrophy in the lower extremity is easily confused with vascular disorders. Presence or absence of pulses is noted and recorded. Differential diagnosis includes, as in the upper extremity, other neurovascular disorders, such as Raynaud's phenomenon and scleroderma. As in the upper extremity, "trigger pain points," especially from nerve injury, are looked for and appropriately treated if present. Lack of response after an adequate trial period or a marginal response is an indication for a trial of paravertebral lumbar sympathetic blocks.

Paravertebral Lumbar Sympathetic Block

Technically, a lumbar sympathetic block is more difficult than a stellate block (Moore, 1973). Three separate injection sites are required. Some feel that only the lower two ganglia need be blocked for lower leg pain. However, for completeness, certainly all three ganglia should be blocked. Not only is the block more difficult to perform, it is also more difficult to evaluate the adequacy or success of the block. This difficulty has led some to discredit the value of the block as a predictor of success of sympathectomy. The sine qua non is, of course, objective vasodilatation and relief of symptoms. Vasodilatation without relief of symptoms always raises questions as to the completeness of the block. If, after several objectively successful blocks there is no improvement in symptoms, then another diagnosis should be sought. If relief of symptoms is good but only transient, lumbar sympathectomy may be advised.

The block is performed in a hospital outpatient facility as a precaution against untoward reactions. The patient is monitored several hours later to observe and evaluate his response. Intraspinal injection of the anesthetic is rare yet upsetting even though only transient.

The patient is placed in the prone position with a pillow under the abdomen to flatten the lumbar curvature. The midline is marked, and a transverse line is drawn through the spaces of the lumbar vertebrae of the ganglia to be blocked. A second line is drawn 4.5 to 5 cm lateral to the midline on the affected side. The intersections of this lateral line and the transverse lines mark the sites of injection (Fig. 17–8). After skin preparation, local anesthetic wheals are raised. A 10 cm, 22 gauge spinal needle is inserted through the wheals at an 85 degree angle to the skin, inclining toward the midline for a distance of 4 to 5 cm. If the needle does not strike the vertebral body, it should be partially withdrawn and re-angled to do so. The needle point is walked off the vertebral body. At the point where it just misses the vertebral body, 10 cc of 0.5 per cent Marcaine may be injected after one is certain that no blood can be aspirated. The process is repeated at L2 and L3 levels (Fig. 17–9).

Lumbar Sympathectomy

If transient good relief of pain is obtained only to recur after a series of successful blocks, lumbar sympathectomy should be considered. As with the upper extremity, where the indications for sympathectomy are more controversial, such as cold injury, hyperhidrosis, and vascular insufficiency secondary to either trauma or disease, sound clinical judgment is of prime importance. The psychologic overlay in these patients is evaluated and considered before embarking on an operative course.

An intravenous pyelogram is particularly useful in the preoperative evaluation of the patient, in addition to routine laboratory studies to locate any vascular or urogenital anomalies that may complicate the dissection.

There are several approaches to the lumbar sympathetic chain. The retroperitoneal flank approach through either a transverse or an oblique inci-

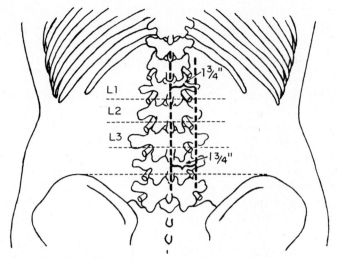

Figure 17–8 Lumbar sympathetic block – topographical anatomy. Midline is marked; transverse lines are drawn through the spaces between the transverse processes. A second line 4 to 5 cm lateral to the midline and transecting the transverse line will mark the site of injection.

sion produces adequate visualization of the chain with minimal postoperative ileus or pain and a shorter period of hospitalization. Unfortunately, it is difficult to deal with hemorrhage from lumbar veins or the vena cava with this approach. The rapid conversion to a transabdominal approach is possible should the need arise. The transabdominal approach has the advantages of allowing simultaneous bilateral sympathectomies, good exposure, and good

Figure 17–9 A 22 gauge needle is inserted. When the tip strikes the body of the vertebra, the needle is partially withdrawn and walked around the vertebral body.

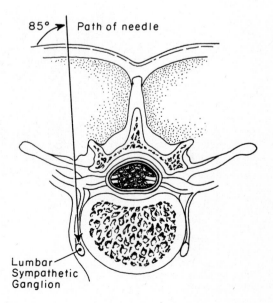

vascular control. However, a more prolonged ileus, intra-abdominal adhesions, and increased incisional discomfort are more likely to occur.

Operative Technique

The patient is placed in the lateral jackknife position, with appropriate padding between the bent knees and between chest and arm. An incision is made obliquely in the flank, beginning near the anterior superior iliac crest and extending superior and lateral to the tip of the twelfth rib. The incision is carried to the muscle layer. After hemostasis is achieved, the internal and external oblique muscles are divided and the transversalis muscle and fascia are opened in the direction of their fibers. The peritoneum is gently separated by blunt dissection from the lateral abdominal wall and retracted anteriorly. The dissection is carried along the anterior surface of the quadratus lumborum and psoas muscles. The kidney is elevated anteriorly while avoiding injury to the ureter and genital vessels.

On the right side, the lumbar sympathetic chain lies at the junction of vertebrae and the medial margin of the psoas muscles. The chain is located posterior to the inferior vena cava, and it may be necessary to divide several lumbar veins to visualize it (Fig. 17–10). On the left, the chain lies in the grooves between the psoas muscles and the vertebral body, with the aorta usually anteromedial to it, making dissection somewhat easier. The chain is usually palpable as a bowstring on the vertebral body.

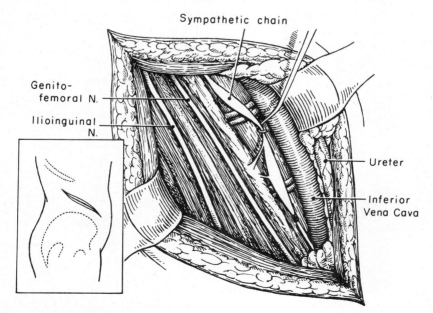

Figure 17–10 Right side—The sympathetic chain is located posterior to the inferior vena cava, which is gently retracted anteriorly for maximum exposure. Usually ganglia L2, L3, and L4 are excised for complete lower extremity sympathectomy. Avoid L1 in the male.

After exposing the sympathetic chain, a blunt nerve hook is used for tension and the chain is excised. Usually two to three ganglia are removed after first dividing the rami between silver clips. There may be fusion and attenuation of ganglia, making distinct identification difficult. In males, the first lumbar ganglion is usually left in place, since impotence may follow its removal, especially bilateral removal (Artz, 1975). Preganglionic sympathectomy is now preferred to the older, less reliable periarterial or postganglionic types (Sunderland, 1972). After hemostasis is secured, any rents in the peritoneum are repaired and the peritoneum is allowed to fall back into position. The muscle layers are sequentially reapproximated with interrupted 4-0 polyglycolic acid sutures and the skin edges with a 4-0 nylon pullout subcuticular suture.

The nasogastric tube is usually removed on the first or second postoperative day, and early ambulation is encouraged. While the potential for renal and ureteral damage exists, it is not likely and can be avoided by careful dissection and gentle retraction in a bloodless field. Incisional discomfort is usually the principal postoperative complaint.

As is true with the upper extremity, recurrence of lower extremity pain requires re-evaluation of the cause for pain and the completeness of the sympathectomy. Pain after adequate sympathectomy indicates either an incorrect or incomplete diagnosis. Pain after incomplete sympathectomy suggests that reoperation by the transabdominal approach should be considered if the diagnosis of sympathetic dystrophy was originally correct.

CONCLUSION

Sympathetic dystrophy is a devastating complication of trauma or elective surgery. Its cause is obscure and its course insidious. Early diagnosis and treatment are essential to a successful outcome. Prompt conservative management can often restore function to the disabled extremity and avoid the necessity of operative sympathectomy.

With experience, the clinician will often suspect the patient who will develop sympathetic dystrophy and thus can make the diagnosis early in its course. Frequently, such patients (or those with a previous history of dystrophy), when undergoing additional surgery, can be given sympathetic blocks in the immediate postoperative period to break the cycle of dystrophy development.

Surgical sympathectomy should be considered only for those patients with continuing moderate to severe dystrophy who have an objective, however temporary, response to multiple repeated sympathetic blocks and adjunctive therapy.

REFERENCES

Adson, A. W., and Brown, G. E.: The treatment of Raynaud's disease by resection of the upper thoracic and lumbar sympathetic ganglia and trunks. Surg. Gynecol. Obstet. *48*:577, 1929.
Artz, C., and Hardy, J. D.: Management of Surgical Complications. Philadelphia, W. B. Saunders Co., 1975, p. 432.

deTakats, G.: Causalgic states following injuries to the extremities. Arch. Phys. Therapy *24*:647, 1943.

Homans, J.: Treatment of peripheral vascular diseases. Med. Clin. North Amer. *26*:1457, 1942.

Kleinert, H. E., and Hyland, W. T.: Transaxillary transpleural thoracic sympathectomy. Surg. Techniques Illus. *2*(3):29, 1977.

Kleinert, H. E., Cook, F. W., and Kutz, J. E.: Neurovascular disorders of the upper extremity. Arch. Surg. *90*:612, 1965.

Kleinert, H. E., Cole, N. M., Wayne, L., Harvey, R., Kutz, J. E., and Atasoy, E.: Post-traumatic sympathetic dystrophy. Orthop. Clin. North Amer. *4*:917, 1973.

Mitchell, S. W., Morehouse, G. R., and Keen, W. W.: Gunshot Wounds and Other Injuries of Nerves. Philadelphia, J. B. Lippincott Co., 1864.

Moore, D. C.: Regional block. 4th ed., Springfield, Charles C Thomas, 1973.

Palumbo, L. T.: Anterior transthoracic approach for upper thoracic sympathectomy. Arch. Surg. *72*:659, 1956.

Skoog, T.: Ganglia in communicating rami of the cervical sympathetic trunk. Lancet *28*:457, 1947.

Sunderland, S.: Nerves and Nerve Injuries. London, Churchill Livingstone, 1972.

Urschel, H. C., and Razzuk, M. A.: Posterior thoracic sympathectomy. Surg. Techniques Illus. *2*(3):39, 1977.

18

CENTRAL SURGICAL PROCEDURES FOR PAIN OF PERIPHERAL NERVE ORIGIN

PHILIP L. GILDENBERG

It is not uncommon for peripheral nerve lesions to cause chronic pain even after appropriate peripheral nerve repair or treatment. After all attempts at treatment of nerve pain by peripheral or sympathetic procedures have been tried, it may be necessary to turn to the central nervous system in an attempt to alleviate pain resulting from peripheral nerve injury.

SELECTION OF PATIENTS

Which patients with pain of peripheral nerve origin may be considered for central procedures? Certainly no patient for whom another treatment opportunity exists (Gildenberg and DeVaul, 1978). No patient should be considered for a central procedure until the pain has persisted for sufficiently long to be sure that it will not spontaneously resolve. Generally, several months is allowed, during which an exhaustive attempt at pain treatment has been under way, at which point the pain may be defined as being chronic rather than acute.

The approach to patients with chronic pain generally must be more comprehensive than the approach to patients with acute pain, and the orientation of the doctor–patient relationship is significantly altered (DeVaul et al., 1977a). In an acute problem, the patient presents himself as a passive participant. He is

303

encouraged to rest to allow time for the healing process and to allow the physician to treat actively. It is appropriate to treat the patient with strong analgesics or narcotics, in anticipation that the pain will soon go away and that medication can be discontinued.

However, in the chronic pain state, it must be recognized that pain may not go away. Analgesics and narcotics are ineffective for chronic pain. The patient must actively participate in the treatment program, and should use whatever resources he has despite the persistence of the pain. It is no longer appropriate to sit and wait for a cure. Activity and resocialization should proceed despite the patient's symptoms. During the initial months of a painful or disabling condition, many psychological problems develop, especially in the patients whose preexisting personality predisposes toward the development of such factors (Engel, 1959; Fordyce, 1974; DeVaul et al., 1977b; Gildenberg and DeVaul, 1978).

In evaluating whether a patient is a candidate for a central pain relieving procedure, it may be helpful to consider pain as having three components.

Physiologic pain, in this definition, is pain from some condition which produces noxious stimulation. The intact nervous system perceives this stimulation appropriately and the patient feels pain.

Pathologic pain, in this definition, occurs when no noxious peripheral stimulus is applied. However, the central or peripheral nervous system is not functioning properly, as often occurs after peripheral nerve injury. Even a non-noxious stimulus may be perceived as being painful. Treatment is directed not toward removal of a peripheral pathologic stimulus, which may not be present, but toward altering the nervous system to diminish the misinterpretation of incoming sensory information.

Psychologic pain originates within the thought processes. Chronic psychologic pain may be obscured when it coexists with organic physiologic or pathologic pain. It is extremely important for the physician to recognize that most patients with chronic pain are depressed, and that depression decreases pain tolerance and may adversely affect the response to the treatment program. Other psychologic factors provide the patient with secondary gain. There may be considerable secondary emotional gain from, for instance, a too supportive spouse. It is not difficult for the patient to convince himself that *any* remaining discomfort is overwhelming and disabling, and chances for successful treatment are minimized. It is necessary to consider psychological factors before embarking on a treatment program for any patient with chronic pain, particularly pain of peripheral nerve origin (Gildenberg and DeVaul, 1978).

Prior to any central procedure for the treatment of intractable pain, a thorough psychological inquiry should be made, since patients with a large emotional component to their pain require concurrent treatment of the emotional factors. Even patients whose pain is secondary to obvious organic causes frequently develop significant secondary psychopathology to the extent that no pain relieving procedure in itself would affect either the patient's disability or perception of pain. Perhaps the most significant factor in the failure of surgical procedures to alleviate chronic pain is the failure to recognize and treat the profound emotional distress that can accompany any chronic pain state.

Classically, an experimental animal may be conditioned by reward for behaving in a certain way and by punishment for behaving otherwise. When a patient receives secondary gain (rewards) for having chronic pain over a period of months, but faces the loss of rewards and a return to responsibility (punishment) if he were not to have pain, one can see that with time the patient may become firmly conditioned not only to behave as if he has pain but also actually to perceive pain. Surgical intervention at that point may interrupt the peripheral input involved with pain sensation but may not influence the perception which the patient experiences from the conditioning process (Fordyce, 1974).

It is natural that a patient does not usually appear for neurosurgical intervention for pain until he has had his pain for some months (and rightly so), but, at that point, the surgeon must be cognizant of the psychological and conditioning factors which have developed and which may doom the response to treatment. Patients are not candidates for surgical intervention for pain while these factors remain.

The problem of addiction is not always obvious. The patient who takes narcotics out of proportion to the pain complaint can often be identified as having a primary addiction problem. However, one must sadly recognize that we have no acceptable medication for chronic pain. All commonly used analgesics are not only useless on a long-term basis but are also highly addicting, including many heavily advertised as non-narcotics.

It is quite common for patient and physician alike to confuse alleviation of withdrawal symptoms with alleviation of pain. As patients develop tolerance to their analgesics, they require larger doses at more frequent intervals. Withdrawal may set in just before the time for each dose. One of the manifestations of withdrawal is decreased tolerance to pain, so that the patient's pain may become magnified every few hours. This increased pain perception (which is actually withdrawal) is alleviated by the addicting drug, so that both physician and patient interpret this phenomenon as the drug successfully alleviating the patient's pain which has increased in severity over the months. It is not uncommon to find, however, that both the addiction and the pain are effectively treated when the patient is successfully withdrawn from the drug.

With these considerations, it is not surprising that an average of only 5 per cent of patients referred to chronic pain units eventually have invasive neurosurgical procedures to treat their pain. The figure may be somewhat higher for patients with pain of peripheral nerve origin, since the etiology is often well defined and more non-destructive treatments are available.

In summary, in patient selection for central procedures for the treatment of intractable pain secondary to peripheral nerve lesions one must first consider that the duration and severity of the pain must be sufficient to justify the risk of surgical intervention. There must be no psychiatric factor which contraindicates such treatment, or a program to manage the psychiatric factors must precede or run concurrent with evaluation and surgical treatment of the pain.

SELECTION OF PROCEDURES

Pain following a peripheral nerve injury is perhaps the most common cause for persistent pain of peripheral nerve origin. The first consideration is whether a procedure at the site of the nerve injury may be indicated. Only after it has been demonstrated that a local procedure or sympathectomy would not be effective would one consider a central procedure for the treatment of pain.

As a general rule, central procedures should not be considered until all peripheral procedures have been exhausted. Then the most distal procedure should be considered before those that concern manipulation higher in the nervous system.

Nondestructive treatment, such as temporary blocks or stimulation, should be considered before destructive lesions which interrupt nervous system pathways. Pain tends to recur weeks, months, or even years after destructive lesions for the treatment of chronic pain of benign origin, presumably as a reflection of the plasticity and redundancy built into the nervous system (Spiegel and Wycis, 1962; Spiegel et al., 1966).

Transcutaneous, peripheral nerve and dorsal column stimulation techniques are based on the Melzack–Wall gate theory (Melzack and Wall, 1965). In general, the application of a non-painful stimulus inhibits the firing of neurons in the pain pathways, as is naturally done when one rubs a painful area to make it feel better.

Transcutaneous stimulation may be useful as an initial screening procedure or as a treatment in itself. It is simple and noninvasive, and may afford a gratifying amount of long-term relief to 12.5 per cent (Loeser et al., 1975) to 50 per cent (Long, 1974; Shealy, 1974; Long, 1975) of patients with pain secondary to peripheral nerve injury.

The selection of the optimal site of application of the transcutaneous electrodes varies between patients (Burton and Maurer, 1974; Loeser, 1975). The patient should be instructed by one familiar with the use of the apparatus, since anxiety about the stimulator may override potential benefit. The initial site of electrode placement might be over the nerve just proximal to the site of injury so that sensation is projected into the distribution of the nerve (Wall and Sweet, 1967; Campbell and Taub, 1973). This may or may not project a sensation into the distribution of the nerve, but pain relief can occur in either circumstance. If that is not successful, stimulation might be tried with one electrode above and one below the site of the peripheral nerve injury, in effect stimulating across the injury. The next step would be to apply the electrodes adjacent to and then within the area of pain. Causalgia pain appears to respond particularly well to transcutaneous stimulation (Meyer and Fields, 1972; Sternschein et al., 1975), at least initially (Loeser et al., 1975).

Those patients who may obtain some but not sufficient relief might be evaluated for the implantation of a peripheral nerve stimulator. Transcutaneous stimulation helps screen patients for implanted stimulators in that it allows one to assess the patient's tolerance to electronic stimulating devices and to exclude those patients whose tolerance to the use of electronic apparatus would contraindicate the use of an implanted system.

Patients who are candidates for peripheral nerve stimulation can be further evaluated by the use of a percutaneous stimulating electrode (Long, 1973; Erickson, 1975). The commercial electrodes used for percutaneous dorsal column stimulation can be employed. A needle is inserted parallel to the nerve proximal to the site of injury, care being taken not to traumatize the nerve. The electrode is inserted through the needle, which is then withdrawn. A stimulus is applied at a frequency between 30 and 120 Hz at a pulse width of 0.1 to 0.2 milliseconds (Sweet and Wepsic, 1969). Sufficient voltage is employed so that the sensation is discernible but not painful. Ideally, the sensation is projected to the cutaneous distribution of the nerve, but this is not essential for pain relief.

If the patient responds to the percutaneous trial of peripheral nerve stimulation, a permanent peripheral nerve stimulator may be surgically implanted, if there is a normal proximal portion which can be isolated. In upper extremity injuries, it can be applied to the entire brachial plexus if necessary. The implanted portion consists of an electrode pair embedded in a silastic leaf which can be wrapped around the nerve. Leads are tunneled subcutaneously to a radio receiver which is implanted at a convenient location, usually just below the clavicle for the upper extremity or just above the belt line for the lower extremity. The implanted portion is passive with no power supply of its own, so that it is not necessary to replace batteries surgically. The power is conveyed through a radio frequency signal from a small radio transmitter (slightly larger than a pack of cigarettes and operated by standard 9-volt batteries), which the patient can wear clipped to his clothing. The signal is conveyed through an antenna taped over the radio receiver. The patient can control the transmitter so that pulse rate, pulse width, or voltage can be varied independently.

It should be noted that successful pain relief after a nerve block is not a reliable indicator for pain relief by stimulation. Although in one study 90 per cent of patients with pain of peripheral nerve origin obtained relief by a nerve block, only 25 per cent of those patients obtained long-term relief by use of a peripheral nerve stimulator (Sweet, 1976). Other series report up to 80 per cent of patients with peripheral nerve injury who received significant pain relief (Long, 1973; Long and Hagfors, 1975; Campbell and Long, 1976). As with any other treatment, the success rate with peripheral nerve stimulation diminishes with time (Sweet and Wepsic, 1973; Nielson et al., 1976; Picaza et al., 1977/78.

If peripheral nerve stimulation is not successful, or if multiple nerves or nerve roots are involved so that peripheral nerve stimulation is not feasible, dorsal column stimulation may be employed. The theory behind stimulation of the dorsal spinal cord for the treatment of pain is the gate theory of Melzac and Wall (1965). When large fibers, those ordinarily conveying touch and proprioception, are stimulated, they compete with the small neurons within the nervous system which respond to pain. Whether or not pain is perceived depends on the balance between large and small fiber firing. The large axons are stimulated at a lower threshold than the small, so it is possible to adjust the voltage according to the sensation the patient perceives. When a non-painful tingling or vibration sensation is felt, the large fibers are being stimulated preferentially. This tips the balance to close the gate, inhibiting the transmission of pain impulses.

The dorsal columns of the spinal cord consist almost exclusively of large fibers concerned with proprioception and touch. When the dorsal columns are stimulated, the impulse travels both up and down the spinal cord. The descending impulse causes the collateral large fibers at the spinal segments concerned with the patient's pain to fire, so that at multiple spinal levels the balance is tipped in favor of the large fibers, and the pain is inhibited (Shealy et al., 1967, 1970). Although this theory is not above criticism, it has provided a useful concept for the development of stimulation techniques as means of alleviating intractable pain.

Dorsal cord stimulation can be evaluated non-surgically with percutaneous electrodes similar to those used for percutaneous peripheral nerve stimulation (Hosobuchi et al., 1972). A flexible wire electrode is inserted through a needle either into the subarachnoid space through a lateral approach at the C2 level or into the epidural space at least several levels above the nerve roots conveying the pain sensation. The presently preferred procedure is to employ two epidural electrodes in the midline one or more levels apart. The percutaneous electrodes are connected to a stimulator so that stimulation identical to that in dorsal column stimulation can be applied to the spinal cord. Over a several day trial period, the electrodes can be repositioned until the optimal localization has been determined.

If the patient obtains satisfactory relief from the percutaneous dorsal column stimulating electrodes, they can be converted into a permanent system by connection through subcutaneous leads to an implanted radio receiver identical to the one described for peripheral nerve stimulation (Hoppenstein, 1975; North et al., 1977/78). However, some neurosurgeons prefer to implant permanent stimulating electrodes surgically. A laminectomy is performed and the electrodes are sutured to the outside of the dura, in the subdural space, or in a pocket made at the time of surgery within the layers of the dura (Sweet and Wepsic, 1974; Long and Erickson, 1975; Burton, 1976).

Up to 57 per cent of patients with pain of peripheral nerve origin of all types have responded satisfactorily to dorsal column stimulation (Sweet and Wepsic, 1974), as have 80 per cent of patients with phantom limb pain (Hosobuchi et al., 1972; Miles et al., 1974). It has been particularly helpful in the management of phantom limb pain (Miles et al., 1974; Nielson et al., 1975). One problem with the use of this procedure in benign conditions is that with time the stimulation may become less effective, possibly due to the formation of fibrous tissue around the electrode (Pineda, 1975).

Although deep brain stimulation is still in an investigational state, it represents an encouraging and efficient means of nondestructive pain relief. Stimulation of the periventricular area or upper periaqueductal gray area can produce alleviation of chronic pain (Richardson and Akil, 1977a, 1977b; Adams, 1977/78) or analgesia (Liebeskind et al., 1974; Mayer and Liebeskind, 1974; Liebeskind, 1976) over large areas of the body. This procedure is ordinarily reserved for pain which is disabling enough to justify a central procedure, which may be of a distribution so that other stimulation procedures are not appropriate (as in upper extremity pain), or which may not have responded to other non-ablative treatments. A multicontact electrode is stereotactically inserted to the target point described above, usually unilaterally. A trial period of several days involves stimulating through wires protruding through the scalp. If a satisfactory stimulation is found, the device can be internalized, that is, connected via a subcutaneous lead to an implanted radio receiver. Again, the patient controls the stimulus himself, turning it on and adjusting the voltage to suit the requirements for alleviation of pain. Three of the first five patients reported to obtain relief from this type of stimulation had pain secondary to injury of peripheral nerves (Richardson and Akil, 1977a, 1977b).

It is only after stimulation procedures have been found unsuccessful that ablative procedures might be considered.

As with stimulation procedures, one considers the most peripheral procedure first. If there is no chance that the peripheral nerve will ever function normally, as after amputation, section of the peripheral nerve proximal to the site of injury may be sufficient for pain relief.

Although the classical three neuron chain pain pathway has proven to be an inadequate physiological concept, it has been the basis for most ablative procedures. A small, usually unmyelinated peripheral nerve synapses with a second order neuron, which decussates within one or two segments and ascends in the contralateral lateral spinothalamic tract to end in the ventral posterolateral nucleus of the thalamus. The third order neuron which originates in that structure carries the information to the cortex. Interrupting this classical pathway anywhere along its course below the thalamus can interrupt pain perception in selected areas of the body. Interruption of the peripheral nerve, with a resultant loss of motor function and all types of sensation, includes such procedures as neurectomy, either surgical or chemical, or resection of the proximal portion of a divided nerve, usually to isolate a traumatized peripheral nerve or a peripheral neuroma. Section of the second order neuron within the anterolateral quadrant of the spinal cord or brain stem results in a loss specifically of pain perception, but not a loss of other modalities or motor function. Interruption of the third order neurons between the thalamus and the cortex results in a loss of appreciation of the characteristics of the specific pain but generally not good pain relief, and is for the most part no longer in use. Interruption of the limbic system, as in centrum medianum lesions, results in loss of the distress of chronic pain but not in actual loss of pain perception.

If peripheral nerve section is not feasible, either because of the anatomical location or to preserve motor function, one might consider rhizotomy, sectioning of selected dorsal roots, which causes a loss of all sensory modalities but preserves motor function. Each peripheral nerve is the product of more than one nerve root, so that it is necessary to section multiple dorsal roots in order to denervate a single peripheral nerve. Particularly in the extremities, the patient may have an insensitive area which may be subject to trauma. It is extremely important that an entire extremity not be completely denervated, since the loss of proprioception will result in a flail extremity entirely out of control of the individual. Usually, such an extremity becomes not only useless but also dangerous to the patient and must later be amputated.

These factors limit the usefulness of dorsal rhizotomy in treatment of pain secondary to nerve trauma. Nevertheless, occasionally a dorsal rhizotomy is a help in managing patients with pain that persists following peripheral neurectomy. The procedure involves a multilevel laminectomy with exposure of the spinal cord and nerve roots at the appropriate levels. It is advisable to verify the level either roentgenographically or by stimulation of the motor roots. Radicular arteries should be separated from the nerve root and spared to avoid ischemia to the spinal cord. Prior to section, the dorsal roots are crushed or clipped to prevent oozing from small accompanying vessels. Regeneration does not occur.

Anterolateral cordotomy was first described by Spiller and Martin in 1912, and the basic precepts have not changed significantly. Since the lateral spinothalamic tract which is interrupted by this procedure carries only pain and temperature sensations, other sensory modalities are left intact. Also, since motor fibers run more dorsally in the spinal cord, it is possible to obtain analgesia over large portions of the body with no motor deficit.

Unfortunately, it is quite common for pain of peripheral origin to recur weeks or months after an anterolateral cordotomy; this is in part due to the redundancy of the pain pathways. A diffuse multisynaptic pathway surrounding the central gray of the spinal cord transmits vaguely defined pain associated with chronic aching or burning dysesthesia which is not interrupted by cordotomy. Nevertheless, cordotomy can be beneficial in selected patients, particularly those whose pain is due to malignancy, even if the pain is caused by metastatic involvement of the peripheral nerves (Joyner et al., 1966; Gildenberg, 1974).

As classically performed, cordotomy involves a laminectomy and incision of the anterolateral quadrant of the spinal cord under direct vision. This has particular disadvantages in that it is necessary to perform a surgical procedure under general anesthesia. There is considerable variability of the distribution of the pain fibers within the anterolateral quadrant of the spinal cord, so that it is necessary to denervate a large portion of the body in order to ensure pain relief. When the spinal cord is rotated under direct vision to gain access to the antero-lateral quadrant, there may be some distortion of the internal anatomy, further compromising the effectiveness of the procedure.

However, many of these problems have been overcome by the development of percutaneous cervical cordotomy. A fine wire electrode is inserted into the anterolateral quadrant of the spinal cord under x-ray guidance, and the pain fibers are interrupted by a radiofrequency current. As originally described (Mullan et al., 1965; Rosomoff et al., 1965; Crue et al., 1968), a spinal puncture needle is introduced laterally at the C2 level. A thin wire electrode is passed through the needle to lie in the pain fibers in the anterolateral quadrant of the cord. Since this can be done under local anesthesia, the patient is awake and able to respond to the effects of stimulation to further localize the tip of the needle. The lesion is made by applying short bursts of radiofrequency current. The development of analgesia can be tested between each short burst and the lesion tailored to the needs of the individual patient.

A further refinement of this technique was evolved to avoid interruption of the fibers at the upper cervical levels of the spinal cord concerned with respira-tion (Rosomoff et al., 1969). The needle electrode is introduced diagonally through an intervertebral disc in the lower cervical spine. The tip enters the anterolateral quadrant of the spinal cord, and a lesion is made with a radio-frequency current, similar to the C2 technique (Lin et al., 1966; Gildenberg et al., 1968, 1969, 1971, 1974).

Relief of pain of benign origin may not be permanent with either surgical or percutaneous cervical cordotomy. To further limit the usefulness of cordotomy, one must consider that in pain of peripheral nerve origin the extremity supplied by the pathologic nerve may have motor impairment. Since the cordotomy lesion is made on the side contralateral to the pain, the most worrisome complication because the pain fibers decussate, is temporary or permanent weakness or paralysis of the good extremity. At the end of three years only about one third of patients thus treated remain pain free (Gildenberg, 1974).

In cases of pain of peripheral nerve origin where profound painful disabili-ty might warrant, some ablative procedures involve interrupting pathways within the brain itself, ordinarily by stereotactic surgery. The patient's head is supported in an apparatus which contains an electrode-carrying device to aim the electrode accurately to a specific target point within the brain. X-rays are taken, using contrast material within the ventricular system, and calculations are made to guide the electrode to the target at a precisely given location in relation to the visualized ventricular system. The procedure is usually done with the patient awake, so that physiologic recordings or response to stimulation can further verify the accuracy of electrode placement (Spiegel and Wycis, 1962).

There are several targets associated with the alleviation of pain. The original target involved the pain pathway of the lateral spinothalamic tract as it ascends through the mesencephalon (Nashold et al., 1969). Interruption of this pathway alone can provide analgesia or relief from chronic pain or analgesia to a large area of the contralateral body. By extending the lesion slightly more medially, it is sometimes possible to interrupt also the connections to the limbic system to alleviate some of the emotional distress associated with chronic pain. Because the procedure may lead to difficulty in control of extraocular movements, the lesion is commonly placed somewhat higher as the spinothalamic fibers enter the thalamus (Hawkinson et al., 1969; Spiegel et al., 1964, 1966; Albe-Fessard et al., 1970). Rather than concentrating on the spinothalamic pathway itself, however, which would cause analgesia to the contralateral body, the lesion may be made more medially in the intralaminar area of the thalamus (Spiegel et al., 1964, 1966). The lesion can be further extended medially into the dorsomedian nucleus, which is directly concerned with the emotional response to chronic pain. Other neurosurgeons make the lesion primarily in the centrum median-um, which is part of the limbic system (Watkins, 1966; Foltz and White, 1968). By affecting only the emotional response to chronic pain, it is often possible to alleviate the pain and especially the suffering without the loss of pain sensation. This procedure is generally reserved for pain that originates from malignancy.

One peripheral nerve condition that produces chronic pain which defies usual treatments is that of post-herpetic neuralgia. This viral disease attacks the dorsal root ganglion, so that interruption of the nerve distal to the ganglion is completely ineffective. However, once the pain has become established, even cordotomy proximal to the ganglion may not alleviate the pain. Approximately 50 per cent of patients with such pain respond to transcutaneous stimulation (Long, 1974, 1975; Shealy, 1974). Because the area of involvement is very often hypersensitive, the electrodes may be placed immediately adjacent to the painful area.

For those patients who are extremely disabled from post-herpetic neuralgia and who do not respond to transcutaneous stimulation, a procedure has been reported recently which may offer hope for this as well as other types of intractable pain involving wide areas of the body or extremities. Central myelo-tomy involves the stereotactic insertion of an electrode into the central area of the spinal cord where it meets the medulla. The precise pathway that is interrupted has not been verified anatomically, but it appears to be the multisynaptic pathway which ascends along the medial brain stem to the thalamus and limbic areas. Although this procedure is still in the investigational stages, it has proven to be effective in some types of pain which defy other treatment (Hitchcock, 1970; Schvarcz, 1976, 1978).

The pain of peripheral neuritis does not generally respond well to central ablative procedures. Chronic stimulation of the brain at or just below the thalamus has been effective in several cases, but its role in the treatment of such pain has yet to be determined.

Amputation stump pain is generally better treated with peripheral procedures, but phantom limb pain does not always respond to such treatment. Again, although it is still investigational, chronic electrical stimulation of the internal capsule has been of help in several patients with such pain (Adams, J. E., 1977/78).

In summary, there is presently only a modest role for the use of central procedures in the treatment of pain of peripheral nerve origin, with the exception of pain secondary to malignancy. However, some of the newer investigational procedures may prove to be of benefit in several types of pain which defy treatment by any other means.

REFERENCES

Adams, J. E.: Techniques and technical problems associated with implantation of neuroaugmentive devices. Appl. Neurophysiol. 40:111, 1977/78.

Albe-Fessard, D., Dondey, M., Nicolaidis, S., and LeBeau, J.: Remarks concerning the effect of diencephalic lesions on pain and sensitivity with special references to lemniscally mediated control of noxious afferences. Confin. Neurol. 32:174, 1970.

Burton, C.: Dorsal column stimulation: Optimization of application. Surg. Neurol. 4:171, 1976.

Burton, C., and Maurer, D. D.: Pain suppression by transcutaneous electronic stimulation. IEEE Trans. Biomed. Engineer., 21:81, 1974.

Campbell, J. N., and Long, D. M.: Peripheral nerve stimulation in the treatment of intractable pain. J. Neurosurg. 45:692, 1976.

Campbell, J. N., and Taub, A.: Local analgesia from percutaneous electrical stimulation. Arch. Neurol. 28:347, 1973.

Crue, B. L., Todd, E. M., and Carregal, E. J.: Posterior approach for high cervical percutaneous radiofrequency cordotomy. Confin. Neurol. 30:41, 1968.

DeVaul, R. A., Zisook, S., and Lorimer, R.: Patients with chronic pain. Med. J. St. Joseph Hosp. Houston 12:59, 1977a.

DeVaul, R. A., Zosook, S., and Stuart, J. H.: Patients with psychogenic pain. J. Fam. Pract. 4:53, 1977b.

Engel, G. L.: Psychogenic pain and the pain-prone patient. Am. J. Med. 26:899, 1959.

Erickson, D. L.: Percutaneous trial of stimulation for patient selection for implantable stimulating devices. J. Neurosurg. 43:440, 1975.

Foltz, E. L., and White, L. E., Jr.: The role of rostral cingulumotomy in "pain" relief. Int. J. Neurol. 6:353, 1968.

Fordyce, W. E.: Pain views as learned behavior. In Bonica, J. J.: Pain: Advances in Neurology. New York, Raven Press, 1974.

Gildenberg, P. L.: Angle-meter to indicate the proper angle of insertion in anterior percutaneous cervical cordotomy. Technical note. J. Neurosurg. 34:244, 1971.

Gildenberg, P. L.: Percutaneous cervical cordotomy. Clin. Neurosurg. 21:246, 1974.

Gildenberg, P. L., and DeVaul, R. A.: Management of chronic pain refractory to specific therapy. In Youmans, J. R.: Neurological Surgery 2nd ed., Philadelphia, W. B. Saunders Company, 1978.

Gildenberg, P. L., Lin, P. M., Polakoff, P. P. II, and Flitter, M. A.: Anterior percutaneous cervical cordotomy: Determination of target point and calculation of angle of insertion. Technical note. J. Neurosurg. 28:173, 1968.

Gildenberg, P. L., Zanes, C., Flitter, M., Lin, P. M., Lautsch, E. V., and Truex, R. C.: Impedance measuring device for detection of penetration of the spinal cord in anterior percutaneous cervical cordotomy. Technical note. J. Neurosurg. 30:87, 1969.

Hankinson, J., Pearce, G. W., and Rowbotham, G. F.: Stereotaxic operations for the relief of pain. J. Neurol Neurosurg. Psychiatry 23:352, 1960.

Hitchcock, E. R.: Stereotactic cervical myelotomy. J. Neurol. Neurosurg. Psychiatry 33:224, 1970.

Hoppenstein, R.: Percutaneous implantation of chronic spinal cord electrodes for control of intractable pain. Preliminary report. Neurology 4:195, 1975.

Hosobuchi, Y., Adams, J. E., and Weinstein, P. R.: Preliminary percutaneous dorsal column stimulation prior to permanent implantation. Technical note. J. Neurosurg 37:242, 1972.

Joyner, J., Merley, J., Jr., and Freesman, L. W.: Cordotomy for intractable pain of nonmalignant origin. Review of twenty cases. Arch. Surg. 93:480, 1966.

Liebeskind, J. C.: Pain modulation by central nervous system stimulation. *In* Bonica, J. J. and Albe-Fessard, D.: Advances in Pain Research and Therapy. New York, Raven Press, 1976, Vol. 1.

Liebeskind, J. C., Mayer, D. J., and Akil, H.: Central mechanisms of pain inhibition: Studies of analgesia from focal brain stimulation. *In* Bonica, J. J.: Pain: Advances in Neurology. New York, Raven Press, 1974, Vol. 4.

Lin, P. M., Gildenberg, P. L., and Polakoff, P. P.: An anterior approach to percutaneous lower cervical cordotomy. J. Neurosurg. *25*:553, 1966.

Loeser, J. D., Black, R. G., and Christman, A.: Relief of pain by transcutaneous stimulation. J. Neurosurg. *42*:308, 1975.

Long, D. M.: Electrical stimulation for relief of pain of chronic nerve injury. J. Neurosurg. *39*:718, 1973.

Long, D. M.: Cutaneous afferent stimulation for relief of chronic pain. Clin. Neurosurg. *21*:257, 1974.

Long, D. M., and Erickson, D. E.: Stimulation of the posterior columns of the spinal cord for relief of intractable pain. Surg. Neurol. *4*:134, 1975.

Long, D. M., and Hagfors, H.: Electrical stimulation in the nervous system: The current status of electrical simulation of the nervous system for relief of pain. Pain, *1*:109, 1975.

Mayer, D. J., and Liebeskind, J. C.: Pain reduction by focal electrical stimulation of the brain: An anatomical and behavioral analysis. Brain. Res. *68*:73, 1974.

Melzack, R., and Wall, P. D.: Pain mechanisms: A new theory. Science *150*:971, 1965.

Meyer, G. A., and Fields, H. L.: Causalgia treated by selective large fibre stimulation of peripheral nerve. Brain *95*:163, 1972.

Miles, J., Lipton, S., Hayward, N., Bowsher, D., Mumford, J., and Molony, V.: Pain relief by implanted electrical simulators. Lancet *1*:777, 1974.

Mullan, S.: New techniques in neurosurgery. Postgrad. Med. *37*:636, 1965.

Nashold, B. S. Jr., Wilson, W. P., and Slaughter, D. G.: Stereotactic midbrain lesions for central dysesthesia and phantom pain. J. Neurosurg. *30*:116, 1969.

Nielson, K. D., Adams, J. E., and Hosobuchi, Y.: Phantom limb pain. Treatment with dorsal column stimulation. J. Neurosurg. *42*:301, 1975.

Nielson, K. D., Watts, C., and Clark, W. K.: Peripheral nerve injury from implantation of chronic stimulating electrodes for pain control. Surg. Neurol. 5:51, 1976.

North, R. B., Fischell, T. A., and Long, D. M.: Chronic dorsal column stimulation via percutaneously inserted epidural electrodes: Preliminary results in 31 patients. Appl. Neurophysiol. *40*:184, 1977/78.

Picaza, J. A., Hunter, S. E., and Cannon, B. W.: Pain suppression by peripheral nerve stimulation: Chronic effects of implanted devices. Appl. Neurophysiol. *40*:223, 1977/78.

Pineda, A.: Dorsal column stimulation and its prospects. Surg. Neurol. *4*:157, 1975.

Richardson, D. E., and Akil, H.: Pain reduction by electrical brain stimulation in man. Part 1: Acute administration in periaqueductal and periventricular sites. J. Neurosurg. *47*:178, 1977*a*.

Richardson, D. E., and Akil, H.: Pain reduction by electrical brain simulation in man: Part 2: Chronic self-administration in the periventricular grey matter. J. Neurosurg. *47*:184, 1977*b*.

Rosomoff, H. L., Brown, C. J., and Sheptak, P.: Percutaneous radiofrequency cervical cordotomy: Technique. J. Neurosurg. *23*:639, 1965.

Rosomoff, H. L., Kriger, A. J., and Kupman, A. S.: Effects of percutaneous cervical cordotomy on pulmonary function. J. Neurosurg. *31*:620, 1969.

Schvarcz, J. R.: Stereotactic extralemniscal myelotomy. J. Neurol. Neurosurg. Psychiatry *39*:33, 1976.

Schvarcz, J. R.: Spinal and stereotactic techniques re trigeminal nucleotomy and extralemniscal myelotomy. Appl. Neurophysiol. *41*:99, 1978.

Shealy, C. N.: Transcutaneous electrical stimulation for control of pain. Clin. Neurosurg. *21*:269, 1974.

Shealy, C. N., Mortimer, J. T. and Hagfors, N. R.: Dorsal column electroanalgesia. J. Neurosurg. *32*:560, 1970.

Shealy, C. N., Mortimer, J. T. and Reswick, J. B.: Electrical inhibition of pain by dorsal column stimulation: Preliminary clinical report. Anesth. Analg., *46*:489, 1967.

Spiegel, E. A., and Wycis, H. T.: Stereoencephalotomy. Part II. Clinical and Physiological Applications. New York, Grune and Stratton, 1962.

Spiegel, E. A., Wycis, H. T., Szekely, E. G., and Gildenberg, P. L.: Medial and dorsal thalamotomy in so-called intractable pain. *In* Knighton, R. S. and Dumke, P. R.: Pain. Boston, Little Brown and Company, 1966.

Spiegel, E. A., Wycis, H. T., Szekely, E. G., Gildenberg, P. L., and Zanes, C.: Combined dorsomedial, intralaminar and dorsal thalamotomy for the relief of so-called intractable pain. J. Int. Coll. Surg. *42*:160, 1964.

Spiller, W. G., and Martin, E.: The treatment of persistent pain of organic origin in the lower part of the body by division of the anterolateral column of the spinal cord. J.A.M.A. 58:1489, 1912.

Sternschein, M. J., Myers, S. J., Frewin, D. B., and Downey, J. A.: Causalgia. Arch. Phys. Med. Rehabil. 56:58, 1975.

Sweet, W. H.: Control of pain by direct electrical stimulation of peripheral nerves. Clin. Neurosurg. 23:103, 1976.

Sweet, W. H., and Wepsic, J. G.: Control of pain by focal electrical stimulation for suppression. Ariz. Med. 26:1042, 1969.

Sweet, W. H., and Wepsic, J. G.: Electrical stimulation for suppression of pain in man. *In* Fields, W. S.: Neural Organization and Its Relevance to Prosthetics. New York, Intercontinental Medical Book Corp., 1973.

Sweet, W. H., and Wepsic, J. G.: Stimulation of the posterior columns of the spinal cord for pain control: Indications, techniques and results. Clin. Neurosurg. 21:278, 1974.

Wall, P. D., and Sweet, W. H.: Temporary abolition of pain in man on stimulation of large diameter cutaneous afferent fibers. Science 155:108, 1967.

Watkins, E. S.: Stereotaxic thalamotomy for intractable pain. Presented at the meeting of The Harvey Cushing Society, April 19, 1966.

Anatomical
Exposures

III

19

SURGICAL EXPOSURE OF PERIPHERAL NERVES

ALLAN E. INGLIS

Surgical anatomy is a science of locational percentages. In the beginning the student or physician learns the name, position and function of all the various anatomical parts; and with some gratitude he learns that the *name* and *function* of the parts remain consistent. However, it is with some chagrin that he notes that the *positions* of the parts may vary from specimen to specimen. It is this variation that stimulates the surgeon to carefully plan his incision for exposure to cover the various anatomical variations. One of my early surgical teachers advised, "If you don't know the anatomy cold you do not have the right to operate." The well worn anatomical texts and atlases in the dressing rooms outside operating rooms attest to the surgeon's respect for this fundamental concept. The surgical exposure should always embody what Dr. Ernest Lampy called the first rule for incisions: "Place the incision directly over the pathology." This statement seems obvious; however, all too often the surgeon will find himself tunneling beneath muscles or working beneath the flaps of a "lazy S" incision rather than directly over the area in question. These curving incisions over the antecubital fossa or in the popliteal fossa provide less than satisfactory exposures for the radial and peroneal nerves. A straight longitudinal incision over these nerves, which can later be closed with a "Z-plasty" at the joint crease, will allow both excellent exposure of the nerves and good healing without contracture. Whenever possible in peripheral nerve surgery a tourniquet should be employed. This will permit rapid accurate exposure of the anatomical parts with maximum safety during the exposure. The tourniquet can be released when desirable after the development of the anatomical field. The tourniquet also provides an excellent margin for safety during the location of the anatomical parts, particularly in areas where variations in the anatomical parts and locations are high.

EXPOSURE OF THE BRACHIAL PLEXUS

There are two considerations involved in exposure of the brachial plexus: does the plexus require exposure above the clavicle or is the plexus to be explored only below the clavicle. In exposure of the plexus below the clavicle it is necessary to carry the incision from the mid-axilla to an area 5 cm or more above the clavicle. The pectoralis major muscle is divided not at its insertion into the humerus but directly over the brachial plexus. This is usually 5 cm from its insertion into the humerus. As the pectoralis major muscle is divided the clavipectoral fascia will be identified. The dissection is then continued medial to the coracobrachialis and short head of the biceps muscles. The axillary vein, axillary artery, and cords of the brachial plexus will be easily identified. The arterial branches of the thoracoacromial axis will be noted and can be ligated as necessary. The pectoralis minor muscle can be released from the coracoid process, providing further exposure. If the dissection is continued above the clavicle, then the clavicle is incised along with the subclavius muscle. Meticulous

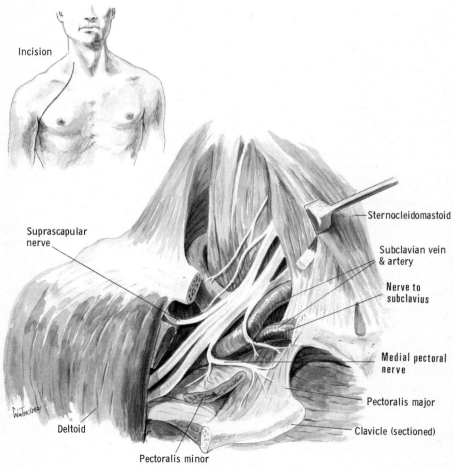

Figure 19–1   Brachial plexus exposed with the clavicle sectioned.

attention must be given to ligation of the various branches of the axillary artery and vein as well as the subclavian artery and vein, as they block exposure. Osteotomy of the clavicle usually facilitates exposure of the lower trunk portions of the plexus. Osteotomy of the coracoid process following release of the pectoralis minor muscle will allow lateral retraction of the coracobrachialis and the short head of the biceps brachii muscle. At closure the clavicle is realigned and stabilized with a threaded Steinman pin, and the pectoralis minor muscle is replaced to the coracoid process. If the coracoid process has been osteotomized, it may be replaced with a small screw or wire suture. If the reattached coracoid is very secure, the pectoralis minor can be sutured to the fragment; however, it can be left unattached. The pectoralis major muscle is easily repaired with multiple epimysial sutures, and the arm is then maintained in internal rotation. Shoulder motion is initiated in about 10 days.

Exposure of the brachial plexus above the clavicle is accomplished through an incision along the posterior border of the sternocleidomastoid muscle. The incision begins just below the mastoid process and stops at mid-clavicle. If need be, preparation should be made to extend the incision distally, as previously described. The platysma is opened, exposing the external jugular vein. The vein should be ligated and removed for clear exposure. The dissection is continued posteriorly until the scalene anterior muscle is observed. The phrenic nerve is identified and traced cephalad to the C4 root. The trunks and roots can then be exposed as needed. The suprascapular nerve will be seen arising from the junction of the C5 and C6 roots or a short distance down the upper trunk. The roots of the plexus can be traced back through the scalene anterior muscle to the transverse processes of the cervical vertebrae. Extreme care should be taken in this area to avoid injury to the vertebral artery. Exposure of the lower roots below C6 is difficult without osteotomy of the clavicle; however, the trunks can be exposed for decompression if necessary (Fig. 19–1).

The Musculocutaneous Nerve

The musculocutaneous nerve is exposed through an incision beginning halfway between the coracoid process and the base of the concavity in the axillary fold. The incision is carried from this point across the anterior axillary fold into the axilla and when necessary down the inner aspect of the arm along the coracobrachialis muscle. The deltopectoral groove is then located by noting the cephalic vein. These two muscles are then separated and retracted. As they are retracted a fascial sheath will be observed covering the floor of the deep portion of the wound. This is the clavipectoral fascia. The clavipectoral fascia lying along the medial border of the coracobrachialis muscle is carefully exposed. An incision is then made in this fascia, exposing the coracobrachialis muscle. The musculocutaneous nerve has a highly variable penetration of the coracobrachialis muscle. It may penetrate the muscle very high or in multiple branches or quite low. Therefore, the inner border of the coracobrachialis muscle is carefully exposed and then incised longitudinally to identify the branches of the musculocutaneous nerve. Alternatively, the musculocutaneous nerve may be located by retracting the coracobrachialis muscle laterally, incising the clavipectoral fascia, and locating the lateral cord of the brachial plexus. The

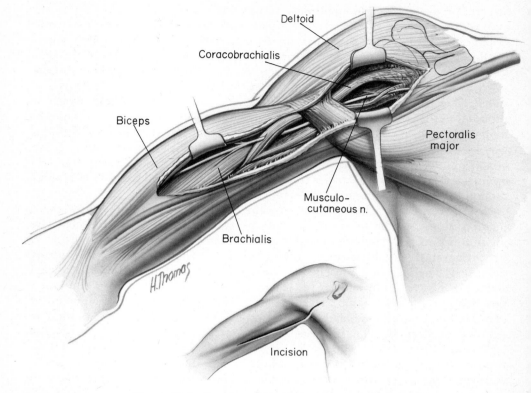

Figure 19–2 Exposure of the musculocutaneous nerve.

musculocutaneous nerve will be observed leaving the lateral cord and entering the coracobrachialis muscle and traced distally within the muscle. As these branches are identified they may be traced distally in the substance of the muscle and, as they leave the muscle, entering the mid-portion of the arm between the coracobrachialis muscle and the biceps brachii. The coracobrachialis muscle may be incised with impunity to provide the necessary exposure of the nerve. When the nerve has been identified in or entering the muscle, it can be traced proximally toward the lateral cord of the brachial plexus (Fig. 19–2).

The Axillary Nerve

The axillary nerve is best exposed posteriorly through the quadrilateral space. Normally the axillary nerve is quite large and remains as a single major nerve as it passes around the neck of the humerus within the substance of the deltoid muscle. It is slow to arborize, having many small branches passing from the major trunk of this peripheral nerve. Exposure of the axillary nerve is difficult unless the posterior aspect of the deltoid muscle is elevated from the spine of the scapula as far as the acromion process or unless the deltoid muscle is partially divided. Incision, therefore, is along the spine of the scapula, passing through the middle of the concavity of the posterior axillary fold into the axilla.

As the deltoid muscle is retracted laterally and superiorly, the infraspinous fascia will be observed. This fascia must be incised to allow exposure of the upper border of the teres major muscle. As the infraspinous fascia is elevated the nerve can be observed exiting through the quadrilateral space and entering the deltoid muscle. If further exposure of the axillary nerve is required, the teres major and latissimus dorsi muscles must be carefully dissected free and incised. These muscles can be readily reapproximated if they are exposed carefully before they are released. The arm can then be abducted more fully, giving complete exposure of the nerve as it passes close by the capsule of the shoulder toward the posterior cord of the brachial plexus. In addition to this posterior approach to the axillary nerve, it is additionally necessary to expose the nerve anteriorly. This is accomplished through the deltopectoral groove. The clavipectoral fascia is exposed deep between these separated muscles. The coracobrachialis and short head of the biceps brachii are identified, the clavipectoral fascia incised medially,

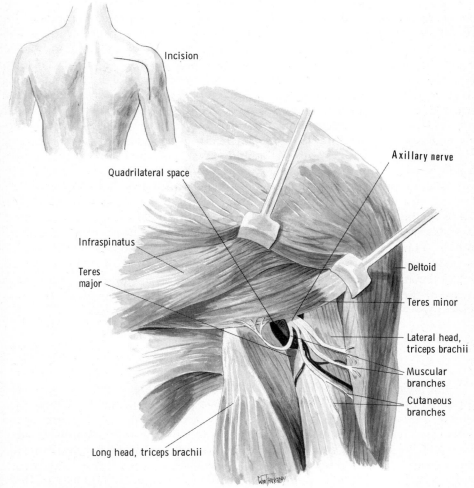

Figure 19–3 Exposure of the axillary nerve in the posterior aspect of the shoulder.

and these muscles retracted laterally. This will expose the axillary artery and vein, and the cords of the brachial plexus, the artery, and the vein can be carefully retracted medially, exposing the posterior cord of the brachial plexus. The posterior humeral artery and vein along with the axillary nerve can be exposed as they descend to pass deep around the neck of the humerus. The nerve can then be freed up for grafting or decompression as needed. The latissimus dorsi and teres major muscles must be carefully closed during closure of the wound (Fig. 19–3).

UPPER EXTREMITY

The Radial Nerve in the Arm

The nerve is best identified in the proximal half of the humerus by locating the nerve as it passes through the lateral intermuscular septum. At this level the lateral intermuscular septum is incised, providing wider exposure of the triceps muscle. The radial nerve is then seen passing between the medial and lateral heads of the triceps muscle covered by the long head of the triceps muscle. Accompanying the nerve will be the profunda brachii and its accompanying veins. If further exposure is required, the long head of the triceps muscle can be released and subsequently sutured. The radial nerve in the distal half of the arm is best identified through an anterolateral exposure, with the dissection proceeding between the brachioradialis and brachialis muscles. The nerve will lie deep between these structures with the accompanying terminal portion of the profunda brachial artery and its vena comitans. These veins can be rather large. Further exposure of the radial nerve as it passes toward the elbow is accomplished with an incision along the border of the brachioradialis muscle. The nerve can be observed in its relationship to the brachialis muscle and distally as the posterior interosseous nerve passes between the two heads of the supinator muscle. The nerve lies quite deeply in the cubital fossa, and a generous incision must be employed for good visualization. This is particularly true in a well-muscled patient. This wound should be closed with a Z-plasty in the flexion crease of the elbow, thereby preventing contracture of the skin and subcutaneous tissues (Fig. 19–4).

The Median and Ulnar Nerves in the Arm

The median nerve in the arm is best seen through a medial incision just anterior to the intramuscular septum and just posterior to the coracobrachialis muscle. The nerve is identified along with its accompanying brachial artery and veins. The nerve will lie medial to the biceps brachii and on the medial edge of the brachialis muscle. The median and ulnar nerves in the arm have no branches and are easily mobilized for repair. The ulnar nerve is exposed through a medial incision in the arm. The upper end of the incision should be parallel and above the intramuscular septum and just beneath the coracobrachialis muscle. The nerve will accompany the brachial artery and vein as far as the middle of the

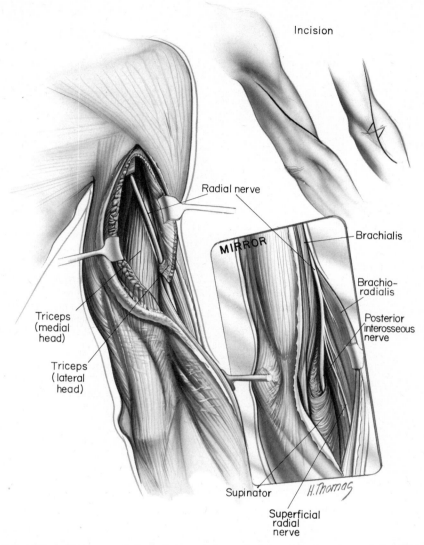

Figure 19-4 Exposure of the radial nerve through the arm. In the mirror, the radial nerve is seen passing anteriorly in the distal humerus; in the proximal forearm the posterior interosseous nerve penetrates the supinator.

arm (Fig. 19-5). A distal exposure of the ulnar nerve in the arm requires an incision in the intramuscular septum as the nerve passes through the intramuscular septum in the mid-arm. The ulnar nerve will then be noted beneath and within the epimysium of the triceps muscle. The ulnar collateral artery will join and accompany the nerve distally in the arm. More distally the ulnar nerve usually lies in the groove for the ulnar nerve in the humerus. Occasionally it has been displaced out of the groove by the triceps muscle or by the cutaneous ligament. It then penetrates the two heads of the flexor carpi ulnaris and passes into the forearm. The two heads of the flexor carpi ulnaris can be safely separated for approximately 5 cm, providing a proximal exposure of the ulnar nerve in the

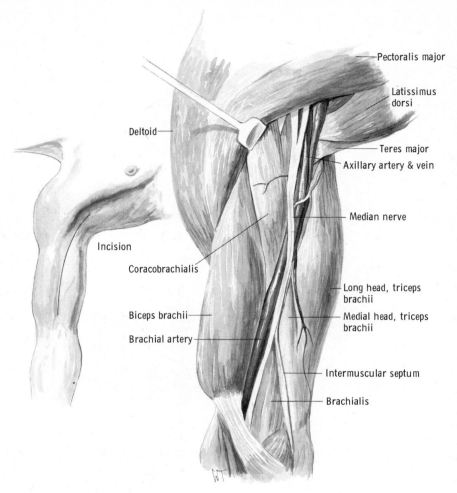

Figure 19–5   Exposure of the median nerve in the arm.

forearm. The branches from the ulnar nerve all emanate from the deep surface of the nerve to innervate the flexor carpi ulnaris and the flexor digitorum profundus muscles, hence the muscle can be split without risk, thereby obtaining wider exposure of the ulnar nerve.

The Median Nerve in the Elbow

The median nerve is best exposed through a longitudinal incision along the medial border of the biceps brachii in the distal arm passing into the forearm along the inner border of the pronator teres muscles. The antebrachial fascia and the lacertus fibrosus are incised, thereby providing wide exposure of the median nerve. The median cubital vein may be ligated, providing improved exposure. The median nerve usually passes between the ulnar and humeral

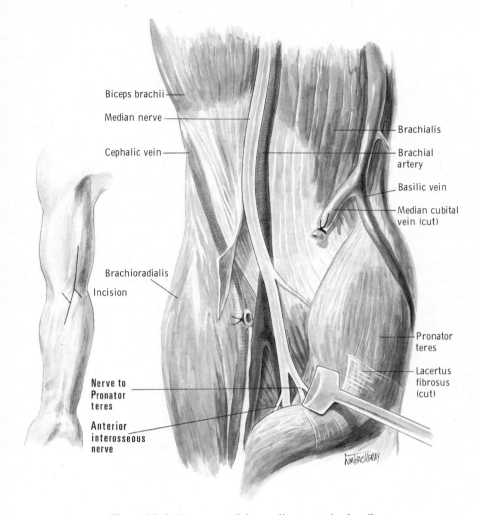

Biceps brachii

Median nerve

Cephalic vein

Brachioradialis

Incision

Nerve to
Pronator
teres

Anterior
interosseous
nerve

Brachialis

Brachial
artery

Basilic vein

Median cubital
vein (cut)

Pronator
teres

Lacertus
fibrosus
(cut)

Figure 19–6 Exposure of the median nerve in the elbow.

heads of the pronator teres. When necessary, the humeral head of the pronator teres may be incised to provide better exposure of the median nerve. Just beyond the exit of the median nerve from between the heads of the pronator teres, the anterior interosseous nerve can be seen passing forward to supply the deep muscles of the forearm. It continues distally to the pronator quadratus muscle (Fig. 19–6).

The Ulnar Nerve in the Forearm

The ulnar nerve enters the forearm between the two heads of the flexor carpi ulnaris muscle. After penetrating the flexor carpi ulnaris muscle, it continues throughout the entire forearm lying between the flexor carpi ulnaris and the flexor digitorum profundus muscles. It is joined approximately halfway down the forearm by the ulnar artery and veins. Exposure of the ulnar nerve is best accomplished through an incision along the ulnar border of the forearm about 5 cm volar to the palpable portion of the ulnar bone. After opening the antebrachial fascia, the nerve should be approached first by separating the flexor carpi ulnaris from the flexor digitorum superficialis muscle. This separation is best accomplished anteriorly and not through the interval between the flexor digitorum profundus and flexor carpi ulnaris. The interval between the flexor carpi ulnaris and the flexor digitorum superficialis is easily found. This interval can be opened briefly and a clamp passed around the flexor carpi ulnaris, thereby elevating it deeply from the flexor digitorum profundus. After this has been accomplished the interval between the flexor digitorum profundus and the flexor carpi ulnaris can be completed. Attempting to open this interval directly is difficult, as the exact boundaries of the flexor digitorum profundus are difficult to identify. As the flexor carpi ulnaris is elevated anteriorly from the flexor digitorum profundus the ulnar nerve can be exposed through the entire aspect of the forearm. If necessary, the origin of the flexor carpi ulnaris from the olecranon process can be incised, providing even greater exposure of the nerve proximally. The numerous branches of the ulnar nerve as they innervate the flexor digitorum profundus and the flexor carpi ulnaris can be noted and preserved. Distally in the forearm, the dorsal cutaneous branch of the ulnar nerve can be seen as it separates and passes toward the dorsal aspect of the wrist and hand.

The Median Nerve in the Forearm

There are two exposures to the median nerve in the forearm. The first is the most utilitarian and provides excellent exposure of the nerve through the distal two thirds of its passage in the forearm. An incision along the anterior medial aspect of the forearm is used. The antebrachial fascia is incised throughout the length of this incision. The palmaris longus is retracted medialward. This provides exposure of the median nerve in the distal part of the forearm. The median nerve then passes proximally beneath the flexor digitorum superficialis muscle. As this dissection is continued proximally, the flexor digitorum superficialis muscle is retracted radialward, providing exposure of the median nerve along its undersurface. Throughout the middle third of the forearm the median nerve will be seen not between the flexor digitorum profundus and the flexor superficialis muscle but within the deep portion of the epimysium of the superficialis muscle. Exposure of the median nerve in this area involves incising the epimysium and carefully elevating the median nerve. This exposure is ideal for neurolysis of the median nerve as required in a Volkmann's ischemic contracture. It is also useful in mobilizing cut ends of the median nerve for graft repair. More proximally, the median nerve will pass under the proximal arch or bridge of the flexor digitorum superficialis muscle and pierce the pronator teres muscle passing into the elbow. Exposure in this area is best accomplished with the second exposure of the median nerve (Fig. 19–7).

The second exposure is on the radial side of the flexor digitorum superficialis. This interval is identified by incising the fascia along the edge of the brachioradialis muscle. Just beneath the brachioradialis muscle is the insertion of the

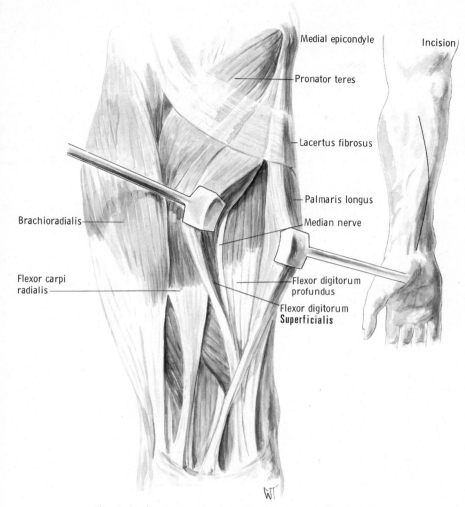

Figure 19–7 Exposure of the median nerve in the forearm.

pronator teres. This muscle can be partially or completely incised, providing good exposure of the origin of the flexor digitorum superficialis muscle at the anterior oblique line of the radius. As the anterior oblique line of the radius is noted and the origin of the flexor digitorum superficialis muscle identified, this origin can be incised. As the flexor digitorum superficialis muscle is incised, elevated, and retracted the median nerve can be seen directly beneath this structure. Continuing proximally, one can see the median nerve piercing the pronator teres muscle. The pronator teres muscle can be incised as needed, providing good exposure of the median nerve proximally. Regrettably, this approach is not easily combined with the previously described medial approach to the median nerve. When in doubt as to the choice of exposures, one should go to the medial approach unless one is certain that the lesion is proximal to the origin of the anterior interosseous nerve. If the lesion is known to be proximal to the anterior interosseous nerve, then the simplest approach is to identify the median nerve in the antecubital fossa and trace it through the pronator teres and flexor bridge of the flexor digitorum superficialis, opening and retracting these muscles as needed.

Combined Median and Ulnar Nerves in the Forearm

The median and ulnar nerves can be exposed through a single incision when necessary. This incision should begin at a point midway between the median and ulnar nerves and continue along the anterior medial aspect of the forearm. The antebrachial fascia is opened and the interval developed between

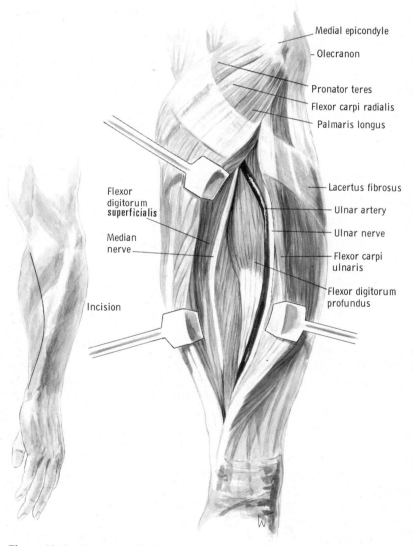

Figure 19–8   Exposure of both the median and ulnar nerves in the forearm.

the palmaris longus and the flexor carpi ulnaris muscles. The ulnar nerve can be observed throughout the entire length of the forearm in the interval between the flexor carpi ulnaris and flexor digitorum profundus muscles. Similarly, the median nerve can be observed as it lies within the fascia of the flexor digitorum superficialis muscles. At times a communicating nerve branch between the ulnar and median nerves (Martin–Gruber) will be observed. This exposure provides excellent visualization of the ulnar nerve throughout the distal half of the forearm. However, in the proximal half of the forearm the nerve becomes more difficult to expose because of the tightness of the flexor carpi ulnaris and flexor digitorum superficialis muscles. Nevertheless, these muscles can be retracted sufficiently to provide good exposure of both the median and the ulnar nerve in the distal two thirds of the forearm (Fig. 19–8).

Radial Nerve in the Forearm

There is one utility approach to the posterior interosseous nerve in the forearm. This approach is improved by partially releasing the adjacent origin of the bordering muscles. The approach is on the radial border of the forearm in the interval between the extensor digitorum communis and the extensor carpi radialis brevis. After this interval is developed, the extensor carpi radialis brevis is retracted, exposing the surface of the supinator muscle. The posterior interosseous nerve will be noted penetrating the substance of the supinator and at its exit from this muscle has major branches which supply the extensor digitorum communis, the extensor digiti quinti, the extensor carpi ulnaris, the extensor indicis proprius, the abductor pollicis longus, and the extensor pollicis longus and brevis. These essential nerve branches must be protected (Fig. 19–9).

The radial nerve in the forearm is in constant relationship with the brachioradialis muscle. As the radial nerve crosses the elbow joint it can be noted to be intermittently associated with the brachioradialis muscle. The radial nerve will divide at the level of the radiocapitellar joint into the posterior interosseous nerve and into the motor branches for the extensor carpi radialis brevis and the superficial radial nerve. The superficial branch of the radial nerve will then continue down the forearm under the cover of the brachioradialis muscle. The relationship of the branches at the level of the supinator muscle is inconsistent; therefore, care must be exercised in identifying the appropriate branches during decompression of the posterior interosseous nerve as it enters the supinator muscle. The exposure for the superficial branch of the radial nerve is along the border of the brachioradialis muscle in the forearm. The antebrachial fascia must be incised and the brachioradialis muscle identified and retracted. The superficial branch of the radial nerve courses along the deep surface of this muscle at the level of the juncture between the lower one fourth and upper two thirds of the forearm. The superficial branch of the radial nerve passes under the brachioradialis and then continues along the tendinous insertion of this muscle into the distal radius. At this level the nerve will branch into three or more large sensory nerves.

Any of these three sensory branches that has been damaged during other surgery should be immediately repaired. Traumatic neuromas of the superficial branch of the radial nerve are extremely difficult to treat at subsequent, second-

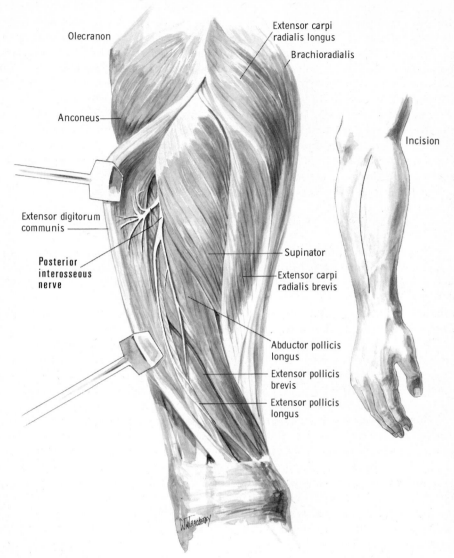

Olecranon

Extensor carpi
radialis longus

Brachioradialis

Anconeus

Incision

Extensor digitorum
communis

Posterior
interosseous
nerve

Supinator

Extensor carpi
radialis brevis

Abductor pollicis
longus

Extensor pollicis
brevis

Extensor pollicis
longus

Figure 19–9   Exposure of the posterior interosseous nerve in the forearm.

ary procedures. Repair of this nerve at the time of initial laceration provides
excellent recovery of this purely sensory nerve without the dread risk of neuroma in this highly visible and palpable area. Incisions for carpal tunnel syndrome
which extend around the thenar eminence toward the area of the flexor carpi
radialis have a propensity to injure the palmar cutaneous branch of the *median*
nerve and occasionally the palmar branch of the nuchal nerve. In patients who
have sustained an injury to this nerve and who have long-standing neuropathy
with symptoms in the thenar area of the hand and who have had multiple
procedures to correct this problem, it is occasionally the volar branch of the

radial nerve that causes the problem. The diagnosis can easily be established by a simple anesthetic block of the radial nerve in the area of the insertion of the brachioradialis muscle.

Branches of the radial nerve beyond the wrist are quite small. The nerve can be identified easily as far as the midshaft of the metacarpal bones. Beyond this, the fibers become quite small and there is substantial overlap from the ulnar nerve sufficient that repair of these nerves beyond the mid-carpal area is usually not practical. However, any of the branches that are more proximal and visible should always be repaired. They lie free in the subcutaneous tissues. Repair of these nerves is important for two reasons: first, there is a high propensity for these radial nerve branches to form painful neuromata in an area which is constantly in use by the patient. Second, the area of reduced sensation will be apparent and disturbing to the patient.

Ulnar Nerve in the Wrist and Hand

Exposure of the ulnar nerve is accomplished through an incision directly over the tendon of the flexor carpi ulnaris. As the incision continues distally it should cross the two flexion creases of the wrist at 45 degrees and then continue around the hypothenar eminence. As the incision passes over the flexor retinaculum it should continue distally toward the fourth web space. The incision should cross the two flexion creases at an angle to prevent contracture across these lines. The ulnar nerve can be identified beneath the flexor carpi ulnaris tendon. The dorsal cutaneous branch of the ulnar nerve leaves the nerve at variable levels and must be carefully protected. This dorsal branch always leaves the main nerve in an ulnar direction; therefore, if the dissection is maintained on the radial side of the nerve it will be protected. The ulnar nerve is relatively unprotected except by a layer of fat at the level of the distal crease of the wrist. Here the nerve passes from a protected area beneath the flexor carpi ulnaris passing toward the canal of Guyon (Fig. 19–10). The nerve is protected by a mass of fatty tissue that resembles a lipoma. When a modest increase in length is needed for nerve repair, the incision can be carried proximally and the nerve carefully elevated on its vascular pedicle and advanced distally. If greater length is needed, particularly in children, the nerve can be elevated to the elbow. The additional length required is achieved by transposing the ulnar nerve over the medial epicondyle and *beneath* the flexor pronator muscle origins. Care must be taken during this procedure to preserve the blood vessels of the nerve. This transposition for additional length is of particular value in small children for whom only a moderate added length is required, thereby avoiding nerve grafting.

The ulnar nerve branches within the canal of Guyon form the deep motor branch of the ulnar nerve and the more superficial proper volar digital branches. The exposure for this position is accomplished in the mid portion of the incision. The subcutaneous tissues can be elevated from the fascia overlying the hypothenar eminence. The canal of Guyon can be opened, exposing the branches of the ulnar nerve. The deep branch of the ulnar nerve can be traced into the fascia of the carpal canal. It is essential to have proper exposure for evaluation and repair of these nerves in the palm. The motor and sensory branches of the ulnar nerve can be traced proximally by opening the epineurium

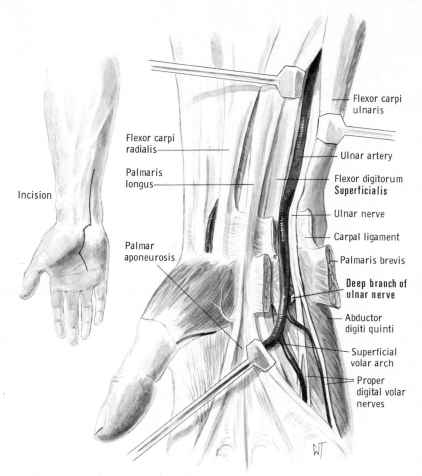

Incision

Flexor carpi
radialis

Palmaris
longus

Palmar
aponeurosis

Flexor carpi
ulnaris

Ulnar artery

Flexor digitorum
Superficialis

Ulnar nerve

Carpal ligament

Palmaris brevis

**Deep branch of
ulnar nerve**

Abductor
digiti quinti

Superficial
volar arch

Proper
digital volar
nerves

Figure 19–10 Exposure of the ulnar nerve in the wrist and hand.

and separating the various fascicles proximally. The motor fascicle is usually located medially in the distal portion of the ulnar nerve. This procedure is particularly useful when there is a laceration at the wrist joint level. With this technique the motor branch can be easily identified, separated, and prepared for repair. The proximal branch of the nerve can then be opened by dividing the epineurium, and the nerve endings can be matched up with those of the distal nerve. The distal dissection should always be completed, thereby allowing the surgeon to observe the general size and distribution of the sensory and motor bundles. With this information, dissection and separation of the proximal nerve are much easier. The sensory and motor branches can then be repaired either with an epineurial suture or by perineurial sutures of the separate groups of fascicles. Additional length can be achieved by transposing the motor fascicles from the canal of Guyon into the carpal canal.

Exposure of the deep branch of the ulnar nerve after its division from the sensory branches should be done carefully. The fascia and lining of the carpal canal must be incised, allowing the nerve to be elevated into the carpal canal. Once the nerve has been elevated into the carpal canal, it can be dealt with appropriately. Considerable care must be exercised as the nerve is mobilized, as there are numerous small motor branches to the lumbrical muscles and to the interosseous muscles. The sensory branches will be noted to be passing distally beneath the small muscles of the thenar eminence. These muscles may be either mobilized or incised to provide good exposure of the proper volar digital nerves.

Median Nerve in the Wrist and Hand

The surgical exposure for the median nerve in the hand is best accomplished by an incision paralleling the thenar eminence in the distal portion of the wound and the hypothenar eminence proximally. The incision should be distal to the recurrent branch of the median nerve and continued along the hypothenar eminence to the area of the proximal flexion crease of the wrist. At this point the incision should cross the flexion creases of the wrist at a 45 degree angle, thereby preventing contractures. Incision can then be carried up toward the mid-portion of the forearm. This flap can then be carefully elevated and the median nerve identified just beneath the palmaris longus tendon. The attachment of the palmaris longus tendon to the palmar aponeurosis can be divided to provide exposure of the nerve at the wrist joint level. The flexor retinaculum should be divided to provide exposure of the nerve from the level of the recurrent branch of the median nerve to the wrist. It is not possible to obtain much additional length in the median nerve distally because of the sharply angulated recurrent motor branch of the median nerve as it passes around or at times through the flexor retinaculum (Fig. 19–11).

The palmar cutaneous branch of the median nerve should be watched for and protected if observed as it passes radially toward the thenar eminence. At times it can be seen passing radially and then branching, with a filament crossing the incision going toward the hypothenar area. If a modest amount of additional length is required, the incision can be continued proximally up the forearm, as previously described. If nerve grafting is required the epineurium can be opened and the various motor and sensory fascicles of the nerve identified. These should be carefully sorted out and an epineurotomy of the proximal nerve performed sufficient that the fascicles or groups of fascicles can be matched with those distally. The nerve graft can then be employed appropriately. If an epineurial suture is employed, the motor and sensory branches of the median nerve can be identified proximally and matched with those of the proximal limb. Frequently, it is wise to repair these two groups separately, thereby increasing the opportunity for optimal motor and sensory neuron matchup.

Repair of the median nerve in the palm usually involves exposure of one or more of the distal branches of the median nerve. The exposure is the same as for the wrist; however, the incision is carried more distally, depending upon the involved distal nerve branches. Considerable time is required to sort out the various branches of the median nerve at the level of the distal portion of the flexor retinaculum. The sensory branches to the thumb as well as the motor branches to the index finger all arborize in the same area. Assessment of these

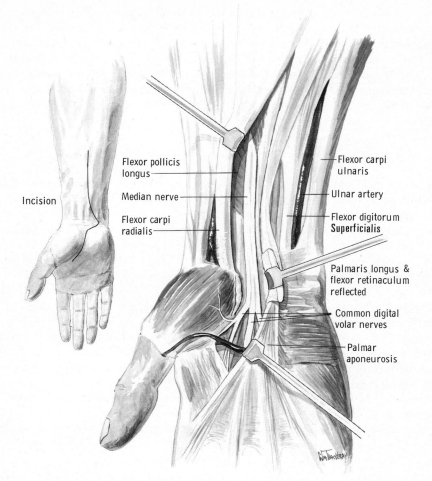

Figure 19–11 Exposure of the median nerve in the wrist and hand.

nerves can be made principally by the lengths of the nerves involved as well as by the size of the fasciculi. Each of these branches should be repaired separately and accurately.

The proper volar digital branches are located directly on the surfaces of the lumbrical muscles. The ends can be identified and repaired in a standard manner. It is difficult to obtain length through immobilization distally or proximally. If the injury has been substantial or if length has been thought to be a problem preoperatively, preparation should be made for nerve grafting. These are, of course, pure sensory nerves and a high level of return can be anticipated.

Digital Nerves in the Hand

Exposure of the digital nerves in the fingers can be accomplished through the classic midaxial incision (Fig. 19–12). However, the darted Bruner incision is

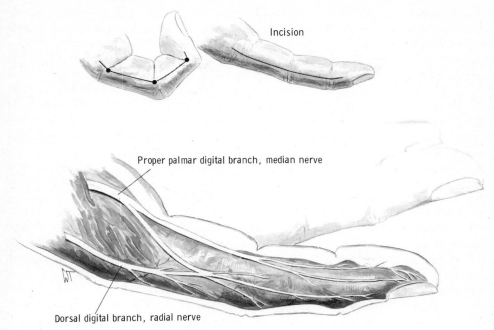

Incision

Proper palmar digital branch, median nerve

Dorsal digital branch, radial nerve

Figure 19–12   Digital nerve exposure.

especially useful, as it provides improved exposure of the nerves, flexor tendons, and pulleys and tendon sheaths. This exposure is especially valuable when grafting both nerves and when there is vascular damage on one side. However, this incision does not provide the best exposure for the digital nerves, as it is difficult to visualize all of the branches of the distal portion of the digital nerves. Additional branches of the digital nerves located more dorsally can be missed. Therefore, when the digital nerve requires exposure the direct lateral approach along the midaxial line is preferred. This incision will allow exposure of all the digital branches. Frequently, between three and five in number, each of these small branches must be repaired to achieve high levels of distal sensation. The nerves must be dissected free from their appropriate cutaneous ligamentous coverings, such as Grayson's ligament at the level of the proximal phalangeal joint. Care and patience are required to carefully dissect out each of the fine sensory branches. A successful repair of all the branches will improve distal two-point sensation.

LOWER EXTREMITY

Exposure of the Obturator Nerve at the Hip

The obturator nerve can be exposed either intrapelvically or extrapelvically. The intrapelvic approach to the obturator nerve may be used when there is isolated spasticity of all adductor muscles. In adults it is considered moderately hazardous, as the approach must be directed lateral to the femoral artery and vein without disturbing the femoral nerve. The incision is placed from the anterior superior iliac spine distally along the inguinal ligament. The lateral femoral cutaneous nerve is observed and retracted laterally. The sartorius muscle and the inguinal ligament are then gently separated, exposing the femoral nerve. The femoral nerve is retracted medially. The dissection is then carried over the surface of the iliopsoas muscle over the pelvic brim. Deep in this section, the terminal branches of the hypogastric artery and vein (that is, the obturator artery and veins) will be noted. The obturator nerve accompanies these structures. The obturator nerve is then dissected free and treated according to the surgical plan.

An alternative method is the extrapelvic approach. A longitudinal incision beginning at the level of the inguinal ligament halfway between the palpable femoral artery and the symphysis pubis is used. This incision should be approximately 5 to 7.5 cm in length. The fascia lata will be encountered. This should be opened to expose the adductor longus and pectineus muscles. The interval between these two muscles is then developed, and deep to the adductor longus will be the adductor brevis. The adductor brevis can be identified specifically by the superficial branch of the obturator nerve, which passes anterior to or over this muscle. The superficial branch can then be traced proximally to the edge of the adductor brevis, at which point the deep branch of the nerve can be observed. The common trunk of the obturator nerve can then be incised or crushed, depending on the surgical plan. Simple division of the superficial branch of the obturator nerve as well as tenotomy of the adductor longus is frequently sufficient to control adductor spasm in those patients suffering upper motor neuron disease with adductor contracture and/or spasm. The key to this approach is the development of the interval between the adductor and the pectineus muscles. Once this interval has been identified, usually about 3.5 cm from the pubis, these two muscles can be separated to expose the deeper adductor brevis and the superficial branch of the obturator nerve.

Exposure of the Femoral Nerve at the Hip

The femoral nerve is located within the fascia of the iliopsoas muscle in the retroperitoneal space within the pelvis. Therefore, it will exit from the pelvis beneath the inguinal ligament intimately associated with the iliopsoas muscle. Frequently the femoral nerve will have already divided into several branches by the time the nerve passes beneath the inguinal ligament. Therefore, one should not search for a single common nerve beyond that point. The nerve is best exposed through a longitudinal incision beginning just distal to the anterior superior iliac spine, curving along the inguinal ligament and then passing down the leg midway between the palpable femoral artery and the anterior superior iliac spine. The incision should be made at the level of the inguinal ligament proximally and extend distally for 10 to 15 cm. This provides adequate exposure of the distal nerve and its numerous branches. The fascia lata should be opened widely so that the content of the lateral aspects of the femoral triangle can be dissected. A moderate amount of fatty areolar tissue and lymph nodes may be noted. The femoral nerve is best identified above the inguinal ligament in the fascia of the iliopsoas muscle. The branches can then be traced distally as they pass beneath the inguinal ligament heading toward the rectus femoris muscle to serve the vastus lateralis and vastus intermedius muscles. The nerve will then pass through the fascial planes to serve the rectus femoris, vastus medialis, and pectineus muscles. Numerous sensory branches will also be noted. The saphenous nerve will pass medially, joining the femoral artery and nerve to pass distally into Hunter's subsartorial canal. If a neurolysis is the designated procedure, the femoral artery and vein should be dissected free from all nerve filaments and retracted medially. The profunda femoris will be noted as it passes deeply toward the adductor longus. The lateral femoral circumflex vessel occasionally is noted deep in the wound. This vessel can be ligated if it blocks the dissection. The medial femoral circumflex will pass posterior toward the hip joint and should not be sacrificed, as this vessel supplies the femoral head. A high incidence of osteonecrosis of the femoral head will occur if this vessel is sacrificed. Dissection of the femoral nerve in this area is tedious because of the numerous cutaneous and muscular branches, all of which arborize very quickly after the nerve has passed beneath the inguinal ligament.

Exposure of the Lateral Femoral Cutaneous Nerve

Exposure of the lateral femoral cutaneous nerve is needed for the resistant case of meralgia paresthetica. It should be recalled that the lateral femoral cutaneous nerve does not pass over the inguinal ligament, nor does it pass under the inguinal ligament, but often passes directly through it. Therefore, entrapment neuropathies of the lateral femoral cutaneous nerve involve decompressing the nerve from its canal through the inguinal ligament. The nerve is best approached through an incision which begins approximately 2.5 cm above the anterior superior iliac spine along the edge of the wing of the ilium. It should then pass around and medial to the anterior superior iliac spine and continue down the thigh, overlying the interval between the sartorius and tensor fasciae latae muscles. The nerve is best identified distally as it passes just beneath the fascia lata and penetrates the fascia lata. When the nerve has been identified distally, it can be easily traced proximally to the area of entrapment within the inguinal ligament. The nerve usually can be released from the inguinal ligament and allowed to rest in the subcutaneous tissues of the thigh. The superficial external iliac vessels are usually noted and require ligation. There is an alternative exposure through the same incision in which the nerve is identified proximally. The fascia of the external oblique muscle is incised from its attachment to the anterior superior iliac spine, thereby exposing the fascia of the iliacus muscle. Within the fascia of this muscle can be seen the nerve. The nerve can be traced distally through the area of entrapment. The distal exposure is more direct; however, if difficulty is encountered, the proximal exposure can be utilized.

Exposure of the Sciatic Nerve at the Hip

Exposure of the sciatic nerve at its exit from the pelvis follows an anatomical dissection route. The incision should be angular in shape and commence approximately 2.5 cm from the posterior superior iliac spine and head directly toward the greater trochanter. At this point it should turn and head posteriorly toward the shaft of the femur. The dissection should begin distally. The iliotibial band should be opened in the direction of its fibers proximally to just above the greater trochanter. The fibers of the gluteus maximus should then be split in the cephalad direction of their fibers to within 4 cm of the pelvis. Splitting the muscle beyond this point may injure the inferior gluteal artery and nerve passing along the edge of the origin of the gluteus maximus. The entire gluteus maximus should then be retracted posteriorly. The gluteus medius and minimus muscles with the trochanteric bursa will be observed anteriorly. The leg can then be internally rotated and the large fascial covering over the small external rotator muscle observed. The sciatic nerve can be readily palpated in the depths of this incision. The gluteus maximus muscle may be firmly retracted posteriorly and out of the way. The nerve can then be dissected proximally toward the piriformis muscle. As the piriformis muscle comes into view it can be retracted cephalad. At this pont the posterior rim of the acetabulum will be directly beneath the sciatic nerve. Further dissection of the nerve into the pelvis is easily accomplished with this exposure. Neurolysis or decompression of the nerve can be carried out without difficulty. If there has been a posterior dislocation of the

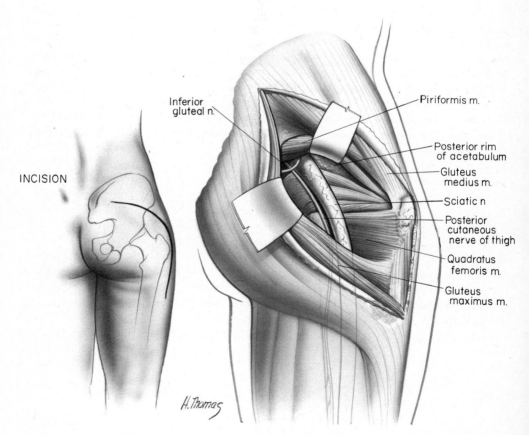

Figure 19–13   Exposure of the sciatic nerve in the buttock.

hip joint, the nerve may be involved in the fracture of the posterior rim of the acetabulum. If this occurs, a moderate amount of scar tissue or callus may be encountered in or surrounding the nerve. This can be dissected free and the nerve moved more medially into a free bed of areolar tissue (Fig. 19–13).

Exposure of the Superior Gluteal Nerve

Exposures of the superior gluteal nerve are occasionally necessary when the nerve has been injured during a fall or when neurolysis is required following an injection. The exposure is similar to that of the sciatic nerve at the hip joint level. However, the superior gluteal nerve will be observed passing, along with its large artery and veins, above the piriformis muscle. At times they are quite close to the wing of the ilium and may have several branches. The vein is usually observed first. This can be traced back to the upper edge of the piriformis muscle. As the piriformis muscle is retracted distally the nerve can be seen exiting from the pelvis. Careful dissection of the nerve is required and particular attention given to avoiding the superior gluteal artery. If this artery is severed it may withdraw into the pelvis and be quite difficult to control. The nerve will pass over the surface of the gluteus medius muscle, sending branches around and anteriorly to innervate the tensor fasciae latae. A neurolysis can be easily carried out if the exposure is developed carefully.

Exposure of the Sciatic Nerve in the Thigh

Exposure of the sciatic nerve is required when there are traumatic lesions of the nerve with distal involvement or when there are contusions of the nerve with peripheral neuropathy and at times for neoplasms of the nerve. The classic "question mark" incision of Henry is the most reliable approach to this nerve. The major landmark is the posterior cutaneous nerve of the thigh. This nerve will lead the surgeon directly down to the area in the fascia lata that may be incised, exposing the biceps femoris and the semitendinosus muscles. The two muscles may be separated, thereby exposing the sciatic nerve. The biceps femoris can be retracted to provide further exposure of the nerve proximally and, if necessary, the muscle can be retracted medially, providing further exposure cephalad of the sciatic nerve. Distally the femoral artery and vein can be observed passing through the small aperture in the muscle of the adductor magnus. If wide exposure of the sciatic nerve is required, the pelvic portion of the biceps femoris may be incised and repaired at the completion of the procedure. Through this exposure the entire sciatic nerve can be observed from the level of the piriformis to the popliteal fossa (Fig. 19–14).

Exposure of the Posterior Tibial Nerve

This nerve is best exposed through the longitudinal incision in the middle of the popliteal fossa. This incision provides excellent exposure of the nerve with minimal traction on the skin. The wound should be closed with a Z-plasty at the

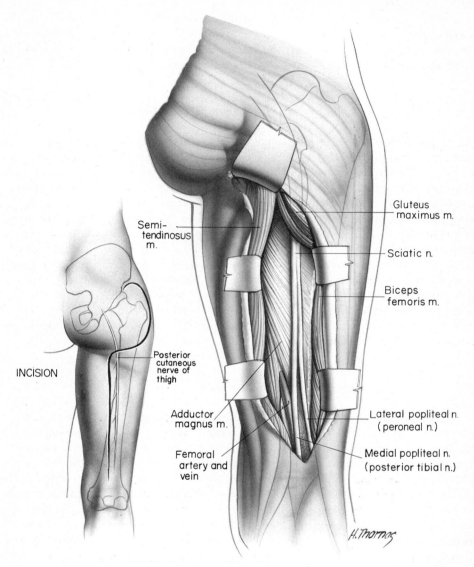

Figure 19–14   Exposure of the sciatic nerve in the thigh.

flexion crease of the knee. Each of the limbs of the Z-plasty should measure 2.5 cm. This incision is preferred over the usual serpentine incision from one side of the knee across the popliteal fossa and down the other side of the leg. The inner corners of that curving incision frequently show signs of vascular embarrassment and heal slowly. Distally, the sural nerve can be identified and traced proximally as an aid in rapid identification of the posterior tibial (medial popliteal) nerve (Fig. 19–15). This maneuver is particularly helpful when there has been scarring about the nerve or in disrupted wounding. Alternatively, the tibial nerve can be seen as one opens the deep fascia of the leg. It is readily identified proximally and then exposed carefully as it supplies the gastrocnemius and

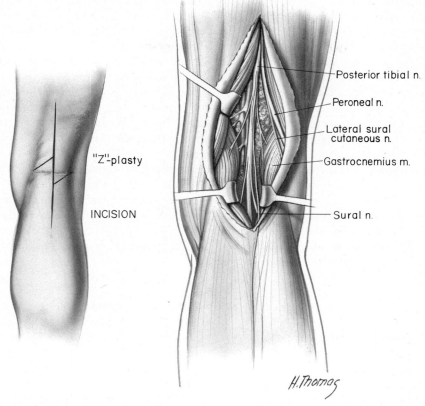

"Z"-plasty

INCISION

Posterior tibial n.

Peroneal n.

Lateral sural cutaneous n.

Gastrocnemius m.

Sural n.

H.Thomas

Figure 19–15 Exposure of the posterior tibial and peroneal nerves.

popliteus muscles. A major consideration in surgery of this nerve in the popliteal fossa is to separate the nerve from the nearby vascular structures and surrounding areolar tissues. The numerous geniculate arteries and nerves can be troublesome as the nerve is mobilized and prepared for surgical therapy.

Exposure of the Saphenous Nerve near the Knee

Surgical exposure of the saphenous nerve is occasionally required following an injury to the inner aspect of the knee or following extensive or repeated surgical exposures along the inner aspects of the knee during which there has been an injury to the nerve. The surgical exposure of this nerve at the knee joint level is best accomplished by placing the patient in the supine position and partially flexing the knee. The incision should be placed in the medial aspect of the knee along the midaxial line and should extend from approximately 7.5 cm above the knee to 7.5 cm below the knee joint. The fascia lata and deep fascia of the leg should be opened over the interval between the vastus medialis and sartorius muscles. The sartorius muscle is the most anterior of the medial hamstring group. This muscle can be dissected free from the vastus medialis.

The saphenous nerve can be identified proximally beneath the sartorius muscle. The saphenous nerve will have departed from the femoral artery and vein at the point where the femoral artery and vein pass through the adductor canal. The highest genicular or descending genicular artery will be seen accompanying the nerve for a short distance before the artery and vein penetrate the vastus medialis muscle. As the nerve is traced distally it will be observed to pierce the fascia lata and deep fascia of the leg to become subcutaneous, joining the greater saphenous vein servicing the lower part of the leg. The nerve is quite large, making identification relatively simple even at the level where the nerve passes between the sartorius and gracilis and on out through the deep fascia of the leg.

As the nerve is dissected from proximal to distal a large infrapatellar branch will be noted. This nerve will pass anteriorly around or through the sartorius muscle and pierce the fascia lata, and will service the anterior and medial aspect of the knee at the level of the patella. This nerve is commonly incised during routine exposures of the knee joint. Fortunately, it rarely forms painful neuro-mata. Therefore, when the nerve is cut during surgery it is not necessary to repair this structure.

Exposure of the Common Peroneal Nerve

Exposure of the peroneal nerve is most commonly required following a closed traumatic incident to the inner border of the knee joint. The patient is most conveniently placed in the lateral decubitus position with the leg draped free. An incision is employed that extends proximally to distally along the inner aspect of the biceps femoris to the level of the neck of the fibula. It is then continued over the peroneal compartment as far distally as necessary. In this incision it is important to keep the distal concavity at the level of the neck of the fibula or further distally rather than across the head of the fibula. This will provide a good flap of tissue that is easily retracted, exposing all of the branches of the common peroneal nerve. This longitudinal incision should be closed with a Z-plasty at the level of the flexion crease of the knee. The limbs of the Z-plasty should measure 2.5 cm in length. The dissection should be carried down to the fascia lata, which is open, exposing the biceps femoris muscle. The exposure of this nerve should be started proximally, as it lies medial and deep to the biceps femoris, eventually passing between the biceps and the lateral head of the gastrocnemius muscle. The nerve is always a bit deeper in this proximal portion of the wound. However, it can be noted easily in the loose areolar tissue of the upper portion of the popliteal fossa. Frequently one will observe the large lateral sural cutaneous nerve departing high from the common peroneal nerve. This nerve will pass down the leg, giving a peroneal anastomotic branch to join the medial sural cutaneous nerve and then continue on as the sural nerve. The lateral sural cutaneous nerve must be protected. There are numerous fine tough fascial layers overlying and securing the peroneal nerve as it passes behind the tendon of the biceps femoris toward the fibular neck. The common peroneal nerve can be noted to divide into the deep peroneal (anterior tibial) nerve, which will pass beneath the extensor digitorum communis aponeurosis into the anterior compartment of the leg. If necessary the origin of the extensor digit-

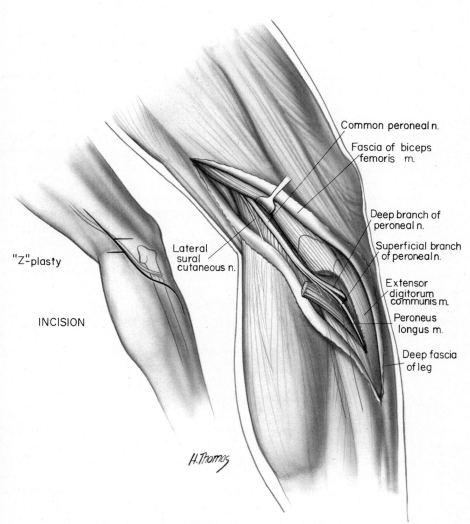

"Z"plasty

INCISION

Lateral
sural
cutaneous n.

Common peroneal n.

Fascia of biceps
femoris m.

Deep branch of
peroneal n.

Superficial branch
of peroneal n.

Extensor
digitorum
communis m.

Peroneus
longus m.

Deep fascia
of leg

H.Thomas

Figure 19–16 Exposure of the common peroneal nerve.

orum may be incised to provide exposure of the nerve. The other branch of the common peroneal nerve, the superficial peroneal nerve, has numerous branches supplying the peroneus longus and brevis and the skin over the lateral aspect of the leg and the dorsum of the foot. Surgery on the peroneal nerve can be made easier if the surgeon will remember to identify the nerve proximally and then continue distally. The dense fibrous layers emanating from and surrounding the nerve make the dissection tedious if approached directly (Fig. 19–16).

Exposure of the Superficial Branch of the Peroneal Nerve

The superficial branch of the peroneal nerve frequently requires exposure when there has been an injury to or about the head of the fibula. The incision is nearly the same as that for the common peroneal nerve. The incision should start proximal to the flexion crease of the knee and continue distally toward the neck of the fibula and then over the peroneal compartment. This incision should be closed with a Z-plasty at the level of the flexion crease of the knee. The common peroneal nerve should be identified proximally and the nerve dissected distally into its deep peroneal nerve branch and then the superficial peroneal nerve. The numerous segments of the superficial branch of the peroneal nerve all branch early. The motor branches to the peroneus longus and brevis muscles will be noted to leave within 2.5 to 4 cm of the division between the superficial and deep branches of the peroneal nerve and quickly enter the muscles. The sensory branches will also be noted to divide quickly and then pass down the leg, forming the medial and intermediate dorsal cutaneous nerves of the foot. The deep branch of the peroneal nerve may need to be exposed for traumatic lesions or entrapment neuropathies. The exposure is as before; from proximal to distal, the origins of the peroneus longus and extensor digitorum longus muscles may be incised for exposure of the deep branch. Indeed, part or all of the fibular neck can be removed for exposure and decompression of the nerve (Fig. 19–16).

Exposure of the Anterior Tibial Nerve

The anterior tibial nerve can be exposed throughout its length through an incision beginning at the head of the fibula curving down over the anterior compartment of the leg. By placing the incision over the fibula head the lateral flap of the incision can be retracted, providing easy access to the neck of the fibula. The anterior tibial nerve is best exposed proximally through the interval between the extensor digitorum communis muscle and the anterior tibial muscles. The tendency to approach this nerve through the interval between the tibia and the anterior tibial muscle is incorrect, as this compels the surgeon to elevate the anterior tibial muscle from the interosseous membrane and then work underneath this muscle. The deep fascia of the leg is incised throughout its length, exposing the anterior tibial and extensor digitorum communis. This interval is best developed in the mid-diaphyseal area and then the muscles separated proximally. The anterior tibial nerve can be seen passing along between these structures. If necessary, the extensor digitorum communis muscle can be incised, providing exposure of the anterior tibial nerve as it passes over

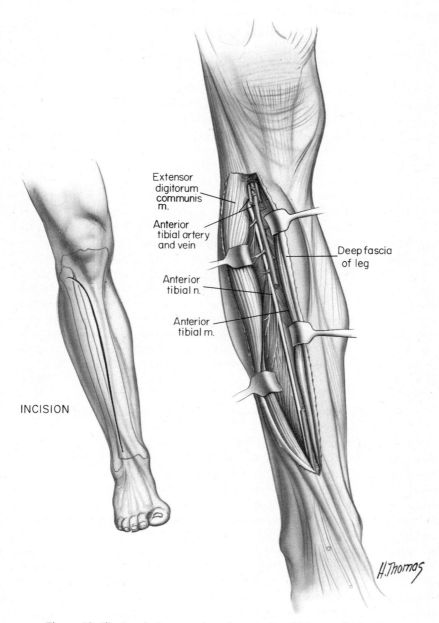

Extensor
digitorum
communis
m.

Anterior
tibial artery
and vein

Anterior
tibial n.

Anterior
tibial m.

Deep fascia
of leg

INCISION

H.Thomas

Figure 19–17   Surgical approach to the anterior tibial nerve in the leg.

the neck of the fibula. The muscle is closed at the completion of the procedure without loss in muscle power. In the distal part of the incision the extensor hallucis longus will be noted to cross the neurovascular bundle. The muscle can be retracted for improved exposure (Fig. 19–17).

Exposure of the Sural Nerve in the Calf

Exposure of the sural nerve is frequently required, as it may be needed elsewhere for nerve grafting. This nerve can be removed with only a modest loss of distal sensation. Exposure may also be needed for neurolysis when this nerve has been either directly injured or involved in an old hematoma or soft tissue injury. If possible, the patient should be placed in the prone position. This is frequently not practical when nerve grafting is required and the patient is required to be in the supine position. The nerve may be approached either with a continuous incision from approximately 7.5 cm below the flexion crease of the knee to the medial malleolus or through a series of 5 cm transverse incisions. The 5 cm transverse incisions are particularly useful when the nerve is required for grafting. These transverse incisions heal with a thin narrow scar, whereas the longitudinal incision tends to spread. The nerve is usually best located by identifying the lesser saphenous vein in the subcutaneous tissues near the lateral border of the ankle. As the nerve is identified, it can be carefully dissected proximally. Peculiarly, this nerve is quite adherent to the subcutaneous tissues and care must be exercised when a graft of high quality, minimally traumatized nerve is needed. The nerve can be dissected proximally to the point where the lateral and medial sural nerves join. If additional length is required, a little extra can also be obtained by dissecting these nerves proximally.

Exposure of the Posterior Tibial Nerve in the Calf

Exposure of the posterior tibial nerve in the calf is frequently required following penetrating wounds of the calf in which the nerve is damaged. It is also required for neurolysis when the nerve has been injured by a fracture of the tibia or following compression syndromes in which the nerve has been compressed. Exposure of the nerve is accomplished without difficulty. The patient is placed in the supine position and the involved leg allowed to cross the uninvolved leg in full external rotation with the knee flexed slightly. The contralateral hip can be elevated if the patient does not possess good external rotation of the involved hip. A tourniquet is always needed. The incision should be along the entire inner border of the tibia. It should start a few inches below the knee and continue to just above the ankle. The deep fascia should be incised throughout the length of the incision. In this dissection the key to success is release of the soleus muscle from its origin along the inner border of the tibia. As the soleus muscle is elevated from its origin, the entire deep compartment of the leg will be apparent. The soleus muscle can then be elevated and the dissection continued further in a proximal direction. This will lead the surgeon along the so-called "popliteal line" of the tibia. The soleus muscle should be elevated from this line all the way to the tendinous arch between the two origins of this muscle. The entire posteri-

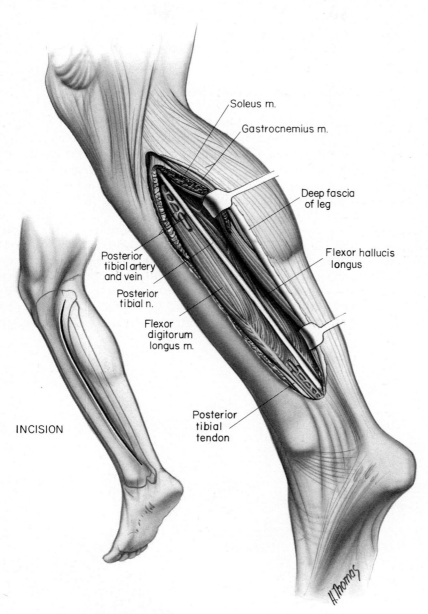

Soleus m.

Gastrocnemius m.

Deep fascia
of leg

Flexor hallucis
longus

Posterior
tibial artery
and vein

Posterior
tibial n.

Flexor
digitorum
longus m.

Posterior
tibial
tendon

INCISION

Figure 19–18 Exposure of the posterior tibial nerve in the leg.

or tibial nerve will now be in view, extending from the popliteal space to the posterior aspect of the ankle (Fig. 19–18). The peroneal artery and posterior tibial artery and veins will be noted and should be protected. The nerve can be dissected free from its position in the deep compartment of the leg. Neurolysis repair, or grafting can be carried out through this wide exposure. If nerve grafting is required, the sural nerve should be harvested from the opposite leg.

Exposure of the Posterior Tibial Nerve at the Ankle

Exposure of the posterior tibial nerve at the ankle joint level is frequently needed for entrapment neuropathies as well as traumatic problems along the inner border of the ankle and foot. The patient is best placed in the supine position and the foot placed on a pillow crossing the opposite leg. A tourniquet is extremely useful, as there are numerous small nerve filaments that require identification and protection. The incision is carried along the inner border of the ankle well posterior to the medial malleolus. The incision should begin approximately 5 to 7 cm above the ankle and then continue down around the malleolus at least another 4 to 5 cm. The skin and subcutaneous tissues should be carefully elevated to provide good exposure of the retinacular or cruciate crural ligaments passing over the neurovascular structures. The nerve is best identified proximally in the deep compartment of the leg. As this compartment is opened the neurovascular structures will be evident. The medial calcaneal nerve will be noted branching rather high and continuing in a more linear

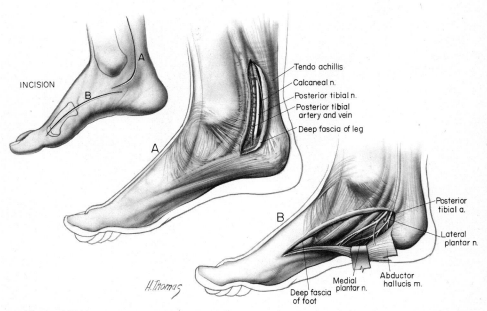

Figure 19–19   *A*, Exposure of the posterior tibial nerve at the ankle. *B*, Exposure of the medial and plantar nerves of the foot.

direction toward the calcaneus (Fig. 19–19A). Numerous small fascial bands secure the neurovascular structures to the adjacent bony structures. The medial and lateral plantar nerves can be separated if necessary. Occasionally fascial bands will run between these two nerves, producing entrapment problems distally in the foot. As the nerve passes toward the plantar surface of the foot it will be in direct contact with the deep border of the abductor hallucis muscle.

Exposure of the Medial and Lateral Plantar Nerves

Exposures of the medial and lateral plantar nerves are occasionally required for nerve repair following penetrating injuries to the bottom of the foot. Usually these penetrating injuries produce painful neuromata. Late repair of the nerves is possible at times; however, it is often difficult to mobilize these nerves sufficiently to suture them primarily without excessive tension, and grafting may be necessary. In any case, the neuromata and scar tissue can be appropriately treated. The incision should be placed along the medial border of the foot, extending from the medial malleolus as far medially as possible while still avoiding the weight-bearing area of the lateral border of the foot. The incision should then be brought back more medially again to the area of the neck of the first metatarsal. The skin and subcutaneous tissues should be preserved as a single layer, thereby protecting the valuable padding tissue on the plantar surface of the foot. The point of entry into the deeper structures should be between the abductor hallucis and the flexor digitorum brevis muscles. As this interval is developed the deeper structures will be apparent. The medial and lateral plantar nerves both lie between the flexor digitorum brevis and the quadratus plantae muscles, the inner border of this area being the abductor hallucis. If the dissection has been started proximally then the lateral and medial plantar nerves can be identified and traced distally into the area of the pathologic problem. If necessary, the flexor digitorum brevis can be incised and elevated, providing a wide exposure of these nerves on the plantar surface of the foot. The medial and lateral plantar arteries and veins will be noted and should be protected (Fig. 19–19B).

REFERENCES

Banks, S. W., and Laufman, H.: Atlas of Surgical Exposures of the Extremities. Philadelphia, W. B. Saunders Co., 1953.

Cosentiono, R.: Atlas of Anatomy and Surgical Approaches in Orthopaedic Surgery: Upper Extremity. Springfield, Ill., C. C Thomas, 1960, Vols. 1 and 2.

Goss, C. M. (ed.): Gray's Anatomy of the Human Body. 29th American ed., Philadelphia, Lea & Febiger, 1973.

Henry, A. K.: Extensile Exposure: Applied to Limb Surgery. Baltimore, Williams & Wilkins, 1945.

Hollinshead, W. H.: Anatomy for Surgeons: The Back and Limb. 2nd ed., New York, Harper & Row, 1969.

Hollinshead, W. H.: Textbook of Anatomy. 3rd ed., New York, Harper & Row, 1974.

Kaplan, E. B.: Functional and Surgical Anatomy of the Hand. Philadelphia, Lippincott, 1965.

Lanz, T. von: Praktische Anatomie. Berlin, Springer Verlag, 1953.

Last, R. J.: Anatomy: Regional and Applied. 5th ed., London, Longmans, 1972.

Lyons, W. R., and Woodhall, B.: Atlas of Peripheral Nerve Injuries. Philadelphia, W. B. Saunders Co., 1949.

Nicola, T.: Atlas of Orthopaedic Exposure. Baltimore, Williams & Wilkins, 1976.

Sobotta, J. J.: Atlas of Human Anatomy. Ed. by F. J. Figge. 9th English Edition, 3 vols. Munich, Urban & Schwartzenberg, 1974.

Suture Techniques

IV

20

THE HISTORY
OF
NERVE REPAIR

CLIFFORD C. SNYDER

In an era abounding in surgical fascinations and infatuating scientific innovations, we must not allow our pride in contemporary brilliance to let us forget the valiant and courageous feats of our medical predecessors. The cornucopia of notable achievements that we presently enjoy is derived from an earlier, exasperating, but fruitful surgical time.

Recent findings lead us to believe that medicine had its beginnings possibly 1,000,000 years ago when Stone Age man first exhibited concern over an injured or ailing member of his family. From Sumerian writings, it has become evident that medical knowledge existed at least 4000 years before Christ (Garrison, 1929). Artifacts, bas-reliefs, hieroglyphics, and medical papyri dating back to around 3000 B.C. indicate that medicine and rudimentary surgery were already being practiced by temple priests in Egypt. Although the nerve unit was yet to be discovered, the value of the nervous system at this early era was understood, and this understanding was demonstrated by decompressive trephining for such neuropathies as epilepsy and melancholia.

Somewhat later, during the Chow dynasty (1123-256 B.C.), the Chinese resorted to moxa (small combustible cones applied to the skin and ignited) and acupuncture in combating neuralgia, neuritis, and various nerve disorders (Morse, 1934).

During the classic period (460-136 B.C.), Hippocrates of Cos (by common consent the "Father of Medicine") separated the practice of medicine from that of religion. A great diagnostician, especially skilled in the art of scientific observation and inspection, he still failed to appreciate the differences between nerves and tendons (Adams, 1886). This distinction was made by still another Greek, Clarissimus (Claudius) Galen (131–201 A.D.), who dissected the bodies of many apes (and two humans), after which he wrote his famous nine books of anatomy (Brock, 1939). Galen's knowledge of neurology is the finest feature of his monumental anatomical labors. He distinguished for the first time the dura and

353

pia mater, the third and fourth ventricles, the hypophysis, and seven of the twelve cranial nerves. Galen was a physician for the Roman gladiators. He traveled and lectured throughout Europe, and was the most voluminous contributor of all the ancient writers, producing 81 books and 16 essays. Unfortunately, Galen harbored a belief that "nature makes nothing in vain," and this obsession propelled him into superstitions and errors. Because his works were read everywhere, he actually hindered the advancement of medical science for the next 250 years.

With the decline of the Eastern Roman Empire, Arabian medicine emerged and reached its most prestigious level. This was partly achieved by the intense desire of the erudite to study, to learn, and to translate literature from other countries. Through the efforts of the Arabian physician-authors the earlier Egyptian, Greek, and Roman medicine has been translated, stored, and transmitted for our current interest. During this time, it was the consensus that severed nerves were responsible for many convulsive disturbances, and that injured nerves never regained a functional level, regardless of treatment. Therefore, divided nerves were not sutured until the great Arabic clinician of Baghdad, Rhazes the Experienced, dared the critics of the ninth century and sutured the two ends of a severed nerve. Unfortunately, the result of this exercise remains an enigma (Rhazes, 1511).

Avicenna, another Arabian physician, further challenged the non-surgical nerve dilemma in his celebrated medical text, the *Canon,* in the first half of the 11th century, by advocating the coaptation of nerves by direct suturing (Greener, 1930). This "Prince of Physicians" was not only physician but also vizier to his caliphs. He wrote over 100 works of great value. Avicenna is known to medical historians as the "Persian Playboy," a person who enjoyed the pleasures of life, defying the codes of nature, and dying at 57, at the most productive time of life.

Ambroise Paré (1510–1590), the greatest French army surgeon of his time, in 1551 particularized the "phantom limb" phenomenon as well as that of "causalgia," by writing ". . . Patients imagine they have their members yet entire, and yet doe complaine thereof . . . the cut nerves retire themselves towards their originall, and thereby cause a paine like to convulsions. . ." (Singer, 1924). (It was over 300 years later that the Civil War neurologist Silas Weir Mitchell introduced the term "phantom limb" to describe the phantasm that lingers following the separation of a limb from its host [Mitchell, 1864]). Paré also supported the popular attitude that partially severed nerves should be totally divided to inhibit the likelihood of convulsions. In 1608, the Italian Gabriele Ferrara dissected the leg tendons of a tortoise, tediously split them longitudinally into fine filaments, dipped them into hot red wine, and, after threading the tendrils on needles, coapted the ends of severed nerves (Ferrara, 1608). Ferrara's report was the first detailed account of an operative procedure for the suturing of severed nerves. Although hot wine was a favorite "antiseptic" throughout the medieval period, its "intoxication" of the nerve endings in Ferrara's case never merited further investigation.

From the early part of the seventeenth to the mid-nineteenth century, a period of 250 years, the preferential approach to traumatic peripheral nerve discontinuity was either to abstain from any surgical approximation or to sacrifice the useless extremity. This was an era in which many nations were continuously engaged in military conflicts leading to a multiplicity of nerve injuries in the armed service personnel. Many limbs were purposely amputated, especially lower extremities with severed sciatic nerves. The thinking behind the concept of "no repair" was that the interspersed suture material at the anastomotic site served as a barrier to nerve growth, and that most surgeons of the time assumed that spontaneous recovery would ensue regardless of whether the nerves were touched. Such assurances expressed by such men as the English authority Joseph Swan (1820), the Scotsman Wood (1829), the Frenchman Velpeau (1841), and the Irishmen Smith and Adams (Smith, 1849, Adams, 1848) were convincing to most practicing physicians. And with the blessings of the Pomeranian Rudolf Virchow, who commented that "nerve gaps over 10 cm. long may not completely regenerate, but in time, function return sometimes is unbelievable" (1846), nerves were left to wither. Other writers compounded the confusion by reporting such postsurgical neurorrhaphy complications as neuralgia, neuritis, erysipelas, lung abscesses, tetanus, and septicemia. Is there any wonder that attempts to repair nerves were severely criticized, when injured blood vessels could be repaired with immediate results but nerve repair evaluation would be wanting for months!

Some clinicians defied the sutureless approach to nerve injuries and were courageous enough to bring the separated ends into apposition with sutures (Arnemann, 1787). Unfortunately, many lacked the understanding of neuroanatomy and neurophysiology and, through this inexperience, abutted the divided nerve tips in many bewildering ways. The comparison of nerves to tendons was deceptive and added further confusion to the already prevailing dilemma of neurorrhaphy. Among the illegitimate maneuvers were Markoe's tangential prepared ends to increase the contact surfaces (Fig. 20–1), which upon the first postoperative limb stretch wrenched the repair apart (Markoe, 1885); Létiévant's double flap (Fig. 20–2) (Létiévant, 1873); and Lanfrank's nerve-to-skin suture

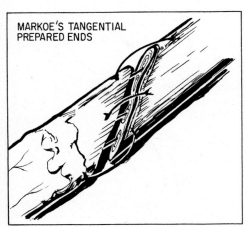

MARKOE'S TANGENTIAL PREPARED ENDS

Figure 20–1

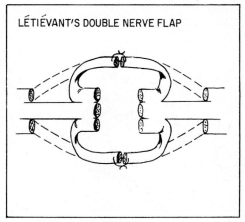

LÉTIÉVANT'S DOUBLE NERVE FLAP

Figure 20–2

Figure 20–1   To increase the anastomotic surface, Markoe in 1885 cut the nerve ends tangentially. This illegitimate method was unsuccessful.

Figure 20–2   Létiévant's double nerve flap, designed to bridge gaps, sacrificed more axis cylinders than were salvaged.

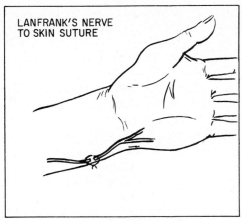

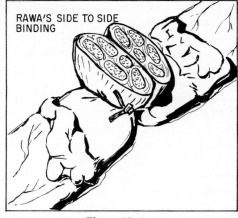

Figure 20–3   Figure 20–4

Figure 20–3   The purpose of the nerve-to-skin suture of Lanfrank was to abolish suture interference at the anastomotic line, acting as a pull-out; but this spurious technique left much to be desired.

Figure 20–4   Rawa's side to side bundle was a poor surrogate to achieve fascicular continuity, even in 1885.

(Fig. 20–3) (Spurling, 1943). Another well-intended but outrageous procedure was Rawa's side-to-side binding (Fig. 20–4) (Rawa, 1885). The transfixion suture (Fig. 20–5), the transposition suture (Fig. 20–6), and the suture "à distence" (Fig. 20–7) methods were three of many more drawing board designs that were as useless as cataracts in an artist's lens.

The uncertainty of nerve repair by suturing remained a perplexity, and this was partly due to complicating infections, hematomas, ischemia, fibroblastic

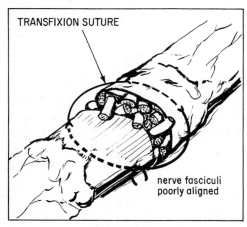

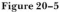

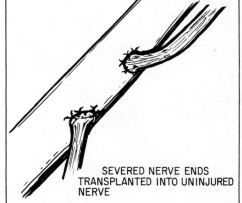

Figure 20–5   Figure 20–6

Figure 20–5   The transfixion suture is one of desperation both for the surgeon and the unguided fascicles, like spaghetti on a chopstick.

Figure 20–6   Transposition is more applicable to hollow organs and vessels than to nerves, but with current adroit fasciculoplasties, axons may find their way into inviting kindred axons.

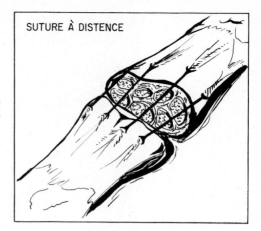

SUTURE À DISTENCE

Figure 20–7 Suture à distence is a lazy man's fantasy of governing undisciplined funiculi—as useless as shoes on a snake.

intrusions, and technical deficiencies, but also to the unknown complexity of the factors which influence functional recovery of an injured nerve. Unfortunately, in the nineteenth and early twentieth centuries there were not enough surgical researchers or instruments for adequate analyses of nerve degeneration and regeneration; and very few physicians were interested in the number of regenerating fasciculi that would reach the appropriate peripheral end organs — muscle motor units and sensory receptors (Holmes, 1942; Terzis, 1976). Over the years, but especially since World War I, methods of neurorrhaphy have varied according to the surgeon's caprice or his serious research, and among these techniques may be considered the interrupted suture of the epineurium (Edshage, 1964; Kleinert, 1973; Orgel, 1977), the intraneural monosuture (Snyder, 1968), the intrafascicular suture (Bora, 1967; Langley, 1917; O'Brien, 1977, Stoffel, 1913) and the interfascicular suture (Kurze, 1965, Samii, 1975, Smith, 1964), the sheathing (Ducker, 1968; Kline, 1964; Midgley, 1968; Weiss, 1943), the adhesives (Ferlitsch, 1964; Freeman, 1969), the plasma clot (Tarlov, 1950), and the epineurial sleeve technique (Fig. 20–8).

Many of the early misconceptions of nerve repair results were partially rectified through the adept efforts of such investigations as the identification of the cross-conduction of peripheral nerves (Mitchell, 1872); the description of catabolism of the severed distal nerve segment, now known as wallerian degeneration (Waller, 1852); the demonstration of histological axonal regeneration (Ranvier, 1875); the establishment of the axis cylinder as a component of the nerve cell (His, 1890); the description of the medullated nerve fiber (von Kolliker, 1879); the dissertation on the pear-shaped ganglionic cells in the cerebellum (Purkinje, 1837); the illustration that severed nerve ends did grow together and that there was a recovery time before nerve function was re-established (Cruickshank, 1795); the initiation of specific methods for staining nervous tissues (Cajal, 1928); and the research of clinical tests for sensation (Moberg, 1975).

One of the earliest recorded attempts to suture a severed nerve was that described by Arnemann (1787). Another was that by Jacques Baudens, who in 1836 encountered a patient with saber wounds of the brachial plexus involving the median and ulnar branches (Baudens, 1836). He repaired the nerves by

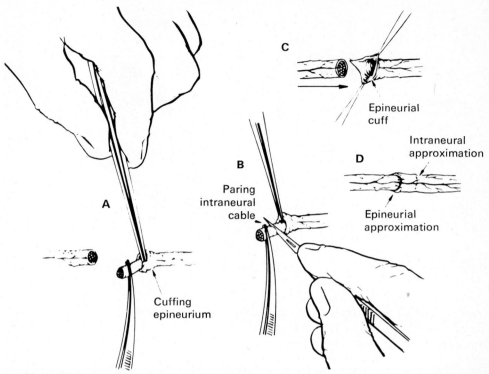

Figure 20-8   For those who believe the epineurium has a function, the epineurial sleeve serves purposefully to direct lost fasciculi to a functioning end-organ without escape into ectopic fibrous tissue.

approximating the adjacent tissues; unfortunately, when the man succumbed to his injuries eight days later, Baudens found the nerve endings unattached. In 1854, Bernard von Langenbeck, the greatest clinical surgeon and teacher of his day in Germany, repaired a severed median nerve using Baudens' technique, and a year later complete return of hand function was achieved (von Langenbeck, 1876). In a dissertation before the Paris Academy of Sciences on June 27, 1864, C. Laugier described his technique of primary suture of nerves with a single silk thread through the severed segments 12 millimeters from the ends, with motor and sensory recovery (Laugier, 1864). E.F.A.Vulpian, who held the Chair of Pathology in Paris at that time, employed a single linen suture through the central portion of the nerve to approximate the cut ends (Philipeaux and Vulpian, 1870). Snyder and his colleagues have used this same technique in over 200 peripheral nerve repairs with excellent success (Fig. 20–9) (Snyder, 1968). In 1882, Johann von Mikulicz-Radecki, a Polish surgeon who had enjoyed professorships of surgery at Konigsburg and Breslau, instituted the "sling" suture, which pierced through the nerve segments and pulled the ends together under tension (Daniel, 1977). This was followed by three epidermal sutures of chromic catgut to align the nerve endings (Schramm, 1883). The stretching of nerve ends to achieve approximation was the universal technique until recently and was advocated by Richardson (1886), Schüller (1888), Bolby (1890), and others. But B. Stookey voiced strong opposition to nerve approximation by tension because it caused intraneural hematomas and subsequent scarring (Stookey, 1922). Dur-

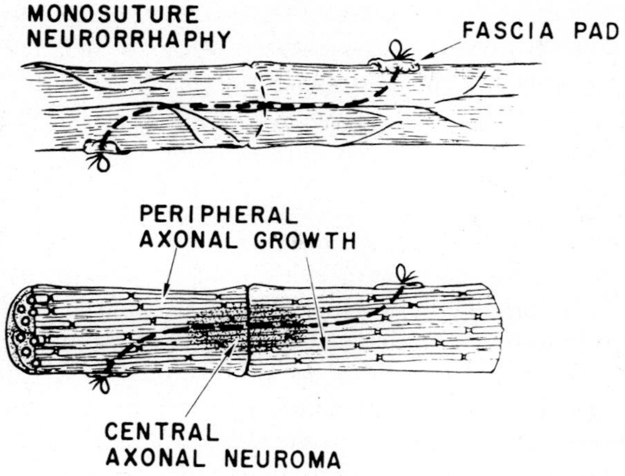

MONOSUTURE
NEURORRHAPHY   FASCIA PAD

Figure 20–9 The monosuture
type of neurorrhaphy has been used
in over 200 peripheral nerve severances with excellent success.

PERIPHERAL
AXONAL GROWTH

CENTRAL
AXONAL NEUROMA

ing World War I, neuroma or bulb suturing was popular, but this method of
neurorrhaphy necessitated secondary operations, and during the interim the
denervated muscles and many end-organs atrophied and degenerated (Kirklin,
1949; Weckesser, 1969). Sterling Bunnell is credited with the first successful
facial nerve anastomosis within the temporal bone (Bunnell, 1927).

Surgeons then, as now, preferred specific suture materials for nerve repairs
(Guttmann, 1943). Although personal preferences varied, among the favorite
materials were split tortoise tendon (Bora, 1967), animal and human hair shafts
(Verne, 1941), kangaroo tendon (Philipeaux, 1870), linen and silk (von Kolliker,
1879), fascia (Sargent, 1919), tantalum (Spurling, 1943), cotton, and polyesters.
Because nerve roots differ from peripheral nerves in that the former lack an
epineurium and a perineurium, they are sometimes difficult to suture. For this
reason aqueous or gel media were employed to adhere the cut nerve terminations; among these were autologous, homologous, and heterogenous plasma
(Velpeau, 1841; Young, 1940). Another method of coapting nerve tips is by
conduit or tube. These have been constructed from bone, blood vessels (von
Bungner, 1894), Cargile membrane (Huber, 1895), parchment (Verne, 1941),
metals (Payr, 1900), and other materials. Tubulization procedures for repairing
nerve gaps have become less popular, yet some surgeons use silicone cuffs today
(Ducker, 1968). Snyder and his co-workers use a silicone trough for the nerve to
regenerate in where there is a scar-infested bed (Fig. 20–10).

There is an occasional need to repair nerves by use of a segment of an
adjacent nerve; this method is known as nerve crossing or nerve pedicle flap.
Flourens, in 1827, reported successful function after interchanging the proximal
and distal ends of severed median and musculospiral nerves in fowl (Flourens,

GRAFT   FASCIA PAD

Figure 20–10 When the neurorrhaphy lies in an intolerable bed of scar
tissue, protect the succulent nerve or
graft with a trough which resists contracting cicatrix.

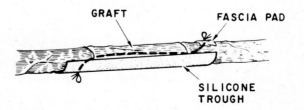

SILICONE
TROUGH

1828). Létiévant prescribed nerve crossing in humans, and in 1872 he corrected a 4 cm median nerve deficit using the nerve pedicle flap technique — it failed (Majno, 1975). Although the nerve cross procedure initially met with success, it fell into disuse because one nerve was sacrificed for another and it also was a multiple surgical procedure. Byron Stookey, a United States Army officer, at the time on special detail relative to experimental nerve surgery, critically reviewed the world literature through the year 1915 on bridging nerve defects by means of nerve flaps. He refuted one report after another stating that, "In no such case was there convincing evidence that as a result of the nerve flap operation any real improvement was established" (Stookey, 1919). Stookey's condemnation of nerve flaps may have convinced many, but in 1947, Strange reported his nerve pedicle operation and in 1950 published his successful results (Strange, 1950). Snyder, in 1966, presented a similar nerve crossing technique with two successes (Snyder, 1966). It is important to preserve the blood supply of the donor nerve and correctly determine the length of nerve flap needed (Fig. 20–11). Reinnervation is usually incomplete and success not total, probably because of poor adaptive readjustments from the central nerve centers, and reasoning that a distal nerve stump is innervated by a "foreign" donor. Facial nerve severances usually respond very well to this maneuver of nerve crossing or pedicle flaps.

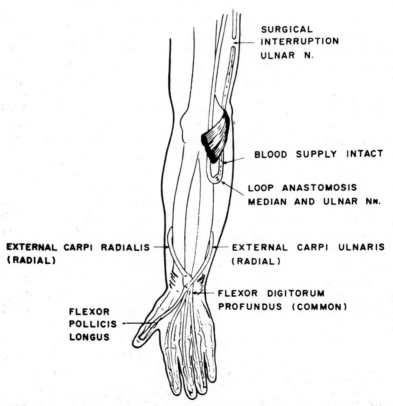

SURGICAL
INTERRUPTION
ULNAR N.

BLOOD SUPPLY INTACT

LOOP ANASTOMOSIS
MEDIAN AND ULNAR Nn.

EXTERNAL CARPI RADIALIS
(RADIAL)

EXTERNAL CARPI ULNARIS
(RADIAL)

FLEXOR DIGITORUM
PROFUNDUS (COMMON)

FLEXOR
POLLICIS
LONGUS

Figure 20–11   Do not build a coffin when two long sections of a nerve are missing; a nerve flap may eliminate the hearse. Preserve the blood supply and correctly determine the nerve length needed.

Three world wars, numerous nation to nation conflicts, and an increase in peripheral nerve injuries in civilians confirm the successful results of end-to-end nerve repair, and to this date all other methods of neurorrhaphy have been inferior. However, when it is impossible to adjust the body parts in an effort to approximate the separated nerve ends, consideration of other therapeutic means is necessary. The bridging of nerve gaps with nerve grafts is an augmentation to be evaluated. Nerve grafts became very popular during World War II and have continued so. The ideal nerve graft is transposed from the same host to the recipient site. Early pioneers noteworthy of mention were Philipeaux and Vulpian, who successfully filled a hypoglossal nerve gap with a lingual nerve graft (Philipeaux and Vulpian, 1870); Albert was not so successful with his nerve homograft (Albert, 1885); Assaky inquisitively tried a fresh nerve heterograft and also popularized the "suture à distence" (Assaky, 1886); and Mayo-Robson used a section of spinal cord to bridge a median nerve gap (Mayo-Robson, 1896). Among the more recent researchers are Delagéniere (1924), Bunnell and Boyes (1939), Millesi (1967), Sunderland (1972), and Seddon (1975). This body of experimenters and clinicians delved into the problem of bridging gaps in peripheral nerves using autografts, homografts, cable grafts, predegenerated grafts, and inlay grafts. To these trailblazers we owe much.

OPTICAL MAGNIFICATION

The renaissance of peripheral nerve repair began with the advent of magnification. But to specify an absolute time or incident of the first success of magnifying instruments and attach a letter of authority would be as sacrilegious as to request exemption from death. Magnification is older than man. Both secular and monastic historiographers have attempted to immortalize specific individuals by honoring them as creators or inventors of the magnifying lens and spectacles. In researching the subject, it becomes obvious that many of the chronicler's recordings are anachronisms fraught with inconsistencies.

Many forest fires have been ignited by the optical convergence of the sun's rays through earth quartz crystals. The Chinese and Egyptians utilized transparent minerals to magnify objects (Morse, 1934). Many are acquainted with the exciting incident of Sir John Layard unearthing a plano-convex lens of rock crystal during his excavations at Nineveh, which would indicate that it was ground between 720 and 705 B.C. (Munoz, 1943). It is a fact that in the Middle Ages the Arabians were more enthusiastic in the science of optics than any other nation. Ibn al Hatham, customarily known as Alhazan (996–1038), in his *Thesaurus of Optics,* described his fascination with magnification and the bending of light rays through portions of glass spheres (refraction) (Garrison, 1929). The actual science of grinding glass lenses may have developed on the small Venetian island of Murano, where in 1200 the celebrated glass blowers processed spectacles as a profession. Pliny the Elder (Major, 1954), a fluent Roman author, mentioned that Nero observed gladiator competitions through a flat emerald lens, which most likely was fashioned by this personal Murano optician. The greatest scientific investigator of the thirteenth century, the English Franciscan Roger Bacon wrote a text and sent it to the Pope in 1267, in which he anticipated the telescope and also proposed a reading glass for the elderly and poor-sighted

(Adams, 1849). Among the distinguished persons who have been credited with the early development of the magnifying lens were the monk Alessandro della Spina of Pisa (1305), Salvino D'Armato of Florence (1315), Nicolas Copernicus, the Polish physician-astronomer (1542), Cornelius Drebbel, the Hollander of perpetual motion notoriety (1621), and Jean Zahn of Nuremberg (1702).

THE MICROSCOPE

There are few medical instruments whose history can equal the long and fascinating one of the microscope. Was it invented by a single person or a group, or did it develop by spontaneous evolution? There are so many contradictory references that searching for *the* creator of the microscope is futile; it is discouraging to try to designate with authenticity any specific individual as the inventor and developer of this instrument. Many reliable medical historians credit the Dutch brothers Hans and Zaccharias Janssen with the invention of the compound lens microscope in 1590 (Major, 1954). This may satisfy some, but there are others who contradict these conclusions. In 1542, Nicolas Copernicus, while a medical professor at Bologna, used a crude instrument of his own making to study the planets (Clendening, 1942). The following year he published his famous treatise on the revolution of planets around the sun. He spoke of his mechanism as a "telescope," and some analysts credit it as the predecessor to the microscope. The instrument apparently influenced the thinking of Galileo, the inventor of the telescope (1609). Another Hollander, who is better recognized for his theories of perpetual motion, Cornelius Drebbel, has also been credited with constructing the first microscope, in 1621; however, many historians dispute this. Robert Hooke (1635–1703), one of England's multitude of native geniuses, claimed many inventions, including the microscope. So, down through history many have been given the honor of inventing the microscope, while others have bestowed it upon themselves — far too many to discuss here.

MICRONEUROSURGERY

The introduction of the operating microscope has permitted the surgeon to cleave and align intraneural components and restore a functional capacity to the peripheral nerve that had never been experienced previously. Employment of the microscope in clinical surgery was first recommended by Carl Olaf Nylen in 1921 while he was assisting Gunnar Holmgren (Nylen, 1954). Later in the same year Nylen used a Brunell monocular microscope for temporal bone surgery of both humans and animals. Gunnar Holmgren, working with Carl Zeiss, in 1923 constructed the first binocular surgical microscope (Holmgren, 1923). Designs improved through the years as the requirements of luxury became those of necessity. The Littman-Zeiss instrument permitted an assistant to view the operation (Nylen, 1954), and the O'Brien triploscope provided the surgical nurse with a view also (O'Brien, 1977). The Urban head addition allowed two surgeons to simultaneously operate in the same field (Daniel, 1977). Table model, portable, and zoom microscopes with foot controls and up to 40 power magnification are now available for every surgical specialty (Jacobson, 1963). Microneurosurgery demands that the surgeon have absolute control of his own nerves as well as those of his patients. Microinstruments and microsutures are prepared for these skilled procedures. There remain numerous differences of opinion relative to the type of nerve repair that is most successful — epineurial, perineurial, intrafascicular, or other — and these deserve time for evaluation (Sunderland, 1954; Spinner, 1972).

Interest in nerve repair lay dormant for centuries, reviving during times of war only to succumb again. For the past three decades interest has been intense. Although currently it may seem that research has reached a plateau and that there remain few problems to solve, thoughts must be directed to progress toward perfecting our present methodology. The teaching of microstructure repair by such scientists as Harry Buncke, and the instruction of modern limb rehabilitation by such surgeons as George Omer will give driving force toward perfection. On the horizon, there appears to be a need for accurate timing of nerve repair, for improvement in anastomosis techniques, for nerve augmentation by substitution (grafts, chemical and mechanical artifices), for a study of vascular improvement, for restrictions on fibrous trespassing, and especially for ways to enhance our knowledge of nerve degeneration and regeneration. The success of nerve repair and refunction will never be the property of one or a few individuals, but, rather, will be the product of continuous efforts by pioneering scientists and surgeons — a sort of axonal transmission.

REFERENCES

Adams, F.: The Genuine Works of Hippocrates. New York, Wood, 1886.

Adams, J.: The nervous system. Dublin Quart. J. Med. Sci. 5:548, 1858.

Albert, E.: Einige Operationen an Nerven. Wein Med. Presse 26:1285, 1885.

Arnemann, J.: Versuche über die Regeneration der Nerven. Göttingen, Vandenhoeck et Ruprecht, 1787.

Assaky, G.: De la suture des nerfs à distence. Arch. Gen. Med. 17:529, 1886.

Ballance, C. A., and Duel, A. B.: The operative treatment of facial palsy. Arch. Otolaryngol. 15:1, 1932.

Bateman, J. E.: Plasma silk suture of nerves. Ann. Surg., 127:456, 1948.

Baudens, J. B. L.: Clinique des Plaies d'Armes à Fèu. Paris, Baillière, 1836.

Bolby, A. A.: Injuries and Diseases of Nerves and Their Surgical Treatment. Philadelphia, P. Blakiston Son & Co., 1890.

Bora, F. W., Jr.: Peripheral nerve repair in cats. The fascicular stitch. J. Bone Joint Surg. 49A:659, 1967.

Brock, A. J.: Greek Medicine. New York, J. M. Dent and Sons, 1929.

Bunnell, S.: Suture of facial nerve within temporal bone with report of first successful case. Surg., Gynecol. Obstet. 45:7, 1927.

Bunnell, S., and Boyes, J. H.: Nerve grafts, Am. J. Surg. 44:64, 1939.

Clendening, L.: Source Book of Medical History. New York, Dover Inc., 1942.

Cruickshank, W.: Experiments on the nerves, particularly on their reproduction; and on the spinal marrow of living animals. Philos. Trans. Royal Soc. London, 85:177, 1795.

Daniel, R. K., and Terzis, J. K.: Reconstructive Microsurgery. Boston, Little, Brown and Co., 1977.

Delagéniere, H.: A contribution to the study of the surgical repair of peripheral nerves; based on three hundred and seventy-five cases. Surg., Gynecol. Obstet. 39:543, 1924.

Ducker, T. B., and Hayes, G. J.: Experimental improvements in the use of silastic cuff for peripheral nerve repair. J. Neurosurg. 28:582, 1968.

Edshage, S.: Peripheral nerve suture. A technique for improved intraneural topography. Acta Chir. Scand. (Suppl.) 331:1, 1964.

Ferlitsch, D., and Goldner, L.: Evaluation of the effect of methyl-2-cyanoacrylate in peripheral nerves. South. Med. J. 58:679, 1964.

Ferrara, G.: Nuova Selva di Cirurgia Divisia in tre Parti. Venice, S. Combi, 1608.

Flourens, P.: Expériences sur la réunion on cicatrisation des plaies de la Moelle épinere et des nerfs. Ann. d. Sc. Nat. *13*:113, 1828.

Freeman, B. S., Perry, J., and Brown, D.: Experimental study of adhesive surgical tape for nerve anastomosis. Plast. Reconstr. Surg. *43*:174, 1969.

Garrison, F. H.: History of Medicine. Philadelphia: W. B. Saunders Company, 1967.

Gluck, T.: Ueber Neuroplastick auf dem Wege der Transplantation. Arch. Clin. Chir. *25*:606, 1880.

Greener, O. C.: A Treatise on the Canon of Medicine of Avicenna, Incorporating a Translation of the First Book. London, Luzac and Co., 1930.

Guttmann, L.: Experimental study of nerve suture with various suture materials. Brit. J. Surg. *30*: 370, 1943.

His, W.: Histogenesis of nerve articulations. Arch. Anat. Physiol. (Anatomical Classification Supplement) *95*:117, 1890.

Holmgren, G.: Some experiences in surgery of otosclerosis. Acta Otolaryngol. *5*:460, 1923.

Holmes, W., and Young, J. Z.: Nerve regeneration after immediate and delayed suture. J. Anat. *77*:63, 1942.

Huber, G. C.: A study of the operative treatment for loss of nerve substance in peripheral nerves. J. Morphol. *11*:629, 1895.

Jacobson, J. H.: Microsurgical technique in repair of the traumatized extremity. Clin. Orthop. *29*:132, 1963.

Kirklin, J. W., Murphey, F., and Berkson, J.: Suture of peripheral nerves. Factors affecting prognosis. Surg., Gynecol. Obstet. *88*:719, 1949.

Kleinert, H. E., and Griffin, J. M.: Technique of nerve anastomosis. Orthop. Clin. North Amer. *4*:907, 1973.

Kline, D. G., and Hayes, G. J.: The use of a resorbable wrapper for peripheral nerve repair. Experimental study in chimpanzees. J. Neurosurg. *21*:737, 1964.

Kurze, T.: Microscopic fix on fine nerves. Med. World News *6*:(No. 42) 50, 1965.

Langley, J. N., and Hashimoto, M.: On the suture of separate nerve bundles in a nerve trunk and on internal nerve plexuses. J. Physiol. (Lond.) *51*:318, 1917.

Laugier, C.: Séance de l'Académie des Sciences, Paris. Gaz. des Hôp. *37*:297, 1864.

Létiévant, E.: Traité des Sections Nerveuses. Paris, J. B. Baillière et Fils, 1873.

Majno, G.: The Healing Hand. Man and Wound in the Ancient World. Cambridge, Harvard University Press, 1975.

Major, R. H.: A History of Medicine. Springfield, Charles C Thomas, 1954.

Markoe, T. M.: Secondary nerve suture. Ann. Surg. *2*:181, 1885.

Mayo-Robson, A. W.: A case in which the spinal cord of a rabbit was successfully used as a graft in the median nerve of man. Br. Med. J. *2*:1312, 1896.

Moberg, E.: Future hopes for the surgical management of peripheral nerve lesions. *In* Michon, J., and Moberg, E.: Traumatic Nerve Lesions of the Upper Limb. Edinburgh, Churchill Livingstone, 1975.

Midgley, R. D., and Woolhouse, F. M.: Silastic sheathing technique for the anastomosis of nerves and tendons. Canad. Med. Assoc. J. *98*:550, 1968.

Millesi, H., Ganglberger, J., and Berger, A.: Erfahrungen mit der Mikrochirurgie peripherer Nerven. Chir. Plast. Reconst. *3*:47, 1967.

Mitchell, S. W.: Injuries of Nerves and Their Consequences. Philadelphia, J. B. Lippincott Co., 1872.

Mitchell, S. W., Morehouse, G. R., and Keen, W. W.: Gunshot Wounds and Other Injuries of Nerves. Philadelphia, J. B. Lippincott, 1864.

Morse, W. R.: Chinese Medicine. New York, Paul B. Hoeber, Inc., 1934.

Munoz, F. J., and Charipper, H. A.: The Microscope and Its Use. Brooklyn, Chemical Publishing Co., Inc., 1943.

Nylen, C. O.: The microscope in aural surgery, its first use and later development. Acta Otolaryngol. *116*:226, 1954.

O'Brien, B.: Microvascular Reconstructive Surgery. Edinburgh, Churchill Livingstone, 1977.

Orgel, M. G., and Terzis, J. K.: Epineural vs. perineural repair: An ultrastructural and electrophysiological study of nerve regeneration. Plast. Reconstr. Surg. *60*:80, 1977.

Payr, R.: Beiträge zur Technik der Vlutegefäss—und nerveuncht nebst mittheilungen über die Verevendung eines resorbibaren Metalles in der Chirurgie. Arch. f. klin. Chir. *62*:67, 1900.

Philipeaux, J. M., and Vulpian, E. F. A.: Note sur des essais de greffe d'un troncon du nerf lingual entre les deux bouts du nerf hypoglosse, apres excision d'un segment de ce dernier neft. Arch. Physiol. Norm. Path. *3*:618, 1870.

Purkinje, J. E.: Ber. d. Versamml. Deutsch. Prague, Naturf. u. Aerzte, 1837.

Ramón Y Cajál, S.: Degeneration and Regeneration of the Nervous System. New York, Hafner, 1928.

Ranvier, L. A.: Traité Technique d'Histologie. Paris, Savy, 1875.

Rawa, A. L.: Ueber die nervennaht. Wein Med. Wchnschr. *35*:358, 1885.

Rhazes: Continens. Lugduni, J. de Ferrarüs, 1511.

Richardson, M. H.: Operations on nerves. Boston Med. Soc. J. *115*:368, 1886.

Samii, M.: Use of microtechniques in peripheral nerve surgery—experience with 300 cases. *In* Handa, H.: Microneurosurgery. Baltimore, University Park Press, 1975.

Sargent, P., and Greenfield, J. G.: An experimental investigation of certain materials used for nerve suture. Brit. Med. J. *2*:407, 1919.

Schramm, H.: Bieträge zur Kasuistik und Technik der Nervennaht. Wien. Med. Wchnschr. *33*:1161, 1883.

Schüller, A.: Die Verwendung der Nervendehnung zur operativen Heilung von Substanzverlusten am Nerven. Wien. Med. Presse No. 5 Jahrg. *29*:146, 1888.

Seddon, H.: Surgical Disorders of the Peripheral Nerves. Edinburgh, Churchill Livingstone, 1975.

Singer, D. W.: Selections from the Works of Ambroise Paré, with Short Biography. Oxford, John Bale Sons and Danielsson, 1924.

Smith, J. W.: Microsurgery of peripheral nerves. Plast. Reconstr. Surg. *33*:317, 1964.

Smith, R. W.: A Treatise on the Pathology, Diagnosis, and Treatment of Neuroma. Dublin, Hodges and Smith, 1849.

Snyder, C. C.: The hand injured by electricity. *In* Wallace, A. B.: Transactions International Society of Plastic Surgeons. London, E. and S. Livingstone, Ltd., 1960.

Snyder, C. C., Webster, H. D., Pickens, J. E., Hines, W. A., and Warden, G. D.: Intraneural neurorrhaphy: A preliminary clinical and histological evaluation. Ann. Surg. *167*:691, 1968.

Spinner, M.: Injuries to the Major Branches of Peripheral Nerves of the Forearm. Philadelphia, W. B. Saunders Co., 1978.

Spurling, R. G.: Tantalum repair of peripheral nerves. Med. Clin. North Amer. *23*:1491, 1943.

Stoffel, A.: Beitrage zur einer rationellen Nervenchirurgie. Munich, Med. Wchnschr. *60*:175, 1913.

Stookey, B.: The futility of bridging nerve defects by means of nerve flaps. Surg. Gynecol. Obstet. *29*:287, 1919.

Stookey, B.: Surgical and Mechanical Treatment of Nerves. Philadelphia, W. B. Saunders Co., 1922.

Strange, F. G. St. C.: Case report on pedicled nerve graft. Brit. J. Surg. *37*:331, 1950.

Sunderland, S.: Funicular suture and funicular exclusion in the repair of severed nerves. Brit. J. Surg. *40*:580, 1954.

Sunderland, S.: Nerves and Nerve Injuries. Edinburgh, Churchill Livingstone, 1972.

Swan, J.: A Dissertation on the Treatment of Morbid Local Affections of Nerves. London, J. Drury, 1820.

Tarlov, I. M.: Plasma Clot Suture of Peripheral Nerves and Nerve Roots. Springfield, Charles C Thomas, 1950.

Terzis, J. K., Dykes, R. W., and Hakstian, R. W.: Electrophysiological recordings in peripheral nerve surgery: A review. J. Hand Surg. *1*:52, 1976.

Velpeau, A. A. L. M.: Neuromas. Leçons orales de clinique chirurgicale. *3*:408, 1841.

Verne, J., and Iselin, M.: Réflexions sur deux picèls de réparation nerveuse sur l'homme prélevées dix semaines et six mois l'operation. Presse Med. *49*:789, 1941.

Virchow, R.: Die Krankhaften Geschwulste. Berlin, A. Hirschwold, 1846; 3 vols.

Von Büngner, O.: Ueber die Degenerations- und Regenerationsvorgänge am Nerven nach Verletzungen. Beitr. Path. Anat., *10*:321, 1894.

Von Kolliker, A.: Comparative Embryology of the Higher Animal. Leipzig, W. Engelman, 1879.

Von Langenbeck, B.: Verhandl. d. deutsch. Gesselsch. f. chir. (Funfter Congress), p. 111, 1876.

Waller, A.: The reproduction of nerves and the structure and function of the spinal ganglions. Arch. Anat. Physiol. Med. *92*:401, 1852.

Weckesser, E. C.: The repair of nerves in the palm and the fingers. Clin. Orthop. *19*:200, 1961.

Weiss, P.: Nerve reunion with sleeves of frozen-dried artery in rabbits, cats and monkeys. Proc. Soc. Exp. Biol. *54*:274, 1943.

Wood, W.: Observation on neuroma. Tr. Med-Chir. Soc. *3*:367, 1829.

Young, J. Z., and Medawar, P. B.: Fibrin suture of peripheral nerves. Lancet, *2*:126, 1940.

21

EPINEURIAL NERVE REPAIR

RICHARD M. BRAUN

It is obvious that the practical working surgeon must develop a method of nerve repair that is successful in his own hands and is dependent on the technology available to him. This discussion of epineurial nerve repair and the technology employed by the author to achieve reasonable results is determined by today's standards. The methods to be described have been found to be practical and predictable, and have returned patients to useful states of hand function.

Many methods of nerve repair are discussed in the surgical literature. At present, there is no single definitive human clinical study that can conclusively prove that one method is superior to the others. Two recent studies have given support to epineurial repair. Mutz and co-authors (1976) showed that improved nerve function followed experimental epineurial repair of the ulnar nerve in the cat. Parameters measured in the study included nerve fiber counts, muscle weight, and volume measurement, as well as motor and sensory testing. Bora and associates (1976) confirmed these conclusions chemically with studies of myelin regeneration. They reported that improved results occurred with early epineurial suture compared to intrafascicular perineurial repair. The field is presently in flux and obviously requires continued investigation.

At this time I prefer epineurial nerve suture for civilian injuries that transect nerves in the upper limb. This preference may change in the future because of improved technology and continuing clinical studies. Each surgeon should evaluate the technology that is comfortable for him and that produces acceptable results with standard measurements published in the surgical community.

If there is any question about appropriate instrumentation, proper operating room environment, or physical fatigue status of the surgical team, delayed primary repair is electively performed within a few days of the injury, after a primary skin closure and an antibiotic regimen has rendered the wound clean and ready for this type of surgical approach. Eye loupes providing magnification of 4.5 × are used routinely by the surgeon and his assistant.

366

It should be emphasized that the surgeon who chooses to do epineurial nerve repair *without* the aid of a surgical microscope does so because he prefers to do so, not because he is incapable of performing a microscopic repair, or because other operative methods are not available, or because his surgical team is inexperienced in sophisticated surgical technology. It is simply a matter of personal preference.

A surgeon who performs nerve repair of any type should be familiar with those anatomic and physiologic aspects of nerve repair that will assist him in performing better surgery, oriented toward assisting the biology of nerve wound healing. Original studies by Weiss (1944) described the physiology of peripheral nerve repair and showed the importance of appropriate nerve fiber alignment, with particular reference to tension. Neural elements extruded into a gelatinous environment may take a branching, random, confused pattern that can be longitudinally oriented by a slight distraction force at the neurorrhaphy site. Weiss produced this environment by using an elastic arterial cuff around the nerve edges. This method has not proved to be practical for clinical work, but did demonstrate that nerve edges that were impacted tightly together caused confused fiber patterns, increased fibrosis, and produced obviously inferior results. If one is to use any suture technique, then, it is imperative that appropriate tension be developed at the neurorrhaphy site. For practical purposes, this means that the edges of the fascicles must gently touch the distal stump of the receiving nerve. Impaction is disastrous, as is a loose anastomosis that allows the nerve edges to lose alignment with distraction. The latter problem led to the abandonment of clot techniques developed by Tarlov (1944). It is difficult to quantitatively describe the desirable tension for nerve repair, and the technology cannot be learned in the middle of the night on a patient who has transected his median nerve. It is much better for the inexperienced surgeon to spend time in the laboratory performing nerve repairs on animals and preparing his own histological sections to learn the technique that is best suited to him. It is unfair to the patient for the surgeon to "see one — do one — teach one."

Optical magnification is presently available in virtually all operating rooms. Eye loupes are now constructed with an appropriate intraocular space and working distance. They provide 2.5 to 6× magnification. My own preference for standard use in a 4.5× eye loupe focused at a working distance of 14 inches. It should be understood how these loupe magnifications relate to the surgical microscope with standard microscopic optics. Loupe magnification of 4.5× equals nine power magnification on the microscope. This means that under usual circumstances eye loupes can furnish magnification equal to 12 power in the optical microscope. There is really very little difference in magnification between the large eight power microscope, which stands on the floor, and the small 4.5× loupe, which attaches to the operator's head. The best place for the individual surgeon to develop a feeling for the magnification that is comfortable to him is the laboratory. Various techniques can be worked out in laboratory animals for nerves of different diameters, and these can be duplicated in fresh cadaver specimens, if available. My personal preference is to have a surgical microscope available, although it is rarely used in peripheral neurorrhaphy. Occasionally, fascicular arrangement requires examination at higher magnification if there is a question about alignment or fascicular intraneural injury in perforating wounds. The degree of magnification that is needed to do the job must be readily available for the operating team.

Suture technique requires appropriate instrumentation. I use a series of forceps, ranging from a standard Adson forceps with small teeth to smooth, small jeweler's forceps suitable for microsurgery. Selection of instruments that are too small merely prolongs the surgical procedure. Efficiency of motion and selection of proper sized instruments is important, and the surgeon must be familiar with his instruments. It is obviously more efficient to be completely familiar with a few, frequently used, effective instruments than to have a hundred randomly selected useless pieces on the back table. Suture holders of the Castroviejo type allow for the placement of sutures with a well controlled rotational movement between the thumb and index finger. This is far more accurate than the usual needle holder, which requires rotation of the forearm and wrist for appropriate use. Rounded handles facilitate the rotational thumb–finger action required for the placement of fine suture material. The selection of suture material includes low reactivity sutures of 7–0 or 8–0 Prolene and the standard microsurgical material of 9–0 and 10–0 nylon. Epineurial nerve repair rarely requires the use of 10–0 suture, but in digital nerves or other small branches, this monofilament material is invaluable for edge approximation. Nerve repair is not a contest for the placement of the greatest number of small caliber sutures in a biologic structure. It is an attempt to restore the physiology of the nerve by gentle and accurate approximation of the nerve edges, with minimal trauma to the intraneural connective tissue that sustains the intraneural vascular supply of the nerve and with minimal trauma to the surrounding extraneural tissue.

Epineurial nerve repair without the use of nerve grafts requires that the surgeon be aware of the anatomy of the limb so that the nerves may be advanced for suture at appropriate tension. Controversy exists about the efficacy of nerve mobilization. It has been my experience that a nerve may be mobilized by external dissection over extremely long distances without impairment to the internal blood supply. Experimental studies on primates would confirm this clinical impression. Mobilization of the ulnar nerve for suture in the forearm may require external dissection to a level well above the elbow for anterior transposition. On one occasion, it was my unfortunate experience to achieve what appeared to be a good mechanical neurorrhaphy in such a case only to release the tourniquet and find that profuse bleeding from the proximal stump of the ulnar nerve was so intense that the neurorrhaphy had to be taken down, the fascicles separated slightly at the nerve edges, and the bipolar electrocoagulator used to achieve intraneural hemostasis. A gap in the median nerve of 4 cm can be bridged by elevating the nerve from the antecubital space and the pronator muscle. This method has been presented by Ashworth (1971) and has been known to peripheral nerve surgeons for many years. Despite lengthy mobilization, the surgeon will frequently observe bleeding from the cut distal end of the nerve when the tourniquet is released. Hemostasis can usually be accomplished with direct gentle digital pressure. Observation of the median or ulnar nerve during elevation and advancement will convince the operator that vascularity is present if the nerve remains pink. If a major nerve in the forearm is externally dissected for advancement and the tourniquet is released, one may place the nerve on a moist pad and irrigate the surface of the nerve to observe its color. It will usually remain quite pink and unaffected by separation from the surrounding tissue. If the nerve is gently compressed between the fingers and the fingers moved proximally so that the nerve blanches, it is possible to maintain very gentle pressure on the nerve between the thumb and index finger and prove that the blood supply is coming from a point that is proximal to the digital tourniquet. The distal edge of the cut nerve, which has now been stripped of its external blood supply and prevented from receiving its internal blood supply, is quite white and relatively avascular. It is also interesting to observe during an intrafascicular dissection whether or not the area surrounding the internal neural surgery has been devascularized. If the tourniquet is released and the nerve is irrigated with a saline solution and examined, the fascicles frequently appear white and avascular. It may well be that this internal dissection (which may or may not be associated with external neural dissection) has turned the fascicles into nerve grafts by destroying the blood supply which is found in the interfascicular, intraneural, connective tissue. The practical suggestion that stems from this discussion is that the internal neural blood supply must be considered in performing neurorrhaphy. The tourniquet should be released at some time during the operation so that the surgeon has an idea of the vascular status of the anastomosis. An internal neural hemorrhage of significant magnitude to cause intraneural fibrosis may be discovered at this point. It is obvious that the most meticulous and mechanically accurate repair can be foiled by this type of occurrence. Condemnation of a procedure because of failure to consider each technical entity with its appropriate management technique is less than fair to the method under consideration.

Mobilization of transected nerves is usually required following secondary resection of a neuroma. Primary, sharp civilian injuries do not usually require major nerve dissection. Moderate flexion of adjacent joints, release of the median nerve in the carpal tunnel, and similar local operative maneuvers will usually allow the neurorrhaphy to be performed with minimal external nerve dissection. The remaining technique that should be discussed is surgical transection for debridement of the nerve edge. It has been shown experimentally that this one factor is of major importance in aligning the fascicles when completing a satisfactory epineurial nerve repair (Edshage, 1964). Miter boxes, neurotomes, and other special instruments are available in some centers, but generally the surgeon must discover some extemporaneous method for performing nerve debridement transection. The classical technique of placing a nerve on a tongue blade and cutting it with a razor blade can be improved upon without any special equipment. This improved method consists of circumferentially wrapping the nerve with a soft membrane such as moistened paper, soft plastic strips, or even the plastic wrapper from a package of suture material. The important thing is to circumferentially hold the nerve together and gently compress it. This will turn the loose gelatinous nerve into a firm, semi-solid object which can be cut across with a regular surgical blade to yield a flush cut across the surface. If small, irregular fascicles are occasionally seen then they may be trimmed with microsurgical scissors and the edges of the fascicle everted, as the scissor blades will usually bend these small perineurial membranes inward. This method, which produces a flush face of the nerve, is invaluable in performing accurate epineurial nerve repair and can be used without such special equipment as the surgical miter box (Fig. 21–1).

It remains at this time to carefully describe the epineurial technique routinely used in acute cases of trauma leading to transection of nerves. This method can be used without difficulty in those cases in which nerve substance has been lost up to a length of about 4 cm in the median nerve and up to a length of about 5 cm in the ulnar nerve. The basic principles previously described apply in all

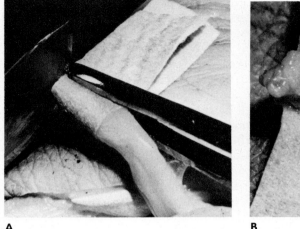

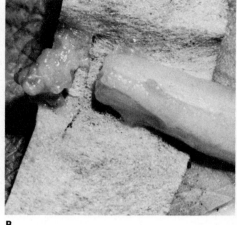

A

B

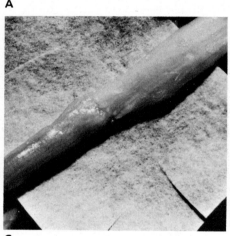

Figure 21–1 *A*, Initial debridement of the nerve edge is performed by circumferentially wrapping a soft substance around the nerve so that the nerve becomes firm enough to cut with an ordinary scalpel, which is passed through the paper wrapper and through the nerve to form a flush face when the wrapper is opened. The wrapper may be held against the side of the nerve by an instrument, as shown, or by the operator's fingertips. *B*, The flush face of the cut nerve is seen. The incision through the irregular nerve bundles and through the wrapper is also noted. Any irregular fascicles may be trimmed selectively with microsurgical scissors. *C*, A smooth butt joint is seen as the nerve lies on a soft background material to facilitate suture placement and retrieval during epineurial neurorrhaphy.

C

cases. The surgical microscope stands in readiness if there is any question that appropriate progress is not being made with routine epineurial repair.

Basic surgical wound technique requires debridement of all devitalized tissues, adequate surgical hemostasis, stabilization of bony architecture, consideration of soft tissue closure, and repair of such other anatomic structures as vessels or tendons in a complex wound. We will assume that the injury is a nerve transection treated as a primary or delayed primary repair in a relatively clean wound that can be closed primarily. Dissection of the forearm is carried out to allow complete exposure of the nerve. Most civilian injuries occur at about the junction of the middle and distal thirds of the forearm. In most of these cases, the median nerve may be relaxed by longitudinally severing the transverse and volar carpal ligaments and allowing the wrist to flex about 30 degrees. The nerve has a normal elasticity that allows an excursion amplitude of about 4 cm. If the nerve did not have this natural elasticity, it could not participate in the proximal and distal excursion required when the wrist is placed in a full range of motion. When the nerve is transected, its peripheral attachments may not allow it to retract this full distance, but the potential for movement is there. Restoring the nerve to its natural length should not be thought of as a traumatic episode, and removing 1 cm from the nerve will not impair its function. If the wrist is held at neutral, 2 cm of nerve may be sacrificed without any change in tension on the nerve from the state that existed prior to the injury. We have seen no case of diminished nerve function when the wrist is extended from a neutral position to 60 degrees of dorsiflexion over a period of several months after injury, which would refute the concept that any removal of nerve tissue from the forearm will cause undue stretching on the nerve when a full range of motion is re-established at a later date. Decompression of the median nerve at the wrist or of the ulnar nerve at the canal of Guyon will allow mobilization of the nerve and will frequently prevent the possibility of a carpal tunnel syndrome occurring during the postoperative phase, when swelling in the area causes a reduction in the volume available for the nerve in the carpal canal. Proximal dissection depends completely on the amount of nerve tissue sacrificed. This is minimal in a primary sharp laceration, but may increase to 5 cm with resection of a large neuroma or with other procedures requiring major proximal mobilization. The techniques basically consist of transposition of the ulnar nerve anterior to the elbow and extraneural dissection in the forearm for release of the median nerve beneath the lacertus fibrosus in the antecubital area and elevation of the nerve through the substance of the pronator muscle in the forearm. These procedures should be done carefully by an experienced surgeon. An understanding by the operating surgeon of peripheral nerve anatomy in the forearm, including common abnormalities that occur in these nerves, is essential.

The nerve edges are then inspected so that an appreciation of the fascicle bundles can be noted. The two major areas of concern at this stage of the procedure are rotation for appropriate fascicle matching and the proper relationship between distraction and impaction forces. Rotational alignment can frequently be attained by observation of the blood vessels which lie on the surface of the epineurium. Fascicular orientation may be determined after the edges of the nerves are transected by the method described, which leaves the nerve with a flush face for observation. In the distal forearm, the median nerve has four or five major bundle components, and the ulnar nerve has divided into a fascicular motor bundle, which curves under the radial bundle at the wrist and then proceeds to innervate muscles of the hand. If malrotation occurs during neurorrhaphy and the suture line is placed so that impaction of the nerve edges results, then the repair will be compromised. Condemnation of epineurial repair is clearly unfair if these technical points are not carefully considered. After orientation of rotation is completed, placement of the sutures begins at 180 degree angles along the periphery of the nerve. At this point, the surgeon should decide if the tension at the edges of the neurorrhaphy is appropriate. If there is any question about the orientation or if there appears to be a tendency toward distraction of the nerve edges, peripheral holding sutures may be placed through peripheral tissue 2 cm away from the neurorrhaphy site and severed after the neurorrhaphy has been partially completed. A pliable background material of a suitable color, such as the green used in microsurgery, will allow for ease in defining the details of the anastomosis and for picking up fine suture material. Eight–0 Prolene suture can be handled easily for epineurial repair. This material may vary from 7–0 to 9–0 at the discretion of the surgeon or may be replaced by 9–0 monofilament microsurgical nylon. Under usual conditions,

10–0 nylon is not used for epineurial repair of this type. The object of the initial epineurial suture placement is to create a trough for the nerve fascicles and interfascicular connective tissue to lie in during the healing process. It has been shown experimentally that nerves will grow together with excellent histology of regeneration if the two cut edges are placed opposite each other in a preformed trough. Sutures are not required for this type of nerve repair, which can be performed in experimental animals. Extrapolation of this data to epineurial repair would indicate that the nerve sheath itself may be used to fashion a cylindrical trough into which the fascicles and connective tissue are placed in optimal rotation and appropriate coaptation for regeneration. The sutured neural sheath is usually strong enough to accomplish this. After a reasonable portion of the suture line has been completed, it is possible for the surgeon to observe the intraneural anatomy and determine whether or not appropriate rotation and fascicular orientation has occurred. It is obvious that one should attempt to prevent fascicular overlap, impaction, or malrotation, and at this point, the surgeon may elect to consider trimming or reorienting individual fascicles appropriately.

Although a preference has been expressed for epineurial nerve repair, dogmatic insistence on this method is unnecessary, and if improved magnification will allow the surgeon to be more comfortable in what he is doing, then it is obvious that the microscope may be used. This is seldom necessary.

At some time during the procedure of suture repair, release of the tourniquet is recommended to ensure hemostasis at the anastomosis site. Hematomas that appear within the nerve sheath are unacceptable and impair healing. Complete nerve closure with peripheral interrupted sutures may be accomplished for a smooth butt joint without impaction. Stay sutures at a distance may be released at this time if the surgeon feels they are no longer necessary.

Evaluation of the anastomosis site is then made with the wrist and elbow in various positions of flexion to determine the adequate position of relaxation that should be maintained for three weeks following nerve repair. It is also reasonable to determine the excursion necessary to allow for full joint motion and to determine a plan for joint mobilization that will follow three weeks of immobilization. Appropriate wound closure, suction drainage, and antibiotics are used in the usual fashion for these injuries. Full joint ranging exercises commence at six weeks postoperatively.

Acute cases usually involve minimal nerve gaps. An exercise program may begin after 3 weeks of immobilization. Splints should be used to prevent rapid stretching. The patient and his therapist should know that extension of 10 to 15 degrees per week is sufficient. A wrist that is flexed to 30 degrees for three weeks may attain 15 degrees of protected extension within six weeks from the date of surgical repair. Unprotected use and more strenuous exercises may be permitted after this six week period. Delayed repairs, or cases with loss of nerve tissue, may require 60 degrees of wrist flexion for appropriate neurorrhaphy. These patients require a longer period of exercise to gradually attain a neutral wrist position about six weeks postoperatively. They may begin moving in protective splints at three weeks after surgery and progress at about 10 to 15 degrees per week. A similar rate of elbow extension is used in cases where flexion of this joint is required to attain neurorrhaphy without tension. At

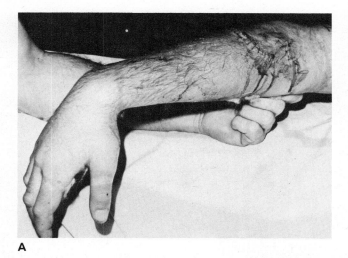

A

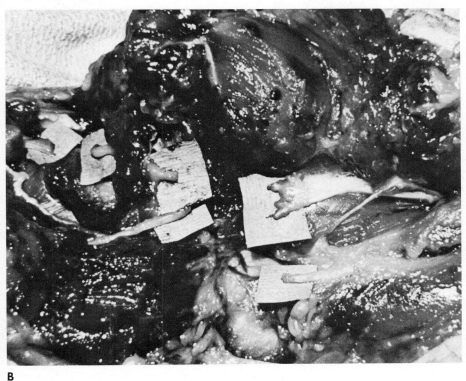

B

Figure 21–2 *A,* This young adult man sustained a deep laceration to the forearm in a fall through a plate glass window. Primary wound lavage and closure was followed by delayed primary nerve repair 48 hours after injury when the surgical team was fresh and instrumentation appropriate. Complete loss of radial nerve function was present prior to surgery. *B,* Exploration of the forearm showed multiple segmental lacerations of the radial nerve. The edges of the nerve were trimmed using the technique showin in Figure 21–1.

Illustration continued on the following page

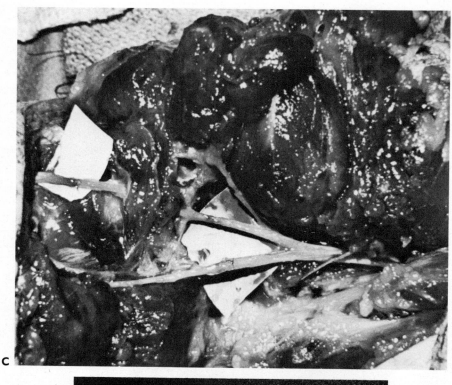

C

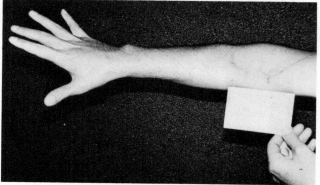

D

Figure 21–2 *Continued*   *C*, Repair of the multiple branches of the radial nerve by epineurial suture with 9-0 monofilament nylon was accomplished. Each identified segment was repaired. *D*, One year following surgery the patient demonstrates excellent extension at the wrist, fingers, and thumb.

Illustration continued on the opposite page

this rate, an elbow that is flexed 60 to 80 degrees may be fully extended within about two months following surgery. Clinical judgment is important in each case, especially if pain or other untoward responses are encountered.

Illustrations are presented to demonstrate the results of this method of peripheral nerve repair (Figs. 21–2 to 21–5).

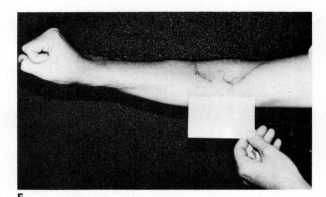

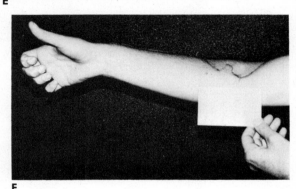

Figure 21-2 *Continued E,* Individual selective wrist extension has returned one year following surgery. *F,* Individual selective thumb extension is demonstrated at one year followup examination.

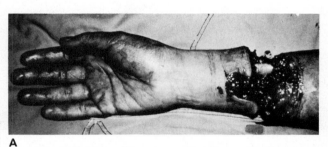

Figure 21-3 *A,* A severe transection injury of the forearm which severed all flexor tendons, both major arteries, and both the median and ulnar nerves is noted. This complex injury destroyed about 2 to 3 centimeters of tissue in a wedge down to the level of the intraosseous membrane and partially through the radius. *B,* Examination four years after injury and repair of all tendons, the radial artery, and both the median and ulnar nerves shows good balance of intrinsic and extrinsic muscles in the hand.

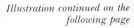

Illustration continued on the following page

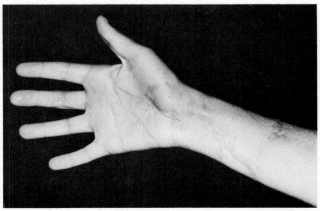

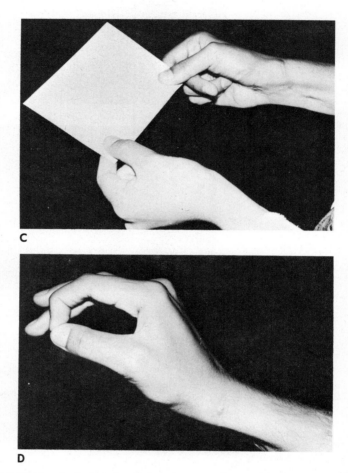

Figure 21–3 *Continued C*, Return of ulnar innervated intrinsic musculature has occurred. The patient does not demonstrate weakness in pinch or Froment's sign. *D*, Good pinch attitude and thumb-index control are demonstrated. Some minimal weakness in the median and ulnar intrinsic musculature is present, but the patient's pinch and grasp are completely functional, and sensibility is good. Dextrous activities handling small objects present no major problem for this patient.

Illustration continued on the opposite page

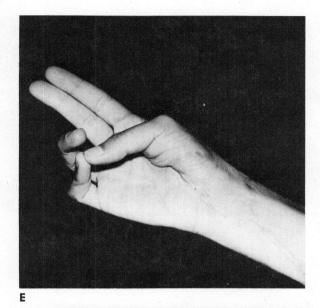

E

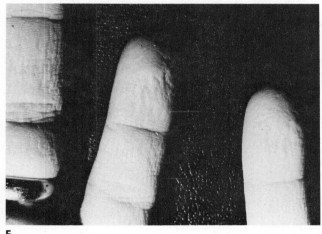

F

Figure 21–3 *Continued* *E*, Return of thenar function is noted. The patient does not require tendon transfer. *F*, Return in normal puckering of the fingertip touch pads following immersion in warm water is noted. Sweating has also returned to the fingertips.

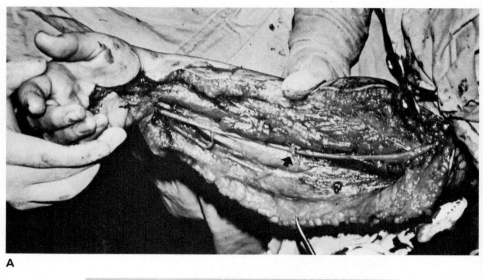

A

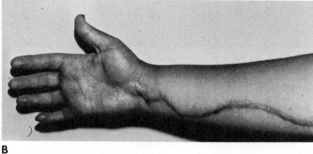

B

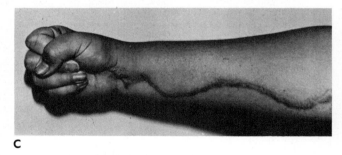

C

Figure 21–4   *A*, Advancement of the ulnar nerve throughout the length of the forearm is seen in a 16-year-old boy, who sustained an injury which required resection of 5 cm of the ulnar nerve. The neurorrhaphy site is marked by the arrow. Fresh bleeding from the tip of the proximal stump was noted following release of the tourniquet. *B*, Good balance of the intrinsic musculature of the hand, absence of clawing, and normal posture are noted three years following surgery. *C*, Full hand function has returned. Muscle balance between intrinsic and extrinsic musculature is good. Tendon transfer is not required. The patient shows no evidence of weakness in the intrinsic muscles innervated by the ulnar nerve.

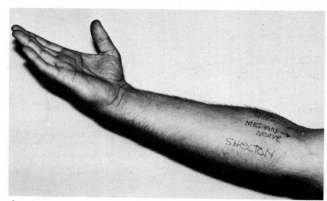

Figure 21-5 *A,* The patient's **A**
hand is seen five years following
transection of the median nerve
and brachial artery at the antecubital space caused by a sharp glass
laceration. Primary epineurial repair and brachial artery repair were
performed. Good balance in the
hand and restoration of forearm
musculature are noted. *B,* Thenar
function has returned. Opponensplasty or similar tendon surgery is
unnecessary. *C,* Full function of the
forearm flexor musculature is noted
as the patient makes a tight fist. His
grip strength is good. He is right-
handed and works in strenuous employment using his injured domi-
nent right hand without restriction.

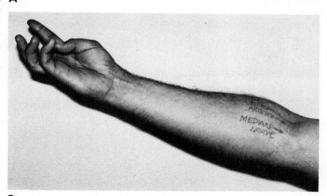

B

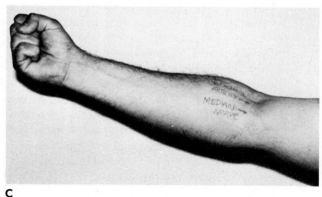

C

REFERENCES

Ashworth, C. R., Boyes, J. H., and Stark, H. H.: A method of overcoming a gap in the median nerve.
J. Bone Joint Surg. *53(A)*:813, 1971.

Bora, F. W., Pleasure, D. E., and Didizan, N. A.: A study of nerve regeneration and neuroma
formation after suture by various techniques. J. Hand Surg. *1*:138, 1976.

Cabaud, H. E., Rodkey, W. G., McCarroll, H. R., Mutz, S. B., and Neibauer, J. J.: Epineurial and
perineurial fascicular nerve repairs: A critical comparison. J. Hand Surg. *1*:131, 1976.

Edshage, S.: Peripheral nerve suture. A technique for improved intraneural topography. Acta Chir.
Scand. Suppl 331:1, 1964.

Tarlov, I. M.: Plasma clot suture of nerves. Surgery *15*:257, 1944.

Weiss, P.: The technology of nerve regeneration: A review. Sutureless tubulation and related
methods of nerve repair. J. Neurosurg. *1*:400, 1944.

22

FASCICULAR NERVE REPAIR

JACK W. TUPPER

Within a peripheral nerve, the nerve fiber (axon and its sheath) is the smallest functional unit (see Fig. 22–1). Bundles of these fibers, contained by specialized tubular membrane, the perineurium, form the smallest surgical unit, the fasciculus (funiculus) (see Figs. 22–2 and 22–3). This may vary from less than 0.1 millimeters to several millimeters in diameter. The funicular contents are under axoplasmic pressure and are therefore always round in cross section. In contradistinction to the epineurium, the perineurium forms not only a physical but also a physiological barrier, allowing preferential passage of some materials. Capillaries form the only true intrafunicular vessels.

Fasciculi may pass singly along the nerve or may be arranged in groups (fascicular bundles). Surrounding fasciculi and fascicular groups, and binding all together, is a loose areolar tissue, the epineurial connective tissue. In this tissue are the blood and lymph vessels and sympathetic fibers to the arterioles. Surrounding all of this to form the outer layer of the peripheral nerve is a condensed membrane of the same material, the epineurial sheath (Fig. 22–1).

At the present time, the nerve fibers within the fasciculus, the lymphatics and sympathetic fibers to the intraneural arterioles, are not readily identifiable to the operating surgeon. It is the perineurium of the fasciculus, the condensed epineurial connective tissue about the fascicular bundle and the epineurial sheath, that the peripheral nerve surgeon has best access to and can best suture.

From an anatomic standpoint, nerve repairs may be of several types:

1. Epineurial — sutures through the epineurial sheath only.
2. Epineurial plus a few sutures in funiculi or funicular bundles (in large nerves).
3. Large bundle repair — removal of epineurial sheath and suturing of large bundles (in large nerves).
4. Perineurial (funicular, fascicular) — both epineurial sheath and loose areolar epineurial connective tissue are discarded at the repair site. Funiculi are repaired with sutures in the perineurium only. Even in this type, fascicular bundle groups of very small funiculi (less than 0.2 mm) are usually sutured as a unit.

380

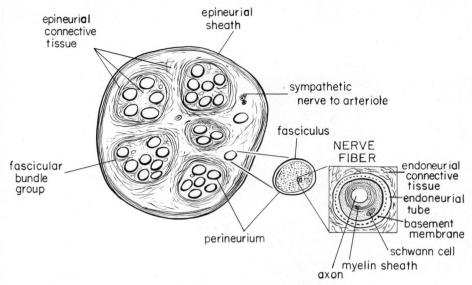

epineurial
connective
tissue

epineurial
sheath

sympathetic
nerve to arteriole

fasciculus

NERVE
FIBER

endoneurial
connective
tissue

endoneurial
tube

basement
membrane

fascicular
bundle
group

schwann cell

perineurium

myelin sheath

axon

Figure 22–1   Composite peripheral nerve represented diagrammatically.

There are approximately 25 funiculi in the median nerve at the wrist and five in a proper digital nerve (see Figs. 22–7 and 22–8).

If an epineurial repair is done, there is a gross orientation of the nerve ends but poor funicular coaptation. A tight closure inhibits escape of budding axons but may make intraneural hematoma more likely. Since a peripheral nerve is often 50 per cent interfunicular tissue (Fig. 22–4), it would follow that regenerating axons would have a significant chance of not growing down a distal perineural tube but, rather, into the tissue between the neural tubes. At a specific

Figure 22–2 The two forceps hold the epineurial sheath. The median nerve at the wrist is seen trifurcating at the distal end of the carpal tunnel.

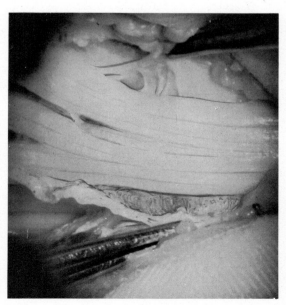

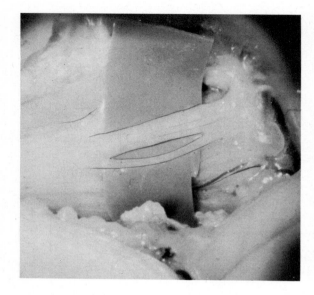

Figure 22-3 This median nerve is seen with both a funiculus and a funicular group dissected. A latex background is in place.

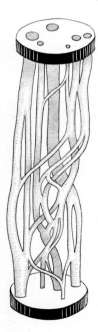

Figure 22-4 Funicular pattern in peripheral nerves. (From Sunderland, S.: Nerves and Nerve Injuries. Baltimore, Williams and Wilkins, 1968.)

funicular juncture, if motor and sensory fibers could be identified accurately, theoretically, a larger number of functioning nerve fibers could regenerate following repair.

Accurate funicular matching can be done only in primary repair of sharply divided nerves. At the wrist level, the motor funiculus is separate and can usually be identified, but proximally funiculi will be mixed in their motor-sensory content (Fig. 22–4).

If a graft is to be used, the repair may be either epineurial or perineurial. The sural nerve is the usual donor. If a funicular graft is to be performed, the epineurium must be removed and the funiculi dissected into lengths determined initially by the distance between branching funiculi so that the length of funicular graft is essentially one fairly homogeneous strand. Not all funiculi within a nerve are useful, many being too small. These funicular grafts may then be sutured to bridge the gap between proximal and distal funiculi in the injured nerve.

TECHNIQUE OF FASCICULAR REPAIR

A piece of ordinary light-blue latex balloon serves nicely as a background. It is readily available, cheap, and does not give a light reflection. Frequent flushing using a plastic BSS bottle* with a blunt needle allows easier identification of tissues to be discarded. The irrigating solution is heparinized saline, which keeps the fine suture materials from sticking to the wound surface. The author's preference in suture material is the S & T 50 micron (5-V) *short* (3 mm), straight needle swaged onto 18 micron nylon.** It is difficult to carry out accurate perineurial sutures with larger needles (Fig. 22–11).

1. Dissect away the epineurial sheath from the end of the nerve for a distance approximately equal to the diameter of the nerve.

2. When dealing with a large nerve, identify the fascicular bundles and dissect them initially as bundle groups, proximally and distally. Match them with what appear to be corresponding units and, temporarily, loosely suture them together. Then, one bundle at a time, dissect all funiculi from each other, removing all the loose areolar epineurial connective tissue. Frequent flooding of the field will aid in cleanly preparing the funiculi. Each funiculus shows a spiral pattern in the perineurium (Fig. 22–5); these are pleats which disappear on axial stretch and reappear when tension is relaxed. The funiculi from the two paired bundles are arranged in a fan-shaped pattern on a flat surface facing each other (Figs. 22–7A and 22–8A). These are then matched one to another by size. Protruding from the perineurial cuff are the gelatinous intrafunicular contents (Fig. 22–6). This is trimmed flush with the perineurium (Fig. 22–5), and two sutures are then placed at 180 degrees from each other. Axoplasmic leak will then usually cease. If only one suture is used, there is a possibility of torsion of the funiculus with loss of contact (Fig. 22–9A). The rest of the funiculi in the

---

*Alcon Co., P. O. Box 2664, Forth Worth, Texas 76101.
**S & T Chirurgische Nadeln, 7893 Jestetten (B.R.D.), West Germany.

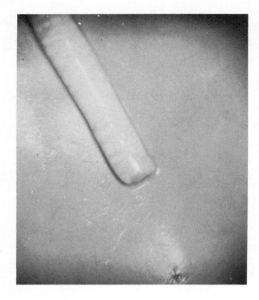

Figure 22–5 Single funiculus from a sural nerve. Note the spiral markings in the perineurium.

bundle are then matched and sutured in like manner. Then the next bundle is dealt with in similar fashion until repair is complete (Fig. 22–7).

In smaller nerves such as the digital, there are only three to five funiculi, which are not formed into bundles but pass singly through the nerve (Fig. 22–8).

A delay of only a few days will result in shrinking of the distal perineurial tubes and make repair slightly more difficult.

A secondary repair after scar and neuroma formation have occurred requires a resection of the scar regardless of whether the nerve repair is to be perineurial or epineurial. If a funicular juncture is to be used, then the multiple new funicular sprouts must be removed until a normal funicular anatomy is reached. This may leave a sufficient gap so that a graft is required.

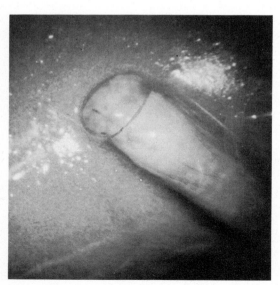

Figure 22–6 The intrafunicular contents of the funiculus are protruding.

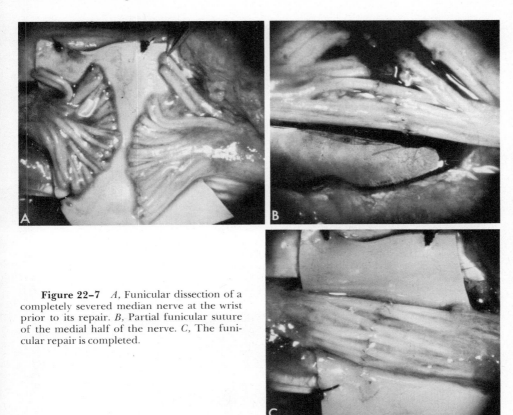

Figure 22–7   *A*, Funicular dissection of a completely severed median nerve at the wrist prior to its repair. *B*, Partial funicular suture of the medial half of the nerve. *C*, The funicular repair is completed.

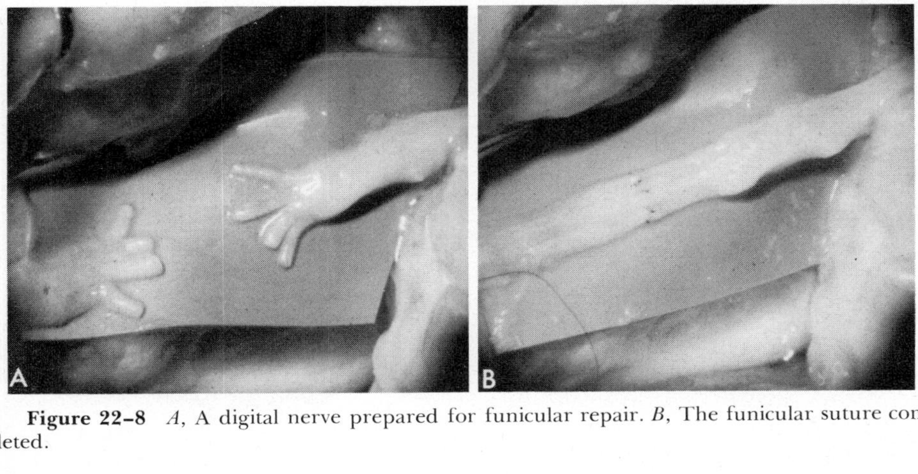

Figure 22–8   *A*, A digital nerve prepared for funicular repair. *B*, The funicular suture completed.

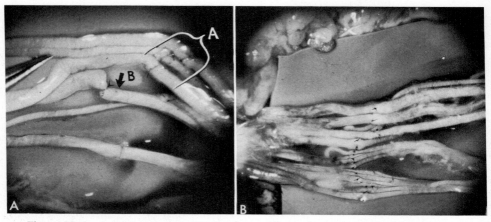

Figure 22-9 *A,* Funicular graft. Graft segments (forceps) are sutured individually (A). Note one funiculus (B) with only one suture in place has poor approximation. *B,* Completed funicular graft of ulnar nerve. Note the varying sizes of the funiculi.

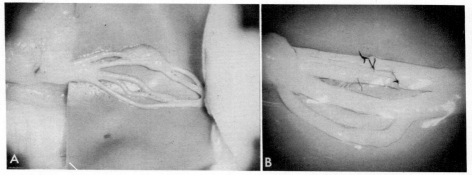

Figure 22-10 *A,* Partially divided digital nerve with some sensory loss and a painful neuroma. Two funiculi had been severed. *B,* Repair of the two severed funiculi resulted in improved sensation and loss of neuroma tenderness.

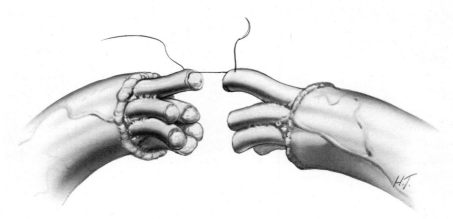

Figure 22-11 Perineurial suture of a typical nerve.

FUNICULAR GRAFT TECHNIQUE

The sural nerve is the best donor. It may be removed while the patient is supine, but this is carried out more easily in the prone position, particularly if both 'sural nerves are to be removed. Frequently, the grafts are removed and prepared the day prior to insertion if the necessity for grafting is known. These may then be stored at 4° C overnight. Blood storage refrigerators are kept at this temperature.

On a moist plastic surface, each funiculus is dissected free from the others. The funiculus is kept as a unit until branching occurs, at which spot it is transected. Usually the larger funiculi in the nerve are the ones most suitable. These funicular lengths are then stored overnight in a sealed jar with a lightly moistened sponge. Then, after preparation of the proximal and distal nerve stumps in the manner described above, these funiculi are trimmed to the necessary length and suturing is carried out (Fig. 22–9).

The original proximal–distal orientation of the graft funiculi is thought to be not important. The proximal nerve stump will usually have more funiculi than the distal and, therefore, all distal junctures are made first. These are then covered with a piece of plastic to prevent them from sticking to gloves or gowns, and then the proximal junctures are carried out. An attempt is made to place grafted material in a vascular bed of muscle, fat, or areolar tissue.

It is not yet possible to define the usefulness of fascicular repair because, at the present time, insufficient nerves have been repaired and followed. Preliminary results are as follows. In digital nerve repairs on a funicular basis, there were 14 cases, age over 21, followed for one year or more. In these cases, the Von Frey tests were 2.57 compared with a normal of 1.65. Two-point discrimination was 9.82 (if all patients with no two-point at all were measured as 15 for purposes of obtaining an average).

There were 27 patients with epineurial repairs with the same qualifications. In these, Von Frey tests equaled 2.55 and two-point discrimination 7.63. This indicates that there is approximately the same result from each. In nerve grafts with the same qualifications, there were two cases which had epineurial grafts and these both had a Von Frey of 1.65 and a two-point of 15 (no two-point discrimination at all). There were six fascicular nerve grafts done on digital nerves; these had a Von Frey of 1.9 and a two-point of 9.5.

There have been insufficient numbers of median and ulnar nerves above the wrist to draw general conclusions. Nevertheless, in my opinion, at the present state of the art of repair of complete nerve injury, there is no conclusive evidence that an isolated fascicular suture produces a better result than an epineural repair. When possible, I prefer suture of single large fasciculi and groups of small fasciculi. Fascicular repair has a distinct role when repairing partial nerve lesions and complete lesions located at sites of branching of peripheral nerves. With partial lesions uninjured funiculi can be preserved while the specific injured fasciculi can be mended (Figs. 22–10*B* and 22–11).

REFERENCES

Bora, F. W.: Peripheral nerve repair in cats: The fascicular stitch. J. Bone Joint Surg., *49A*:659, 1967.
Sunderland, S.: Nerves and Nerve Injury. Baltimore, Williams & Wilkins Co., 1968, Chaps. 7, 8, 29, 30, 45.

23

MANAGEMENT OF NERVE GAPS

ROBERT J. SCHULTZ

A nerve gap may be defined as a break in the continuity of a nerve with actual loss of nerve substance, replacement of neural tissue by a non-functional segment, or retraction of the divided nerve ends. The extent of a gap may vary from a few millimeters to many centimeters.

Nerve gaps can occur at any level from the origin of the roots which emerge from the spinal cord to the distal aspect of the digits. One must, therefore, consider methods of closing gap lesions in each of these areas. Although it is impossible to anticipate or describe every possibility of nerve injury and gap, it is important to realize that lesions involving either the upper or the lower extremity frequently have pathological features in common. Thus it becomes necessary to establish basic principles which can be applied whatever the location or nature of the injury. The techniques available to bridge gaps include nerve stretching, nerve mobilization, epineurial or intraneural neurolysis, joint positioning, nerve transposition, nerve pedicles, nerve transfers, bone resection, soft tissue excision or release, and nerve grafting.

Aim of Reparative Technique

The aim of the technique of bridging a gap is to restore functional continuity to an injured nerve without producing tension at the suture line.

Etiology of Nerve Gap

The etiology of nerve gaps is varied. Most commonly, gaps are caused by the retraction of apposing ends of a severed nerve; however, they also result from crush injuries, missile injuries, nerve avulsion, and other forms of extensive trauma in which a large segment of a nerve is damaged or lost. In addition, resection of nerve tumors or neuromas that are in continuity with the nerve, or resection of terminal neuromas and gliomas at the time of secondary repair, can also cause nerve gaps.

388

As opposed to gaps caused by a physical break in the nerve, electrical injuries, injection injuries, ischemic injuries, and traction injuries can produce gaps in nerves that are still in continuity.

Whatever the etiology, the method of repair is essentially the same, and consists of resecting the scar, freshening the severed ends as in a primary repair, bringing together the apposing surfaces without tension, and, finally, neurorrhaphy.

Methods of Gap Closure

The choice of surgical procedure to bring about gap closure depends on many features: the extent of the gap; the anatomic location of the injury; the mechanism of injury; the particular nerve involved; the presence of associated injuries, such as an accompanying fracture or loss of bone stock at the same location; extensive soft tissue damage; multiple nerve loss; amputation or severe injury to distal parts; and the status of the opposite extremity as well as the pre-injury status of the involved extremity. Following neurorrhaphy, a nerve can be stretched without producing nerve damage, but one must have an understanding of the tensile strength and elasticity of nerves.

After thorough physical examination and accurate evaluation of motor and sensory deficits, surgical exploration of the injured nerve is the first step toward locating and evaluating the magnitude of the lesion. At surgery, the length of the gap is determined, which is the sum of nerve loss at the time of the original injury plus the resection of neuroma and glioma necessary to visualize the fascicular pattern.

Gap closure is generally accomplished either by producing an apparent increase in the length of the nerve or by decreasing the distance the segment of nerve has to transverse. Substitution or short-circuiting procedures are reserved for large defects or lesions in which the anticipated regeneration would require a prolonged period of time, resulting in significant functional loss.

1. Increasing apparent length
   a. Nerve stretching
   b. Nerve mobilization
   c. Nerve pedicles
   d. Nerve grafts
2. Decreasing distance the segment has to traverse
   a. Positioning of joints
   b. Nerve transposition from normal anatomic locations
   c. Shortening of long bones (especially when fracture or non-union coexists)
   d. Resection of transfixing bone
   e. Release or resection of restraining soft tissues

GENERAL CONCEPTS

Although it is necessary when writing a text to list procedures separately, more frequently than not in the actual management of nerve gaps, several methods are used concurrently and in different combinations. The selective choice of technique should proceed from the simplest to the most complex. It is also necessary to remember that nerve grafting, which will be covered in detail in another section, is an effective alternative (Chapter 24).

The ideal method of nerve gap closure is by direct suturing after fashioning the sectioned ends. This is only possible, however, in fresh injuries with a relatively short gap.

Nerve Stretching

The irregular course, natural undulations, and natural elasticity of a peripheral nerve permit a certain amount of length to be gained by stretching. This gain is relatively small, since the undulations and elasticity of the nerve soon reach their limit. This method used alone is useful for small gaps only.

Nerve Mobilization

Nerve mobilization, perhaps the commonest technique utilized for gaining length, is performed to some extent in almost every nerve repair procedure, since it takes advantage of the nerve's natural slack as it passes along its course. When mobilizing a nerve, magnification and fine dissecting instruments should be utilized. In addition to epineurial dissection, intraneural neurolysis can also be performed.

Nerve mobilization can be done over any segment along the course of the nerve, both distally and proximally, despite the anatomic location of the injury, the particular nerve involved, or the size of the defect. This technique can be accomplished beneath bridging muscles and, if necessary, muscles, ligaments, or restraining tissues can be released. An increase in the length of long nerves by as much as two to three centimeters can be obtained by this method alone.

There are, however, factors that limit the extent of nerve mobilization. These are the origin of branches from the nerve trunk and the ischemic effects secondary to loss of the epineural vessels as a consequence of extensive nerve stripping.

The presence of muscular branches limits nerve mobilization because of the relatively short course from the origin of the branch to the myoneural junction. When gaps occur in these locations, additional slack can be gained by intraneural dissection. The extent of intraneural dissection of a muscular branch, however, is extremely variable, being dependent upon the fascicular pattern of the nerve. Some fasciculi ascend only a short distance before losing their identity and intermingle with other fasciculi, limiting the length of permissible stripping; others may continue as independent fasciculi for greater distances.

In certain locations, muscular and/or articular branches can be sacrificed to gain length. Whether or not a branch should be sacrificed is determined by the judgment of the surgeon and the importance of the branch. Care must be taken, however, to prevent inadvertent laceration or avulsion of muscular branches during nerve mobilization at the gap area. Relaxation is obtained more easily by nerve mobilization when the lesions have occurred distal to muscular branches rather than proximal to their emergence from the main trunks (Fig. 23–1).

Neural ischemia can result from nerve stripping during mobilization. The vascularity of nerves is derived through longitudinal intra- and extraneural blood vessels. Peripheral nerves have a mesoneurium in which all vessels carrying blood to and from the nerve lie. This mesoneurium permits the blood to be transported from a fixed underlying bed to the nerve, while allowing the nerve to accommodate for changes in position and alterations in tension. A series of arcades within the mesoneurium provides a segmental circulation that supports the longitudinal vessels within the nerve. When nerves are isolated or separated from the mesoneurium over a distance greater than 6 to 8 cm, adequate circulation may not be maintained. Thus extensive stripping may cause a segment of nerve freed at surgery to function essentially as a free graft.

The extent of mobilization, therefore, should be limited to avoid significant vascular injury to the nerve. Technically, where possible, the vascular mesentery should be defined and the areolar tissue surrounding the neurovascular bundle containing the arteries, the capillaries, and the segmental muscular and direct

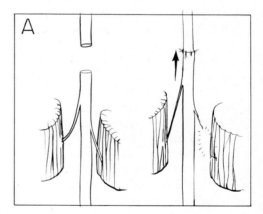

Figure 23–1 *A,* Closure of gap proximal to muscular branches produces traction on muscular branch and may even result in avulsion of branch. *B* Gap closure distal to muscular branches is more easily performed, since it produces relaxation of muscular branches.

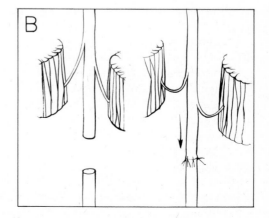

arterial branches preserved. In closing a gap, the traction necessary to take advantage of the natural slack in a nerve should be gentle and delicate, and not produce blanching of the vascular supply to the nerve.

Gap closure by nerve mobilization has these advantages: it permits good matching of the fascicular pattern; it produces only one suture line to be crossed by axonal tissue; and, if of limited length, it does not jeopardize the longitudinal intraneural blood supply.

Joint Positioning

Since extensive nerve stripping may produce ischemia, additional modalities should be employed, depending on the site of injury.

When the nerve gap occurs at or about an articulation that is not ankylosed, joint positioning can be performed to decrease the distance the nerve segment must traverse. When joint flexion is used in combination with nerve mobilization, less neural dissection is required, thus decreasing the potential damage to the vascular supply of the nerve. The joint should be displaced in the direction of the involved nerve but excessive flexion or extension is to be avoided.

The limiting factors in joint positioning are the amount of flexion needed to close the gap and the response of the nerve to the gradual stretching to which it will be subjected when postoperative extension of the joint is instituted. In general, it is not advisable to flex the elbow or knee more than 90 degrees, the wrist more than 40 degrees, and the ankle more than 10 degrees. If at all possible, it is better to flex the joint that is furthest from the suture line.

Stretching the nerve after suture causes increasing tension and possible intraneural fibrosis. Injudicious stretching, therefore, should be avoided, and other modalities employed to prevent the joint from being placed in extreme positions. As an example of the amount of gap that can be bridged by joint positioning, wrist flexion will permit a gain of 2.5 cm, and wrist flexion combined with elbow flexion will allow up to a total of 7.5 cm. Nine to 10 centimeters is the maximum distance over which a long nerve can be sutured and stretched without serious damage to both its proximal and distal stumps. The distal stump has more chance of being damaged by stretching than the proximal one.

Two important factors must be considered when stretching a nerve: (a) the magnitude of the force applied, and (b) the time over which the force acts on the nerve. Once the natural slack in a human nerve is taken up, the elastic limit of the nerve will be reached when it is elongated from 6 to 20 per cent of its mobilized length. Greater stretch will cause mechanical failure. Since at the time of surgery there is no way to evaluate the elastic limit of a damaged nerve in a given patient, stretch should not exceed 6 per cent in order not to jeopardize the final result.

Greater degrees of stretch can be more safely attained when the deformation is accomplished slowly over a prolonged period of time. With rapid stretch, the elastic limit of the nerve is rapidly exceeded. Thus, controlled return of the joint to its natural position, with the position being maintained by a brace or plaster splint, is recommended. Following suture line healing, the joint should be extended no more than 10 degrees per week.

Nerve Transposition

At times, nerves pass over the extensor (convex) surface of an articulation that bends only in one direction; for example, the ulnar nerve at the elbow. In these instances, joint flexion would produce not additional relaxation but the opposite effect: increased tension in the nerve. In these locations, nerve length can be obtained by transposition of the nerve from the extensor to the flexor surface. Large gaps can be closed by this method, since the slack now obtained is the total not only of nerve transposition but also of nerve mobilization plus joint flexion.

Nerve transposition is not limited to the extensor surfaces of joints. Nerves can be transposed about muscles (e.g., the median nerve can be rerouted anterior to the pronator teres), transposed about bones, whether the bone has been fractured or not (e.g., the radial nerve can be transposed anterior to the shaft of the humerus); and about ligaments (e.g., the motor branch of the ulnar nerve routed into the carpal canal).

Bone Shortening and Resection

In certain anatomic locations, fractures frequently accompany nerve injury. In these instances, especially when the fracture occurs in the shaft of a long bone where good approximation of bone ends can be obtained and good fixation anticipated, resection of bone can be performed to decrease the distance the nerve has to travel. This procedure is particularly suitable in old lesions when the nerve gap is associated with a non-union of the fracture. The amount of resection must be individualized in each case. Seddon has recommended up to 5 cm, while Massie has noted that the humerus could be shortened by one fifth of its length.

Nerve transposition can be performed in conjunction with bone shortening or prior to fracture reduction. These procedures can be employed even when the gap is at a distance from the fracture site.

At times, the anatomic position of a bone, or a bony protuberance, crosses the path of a nerve, as may be seen with the clavicle and brachial plexus, the supracondyloid process and the median nerve, or an osteocartilaginous exostosis of the proximal fibula and the peroneal nerve. In these instances, excision or resection of bone can be done to decrease the distance the nerve must travel and thus gain additional slack.

Soft Tissue Release

Soft tissues such as muscles, fascia, or transfixing ligaments frequently extend across the course of nerves. For example, the median nerve courses beneath the transverse carpal ligament and between the two heads of the pronator teres. At these locations, additional slack can be obtained by transection, excision, or release of crossing ligaments or muscles. This will be covered further in the ensuing pages.

MANAGEMENT OF LARGE GAPS

The term large gaps can be considered to encompass those lesions that cannot be bridged with the modalities presented. These injuries present special problems, and the prognosis for recovery is poor. The goal of treatment, in most instances, is the return of sensation.

Sensibility is altered, but can usually be regained; however, restoration of motor function is a bit more variable. Nerves which innervate large muscle masses and in which the level of injury is only a short distance from the site of innervation can be expected to give better results than those which innervate small muscles and the regenerative process must travel a greater distance to the motor end plates. Thus, for example, radial nerve injuries will produce better results than ulnar nerve injuries occurring at the same level in the arm.

The techniques utilized to bridge large defects are nerve pedicle procedures, nerve transfer procedures, and substitution procedures in which the nerve gap is short-circuited.

Nerve Pedicle Procedures

Nerve pedicle procedures were the product of the era when there was gloom over the results of free nerve grafts, which were believed to fail because of central necrosis and collagenization of the grafts from loss of vascularity. Nerve pedicle procedures were designed to transfer large segments of nerve from their original beds to another location while maintaining the blood supply.

Strange Procedure

In 1947, Strange described a method of gap closure for lesions greater than 12 cm utilizing a vascularized nerve pedicle. The aim of the procedure was to maintain the blood supply to the grafts through longitudinal intraneural vasa nervorum, comparable to the principle of full thickness skin pedicle grafting. Strange utilized the technique to bridge a 12 cm gap in the median nerve with a graft of the ulnar nerve which had been cut at the same level and had a similar gap. Since then, the technique has been used to bridge large gaps in other major nerves by utilizing an adjacent nerve.

Technique

The procedure requires two stages. The first consists of suturing the distal ends of both proximal segments of the two nerves together after resection of the terminal neuromas. Once the repair is complete, the donor nerve is incompletely sectioned proximally so that the segment from incomplete section to suture will be 2.5 to 5 cm longer than the gap to be spanned. The partial sectioning leaves intact a segment of epineurium containing the longitudinal vessels (Fig. 23–2A and B). This step permits the donor nerve to retain its blood supply and maintain suitable Schwann tubes for the axons to enter from the proximal stump of the primary nerve.

In the second stage, six weeks later, the proximal laceration in the donor

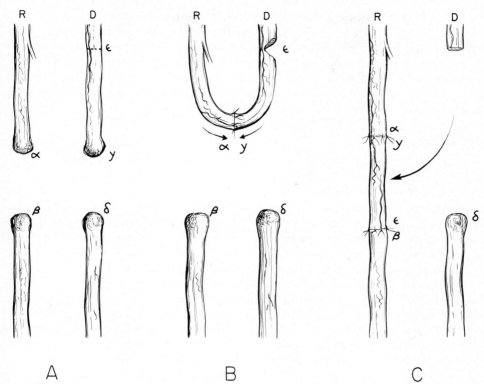

A   B   C

Figure 23–2 *A* and *B*, After resection of the neuromas, the proximal segments of both donor and recipient nerves are sutured together (points α–γ) and the donor nerve sectioned proximally, leaving intact a segment of epineurium containing longitudinal blood vessels (point ε). *C*, Six weeks later, the proximal laceration of the donor nerve (point ε) is completed and sutured to the distal stump of the recipient nerve (point ε–β). (After Strange, F.G. St.C.: Brit. J. Surg., *37*:574, 1959.)

graft is completed. The nerve is then mobilized, leaving the anastomosis intact, threaded through the subcutaneous tissue and sutured to the distal stump of the recipient nerve (Fig. 23–2*C*). In this technique, the gap is bridged while the graft retains its blood supply across the first suture line. The procedure is designed to avoid any period of ischemia, thus preserving the viability of Schwann cells and allowing the axons to traverse a vascularized graft.

Indications

Since the procedure involves sacrifice of one major nerve to regain function of a more important nerve, its application is limited. The principle, however, is applicable in the treatment of extensive combined nerve injuries, so that, for example, a damaged ulnar or radial nerve can be used for the median nerve, and a damaged lateral popliteal nerve for the medial popliteal nerve. The procedure can also be utilized where there is loss of the terminal digits and the sensibility supplied by the donor nerve is no longer needed.

Edgerton Procedure

In a modification of the Strange procedure, proposed by Edgerton (1968), the contralateral extremity is utilized to supply the donor nerve. This procedure is designed to transfer the nerve pedicle while maintaining its longitudinal intraneural blood supply through its entire length and its peripheral circulation to one half its length at all times during transfer. In this procedure, the graft receives its longitudinal intraneural blood supply through the anastomosis and maintains its peripheral blood supply from the surrounding tissues, which envelop one half its total length. The method utilizes cross arm pedicles and requires two stages. Proper skin coverage must be present before attempting pedicle transfer.

Technique

Stage I. The injured left median nerve is exposed and the length of its defect determined. Following this step the donor right ulnar nerve is exposed and freed to one half of the appropriate graft length. The right ulnar nerve is then severed at its distal end, introduced into the left forearm through a subcutaneous tunnel, and sutured to the proximal stump of the median nerve. Upon completion of the anastomosis, the donor right ulnar nerve is sectioned at its proximal end, leaving the mesoneurium intact. The skin incisions are closed and both forearms are immobilized together in a crossed position (Fig. 23–3*A*).

Stage II. Four weeks later, the skin bridge between the two forearms is released. The remaining segment of the ulnar nerve graft is dissected free from the donor forearm to the level of the previous partial neurectomy and the neurectomy completed. The graft is then routed through a subcutaneous tunnel in the distal forearm and wrist and sutured to the distal stump of the recipient median nerve (Fig. 23–3*B*).

Indications

The indications for this technique are extremely limited, being reserved for large defects in a major nerve when there is significant injury to two extremities.

In addition to arm to arm transfers, lower to upper extremity transfers can also be performed; for example, an uninjured ipsilateral lateral popliteal nerve can be used to bridge a defect of the median nerve, if the distal portion of the ipsilateral foot is severely injured and beyond salvage.

Nerve Transfer Procedures

Nerve transfer procedures can be utilized to restore motor or sensory function by direct anastomosis of the proximal segment of an available nerve to the distal stump of the injured nerve. As with nerve pedicles, the sacrificed nerve should be one whose absence will not result in significant disability, and the need to restore function to the recipient nerve should be important enough to be worth the sacrifice. This, of course, limits the use of the procedure, since a suitable donor nerve that can be sacrificed is not always adjacent to the distal stump of the injured nerve, permitting the cross anastomosis. This can, however, be overcome by tapping the donor nerve into the recipient nerve at a more distal level, as described in the lumbrical nerve transfer.

To restore nerve function in the extremities, Lurje (1948) transferred a musculocutaneous nerve, which was sectioned between the innervation of the biceps and the brachialis muscle to an irreparable radial nerve. To provide sensa-

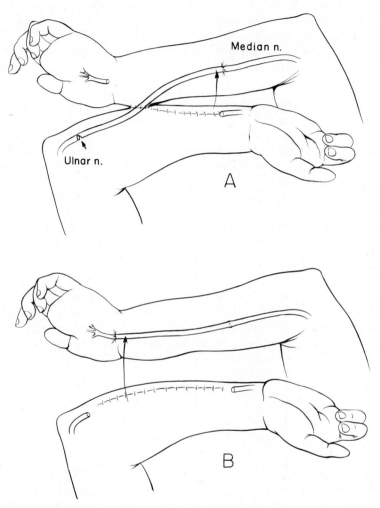

Figure 23–3 *A,* The distal end of donor ulnar nerve is sutured to the proximal segment of the recipient median nerve. Note that the longitudinal blood supply remains intact, as does one half of the peripheral blood supply. *B,* Four weeks later, the segment of ulnar nerve is freed and sutured to distal stump of recipient median nerve. (After Edgerton, M. T.: Surgery, *64*:1, 1968, p. 251.)

tion in the palm, Turnbull (1948) transferred the superficial radial nerve to the distal stump of the median nerve. Similarly, Sunderland (1968) has recommended transfer of the dorsal cutaneous branch of the ulner nerve to restore sensation to an irreparable median nerve. Nerve transfers have also been useful in the restitution of facial nerve function.

In high nerve lesions, or when large gaps are present, sensation can frequently be restored by some procedure; however, motor function, especially of the small muscles, does not return. A nerve transfer utilizing branches from an intact nerve close to the myoneural junction can produce an anastomosis so that muscle reinnervation can occur early.

Lumbrical Nerve Transfer (Motor Transfer)

Schultz and Aiache (1972) described a nerve transfer procedure in which a motor branch of the ulnar nerve supplying the ring finger lumbrical muscle is transferred to the thenar motor branch of the median nerve. The procedure is designed to restore thumb opposition in high median nerve injury or when an extensive gap along the course of the median nerve exists and motor function to the thenar muscles is not expected to be restored.

In the presence of a gap, only a small segment of the distal stump of the motor median nerve need remain.

Technique

The motor branch to the ring finger lumbrical muscle is identified and dissected from the muscle to gain as much length as possible. The branch to the interosseous muscle is left intact. The motor median nerve is then identified and transected as close to the thenar muscles as the length of the lumbrical nerve will permit. A direct anastomosis is then performed (Fig. 23–4).

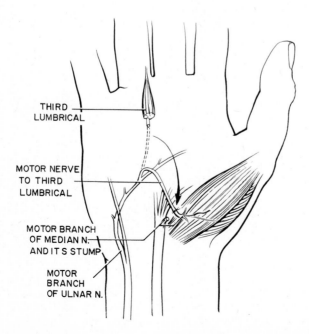

THIRD
LUMBRICAL

MOTOR NERVE
TO THIRD
LUMBRICAL

MOTOR BRANCH
OF MEDIAN N.
AND ITS STUMP

MOTOR
BRANCH
OF ULNAR N.

Figure 23–4 The motor branch to the ring finger lumbrical is severed as distally as possible and a direct repair is made to the motor median nerve close to the myoneural junction. (After Schultz, R. J., and Aiache, A.: Arch. Surg., *105:* 777, 1972.)

Indications

The indications for the procedure are high nerve injuries or the presence of nerve gaps where critical muscle function will be lost. It is, of course, important to have the donor and recipient nerves in close proximity.

Innervated Skin Island Flap Transfers (Sensory Transfer)

The maintenance of median nerve sensation is critical. Where an extensive median nerve gap exists and sensation is not expected to return, a neurovascular skin island flap transfer from nearby innervated dermatomes offers a sensory function substitute for the pinching and grasping areas of the thumb and index finger.

Technique

One half the pulp with the complete neurovascular bundle is dissected free of the donor finger. The free island of skin with its intact neurovascular bundle is taken to the thumb and index finger through a tunnel under the skin, spanning between the donor and the recipient areas. (Chapter 48.)

MANAGEMENT OF INDIVIDUAL NERVE PROBLEMS

The principles of bridging gaps have been presented, and we can now apply these principles to individual nerve problems. Every nerve has an area that is particularly vulnerable to injury and where most of the lesions occur. To apply the techniques of nerve gap closure, knowledge of the anatomic course of the nerve and of the level of muscular branches is of paramount importance.

Brachial Plexus

Nerve Course

The brachial plexus is formed by the junction of the roots of the anterior primary divisions of the last four cervical and the first thoracic nerves. These roots then combine to form trunks, followed by divisions, cords, branches, and finally the terminal nerves. The brachial plexus spans the posterior cervical triangle, passing to the axilla and then distally, in the form of peripheral nerves, to the extremities.

In addition to its major peripheral nerves, the brachial plexus also has collateral branches, namely the suprascapular, anterior thoracic, scapular, and axillary nerves.

Methods of Nerve Gap Closure

Unfortunately, the results of surgery in this region are still disappointing. Surgery is usually not indicated in traction injuries when the continuity of the nerve is intact because of the possibility of spontaneous functional recovery. Nerve gaps, however, which are the result of division of the nerve roots, trunks, divisions, or cords, should be repaired by direct end to end neurorrhaphy whenever possible. The method utilized to close these nerve gaps is a combination of nerve mobilization and proper positioning of the neck and shoulders to shorten the distance. Nerve grafting, which perhaps is a better technique in this location, will be covered in another section.

The initial gain in length is obtained by nerve mobilization. The collateral branches of the plexus (suprascapular, anterior thoracic, subscapular, and axillary nerves), however, limit mobilization in this region. When this occurs, and more length is needed, careful intraneural neurolysis of the collateral nerves proximally permits some additional length to be obtained.

If a gap still exists, then shortening the distance the nerve must traverse can be accomplished by bending the neck toward the side of the lesion and placing the shoulder into internal rotation and adduction with the arm across the chest. Elevation of the shoulder along with flexion of the elbow is also of assistance.

Median Nerve

Etiology of Nerve Gap

A nerve gap may be produced in any region along the course of the nerve. Most commonly, however, the median nerve is injured at the wrist by sharp trauma. Fractures about the elbow can produce involvement of the median nerve secondary to Volkmann's ischemic contracture.

Nerve Course

The median nerve originates from the brachial plexus and is composed of fibers from C6, C7, C8, and T1. In the arm, it accompanies the brachial artery; as it passes into the cubital fossa, it leaves the artery to pass between the two heads of the pronator teres, descending the forearm in the midline between the flexor digitorum superficialis and profundus. It becomes superficial in the distal forearm and enters the palm through the carpal tunnel to end as a motor branch to the thenar and radial two lumbrical muscles, and cutaneous sensory branches to the radial three and one half digits.

The median nerve gives no motor branches in the arm. The branches to the pronator teres, flexor carpi radialis, palmaris longus, and flexor digitorum superficialis arise in the cubital fossa and the forearm. The flexor pollicis longus, pronator quadratus, and radial half of the flexor digitorum profundus are innervated through its anterior interosseous branch.

Methods of Nerve Gap Closure

The median nerve is perhaps the most important nerve of the upper limb, since it provides critical sensation to the thumb, index and long fingers and in addition, it provides the thumb with its essential movement of opposition. Since hand function is severely curtailed in the absence of the median nerve, all efforts should be directed to restoring the continuity of this nerve.

Gap closure of the median nerve utilizes many of the techniques previously described, with the level of injury as well as the length of gap dictating the procedure. Mobilization of the nerve with proximal stripping of its muscular branches produces approximately 2.5 cm of length. Approximately 5 cm of additional slack can be gained by elbow flexion, and 2.5 cm by wrist flexion, while transposition of the nerve anterior to the pronator teres provides another 1 to 2 cm. Release of the tendinous origin of the deep head of the pronator teres alone can yield 1 cm of length.

Level of Injury

GAPS IN THE ARM. The median nerve forms from the branches of the plexus at about the level of the pectoralis minor and descends in close relation to the brachial artery. Gaps in this region are usually the result of severe trauma and are frequently associated with laceration of the brachial artery. Since the median nerve has no muscular branches in the arm, nerve mobilization can be effectively utilized. If a gap still exists, elbow flexion and release of the deep head of the pronator teres can be employed to bring the ends together, especially in lesions involving the distal arm.

Since nerve gaps in this region are commonly the result of severe trauma, fracture of the humerus may coexist. In these instances, shortening of the humerus, especially if the fracture involves the mid-humerus, can produce additional relaxation in order to close the gap.

GAPS ABOUT THE ELBOW. Nerve mobilization is limited in lesions in the antecubital fossa or proximal forearm because of the presence of the multiple muscular branches that innervate the forearm flexor muscles of the wrist and fingers. To reduce the postoperative stretching that accompanies joint positioning when motion is instituted, short gaps that remain after nerve mobilization should be closed by intraneural dissection of the muscular branches whenever possible. Larger gaps, however, will require varying degrees of elbow flexion as well as release of the pronator teres with anterior transposition of the nerve. Bone resection must be judiciously considered in this region because of the altered configuration of the distal humerus and difficulty in obtaining good end to end approximation.

GAPS IN THE FOREARM. In the forearm, the nerve runs a straight course deep to the flexor digitorum superficialis, and nerve mobilization can be effectively used. If necessary, positioning of the elbow and wrist into flexion can be utilized to gain additional length.

GAPS AT THE WRIST AND PALM. The wrist is the most common site of median nerve laceration, and gaps are usually the result of delayed repair for a laceration or trauma inflicted by blunt objects or crush injuries. As in all other areas, gaps are first bridged by local nerve mobilization. An additional 2.5 cm can be gained by wrist flexion. Excessive wrist flexion should be avoided, since it results in poor drainage and venous return as well as in placing the hand in poor position for finger flexor function.

Gaps occurring in the motor median nerve or involving a segment of the main trunk of the median nerve which, because of fixation by the motor median nerve, limit mobilization, can be overcome by intraneural proximal dissection of the fascicles of the motor median nerve.

Large Defects

When extensive injuries of the median nerve accompany concomitant extensive injuries of the ulnar or radial nerve, or both, a nerve pedicle graft utilizing either of these nerves as a donor may be considered. Nerve pedicles from the ulnar nerve may also be indicated when a large gap in the median nerve exists and there has been concomitant loss of the distal ulnar rays of the hand and palm. The Strange procedure or, in selected instances, the Edgerton procedure may be used to bridge the gap in the median nerve.

In high injuries or severe lesions of the median nerve where the possibility of thenar muscle function return is doubtful, the lumbrical nerve transfer may be considered.

Ulnar Nerve

Etiology of Nerve Gap

The ulnar nerve can be injured in any area along its route; however, like the median nerve, it is most commonly injured by lacerations at the wrist, usually proximal, but at times through Guyon's canal.

Nerve Course

The ulnar nerve is the terminal continuation of the medial cord of the brachial plexus, arising from C7-T1. It traverses the axilla medial to the axillary artery and passes into the arm accompanied by the brachial artery. In the middle third of the arm, the nerve pierces the medial intermuscular septum and descends behind the medial humeral epicondyle. In the forearm, it assumes a volar course, passing first between the two heads of the flexor carpi ulnaris and then deep to it. Accompanied by the ulnar artery, it enters the palm through Guyon's canal, where it divides to terminate into its superficial cutaneous and deep motor branches.

Branches arise behind the medial epicondyle passing to the elbow joint and the flexor carpi ulnaris, and distal to the medial epicondyle going to the ulnar half of the flexor digitorum profundus and flexor carpi ulnaris.

Methods of Nerve Gap Closure

Of all the nerves, the ulnar is perhaps the most amenable to the bridging of gaps. Mobilization of the nerve along with stripping of the motor branches will permit closure of gaps up to 2.5 cm. Further relaxation of 2.5 to 5 cm. can be gained by transposition of the nerve anteriorly from behind the medial epicondyle. Flexion of the elbow after anterior transposition adds a further 5 cm., while flexion of the wrist slackens the nerve by another 2.5 cm.

Level of Injury

GAPS IN THE ARM.   The ulnar nerve gives no branches in its course through the arm. It descends from the branches of the brachial plexus, piercing the medial intramuscular septum to arise posterior to the medial epicondyle of the elbow. As with the median nerve, it is usually injured in this region as a result of severe trauma.

Gaps in the ulnar nerve at the level of the arm are closed primarily by nerve mobilization. If further relaxation is necessary, transposition of the ulnar nerve anterior to the medial epicondyle, followed by elbow flexion, can then be employed. Should a humeral fracture accompany an extensive defect in the nerve, resection and shortening of the humerus can be performed in order to produce additional relaxation to close the gap.

GAPS ABOUT THE ELBOW.   At the level of the elbow, the ulnar nerve begins to give off its muscular and articular branches. Gaps at the distal arm, proximal forearm, and elbow can be closed by nerve mobilization as well as by anterior nerve transposition and elbow flexion. The articular branches to the elbow may be sacrificed and the branch to the flexor carpi ulnaris dissected by intraneural neurolysis, if necessary. Release of the humeral head of the flexor carpi ulnaris will provide additional length. Further nerve mobilization can be performed by dissection between the two heads of the flexor carpi ulnaris. Extensive gaps can be closed by these methods without tension at the sutured ends.

GAPS IN THE FOREARM.   Gaps at this level are difficult to bridge by just utilizing joint positioning in addition to nerve mobilization. Nerve transposition at the elbow frequently is necessary to gain enough slack to close the gap. If a fracture of both bones of the forearm occurs, bone shortening can also be utilized.

GAPS AT THE WRIST AND PALM.   As with the median nerve, this is the most common location for laceration of the ulnar nerve. Gaps in this location can be closed by nerve mobilization and wrist flexion. The unroofing of the volar carpal ligament overlying the Loge de Guyon can help produce additional length. Resection of the tendinous component of the flexor carpi ulnaris as it passes to its insertion will also produce additional slack, if necessary.

After the Loge de Guyon, the deep branch of the ulnar nerve becomes a pure motor nerve as it passes across the palm. In this area, nerve mobilization is extremely difficult and can only be used to close small defects. A technique that can be employed has been described by Boyes. In this technique, the motor branch is mobilized and transposed into the carpal tunnel in order to shorten the distance it must traverse in order to accomplish the repair (Fig. 23–5).

Radial Nerve

Etiology of Nerve Gap

The radial nerve is most commonly injured in association with the fractures of the humeral shaft, since it is in intimate contact with the bone running in the spiral groove. Simple lacerations usually involve the superficial sensory branch and can also arise iatrogenically during surgical procedures on the forearm and wrist.

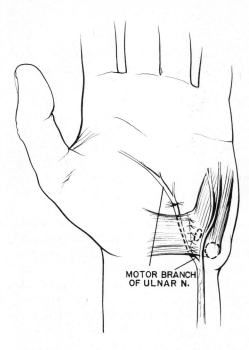

Figure 23–5 The motor branch of the ulnar nerve has been rerouted into the carpal canal in order to overcome a neural gap. (After Boyes, J. H.: J. Bone Joint Surg., *37A*:921, 1955.)

MOTOR BRANCH
OF ULNAR N.

Nerve Course

The radial nerve is the continuation of the posterior cord of the brachial plexus and is composed of fibers from C5, C6, C7, C8, and sometimes T1. In the arm, it is in intimate contact with the posterior humeral spiral groove and appears anterolaterally in the lower third of the arm after piercing the lateral intermuscular septum. It crosses the cubital fossa anterior to the lateral epicondyle and divides into a superficial cutaneous and deep motor branch called the posterior interosseous nerve. The superficial branch of the radial nerve runs along the lateral border of the forearm under cover of the brachioradialis, and, in the lower third of the forearm, angles toward the dorsum of the wrist to divide into cutaneous branches. The posterior interosseous nerve courses about the proximal radius, traversing between the two heads of the supinator muscle to appear on the extensor surface of the forearm where it arborizes to innervate the muscles of the extensor compartment.

Muscular branches arise from the radial nerve in the axilla to supply the medial and long heads of the triceps. In the spiral groove motor branches also appear to supply the medial and lateral heads of the triceps and the anconeus.

Methods of Gap Closure

GAPS IN THE ARM. A nerve gap involving the radial nerve in the axilla and upper arm proximal to its muscular branches to the triceps can be closed to a limited extent by nerve mobilization. Additional length, if needed, can be gained by placing the shoulder in adduction and external rotation. Distal to the motor branches to the triceps, nerve mobilization can gain about 2.5 cm. in length. If necessary, an additional 2.5 cm. can be obtained by transposing the nerve anterior to the humerus, followed by neurorrhaphy. Once the nerve is transposed anteriorly, a further gain of 2.5 cm. can be obtained by flexion of the elbow joint.

Since fractures of the midshaft of the humerus frequently accompany radial nerve disruption, shortening the humerus at the fracture site can be utilized to bring the gap edges together.

GAPS AT THE ELBOW.   At the elbow, the radial nerve passes anterior to the lateral condyle of the humerus, and shortly thereafter pierces the supinator muscle, dividing into its superficial sensory branch and the posterior interosseous nerve.

Lacerations that occur at the level of the elbow can be closed by nerve mobilization and elbow flexion.

The posterior interosseous nerve can be mobilized by dissecting it free as it traverses the supinator muscle. Since there are numerous muscular branches in its course, both proximal to and distal to the supinator, as well as to the supinator, intraneural neurolysis may be necessary in order to gain enough slack to close the gap.

GAPS IN THE FOREARM.   As the superficial branch of the radial nerve passes in a straight course and gives no branches in the forearm, gaps can usually be closed by nerve mobilization. Extensive dissection to bridge the gap is not necessary and is contraindicated, since this nerve is purely sensory to the extensor surface of the hand. The main disability when the nerve is severed is painful neuroma formation.

Femoral Nerve

Etiology of Nerve Gap

The femoral nerve is most often injured by penetrating wounds of the lower abdomen, which frequently accompany injury to the femoral or iliac vessels.

Nerve Course

The femoral nerve is the largest branch of the lumbar plexus and is formed by union of posterior divisions of L2, L3, and L4 roots. It accompanies the iliac artery and then enters the anterior aspect of the thigh deep to the inguinal ligament where it accompanies the femoral artery on its lateral side. Just distal to the inguinal ligament, it divides into cutaneous sensory branches and muscular branches to the anterior muscles of the thigh. Muscular branches to the iliacus muscle are given off within the abdomen.

Methods of Closing Nerve Gap

Large gaps can be closed by mobilization of the nerve both proximally and distally in conjunction with flexion of the hip. This method can produce enough length to bridge an 8 to 10 cm gap.

Level of Injury

Intrapelvic lacerations are usually the result of penetrating injuries. These lesions can be closed by nerve mobilization, and, if necessary, additional length can be gained by hip flexion. At the level of the inguinal ligament, nerve mobilization is less effective, since the nerve soon divides into its terminal branches. (Hip flexion can be used if necessary to enact gap closure.)

Sciatic Nerve

Etiology of Nerve Gap

The sciatic nerve is usually injured by penetrating wounds of the thigh or buttocks; damage can also be associated with posterior fracture dislocations of the hip.

Nerve Course

The sciatic nerve, the largest nerve in the body, is the continuation of the greatest part of the sacral plexus and is composed of fibers from L4, L5, S1, S2, and S3. Although variations do occur, it usually leaves the pelvis through the sciatic notch and descends in the posterior thigh deep to the gluteus maximus, midway between the ischial tuberosity and the greater trochanter. The muscular branches to the hamstrings arise in the gluteal region and the proximal thigh. The nerve terminates in the distal third of the thigh as the common peroneal and tibial nerves.

Methods of Nerve Gap Closure

As with the nerves of the upper extremity, gap closure in the sciatic nerve utilizes a variety of the techniques previously described.

Mobilization of the nerve, especially distal to its muscular branches, accompanied by proximal intraneural neurolysis of muscular branches, can produce approximately 3 cm of slack. Extension of the hip gives an additional nerve length of 2 cm, and flexion of the knee a further slack of 5 cm. Femoral shortening may be utilized to gain further length in the presence of a fresh fracture or non-union of a femoral fracture.

Level of Injury

GLUTEAL REGION. Since the sciatic nerve gives off muscular branches in the hip and gluteal region, mobilization of the nerve can be extremely limited, and requires intraneural neurolysis. Release of the piriformis muscle as well as the internal obturator and gemellus muscles may assist in producing additional length. Extension of the hip can be utilized; however, this position may be extremely uncomfortable for the patient.

THIGH. Since this nerve is extremely important in providing sensation to the sole of the foot, and muscle function to the entire leg and foot, gap closure is extremely important. Mobilization of the sciatic nerve in the thigh can be effectively utilized to gain length, since the muscular branches arise more proximally. Flexion of the knee will produce additional length if necessary.

If, by chance, a fracture accompanies the nerve laceration, bone shortening of 1 to 2 cm may be utilized to gain nerve closure without producing significant alterations in gait due to leg length discrepancy.

Posterior Tibial Nerve

Etiology of Nerve Gap

The posterior tibial nerve can be injured by penetrating wounds of the leg, by fractures of the upper end of the tibia, and by ischemia.

Nerve Course

The posterior tibial nerve, the larger of the two terminal branches of the sciatic nerve, begins its course in the distal third of the thigh and passes through the middle of the popliteal fossa. At the distal angle of the popliteal fossa, it disappears beneath the soleus muscle, descends straight down on the posterior tibial muscle, and finally enters the sole of the foot beneath the medial deltoid ligament where it divides into the medial and lateral plantar nerves supplying the skin and the muscles of the plantar surface of the foot.

Muscular branches arise in the popliteal fossa for both heads of the gastrocnemius, plantaris, soleus, and popliteal muscles. A second set of branches, arising more distally, supplies the soleus, posterior tibial, flexor digitorum longus, and flexor hallucis longus muscles.

Methods of Nerve Gap Closure

The posterior tibial nerve supplies the greatest area of sensation to the sole of the foot and, in this respect, assumes the same importance in the foot as the median nerve does in the hand.

Gaps up to 10 cm can be closed by a combination of mobilization of the nerve and flexion of the knee joint. For larger gaps that cannot be bridged by the common methods, the lateral popliteal nerve can be used as a pedicle graft, utilizing the Strange technique, providing the criteria of damage to both nerves has been met.

Common Peroneal Nerve

Etiology of Nerve Gap

The common peroneal nerve is more prone to injury than the posterior tibial nerve because it is more prone to stretch between its two anchor points, the sciatic notch and the fibular neck.

Nerve Course

The common peroneal nerve is the smaller of the two terminal divisions of the sciatic nerve and separates from the sciatic nerve approximately at the distal third of the thigh. Here it deviates laterally in the popliteal fossa; passing in intimate contact with the fibular neck, entering the anterior compartment of the leg where it divides into the superficial and deep peroneal nerves.

The common peroneal nerve does not give any muscular branches in the popliteal fossa.

Methods of Nerve Gap Closure

Mobilization of the nerve produces about 5 cm of slack, while flexion of the knee permits an additional 5 cm. In the region of the fibular neck, where the nerve passes in intimate contact to the bone, excision of the upper end of the fibula will contribute to an increase in nerve slack in order to produce gap closure.

Gain in length distal to the fibular neck is limited because of its division into branches. Bridging of this nerve is not absolutely necessary, since substitution procedures such as tendon transfers are available.

REFERENCES

Babcock, W. W.: A standard technique in operations on peripheral nerves with special reference to the closure of large gaps. Surg. Gynecol. Obstet. *45*:364, 1927.

Boyes, J. H.: Repair of the motor branch of the ulnar nerve in the palm. J. Bone Joint Surg. *37A*:920, 1955.

Dandy, W. E.: A method of restoring nerves, requiring resection, shortening of humerus by oblique osteotomy and wiring. J.A.M.A. *122*:35, 1943.

Edgerton, M. T.: Cross arm nerve pedicle flap for reconstruction of major defects of the median nerve. Surgery *64*:248, 1968.

Finseth, F., Constable, J. D., and Cannon, B.: Interfascicular nerve grafting. Early experience at the Massachusetts General Hospital. Plast. Reconstr. Surg. *56(5)*:492, 1975.

Highet, W. B., and Sanders, F. K.: The effect of stretching nerves after suture. Br. J. Surg. *30*:355, 1943.

Hoen, T. I., and Brackett, C. I.: Peripheral nerve lengthening. J. Neurosurg. *13*:43, 1956.

Holmes, W., Highet, W. B., and Seddon, H. J.: Ischaemic nerve lesions occurring in Volkmann's contracture. Br. J. Surg. *32*:259, 1944.

Learmonth, J. R.: Technique for transplanting the ulnar nerve. Surg. Gynecol. Obstet. *75*:729, 1942.

Littler, J. W.: Neurovascular skin island transfer in reconstructive hand surgery. Trans. Intl. Soc. Plast. Surg. 2nd Congress, London, 1959, p. 175.

Liu, C. T., Benda, C. E., and Lewey, F. H.: Tensile strength of human nerves: Experimental, physical and histological study. Arch. Neurol. Psychiat. *59*:322, 1948.

Livingston, W. K., Davis, E. W., and Livingston, K. E.: "Delayed recovery" in peripheral nerve lesions caused by high velocity projectile wounding. J. Neurosurg. *2*:170, 1945.

Llunch, A. L.: Ulnar entrapment after anterior transposition at elbow. N.Y. State J. Med. *75(1)*:75, 1975.

Lurje, A. S.: Use of N. musculocutaneus for neurotization of N. radius in cases of very large defects in the latter. Ann. Surg. *128*:110, 1948.

Millesi, H., Meissl, G., and Berger, A.: Further experience in interfascicular grafting of the median, ulnar and radial nerves. J. Bone Joint Surg. *58A(2)*:209, 1976.

Puckett, W. O., Grundfest, H., McElroy, W. D., and McMillen, J. H.: Damage to peripheral nerves by high velocity missiles without direct hit. J. Neurosurg. *3*:294, 1946.

Sanders, F. K.: The repair of large gaps in peripheral nerves. Brain *65*:281, 1942.

Schultz, R. J., and Aiache, A.: An operation to restore opposition of the thumb by nerve transfer. Arch. Surg. *105*:777, 1972.

Smith, J. W.: Factors influencing nerve repair. Blood supply of peripheral nerves. Arch. Surg. 93:335, 1966.

Smith, J. W.: Factors influencing nerve repair. Collateral circulation of peripheral nerves. Arch. Surg. 93:433–437, 1966.

Strange, F. G. St. Clair: An operation for nerve pedicle grafting, preliminary communication. Br. J. Surg. 34:423, 1947.

Strange, F. G. St. Clair: Case report on pedicled nerve graft. Br. J. Surg. 37:331, 1950.

Sunderland, S.: Nerves and nerve injuries. Baltimore, Williams & Wilkins, 1968.

Taylor, G. I., and Ham, F. J.: The free vascularized nerve graft. A further experimental and clinical application of microvascular techniques. Plast. Reconstr. Surg. 57(4):413, 1976.

Turnbull, F.: Radial median anastamosis. J. Neurosurg. 5:562, 1948.

24

NERVE GRAFTS: INDICATIONS, TECHNIQUES, AND PROGNOSIS

HANNO MILLESI

BASIC CONSIDERATIONS

The logical technique for the repair of a transected peripheral nerve is end-to-end neurorrhaphy. In this procedure there is only one gap and one suture site that the regenerating axon sprouts must cross to immediately reach the distal stump. In an ideal situation, with no nerve defect, the fascicular structures of the proximal and distal stumps are equal, and there is no jump in the fascicular pattern. If there is a defect caused by the changing fascicular pattern (Sunderland, 1952), a difference of the pattern exists which makes it more difficult for the axon sprouts to reach their proper peripheral destination. Having crossed the suture line, into the endoneurium of the distal stump, the axons immediately find an optimal environment within the Büngner bands, which are columns, or tubes, of proliferated Schwann cells. These Büngner bands represent the end stage of wallerian degeneration caused by the nerve injury.

If the distance between the two nerve stumps is bridged by a nerve graft, the regenerating axons must cross two suture lines, one at the proximal end and one at the distal end of the nerve graft. There are thus two jumps of the fascicular pattern. The environments that the axon sprouts meet within the

410

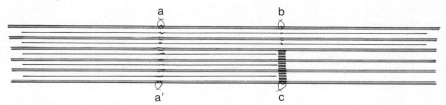

Figure 24–1 Schematic representation of nerve grafting. The proximal coaptation (a-a′) is crossed by axons. At the distal end only a part of the axons reaches the distal nerve stump (b). At (c) scar tissue blocks the further outgrowth of the axons. In this case the distal site of coaptation is to be resected in a second stage with a new coaptation.

nerve graft may be different, depending upon the survival of the graft. If graft survival is optimal, the environmental conditions are identical as in both nerve stumps. If graft survival is not optimal, fibrotic changes may impede the neurotization of the graft. The distal suture site may be blocked by scar tissue when the axon sprouts arrive (Fig. 24–1).

There is general agreement that under optimal conditions an end-to-end nerve repair offers the best chances of functional recovery. However, under less than optimal conditions, if end-to-end repair is impossible or unsuitable, nerve grafting offers excellent chances, provided that the unfavorable factors can be minimized. As these unfavorable factors play different roles in different techniques, we cannot discuss nerve grafts in general but, rather, must consider the value of a specific nerve grafting procedure.

Among the many factors to be considered, the following are the most important.
1. Survival of the nerve graft.
2. Optimal coaptation.
3. Optimal imitation and restoration of the fascicular pattern of the nerve to be repaired by the nerve grafts.
4. Minimal surgical trauma to reduce tissue damage.

Survival of Nerve Graft

Most nerve grafts are free grafts that are without blood supply for a period of time. Restoration of circulation is achieved by vessels ingrowing at the surface of the graft. Optimum survival therefore depends on a soft tissue bed that should contain many vessels and no, or minimal, scar tissue, and on the relation between the surface and the tissue mass of the graft. If a whole mixed nerve trunk is grafted as a free graft, fibrotic changes quite often occur in the center of the graft as a consequence of delayed restoration of blood supply. Thin skin nerves, having a more favorable relation between surface and mass, have a much better chance for complete survival if placed individually, with circumferential contact to the wound bed. This advantage is lost if the skin nerves are packed together to form a cable the size of the nerve to be repaired, as in the old cable graft technique (Seddon, 1947), because a great part of their surface is in contact with other grafts and not with the surrounding tissue.

To solve the problem of optimal survival of trunk grafts, the technique of pedicled nerve grafting (Strange, 1947) was developed, in which blood supply is preserved during the complete grafting procedure. However, this technique can only be used if two parallel running nerves are involved and one is sacrificed to reconstruct and preserve the continuity of the other.

In this era of microsurgery, free grafting of a nerve trunk, including its surrounding connective tissue, and a major vessel by microvascular anastomosis has been performed using the superficial peroneal and superficial radial nerves as donors (Taylor and Ham, 1976).

Optimal Coaptation

Optimal coaptation to achieve the best healing can be obtained only by reducing the tissue reaction at the suture sites. In an average nerve repair, under moderate tension, an unstructured gap develops between the two stumps that must be crossed by regenerating axon sprouts. The epineurium proliferates around the suture site and forms a fusiform thickening (Fig. 24–2). Ideal healing is achieved if the two nerve stumps are coapted exactly, under microsurgical vision, and tension at the suture site is completely avoided. Minimal surgical trauma is required, and minimal suture material is used. To delay the epineural reaction at the suture site, a strip of epineurium is resected at the proximal and distal stumps.

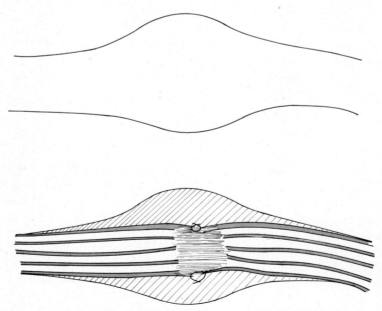

Figure 24–2 Scheme of a nerve repair showing the unstructured tissue between the stumps and the epineurial proliferation.

Restoration of Fascicular Pattern

Each nerve has an individual fascicular pattern. A trunk graft, even one from a corresponding donor nerve (e.g., median for median nerve), has no identical fascicular pattern. The differences in the pattern are much more pronounced if another nerve, such as the ulnar, is used to coaptate with the median nerve in the pedicle grafting technique. This is also true for free grafted nerve trunks with microvascular anastomosis. Optimal restoration of the fascicular pattern cannot be achieved. However, a rough restoration of the pattern may be accomplished after splitting the two nerve stumps into their individual fascicles and fascicular groups, respectively, by individual nerve grafts. The fascicular pattern of the peripheral nerve changes very rapidly at different levels (Sunderland, 1945). The plexiform arrangement of the fascicles within the nerves seems to make any attempt to restore the exact fascicular pattern impossible.

If intraneural dissection of a peripheral nerve is performed, one will note that some fascicles are packed together more closely than others, forming groups. Between these groups the space is somewhat wider than that between the fascicles within the group. In the spaces between the groups course the major vessels of the nerves. Along the course of a peripheral nerve there are certain areas where much interchange between these groups of fascicles occurs. However, there are long distances wherein the group pattern is fairly constant and the interchange of fibers is mostly restricted to the fascicles within the group. It is, therefore, much easier to define corresponding fascicle groups of two nerve stumps after loss of nerve substance than to identify the corresponding individual small fascicles. For this reason, we will attempt to restore a group pattern and not the individual fascicle pattern (Figs. 24–3 and 24–5).

Minimal Surgical Trauma

The intraneural dissection must be performed with a minimum of surgical trauma. Sutures are used to approximate the fascicles to the corresponding fascicle groups of the stumps. As tension is completely avoided, there is no need to use more sutures than are necessary to maintain accurate coaptation. To minimize surgical trauma, microsurgery is essential. An attempt to restore the fascicular pattern in a polyfascicular nerve would require that the graft be split into its individual fascicles, requiring additional trauma, and it is doubtful that this structural improvement would outweigh the increased tissue reaction.

INDICATIONS FOR NERVE GRAFTING

Discussion concerning the indications for nerve grafting continues to the present. There is no question that, if transection is clean, and without defect, end-to-end repair is the optimal solution.

However, there is no question that nerve grafting offers the prospect of an acceptable result, especially in cases in which longstanding defects exist and in which end-to-end neurorrhaphy is impossible. There is a wide gap between these two extremes. The prospect of a good functional recovery deteriorates with increased tension at the suture sites. However, it is evident that, even though two suture sites are necessary, nerve grafts can produce excellent results if performed properly. From this simple consideration we can conclude that nerve grafting is indicated if the defect is long enough that the result of end-to-end nerve repair under such tension will probably be worse than the result following nerve grafting. Therefore, the indications depend very much on the results of nerve graft expected by the surgeon. My personal experience with nerve grafts has become better and better over the years and, therefore, the indication has expanded.

In *primary nerve repair* without loss of nerve substance, I would try end-to-end repair using epineural sutures. Slight tension would be acceptable and neutralized by slight flexion of the adjacent joints. These cases are closely followed and, if after five to six months, no sign of function return can be noted, then exploration is indicated.

Patients who have suffered a loss of nerve substance are scheduled for early secondary repair.

In *secondary nerve repair* an end-to-end neurorrhaphy is done only if, after proper resection, the two nerve stumps can be coapted without tension with the wrist in neutral position and the elbow extended.

TECHNIQUE

Autografts are used only because allografts and heterografts have not proved to be successful.

Exposure

In the forearm, the hand, and the foot, a tourniquet is used. Usually a wide exposure is favored. The incisions follow the principles of plastic surgery. The nerve stumps are exposed proximal and distal to the lesion, in healthy tissue. The dissection then proceeds toward the nerve stumps, and the neuroma and glioma are respectively exposed.

If, from the primary operation, the complete neural transection is known, as is the length of the defect, another approach can be used. The nerve stumps are exposed through small incisions. A tunnel is created between the two incisions, and the nerve grafts are introduced into the tunnel, using a silastic tube, which is removed after passing the grafts.

Preparation of the Stumps

Sufficient resection is very important. To achieve this, an interfascicular dissection is performed. The epineurium is incised proximal to the neuroma. The external layers of the epineurium are undermined and reflected. The superficial fascicles are exposed. In many instances, and especially in the peripheral portion of a nerve, groups of fascicles can be seen which are in closer contact with each other than with other groups. The dissection enters into the spaces between these groups (Fig. 24–3). The vessels of the nerve usually run in these spaces. The nerve can be divided into several preformed fascicle groups by subsequent interfascicular dissection. Each group is followed toward the neuroma. At the exact point at which the fascicle group loses its normal appearance and starts to merge into the neuroma, it is transected. Thus a proper resection is achieved with preservation of as much neural tissue as possible, especially in the case of an oblique border line between fibrotic and normal tissue. Such an interfascicular dissection is not possible in all nerves at all levels. Basically, we can differentiate between four types of intraneural fascicular patterns:

1. *Monofascicular Nerves.* These nerves consist of just one big fascicle surrounded by perineural tissue. An example is the facial nerve at the stylomastoid foramen. If this fascicle has the approximate size of the nerve to be used as a graft, one graft will satisfy the neural cross section. This procedure represents a fascicular grafting if one pays no attention to the fact that the graft usually consists of several fascicles. If the monofascicular nerve is larger than the donor nerve, two, three, four, or even more grafts must be coapted with the nerve stump to cover the cross section (fascicular grafting 1:2, 1:3, 1:4, and so on). If there is a predominance of fibers of a

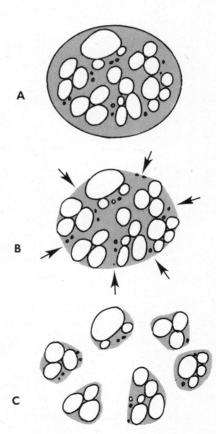

Figure 24–3 *A,* Cross section of a peripheral nerve (polyfascicular nerve with group arrangement). *B,* After removal of the epineurium, *C,* the fascicle groups are separated by interfascicular dissection.

specific function in a particular sector of this nerve, the grafts coapted with these sectors are united with their peripheral ends to the corresponding peripheral branches. In the facial nerve there is actually a predominance of fibers going to the different muscle groups of the facial muscle within the cross section (Meissl, 1976).

2. *Oligofascicular Nerves.* If a nerve consists of only a few larger fascicles, it depends again on the size of the fascicles as to how many grafts must be coapted with each fascicle to satisfy the cross section. Fascicular grafting 1:1, 1:2 must be performed (Fig. 24–4). Typical examples are the radial nerve in the proximal half of the upper arm and the sciatic nerve in the rabbit. If an end-to-end repair can be performed in such nerves, a fascicular coaptation is easily achieved by epineurial suture. Such oligofascicular nerves are consequently not proper models for study of the value of epineurial or fascicular nerve repair.

3. *Polyfascicular Nerves with Group Arrangement.* There are many, rather small fascicles of different sizes in the peripheral portion of the major nerve trunks. Proximal to the division of such a trunk, the fascicles destined for a specific branch are already arranged in a fascicle group. In many cases, this group arrangement is maintained proximally over varying distances. If this occurs, interfascicular dissection, as described above, can be performed. This interneural arrangement is present in most of our peripheral nerves, in the distal portion, which is the most common site of nerve in-

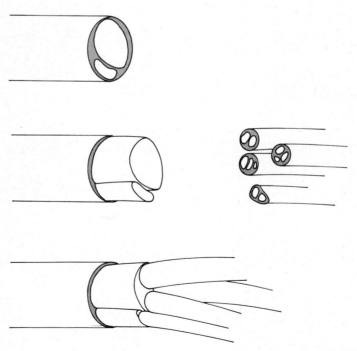

Figure 24–4   Coaptation (oligofascicular nerve). The cross section of the large fascicle is covered by three grafts (fascicular grafting 1:3) and the smaller one by one graft (fascicular grafting 1:1).

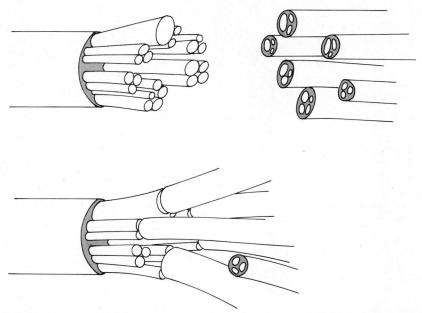

Figure 24–5 Coaptation (polyfascicular nerve with group arrangement). After resection of a strip of epineurium and interfascicular dissection, each fascicle group is coaptated with one graft (interfascicular nerve grafting).

juries. Under these circumstances, the corresponding fascicle groups (Fig. 24–5) are united by individual nerve grafts (interfascicular nerve grafting).

4. *Polyfascicular Nerves Without Group Arrangement.* These are nerves consisting of many fascicles that are not arranged in fascicle groups but are distributed rather diffusely over the cross section. Such fascicular patterns can be met at very proximal levels; for example, at the root level of the brachial plexus. These fascicular patterns are also present at particular levels of peripheral nerves where a major exchange of fibers between the groups occurs. In this case no attempt at interfascicular dissection is undertaken. Each sector of the cross section is covered by a nerve graft (Fig. 24–6) until the whole cross section is satisfied (sectoral nerve grafting).

To perform a fascicular nerve grafting procedure in a polyfascicular nerve with many small fascicles, the nerve grafts themselves must be split into their individual fascicles to get grafts thin enough to be united with the individual fascicles of the nerve stumps (Fig. 24–7). In a procedure of this type the surgical trauma is very much increased, and it has not yet been proved that such a procedure produces better results.

Harvesting the Nerve Grafts

After the stumps have been prepared and the tourniquet removed, precise hemostasis is performed, using bipolar coagulation. The exact length of

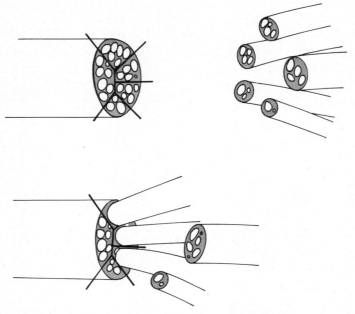

Figure 24–6   Coaptation (polyfascicular nerve without group arrangement). Each sector of the cross section is coaptated with one graft (sectoral nerve grafting).

the defect is measured, and the surgical team must obtain the nerve grafts. The following donor nerves have been used:

Sural Nerve

The sural nerve is ideal for grafting. One can obtain a piece of nerve 30 to 40 cm in length. This nerve divides distally behind the lateral malleolus. The sural nerve is a branch of the posterior tibial nerve arising behind the knee joint. Sometimes it receives an additional branch, the communicating

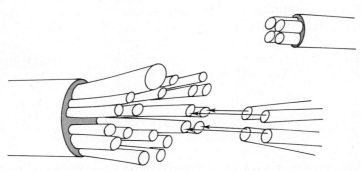

Figure 24–7   To achieve a fascicular coaptation in a polyfascicular nerve each fascicle has to be isolated and the graft split into its individual fascicles.

sural nerve, from the peroneal nerve. This additional source may be destroyed if a nerve stripper is used. The sural nerve can be exposed through a small transverse incision behind the lateral area of the ankle following the lines of Langer. The proximal course of the nerve can be palpated by a gentle pull. A second incision is made 3 or 4 cm proximal, and the sural nerve, which can be found with the short saphenous vein, can be lifted on a tape. After transection of the main trunk of the nerve at the level of the first incision, two or three additional branches can be palpated at this level by gentle longitudinal tugging at the second incision. After these branches have been defined and transected, the nerve can easily be extracted through the second incision. Again the course of the nerve is located by pulling longitudinally and palpating the calf more proximally. Usually two more incisions, one at the lower border of the popliteal fossa and one in the middle of the calf, are sufficient to excise the whole nerve. If a very long graft is needed, the sural nerve can be followed in a proximal direction within the posterior tibial and sciatic nerves. It forms a distinct fascicle group in these nerves and can be excised up to the middle of the thigh without significant damage to other fascicle groups.

Medial Cutaneous Nerve of the Forearm

This nerve is located at the lower border of the axillary groove. After incising the fascia, the nerve is found in close proximity to the brachial vein. Usually through two or more incisions, one in the mid arm and the other at the elbow level, the medial cutaneous nerve of the forearm nerve can be excised. One can obtain about a 20 cm graft.

Lateral Femoral Cutaneous Nerve

This nerve is exposed through a transverse incision below the anterior superior iliac spine. By a gentle pull and distal palpation, the further course of the nerve is defined. The whole nerve is excised through several transverse incisions. About 20 cm of nerve tissue can be obtained. If more is needed, the nerve can be followed into the pelvic cavity and resected there.

Superficial Radial Nerve

This nerve has been sacrificed on a few occasions to cover defects of the brachial plexus, when an enormous amount of nerve grafts were needed. Otherwise, I would not use this nerve, especially if the median or the ulnar nerve of the same extremity is involved, because of increased sensory loss due to overlapping of the cutaneous nerve territories.

Lateral Antebrachial Cutaneous Nerve

This is a terminal branch of the musculocutaneous nerve, and is identified at the lateral border of the biceps tendon. It has been used successfully by McFarlane et al. (1976).

Saphenous Nerve

This nerve has been used in rare instances. It should not be excised if the sural nerve of the same extremity is to be excised also. The loss of sensibility incurred will be greater than the sum of the zone of hypaesthesia after an isolated nerve graft excision.

Dorsal Cutaneous Branch of the Ulnar Nerve

This nerve yields only a rather small nerve graft and has not been used.

Intercostal Nerves

These nerves have the advantage that they contain both motor and sensory fibers, rather than sensory fibers only, as do the other donors. However, since they have many branches along their course, a great number of axons are lost.

Cervical Plexus

The sensory branches of the cervical plexus can be used to restore the facial nerve. After the nerve grafts have been obtained, they should be cut into pieces approximately 20 per cent longer than the actual distance between the two stumps, which may vary because of the following factors:
  a) elastic retraction of the nerve tissue.
  b) defect of nerve tissue caused by loss of nerve substance.
  c) defect caused by resection of the neuroma or the glioma, or both.
The differentiation between the actual distance between the nerve stumps (a + b + c) and real defect of nerve tissue (b + c) is very important. If the actual distance is merely due to retraction (a), the fascicular pattern of the cross section is similar, and the recognition of the corresponding fascicles and fascicle groups, respectively, is rather easy. If there is a marked loss of nerve substance, the fascicular pattern has changed very much, and it is more difficult to get the axons in the correct distal pathways (Fig. 24–8). For this reason, the result of nerve repair by nerve grafting depends on the length of the defect (b + c) and not on the distance caused by retraction (a). There are strong arguments that within certain limits the length of the grafts really do not influence the result. With a given defect of, let us say, 4 cm, the result will not change very much if grafts 4, 5 or 6 cm are used. Because of this we prefer to use a longer graft and to place it in the good soft tissue rather than to select the shortest way, especially if this places the grafts in scar tissue bed. As the length of the graft, within certain limits, is unimportant, the distance between the two stumps after proper resection is measured in extended position rather than flexed position (Fig. 24–9). The minimal advantage of being able to use a shorter graft is heavily outweighed by the fact that the grafts and the two sides of coaptation will be under repeated tension when the limb is subsequently mobilized.

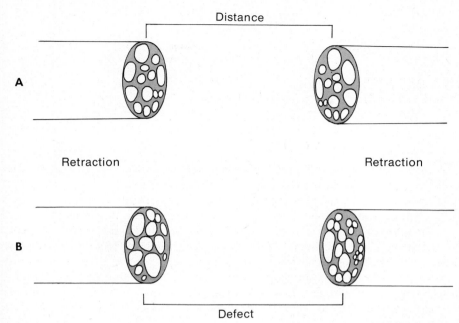

Figure 24–8   A given distance between two nerve stumps can be caused by elastic retraction (*A*). In this case the fascicular pattern corresponds well. The gap can also be due to a loss of nerve substance (*B*). In this case the fascicular pattern differs. In spite of the same length of the grafts the result will be better in *A* than in *B*, if all the other factors influencing nerve regeneration do not differ.

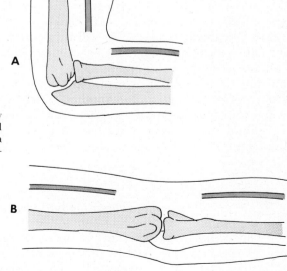

Figure 24–9   A given defect by loss of nerve substance can be decreased by flexion of the adjacent joints to give a minimal defect (*A*) or increased by extension to give a maximal defect (*B*).

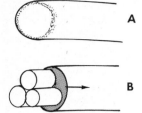

Figure 24-10 The epineurium may overlap the cut end of the graft (*A*). It has to be shifted away before coaptation (*B*).

Transection of the graft must be performed very carefully. We prefer special scissors with serrated blades to avoid shifting of the nerve tissue when cutting. The nerve is transected fascicle by fascicle. Each time the epineurium is shifted slightly away from the cut end (Fig. 24–10). Overlapping of the cut surface by epineurium must be avoided. It is not necessary to resect the epineurium at both ends of the nerve graft. Since the grafts are free grafts, the epineurium will begin to proliferate after circulation of the graft is restored, with a certain delay, depending upon epineurial proliferation of the two nerve stumps. There is no danger that epineurial proliferation originating from the graft will interfere with the neural regenerative process at the site of coaptation.

Definition of Corresponding Fascicles and Fascicle Groups in Proximal and Distal Stumps

As we approach the division of the nerve, we find that more and more nerve fibers of a particular function are arranged in well defined fascicle groups. The end results depend very much on recognition of corresponding fascicle groups. It is essential to unite motor fascicles of the proximal stump with motor fascicles of the peripheral stump. In the future, the further development of electric stimulation (Hakstian, 1968) and of special staining techniques (Freilinger et al., 1975) will help to make this definition easier. At the present, we attempt to get an exact idea of the fascicular pattern of the peripheral stump by exposing the nerve until it branches and then following the individual fascicles in a proximal direction. A sketch is made of the fascicular pattern of the distal stump. Another sketch is made of the fascicular pattern of the proximal stump. By matching the sketches an approximate assumption is made of the corresponding fascicle groups in the proximal stump and the distal stump. The functional result indicates that in the majority of cases the guess has been correct.

Adaptation and Coaptation

The grafts are placed into the defect. A graft is selected for each fascicle group. The fascicular pattern of the sural nerve changes along its course: in the proximal level, it consists of one or a few fascicles, but the number of fascicles increases toward the periphery. Of course, one tries to select the best-fitting graft for each fascicle group. The graft is approximated to the cross-sectional area of the fascicle group with a 10–0 nylon stitch, which catches the epineurium of the graft. This suture is anchored in the remaining interfascicular connective tissue between the fascicles of the group (Fig. 24–11*A*) or in the perineurium of one of the fascicles of this group (Fig. 24–11*B*). After the suture is tied, the graft is approximated to the cut end of the fascicle group. However, if there is tension in a longitudinal direction, the approximation is at the point where the suture is located, and, because of the tension, the opposite perineurial and endoneurial tissues tend to separate (Figs. 24–12*A* and *B*). Thus more stitiches are needed to provide abutment of the cut ends. If tension is avoided completely, good contact of the whole surface of each end can be achieved with one stitch, especially if the stitch is placed at the correct point (Fig. 24–12*C*). If optimal contact is achieved between the whole surface of the two ends, no further attempt need be made to secure the coaptation. Natural fibrin clotting is sufficient to maintain the coaptation if tension is completely avoided. The tensile strength of such a neural juncture is minimal, but sufficient if the graft is long enough and there is no separating force. In this way a grafting procedure can be performed with minimal surgical trauma or foreign body reaction. It cannot be stressed enough that the whole technique is based on coaptation without tension. A compromise in this regard will yield a poor result.

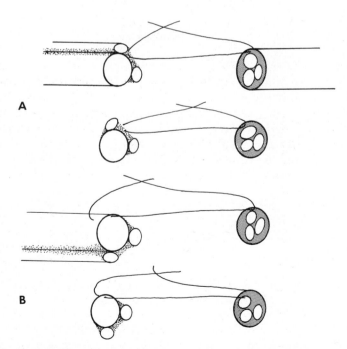

Figure 24–11 Approximation of the graft (*right*) to a fascicle group (*left*). One stitich catches the epineurium of the graft and the interfascicular tissue (*A*) of the fascicle group or the perineurium of one fascicle of the graft and of the fascicle group (*B*).

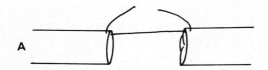

A

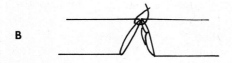

B

Figure 24–12 Coaptation by one stitch (*A*) under slight tension (*B*). The site of the stitch is coapted but the remaining cross-sectional area is still spreading apart. If tension is avoided one loose-stitch is sufficient to achieve a broad contact of the whole cross section (*C*).

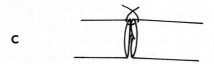

C

Wound Closure

After exact hemostasis the skin wound is closed very carefully to avoid shearing forces, which might dislocate the grafts. No suction drainage is used.

Immobilization

The extremity is immobilized in the exact position it was in during the operation. An exact immobilization is extremely important, especially during the first 24 hours and the first postoperative days. Experiments have shown that the tensile strength after such a grafting operation increases during the first days and after six days reaches a sufficiently high level to allow mobilization. Therefore, from a clinical viewpoint, the plaster cast can be removed after 10 days and free active motion allowed. This additional four day period of immobilization allows an additional safety margin for maturation of the nerve suture site.

PROGNOSIS

Resection of Distal Coaptation

It has already been mentioned that scar tissue formation at the peripheral end of the graft may cause an obstacle for further advancement of the axon sprouts. The frequency of this depends on the amount of connective tissue reaction at the distal end of the graft and on the time elapsed since the grafting procedure, when the axons reach the distal neural junction. In our first 50 cases the scar block at the distal coaptation was observed in seven patients (14 per cent). One gets suspicious that a scar block may have formed if the Tinel-Hoffmann sign, after advancing along a graft, stops with its maximum at the distal end of the graft and does not proceed. If this situation remains unchanged for two or three months, an exploration is indicated. If thickening is detected at the distal suture site, it is resected and a new coaptation performed. In the majority of the cases the Tinel sign reassumes its advancement and useful recovery occurs. In later cases the frequency of the scar block has decreased, and is now between one and two per cent. One must bear this possibility in mind. A lack of understanding is demonstrated by one who reports on failures of nerve grafts and does not even mention the possibility of a block at the distal suture site.

Reasons for Failure Following Nerve Grafting

Many factors influence the quality of nerve regeneration. Advanced age of the patient and a long-term interval following neural injury are unfavorable factors. In some cases the result has been compromised by delayed wound healing and infection. Scars crossing the nerve graft may cause compression and impede regeneration. A plastic surgical procedure before or at the time of nerve grafting can prevent this outcome. In one case a fibrosis of all the grafts, including the proximal and distal coaptation sites, was observed. After new resection of the nerve stumps, the grafting procedure was repeated, and satisfactory regeneration occurred. No reason for the occurrence of the fibrosis could be detected. One might suspect that rupture of one of the suture sites may be the cause of some failures. In fact, this is not so; in none of the cases which were re-explored for any reason was a rupture of one of the suture sites observed.

RESULTS

The results of interfascicular nerve grafting of the median, ulnar, and radial nerve have been reported in full detail elsewhere (Millesi, Meissl, and Berger, 1972 and 1976). For this reason a brief summary might be sufficient.

The results are evaluated according to Highet's scheme (Nicolson and Seddon, 1957) for the median and ulnar nerve. For the other nerves the scale developed by Lovett (Wright, 1912), which was extensively described by Daniels, Williams and Worthingham (1961) was used. It corresponds with the common grading system of motor function (M0 to M5).

Axillary Nerve

Grafting of this nerve is very important. The lesions are mostly of the traction type and involve a long segment of the nerve. If the site of the lesion is in the quadrangular space region, surgical access is very difficult. To per-

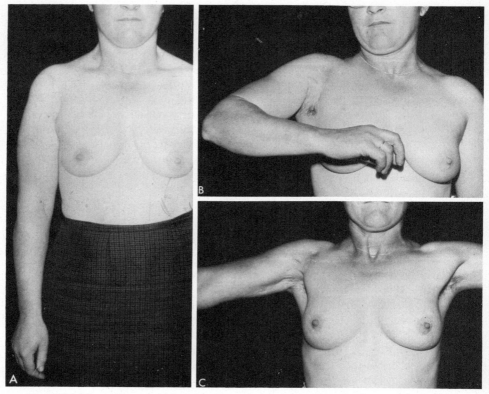

Figure 24–13   A 35-year-old female with open wound at the right shoulder, infection, and incision to evacuate pus. After the incision, complete palsy of the axillary nerve occurred. Fourteen months later there was still a complete paralysis of the muscles innervated by the axillary nerve (*A*). The exploration revealed a complete transection with a distance between the two stumps after resection of the neuroma of 2 cm. Continuity was restored by two nerve grafts (sural nerve) of 2 cm length. *B* and *C*, Result after 8 years.

form an end-to-end nerve repair would be very difficult. In the majority of our five cases both anterior and posterior explorations were performed to define the proximal and distal stumps. The graft was then passed through the quadrangular space, and the proximal coaptation performed. Subsequently, the distal coaptation is completed posteriorly on the dorsal surface of the space through the posterior incision. One or two nerve grafts are sufficient. The axillary nerve is treated as a single fascicle group. In four of the five cases useful recovery was obtained (Fig. 24–13).

Musculocutaneous Nerve

One graft is sufficient for this nerve. Four cases were operated and all four yielded excellent recovery.

Radial Nerve

In 13 cases of radial nerve lesions with defects from 3 to 12.5 cm, a result of M4 to M5 was achieved in 10 patients. In two patients, who were operated late — 12 and 29 months after the original accident — recovery reached M3. In one of these, an additional tendon transfer was performed to improve the strength of a second operation. In one 62-year-old patient the recovery was only M2.

Median Nerve

There were 38 cases of complete transection of the median nerve in this series. In 10 of them the motor function was not completely lost owing to mixed innervation via the ulnar nerve. All these 10 patients had preoperative complete loss of sensibility in the median nerve area. Therefore, 28 cases were available for evaluation of recovery of motor function and 38 for evaluation of restoration of sensibility. In 23 of the 28 cases with complete loss of motor function, a useful recovery (M3 or better) was achieved. If the motor recovery is plotted against the length of the defect, a relationship between quality of regeneration and length of defect becomes clear. Four patients having a defect of 2.5 cm or less achieved an M4 to M5 result. Of 11 cases with a defect between 2.6 and 5 cm, 10 had a result of M3 or better. The same amount of recovery could be observed in five of seven patients who had a defect of between 5.1 and 10 cm. Four of six patients who had a defect of 10.1 cm or more had a result of M3 or better. Fifteen of the 38 patients developed a result of S3$^+$ or S4 with two point discrimination. In 22 patients protective sensibility returned. Only one patient did not have satisfactory return of protective sensibility. Among these cases there were seven patients with high or intermediate median lesions. Six of them achieved a result of M3 or better. Thirteen patients had a combined lesion of the median and ulnar nerve of the same arm, with restoration of the continuity of the median nerve by a nerve graft (Fig. 24–14). In nine cases the result was M3 or better.

Ulnar Nerve

Thirty-nine patients with ulnar nerve lesions were operated during the same period of time. Thirty-one achieved a recovery of M3 or better, according to Highet's grading, and thirty-four had a result of M2$^+$ or better. Of 11 patients with high ulnar nerve lesions the results in six cases was M3 or better, while in five cases it was not satisfactory. Of 13 patients with a combined median and ulnar nerve lesion of the same arm, the ulnar nerve was operated upon the 12 patients, nine of which recovered to a degree of M3 or better.

Femoral Nerve

In four patients the femoral nerve had to be repaired. All four were iatrogenic lesions, with resection of the nerve to perform a radical removal of

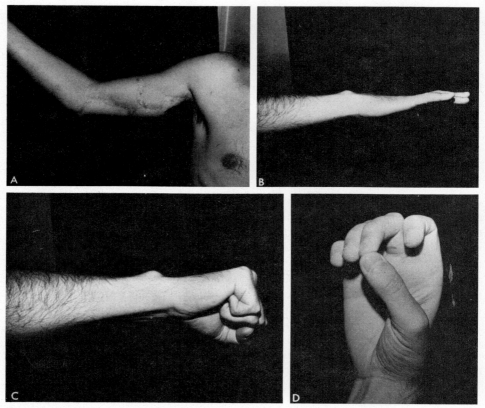

Figure 24–14 This 21-year-old male was injured by broken glass. He received a laceration of the brachial artery and the median and ulnar nerves at the middle of the upper arm. Primary nerve repair was of the median nerve. The ulnar could not be detected. Surgery was unsuccessful. At the second operation, 6 months later, it was found that the first surgeon had sutured the proximal stump of the ulnar nerve to the distal stump of the median nerve. The median nerve had developed a painful neuroma. After resection of the neuroma and the suture site, continuity of the median nerve was restored by five nerve grafts, 7 cm in length, and continuity of the ulnar nerve was restored by four nerve grafts, 7 cm in length (both sural nerves). Full protective sensibility returned by three years.

a hypernephroma in one case and accidental lesion during other operations in the three remaining patients. All four patients demonstrated useful recovery.

Sciatic Nerve

The sciatic nerve has the worst prognosis of all peripheral nerves. It is a thick nerve, requiring many nerve grafts to obtain a satisfactory coverage and bridging of a defect. The two medial cutaneous nerves of the forearm, along with the two sural nerves, are excised to provide a sufficient amount of graft material. Return of sensibility to the plantar aspect of the foot with no trophic changes developing and return of motor function to the tibial nerve innervated muscles of the calf would be regarded as a useful result; indeed such was obtained in three of our five cases. Motor recovery in the peroneal nerve innervated muscles did not occur in these patients.

Posterior Tibial Nerve

Isolated lesions of the tibial nerve have an excellent prognosis, and all four cases operated upon recovered in a useful way.

Common Peroneal Nerve

Lesion of the common peroneal nerve is a complex problem. Even with a healthy peroneal nerve there is a tendency to develop a pes equinus due to inactivity and poor positioning. The peroneal nerve innervates muscles that are much weaker than their antagonists. This impedes regeneration of the muscles and useful recovery, even when reneurotization is successful. For this reason, and for restoration of the continuity of the peroneal nerve, a transfer of the tibialis posterior tendon is performed simultaneously or at a second stage. This transfer improves the muscle balance. It does not really influence the muscle recovery because only dorsiflexion of the ankle is obtained. This has nothing to do with the function of the long extensor of the toes and the function of the peroneus longus and brevis. We have performed surgery in 23 patients in this manner, and in the vast majority useful recovery occurred not only in the tibialis anterior but also in the peroneus and the extensor hallucis longus and the extensor digitorum longus muscles.

Digital Nerves

Digital nerves are also regarded as a single fascicle group, and continuity is restored with only one graft. Many digital nerve repairs have been performed over the years. A series of secondary repair of 30 digital nerves in 17 patients was carefully studied. In six patients whose average age was 27 years and in whom 11 nerve grafts were involved, a two-point discrimination of 6 mm or less was obtained. In nine patients whose average age was 31 years and in whom 12 digital nerves were involved, we achieved results of 7 to 10 mm at two-point discrimination. In three patients whose average age was 37 years and in whom three digital nerves were involved, the two-point discrimination after the repair was 11 to 15 mm. Three patients with four digital nerves involved developed two-point discrimination of 16 mm or more and were regarded as unsuccessful.

REFERENCES

1. Daniels, L. M. Williams and Worthingham, C.: Muscle Testing. 3rd Ed., Philadelphia, W. B. Saunders Co., 1972.
2. Freilinger, G., Gruber, H., Holle, J., and Mandl, W.: Zur Methodik "sensomotorisch" differenzierter Faszilelnaht peripherer Nerven. Handchirurgie 7:133, 1975.
3. Hakstian, H. W.: Funicular orientation by direct stimulation. An aid to peripheral nerve repair. J. Bone Joint Surg. 50A, 1178, 1968.
4. McFarlane, R. M., and Mayer, J. R.: Digital nerve grafts using the lateral antebrachial cutaneous nerve. J. Hand Surg. 1:169, 1976.
5. Meissl, G.: Die Intraneurale Topographie des Extracraniellen N. Facialis. Acta. Chir. Austriaca, Suppl. 1978.
6. Millesi, H., Meissl, G., and Berger, A.: The interfascicular nerve grafting of the median and ulnar nerves. J. Bone Joint Surg. 54A:727, 1972.

7. Millesi, H., Meissl, G., and Berger, A.: Further experience with interfascicular grafting of the median, ulnar and radial nerves. J. Bone Joint Surg. *58A*:209, 1976.
8. Nicolson, O. R., and Seddon, H. J.: Nerve repair in civil practice. Results of treatment of median and ulnar nerve lesions. Br. Med. J. *2*:1065, 1957.
9. Seddon, H. H.: Restoration of function in peripheral nerve injuries. Lancet *1*:418, 1947.
10. Strange, F. G. St. C.: An operation for nerve pedicle grafting. Preliminary Communication. Br. J. Surg. *34*:423, 1947.
11. Sunderland, S.: The intraneural topography of the radial median and ulnar nerve. Brain *68*:243, 1945.
12. Sunderland, S.: Factors influencing the course of regeneration and the quality of recovery after nerve suture. Brain *75*:19, 1952.
13. Taylor, G. I., and Ham, F. J.: The Free Vascularized Nerve Graft. Plast. Reconstr. Surg. *57*:413, 1976.
14. Wright, N. G.: Muscle training in the treatment of infantile paralysis. Boston M. & S. Journal, *167*:567, 1912.

25

THE EVALUATION OF CLINICAL RESULTS FOLLOWING PERIPHERAL NERVE SUTURE

GEORGE E. OMER, JR.

Surgery to repair a peripheral nerve is successful only when there is subsequent pain-free useful function of the involved extremity. A major problem in the evaluation of nerve repair is the definition of a good clinical result. There are no worldwide accepted criteria for evaluation of functional recovery after nerve suture. A minimal evaluation of functional recovery should include: 1) motor strength and range of motion, 2) sensibility level and associated pain interference, and 3) coordination of the extremity.

MOTOR FUNCTION

Techniques to examine muscle strength are based on the use of gravity and resistance. Doctor Robert W. Lovett, Professor of Orthopaedic Surgery at the Harvard Medical School, devised tests for function against gravity in 1912, and in 1916 added a spring balance test for resistance in collaboration with E. G.

Martin, Ph.D. (Daniels, Williams, and Worthingham, 1946). In Doctor Lovett's text on the treatment of infantile paralysis, published in 1917, he listed the combined gravity and resistance tests for "good" and "normal" ratings. In 1932, Arthur T. Legg and Janet B. Merrill listed further development of the tests given in Lovett's book, including tests for a greater number of muscles and adding "poor" and "fair" ratings. A percentage system for recording the results of manual muscle grading was devised in 1936 by Henry O. Kendall and Florence P. Kendall, physical therapists at the Children's Hospital School in Baltimore. The common manual tests for muscle power in use today are based on the Lovett method:

100%	5	N	Normal	Complete range of motion against gravity with full resistance
75%	4	G	Good	Complete range of motion against gravity with some resistance
50%	3	F	Fair	Complete range of motion against gravity
25%	2	P	Poor	Complete range of motion with gravity eliminated
10%	1	T	Trace	Evidence of slight contractility; no joint motion
0%	0	0	Zero	No evidence of contractility

A voluntary muscle test with manual grading demands precise anatomical knowledge and is based on the examiner's ability to grade muscle power by palpation of the involved muscle-tendon unit and resisting movement of a bone-joint lever arm motored by the involved muscle. Trick movements must be detected, and on occasion a local anesthetic is required to block competing innervation. I attempt to quantitate the active range of motion with a goniometer across an appropriate joint and to document strength with resistance instruments such as a grip meter or pinch meter. A double exposure photograph often demonstrates the absent function.

The techniques for testing motor function are discussed in Chapter 2.

The British Medical Research Council introduced a system of grading in 1954 (Seddon, 1954) that attempted to assess the recovery of a peripheral nerve in relation to total extremity function. It is most useful in proximal (high) nerve lesions (Seddon, 1975):

M5	Complete recovery
M4	All synergic and independent movements are possible
M3	All important muscles act against resistance
M2	Return of perceptible contraction in both proximal and distal muscles
M1	Return of perceptible contraction in proximal muscles
M0	No contraction

The peripheral nerve research study group of the United States Veterans Administration modified this scale into seven levels (Woodhall and Beebe, 1956):

M6	Complete recovery
M5	Some synergic and isolated movements possible
M4	All important muscles have sufficient power to act against resistance
M3	Proximal muscles act against gravity; perceptible contraction in intrinsic muscles
M2	Proximal muscles act against gravity; no return of power in intrinsic muscles
M1	Return of perceptible contraction in the proximal muscles
M0	No contraction

Both the British and American reports are concerned with war injuries, and are confusing because they have different levels.

SENSIBILITY LEVEL

Sensibility is even more difficult to evaluate than motor power, because sensibility is subjective, and objective findings may indicate paresthesia rather than useful function. W. B. Highet described an assessment of sensory recovery in 1954 (Wynn Parry, 1973):

S5	Recovery of two-point discrimination within the autonomic zone
S4	Superficial pain and tactile sense in the autonomic zone, with disappearance of over-response
S3	Superficial pain and tactile sense in the autonomic zone
S2	Deep cutaneous pain in the autonomic zone
S1	No sensation

The British Medical Research Council scale has six levels (Seddon, 1975):

S4	Complete recovery
S3+	Some recovery of two-point discrimination within the autonomous area
S3	Return of superficial cutaneous pain and tactile sensibility throughout the autonomous area with disappearance of any previous over-reaction
S2	Return of some degree of superficial cutaneous pain and tactile sensibility within the autonomous area of the nerve
S1	Recovery of deep cutaneous pain sensibility within the autonomous area of the nerve
S0	Absence of sensibility in the autonomous area

Techniques for evaluating sensory recovery during World War II included pinprick, von Frey hairs, the Weber two-point discrimination test, and vague localization tests. However, most tests, other than pinprick and cotton wool, were not performed routinely, and the precise distance for "some" two-point discrimination was not defined.

A precise rating of sensibility was presented by Moberg (1975) for the autonomous areas of the median and ulnar nerves.

Median and Ulnar Sensibility
Two-Point Discrimination Distance

Good	<12 mm
Fair	12–15 mm
Poor	15–20 mm
Bad	>20 mm

Moberg believes that a two-point discrimination distance greater than 12 millimeters provides only decreased functional sensibility because the patient must utilize visual control of hand activities.

The techniques for sensibility testing are discussed in Chapter 1.

When pain dominates the clinical situation, a simple classification has been made according to how the pain interferes with the activities of daily living (Swanson, Goran-Hagert, and Swanson, 1978):

100%	P4	Severe enough to prevent all activity and causes distress
75%	P3	Prevents some activity
50%	P2	Interferes with activity
25%	P1	Annoying

EXTREMITY COORDINATION

Coordination is the end product of the highly specialized motor and sensory systems, and evaluation should include both activities.

The picking-up test was introduced by Erik Moberg in 1958. The patient ". . . should pick up a number of small objects on a table and put them as quickly as he can into a small box. After he has done this a few times, he is asked to do the same thing blindfolded. The test with blindfolding can be made more difficult by asking the patient to identify the objects as he picks them up" (Moberg, 1958). We quantitated the picking-up test by measuring the time required to pick up nine objects of different size and shape (Omer, 1968). Seddon (1975) states that the precursor of the picking-up test is the coin test. The patient, whose eyes must be closed, is given a coin and asked to identify it.

Greenseid and McCormack (1968) designed 12 functional tests requiring the use of pinch, grip, range of grasp, and finger manipulation. Tests are timed with a stopwatch, and the scored result is the fastest time of three performances on each test.

Tactile gnosis can be tested by writing numbers on the patient's digit (Bowden and Napier, 1961) or Porter's letter test (Porter, 1966) in which the patient palpates type set in a block.

Coordination tests are not static, and will change with the level of homeostasis of the extremity or through experience with the test used for the evaluation. Re-education programs following nerve suture include repeated stimulation and repeated motor-sensory activity to improve coordination through experience.

CLINICAL RESULTS

The appropriate time to attain maximum clinical recovery depends upon the level and severity of the nerve lesion. Sunderland (Stromberg et al., 1961) states that improvement after nerve suture will continue slowly and irregularly over several years. Zachary (Seddon, 1954) extended the period to five years in the World War II casualties, and Stromberg et al. (1961) also concluded that maximum recovery requires five years in adults and two years in children. Evaluation studies should demonstrate the functional results in three to five years after nerve suture.

Few clinical reports have followed any standard method for evaluating the clinical result. For example, Bjorkesten (1947) reported the results of 756 nerve sutures between January 1940 and January 1943. The results were judged exclusively from the aspect of motor function, with postoperative observation from six months to five years. A good result denoted an active motility of at least two thirds of normal, medium was active motility about one half to two thirds of normal, poor was minimal active contraction, and negative denoted no contraction. Bjorkesten recorded 16.7 per cent good, 39.3 per cent medium, 29.5 per cent poor, and 14.5 per cent negative results. This quantitative report was a better evaluation than most series previously published during the twentieth century.

Prior to routine magnification, the largest clinical series subjected to motor and sensory evaluation for functional recovery were the military injuries in World War II (Seddon, 1954; Woodhall and Beebe, 1956). These studies indicate that the potential for a "good clinical result" five years after secondary suture in a severe injury is as follows (Woodhall and Beebe, 1956):

Nerve	British Code "Good" Result	Total Nerves U.S.	Brit.	Per cent "Good" U.S.	Brit.
Median	M3 to M5	233	290	51.1	32.7
	S3+ to S4	244	278	17.6	8.6
Ulnar	M4 to M5	433	384	12.9	4.9
	S3 to S4	441	390	31.4	30.8
Radial	M4 to M5	197	114	21.3	36.9
Tibial	M3 to M5	91		24.5	
	S3+ to S4	97	118	2.0	0.0
Common Peroneal	M4 to M5	138		7.2	

Military injuries are often severe, enforcing delayed suture of the involved peripheral nerve. Later studies of delayed suture involve military injuries during the Viet Nam War. During this period, the use of magnification, delicate instruments, and finer, less reactive suture material improved the technique of nerve suture. In addition, there was better battle area evacuation time, and the majority of sutures were performed within the first three months after injury. Omer (1978) reported the results of 143 epineural sutures of upper extremity nerves followed for at least twelve months:

VIET NAM NEURORRHAPHY
RELATED TO ETIOLOGY AND LEVEL OF INJURY

Etiology	Adequate Follow-up	Clinical Return	Percentage
Lacerations			
9 above elbow	8	3	37
90 below elbow	67	30	45
High velocity gunshot			
24 above elbow	21	6	28
24 below elbow	14	6	43
Low velocity gunshot			
19 above elbow	18	9	50
16 below elbow	14	6	43
Fracture — dislocations			
1 above elbow	1	0	0
1 below elbow	0	0	0
184 Totals	143	60	42

Brown (1970) recorded the results of 135 epineural sutures followed six to 24 months.

VIET NAM NEURORRHAPHY SECONDARY SUTURE — SPECIFIC NERVES

Nerve	Number Repaired	No Return Per cent	Some Return Per cent
Ulnar	68	44 (65%)	24 (35%)
Median	38	19 (50%)	19 (50%)
Radial	5	3 (60%)	2 (40%)
Digital	24	10 (40%)	14 (60%)
Totals	135	76 (56%)	59 (44%)

Neither study had adequate follow-up, and the results are not fully graded. Brown states "some return." Omer has two criteria for "clinical return": for the above-elbow lesion — progressive motor return with independent movement and point localization of 3.84 von Frey filament without over-response (M3-S2); for the below elbow lesion — progressive motor return with independent movement and two-point discrimination of 20 millimeters (M3-S3). In addition, Omer noted that none of his patients with above elbow neurorrhaphy had recovery of the intrinsic muscles of the hand during the period of study. The results of the two Viet Nam series were very similar and only indicated that 40 to 45 per cent of sutured nerves result in progressive functional return; final recovery was not complete and therefore not evaluated.

Stromberg and co-authors (1961) reported a series of 150 cases in 1961. The nerve injury level was distal to the mid-third of the forearm, with minimal extremity destruction. The patients were evaluated between one and 24 years following nerve suture. Sweating returned in seven to 12 months. The two-point discrimination distance was 20 mm or less in 13 patients (9 per cent). A similar study was done by Boswick and coauthors in 1965, with two-point discrimination distance of 20 mm or less in 11 patients (13 per cent) of 82 cases.

The "civilian" injury is considered a more likely candidate for immediate suture, although the individual problem may be severe in either circumstance. During the same period as the studies from Viet Nam, Sakellarides (1962) evaluated 205 sutures of 172 nerves in 149 patients. Secondary suture gave better results than primary suture in the median and ulnar nerves. The prognosis for recovery was best for radial nerve lesions, and poorest for the ulnar nerve suture. All patients had been followed for at least two years at the Massachusetts General Hospital:

Nerve	British Code "Good" Result	Total Nerves*	Number "Good"
Median	M3 to M5	85	32
	S3+ to S4	85	3
Ulnar	M4 to M5	107	1
	S3 to S4	107	28
Radial	M4 to M5	13	2

*Totals include resutures.

Seddon (1975) makes the point that the distal injury in a child has the best prognosis for functional recovery. He refers to McEwan's (1962) study that demonstrates a decline with age in the quality of recovery but also firmly adheres to secondary suture as the procedure of choice (Nicholson and Seddon, 1957).

MEDIAN AND ULNAR NERVES AT THE WRIST – PERCENTAGE OF "GOOD" RECOVERY

Series	Median		Ulnar	
	M3 to M5	S3+ to S4	M4 to M5	S3 to S4
McEwan (adult)	60%	67%	23%	84%
(child)	92%	93%	71%	100%
Nicholson and Seddon	65%	25%	35%	69%

Clarkson and Pelly (1962) stated that in only 54 per cent of nerve sutures is there return of independent intrinsic action. They reported return of two-point discrimination distance of less than 10 mm in only 10 per cent of low median sutures. Onne (1962) first reported precise sensibility studies with two-point discrimination distance tests in 32 median and 17 ulnar nerve sutures. The recovery of sensibility decreased with the age of the patient; the regained two-point discrimination distance in millimeters was generally the same as the age of the patient, up to 20 years. Between 20 and 31 years of age the sensibility recovery varied but tended to be poor. Above age 31 years all median and ulnar nerve sutures showed poor sensibility, with two-point discrimination distance near or above 30 mm. However, good results for digital nerve sutures were recorded up to the age of 50 years.

The use of magnification has stimulated better techniques for funicular alignment with minimal suture level tension, both circumferential and longitudinal. Instruments and suture material have been adapted to the more precise techniques utilized with magnification. Elsewhere in this text, Millesi (Chapter 24) and Tupper (Chapter 22) report their results utilizing microsurgical techniques.

Buncke (1972) reported his results in 20 digital nerves in which microsurgical techniques were utilized. Two-point discrimination distance under 10 millimeters was demonstrated in 17 of 20 patients.

DIGITAL NERVE RECOVERY MICROSURGICAL TECHNIQUE

Patients	Age	Repair Prim.	Sec.	2-Point <10 mm.	Discrimination >10 mm
4	20 or less	1		1	
			3	3	
15	20 to 50	6		5	1 (24 mm.)
			8	8	
			1 graft		1 (20 mm.)
1	over 50	1			1 (24 mm.)

RATINGS FOR FUNCTIONAL EVALUATION

Moberg (1978) makes the valid point that all nerve sutures must be evaluated by a single meaningful method to permit proper comparison of techniques. Further, Moberg believes that the sensibility system adopted by the British Research Council in 1954 is inadequate. He believes that there should be additional ratings between S3+ and S4, and that all "lower" ratings are useless to the reconstructive surgeon:

Moberg Scale	British Code	Sensory Grades
	S4	Complete recovery
Good		Tactile gnosis—two-point discrimination distance of 12 mm or less
Fair		Sensibility of 12 to 15 mm
Poor	S3+	Sensibility for gross grip and slow protection—two-point discrimination distance of 15–20 mm
Bad	S3	Sensibility at 20 mm, reaction too slow for good protection
	S2	Hyperesthesia or paresthesia, producing impairment to gripping function
	S1	"Feeling"—the total field reacts to cotton wool and pinprick
	S0	Absent

However, the British Research Council grading system is the only one in general use today.

In order to utilize the British Research Council grading system, one must define "proximal" and "distal" muscles for each nerve:

RADIAL NERVE

Proximal muscles

Brachioradialis
Extensor carpi radialis longus
Extensor digitorum communis
Extensor carpi ulnaris

Distal muscles

Abductor pollicis longus
Extensor pollicis longus
Extensor indicis

MEDIAN NERVE

Proximal muscles

Pronator teres
Flexor carpi radialis
Flexor digitorum superficialis
Flexor pollicis longus

Distal muscles

Abductor pollicis brevis

ULNAR NERVE

Proximal muscles

Flexor carpi ulnaris
Flexor digitorum profundus
  (ring and little)

Distal muscles

Abductor digiti quinti
Interossei

COMMON PERONEAL NERVE

Proximal muscles

Tibialis anterior
Extensor digitorum longus
Extensor hallucis longus
Peronei

Distal muscles

Extensor digitorum brevis

TIBIAL NERVE

Proximal muscles

Gastrocnemius and soleus
Tibialis posterior
Flexor digitorum longus
Flexor hallucis longus

Distal muscles

Intrinsic muscles of sole
Abductor hallucis

The grading system must be flexible enough to combine motor and sensory findings to demonstrate a "good" clinical recovery.

GOOD CLINICAL RECOVERY

Median Nerve

"S" scale according to Moberg:	"M" scale according to Seddon
Good	S4 or S3+:M3
Fair	S3 :M2
Bad	S1 or S2 :M1 or M0

Ulnar Nerve

"S" scale according to Moberg:	"M" scale according to Seddon
Good	S3 :M4
Fair	S2 :M3
Bad	S1 or S0 :M2 or M1

Radial Nerve

"M" scale according to Seddon

Good	:M4
Fair	:M3
Bad	:M2 or M1

Digital Nerve

"S" scale according to Moberg

Good	S4 or S3+:
Fair	S3
Bad	S2 or S1

Common Peroneal Nerve

"M" scale according to Seddon

Good	:M4
Fair	:M3
Bad	:M2 or M1

Tibial Nerve

"S" scale and "M" scale according to Seddon

Good	S4 or S3+:M3
Fair	S3 :M2
Bad	S1 or S2 :M1 or M0

Clinical results should be assessed by clinicians who did not participate in the surgical procedure, if possible. Clinical studies should be done before nerve suture as well as postoperatively. An improved rating system must be developed if an accurate evaluation of clinical results is to be available for comparison studies.

AN "IDEAL" CLINICAL RESULTS STUDY

No one individual has sufficient cases for statistically valid evaluation of all the factors involved in the repair of peripheral nerve injuries. Only the combined results from many surgical centers will provide answers, but to be useful all must be measured on an identical scale with identical techniques.

An "ideal" clinical study would have these features: (1) documentation of motor and sensory impairment, and of associated sudomotor loss, before the surgical procedure; (2) the nerve injury must be at the same level in a similar age patient group; (3) the nerve must be repaired with identical suture techniques at approximately the same time post injury; (4) there should be a continuing study of the effect of spontaneous or planned re-education on the functional activities of the involved extremity; (5) there should be serial and precise motor and sensibility tests to measure the regeneration of the involved nerve; (6) the "final" clinical evaluation should be delayed until three to five years after the nerve suture; and (7) all the nerve sutures should be performed by one surgeon, and all the clinical evaluations should be done by another physician.

Methods to test sensibility are not precise, and need to be more objective (Moberg, 1978). Tactile gnosis is an essential sensory activity, but we have no reliable technique to quantitatively measure the patient's function. Tests for motor function have not really improved since 1912. We need new techniques, precise methods, and pooled information to set standards for the evaluation of clinical results following peripheral nerve suture.

REFERENCES

Boswick, J. A., Jr., Schneewind, J., and Stromberg, W., Jr.: Evaluation of peripheral nerve repairs below elbow. Arch. Surg. *90*:50, 1965.

Bowden, R. E. M., and Napier, J. R.: The assessment of hand function after peripheral nerve injuries. J. Bone Joint Surg. *43(B)*:481, 1961.

Brown, P. W.: The time factor in surgery of upper extremity peripheral nerve injury. Clin. Orthop. *68*:14, 1970.

Buncke, H. J., Jr.: Digital nerve repairs. Surg. Clin. North Am. *52*:1267, 1972.

Bjorkesten, G. af: Suture of war injuries to peripheral nerves. Clinical studies of results. Acta Chir. Scand. *95*:(Suppl. 119)1, 1947.

Clarkson, P. W., and Pelly, A.: The General and Plastic Surgery of the Hand. Oxford, Blackwell, 1962.

Daniels, L., Williams, M., and Worthingham, C.: Muscle Testing: Techniques of Manual Examination. Philadelphia, W. B. Saunders Co., 1946.

Greenseid, D. Z., and McCormack, R. M.: Functional hand testing: a profile evaluation. Plast. Reconstr. Surg. *42*:567, 1968.

McEwan, L. E.: Median and ulnar nerve injuries. Aust. N.Z. J. Surg. *32*:89, 1962.

Moberg, E.: Objective methods for determining the functional value of sensibility in the hand. J. Bone Joint Surg. *40(B)*:454, 1958.

Moberg, E.: Surgical treatment for absent single-hand grip and elbow extension in quadriplegia, principles and preliminary experience. J. Bone Joint Surg. *57(A)*:196, 1975.

Moberg, E.: Sensibility in reconstructive limb surgery. *In* Fredricks, S., and Brody, G. S. (eds.): Symposium on the Neurologic Aspects of Plastic Surgery. Saint Louis, C. V. Mosby, 1978, p. 30.

Nicholson, O. R., and Seddon, H. J.: Nerve repair in civil practice. Results of treatment of median and ulnar nerve lesions. Br. Med. J. *2*:1065, 1957.

Omer, G. E., Jr.: Evaluation and reconstruction of the forearm and hand after acute traumatic peripheral nerve injuries. J. Bone Joint Surg. *50(A)*:1454, 1968.

Omer, G. E., Jr.: Injuries to nerves of the upper extremity. J. Bone Joint Surg. *56(A)*:1615, 1974.

Onne, L.: Recovery of sensibility and sudomotor activity in the hand after nerve suture. Acta Chir. Scand. Suppl. 330, 69 pages, 1962, Stockholm.

Porter, R. W.: New test for fingertip sensation. Br. Med. J. *2*:927, 1966.

Sakellarides, H.: A follow-up study of 172 peripheral nerve injuries in the upper extremity in civilians. J. Bone Joint Surg. *44(A)*:140, 1962.

Seddon, H. J. (ed.): Peripheral nerve injuries. Medical Research Council Special Report Series, No. 282, London, 1954, Her Majesty's Stationery Office.

Seddon, H. J.: Surgical Disorders of the Peripheral Nerves. 2nd ed., Edinburg, Churchill Livingstone, 1975, p. 53.

Stromberg, W. B., Jr., McFarlane, R. M., Bell, J. L., Koch, S. L., and Mason, M. L.: Injury of the median and ulnar nerves. J. Bone Joint Surg. *43(A)*:717, 1961.

Swanson, A. B., Goran-Hagert, C., and Swanson, G. deG.: Evaluation of impairment of hand function. *In* Hunter, J. M., et al. (eds.): Rehabilitation of the Hand, Saint Louis, C. V. Mosby, 1978.

Woodhall, B., and Beebe, G. W. (eds.): Peripheral nerve regeneration, a follow-up study of 3,656 World War II injuries. Veterans Administration Medical Monograph, Washington 25, D.C., U.S. Government Printing Office, 1956, 116 and 257.

Wynn Parry, C. B.: Rehabilitation of the Hand. 3rd ed. London, Butterworths, 1973.

26

SPECIAL SURGICAL TECHNIQUES

Special Suture Technique

KENYA TSUGE

A great deal of study has been devoted in the past to the improvement of techniques for nerve suture. Such studies include efforts toward the removal of irritants from suture material, techniques for achieving good coaptation of the nerve endings, for elimination of tension, for and prevention of stray regenerating nerve fibers and the growth of fibrous scar into nerves. These various methods will be briefly described and the problem areas pointed out. The author will also introduce his recent epineurial anchoring suture method, which involves the use of a needle fitted with looped nylon suture.

PLASMA CLOT METHOD

This method was originally introduced by Young and Medawar (1940) as an experimental technique for performing sutureless nerve repair. It was possible to achieve successful nerve suture by this method, which employs the use of fortified cocktail plasma, clotted with chick embryo extract. However, when using this method, Tarlov and coworkers frequently experienced considerable inflammatory reaction followed by fibrosis (Tarlov et al., 1944a, 1944b; Tarlov, 1945). They employed the autoplasma method, in which autologous plasma is used. This results in very little inflammatory and fibrotic reaction at the suture site. Furthermore, to eliminate some of the technical difficulties, a mold was devised to surround the anastomosis with the plasma clot, which is compressed as it sets.

443

However, the disadvantage of this method is that when there is tension on the suture line, there is risk of separation of nerve ends. Tarlov and others reported that this problem could be resolved by the combined use of very fine tantalum wire tension sutures.

The results of autologous plasma clot suture of nerves are usually good. It is a particularly convenient procedure in repair of small nerves or when tension free coaptation can be achieved by the use of cable grafts. Millesi states that, since there is no tension in interfascicular nerve grafting, the ends of each graft and the corresponding fasciculi remain in contact, and in a few minutes stick together as a result of the normal clotting mechanism (Millesi et al., 1972).

ADHESIVE ANASTOMOSIS

Eastman 910 (Methyl-2-cyanoacrylate) and Aron alpha (ethyl-2-cyano-acrylate) are well known adhesives. Both are prepared in monomer form, and are catalyzed by minute amounts of water. They undergo an extremely rapid anionic polymerization at room temperature, and bind with good shear and tensile strength, as well as solvent resistance. However, severe inflammation and necrosis of the nerve frequently develop, and the adhesives are known to have a toxic effect. This method cannot be recommended as a good procedure for nerve repair.

Three other procedures, one of which is a combination of the clot method and fibrin film (Singer, 1945), one a variation of the plasma glue technique, and one which used a micropore adhesive tape (Freeman, 1964), involve the careful coaptation of the nerve ends and enclosing them in a film that is rolled into a tubular sheath. However, these procedures cannot be employed for nerve suture when there is tension. It can be said, therefore, that the problem with adhesive anastomosis is that it is restricted to small nerves in which there is no tension.

TUBULAR SPLICING

This method involves the wrapping of the nerve suture site in nonirritant material or splicing the nerve ends after pulling them into a closely fitting sleeve or tube. This is referred to as sheathing, tubulation, or cuffing. The objective is to bring about good coaptation of the nerve ends and to allow the nerve fibers to regenerate in straight, parallel courses. These procedures prevent the invasion of fibrous scars from the surrounding area. The advantages of these methods are that, with the use of the tube, it is possible to anastomose nerves without leaving any suture material in the suture site and to retard the direct effects of tensile strength upon the suture line.

The materials that have been used for tubular splicing are live artery (Weiss, 1943), frozen dried artery (Weiss, 1943), tantalum (Weiss, 1944), vein (Takemoto, 1955), millipore (Campbell, 1961), and gelatin and collagen film (Braun, 1966).

Recently, silicone, a biologically inert polymerase, has been used. The method involves the use of a thick silicone tube or a thin walled silicone sheath. Silicone is not absorbable, thus removal of these materials may require a secondary procedure. If the tube is too loose, it will fail to support the suture site; if it is too tight, it may interfere with circulation and restoration or even invade the vessels involved, causing necrosis or disturbance in nerve union. Because of these potential hazards, this method has not been widely adopted.

OTHER METHODS OF ANASTOMOSES

Epineurial Cuff Neurorrhapy

This technique, which was introduced by Snyder and his associates, (Snyder et al., 1974), is described in Figure 26–1. It is a two-level epineurial repair method in which a cuff of epineurium is prepared so that, when the cut ends are approximated, the epineurial sutures are 0.6 centimeter from the point of intraneural severance. However, it is difficult to perform this procedure under tension, and further comparative studies on the end results are required before its general use can be recommended.

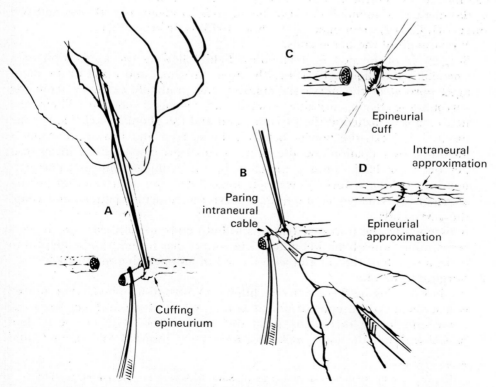

Figure 26–1   Details of the epineurial cuff neurorrhaphy. (Courtesy Dr. Clifford C. Snyder.)

Author's Anchoring Funicular Suture Method

Tension is always a problem in nerve suture. In most of the cases experienced by the author, particularly in old cases, some degree of defect exists between the two nerve ends. Therefore, it is almost always necessary to perform the anastomosis in the presence of tension while simultaneously matching the funicular pattern. Millesi (1972) states that, since it is impossible to perform funicular suture when there is tension, interfascicular nerve graft should be performed, giving consideration to the funicular pattern with the neighboring joints maintained in neutral position. Furthermore, there should be no tension at the time of suturing the nerve ends. This procedure may be theoretically correct, but if carried out as outlined, the following problems will occur: 1) the regenerating axons must cross two suture lines; 2) considerable time is required to obtain nerves and to perform the grafting procedures; 3) the amount of donor nerves available for use is limited. Also, in addition to nerve damage, the injured hand will usually have a number of damaged tendons. Therefore, a large amount of time cannot be devoted to the repair of nerves alone. Consideration must be given to the whole hand at all times, and a balanced allocation of time for the surgical procedure should be planned.

The author's method, called the "anchoring funicular suture," has been found to be quite convenient (Tsuge, 1975). The technique involves the use of a needle fitted with looped nylon suture devised by the author for tendon suture. This is convenient for suturing nerve ends with a gap of 2.0 to 3.5 centimeters in neutral position. The procedure, which is similar in some ways to the method of immobilization of nerve ends by means of a thread and two sinkers (J. Gosset) mentioned by Michon (1975) is described here:

1. Preparation of the nerve ends:

   Surgery is performed in a bloodless field following the application of a pneumatic tourniquet. First, healthy areas proximal and distal to the damaged portion of the nerve are exposed and gradually detached from the surrounding tissue, working toward the damaged portion. Then, the neuroma is detached at the proximal end and the glioma is detached at the distal end. Next, the border between the scarred and healthy portions is identified by palpation and the nerve is cut transversely with a sharp scalpel or razor blade until completely healthy funiculi appear. The epineurium on the reverse side is left intact, with the neuroma and glioma attached. This makes it simple to observe the funicular pattern and coapt the nerve ends.

   Subsequently, the funicular patterns of both ends are studied, and the corresponding funiculi are identified. The author has found it to be helpful to make a sketch of the cut end with the aid of an operating microscope.

2. Surgical technique:

   As shown in Figure 26–2, a needle fitted with 5-0 or 6-0 looped nylon suture* is inserted into the epineurium at points A and B about 1 cm from the nerve end, being careful to avoid the main vessels. The needle is then passed through the loop, making a loop knot, inserted into point C and

---

*Manufactured by Kóno Seisaku–sho, 2-11-10, Soya, Ichikawa–shi. Chiba–Ken, Japan 272.

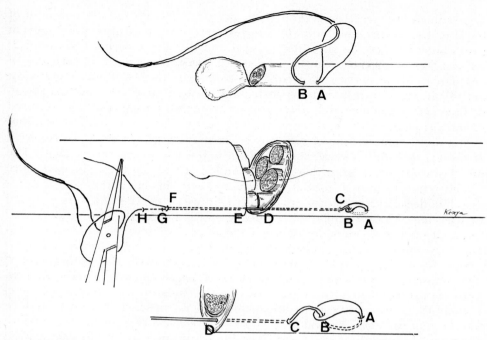

Figure 26–2 The steps of the "anchoring funicular suture," using a needle with a looped nylon suture.

drawn out at point D on the nerve end, which is close to the perineurium of the earlier identified main funiculus. The needle is then inserted at the corresponding point E on the opposite nerve end, and is drawn out at point F about 1 cm from the end. One of the nylon sutures is cut close to the threaded end of the needle, after which the needle is drawn into and out of the epineurium at points G and H taking care to avoid blood vessels. The cut suture is tied, and both nerve ends are drawn together to achieve coaptation. It is important to draw the nerve ends together with the elbow and wrist joints in flexion so that no tension is applied to the nerve. However, no compression should be applied to the nerve ends. This concludes the anchoring suture procedure on one side. If necessary, suturing of the opposite side is performed, following the same steps, but, in this case, the suture is not knotted unless there is considerable tension. Next, a few perineurial sutures are applied to the main funiculi, and, after good coaptation of the funicular pattern is obtained, the anchoring suture on the opposite side is knotted as the final step. Epineurial suture follows the above procedure, but combined suture running from the epineurium to the perineurium may also be used. This concludes the actual procedure.

After releasing the tourniquet, the state of blood circulation at the suture site should be observed. Poor circulation is an indication that the nerve cannot be salvaged by anastomotic procedures, and thus nerve graft is indicated.

The advantages of this suture method are as follows: 1) it is possible to approximate the nerve ends even in the presence of a considerable amount of tension, and at the same time the sutures serve as stay sutures, which permit easy observation of the funicular pattern and simplify suturing operation; 2) tension free anastomosis can be achieved at the suture line; 3) disturbance of circulation at the nerve end occurs less frequently than with other methods; and 4) prevention of hematoma formation is easier. It is felt that this procedure is very convenient for nerve suture in the most frequently encountered clinical situations, where there is a gap of 2.0 to 3.5 cm in neutral position. When the tension at time of suture is great, nerve graft should be considered. If the gap is within several centimeters, it is possible to use this method. The interfascicular nerve graft described by Millesi (1972) can be performed more readily and effectively if used in combination with this method.

The decision to perform either nerve suture or nerve graft is determined by the state of local circulation. Lundborg and Rydevik (1973), on the basis of research on the relationship between the degree of tension and intraneural microvascular circulation, stated that when 5 to 10 per cent stretching is continued for a long period of time, there is a possibility that disturbance of intraneural circulation may occur, resulting in nerve necrosis. Therefore, care must be exercised in suturing nerves that the ends do not become necrotic. Usually the neighboring joints are maintained in sufficient flexion to reduce tension, but the angle should be 20 to 30 degrees less than maximum flexion. Care must be exercised because a hyperflexed position can disturb circulation in the nerve and can result in extensive necrosis and in delay in recovery of muscle power.

The anchoring funicular suture method developed by the author has been described. This method is considered to lie intermediately between the funicular suture method and interfascicular nerve grafting. It can be applied in cases of extensive nerve damage and, since it is a convenient procedure, it is hoped that it will be used widely.

REFERENCES

Braun, R. M.: Comparative studies of neurorrhaphy and sutureless peripheral nerve repair. Surg. Gynecol. Obstet. *122*:15, 1966.

Campbell, J. B., Bassett, C. A. L., Husby, J., Thulin, C-A., and Feringa, E. R.: Microfilter sheaths in peripheral nerve surgery: A laboratory report and preliminary clinical study. J. Trauma *1*:139, 1961.

Ducker, T. B., and Hayes, G. J.: Experimental improvements in the use of Silastic cuff for peripheral nerve repair. J. Neurosurg. *28*:582, 1967.

Freeman, B. S.: Adhesive anastomosis technics for fine nerves. Experimental and clinical technics. Am. J. Surg. *108*:529, 1964.

Lundborg, G., and Rydevik, B.: Effects of stretching the tibial nerve of the rabbit. A preliminary study of the interneural circulation and the barrier function of the perineurium. J. Bone Joint Surg. *55B*:390, 1973.

Michon, J.: Nerve suture today. *In* Michon J. and Moberg, E.: Traumatic Nerve Lesions of the Upper Limb. Edinburgh, Churchill Livingstone, 1975.

Midgley, R. D., and Woolhouse, F. M.: Silicone rubber sheathing as an adjunct to neural anastomosis. Surg. Clin. N. Am. *48*:1149, 1968.

Millesi, H., Meissl, G., and Berger, A.: The interfascicular nerve grafting of the median and ulnar nerves. J. Bone Joint Surg. *54A*:727, 1972.

Morotomi, T., Okazaki, S., and Mizuta, S.: The new method of suturing traumatic peripheral nerve paralysis. Int. Surg. *48*:164, 1967.

Omer, G. E., and Spinner, M.: Peripheral nerve testing and suture techniques. *In* The American

Academy of Orthopaedic Surgeons: Instructional Course Lectures. St. Louis, The C. V. Mosby Co., 1975, Vol. 24.

Singer, M.: The combined use of fibrin film and clot in end to end union of nerves. An experimental study. J. Neurosurg. 2:102, 1945.

Snyder, C. C., Briwnem, E. A., Herzog, B. G., Johnson, E. A., and Coleman, D. A.: Epineural cuff neurorrhaphy. J. Bone Joint Surg. 56A:1092, 1974.

Taketomo, T.: Surgery of peripheral nerves (Japanese). Operation (Tokyo) 9:399, 1955.

Tarlov, I. M., Denslow, C., Swarz, S., and Pineles, D.: Plasma clot suture of nerves. Experimental technic. Arch. Surg. 47:44, 1943.

Tarlov, I. M., and Benjamin, B.: Plasma clot and silk suture of nerves. An experimental study of comparative tissue reaction. Surg. Gynecol. Obstet. 76:366, 1943.

Tarlov, I. M.: Autologous plasma clot suture of nerves. Its use in clinical surgery. J.A.M.A. 126:741, 1944.

Tsuge, K., Ikuta, Y., and Sakaue, M.: A new technique for nerve suture. The anchoring funicular suture. Plast. Reconst. Surg. 56:496, 1975.

Weiss, R.: Nerve reunion with sleeves of frozen-dried artery in rabbits, cats and monkeys. Proc. Soc. Exp. Biol. Med. 54:274, 1943.

Weiss, P.: Nerve regeneration in the rat following tubular splicing of severed nerves. Arch. Surg. 46:525, 1943.

Weiss, P.: Sutureless reunion of severed nerves with elastic cuffs of tantalum. J. Neurosurg. 1:219, 1944.

Young, J. Z., and Medawar, P. B.: Fibrin suture of peripheral nerves. Lancet 2:126, 1940.

27

EVALUATION OF THE NEUROMA IN CONTINUITY

DAVID G. KLINE

One of the greatest challenges to those managing peripheral nerve lesions is the neuroma in continuity. This is because such a lesion may initially be partial, with sparing of a variable amount of important distal function, or when complete may have in some cases the potential for spontaneous regeneration and restoration of important distal function, while having in others no potential for recovery without resection and suture repair. The problem with a neuroma in continuity is its unpredictable future, and the challenge is to develop and use techniques that will accurately predict either recovery without resection and repair or the need for such (Kline and Nulsen, 1972; Woodhall et al., 1957). It is important to realize that at least 60 per cent of nerve injuries, even in civilian practice, do not transect the nerve but leave it with some degree of continuity. Thus, the necessity for careful evaluation of such lesions is not occasional but recurrent. Matters are not so difficult when there is significant sparing of important function distal to such a lesion, for here the clinician can afford to await further return of function to the less significant distal muscular and sensory inputs with the assurance that at least the more important functions have been spared. Indeed, such partial injuries will, with the passage of time, often but unfortunately not always, recover further distal function.

Fascicular assignment for distal function becomes more definite anatomically in the distal segments of the nerve, whereas such assignments are more widely distributed in the proximal course of the nerve (Seddon, 1972). Thus, partial lesions of distal nerves are more likely to damage a fascicle destined for one or more specific distal sites, whereas proximal partial injuries are more likely to damage a cross section of fibers destined for many distal end organs. Thus, if all muscles distal to a proximal lesion are only partially involved, then only a portion of the nerve has been divided, whereas with a distal lesion, a portion of the nerve has been spared if all distal muscular function is completely lost but sensation is spared. An example is provided by a partially injured median nerve at the distal forearm or wrist level where the important and *usually* single sensory fascicle is spared but function of the thenar, abductor pollicis brevis, and opponens pollicis muscles is weak or missing. The clinician can afford to wait three to four months knowing that the important sensory function in this particular nerve is ensured, and only if no further thenar motor recovery occurs does he have to proceed with exploration and differential evaluation and perhaps repair of the motor fascicles of the nerve. Unfortunately, the situation is not so straightforward with a complete lesion in continuity where all function distal to the lesion is lost. Return of function with further time depends on the neuropathology of the lesion, for those with a large neurotmetic element will not recover whereas those with neurapraxia or axonotmetic elements, or both, may (Hubbard, 1972; Seddon, 1972).

Precise knowledge of the wounding agent will be a help in the assessment of potential pathology even though such a history is not always available (Brown, 1972; Buncke, 1972; Seddon, 1972). Glass and knife wounds are likely to lead to transection although 25 per cent of such wounds associated with a complete distal peripheral nerve loss still leave the nerve in gross continuity, and some of these can recover without resection and suture (Kline and Hackett, 1975). Gunshot wounds, severe crush associated with high speed vehicular accidents, and contusion or partial transection due to compound fractures are more likely to be neurotmetic and thus less likely to recover than milder injuries. Nonetheless, the majority of lesions in continuity are unknown quantities, certainly during the early months following injury, and, unfortunately, their course, based on clinical criteria, only becomes evident after many months have elapsed. At this time, resection and repair may be too late, since not only deterioration of distal inputs such as the distal stump as well as muscle replaced with fat and fibrous tissue but also proximal stump changes thwart full functional recovery despite the presence of axons (Ducker et al., 1969; Gutmann and Young, 1944; Guttman and Holubar, 1951). On the other hand, exploration of such a lesion soon after injury may not provide answers, since enough time for measurable regeneration to occur may not have elapsed (Kline and Hackett, 1975). The surgeon is left with inspection and palpation of the lesion, which can, unfortunately, be misleading. A bulbous and firm lesion, perhaps due to a gunshot wound, may be regenerating and the observed deformity may be a result of epineurial and perineurial scar with a relatively organized intrafascicular array of new axons. By comparison, a modeled and sleek-appearing lesion, perhaps resulting from an injection injury, may have severe intrafascicular damage with minimal epineurial and perineurial change and thus, while appearing benign, yet have poor potential for recovery (Clark et al., 1970). As has been pointed out before (Nulsen and Kline, 1973; Woodhall, et al., 1957), one cannot always "tell the contents of the book by its cover." Some of the testing necessary to determine whether or not an injury that is potentially in continuity should be surgically explored is described below.

CLINICAL TESTING

Careful, detailed, and repetitive sensory and motor testing is essential for adequate evaluation of any nerve injury. Clinical testing is useful not only in documenting the original extent of the injury but also in charting any reversal of loss over the early days to weeks when there is a neurapraxic element. Such recovery is too early to ascribe to regeneration, since the latter follows the millimeter-per-day or inch-per-month rule. Autonomic function, such as sweating, is served by fine fibers and, since these regenerate first, it is tempting to use return of sweating as a sign of useful regeneration. Unfortunately, presence of fine fibers even at such distal sites as autonomous sensory zones for the median or ulnar nerve does not guarantee subsequent regeneration of larger sensory and motor axons, although it certainly favors it (Nulsen and Kline, 1973). Of greater significance is the fact that continued absence of sweating does not occur in regeneration. In a similar fashion, return of sensation to autonomous zones suggests further useful regeneration, such as that of motor fibers, but does not guarantee it (Moberg, 1975). Certainly, return of voluntary contraction to muscles that have been totally paralyzed is important. Such recovery should begin in muscle or muscles immediately distal to the injury site and progress by a timetable predicated on the inch-per-month rule to more distal muscles (Seddon et al., 1943; Sunderland, 1947*a* and *b*). In many nerve injuries the wait for motor recovery is, unfortunately, a long one, and if such recovery does not occur at the time calculated that it should, it may be too late for successful resection and repair. This makes other types of testing especially important.

For example, *Tinel's sign* is used by many clinicians to signify regeneration. This test is valuable, but only as long as its limitations are kept in mind. Tinel's test is based on the irritability of fine, regenerating fibers. Tapping over the course of the nerve where such fibers are present produces paresthesias or tingling in the distribution of the nerve, signifies regeneration, and is a positive Tinel's sign. Unfortunately, such fibers may or may not subsequently increase enough in caliber and gain enough myelination to lead to useful distal function. Certainly, a positive Tinel's when tapping over the injury itself is meaningless, for fine fibers almost always reach the injury site where they branch, become disorganized, and become involved in scar. On the other hand, a Tinel's obtained well distal to an injury site tells us that fine fibers have regenerated to that point. If the Tinel's sign progresses down the distal course of the nerve, this suggests further regeneration but again does not guarantee functional recovery (Omer and Spinner, 1975). Indeeed, many patients with an advancing Tinel's sign will need resection and repair of their lesion in continuity (Henderson, 1948; Nulsen and Kline, 1973; Woodhall et al., 1957). On the other hand, when a Tinel's sign cannot be elicited below the injury site three to four months after injury or suture this suggests that not even fine fibers have reached the point being tapped. Thus, absence of a Tinel's sign becomes an important negative finding and suggests the need for exploration (Nulsen and Kline, 1973).

Electrical Tests

Stimulation of a regenerating nerve may produce distal muscular function even though the patient cannot voluntarily contract the same muscles. Such "stimulated function" can antedate voluntary contraction by weeks to a month or so (Grundfest et al., 1957; Nulsen and Lewey, 1947). Nonetheless, a number of months need to elapse between injury and testing, since muscular contraction obtained by stimulation of nerve is predicated not only on axons reaching muscle but also on the occurrence of some degree of axon to motor end-plate reconstruction. For example, with a mid-humeral injury to the radial nerve, stimulation of an axonotmetic lesion, which is of course regenerating, cannot be expected to produce contraction of the brachioradialis until three or four months have passed, since it will take this long for axons to regenerate from the mid-humeral level to this muscle and for some early axon to motor end-plate reconstruction to occur (Nulsen, 1966). Unfortunately, with lesions to other nerves, such as elements of the brachial plexus, or median and ulnar nerves in the upper arm, or the sciatic, time needed for axons to reach musculature distal to the injury site is even greater. For example, six or seven months may have to elapse before there is enough distal regeneration of axons in the upper arm median nerve to allow contraction of the pronator teres or flexor superficialis in response to nerve stimulation. With mid-thigh sciatic nerve injury, nine months to a year may have to elapse before gastrocnemius–achilles contraction or a year to a year and a half before anterior compartment muscular contraction can be expected from stimulation. If enough time has passed that the calculated deadline for axons to reach muscle has elapsed and stimulation of the nerve does not produce contraction, exploration is usually necessary.

Electromyography (EMG) tests the innervation of muscle. Signs of denervation, such as fibrillations and denervation potentials, can be seen two to four weeks after serious injury, the length of interval depending on how far the lesion is from the muscle being tested. If muscles in the distribution of the injured nerve do not show denervational changes, one must make sure that their innervation is not coming from adjacent nerves; this may require special conduction studies or nerve block with a local anesthetic. With re-input of axons into muscle and some motor end-plate reconstruction, the electromyographer finds an increase in insertional activity and a decrease in the number of fibrillations and denervation potentials. In addition, nascent muscle action potentials may be seen (Bowden, 1954). If signs of reinnervation in proximal muscles are seen by EMG, they should progress with time into more distal muscles and not remain relegated to one muscle or one set of muscles. Enough time must elapse for axons not only to traverse the distal nerve stump but also to re-form a nerve to motor end-plate to muscle relationship (Licht, 1961). In the most common injury sites for most nerves, such regeneration usually takes months and this restricts the value of the EMG for documentation of early regeneration. Furthermore, even electromyographic evidence of regeneration does not guarantee subsequent useful clinical function, for electromyography is a physiologic rather than a functional test. Proper electromyography requires thorough sampling of different regions of a number of muscles and thus depends on the perseverance as well as the experience of the electromyographer. Nonetheless, electromyograms done in a careful and serial fashion can provide valuable information as long as the temporal and interpretive limitations of the test are understood.

Conduction studies done in the usual fashion by stimulating nerve and recording from muscle will be useful only in mild or partial injuries, in entrapments, and when there is a question of anomalous or shared innervation, since once again extensive axon to motor end-plate and muscle relationships are necessary in order to evoke a measurable *muscle action potential*. Such studies then find little application in the more serious and more complete nerve injuries until many months later (Kline and Hackett, 1970; Licht, 1961). At this time, clinical recovery is usually already evident, although the question as to how complete such recovery is may be answered in part by such conduction studies.

It is possible by use of a computer to record *Nerve action potentials (NAP's)* noninvasively across some human nerve injuries. Metallic cup electrodes, EEG paste, and tape are used to fix electrodes at the skin level over the dipole or course of the nerve, both above and below the injury. Multiple stimuli are provided by a Grass* S-44 stimulator via an SIU5 stimulus isolation unit. Stimulation is usually done distally and recording proximally in order to minimize muscle action potential artifacts. Sites selected for electrode placement should be in areas where the nerve is relatively close to the skin. Bipolar stimulating and recording electrodes are used and the latter are led to a Grass P55 differential amplifier set at $\times$ 10,000, with the low filter usually at 1 Hz and high filter at 3 kHz. The output from the preamplifiers is then led to the differential amplifier of an oscilloscope so that each sweep can be viewed. Individual sweeps are then summated by a Fabritek computer, which has an input resolution of 9 bits, input level set at $\pm$ 1 volt, filter time constant of .02 milliseconds, and analysis time usually of 20 milliseconds. Trains of 64, 128, 256, 512, or, infrequently, 1024 stimuli are summated by the computer and the resultant trace displayed on an oscilloscope and photographed by a Polaroid camera. This technique not only amplifies the responses, which are only a few microvolts in size by the time they reach the skin level, but, by virtue of the type of summation used, decreases the noise and artifact level associated with such amplification (Dawson, 1956; Gilliat and Sears; Seddon, 1972). Relative amplification used by the technique can be displayed as a digital number, as can the latency between onset of stimulus artifact and onset of evoked response. In this fashion, nerve action potential conduction evidence of early (1½ to 5 months) regeneration can sometimes be recorded. The technique works best for median, ulnar, and some radial nerve lesions but can be used to stimulate and record from elements distal to the injury where the brachial plexus or sciatic nerve are involved. Results with this noninvasive technique are not as accurate as those with operative recording techniques, to be described later in the chapter. There is, in our experience, about a 5 per cent incidence of false negatives and positives. Incidence of misleading results will fluctuate depending on the nerve being tested, level of the lesion, presence of complicating soft tissue wounds, size of the limb and thus distance between nerve and electrode sites, and how much potential regenerative time has elapsed between injury and attempt at recording. This technique is not at present as accurate as the more direct operative assessment of nerve action potentials to be discussed later.

SURGICAL EVALUATION OF A LESION IN CONTINUITY

Careful proximal and distal exposure of a suspected lesion in continuity is essential. Exposure should be generous and dissection of the lesion itself delayed

---

*Grass Instrument Company, Quincy, Massachusetts.

until both proximal and distal elements have been isolated and identified. Longitudinal blood supply to the nerve should be preserved but most collaterals can be sacrificed so that a 360 degree esposure of the nerve itself is gained (Kline et al., 1972; Lundborg, 1975). The lesion in continuity is then inspected. If the neuroma is fusiform, a swelling of up to twice normal diameter can be compatible with either axonotmesis or neurotmesis, whereas swelling larger than that favors neurotmesis, although there are exceptions to this. Firmness or hardness, of course, favors heavy internal scar and neurotmesis. In general, the internal architecture of the neuroma is almost always worse than it appears on inspection or palpation (Seddon, 1972). Lateral neuromas suggest partial transection. If the portion spared with a lateral neuroma or partial transection is known from preoperative clinical examination to go to an unimportant distal structure it can be sacrificed to repair the whole nerve. In partial transection, if more than two thirds of the nerve is divided, complete resection and repair is usually advisable. With more circumferential or fusiform neuromas, some authors have advised trial section, cutting through scar until fascicles are encountered, stopping if they are in continuity (Zachery and Roaf, 1954). We have not had experience with this technique. Injection of saline or other "physiologic" solution into lesions in continuity in an attempt to delineate fascicles does not make anatomic sense, since much of the scar preventing regeneration is intrafascicular rather than perineurial. In the laboratory, injection of a nerve with saline can decrease or eliminate recordable electrical activity, so we do not advise this, even though these physiologic changes are usually temporary.

After inspection and gentle palpation of the lesion, the nerve is stimulated proximal and distal to the lesion itself to see if function of muscle clearly related to the nerve in question and distal to the lesion can be observed. Stimulation, particularly of the proximal stump, will travel retrograde and thus can stimulate muscles with innervation proximal to the lesion. Such function can be misleading unless care is taken to palpate and, if possible, inspect the contracting muscles. This may require special attention to positioning and draping of the extremity before the case is begun. We prefer to use a stimulator with variable voltage and

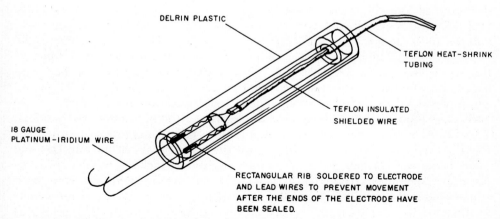

Figure 27–1 Bipolar stimulating or recording electrode. The handle is cut from a Delrin plastic rod 3/5th of an inch in diameter. The center is bored out to accommodate Teflon heat-shrink tubing, which is soldered to 18 gauge platinum-iridium wire. The ends of the handle are sealed with acrylic cement.

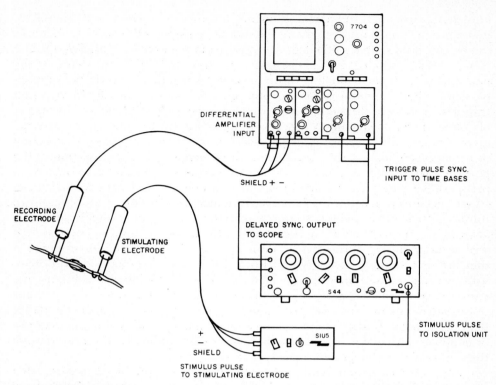

Figure 27–2 Equipment used for stimulating nerve and evoking and recording a nerve action potential (NAP). Stimulator can provide a stimulus of variable voltage, duration, frequency, and onset and interfaces with a stimulus isolator which diminishes chances of ground loop between the equipment and the patient. Responses picked up by the bipolar electrodes are recorded by the differential amplifier of the oscilloscope, displayed on the screen, and photographed by a Polaroid camera. Sweeps on the oscilloscope are synchronized with stimuli to the nerve by the delayed synchronized output from the stimulator, as shown in the drawing.

duration, and currently use a Grass S-44 or S-55 with a SIU-5 stimulus isolation unit. Electrodes are bipolar, with tips made of stainless steel or platinum alloy, and no. 18 in caliber. The end of the electrode is bent like a "shepherd's crook" to fit the nerve. The tips are then soldered to shielded bipolar wire and passed through a Plexiglas or Delrin rod 3/5 inch in diameter whose center has been bored out. The ends of the rods are sealed with acrylic cement (Fig. 27–1).

Since axons may regenerate through a lesion and well into the distal stump and yet be months away from a measurable distal input (Gutmann and Sanders, 1943; Kline et al., 1969), we have attempted to record nerve action potentials (NAP's) across all injuries in continuity for the last 11 years (Kline and DeJong, 1968; Kline and Hackett, 1975). Necessary equipment includes bipolar stimulating and recording electrodes constructed as above. Shielded wire is used for both stimulating and recording electrodes. Once again, a Grass stimulator and stimulus isolation unit are used and recording is done by a differential amplifier and oscilloscope. For a number of years we have used the Tektronix* 565 dual beam

---

*Tektronix Company, Beaverton, Oregon

oscilloscope with two 3A9 differential amplifiers so that we could record a nerve action potential as well as an evoked EMG response on the dual trace scope if we wished. For the last several years we have used the Tektronix 7844 or 7704 dual beam oscilloscope with two differential amplifiers, a 7B70 and a 7B71 time base, a 7M13 readout unit so information about the patient can be displayed on the screen, and a C53 Polaroid camera to record the traces (Fig. 27–2). Whatever components are used it is important that output from the stimulator be interfaced with the oscilloscope so that a trace is triggered across the face with each stimulus. Frequency filters on differential amplifiers are usually set for nerve action potentials at or below 3 kHz for the upper filter and 1 Hz for the lower filter. Amplification necessary to record nerve action potentials will vary between 20 microvolts and .5 millivolts per division, while the time frame is set on 0.5 to 2.0 milliseconds per division. Stimuli need to be brief in duration (.01 to .06 milliseconds) because distance between stimulating and recording electrodes is usually relatively short. As a result, the stimulus artifact is high in amplitude since increased voltage is necessary to evoke a response. This differs from the more physiologic but less clinically applicable methods available for recording nerve action potentials in the experimental literature. Decreasing stimulus duration to

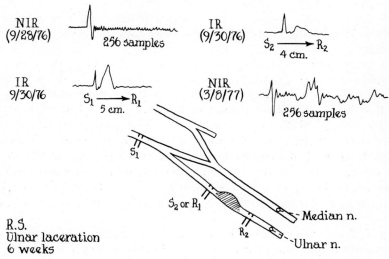

Figure 27–3 Non-invasive and invasive NAP recordings made from ulnar nerve with a proximal upper arm lesion in continuity. Computerized non-invasive recordings (NIR) made preoperatively by taping stimulating electrodes over the olecranon notch region and recording electrodes proximal to skin laceration site showed no NAP after 256 summations. Clinically, this patient had a complete motor loss except for partial sparing of flexor carpi ulnaris function (3/5) and some, but definite, sensory sparing even in the ulnar autonomous zones of the hand. Indeed, at operation 6 weeks post injury, a small invasively recorded NAP (IR-S1-R2) could be obtained across the lesion, while an excellent potential could be recorded proximal to the partial neuroma (IR-S1-R1). Since the retained function was less important than that lost, the lesion was completed by resection of the neuroma and then an epineurial suture repair was done. Histologically, the neuromatous portion of this nerve was neurotmetic in nature. Three relatively small fascicles had not been transected and were responsible for the partially retained function as well as the small invasively recorded NAP. Non-invasive computerized recording 5½ months later shows an excellent NAP across the suture repair. This patient has subsequently made an excellent recovery for a high ulnar lesion (flexor carpi ulnaris, 5/5; flexor profundus, 4/5; hypothenar muscles, 4/5; interossei, 2-3/5; lumbricals, 2-3/5; adductor pollicis, 1/5).

microseconds require a higher voltage but decreases the stimulus artifact runoff, so that the fast-following nerve action potential, if present, can be viewed with minimal interference from the stimulus artifact.

It helps to expose enough of the nerve above the lesion to place both stimulating and recording electrodes proximally. If the stimulating and recording system is working correctly, a nerve action potential should be recorded from the proximal stump. In rare circumstances, stretch and/or lengthy contusion to the nerve extending above the lesion site will make recording of a healthy proximal nerve action potential difficult. Usually, a good proximal potential can be recorded and the recording electrodes moved distal and beyond the lesion to see if a nerve action potential can be evoked through the injury. Voltage may have to be increased to conduct across the neuroma, and amplification will often have to be increased to pick up a small response. Voltage for stimulation at durations of .01 to .06 milliseconds will range from 1 to 125 volts. Stimulus rate can be adjusted, usually somewhere between 1 and 2 per second, so that consecutive traces can be viewed on the oscilloscope screen. A Polaroid camera is then used to make a more permanent record of a single trace.

If a potential is recorded immediately distal to the neuroma in continuity, recording electrodes are moved further down the distal stump to see how far the potential, and thus presumably regenerating fibers of adequate size, has extended (Kline et al., 1969). When stimulation produces muscular contraction, the potential recorded by electrodes placed on the nerve may be mistaken for a nerve action potential. Muscle action potentials will have longer latencies, will require less amplification, and will have a more rounded peak than nerve action potentials.

If a nerve action potential cannot be recorded distal to the injury, voltage and amplification are gradually increased until it is difficult to visualize that portion of the trace following the stimulus artifact. Attention should be paid to electrode contact, and blood should be irrigated away from the region of the electrodes. It is generally best to elevate the nerve away from surrounding soft tissues by means of the electrodes but if need be the nerve can be stimulated and recorded from by isolating short segments on either side of the lesion and placing the electrodes on them. Usually one will want to completely expose the nerve as well as the injury before beginning to record, but occasionally it may be necessary or desirable to stimulate and record with a more limited exposure (Fig. 27–3).

If a NAP can be recorded from a sciatic nerve with a severe distal loss, the nerve should be split into its two divisions. In this setting, it is possible that the potential seen is only from one division and that the other needs resection and repair. If the sciatic injury is close to its natural division into tibial and peroneal nerves, one can accomplish evaluation by stimulating the whole sciatic and recording alternately from each nerve. A similar approach can be used with brachial plexus lesions (Figs. 27–4 and 27–5). For example, lesions of the lateral cord can be handled by stimulating the cord proximal to the region of the injury and recording from the more distal musculocutaneous and lateral cord branch to the median nerve. Medial cord lesions can be evaluated by utilizing for recording sites those portions of the median and ulnar nerves immediately distal to the injury. Lesions to trunks of the plexus may require stimulation of roots and recording from either distal trunks or even their distal divisions or cords. A forearm-

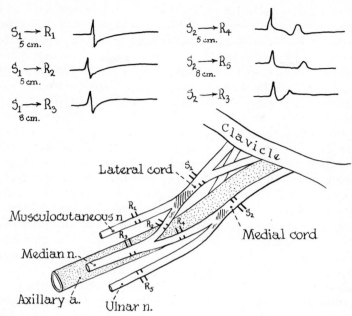

Figure 27–4 Use of stimulation and NAP recording to sort out a severe brachial plexus injury due to GSW. Loss at 3 months post wounding was almost complete, with only deltoid and some triceps sparing. Fortunately, NAP's could be evoked through the medial cord injury in continuity to both median and ulnar nerves while the lateral cord, which is reparable with a better chance of recovery, was severely injured and required resection and repair by interfascicular sural grafts.

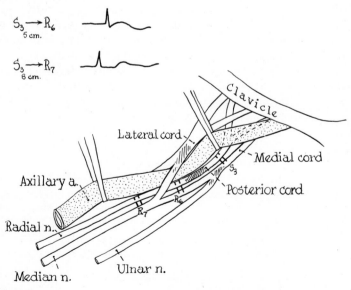

Figure 27–5 Axillary artery has been retracted to expose injured posterior cord, which after neurolysis could be stimulated and recorded from. Stimulation, in addition to producing triceps function, gave an NAP distal to the lesion, so resection was not necessary.

level lesion to the proximal radial nerve can be evaluated by recording from both the superficial sensory nerve and posterior interosseus nerve after stimulation of the whole radial nerve. A similar philosophy on a less macroscopic scale has been used on some partial nerve injuries where we have split the nerve into fascicles and recorded from each fascicle. This variation of our NAP recording technique has been described nicely by Williams and Terzis (1976). Such a technique can be of help when the lesion is known preoperatively to be partial and yet important distal function is absent.

Timing for exploration of a potential neuroma in continuity is most important (Ducker et al., 1969; Engh and Schofield, 1972; White, 1960). In our experience, exploration at 8 to 10 weeks is optimal, since, if adequate recovery is occurring it should be recordable by that time (Kline and Nulsen, 1972; Kline and Hackett, 1975). On the other hand, to delay beyond four months can be deleterious if resection and suture are necessary (Brown, 1972). If the distal deficit is complete and yet an NAP can be recorded, then external neurolysis with perhaps limited internal neurolysis is almost always sufficient, and resection and suture are not necessary. Those lesions in continuity having a nerve action potential have had better than 90 per cent significant recovery with motor and sensory grades of 3 or better. Those not having a nerve action potential and having resection and suture had pathologic changes which one could predict would not have led to recovery, since neurotmesis was present. Most of the neurotmetic lesions (no NAP) were repaired by epineurial end-to-end suture although a few interfascicular sural grafts were necessary in lengthy lesions in continuity, particularly those involving the brachial plexus.

Nerve action potential responses recorded six or more months post injury that require very high amplification (10 microvolts per division) and conduct less than 20 meters per second indicate poor regeneration, and may still need resection and suture despite the presence of an NAP. Lesions in continuity known clinically to be partial will, of course, have a nerve action potential and then its amplitude and duration, as well as conduction velocity of the evoked response, must be taken into account. In partial injuries, presence of a nerve action potential does not necessarily indicate that other more seriously injured portions of the nerve will regenerate, although usually when such a response is recorded they will. Similar criteria in nerves that have had an opportunity to regenerate for many months have to be studied carefully, for a response that might be acceptable at 2 months may not be at 10.

REFERENCES

Bowden, R. E.: Electromyography. *In* Seddon H. J. (ed.): Peripheral Nerve Injuries. Med. Res. Council Spec. Report Series No. 282, p. 263, Her Majesty's Stationery Office, London, 1954.

Brown, P. W.: Factors influencing the success of surgical repair of peripheral nerves. Surg. Clin. N. Am. *52*:1137, 1972.

Buncke, H. J., Jr.: Digital nerve repairs. Surg. Clin. N. Am. *52*:1267, 1972.

Clark, K., Williams, P., Willis, W., and McGavran, W.: Injection injury of the sciatic nerve. Clin. Neurosurg. *17*:111, 1970.

Dawson, G.: Relative excitability and conduction velocity in sensory and motor nerve fibers in man. J. Physiol. *131*:436, 1956.

Ducker, T. B., Kempe, L. G., and Hayes, G. J.: The metabolic background for peripheral nerve surgery. J. Neurosurg. *30*:270, 1969.

Engh, C. A., and Schofield, B. H.: A review of the central response to peripheral nerve injury and its significance in nerve regeneration. J. Neurosurg. *37*:195, 1972.

Gilliatt, R., and Sears, T. A.: Sensory nerve action potentials in patients with peripheral nerve lesions. J. Neurol. Neurosurg. Psychiatry *21*:109, 1958.

Grundfest, H., Oester, Y., and Beebe, G.: Electrical evidence of regeneration. *In* Woodhall, B. and Beebe, G. W. (eds.): Peripheral Nerve Regeneration. V. A. Medical Monograph, U.S. Government Printing Office, Washington, D.C., 1957, p. 203.

Gutmann, E., and Sanders, F. K.: Recovery of fiber numbers and diameters in the regeneration of peripheral nerves. J. Physiol. *101*:489, 1943.

Gutmann, E., and Young, J. Z.: Re-innervation of muscle after various periods of atrophy. J. Anat. *78*:15, 1944.

Gutmann, E., and Holubar, J.: Atrophy of nerve fibers in the central stump following nerve section and the possibilities of its prevention. Arch. Int. Stud. Neurol. *1*:314, 1951.

Henderson, W. R.: Clinical assessment of peripheral nerve injuries. Tinel's test. Lancet *2*:801, 1948.

Hubbard, J. H.: The quality of nerve regeneration: Factors independent of the most skillful repair. Surg. Clin. North Am. *52*:1099, 1972.

Kline, D. G., and DeJong, B. R.: Evoked potentials to evaluate peripheral nerve injuries. Surg. Gynecol. Obstet. *127*:1239, 1968.

Kline, D. G., Hackett, E. R., and May, P.: Evaluation of nerve injuries by evoked potentials and electromyography. J. Neurosurg. *31*:128, 1969.

Kline, D. G., and Hackett, E. R.: Value of electrophysiologic tests for peripheral nerve neuromas. J. Surg. Oncol. *2*:299, 1970.

Kline, D. G., and Nulsen, F. E.: The neuroma in continuity: its pre-operative and operative management. Surg. Clin. North Am. *52*:1189, 1972.

Kline, D. G., Hackett, E. R., Davis, G. D., and Myers, M. B.: Effect of mobilization on the blood supply and regeneration of injured nerves. J. Surg. Res. *12*:254, 1972.

Kline, D., and Hackett, E.: Reappraisal of timing for exploration of civilian peripheral nerve injuries. Surgery *78*:54, 1975.

Licht, S. (ed): Electrodiagnosis and Electromyography, New Haven, Connecticut, E. Licht, Publisher, 1961.

Lundborg, G.: Structure and function of the intraneural microvessels as related to trauma, edema formation, and nerve function. J. Bone Joint Surg. *57A*:938, 1975.

Moberg, E.: Methods for examining sensibility of the hand. *In* Flynn, J. (ed.): Hand Surgery, 1975, p. 295.

Nulsen, F. E., and Lewey, F. H.: Intraneural bipolar stimulation: a new aid in the assessment of nerve injuries. Science *106*:301, 1947.

Nulsen, F. E.: The management of peripheral nerve injury producing hand dysfunction. *In* Flynn, J. E. (ed.): Hand Surgery. Williams & Wilkins, 1966, p. 457.

Nulsen, F. E., and Kline, D. G.: Acute injuries of peripheral nerves. *In* Youmans, J. R. (ed.): Neurological Surgery. W. B. Saunders Co., Philadelphia, 1973, Vol. 2, p. 1089.

Omer, G. E., and Spinner, M.: Peripheral nerve testing and suture techniques. *In* American Academy of Orthopedic Surgeons Instructional Course Lectures. St. Louis, C. V. Mosby & Co., 1975, Vol. 24, p. 122.

Seddon, H. J., Medawar, P. B., and Smith, H.: Rate of regeneration of peripheral nerves in man. J. Physiol. *102*:191, 1943.

Seddon, H. J.: Surgical Disorders of the Peripheral Nerves. Baltimore, Williams & Wilkins Co., 1972.

Sunderland, S.: Rate of regeneration in human peripheral nerves. Arch. Neurol. Psychiat. *58*:251, 1947*a*.

Sunderland, S.: Rate of regeneration in human peripheral nerves: Analysis of interval between injury and onset of recovery. Arch. Neurol. Psychiat. *58*:291, 1947*b*.

White, J. C.: Timing of nerve suture after gunshot wound. Surgery *48*:946, 1960.

Williams, H. B., and Terzis, J.: Single fascicular recordings: an intraoperative diagnostic tool for the management of peripheral nerve lesions. Plast. Reconstr. Surg. *57*:562, 1976.

Woodhall, B., Nulsen, F., White, J., and Davis, L.: Neurosurgical Implications. *In* Peripheral Nerve Regeneration. Washington, D.C., Veterans Administration Monograph, 1957, p. 569.

Zachery, R. B., and Roaf, R.: Lesions in continuity. *In* Seddon, H. J. (ed.): Peripheral Nerve Injuries. Her Majesty's Stationery Office, London, Medical Research Council Special Report, Series 282, 1954, p. 57.

28

INTRAOPERATIVE ASSESSMENT OF NERVE LESIONS WITH FASCICULAR DISSECTION AND ELECTRO-PHYSIOLOGICAL RECORDINGS

JULIA K. TERZIS,
ROLLIN K. DANIEL,
H. BRUCE WILLIAMS

BACKGROUND

Analysis of the excitable properties of the peripheral nerve has had to await the availability of needed instrumentation to achieve the necessary measurements. Throughout the Middle Ages, Galen's doctrine of animal spirits preoccupied the beliefs of the scientific world. In 1791, Galvani, an anatomist and physician, demonstrated in the frog that a nerve–muscle preparation could be easily stimulated by connecting the nerve and the muscle to two dissimilar metals. Volta's invention of the voltaic pile in 1800 offered, for the first time, a source of electricity of great capacity. These developments opened the horizons to the science of electricity. The electrical nature of the action potential was shown conclusively by du Bois-Raymond in 1843. In 1850, Helmholtz reported the first measurement of nerve conduction velocity, in a nerve-muscle preparation in a frog. By altering the distance of the stimulating electrode from the nerve to the muscle, he observed differences in the time intervals between stimulus application and muscular contraction. In his revolutionary experiments, Helmholtz obtained a conduction velocity of 30 M/sec., which, interestingly enough, agrees with today's values. Owing to the lack of rapid recording devices, the action potential itself was not studied accurately. The invention of the vacuum tube in the 1920's, along with major developments in electronics, provided the substrate for present day electrophysiology.

The contributions of Erlanger and Gasser (1937) were essential to the understanding of nerve fiber conduction, the compound action potential, and the refractory period of peripheral nerves. Later, the work of Hodgkin and Huxley provided the first quantitative description of the depolarization process underlying the formation of the action potential (Hodgkin et al., 1952; Hodgkin and Huxley, 1952). These electrophysiological breakthroughs were put into clinical use first by Hodes et al. (1948) in the percutaneous measurement of motor nerve conduction, and a year later, by Dawson and Scott (1949) in sensory nerve conduction studies.

Hakstian (1968) utilized stimulation techniques to deduce the intraneural organization in acute nerve injuries. Motor fascicles were identified in the distal stump within the first four days following trauma by direct nerve stimulation and observation of distal muscular contractions. Identification of sensory fascicles necessitated that the patient remain awake. Thus, stimulation of the proximal stump elicited subjective reports from patients in the case of sensory fascicles. Similar orienting methods were utilized by Vandeputt et al. (1969) in an experimental series in dogs. Improved results were reported by these authors when these stimulation techniques were applied prior to nerve suture.

Clinical assessment of pathological states of the peripheral nerves, using intraoperative whole nerve recordings as diagnostic tools, was offered by Kline (1972). Initial experimental documentation (Kline, 1968, 1969) demonstrated that the compound action potential provided a better indication of function as well as a clearer definition of the injury site. The effectiveness of whole nerve recordings was subsequently verified in the management of neuromas in continuity (Kline and Nulsen, 1972).

INTRAOPERATIVE ASSESSMENT OF NERVE LESIONS WITH FASCICULAR DISSECTION AND ELECTROPHYSIOLOGICAL RECORDINGS

The introduction of magnification in the surgical management of nerve injuries (Smith, 1964) offered opportunities to apply electrophysiological techniques to units smaller than the whole nerve. After several experimental series (Terzis et al., 1975; Terzis and Williams, 1976; Terzis, 1976) in which electrophysiological techniques were utilized to depict the quality of nerve regeneration in the distal stump following various types of nerve suture, these techniques were applied clinically in the intraoperative management of lesions in continuity.

On the basis of the preoperative clinical assessment, we have utilized whole nerve and single fascicular recordings as an intraoperative diagnostic tool in the microsurgical repair of two types of nerve lesions in continuity: localized nerve lesions and diffuse nerve lesions.

Localized Nerve Lesions

The mechanism of injury in all these cases was either a sharp laceration or direct blunt trauma to the nerve. Using Seddon's classification, these lesions included all three types of nerve injury: neurapraxia, axonotmesis, and partial neurotmesis. In all these cases, loss of critical sensibility and cold intolerance was present in the corresponding tactile surface of the hand, along with pain over the neuroma. There was enough residual distal function in the hand that conventional treatment — nerve transection with excision of the neuroma — was considered unjustified, for it would have converted a partial nerve injury into a complete one. Instead, the following intraoperative technique was adopted. With tourniquet control, the nerve lesion was widely explored and the neuroma in continuity freed from underlying tissues. Under magnification, the epineurium was excised from the proximal and distal normal nerve, including any remaining epineurial sheath over the damaged nerve segment. Then, fascicular dissection was started in normal proximal and distal nerve tissue and into the lesion. Single fascicular dissection was greatly facilitated by the use of the diamond knife (Terzis, et al., 1974). Only the fascicles that contributed to the neuroma were subjected to dissection and to physiological testing. After completion of the fascicular isolation, the tourniquet was released and hemostasis achieved. Allowance was made for adequate oxygenation of the extremity prior to the onset of electrical recordings. Gas-sterilized recording and stimulating platinum electrodes were then lowered into the operative field. A nerve microspatula was used to lift each individual fascicle onto the stimulating and recording electrodes. Electrical stimuli were delivered proximally, and the evoked response was recorded distally, amplified, and then visually displayed on an oscilloscope. An audio speaker allowed the action potentials to be heard, while a Polaroid camera provided paper records for instant analysis (Fig. 28–1). Similar recordings were than obtained from the corresponding proximal normal fascicles for intraoperative comparison. Attempts were made to maintain the same distance between recording and stimulating electrodes. On the basis of the latency and amplitude of the evoked responses, as compared to control parameters, a decision was made concerning the surgical treatment of the involved fascicle. If no response was obtained, the involved segment was resected and continuity reestablished by end-to-end fascicular repair or an interposition fascicular nerve graft. If there was a measurable response, an intraneural neurolysis was done without fascicular resection and end-to-end repair.

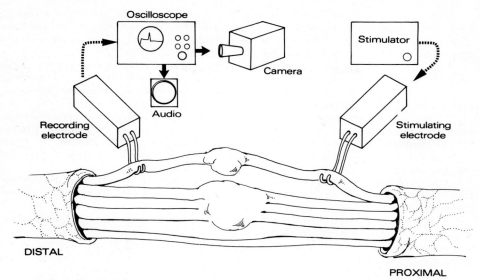

Figure 28–1 Diagrammatic representation of single fascicular recording technique in a localized lesion in continuity.

The long term results in six patients with localized lesions managed with this technique have been very rewarding (Williams and Terzis, 1976).

Diffuse Nerve Injuries

These included nerve lesions resulting from electrical burns of or severe mechanical trauma to the upper extremity. The associated tissue injury that was present in the acute phase in these cases necessitated various reconstructive procedures and, at the same time, considerably delayed the nerve repair. The following case illustrates the valuable diagnostic information that electrophysiological techniques can provide in the management of diffuse nerve injuries. It must be emphasized that physiological testing has a purely adjunctive diagnostic role in peripheral nerve surgery and is not a substitute for careful preoperative clinical examination of the patient.

Case Presentation

A 22-year-old construction worker suffered a severe traumatic ax injury of the right upper limb in 1975. Initial care was undertaken at another center. Subsequently, he was referred to us for definitive reconstruction. His presenting symptoms included inability to work outside due to severe cold intolerance of the right hand, along with pain over the right wrist on contact. Physical examination revealed a painful mass at the right wrist. There was evidence of sweating throughout the palmar aspect of his right hand, and there was minimal pulp atrophy of the digits. The thenar eminence showed some atrophy, and motor examination disclosed inability of the thumb to oppose. Critical sensory testing revealed presence of the sensibilities of pain, pressure, and temperature. However, two-point discrimination over the index pulp was greater than 15 mm.

The gross appearance of the right hand indicated that the patient was making routine use of his hand. There were callouses over the palm and fingers, and the color of the skin was similar to that of the contralateral extremity. There were no burn marks, despite his being a right-handed cigarette smoker.

In view of the minimal symptoms and satisfactory recovery of this patient, exploration of the lesion in combination with intraoperative electrophysiological recordings was planned. The goal was to alleviate the painful neuroma and minimize the severe cold intolerance while preserving existing function.

Under tourniquet control, the right median nerve was widely explored. Following exposure of the nerve for 10 cm proximal in the forearm, a large neuroma in continuity with surrounding scar tissue was found at the level of the wrist. Distally, the transverse carpal ligament was transected and the median nerve exposed up to the level of the proximal palmar crease (Fig. 28–2).

The proximal nerve appeared quite normal under the operating microscope. However, it was decided to first apply physiological testing in the proximal nerve and, only subsequently, across the lesion.

At this point, the tourniquet was deflated and complete hemostasis achieved. Stimulating and recording platinum electrodes were then lowered into the operative field. The median nerve in the proximal forearm was then lifted and placed over the stimulating electrode, and this arrangement was kept constant throughout the recording procedure (Figs. 28–3 and 28–4). The recording electrode was then allowed to make contact with the median nerve, just distal to the stimulating site (Fig. 28–4). Electrical pulses of constant strength and duration were then administered to the nerve at 1 msec intervals via a Grass S$_4$ stimulator. The evoked responses were picked up by the recording electrode, amplified, and displayed on the oscilloscope screen. The tracings depicting the compound responses of the nerve were then photographed with a Polaroid camera. These photographic displays permitted simultaneous comparison of the elicited

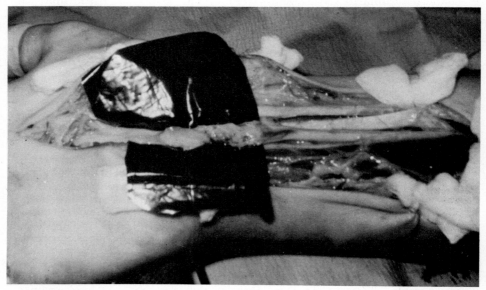

Figure 28–2 Diffuse nerve injury secondary to severe mechanical trauma; note bilobed median nerve neuroma in continuity over dark background.

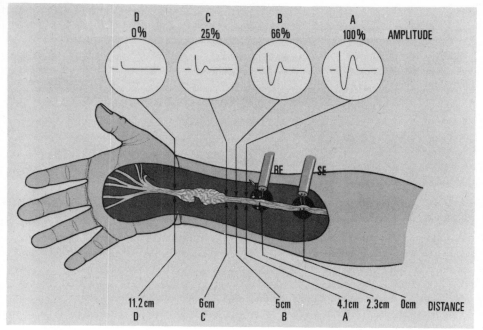

Figure 28–3 Whole nerve recordings of right median nerve to delineate longitudinal extent of neural damage. At 4.1 cm distal to stimulation site, the compound action potential has 100 per cent amplitude. Only 0.9 cm more distally, the evoked response is subject to 34 per cent diminution in height. At the proximal border of the neuroma, 75 per cent of the constituent fibers within the nerve are unresponsive to electrical stimulation. Whole nerve recordings across the lesion reveal no measurable response. (SE = stimulating electrode; RE = recording electrode.)

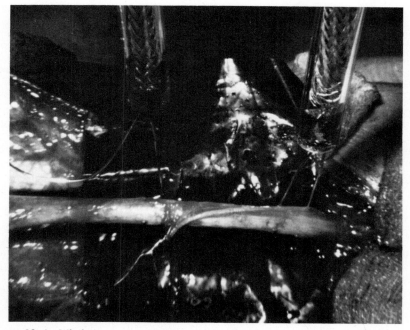

Figure 28–4 Whole nerve recording of the compound action potential. Stimulating electrode is on the right; recording electrode is on the left. Note that this is a monopolar recording arrangement. The active recording electrode is in close contact with the nerve, while the indifferent electrode is placed in surrounding tissue.

467

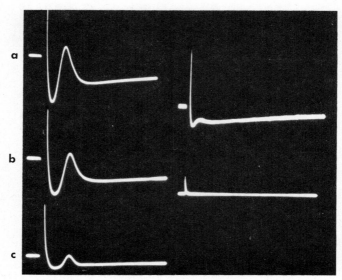

Figure 28–5   These deflections represent the actual intraoperative tracings of the compound action potentials obtained in this case. The three tracings on the left depict: a) the normal compound potential of the median nerve, up to 4.1 cm distal to the stimulation site (upper tracing); b) 66 per cent of the amplitude of the evoked response is present at 5.0 cm (middle tracing); c) proximal border of the lesion; only 25 per cent of the nerve tissue responds to electrical stimulation (lower tracing). The two tracings on the right were obtained from: a) whole nerve recording across the neuroma: note that there is no measurable response (lower tracing); b) fascicular recording from the posterolateral portion of the nerve that was found to be in continuity: note diminished amplitude (upper tracing).

compound action potentials. Thus, measurements of the amplitude of the compound responses were obtained sequentially down the proximal nerve and across the neuroma. It should be emphasized that these whole nerve recordings were conducted monopolarly. This method of measuring potential changes in a peripheral nerve has been described in detail elsewhere (Terzis et al., 1976).

The intraoperative physiological measurements are depicted in Figures 28–3 and 28–5. A full compound response to electrical stimulation was obtained up to 4.1 cm distal to the stimulation site. As the recording electrode advanced to 5.0 cm distally, there was a 34 per cent dropoff in the amplitude of the compound action potential. Just at the proximal border of the neuroma, 75 per cent of the nerve remained unresponsive (Fig. 28–6). Whole nerve recordings across the neuroma revealed no measurable response. The objective information thus obtained was of critical importance in precisely determining the longitudinal extent of the injury, since, even under the highest magnification of the operating microscope, the proximal nerve appeared quite normal.

In view of the preoperative clinical findings of remaining useful sensibility and despite a negative response across the neuroma when whole nerve recordings were carried out, we proceeded with epineuriectomy and fascicular dissection through the neuroma. Only two posterolateral groups of fascicles were found to be in continuity through the lesion.

Fascicular electrophysiological recordings were then carried out. A compound action potential of diminished amplitude was obtained from each of the fascicles that were in continuity (Fig. 28–7). However, no response was elicited when recordings were repeated across the rest of the lesion.

A decision was made to preserve the two groups of posterolateral fascicles, so that the existing sensibility in the hand could be maintained. Thus, only an intraneural neurolysis was performed in that part of the nerve.

The remaining lesion was treated by proximal and distal dissection of the fascicles

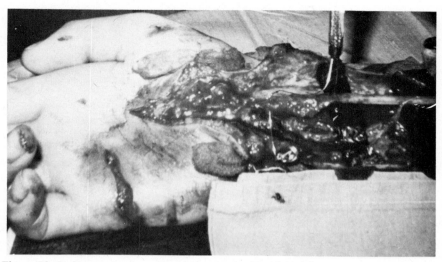

Figure 28–6   Monopolar recording at the proximal border of the neuroma. Note short, active electrode in close contact with the nerve, while longer, indifferent electrode makes contact with adjacent tissue.

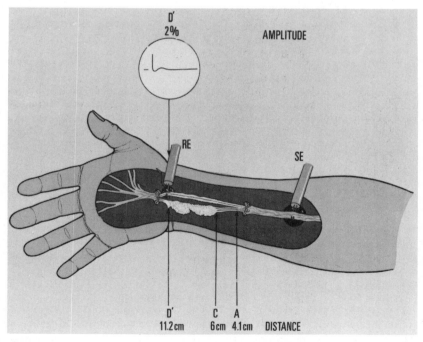

Figure 28–7   Fascicular recording arrangement. Note diminished amplitude of compound action potential at 11.2 cm distal to the stimulating electrode. The actual deflection is shown in Figure 28–5 (right, upper tracing). (SE = stimulating electrode; RE = recording electrode.)

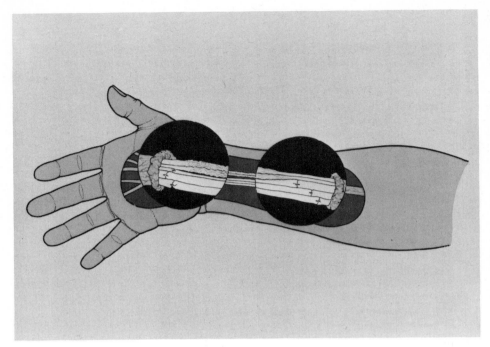

Figure 28–8   Diagrammatic illustration of the final nerve repair procedure performed in this case: interfascicular sural nerve grafting in the medial aspect of the median nerve following fascicular dissection and excision of the neuromatous tissue; intraneural neurolysis with preservation of two posterolateral fascicular groups, which were found to be in continuity.

into groups, resection of the neuroma plus the proximal part of the nerve that demonstrated decreased physiological responses. Finally, three sural nerve grafts were interposed between the corresponding fascicular cut ends in the proximal and distal stumps (Fig. 28–8).

Postoperatively, the patient had similar sensory findings as prior to this procedure, and, in addition, he volunteered that the pain in his wrist had disappeared. At one year following surgery, the patient was pain free and had improved tolerance to cold. The advancing Tinel's sign was positive to the level of the proximal palmar crease, and the two point discrimination varied from 10 to 12 mm in the proximal median nerve distribution over the palm. His hand function continued to be good.

DISCUSSION

Whole nerve recordings can pinpoint the extent, level, and spread of a diffuse nerve injury quite rapidly. However, the technique has definite limitations in its utilization. These recording procedures depend on close contact between nerve tissue and recording electrode. Thus, if the recording electrode is not directly touching the neural tissue, owing to intervening scar, the evoked response may be dissipated in the scar tissue and never reach the recording electrode. It is our impression that this phenomenon explains why initially no measurable response was obtained from whole nerve recordings across the neuroma. When the intervening scar tissue was excised, repeat fascicular recordings revealed a measurable evoked response.

If a diffuse nerve lesion is suspected, electrophysiological recordings can pinpoint the level of normally functioning neural tissue. As repeatedly observed, a relatively normal cross-sectional appearance of the nerve does not necessarily reflect normal function.

The preoperative clinical findings must be kept in mind during such procedures to permit tailoring of the physiological tests to fit the particular clinical situation. Thus, in cases of diffuse nerve injuries where there is complete motor and sensory deficit distally, only whole nerve recordings should be used to delineate the proximal level of neural damage. One is not justified to proceed with fascicular recordings, since the yield will be minimal. In contrast, in cases where there is useful distal function, as in the reported case, one may utilize a combination of whole nerve and single fascicular recordings to obtain maximum information. On the basis of the data obtained, one can tailor the nerve repair procedure according to the presenting injury rather than blindly applying the same technique to a variety of nerve lesions.

SUMMARY

Electrophysiological recordings can provide extremely useful and objective information in the intraoperative management of selected peripheral nerve lesions. Our experience with two types of lesions in continuity, localized and diffuse, is presented. The adjunctive role of these techniques in peripheral nerve surgery is emphasized.

REFERENCES

Dawson, G. D., and Scott, J. W.: The recording of nerve action potentials through skin in man. J. Neurol. Neurosurg. Psychiatry *12*:259, 1949.

Erlanger, J., and Gasser, H. S.: Electrical Signs of Nervous Activity. Philadelphia, University of Pennsylvania Press, 1937.

Hakstian, R. W.: Funicular orientation by direct stimulation. An aid to peripheral nerve repair. J. Bone Joint Surg. *50A*:1178, 1968.

Hodes, R., Larrabee, M. G., and German, W.: The human electromyogram in response to nerve stimulation and the conduction velocity of motor axons. Arch. Neurol. Psychiatry *60*:340, 1948.

Hodgkin, A. L., and Huxley, A. F.: Currents carried by sodium and potassium ions through the membrane of the giant axon of Loligo. J. Physiol. *116*:449, 1952.

Hodgkin, A. L., Huxley, A. F., and Katz, B.: Measurement of current–voltage relations in the membrane of the giant axon of Loligo. J. Physiol. *116*:424, 1952.

Kline, D. G.: Early evaluation of peripheral nerve lesions in continuity with a note on nerve recording. Am. Surg. *34*:77, 1968.

Kline, D. G.: Operative management of major nerve lesions of the lower extremity. Surg. Clin. North Amer. *52*:1247, 1972.

Kline, D. G., Hackett, E. F., and May, P. R.: Evaluation of nerve injuries by evoked potentials and electromyography. J. Neurosurg. *31*:128, 1969.

Kline, D. G., and Nulsen, F.: The neuroma in continuity: Its preoperative and operative management. Surg. Clin. North Amer. *52*:1189, 1972.

Smith, J. W.: Microsurgery of peripheral nerves. Plast. Reconstr. Surg. *33*:317, 1964.

Terzis, J. K.: Functional aspects of reinnervation of free skin grafts. Plast. Reconstr. Surg. *58*:142, 1976.

Terzis, J. K., Dykes, R. W., and Hakstian, R. W.: Electrophysiological recordings in peripheral nerve surgery: A review. J. Hand. Surg. *1*:52, 1976.

Terzis, J. K., Faibisoff, B. A., and Williams, H. B.: A diamond knife for microsurgical repair of peripheral nerves. Plast. Reconstr. Surg. *54*:102, 1974.

Terzis, J. K., Faibisoff, B. A., and Williams, H. B.: The nerve gap: Suture under tension vs. graft. Plast. Reconstr. Surg. *56*:166, 1975.

Terzis, J. K., and Williams, H. B.: Functional evaluation of free nerve grafts. *In* Daniller, A. I., and Strauch, B. (Eds.): Symposium on Microsurgery. St. Louis, C. V. Mosby, 1976, Chap. 16.

Vandeputt, J.; Tanner, J. C., and Huypens, L.: Electrophysiological orientation of the cut ends in primary peripheral nerve repair. Plast. Reconstr. Surg. *44*:378, 1969.

Williams, H. B., and Terzis, J. K.: Single fascicular recordings: An intraoperative diagnostic tool for the management of peripheral nerve lesions. Plast. Reconstr. Surg. *57*:562, 1976.

Trauma: Missiles, Lacerations, Compression, Injections, Traction and Friction

V

29

PATHOPHYSIOLOGY OF PERIPHERAL NERVE TRAUMA

THOMAS B. DUCKER

The central and peripheral nervous systems compose a single functioning unit, the function of which is the processing of information. Impulses travel down the spinal cord and synapse on the anterior horn cell to initiate action throughout the body, or its periphery. Peripheral nerves are simply bundles of axons, the long extensions of neuronal cell bodies located within the spinal cord and brainstem. If the central system is diseased, then inadequate or incorrect information will be passed to and from the periphery. If the peripheral system is diseased, the same principle applies. In addition, if a segment of the system dies, as in poliomyelitis, for example, there not only are central nervous system changes but also degenerative changes in peripheral nerves and muscle.

It is necessary to approach the pathophysiologic factors that occur in the surgery of peripheral nerves in a dual fashion. The normal state will be described first. Then, the changes that are seen in injury or disease will be outlined. These normal and abnormal states will be reviewed stepwise, from central to peripheral along the nerves, starting with the central cell, or the dorsal ganglion cell, and ending with the muscle cell and the sensory end organ.

PATHOPHYSIOLOGY WITHIN THE CENTRAL NERVOUS SYSTEM

Injury to a peripheral nerve axon involves removal of a large portion of the nerve cell volume; however, the biochemical machinery required for repair

475

remains largely intact because it is localized in the soma, or cell body. Because of their unique geometry, nerve cells must synthesize large amounts of structural material and transport these materials over relatively long distances. If the central cell body were the height of an average man, its axon would be one or two inches in diameter and would extend more than two miles. The energy expenditure needed to synthesize structural materials, as well as factors associated with neurotransmission, and transport these over long distances becomes very large and requires markedly enlarged and metabolically hyperactive cell bodies. The mature nerve cell is among the most metabolically active cell types in our bodies (Turner, 1943). In axonal injury or disease even higher metabolic activity occurs, and profound changes take place in the structure as well as in the biochemical and physiological properties of the cell body. Some of these changes may be viewed as particularly appropriate for the repair process. Others are not. After axonal injury, *chromatolysis,* nuclear eccentricity, nucleolar enlargement, and cell swelling are the most conspicuous morphological changes seen during the retrograde response (Lieberman, 1971). For peripheral axons, these changes have been associated with a reorganization and enhanced formation of cytoplasmic ribonucleic acid (RNA) to a more active state directed toward the reconstitution of lost axoplasm and recovery of peripheral connections (Brattgard et al., 1958a, Murray, 1973; Watson, 1965).

Increases in *RNA synthesis,* as expected, have been associated with enhanced cytoplasmic *protein synthesis,* as demonstrated by the incorporation of radioactive amino acid precursors. (Brattgard, et al., 1958b; Engh et al., 1971; Francoeur and Olszewski, 1968; Grafstein and Murray, 1969; Watson, 1965). The changes in protein synthesis are complex and appear to involve a reordering of the various types of proteins synthesized by the injured neuron. Materials required for transmitter function are decreased, while materials required for regeneration of the axon are elevated. For example, in adrenergic neurons there are decreases in dopamine-B-hydroxylase, DOPA decarboxylase, monamine oxidase, and tyrosine hydroxylase activities after axotomy (Cheah and Geffen, 1973; Kopin and Silberstein, 1972; Reis and Ross, 1973; Reis et al., 1974). Similar decreases in acetylcholinesterase and choline acetyltransferase have been reported in axotomized cholinergic neurons (Hebb and Waites, 1956; Lieberman, 1974). In contrast, the activity of glucose-6-phosphate dehydrogenase, a key enzyme by which glucose is converted to precursors required for the biosynthesis of nucleic acids and lipids, is significantly elevated in axotomized neurons (Harkonen and Kauffman, 1974a, 1974b; Watson, 1974).

A number of histochemical and biochemical studies have demonstrated that the activity of glucose-6-phosphate dehydrogenase is increased in axotomized nerve cell bodies. Spinal anterior horn cells, facial nucleus neurons, and sympathetic ganglion cells, all of which direct axons to peripheral structures, show such changes in the *pentose phosphate* pathway (Harkonen, 1964; Hirsch and Obenchain, 1970; Kreutzberg, 1963; Nandy, 1968; Robbins et al., 1961. Increases in this activity are not observed in neuronal perikarya whose axons undergo wallerian degeneration (McCaman and Robbins, 1959). In extended studies of metabolic changes in the axotomized rat superior cervical ganglion, strong evidence has been obtained that increases in glucose-6-phosphate dehydrogenase occurring shortly after axotomy are associated with increased metabolism of glucose via the anabolic pentose pathway (Harkonen and Kauffman, 1974a and *b*). This increase occurs in the absence of any gross alteration in the major energy-yielding reactions such as ATP utilization and oxygen consumption.

Enhanced metabolism via the pentose pathway may have special significance in injured peripheral neurons because two functions of this pathway are to generate NADPH for reductive biosynthetic reactions and to form ribose phosphate required for nucleic acid and ribonucleotide biosynthesis. Studies carried out on non-neuronal tissue provide strong evidence that the formation of NADPH by the pentose pathway is intimately related to the biosynthesis of fatty acids (Banquer et al., 1973). A similar relationship may exist in regenerating neural tissue because significant increases in lipid synthesis begin with the first week after axonal injury (Harkonen and Kauffman, 1974*a* and *b*; Miani, 1962).

The process of regeneration in nerve cell bodies is complicated by the simultaneous occurrence of extensive hydrolytic activity during the period of enhanced biosynthetic activity. A marked increase in acid phosphatase and a corresponding increase in the internal complexity and number of lysosome-like dense bodies has frequently been noted in axotomized nerve cells (Matthews and Raisman, 1972; Sumner, 1974). The former have suggested that the increased hydrolytic activity is related to digestion of transmitter storage granules in axotomized nerve cells. It is not known whether these changes are a necessary prerequisite for axonal sprouting and regeneration.

The regenerative capacity of neurons varies with age. Axonal outgrowth from proximal stumps of transected nerves with reconnection to the denervated end organs appears to be more rapid in younger animals than in older animals (Guth, 1956; Moyer et al., 1953). Pertinent histological and temporal characteristics of the retrograde responses of various classes of neurons in young animals have been recently reviewed by Brodal (1973). Data concerning biochemical differences between young and mature axotomized nerve cells is minimal, and it is not clear what mechanisms account for the greater regenerative capacity of neural tissue from immature animals. Nerve cells from very young mammals tend to degenerate when axonal lesions are introduced at or during the first few days after birth (Grant, 1970). These differences reflect only one aspect of the major biological problem of the nature and control of cellular differentiation, which is itself poorly understood. Nevertheless, these findings have important practical implications for the physician. For example, the neuron's reparative demands may be readily met in a teenager who has a sharp laceration of a digital nerve, and immediate repair is, therefore, indicated. On the other end of the spectrum, a person in his 60's with a proximal blast injury to the ulnar nerve does not have the same significant regenerative power. The neuron may be so busy trying to survive that its regenerative efforts are, in essence, ineffective.

The glial cells form the supportive structure of the central nervous system and are thought to help regulate metabolic events external to the neuronal membrane. They invest the neurons in such a way that sugars, amino acids, and other solutes freely circulating in the extracellular space are made available for the nerve cell's metabolism (Varon, 1975). *Neuroglia* also have comparatively high resting-membrane potentials and a high internal potassium level, which may serve to distribute potassium ions to aid or create surface potentials in active axons (Bunge, 1970; Murray and Grafstein, 1969).

Glial cells in close association with axotomized neuronal perikarya undergo alterations that influence metabolic changes accompanying neuronal regeneration. A proliferation of microglia close to axotomized perikarya occurs shortly after axotomy; in some cases this change is associated with displacement of synaptic boutons from the perikarya and dendrites of axotomized nerve cells. Activation of metabolism in glia surrounding injured neurons is suggested by hypertrophy of astrocytes in the vicinity of axotomized nerve cell bodies (Lieberman, 1971). Literature dealing with glial responses during anterograde and retrograde neuronal responses has been recently reviewed (Brodal, 1976). Relevant to defining those events which take place in glial elements and nerve cells, Watson (1972) has shown that in contrast to neuronal responses the onset of metabolic changes in astrocytes surrounding axotomized nerve cells in the hypoglossal nucleus is independent of the level at which the hypoglossal nerve is injured.

PATHOPHYSIOLOGIC PROCESSES IN THE PERIPHERAL NERVE

Regeneration of a damaged axon requires the restoration of large quantities of axonal lipids and proteins, which are synthesized in the nerve cell body and delivered to the growing axon by transport systems. There is more than one distinct transport process, and materials are transported at different rates. The slow component may be mediated by peristalsis in the nerve trunk plasma, and the fast component involves active participation of microtubules. Inconsistent results have been obtained in studies of the effect of axotomy on fast axonal transport (Carlsson et al., 1971; Frizell and Sjostrand, 1974; Grafstein and Murray, 1969; Ochs, 1974). These inconsistencies may be explained by the recent findings that axotomy produces different responses in different nerves of the same animal (Grafstein, 1975). Griffin, Drachman, and Price (1976) studied fast *axoplasmic flow* in regenerating rat sciatic nerves and demonstrated that the rate of fast flow was not altered in the proximal nerve trunk, and that the rapidly transported proteins were carried past the level of axotomy into the regenerating nerve sprouts. Materials moved down the sprouts at the normal rate of about 400 mm per day. Although rates of axoplasmic flow may not be altered in the regenerating axon, evidence has been obtained that the amount of protein transported is increased (Griffin et al., 1976). Functional adaptation of axoplasmic flow in regenerating axons may also involve a reordering of the types of proteins that are transported. As discussed above, the production of proteins associated with transmitter function seems impaired, while formation of proteins associated with the repair process is enhanced, in nerve cell bodies that have sustained axonal injury.

Within one hour of cutting a peripheral nerve, there is marked proximal swelling from the point of disruption, as much as 1 cm. The amount of swelling is greater than previously realized, for the cross-sectional area of the nerve increases three times (Ducker et al., 1968). The swelling consists of both intracellular and extracellular edema, mostly a gel-like amorphous substance that contains a large quantity of acid mucopolysaccharides (Campbell and Luzio, 1964; Oester and Davis, 1956). It persists for a week or more and subsides slowly thereafter.

Within two or three days after transection of a nerve, there are signs of demarcation of the *nerve stump* or healing over of the open end of the neuron. After a week, there is vigorous sprouting of the axons. In traumatic blast wounds, the axonal sprouting may be 1, 2, or even 3 cm. proximal to the point of the actual severed end. In a clean operative sectioning, this occurs for only a few millimeters retrograde. Between one and three weeks, axon buds begin to advance across the anastomosis of a primary neurorrhaphy (Kline et al., 1964 *a* and *b*). The onset of this budding and regeneration occurs concomitantly with the anabolic hypertrophic phase of the cell body in the spinal cord or dorsal ganglion. Most evidence indicates that there is a delay of a few days before the axon sprouts and crosses a repair site. Thus, it would be ideal to repair an injured nerve when the regenerative efforts of the nerve are at their initial maximum performance.

Neurite elongation and the transduction of chemical energy to sustain this process are central issues in the ongoing nerve regeneration. The process of neurite elongation appears to originate at growth cones situated at the tips of axons (Yamada and Wessels, 1971). *Growth cones* are characterized by a profuse elaboration of microspikes which explore the environment and establish direction for growth (Yamada and Wessels, 1971). The direction and the amount of branching displayed by a growing axon are influenced by adhesion between the cell surface and the substratum upon which it grows (Strassman et al., 1974). Thus, initiation as well as maintenance of neurite elongation may involve changes in the cell surface. Extension of a growing fiber seems to take place at the tip of the fiber (Bray, 1973).

It is unlikely that sustained axonal growth could occur without the enhanced metabolic activity generated in the cell body during the retrograde reaction. This is supported by the finding that the rate of axonal outgrowth is faster after the second of two successive axonal injuries (McQuarrie and Grafstein, 1973). Presumably, the necessary metabolic adaptation for optimal axonal regeneration has taken place prior to the second injury (Grafstein, 1975).

Little information exists concerning the biological signal that initiates nerve sprouting. Considerable evidence exists that *trophic interactions* occur between target tissues and nerves which somehow regulate innervation. One hypothesis that has gained support is that target tissues continually manufacture a substance that stimulates nerves to sprout; this substance is neutralized in a negative feedback manner by the release of neural factors which are carried to nerve endings by axoplasmic flow (Aquilar et al., 1973). This hypothesis explains *"denervation sprouting"* and also explains the phenomenon of collateral sprouting. The recovery of function after sectioning of certain peripheral nerves may be best seen as the collateral sprouting of remaining fibers (Coers and Woolf, 1959).

Within hours after transection of a nerve, the metabolism of the Schwann cells, the perineural epithelial cells, and the epineurium increases. Two to three days after injury, there is a cellular proliferation in both proximal and distal stumps of nearly all elements. After the first week, the most active cell is the Schwann cell, which now has assumed a phagocytic function. The response of these cells is in part proportional to the severity of the wounding. Battle injuries of peripheral nerves are characterized by a marked inflammatory response and retrograde demarcation of the nerve anatomy several centimeters from the actual point of severance of the nerve (Haymaker, 1948). Conversely, a clean operative injury or knife cut is not associated with a marked tissue reaction, and the response of the Schwann cell is less. As the debris is cleared from the injury area, a mesenchymal and neuroectodermal scar is left behind. This tissue is, for the most part, not longitudinally aligned, so that any early axonal regeneration becomes twisted and entangled. In time, a traumatic neuroma may form as the neuronal buds push into a reactive cellular conglomerate that has no anatomic planes.

At the site of injury, supportive cells from both stumps dominate the dynamic and metabolic action in the early post-traumatic period when there are only the earliest signs of axonal budding and regeneration. The orientation of the mesenchyme cells left behind after the debridement of Schwann cells is dependent on the state of the wound and on local geometry rather than on chemotaxis, etc. (Abercrombie et al., 1949; Guth, 1956). There is evidence that indicates that these cellular structures can be longitudinally aligned by mechanical devices such as wraps or tubes (Braun, 1966; Campbell et al., 1963, 1964; Ducker and Hayes, 1968a and b; Gutmann, 1961; Weiss, 1970).

With a *nerve repair,* regardless of the timing, both proximal and distal stumps swell and become edematous. The swelling includes axons in the proximal stump, and the amount of the increase may be two to three times the normal cross-sectional area of the nerve in higher primates and in man (Ducker and Hayes, 1968b). Studies indicate that silicone rubber tubes possess physical properties that can force longitudinal alignment without constricting the nerve (Ducker and Hayes, 1968a). However, larger tubes or cuffs to allow for swelling in the immediate post-repair period are required, and, consequently, their clinical application is limited. Concurrent with the decrease in edema, the neuron bud advances and pushes into the intercellular spaces before the mesenchymal cellular and collagen proliferation becomes impermeable. With the more direct axonal spanning, there should be improvement in functional return (Ducker et al., 1969; Ochs et al., 1969). And with time and maturation, the new nerve trunk returns to approximately 80 per cent of its normal size. Sensory return is benefited the most by external forced longitudinal alignment (Ducker et al., 1969; Weiss, 1970).

It must be stressed (1) that the response to injury of the supportive structures is immediate and that thick collagen is laid down starting three weeks after injury; and (2) that the response of the neuron at the site of injury is often delayed until axonal budding and regeneration take place. Therefore, a properly planned operative repair, pathophysiologically speaking, would place the neurons on more equal footing with the connective tissue supportive elements. Any operative delays depend on the level of the lesion, the severity of the tissue damage in the wound, and the general condition (and age) of the patient.

DISTAL WALLERIAN DEGENERATION

The distal nerve stump can react only with supportive structures. The axonal elements that are separated from their trophic centers die. A *"reactive schwannoma"* or "peripheral glioima" may form from the proliferating supportive elements and can inhibit regenerating axonal penetration. However, these metabolically active and dividing neurolemmal and mesenchymal cells can be cut away at the time of repair. They will react again but in a sequence and with the timing outlined in the previous section of this paper.

Wallerian degeneration of the nerve is defined as the death of all neuronal elements distal to the site of injury. This term should not be applied to any changes in the proximal stump or trunk. After injury, digestive enzymes are present in the axonal segments (Kreutzberg, 1963: Oester and Davis, 1956). Parts of the axonal segments, often near the stump, may isolate themselves into small units that can survive up to two weeks; but the majority of neuronal elements break down within a week. The surrounding myelin undergoes fragmentation and is digested by the Schwann cells. By three weeks, the majority of this cellular debris is phagocytosed by the metabolically active Schwann cells. By six weeks the debridement is complete. Parts of the fascicular anatomy persist in the distal nerve, and the endoneural sheaths become either smaller or nonexistent (Hudson et al., 1970, 1971, 1977; Sjostrand, 1966). The entire nerve shrinks, and in time the shrinkage becomes irreversible and downgrades the prognosis of unduly postponed nerve repair. The neuroectoderm and mesenchymal elements are in part dependent on the nerve fibers to maintain anatomic and metabolic existence.

With penetration of new axons, the Schwann cell again increases its metabolic activity, but not for phagocytic function. Fresh myelin is layered around the the nerves by the Schwann cells. The electron microscopic details of this process have been worked out, as have certain metabolic features. To the surgeon who is repairing a peripheral nerve, the axonal regrowth is the primary concern, and the myelin reconstitution will take place only if regeneration occurs. However, *remyelination* is never as good as the premorbid state; and this fact, along with nerve size and endoneural tube size, accounts for the slower conduction times of the distal nerve trunk after repair.

Practically all the metabolites in the distal peripheral nerve trunk come from the central cell via axoplasmic flow. Enlargement of the central cell is not limited to the immediate post-injury period but also occurs at the end of regeneration when the myoneural junctions are being formed. Engh et al. (1971, 1972) showed that there is a consistent increase in synthetic activity within the central cell which occurs with axonal maturation. The combination of the building of new synaptic end-plates and the return of a trophic perikaryal stimulus to and from the reinnervated peripheral structure can cause a greater increase in metabolism in the central cell than occurs in the immediate post-traumatic period.

Regeneration down most peripheral distal nerve trunks averages about 1 mm per day or 1 inch per month. Initially, however, there is a delay until the neuron is clearly across the anastomosis; then, in some cases, regeneration may occur as fast as 3 mm per day. There is a slowing of the regenerative process with the forming of new connections with the muscle or sensory organs, or both.

PATHOPHYSIOLOGY OF THE DISTAL MUSCLE AND SENSORY ORGANS

The biochemical and electrophysiological properties of skeletal muscles are influenced by peripheral nerves. After nerve injury, the muscle cells shrink, the endomysium and perimysium thicken, and the muscle spindles atrophy. These changes may be ascribed, in part, to a loss of neurotrophic factors supplied to the muscles by nerve. This long term regulatory property of motor neurons is clearly distinct from the more commonly studied electrophysiological properties (Albuquerque and McIsaac, 1970; Deshpande et al., 1976). The early alterations that occur after nerve section or injury include a decline in resting membrane potential, the appearance of extrajunctional acetylcholine sensitivity, and a decrease in muscle phosphocreatine (Albuquerque and McIsaac, 1970; Kauffman and Albuquerque, 1970). The time course of these changes is dependent upon the distance from the muscle at which the nerve is transected as well as the type of muscle denervated, but in general these changes take place over the first three days after nerve section in small mammals. Muscle atrophy begins at two to 16 weeks in animals and somewhat later in man; with time (two years or more), muscle fibers may fragment and disintegrate (Aquilar et al., 1973). Such changes take place despite good physical therapy or intermittent external electrical stimulation, or both. To date, denervation atrophy can be halted only by reinnervation, in which constant stimuli from gamma and alpha fibers as well as delivery of neurotrophic substances result in sufficient drive of the metabolism of the muscle cell. Any denervation atrophy of the muscle is harmful because the thickening of the muscle sheath hinders end-plate formation, and formation of fibrous tissue in and around the muscle interferes with nerve regrowth and muscle contraction. Thus, the sooner a nerve establishes connection with the muscle, the more likely the metabolism and anatomy of the muscle will be normal. If reinnervation is delayed one year, function is very poor. A delay of two years allows irreversible changes to take place in the muscle cells, and any hope of motor return at that time is practically nil.

The sensory end organs are less dependent on nerve innervation for survival. In fact, a World War II study yielded no evidence that the time from injury to nerve repair influenced sensory recovery in any way (Ochs et al., 1969). There are no metabolic studies of these cells to account for the clinical observations, but it is acceptable therapy to perform, for example, a markedly delayed sciatic nerve repair to gain protective sensation of the foot.

SYSTEMIC METABOLIC STATUS

Of all general factors, the age of the patient is the most important. There are no statistical studies to validate the fact that the younger the patient the better he regenerates a peripheral nerve; yet all experienced surgeons have made this observation. Children sometimes have a nearly 100 per cent return after a distal nerve repair. Nerve growth factors found in the laboratory have not been tried in human patients. Clinically, one suspects that growth hormone may be helpful, but it has not been used. There is evidence that thyroid hormone promotes peripheral nerve regeneration; however, the clinical usefulness of thyroid hormone in patients with injured or transected peripheral nerves has not been fully evaluated (Cockett and Kiernan, 1973).

The wound wherein the nerve was injured is important. Massive blast injuries result in thick scar formation and delayed healing. A regenerating nerve may become scarred and entrapped in such injuries, and motor and sensory recovery fails. Or, the blast injury can result in distal ischemia of the limb and irreversible changes in all structures, including the distal nerve trunk and distal muscles. Or, multiple war-inflicted injuries may result in a catabolic state in the patient for two or three months and adversely influence nerve regeneration.

When analyzing studies dealing with nerve regeneration in experimental animals it is important to consider *phylogeny*. Although regeneration of the spinal cord is currently impossible in man, certain lizards regrow segments of spinal cord when the tail is cut off. Rats and dogs can have their nerves severed and not reanastomosed, yet their regenerative efforts are so strong that nerve continuity is restored and motor and sensory return will occur. Monkeys at times will do the same. The nerves of adult baboons and chimpanzees behave more like those of man.

The higher the animal is on the phylogenetic scale the more complex the regeneration process and the less effective is the end result. Consequently, rat experiments cannot be readily applied to the human clinical situation. Within the human nervous system, certain neuronal pathways are phylogenetically older than others. Pain fiber regrowth may exceed proprioceptive fiber regrowth, and leave the patient with pain and no useful function. Consequently, the multiple factors that influence the final result necessitate that one practice the art of medicine (based on clinical experience) as well as the science of medicine.

SUMMARY

Respect for the metabolic changes within the neuron is critical in planning peripheral nerve surgery. Only by understanding the different pathophysiologic responses of the nerve tissue and the supportive tissue can anastomosis be effected when the budding neuron stands its best chance of successfully regenerating across a repair site. When all factors are ideal, good motor function across one joint from the next group of muscles can be counted on. Rarely is there good function across two. Protective sensory function can be achieved distally even under the most adverse metabolic conditions because of the independent metabolic state of these end organs.

REFERENCES

Abercrombie, M., Johnson, M. L., and Thomas, G. A.: Influence of nerve fibers on Schwann cell migration investigated in tissue culture. Proc. Roy. Soc. *136*:460, 1949.

Albuquerque, E. X., and McIsaac, R. J.: Fast and slow mammalian muscles after denervation. Exp. Neurol. *26*:183, 1970.

Aquilar, C. E., Bisby, M. A., Cooper, E., and Diamond, J.: Evidence that axoplasmic transport is involved in the regulation of peripheral nerve fields in salamanders. J. Physiol. (Lond.) *234*:449, 1973.

Banquer, N. Z., Cascales, M., Teo, B. C., and McLean, P.: The activity of the pentose phosphate pathway in isolated liver cells. Biochem. Biophys. Res. Comm. *52*:263, 1973.

Bowden, R. E. M., and Gutmann, E.: Denervation and re-innervation of human voluntary muscle. Brain *67*:273, 1944.

Brattgard, S. O., Edstrom, J. E., and Hyden, H.: The chemical changes in regenerating neurons. J. Neurochem. *1*:316, 1957.

Brattgard, S. O., Edstrom, J. E., and Hyden, H.: The productive capacity of the neuron in retrograde reaction. Exp. Cell. Res. *5*:185, 1958.

Braun, R. M.: Comparative studies of neurorrhaphy and sutureless peripheral nerve repair. Surgery *122*:15, 1966.

Bray, D.: Model for membrane movement in the neural growth cone. Nature (Lond.) *244*:93, 1973.

Brodal, A.: Anterograde and retrograde degeneration of neurons in the central nervous system. *In* W. Haymaker and R. D. Adams (eds.): Histology and Histopathology of the Nervous System. Springfield, Ill., Charles C Thomas, 1976.

Bunge, R. P.: Structure and function of neuroglia: Some recent observations. *In* Schnitt, R. O. (ed.): The Neurosciences (Second Study Program). New York. The Rockefeller Press, 1970, p. 782.

Campbell, J. B., Bassett, C. A. L., and Bohler, J.: Frozen-irradiated homografts shielded with microfilter sheaths in peripheral nerve surgery. J. Trauma *3*:303, 1963.

Campbell, J. B., and Luzio, J.: Symposium: Facial nerve rehabilitation. Facial nerve repair; new surgical techniques. Trans. Am. Acad. Ophthalmol. Otolaryngol. *68*:1068, 1964.

Carlsson, C. A., Bolando, P., and Sjostrand, J.: Changes in axonal transport during regeneration of feline ventral roots. J. Neurol. Sci. *14*:75, 1971.

Cheah, T. B., and Geffen, L. B.: Effects of axonal injury on norepinephrine, tyrosine hydroxylase and monoamine oxidase levels in sympathetic ganglia. J. Neurobiol. *4*:443, 1973.

Cockett, S. A., and Kiernan, J. A.: Acceleration of peripheral nervous regeneration in the rat by exogeneus triiodothyronine. Exp. Neurol. *39*:389, 1973.

Coers, C., and Woolf, A. L.: The Innervation of Muscle; A Biopsy Study. Oxford, Blackwell Scientific, 1959.

Deshpande, S. S., Albuquerque, E. X., and Guth, L.: Neurotrophic regulation of prejunctional and postjunctional membrane at the mammalian motor end plate. Exp. Neurol. *53*:151, 1976.

Diamond, J., Cooper, E., Turner, C., and Macintyre, L.: Trophic regulation of nerve sprouting. Neuron-target interactions and spatial relations control sensory nerve fields in salamander skin. Science *193*:371, 1976.

Ducker, T. B., and Hayes, G. J.: Peripheral nerve injuries: A comparative study of the anatomic and functional results following primary nerve repair in chimpanzees. Military Med. *133*:298, 1968*a*.

Ducker, T. B., and Hayes, G. J.: Experimental improvements in the use of silastic cuff for peripheral nerve repair. J. Neurosurg. *28*:582, 1968*b*.

Ducker, T. B., Kempe, L. G., and Hayes, G. J.: The metabolic background for peripheral nerve surgery. J. Neurosurg. *30*:270, 1969.

Engh, C. A., and Schofield, B. H.: The review of the central response to peripheral nerve injury and its significance in nerve regeneration. J. Neurosurg. *37*:195, 1972.

Engh, C. A., Schofield, B. H., Doty, S. B., and Robinson, R. A.: Perikaryal synthetic function following reversible and irreversible peripheral axon injuries as shown by radioautography. J. Comp. Neurol. *142*:465, 1971.

Francoeur, J., and Olszewski, J.: Axonal reaction and axonplasmic flow as studied by radioautography. Neurology (Minneap.) *18*:178, 1968.

Frizell, M., and Sjostrand, J.: Transport of proteins, glycoproteins and cholinergic enzymes in regenerating hypoglossal neurons. J. Neurochem. *22*:845, 1974.

Grafstein, B.: The nerve cell body response to axotomy. Exp. Neurol. Part 2, *48*:32–51, 1975.

Grafstein, B., and Murray, M.: Transport of protein in goldfish optic nerve during regeneration. Exp. Neurol. *25*:494, 1969.

Grant, G.: Neuronal changes central to the site of axon transection. A method for the identification of retrograde changes in perikarya, dendrites and axons by silver impregnation. *In* W. J. H. Nauta and S. O. E. Ebbesson (eds.): Contemporary Research Methods in Neuroanatomy. New York, Springer-Verlag, 1970, p. 173.

Griffin, J. W., Drachman, D. B., and Price, D. C.: Fast axonal transport in motor nerve regeneration. J. Neurobiol. *7*:355, 1976.

Guth, L.: Regeneration in the mammalian peripheral nervous system. Physiol. Rev. *36*:441, 1956.

Gutmann, E.: Histology of degeneration and regeneration. *In* Licht, S. (ed.): Electrodiagnosis and Electromyography. Baltimore, Waverly Press, 1961, pp. 113.

Harkonen, M.: Carboxylic esterases, oxidative enzymes and catecholamines in the superior cervical ganglion of the rat and the effect of pre- and post-ganglionic nerve division. Acta Physiol. Scand. *63*:(Suppl. 237) 1, 1964.

Harkonen, M. H. A., and Kauffman, F. C.: Metabolic alterations in the axotomized superior cervical ganglion of the rat. I. Energy Metabolism. Brain Res. *65*:127, 1974*a*.

Harkonen, M. H. A., and Kauffman, F. C.: Metabolic alterations in the axotomized superior cervical ganglion of the rat. II. The pentose phosphate pathway. Brain Res. *65*:141, 1974*b*.

Haymaker, W.: Pathology of peripheral nerve injuries. Military Surg. *102*:448, 1948.

Hebb, C. O., and Waites, G. M. H.: Choline acetylase in antero- and retrograde degeneration of a cholinergic nerve. J. Physiol. *132*:667, 1956.

Hirsch, H. E., and Obenchain, T.: Acid phosphatase activity in individual neurons during chromatolysis: A quantitative histochemical study. J. Histochem. Cytochem. *18*:828, 1970.

Hudson, A., Morris, J., Redman, F., and Waddell, G.: An electron microscopic study of regeneration in severed rat sciatic nerves anastomosed with Silastic cuffs. Current Topics Surg. Res. *3*:187, 1971.

Hudson, A., Morris, J., and Waddell, G.: An electron microscopic study of regeneration in sutured rat sciatic nerves. Surg. Forum *21*:451, 1970.

Hudson, A., Morris, J., Waddell, G., and Drury. A.: Peripheral nerve autographs. An electron microscopic study. Surg. Res. *12*:267, 1972.

Kauffman, F. C., and Albuquerque, E. X.: Effect of ischemia and denervation on metabolism of fast and slow mammalian skeletal muscle. Exp. Neurol. *28*:46, 1970.

Kline, D. G., Hayes, G. J., and Morse, A. S.: A comparative study of response of species to peripheral-nerve injuries. I. Severance. J. Neurosurg. *21*:968, 1964*a*.

Kline, D. G., Hayes, G. J., and Morse, A. S.: A comparative study of response of species to peripheral-nerve injury. II. Crush and severance with primary suture. J. Neurosurg. *21*:980, 1964*b*.

Kopin, I. J., and Silberstein, S. D.: Axons of sympathetic neurons: Transport of enzymes *in vivo* and properties of axonal sprouts *in vitro*. Pharmacol. Rev. *24*:245, 1972.

Kreuzberg, G. W.: Changes of coenzyme (TPN diaphorase and TPN linked dehydrogenases during axonal reaction of the nerve cell. Nature *199*:393, 1963.

Lieberman, A. R.: The axon reaction: A review of the principal features of perikaryal responses to axon injury. Int. Rev. Neurobiol. *14*:49, 1971.

Lieberman, A. R.: Some factors affecting retrograde neuronal responses to axonal lesions. *In* R. Bellairs and E. G. Gray (eds.): Essays on the Nervous System. Oxford, Clarendon Press, 1974, p. 71.

Matthews, M. R., and Raisman, G.: A light and electron microscopic study of the cellular response to axonal injury in the superior cervical ganglion of the rat. Proc. Roy. Soc. Lond. (Biol.) *181*:43, 1972.

McCaman, R. E., and Robbins, E.: Quantitative biochemical studies of wallerian degeneration in the peripheral and central nervous systems. II. Twelve enzymes. J. Neurochem. *5*:32, 1959.

McQuarrie, I. G., and Grafstein, B.: Axon outgrowth enhanced by a previous nerve injury. Arch. Neurol. *29*:53, 1973.

Miani, N.: Metabolic and chemical changes in regenerating neurons, III. The rate of incorporation of radioactive phosphate into individual phospholipids of the nerve cell perikaryon of the C-8 spinal ganglion *in vitro*. J. Neurochem. *9*:537, 1962.

Moyer, E. K., Kimmel, D. L., and Winborne, L. W.: Regeneration of sensory spinal nerve roots in young and senile rat. J. Comp. Neurol. *98*:283, 1953.

Murray, M., and Grafstein, B.: Changes in the morphology and amino acid incorporation in regeneration of goldfish optic neurons. Exp. Neurol. *23*:544, 1969.

Murray, M.: ³H-uridine incorporation by regenerating retinal ganglion cells of goldfish. Exp. Neurol. *39*:489, 1973.

Nandy, K.: Histochemical study on chromatolytic neurons. Arch. Neurol. *18*:425, 1968.

Ochs, S.: Systems of material transport in nerve fibers (axoplasmic transport) related to nerve function and trophic control. Ann N.Y. Acad. Sci. *228*:202, 1974.

Ochs, S., Sabri, M. I., and Johnson, J.: Fast transport system of materials in mammalian nerve fibers. Science *163*:680, 1969.

Oester, Y. T., and Davis, L.: Recovery of sensory function. *In* B. Woodhall, and G. W. Beebe (eds.): Peripheral Nerve Regeneration. Washington, D.C., U.S. Government Printing Office, 1956, p. 241.

Reis, D. J., and Ross, R. A.: Dynamic changes in brain dopamine B-hydroxylase activity during anterograde and retrograde reactions to injury of central noradrenergic axon. Brain Res. *57*:307, 1973.

Reis, D. J., Ross, R. A., and Joh, T. H.: Some aspects of the reaction of central and peripheral noradrenergic neurons to injury. *In* K. Fuxe, L. Olson, and Y. Zotterman (eds.): Dynamics of degeneration and growth in Neurons. (Wenner-Cren Symposium XII), Oxford, Pergamon, 1974.

Robbins, E., Kissane, J. M., and Lowe, I. P.: Quantitative biochemical studies of chromatolysis. *In* J. Folch-Pi (ed.): Chemical Pathology of the Nervous System. Oxford, Pergamon Press, 1961, p. 244.

Sjostrand, J.: Morphological changes in glial cells during nerve regeneration. Acta Physiol. Scand. *67*(Suppl. 270):19, 1966.

Strassman, R. J., Letourneau, P. C., and Wessells, N. K.: Elongation of axons in an agar matrix that does not support cell locomotion. Exp. Cell Res. *81*:482, 1974.

Sumner, B. E. H.: The effects of injury on two hydrolases in the hypoglossal nucleus, with quantitative data on N-acetyl-B-glucosaminidase. Brain Res. *68*:157, 1974.

Torvik, A., and Heding, A.: Effect of actinomycin D on retrograde nerve cell reaction. Further observations. Acta Neuropath. *14*:62, 1969.

Turner, R. S.: Chromatolysis and recovery of efferent neurons. J. Comp. Neurol. *79*:73, 1943.

Varon, S.: Neurons and glia in neural cultures. Exp. Neurol. *48*:93, 1975.

Watson, W. E.: An autoradiographic study of the incorporation of nucleic acid precursors by neurons and glia during nerve regeneration. J. Physiol. Lond. *180*:741, 1965.

Watson, W. E.: Observations on the nucleolar and total cell body nucleic acid of injured nerve cells. J. Physiol. Lond. *196*:655, 1968.

Watson, W. E.: Some quantitative observations upon the response of neuroglial cells which follow axotomy of adjacent neurons. J. Physiol. Lond. *210*:321, 1972.

Watson, W. E.: The binding of actinomycin D to the nuclei of axotomized neurons. Brain Res. *65*:317, 1974.

Weiss, P. A.: Neuronal dynamics and neuroplasmic flow. *In* Schnitt, F. O. (ed.): The Neurosciences (Second Study Program). New York, The Rockefeller Press, 1970, p. 840.

Yamada, K. M., and Wessels, N. K.: Axon elongation: Effect of nerve growth factor on microtubule protein. Exp. Cell Res. *66*:346, 1971.

30

NERVE FIBER PATHOLOGY IN ACUTE AND CHRONIC COMPRESSION

JOSÉ OCHOA

INTRODUCTION

Many adults, both ill and healthy, harbor subclinical local lesions of one kind or another within their peripheral nerves or spinal nerve roots. Many of us now suffer or will develop clinical manifestations from such lesions: muscle weakness and atrophy, numbness, or pain and paresthesiae in various combinations. Such symptoms represent an important proportion of neurological and orthopedic consultations.

When one knows nothing about the pathology of local nerve lesions, one somehow tends to assume that the nerve looks thickened (or narrowed) and contains the carcasses of nerve fibers asphyxiated in collagen. The real picture is not as tragic, and is certainly not uniform. There are nerve lesions and nerve lesions, with different mechanisms of production, different structural changes, different electrophysiology, different clinical manifestations, and different prognoses. Since the application of electron microscopy to the study of abnormal nerves, the histopathology behind local nerve injuries is no longer a dull chapter in the story of nerve disease. What follows is an attempt to describe the more lively aspects of the subject, emphasizing those areas that allow correlation with abnormal physiology and with clinical manifestations.

487

ACUTE NERVE LESIONS WITH ANATOMICAL
INTERRUPTION OF AXONS

When a nerve is cut or crushed or infarcted, the distal stump dies. However, until about the third or fourth day after injury, the structure of the disconnected distal nerve fibers remains grossly preserved. Then they become fragmented into ovoids, and the distal stump becomes inexcitable when stimulated directly distal to the lesion. In other words, before three or four days one cannot tell whether paralysis following nerve injury is due to physiological block (neurapraxia) or to anatomical interruption of nerve fibers (axonotmesis and neurotmesis). Nerve fibers in the distal stump undergo a series of changes involving active disintegration of axons and myelin together with proliferation of Schwann cells. Such changes, best described by Cajal (1928) and by Williams and Hall (1971a, 1971b), culminate with the organization of solid columns made of Schwann cells which eventually welcome regenerated axons and direct them to the appropriate peripheral tissues. Meanwhile, the neuronal cell body is engaged in synthesis of macromolecules (chromatolysis), which are transported at various rates down the axon and added at the tip of the stump to build new nerve fibers. Elongation of regenerating axons in tissue culture requires a certain dynamics at the tip of the growth cones which involves ameboid movements dependent upon a contractile apparatus of actin microfilaments (Yamada et al., 1970, 1971). Despite adequate synthesis and transport, nerve regeneration might become arrested if growth cone dynamics is interfered with (Yamada et al., 1971; Wessells et al., 1971). "Gigantic clubs" attest to arrested progress of regeneration (Cajal, 1928; Ochoa and Morgan-Hughes, 1975). An example is given in Figure 30–1.

Each parent axon regenerates several thin branches, like a pruned tree. Anatomical and functional restitution following a nerve lesion characterized by axonal division is much more complete when the nerve trunk retains conti-

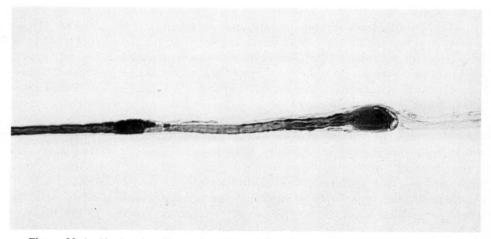

Figure 30–1 Single microdissected myelinated fiber from rat sciatic nerve, many weeks after onset of acrylamide intoxication. Acrylamide causes a "dying back" type of neuropathy. The fiber shows neither signs of active degeneration nor regenerating axon sprouts. Its features are similar to those of the "gigantic clubs" described by Cajal (1928) in arrested regeneration.

nuity (axonotmesis) than when interrupted (neurotmesis). The decisive factors are the helpful guidance of regenerated fibers toward appropriate terminals along the scaffold provided by surviving endoneurial tubes, and the reduced opportunity for fibers to escape their endoneurial and perineurial continents (Gutmann and Sanders, 1943; Young, 1949; Thomas, 1964). After functional contact with the periphery is re-established, only select fibers will mature in diameter and will therefore approach normal conduction velocity. Failure to establish peripheral contact results in an overproduction of regenerated fibers, which remain of immature caliber (Weiss and Taylor, 1944; Weiss et al., 1945; Sanders and Young, 1946; Aitken et al., 1947; Evans and Murray, 1956). Regenerated fibers may go astray and end in the wrong target, especially when they have to grow across a gap in a divided nerve, or across a scar. The consequences of aberrant reinnervation are particularly dramatic in facial muscles. It is common knowledge that in man regenerating fibers advance about 1 mm per day. The progress of sensory fiber regeneration can be roughly monitored clinically by following the advance of the Tinel sign with the passage of time.

Such are some of the events that follow anatomical interruption of nerve fibers, which is, of course, the major pathological catastrophe facing the nerve fiber, leading to prolonged paralysis with atrophy and anesthesia. Recovery is slow and incomplete.

TRANSIENT ISCHEMIC NERVE BLOCK

On the other side of the spectrum of severity is the transient paralysis and anesthesia that may follow acute compression of a nerve, as, for example, when an arm or a leg "go to sleep" or 20 to 30 minutes after application of a suprasystolic cuff to a limb. In the latter case, the deficit is almost immediately reversible on release of the cuff and there is no recognizable microscopic nor ultramicroscopic pathology (Ochoa, unpublished observations). From the classic experiments by Lewis, Pickering, and Rothschild (1931), we all accept that such an immediately reversible defect is the result of nerve ischemia. A significant experiment involved reversible paralysis and anesthesia in the upper limb of human volunteers by means of a pneumatic cuff inflated above systolic pressure, but just before releasing the cuff, a second suprasystolic cuff was placed further proximally. Thus the original pressure on the nerves was removed but the circulation remained arrested. In contrast to the single cuff experiment, paralysis and anesthesia did not recover until the second cuff, maintained for various periods of time, was released. This indicates that ischemia of the limb and not direct local mechanical pressure at one point is responsible for such type of transient nerve dysfunction.

NEURAPRAXIA

We have referred to the two extremes of severity of acute local nerve disorders. A fascinating intermediate level was defined electrophysiologically a century ago by Erb (1876).

Following some forms of acute nerve injury, particularly in "Saturday night paralysis" and "tourniquet paralysis," there is motor deficit with only mild sensory loss and little or no muscle atrophy. The nerve distal to the site of the injury remains excitable throughout. In the terminology of Sir Herbert Seddon (1943) this is "neurapraxia."

This type of intermediate lesion caught the imagination of Denny-Brown and Brenner in the 1940's. They demonstrated that in experimental tourniquet paralysis the local nerve lesion was selective to the myelin sheaths, sparing axons. That was probably the first revival of the idea of demyelinating disease in the twentieth century. In 1880, Gombault had described demyelination in experimental lead poisoning, but the phenomenon was then forgotten. Transcendental as it was, the work of Denny-Brown and Brenner (1944a, 1944b) reached an equivocal conclusion for reasons that in retrospect can be qualified as misleading coincidences. Their conclusion was that the local demyelinating lesion which follows local nerve compression is a result of ischemia and would merely represent a complication of the immediately reversible ischemic nerve block of Lewis et al. (1931). In support of their hypothesis, and against the alternative of a direct mechanical effect, Denny-Brown and Brenner cited the experiment of Grundfest (1936), who had, for different purposes, compressed portions of nerve within pressure chambers. Grundfest had found that, even under enormous pressures, nerves continued to conduct provided there was oxygen within the chamber. From the data to be described below we will see why the apparently legitimate extrapolation by Denny-Brown and Brenner was inaccurate.

In a series of papers from Queen Square, Gilliatt, Fowler, Rudge and Ochoa re-examined demyelinating lesions caused by acute nerve compression in the baboon. Using the tourniquet paralysis model and also a model akin to "Saturday night paralysis," the authors confirmed demyelination but failed to confirm three important features of the lesion described originally by Denny-Brown (Ochoa et al., 1971, 1972, 1973; Rudge et al., 1974; Fowler, 1975).

First, it was found that small diameter fibers were spared (the original description implicated fibers of all diameters). The sparing of small fibers is a very consistent feature and affords an excellent explanation for sparing of pain and temperature sensation and of autonomic function in tourniquet paralysis (Moldaver, 1954). Second, it was found that the nerve fiber defects did not extend throughout the compressed area. Instead, they were concentrated under the edges of the cuff, with sparing under the center. In the narrower

---

Figure 30-2 *A*, Normal microdissected myelinated fiber showing node of Ranvier. Baboon tibial nerve. (Bar = 10 μm.) *B*, Abnormal fiber, early after acute compression. The nodal gap is occluded due to intussusception from right to left. An indentation (pseudonode) marks the original site of the node. (Bar = 10 μm.) *C*, Low power electron micrograph of abnormal myelinated fiber, cut longitudinally after microdissection. Note indentation at Schwann cell junction, J, and new position of the node, N, under infolded myelin (From Rudge, P., Ochoa, J., and Gilliatt, R. W.: J. Neurol. Sci. *23*:403, 1974.) *D*, Diagram of affected fiber showing invagination of one paranode by the adjacent one, movement occurring from right to left. (From Ochoa, J., Fowler, T. J., and Gilliatt, R. W.: *In* Desmedt, J. E. (ed.): New Developments in Electromyography and Clinical Neurophysiology. Basel, Karger, 1973, Vol. 2, pp. 166–173.)

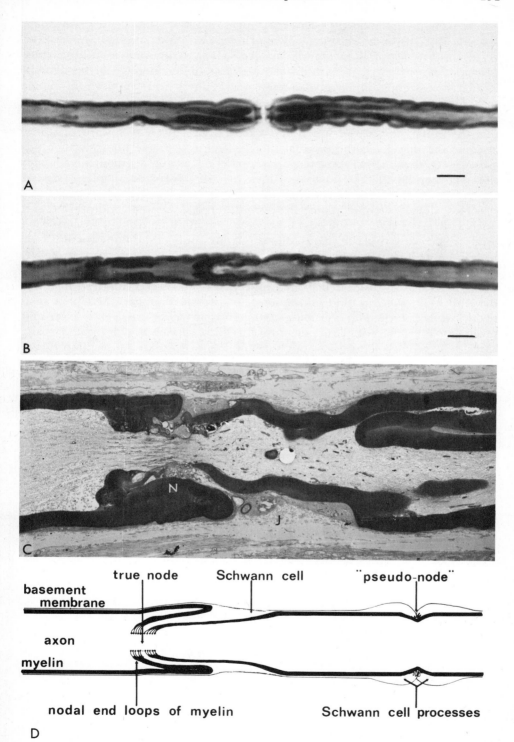

Figure 30–2 *Legend on opposite page*

lesion seen in the model of Saturday night paralysis, the center was again spared. But the most dramatic incongruence with the original report concerned the nodes of Ranvier, which were said to be normal soon after compression; nevertheless, a spectacular distortion of the nodes can be demonstrated consistently in large diameter nerve fibers with modern histologic techniques. In myelinated nerve fibers fixed for electron microscopy, osmicated and microdissected in fluent epoxi-resin, one can see by light microscopy that the nodal gaps are occluded and a dark area is present, toward one side, at some distance from the original site of the node. Single fiber electron microscopy (Ochoa, 1972) explains the lesion: one myelin segment invaginates the next (Fig. 30–2). The polarity of invagination is reversed on either edge of the compressed region (Fig. 30–3).

How does this come about? Pressure differences between compressed and uncompressed nerve, at the edges, generate longitudinal driving forces which tend to extrude axoplasm like toothpaste from a tube. The nodes of Ranvier, where the axon is normally narrowed, offer resistance to axoplasmic prolapse, but progressively the axon becomes stretched at the paranodal region and the node of Ranvier is dislocated from a few microns to several hundred microns, depending on the duration and amount of pressure applied. Myelin is relatively firmly attached to the axon and hence stretches passively. Axon and myelin in the adjacent paranode infold as they receive the dislocated structures. The whole picture is strongly reminiscent of an intussusception of the bowel. Unlike myelin, the Schwann cells do not follow the dislocated axon; they seem to be more firmly tethered to the basal lamina and surrounding collagen than to the myelin and axon. Thus, both the infolded and the stretched paranodal myelin become extracellular with respect to their static Schwann cells. The Schwann cell junction retains its original position and indents the underlying nerve fiber (pseudo-node), giving us a point of reference to measure the extent of nodal dislocation. No such longitudinal forces are generated under the middle of the compressed region because there are no pressure gradients there. Grundfest's experiment compressing segments of nerves within a pressure chamber does not apply, since pressure gradients could not develop under his experimental conditions.

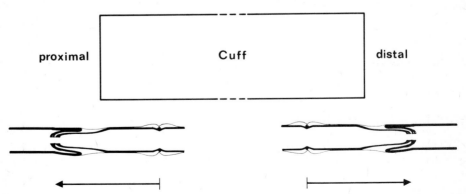

Figure 30–3 Diagram describing the direction of dislocation of the nodes of Ranvier in relation to the compressed zone. (From Ochoa, J., Fowler, T. J., and Gilliatt, R. W.: J. Anat., *113*:433, 1972.)

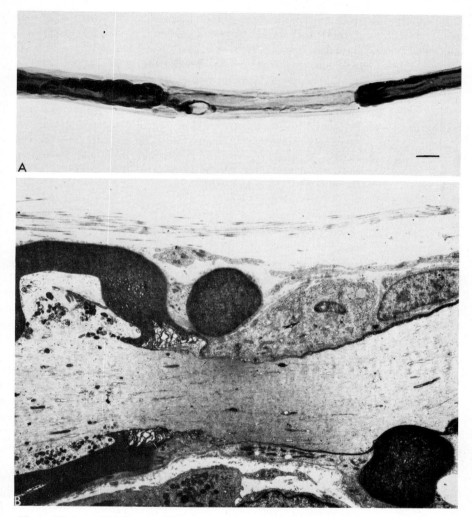

Figure 30-4 *A*, Thinly remyelinated segment intercalated in fiber microdissected from baboon sciatic nerve during repair of paranodal invagination and demyelination (Bar = 10 μm.) *B*, Low power electron micrograph after ultrathin sectioning of the fiber above. It shows detail of the node on the left. (× 5500) (From Ochoa, J.: J. Neurol. Sci. *17*:103, 1972.)

Small fibers are spared because more and more force is required to displace the viscous contents of smaller and smaller diameter tubes: nerve fibres are probably crushed before the required force is met. Indeed, if pressure is excessive, or is sustained for too long, then axons get crushed or overstretched and degenerate: the wallerian component becomes prominent (Ochoa et al., 1972; Fowler and Ochoa, 1975).

Paranodal demyelination and, occasionally, demyelination of complete segments follow within a few days after the injury, the peak occurring during the second week. Repair is achieved by Schwann cells which proliferate, migrate toward the injured paranodes, and intercalated remyelinated segments are formed (Fig. 30-4).

Remyelination parallels clinical and electrical recovery, which are usually fastest between the third and the sixth week (Fowler et al., 1972). Onset of recovery may be delayed and its time course protracted following severe compression. Under these circumstances, the development of intramyelin and periaxonal edema, perhaps due to anoxia, complicates recovery (Ochoa et al., 1972).

How does the early lesion (invagination of myelin segments) cause nerve conduction block? Presumably through occlusion of the nodes of Ranvier and blockade of ionic currents; however, this remains to be explored. Subsequent demyelination, of course, can also produce a conduction block; its mechanism has been elucidated by McDonald (1963) and by Rasminsky and Sears (1972).

CHRONIC NERVE ENTRAPMENT

Is chronic entrapment the result of cumulative subclinical acute compressions? In other words, is the pathogenesis of acute compression similar to that of chronic entrapment? The answer, which is no, emerges from plain histopathology. Indeed, in chronic entrapment we also have a peculiar anatomical lesion, with a fine structure that practically reveals its pathogenesis.

In 1913, Pierre-Marie and Foix discovered that a cause for some forms of thenar wasting was an anatomical lesion of the median nerve at the wrist. Using vintage stains, they noticed that myelin disappeared under the carpal tunnel, but they did not examine the nerves distal to the wrist. Fifty years later, in London, Thomas and Fullerton (1963) obtained another postmortem specimen from a proven carpal tunnel syndrome. Again, myelin disappeared in the region under the tunnel but reappeared distally. Thus, there was an element of focal demyelination in the lesion, which accounts for focal slowing of nerve conduction.

In the 1960's, Fullerton and Gilliatt and their associates discovered that guinea pigs aged two years and over suffer from the carpal tunnel syndrome (Fullerton and Gilliatt, 1967; Anderson et al., 1970). They confirmed local demyelination under the wrist in guinea pigs and also described a peculiar distortion of the myelin segments proximal to the wrist, but, like Marie and Foix, they did not pay attention to the changes distal to the wrist.

While working with Gilliatt at Queen Square, Ochoa and Marotte (1973) adopted the guinea pig model of chronic nerve entrapment, expecting to find evidence of invagination of nodes of Ranvier, as seen following acute compression. Acute changes were never found. However, the authors confirmed that, along stretches of up to 20 mm or more, proximal to the wrist, myelin segments were deformed, resembling tadpoles, being bulbous at one end and tapered at the other. The abnormal segments were consistently polarized, the bulb pointing away from the wrist. Interestingly, distal to the carpal tunnel the same distorted internodes were present as found proximally, but with a reversed polarity. In young animals there is merely asymmetry without demyelination, and the turning point can be shown under the tunnel. With age, the lesions become grotesque, and demyelination and remyelination follow. Eventually axons get interrupted and their distal portions degenerate (Fig. 30–5).

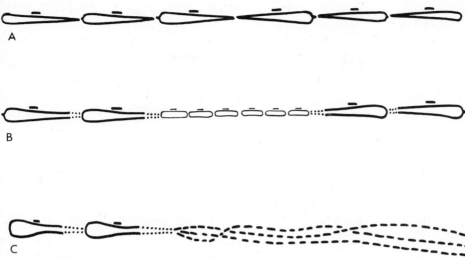

Figure 30–5 *A*, Diagram showing distorted myelin segments from median nerve of young guinea pig. Note reversal of polarity at the wrist. *B*, Further distortion and exposure of the axon proximal and distal to the site of entrapment. The median nerve under the carpal tunnel has lost its original myelin segments. Multiple, short remyelinated internodes repair the lesion. *C*, Advanced lesion with massive bulbs and axonal wallerian degeneration and regeneration.

Examining the abnormal myelin segments by electron microscopy revealed that internal myelin lamellae had slipped away at the tapered ends, and that these displaced lamellae had "buckled" at the bulbous ends (Fig. 30–6). Ochoa and Marotte (1973) suggested that there is nothing peculiar about demyelination in this model: initially it is simple slippage of myelin lamellae followed by disintegration of the contorted myelin at the bulbs. In support of this is the observation that loss of myelin is initially confined to the tapered ends. Sunderland (1976) believes that nerve fiber damage in the carpal tunnel syndrome is due to ischemia caused by local obstruction of venous return resulting from increased pressure in the tunnel. We believe that repeated minor trauma, or perhaps repeated stretching or friction against flexor tendons, elicits pressure waves that propagate in opposite directions, causing detachment of myelin lamellae, which slip away. The unrolled myelin sheath, which is normally symmetrical, becomes skewed (Fig. 30–7).

Neary, Ochoa, and Gilliatt (1975) confirmed, in human median nerves at the wrist and ulnar nerves at the elbow, all the findings described earlier in the guinea pig; identical changes have been found recently in the lateral cutaneous nerve of the thigh under the inguinal ligament in a case of meralgia paresthesica (Ochoa, 1977, unreported), which seems to consolidate the lesions described by Ochoa and Marotte (1973) as the primary pathology of myelinated fibers underlying chronic entrapment in general. Unmyelinated fibers resist until late in the course of entrapment, when evidence of their degeneration and regeneration becomes increasingly apparent (Marotte, 1974). It is conceivable that similar lesions occur at other common sites of local entrapment, the posterior interosseus nerve being strongly suspect at the elbow in the vicinity of the supinator muscle (Spinner, 1968), where it may be

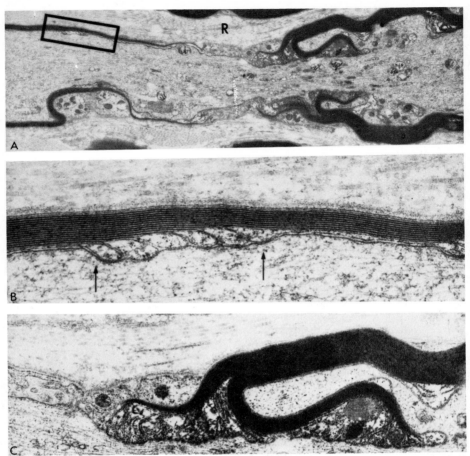

Figure 30–6   *A*, Low power electron micrograph of a moderately abnormal fiber taken from a guinea pig median nerve above the wrist. The paranode on the left is tapered. The bulbous paranode on the right shows inturning of a group of inner lamellae. (R = node of Ranvier.) (× 7000.) *B*, Enlargement of the area enclosed in the rectangle in *A*. Six myelin lamellae end in cytoplasmic loops between the arrows. (× 48,000.) *C*, Detail of the bulbous paranode. (× 20,000.) (From Ochoa and Marotte, J. Neurol. Sci. *19*:491, 1973.)

macroscopically enlarged and microscopically so modified that distinction from neoplasm may be difficult (Ochoa and Neary, 1975).

There should be no doubt that severe acute and chronic ischemia can cause primary damage to nerves (Gairns et al., 1960; Eames and Lange, 1967; Asbury, 1970; Korthals and Wisniewski, 1975). Further, ischemia can contribute to modified function in diseased nerves, both in diabetic polyneuropathy (Seneviratne and Peiris, 1968) and in mononeuropathies, particularly in the carpal tunnel syndrome where ischemia is known to precipitate or exaggerate symptoms (Gilliatt and Wilson, 1954; Fullerton, 1963). It is also conceivable that chronic ischemia may play some role in the pathogenesis of chronic entrapment, since vasa nervorum eventually suffer prominent local damage in plantar neuromas (Lassman et al., 1976). Vascular damage in chronic entrap-

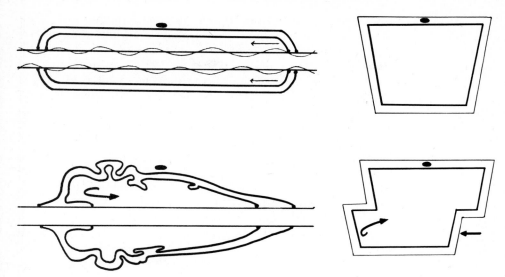

Figure 30–7 *A*, Normal myelin segment and unrolled myelin sheath (right) which is trapezoid shaped. Hypothetical pressure waves in the direction of the arrows along the axon. *B*, Distorted segment with tapered end caused by myelin slippage, and bulbous end containing inturned redundant myelin lamellae. If the myelin were unrolled it would be altered as indicated (right).

ment may be more frequent than it would appear from the study of epineurial arterioles and venules along. Endoneurial vessels appear to be reduced in numbers locally, and it seems likely to the author that Renaut bodies (Asbury, 1973) may represent the residue of injured small caliber endoneurial vessels. Although there are good grounds to suspect a secondary role for ischemia in the pathogenesis of the nerve lesion underlying chronic entrapment, it seems overwhelmingly clear that the polarized changes described in myelinated fibers, involving graded displacement of structures away from the site of entrapment, must be mechanical in origin.

PAINFUL NERVE LESIONS

Too many patients suffer chronic pain from local nerve lesions, and yet we know little about the mechanisms involved, and even less about the underlying histopathology in man. This is not a trivial subject, since current conflicting theories to explain neuralgia presuppose quite different pathological substrates.

For example, Noordenbos (1959) believes that selective loss of large diameter afferents releases the inputs from small fibers which conduct impulses related to pain. Noordenbos' concept was based upon clinical and histological observations in post-herpetic neuralgia and inspired by Henry Head's ideas of two conflicting peripheral sensory systems. Such is the fiber dissociation theory, subsequently embraced by the gate control theory of pain (Melzack and Wall, 1965). Another theory, not individually championed but in "vox populi," implicates an "artificial synapse" created at the level of the injury, where pain fibers would be ephaptically cross-excited by normal, ongoing ascending or descending (somatic or autonomic) impulses. Ephaptic excitation at the artificial synapse has been shown electrophysiologically in acute experimental local nerve injuries in animals (Granit and Skoglund, 1945) and in dysmyelinated spinal roots of dystrophic mice (Rasminsky, 1976), but Wall et al. (1974) failed to confirm longlasting cross-excitation following acute experimental local nerve injury. No comparable studies are available in painful nerve lesions in man. On the morphological side, there has been no serious attempt to identify the structural correlates of "artificial synapses." A third relevant theory to explain neuralgia incriminates the spontaneous generation of impulses in abnormal nerve fibers. For Wall and Gutnick (1974a, 1974b) the abnormal generators would be immature axon sprouts from small diameter afferent fibers. Their electrophysiological studies on experimental amputation neuromas in the rat are convincing and invite extrapolation to human disease. Similarly, Rasminsky (1976) has claimed spontaneous impulse generation in nerve fibers with defective myelin, and it is conceivable and theoretically sound that other structural deviations in nerve fibers may also behave as abnormal pacemakers (Calvin et al., 1977).

Since only a small proportion of local nerve lesions cause chronic pain, any attempt to define the elusive histopathology underlying painful nerve lesions must utilize human material because we still depend on communication of the sensory experience as the single measure of pain. Obviously, a morphological study is unlikely to provide answers on mechanisms but should contribute toward the authentication of current theories to explain neuralgia.

Painful amputation neuromas in man, studied by classic histology, are characterized by focal increase in volume, largely due to deposition of fibrous tissue, and the presence of many tangled nerve fibers. Fiber counts and size frequency histograms obtained from various levels are not available, and it remains unknown whether *non*-painful neuromas show any distinctive features when compared with painful neuromas. Amputation neuromas in experimental animals have been thoroughly studied by Spencer (1971), who has emphasized the formation of small fascicles within or outside the original perineurial limits, as well as nerve fiber branching, the predominance of small sized axons, and the swollen growth cones and retrograde regenerated fibers previously described by Cajal (1928).

Preliminary quantitative studies from human painful nerve lesions in continuity are available (Ochoa, 1977; Ochoa and Noordenbos, in preparation). In selected cases where samples of the whole nerve trunk could be examined proximal to, at, and distal to the local lesion, the common denominator was the presence of an increased total number of fibers, many of them immature, confined to the level of the lesion itself (Fig. 30–8). The myelinated fiber spectrum distal to the lesion was often distorted but not universally so (Fig. 30–9). A similar pattern applied to unmyelinated fibers. If sprouts from small diameter afferents concerned with nociceptive (painful) impulses are represented in the local fiber excess (and this is likely), then such excess of fibers demonstrated at the level of the painful lesions would support the theory of abnormal pacemakers in preference to "fiber dissociation." As to the "artificial synapse," current morphological techniques are not suited for its assessment.

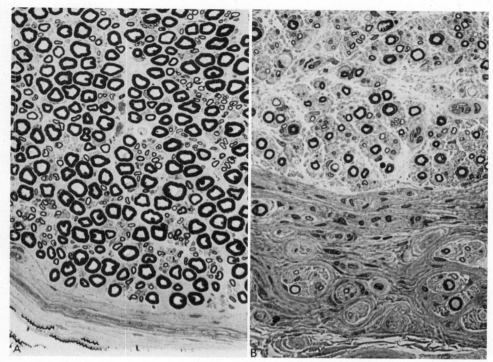

Figure 30–8 *A*, Normal portion of human superficial radial nerve, above the site of the injury. *B*, At the site of the lesion note the drop out of the large diameter fibers. Miniature fascicles are seen external to the perineurium. Magnification is similar for *A* and *B*.

MYELINATED FIBERS

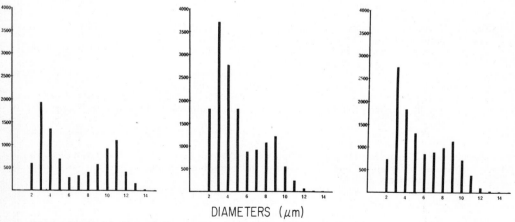

DIAMETERS (μm)

Figure 30–9 Myelinated fiber spectra of a painful neuroma in continuity after total counts proximal to the lesion (*left*), at the level of the lesion (*center*), and distal to the lesion (*right*). Note the increase in the number of small fibers at the level of the lesion: many were immature sprouts. Note further, that in this case there is no selective loss of large diameter fibers.

REFERENCES

Aitken, J. T., Sharman, M., and Young, J. Z.: Maturation of regenerating nerve fibers with various peripheral connections. J. Anat. *81*:1, 1947.

Anderson, M. H., Fullerton, P. M., Gilliatt, R. W., and Hern, J. E. C.: Changes in the forearm associated with median nerve compression at the wrist in the guinea-pig. J. Neurol. *33*:70, 1970.

Asbury, A. K.: Ischemic disorders of peripheral nerve. *In* Vinken, P. J., and Bruyn, G. W. (eds.): Handbook of Clinical Neurology. Amsterdam, Holland, North-Holland Publishing Co., 1970, Vol. 8, p. 154.

Asbury, A. K.: Renaut bodies: A forgotten endoneurial structure. J. Neuropath. Exp. Neurol. *32*:334, 1973.

Cajal, S. R.: Degeneration and Regeneration of the Nervous System. Oxford University Press, 1928.

Calvin, W. H., Loeser, J. D., and Howe, J. F.: A neurophysiological theory for the pain mechanism of tic douloureux. Pain *3*:147, 1977.

Denny-Brown, D., and Brenner, C.: Paralysis of nerve induced by direct pressure and by tourniquet. Arch. Neurol. Psych. *51*:1, 1944*a*.

Denny-Brown, D., and Brenner, C.: Lesion in peripheral nerve resulting from compression by spring clip. Arch. Neurol. Psych. *52*:1, 1944*b*.

Eames, R. A., and Lange, L. S.: Clinical and pathological study of ischaemic neuropathy. J. Neurol. Neurosurg. Psychiatry *30*:215, 1967.

Erb, W.: Diseases of the peripheral cerebrospinal nerves. *In* Ziemssen, H. von. (ed.) Cyclopedia of the Practice of Medicine. London, Samson Low, Marston, Searle and Rivington, 1876, Vol. XI.

Evans, D. H. L., and Murray, J. G.: A study of regeneration in a motor nerve with unimodal fiber diameter distribution. Anat. Rec. *126*:311, 1956.

Fowler, T. J.: Tourniquet Paralysis in the Baboon. D.M. Thesis. University of Oxford, 1975.

Fowler, T. J., and Ochoa, J.: Unmyelinated fibers in normal and compressed peripheral nerves of the baboon; a quantitative electron-microscopic study. Neuropath. Applied Neurobiol. *1*:247, 1975.

Fowler, T. J., Danta, G., and Gilliatt, R. W.: Recovery of nerve conduction after a pneumatic tourniquet: Observations on the hind-limb of the baboon. J. Neurol., Neurosurg. Psychiatry *35*:638, 1972.

Fullerton, P. M.: The effect of ischaemia on nerve conduction in the carpal tunnel syndrome. J. Neurol. Neurosurg. Psychiatry *26*:385, 1963.

Fullerton, P. M., and Gilliatt, R. W.: Median and ulnar neuropathy in the guinea-pig. J. Neurol. Neurosurg. Psychiatry *30*:393, 1967.

Gairns, F. W., Garven, H. S. D., and Smith, G.: The digital nerves and the nerve endings in progressive obliterative vascular disease of the leg. Scot. Med. J. *5*:382, 1960.

Gilliatt, R. W., and Wilson, T. G.: A pneumatic-tourniquet test in the carpal tunnel syndrome. Lancet *2*:595, 1953.

Gombault, A.: Contribution a l'etude anatomique de la nevrite parenchymateuse subaigue et chronique — nevrite segmentaire periaxile. Arch. Neurol. *1*:11, 1880.

Gutmann, E., and Sanders, F. K.: Recovery of fiber numbers and diameters in the regeneration of peripheral nerves. J. Physiol. *101*:489, 1943.

Granit, R., and Skoglund, C. R.: Facilitation, inhibition and depression at the artificial synapse formed by the cut end of a mammalian nerve. J. Physiol. *103*:435, 1945.

Grundfest, H.: Effects of hydrostatic pressures upon the excitability, the recovery, and the potential sequence of frog nerve. Cold Spring Harbor Symposia on Quantitative Biology, *4*:179, 1936.

Korthals, J. K., and Wisniewski, H. M.: Peripheral nerve ischemia: Part 1. Experimental model. J. Neurol. Sci. *24*:65, 1975.

Lassmann, G., Lassmann, H., and Stockinger, L.: Morton's Metatarsalgia: Light and electron microscopic observations and their relation to entrapment neuropathies. Virchows Arch. A. Path. Anat. Histol. *370*:307, 1976.

Lewis, T., Pickering, G. W., and Rothschild, P.: Centripetal paralysis arising out of arrested bloodflow to the limb, including notes on a form of tingling. Heart *16*:2, 1931.

McDonald, W. I.: The effects of experimental demyelination on conduction in peripheral nerve: a histological and electrophysiological study. I. Clinical and histological observations. Brain *86*:481, 1963. II. Electrophysiological observations. Brain *86*:501, 1963.

Marie, P., and Foix, C.: Atrophie isolée de l'éminence thénar d'origine névritique, Rôle du ligament annulaire antérieur du carpal dans la pathogénie de la lésion. Rev. Neurol. *26*:647, 1913.

Marotte, L. R.: An electron microscope study of chronic median nerve compression in the guinea-pig. Acta Neuropath. *27*:69, 1974.

Melzack, R., and Wall, P. D.: Pain mechanisms: A new theory. Science *150*:971, 1965.

Moldaver, J.: Tourniquet paralysis syndrome. Arch. Surg. *68*:136, 1954.

Neary, D., Ochoa, J., and Gilliatt, R. W.: Sub-clinical entrapment neuropathy in man. J. Neurol. Sci. *24*:283, 1975.

Noordenbos, W.: Pain. Amsterdam, Elsevier, 1959.

Ochoa, J.: Neuralgia and hyperalgesia from local nerve lesions: Pathophysiology. Electroenceph. Clin. Neurophysiol. *43*:597, 1977.

Ochoa, J.: Ultrathin longitudinal sections of single myelinated fibres for electron microscopy. J. Neurol. Sci. *17*:103, 1972.

Ochoa, J., and Marotte, L.: Nature of the nerve lesion underlying chronic entrapment. J. Neurol. Sci. *19*:491, 1973.

Ochoa, J., and Morgan-Hughes, J. A.: Arrested peripheral nerve regeneration in acrylamide neuropathy — an ultrastructural study. Excerpta Medica. International Congress Series, 1974. VIIth International Congress of Neuropathology — Budapest.

Ochoa, J., and Neary, D.: Localised hypertrophic neuropathy, intraneural tumour, or chronic nerve entrapment? Lancet March 15, 1975.

Ochoa, J., Danta, G. Fowler, T. J., and Gilliatt, R. W.: Nature of the nerve lesion caused by a pneumatic tourniquet. Nature *233*:265, 1971.

Ochoa, J., Fowler, T. J., and Gilliatt, R. W.: Anatomical changes in peripheral nerves compressed by a pneumatic tourniquet. J. Anat. *113*:433, 1972.

Ochoa, J., Gilliatt, R. W., and Fowler, T. J.: Tourniquet paralysis in the baboon. Trans. Am. Neurol. Assoc. *97*:52, 1972.

Rasminsky, M.: Abstract 595. Neurosci. Abstracts. Vol. 2, Part 1, 1976.

Rasminsky, M., and Sears, T. A.: Internodal conduction in undissected demyelinated nerve fibers. J. Physiol. *227*:323, 1972.

Rudge, P., Ochoa, J., and Gilliatt, R. W.: Acute peripheral nerve compression in the baboon. Anatomical and physiological findings. J. Neurol. Sci. *23*:403, 1974.

Sanders, F. K., and Young, J. Z.: Effect of peripheral connection on diameter of nerve fibers. Nature *155*:237, 1945.

Seddon, H. J.: Three types of nerve injury. Brain *66*:237, 1943.

Seneviratne, K. N., and Peiris, O. A.: The effect of ischaemia on the excitability of sensory nerves in diabetes mellitus. J. Neurol. Neurosurg. Psychiatry *31*:348, 1968.

Spencer, P. S.: Light and electron microscopic observations on localised peripheral nerve injuries. Thesis. 1971.

Spinner, M.: The arcade of Frohse and its relation to posterior interosseous nerve paralysis. J. Bone Joint Surg. *50B*:809, 1968.

Sunderland, S.: Nerve lesion in the carpal tunnel syndrome. J. Neurol., Neurosurg. Psychiatry *39*:615, 1976.

Thomas, P. K.: Changes in the endoneurial sheaths of peripheral myelinated nerve fibers during Wallerian degeneration. J. Anat. *98*:175, 1964.

Thomas, P. K., and Fullerton, P. M.: Nerve fiber size in the carpal tunnel syndrome. J. Neurol. Neurosurg. Psychiatry *26*:520, 1963.

Wall, P. D., and Gutnick, M.: Ongoing activity in peripheral nerves: The physiology and pharmacology of impulses originating from a neuroma. Exp. Neurol. *43*:580, 1974*a*.

Wall, P. D., and Gutnick, M.: Properties of afferent nerve impulses originating from a neuroma. Nature *248*:740, 1974*b*.

Wall, P. D., Waxman, S., and Basbaum, A. I.: Ongoing activity in peripheral nerve: Injury discharge. Exp. Neurol. *45*:576, 1974.

Weiss, P., and Taylor, A. C.: Further experimental evidence against "neurotropism" in nerve regeneration. J. Exp. Zool. *95*:233, 1944.

Weiss, P., Edds, M. V., and Cavanaugh, M.: The effect of terminal connections on the caliber of nerve fibers. Anat. Rec. *92*:215, 1945.

Wessells, N. K., Spooner, B. S., Ash, J. F., Bradley, M. O., Luduena, M. A., Taylor, E. L., Wrenn, J. T., and Yamada, K. M.: Microfilaments in cellular and developmental processes. Science *171*:135, 1971.

Williams, P. L., and Hall, S. M.: Prolonged in vivo observations of normal peripheral nerve fibers and their acute reactions to crush and deliberate trauma. J. Anat. *108*:397, 1971*a*.

Williams, P. L., and Hall, S. M.: Chronic Wallerian degeneration — an in vivo and ultrastructural study. J. Anat. *109*:487, 1971*b*.

Yamada, K. M., Spooner, B. S., and Wessells, N. K.: Axon growth: Roles of microfilaments and microtubules. Proc. Nat. Acad. Sci. *66*:1206, 1970.

Yamada, K. M., Spooner, B. S., and Wessells, N. K.: Ultrastructure and function of growth cones and axons of cultured cells. J. Cell Biol. *49*:614, 1971.

Young, J. Z.: Factors influencing the regeneration of nerves. Adv. Surg. *11*.165, 1949.

31

THE RESULTS
OF
UNTREATED
TRAUMATIC
INJURIES

GEORGE E. OMER, Jr.

The more extensive and severe the injury to the involved extremity the longer the time required for homeostasis of the tissues. Nerves are only as functional as the pertinent sensory receptors and muscle–tendon motors. Multiple nerve involvement is a more serious problem to functional recovery of the entire extremity than is an isolated nerve injury. Severe vascular deficiency, chronic osteomyelitis, and skeletal non-union all contribute to fibrotic infiltration and decreased function. Clinical studies of nerve recovery in the human show considerable variation because return of useful function depends as much on the total response of the extremity to the injury as on the regeneration of the injured nerve (Bowden, 1951).

Seddon (1943) introduced a simple classification of traumatic nerve injuries during World War II. In this classification, minimal injury is termed neurapraxia and may be secondary to localized ischemic demyelination. Moderate injury is termed axonotmesis and is characterized by interruption of the axons and their myelin sheath; but the endoneurial tubes remain intact and guide the regenerating axons to their proper peripheral connections. Severe injury is termed neurotmesis and describes a nerve that has either been completely severed or is so seriously disorganized that spontaneous regeneration is impossible. Most traumatic accidents, including fractures, traction, and gunshot wounds, can result in any one of the three types of injury. It is clinically important to know the percentage of nerves that will recover from various types of accidents, and the time required for return of function. Lacerations usually result in neurotmesis, and total loss of nerve function following this injury demands exploration and suture of the affected nerve.

MISSILE INJURIES

The distinguishing feature of gunshot wounds is the pressure disturbance in the tissues, which often results in loss of function without disruption of the nerve. Foerster (1929) reported 2915 cases of motor paralysis during World War I, of which 1980 (67 per cent) improved sufficiently under conservative treatment to obviate operative treatment. Sunderland (1972) studied a series of military patients during World War II and documented spontaneous recovery in 68 per cent of the cases. Rakolta and Omer (1969) noted that spontaneous regeneration may be delayed up to 11 months without excluding the possibility of complete recovery (Table 31–1). Omer (1974) developed a prospective study of 595 gunshot wounds during the war in Vietnam to determine the percentage of spontaneous recovery and the time required for clinical function. Spontaneous recovery occurred in 227 of 331 (69 per cent) low-velocity gunshot wounds and 183 of 264 (69 per cent) high-velocity gunshot wounds.

Prognosis is improved if the time required for return of clinical function is known. Omer (1974) selected two parameters for a time frame: (1) the interval after injury at which one half of the nerves had recovered function, and (2) the interval after injury after which only 10 per cent of the nerves recovered function. This established the time scale expected for spontaneous recovery in 90 per cent of cases. The time scale for spontaneous function in the 410 nerve lesions recovering from gunshot wounds was three to nine months (Table 31–2). Proximal (high) extremity injuries took longer to show clinical function than did distal (low) extremity injuries. Extensive injuries producing multiple nerve lesions needed a longer time period for return of clinical function than did injuries producing isolated nerve injuries. The prognosis for spontaneous recovery of clinical function is the same for high-velocity and low-velocity gunshot wounds. Neurapraxia and axonotmesis injuries are approximately equal in gunshot wounds, with the clinical time scale for spontaneous recovery being one to four months for neurapraxia and four to nine months for axonotmesis (Table 31–2).

Table 31–1   Interval Between Injury and Spontaneous Recovery in Gunshot Wounds*

NERVE	(NEURAPRAXIA) 0–4 months	(AXONOTMESIS) 4–9 months	(AXONOTMESIS) 9 + months
Radial	20	9	2
Median	10	7	
Ulnar	9	13	4
Sciatic and popliteals	14	14	3
Femoral	1	4	1
Total (111)	54	47	10

*Data from Rakolta and Omer, 1969, and Sunderland, 1972.

Table 31-2   Time Scale in Months for Spontaneous Recovery
in Gunshot Wounds*

| | ISOLATED NERVE LESIONS | |
	Above Elbow	*Below Elbow*
Low-velocity	4–7 mo. (48)	3–6 mo. (90)
High-velocity	3–6 mo. (31)	3–6 mo. (32)
	MULTIPLE NERVE LESIONS	
	Above Elbow	*Below Elbow*
Low-velocity	5–8 mo. (41)	3–7 mo. (48)
High-velocity	5–9 mo. (65)	5–8 mo. (55)
Totals (410)	(185)	(225)

*Data from Omer, 1974.

FRACTURES, DISLOCATIONS, TRACTION INJURIES

The radial nerve is injured more often than any other major nerve (Sunderland, 1972). Approximately 11 per cent of fractures of the shaft of the humerus are complicated by immediate radial nerve paralysis (Barton, 1973). The incidence is about the same in closed and open fractures, and Bristow reported spontaneous recovery in 70 per cent of these nerve injuries (Sunderland, 1972). Garcia and Maeck (1960) reported a series of 23 immediate explorations of radial palsy, and the nerve was found to be divided in only one case. Barton (1973) states that the average onset of spontaneous recovery in complete lesions is five weeks.

The incidence of nerve injury is higher in dislocations than in fractures. The sciatic nerve is often contused in posterior dislocation of the hip, and traction injury of the common peroneal nerve occurs with varus dislocation of the knee. Shoulder dislocations are associated with axillary nerve stretching, and the posterior interosseous nerve may be injured in dislocation of the radial head.

The sciatic nerve or its peroneal component is injured in approximately 10 per cent of patients with posterior dislocation or posterior acetabular fracture of the hip. Hunter (1969) reported 83 per cent spontaneous recovery of sciatic nerve lesions, but Seddon (1975) recorded that only 73 per cent of 22 cases had normal or slightly impaired spontaneous recovery. Nerve problems occur in 25 to 35 per cent of knee dislocations, usually traction injuries that vary from neurapraxia to neurotmesis. Common peroneal nerve palsy should be suspected in any adduction injury to the knee in which there are signs of damage to the lateral ligament and capsule structures. Highet and Holmes (1943) reported eight cases; of these, four had complete rupture and four had macroscopic changes. Repair was not possible in two nerves, and only one of the six sutured nerves regained any function. However, White (1968) collected six cases: two nerves were sutured with functional recovery; the other four nerves had spontaneous recovery with onset between two and six months and complete function between four and 12 months.

Omer (1974) reported a prospective study of 53 fractures and stretch injuries, in which 83 per cent had spontaneous recovery. The nerve lesion

Table 31–3   Time Scale in Months for Spontaneous Recovery in Fractures and Stretch Injuries*

	ISOLATED NERVE LESIONS	
	Above Elbow	*Below Elbow*
Fractures	2–4 mo. (11)	1–4 mo. (22)
Stretch Injuries		
	MULTIPLE NERVE LESIONS	
	Above Elbow	*Below Elbow*
Fractures	1–4 mo. (2)	1–4 mo. (3)
Stretch Injuries	3–6 mo. (6)	
Totals (44)	(19)	(25)

*Data from Omer, 1974.

associated with a fracture-dislocation is less likely to have spontaneous return of function than the nerve lesion associated with a mid-shaft fracture. The time scale for spontaneous recovery in 38 fractures was one to four months. A fracture is usually a neurapraxia injury, while a stretch injury can demonstrate spontaneous recovery following either a neurapraxia or an axonotmesis injury (Table 31–3).

MANAGEMENT PROGRAM

Nerve injuries associated with fractures of the shafts of long bones should be observed for four to five months because approximately 85 per cent of these lesions have spontaneous recovery within four months. The radial nerve has a lower percentage of spontaneous recovery in the humeral fracture, especially in the distal third of the bone. Nerve injuries associated with a dislocated joint or a fracture adjacent to a joint are suspect because fascial envelopes hold nerves close to the bone near joints. These fracture-dislocation accidents often stretch the nerve, and spontaneous recovery may require four to nine months.

Gunshot wounds require debridement and observation of neurovascular structures. Nerve palsies without disruption of the nerve may be observed for nine to 10 months because approximately 70 per cent of these lesions have spontaneous recovery within nine months. The proximal (high) injury presents a difficult problem. It may be a considerable distance from the site of the nerve lesion to the first motor point to be reinnervated. From the time of injury, there is progressive distortion and degeneration of the distal motor and sensory end-organs, with associated slowing of the regenerative process for axon regrowth. Expectant management could be prolonged to the time when suture of a previously unrecognized severed nerve would be without hope of functional recovery.

It is appropriate to explore at three to four months the clinically complete nerve lesion in gunshot wounds above the elbow or knee, stretch injuries from dislocated joints, and fractures adjacent to joints. However, approximately 50 per cent of these nerves will have a neuroma in continuity, and a decision concerning resection of the neuroma can be very difficult. Kline (1975) developed an operating room technique for stimulating the involved nerve proximally and recording distal to the neuroma in continuity. The nerve action potential is related to axon population and myelin return. Significant spontaneous recovery is gained in approximately 90 per cent of those nerves when a normal nerve action potential is recorded across a neuroma in continuity at three months after injury.

Lacerations require exploration and suture of disrupted nerves at the time of injury.

REFERENCES

Barton, N. J.: Radial nerve lesions. Hand 5:200–208, 1973.

Bowden, R. E. M.: The factors influencing functional recovery of peripheral nerve injuries in man. Ann. R. Coll. Surg. Engl. 8:366, 1951.

Foerster, O.: Handbuch der Neurologie. Berlin, Julius Springer, 1929, Part 2.

Garcia, A. Jr., and Maeck, B. H.: Radial nerve injuries in fractures of the shaft of the humerus. Am. J. Surg. 99:625, 1960.

Highet, W. B., and Holmes, W.: Traction injuries to the lateral popliteal nerve and traction injuries to peripheral nerves after suture. Br. J. Surg. 30:212, 1943.

Hunter, G. A.: Posterior dislocation and fracture-dislocation of the hip, a review of fifty-seven patients. J. Bone Joint Surg. 51B:38, 1969.

Kline, D. G., and Hackett, E. R.: Reappraisal of timing for exploration of civilian peripheral nerve injuries. Surgery 78:54, 1975.

Omer, G. E. Jr.: Injuries to nerves of the upper extremity. J. Bone Joint Surg. 56A:1615, 1974.

Rakolta, G. G. and Omer, G. E. Jr.: Combat-sustained femoral nerve injuries. Surg. Gynecol. Obstet. 128:813, 1969.

Seddon, H. J.: Three types of nerve injury. Brain 66:237, 1943.

Seddon, H.: Surgical Disorders of the Peripheral Nerves. 2nd ed., Edinburgh, Churchill Livingstone, 1975.

Sunderland, S.: Nerve and Nerve Injuries. Edinburgh, Churchill Livingstone, 1972.

White, J.: The results of traction injuries to the common peroneal nerve. J. Bone Joint Surg. 50B:346, 1968.

32

NERVES OF
THE HEAD
AND NECK

MADJID SAMII

The introduction of the operating microscope into peripheral nerve surgery (Jacobson, 1963; Smith, 1964, Michon, 1964) brought a new dimension into the surgical treatment of cranial nerves. The satisfying results derived from the microsurgical techniques of neurolysis, nerve suture, and nerve graft following peripheral nerve lesions considerably enlarged the indication of operative treatment of cranial nerve lesions (Millesi 1968, Samii 1970). During the last 10 years, previously existing operative methods were refined and new approaches put into practice.

With increasing experience the preservation and functional reconstruction of cranial nerves became an important component of the operating concept of tumor surgery in the region of the cerebellopontine angle, the base of the skull, and the neck.

In this chapter an attempt is made to review subject *surgical possibilities* with regard to specific cranial nerves. A systematic record of the etiology of lesions, topographic anatomy, and clinical symptomatology in this chapter would be too comprehensive. Special attention is given to the surgical methods of preserving and repairing cranial nerve function through nerve decompression, neurolysis, nerve suture, and nerve grafting.

OLFACTORY NERVE (FIRST CRANIAL NERVE)

The olfactory nerve may be damaged by frontobasal injuries with fractures in the region of the cribriform plate and by space-occupying processes in the region of the anterior cranial fossa. The neurosurgical approach to the anterior cranial fossa and the sella region may involve sectioning of the fila olfactoria, the bulb, or the tractus olfactorius. Therefore, in cases of frontobasal CSF fistulas without loss of the sense of smell the question arises whether or not the rhinosurgical approach would be more advisable than the subfrontal in order to repair a dura leak and at the same time preserve the olfactory nerve. In pituitary gland surgery one has to think of similar aspects. Olfactory function can be saved by choosing either the subfrontal, the trans-septosphenoidal, or the transethmoidosphenoidal approach. Until the present there has been no report on surgical restoration of a damaged olfactory nerve. For this reason, before each surgical procedure in the region of the anterior fossa, the surgeon should be certain that craniotomy is really the best available method.

OPTIC NERVE (SECOND CRANIAL NERVE)

The optic nerve as a rostrally situated part of the brain has no regeneration power after interruption of continuity; therefore, surgical efforts are restricted to decompressive relief operations. The subfrontal approach may be given preference in cases of traumatic swelling within the bony canal, hematoma of the optic sheath, or retrobulbar hemorrhage. Early diagnosis and immediate surgical intervention may be of great significance for the prognosis (Fig. 32–1). The transethmoidal route to decompression of the optic canal has been favored by Japanese authors.

It is possible to preserve existing visual function. Microsurgical technique is mandatory in the transsphenoidal procedure and is a great help in subfrontal procedures for the removal of inflammatory space-occupying processes or tumors in the sella region and orbit.

Functional improvement of visual power and in the field of vision is frequently observed following decompression of the optic apparatus by any surgical approach (Fig. 32–2A and B). This occurs particularly when edema is the main cause of the optic nerve fiber dysfunction.

Among 155 treated cases of pituitary tumors we found disturbances of the visual field in five patients, although the adenoma of the pituitary gland did not produce any compression of the optic nerve or the optic chiasm (Samii and Schürmann, 1976). In one patient, who showed the clinical picture of a bitemporal hemianopsia, there was a vascular compression of the optic chiasm caused by anomalies of both anterior cerebral arteries (Fig. 32–3).

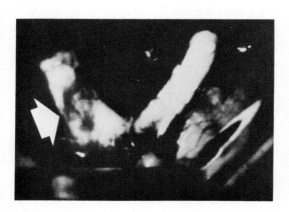

Figure 32–1 20-year-old patient. Amaurosis three hours after a head injury with fracture of the left optic canal. Decompression of the considerably swollen left optic nerve (arrow) in the optic nerve canal 3½ hours after the beginning of the amaurosis. Postoperatively, the patient had a satisfactory recovery.

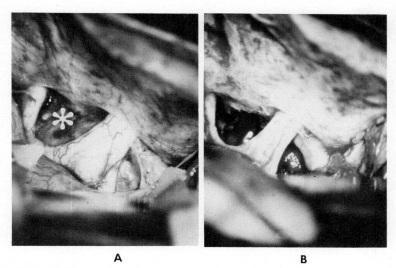

A   **B**

Figure 32–2 *A*, Compression of optic nerves and optic chiasm due to an intra- and suprasellar pituitary gland tumor (asterisk). *B*, Decompression of the optic nerves and the optic chiasm after removal of the pituitary gland tumor.

According to our cisternotomographic investigations, the position and course of the optic nerve in the craniocaudal direction showed considerable variations. These variations were revealed by study of 50 normal pneumoencephalotomograms. The optic chiasm is located close to the diaphragma sellae or up to 10 mm from it. Knowing the possible variations in the course of the optic nerves to the craniocaudal line, we have once again studied the pneumoencephalographic films of 19 patients with visual disturbances in which an intracranial space-occupying process could be excluded with certainty. In three patients with visual field defect (temporal or bitemporal upper quadrantanopia) we found a low projection of the optic chiasm in the cistern picture. A noticeable compression of the optic chiasm was caused by the dorsum sellae (Samii, 1972). However, these examinations were retrospective studies and therefore the patients could not be called upon for operative treatment. In these cases a partial

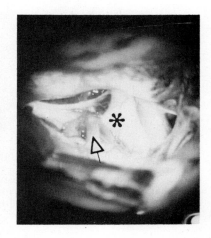

Figure 32–3 Vascular compression of the optic chiasm (asterisk) with the clinical picture of a bitemporal hemianopsia caused by an anomaly of both anterior cerebral arteries (arrow).

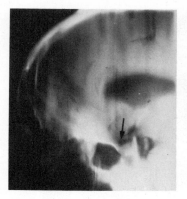

Figure 32–4 Midline pneumoencephalotomogram of a patient with bitemporal upper quadrantanopsia. The soft tissue shadows of the optic chiasm (arrow) are distinctly visible. The chiasm is located very low and is compressed by the dorsum sellae.

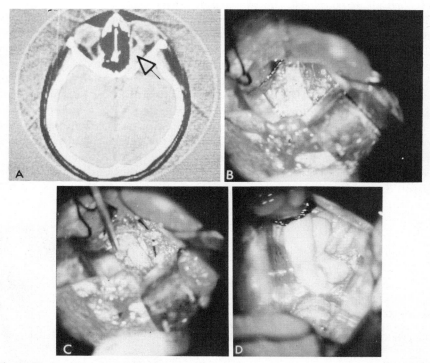

Figure 32–5 *A*, Computed tomogram of a retrobulbar optic nerve sheath meningioma. In contrast to a normal optic nerve on the left side, the nerve on the right side is encircled by the tumor (arrow). *B*, Transfrontal orbitotomy and exposure of the retrobulbar optic nerve sheath meningioma. *C*, After transfrontal orbitotomy and partial removal of the tumor, the optic nerve is partially exposed. *D*, Total removal of a retrobulbar optic nerve sheath meningioma. Exposure of the optic nerve from the optic canal up to the bulb.

resection of the dorsum sellae possibly would have also led to a functional improvement of the clinical syndrome (Fig. 32–4). Retrobulbar tumors in the region of the orbit, with increasing size, may cause a slow and progressive reduction of the visual power due to a compression of the optic nerve. This, especially, may occur if the optic sheath meningioma is compressing the nerve, because the tumor grows all around it and continually constricts the nerve (Fig. 32–5*A* and *B*). Using microsurgical technique after transfrontal orbitotomy for the removal of the tumor, it is possible to free the optic nerve without injuring the bulb or other intraorbital structures (Fig. 32–5*C* and *D*).

OCULOMOTOR, TROCHLEAR, AND ABDUCENT NERVES (THIRD, FOURTH, AND SIXTH CRANIAL NERVES)

Lesions of these nerves, as long as they are not nuclear in origin, often show complete regression following surgical intervention during the optimal time period. Supratentorial intracranial space-occupying processes of a different etiology lead to compression in the tentorial notch, the consequence of which is strain of the oculomotor nerves near the brain stem. An early elimination of the cause of the compression permits complete return of function. Direct compression of the oculomotor nerve in the tentorial notch may also occur due to a tumor or aneurysm (Figs. 32–6*A* and *B*).

The very close relation of the oculomotor nerves to the sinus cavernosus explains their involvement in traumatic processes (e.g. carotid cavernosus fistula), inflammatory thrombosis of sinus cavernosus, and parasellar tumors. Retrobulbar tumors with increasing volume may lead to a neurogenic oculomotor lesion. Although previous experiences regarding relieving and decompressive interventions on the oculomotor nerves were judged to be satisfactory, to our knowledge no one has succeeded to date in reconstruction (nerve grafting) after interruption of continuity. Yasargil has been the only one to date to observe functional recovery of a severed oculomotor nerve as a result of an end-to-end anastomosis. In the future there should be more thought given to the reconstruction of injured cranial nerves III, IV and VI.

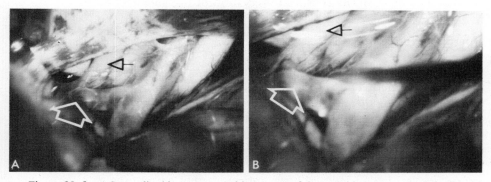

Figure 32–6   *A*, Supraclinoid aneurysm (white arrow) of the carotid artery on the left side with compression of the oculomotor nerve (black arrow). *B*, The aneurysm (white arrow) is kept away with an instrument from the oculomotor nerve (black arrow).

TRIGEMINAL NERVE (FIFTH CRANIAL NERVES)

There have been new indications for the surgical treatment of a traumatized trigeminal nerve (Samii, 1972). Severe facial injuries may be accompanied by lesions of different branches of the trigeminal nerve, most of all at the forehead in the area of the frontal branches or in fractures of the mandible where the inferior alveolar nerves are located. Fractures of the base of the skull or intracranial space occupying processes may lead to a lesion of the trigeminal nerve with partial or total loss of sensation on one part of the face and paralysis of the masticatory muscles.

Radical tumor extirpation of the lower jaw often requires the resection of the inferior alveolar nerve. The consequence is loss of sensation in the region of the mucosa, the lip, and the chin. Nowadays we are able to perform an exact restoration of the trigeminal nerve.

Transection of the *frontal nerve* caused by an incised wound produces a hypesthesia in the region of the forehead which is of relatively minor significance. A trigeminal neuralgia resistant to any therapy may also appear, owing to the formation of a neuroma, and is of greater clinical importance. The technique of neurolysis has only been successful in rare cases. Dissection of the trigeminal nerve in this region in order to re-establish the continuity of the nerve through an end-to-end suture or a nerve graft can be performed. As a result, not only is the pain relieved but also the restoration of sensation can be observed.

The loss of function of the *ophthalmic nerve* constitutes a special problem and can have serious consequences. Keratitis neuroparalytica can lead to ulcer of the cornea and even to blindness of the patient, a possible result of sensory and trophic disorder of the cornea.

Disorders of the ophthalmic nerve occur in connection with retroganglionic injury or after surgical treatment of a trigeminal neuralgia, which may result in a complete loss of sensation. In this case restoration of sensation in the cornea must be the surgical goal. A direct surgical approach to intracranial damage of the trigeminal nerve was until now technically impossible. The only possible method of reconstruction is an anastomosis between the ophthalmic nerve and a cutaneous nerve. The major occipital nerve seems to be most suitable, as it is of the same diameter as the ophthalmic nerve and participates, as does the major ophthalmic nerve, in the sensory innervation of the galea.

Operative Technique

After exposure of the major occipital nerve, an osteoplastic frontal craniotomy is performed. The anterior cranial fossa is epidurally exposed, the roof of the orbit is opened, and, through an incision of the periorbital capsule, the ophthalmic nerve is exposed and proximally transected. The peripheral stump of the ophthalmic nerve is then anastomosed with a sural nerve graft. The transplant is led out of the skull and anastomosed with the major occipital nerve in the subgaleal layer (Figs. 32–7A and B). Recovery of sensation in the region of the cornea has been observed after approximately six months.

Resection of the inferior alveolar nerve is often unavoidable during surgery of benign or malignant tumors of the mandible (Fig. 32–8).

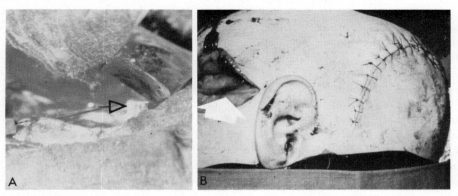

Figure 32–7 *A*, Transfrontal orbitotomy. Exposure of the ophthalmic nerve (arrow) in a patient with retroganglionic trigeminal lesion. Amaurosis caused by a keratitis. *B*, After anastomosis of a 17 cm long autologous nerve graft between the ophthalmic nerve and the major occipital nerve. The right-sided frontal craniotomy is closed again. The nerve graft is still visible behind the ear (arrow).

Anesthesia of the affected side of the lower lip is often a serious problem for the patient because of the uncontrolled drooling and the difficulty in drinking. Ulceration of the lower lip may appear when the anesthetic lip is traumatized between the teeth while chewing. Although for some patients this may not be irritating, others seem to suffer tremendously from this loss of sensation. For this reason all attempts should be made to preserve this nerve, at least in cases of benign tumors of the lower jaw (Becker, 1967, 1970, 1972). This, however, is only possible in cases in which the nerve lies apart from the tumor.

The inferior alveolar nerve is endangered in a group of lower jaw fractures, when the fracture lines cross the nerve canal. Because of its elasticity the nerve may in many cases not be totally affected. The damage may be restricted to

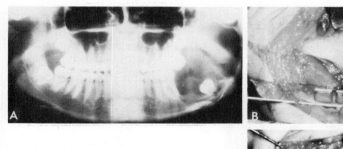

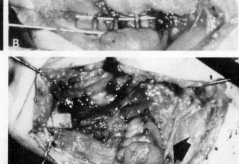

Figure 32–8 *A*, X-ray of the lower jaw of a cystic adamantinoma on the left side. *B*, Exposure of the left lower jaw tumor (asterisk). *C*, Total removal of the lower jaw along with the inferior alveolar nerve. Bridging of the defect by means of a 12 cm long autogenous nerve graft (arrows). Six months postoperatively complete return of sensation in the region of the lower lip, the mucosa and the chin.

tension, contusion, or an edematous compression with temporary loss of sensibility. If there is a compound comminuted fracture or fracture defect, a loss of continuity of the nerve and a total sensory deficit is the rule (Greve, 1927; Hermann, 1958; Simpson, 1958).

For the reconstruction of the inferior alveolar nerve after resection of the lower jaw, it is advisable (Samii, 1972; Hausamen, Samii, and Schmidseder, 1973) to mark and cut the proximal and distal nerve stumps at the mandibular and mental foramina. Thereafter, the tumor resection and the osteoplastic reconstruction may be performed. To restore the continuity of the inferior alveolar nerve, a neural graft is necessary. The sural nerve is the most suitable for bridging the defect. The transplant should be 12 to 15 cm long. The transplant needs to re-establish its connection with the blood circulation. Initially, it remains dependent upon its surroundings via diffusion for nutrition. For this reason we do not place the nerve graft in the avascular bony transplant but at a distance to it.

LINGUAL NERVE (A MAJOR BRANCH OF THE TRIGEMINAL NERVE)

The course of the peripheral part of the lingual nerve in the floor of the mouth is of special interest. After leaving the pterygomandibular space, the lingual nerve establishes very close contact with the mandible at the level of the third molar. Its branches are to be found under the mucosa before they enter the tongue. The nerve supplies the sensory innervation of the anterior two thirds of the tongue and the floor of the mouth, as well as the lingual side of the mandibular gingiva. In addition, it sends out the afferent and efferent parasympathetic fibers for the submandibular and sublingual glands.

The lingual nerve can be traumatized by careless extraction of the lower third molar, by improper intraoral incision of a sublingual abscess, and by injuries with drills during preparation of cavities of the lower molars. Furthermore, the lingual nerve has to be sacrificed in cases of tumors of the floor of the mouth which have invaded the nerve (Fig. 32–9). The sensory disorder of the tongue can lead to repeated bite injuries. In some cases taste may be impaired.

Reconstruction of the lingual nerve may be successful if performed near its

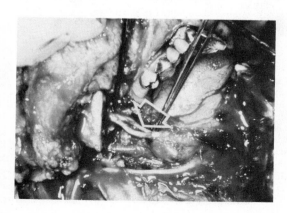

Figure 32–9 Reconstruction of the lingual nerve with two nerve grafts (arrow) after total removal of a large tumor of the floor of the mouth and the mandible.

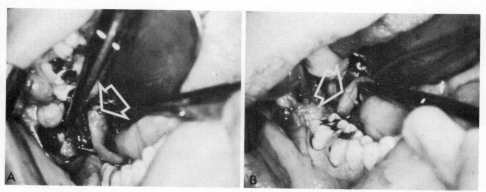

Figure 32–10   *A*, Lesion of the lingual nerve (arrow) after extraction of the right wisdom tooth. *B*, The lingual nerve has been reconstructed by means of a nerve graft (arrow).

trunk and proximal to its divisions in the floor of the mouth. If an extraoral approach is used to resect the mandible, identification of the proximal and peripheral stumps and performance of nerve grafting do not present any special problem.

The intraoral approach to the nerve stumps of the pterygomandibular space and in the floor of the mouth is also not particularly difficult (Fig. 32–10*A* and *B*).

In contrast, the nerve grafting is technically difficult, especially in patients with full dentition because of the very narrow surgical field. Because of the superficial course of the lingual nerve, the transplant has to be bedded directly underneath the mucosa and an exact wound closure is all-important.

FACIAL NERVE (SEVENTH CRANIAL NERVE)

In comparison with other cranial nerves, the facial nerve is the one most frequently afflicted by different types of lesions such as tumors, trauma, and different processes in the area of the skull base and the face. The resulting paralysis of the muscles of the face results in a tragic situation for the patient.

Facial nerve paresis caused by tumors develops slowly. They are either tumors of the cells of the neurilemma or tumors in the environment that lead to compression of the nerve, as is the case with cerebellopontine angle tumors, those found in the region of the petrous bone (e.g., epidermoid, cholesteatoma, chordoma, carcinoma), and those of the parotid. Some malignant tumors can infiltrate the facial nerve.

Facial nerve paresis can also be due to viral or bacterial infection. In particular, it can occur in meningitis and in acute or chronic middle ear infection.

Facial nerve paresis of traumatic origin is caused mostly by laterobasal fractures of the skull or severe facial injuries.

The etiology of Bell's palsy is not well understood. According to Hilger (1949) and other authors, it may be due to a spasm of the facial branch of the external carotid artery. The arterial spasm is followed by disturbances at the capillary level with ischemia and edema of the nerve. The edema itself causes a compression of the nerve, and this leads to an obstruction of the lymphatic and venous circulation, which again increases the edema. With that a vicious circle is completed (Jongkees, 1958, 1961).

According to recent studies a vascular dysfunction does not appear to be the definitive cause. More favored is the hypothesis of an acute benign cranial neuritis caused by a neurotropic herpes simplex virus (Adour, 1977).

Since Jannetta (1977) was able to achieve good results in cases of Bell's palsy after exposure of the cerebellopontine angle and getting the nerve free from compression of a vascular loop, he holds the opinion that a sudden pathological change of the position of an artery loop within the cerebellopontine angle brings about a stretching of the nerve with resulting paresis.

Hemifacial spasm represents another still unsolved problem. Opinions differ with regard to the etiology. Miehlke (1973) argues that the true cause of the idiopathic facial spasm can not yet be explained satisfactorily. In his opinion, the therapy has to be symptomatic as long as the cause is unknown. According to Gardner and Sava (1962), Jannetta (1970, 1975), and Bertrand and co-workers (1977) the facial spasm is to be attributed to a vascular loop compressing the intracranial segment of the facial nerve at the brain stem. In other cases, however, a tumor may be the cause of the facial spasm. During regeneration of a damaged facial nerve a spasm is possible due to scar strangulation of the nerve fibers. This type of facial spasm may occur after nerve suture, nerve grafting, or blunt trauma, or during regeneration with incomplete recovery.

Surgical Treatment of the Facial Nerve

The present standard of surgical treatment of the facial nerve would not be conceivable without the pioneer work of Bunnel (1927), Martin (1931, 1936), Ballance (1932), Duel (1934), Cawthorne (1951, 1963, 1965), Maxwell (1951, 1954), Kettel (1957, 1959), Lathrop (1953, 1956, 1962), Conley (1955, 1961), Clerc and Batisse (1954), Dott (1958), Jongkees (1958, 1961), Wullstein (1958), Miehlke (1960, 1961), House (1961, 1963), and Fisch (1969, 1970) among others. In consideration of the anatomical course of the facial nerve one can distinguish among three different regions for surgical treatment:
1. The intracranial region.
    a. Surgical treatment of hemifacial spasm in the cerebellopontine angle.
    b. Preservation or reconstruction of the facial nerve in the cerebellopontine angle.
2. The intratemporal region.
3. The extratemporal region.
In addition, the surgical treatment of Bell's palsy will be discussed.

Surgical Treatment of the Facial Nerve in the Intracranial Region

Surgical Treatment of Hemifacial Spasm in the Cerebellopontine Angle

Previous surgical methods for the correction of hemifacial spasm consisted of traumatizing the facial nerve at different levels. All these methods failed to produce satisfactory results. In eight patients treated by resection of the peripheral branches of the facial nerve, permanent healing was not achieved; although none of the patients showed immediate postoperative signs of a recurrent facial spasm, this occurred few months later. The longest symptom-free interval was 18 months.

Vascular compression of the facial nerve in the cerebellopontine angle as a possible etiology of the facial spasm was mentioned in 1947 by Campbell and Keedy and in 1962 by Gardner. In 1970, Jannetta reported on the microsurgical vascular decompression of facial spasm in the cerebellopontine angle. His long-term results in 47 patients operated on between 1966 and 1974 were published in 1977. The result was excellent in 38 cases, good in two, fair in three, and poor but improved in two (Cases 3 and 16 — persistent clinical spasm). Of great importance is the fact that the motor disorders in the region of the facial muscles preoperatively ascertained by electromyography were postoperatively reversible in many cases.

The operative technique consists of suboccipital craniotomy and exposure of the cerebellopontine angle. After incision of the dura, the cerebellum is elevated, with the help of a retractor blade, and the facial nerve is exposed at the internal auditory meatus. Dissection of the facial nerve has to be carried out up to the brain stem. Attention must be paid to the fact that after craniomedial elevation of the cerebellar hemisphere the chorioid plexus of the lateral recess of the fourth ventricle and the flocculus of the cerebellum are to be held cautiously away with a retractor blade to expose the central part of the facial nerve. It is essential to expose the exit area of the nerve at the brain stem where the vascular decompression has to be carried out. All vessels in the region of the cerebellopontine angle — the vertebral, basilar, inferior posterior cerebellar, inferior anterior cerebellar, and cochlear arteries — may cause the vascular compression. Vascular compression may also be due to dilated veins or arteriovenous angiomas. Other etiologic factors of facial spasm are small neurinomas or cholesteatomas. Decompression of the facial nerve is performed by changing the axis of the arterial loop and its relationship with the nerve root exit zone at the brain stem. The new position is maintained by placing a segment of muscle between the proximal and distal limbs of the vascular loop and the brain stem. The position of the muscle segment must not be changed by later rotations of the head. In order to ensure its firm position between the brain stem and the vascular loop, the head is turned intraoperatively in different directions. Jannetta's technique seems to be the operative treatment of choice for facial spasm, although the risk of inducing deafness has to be discussed with the patient. An essential prerequisite for the performance of such a surgical intervention is the mastery of the microsurgical technique.

Preservation and Reconstruction of the Facial Nerve in the Cerebellopontine Angle

The portion of the facial nerve in the cerebellopontine angle, with a length of 23 to 24 mm, is endangered by space-occupying processes. About 71 per cent of all tumors of the cerebellopontine angle are acoustic neurinomas. Meningiomas, epidermoids, and, occasionally, metastases occur. During the growth of a cerebellopontine angle tumor the function of the facial nerve remains intact for a long time. Primary intrameatal tumors with extension into the cerebello-pontine angle cause early paralysis, especially when arising from the facial nerve itself. In the cerebellopontine angle, the position and course of the facial nerve may be displaced in different directions by space-occupying processes. Identification of the facial nerve may prove extremely difficult during tumor surgery. Accurate exposure and preservation of the continuity of the facial nerve through microsurgical technique during the removal of cerebellopontine angle tumors should be part of the modern surgical concept.

The *neurosurgical suboccipital approach* of the cerebellopontine angle permits either dorsolateral or dorsocaudal exposure of the tumor. After retracting the cerebellum craniomedially, the caudal cranial nerves, often slightly compressed by the tumor, must be identified and freed from the tumor capsule. An immediate identification of the facial nerve in the cerebellopontine angle will be possible only in those cases in which the tumor is relatively small and, especially, when the tumor compresses the nerve in a more dorsal direction (Fig. 32–11).

The facial nerve is not visible at the brain stem or in the internal auditory meatus when the tumor is large (Fig. 32–12*A*). Starting from a 5 to 10 mm opening of the tumor capsule, the reduction of the tumor is performed under the operating microscope. Thus the tumor capsule loses its primary tension (Fig.

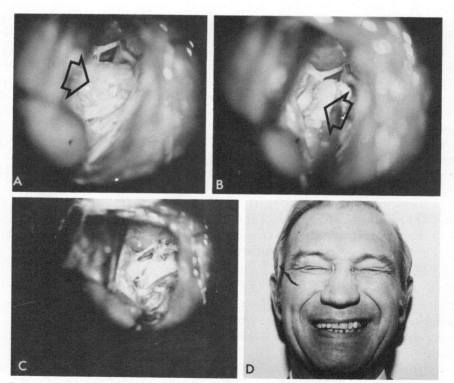

Figure 32–11   *A*, Small neuroma (arrow) of the cerebellopontine angle on the right side. The facial nerve is already visible when the tumor is exposed. *B*, The tumor (arrow) from the brain stem. *C*, Total removal of the neuroma of the cerebellopontine angle after opening the internal meatus. The facial nerve is preserved. *D*, Three months postoperatively.

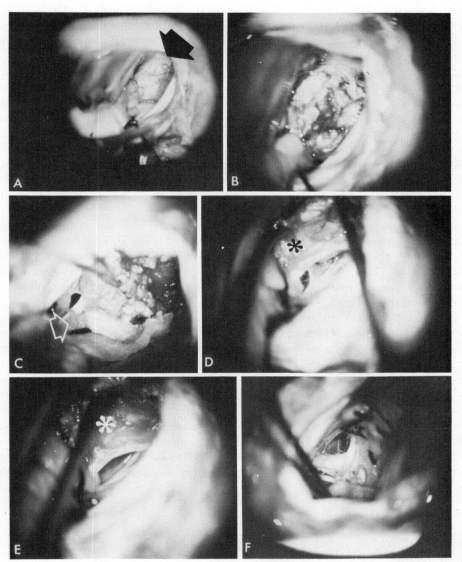

Figure 32–12   *A*, Large acoustic neuroma (arrow) of the right cerebellopontine angle. *B*, Opening of the tumor capsule and partial resection of the tumor. *C*, The facial nerve (arrow) is exposed at the brain stem. The nerve is extensively adherent to the capsule of the tumor. *D*, By gradual further reduction of the tumor (asterisk), the facial nerve is partially exposed in the direction of the internal auditory meatus. *E*, Extensive removal of the tumor. The facial nerve is rolled out to a broad surface caudally. The rest of the tumor (asterisk) is lifted up with a spatula. *F*, The facial nerve is exposed. The forceps is lifting the remaining portion of the tumor. The facial and acoustic nerves are seen in continuity.

32–12*B*). By gradual resection of the tumor capsule, the facial nerve can be identified at the brain stem (Fig. 32–12*C*).

Any direct manipulation of the facial nerve in the cerebellopontine angle will most probably lead to postoperative loss of function, although the continuity of the nerve may be preserved. The facial nerve, therefore, must be pursued from the brain stem to the internal auditory meatus under highest magnification and with extreme patience and caution (Fig. 32–12*D*).

The nerve may not be detached from the tumor capsule, but the tumor capsule itself must be dissected carefully, using microsurgical instruments, from the nerve. Stretching of the nerve, with its adhesion to the tumor capsule, must be strictly avoided. The tumor capsule may be slightly stretched with one hand while with a microsurgical scissor in the other hand the membrane between the tumor capsule and the nerve is precisely transected. Not infrequently the nerve, owing to an expansion compression, is rolled out around the tumor capsule in a thin, broad surface of approximately 2 to 3 cm (Fig. 32–12*E*). The preservation of the facial nerve in such a case is quite difficult; however, it is technically possible (Fig. 32–12*F*).

Most frequently the facial nerve is injured at the internal auditory meatus, when the tumor grows in a cone shape into the internal auditory meatus. Removal of the tumor from this region, likewise, must be performed under direct vision. The internal auditory meatus is exposed by cutting away the posterior lip of the internal auditory meatus with the help of refined punches or a diamond drill (Fig. 32–13).

The facial nerve may remain preserved in its continuity in two thirds of all cerebellopontine angle tumors by using the microsurgical technique and observing the mentioned principles (Drake, 1973; Koos and co-workers, 1973; Yasargil, 1973; Hitselberger and House, 1973). If the facial nerve is injured in one area, the surgeon should not discontinue the preparation of the nerve. Because of the tumor growth in the region of the cerebellopontine angle, the nerve apparently stretches in length, so that in the event of interruption of continuity and loss of substance of about 1 to 1.5 cm during tumor extirpation, one is still able to perform an end-to-end suture without any tension. Because the results of suture of the facial nerve in the cerebellopontine angle are satisfactory and are superior to any other intervention, the effort toward reconstruction of the

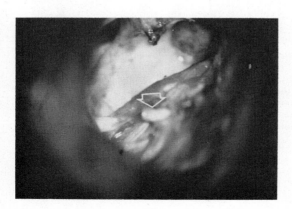

Figure 32–13 Exposure of the facial nerve (arrow) in the internal auditory meatus by the suboccipital approach and removal of the posterior lip of the internal auditory meatus after total extirpation of an acoustic neuroma.

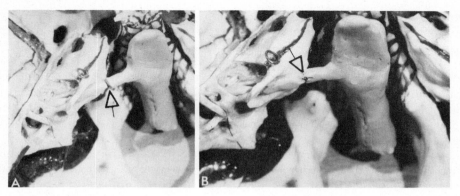

Figure 32–14 *A*, Model of the facial nerve in the cerebellopontine angle after interruption of continuity (arrow). *B*, After end-to-end suture (arrow).

continuity of the facial nerve through nerve suture at the cerebellopontine angle is a rewarding task (Figs. 32–14 and 32–15).

Identification of the distal nerve stump is hardly possible when there is a large defect, and in particular when the tumor extends into the internal auditory meatus. Even electrostimulation cannot help to distinguish the distal stump of the facial nerve from the cochlear nerve. Stimulation of each distal stump of the facial nerve causes a contraction of the face muscles. Dott (1958), therefore, recommended a connection between the central stump of the interrupted facial nerve in the cerebellopontine angle and the extracranial part of the facial nerve in front of the stylomastoid foramen. The method of Dott is as follows.

After removing the acoustic neurinoma, the facial nerve is prepared directly at the brain stem and a 15 to 20 mm sural nerve is obtained to use as a graft. Subsequent to the anastomosis at the brain stem, the nerve graft is led out of the skull through craniotomy. The graft is then passed through a tunnel below the mastoid between the sternocleidomastoid and the splenius capitis muscles. The second end of the graft is marked with a silver clip and is fixed in the retroman-

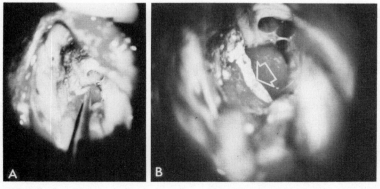

Figure 32–15 *A*, After removal of a very large left-sided acoustic neuroma with interruption of continuity of the facial nerve (forceps). *B*, End-to-end suture of the facial nerve in the cerebellopontine angle (arrow).

dibular fossa. In a second stage, three months later, the distal end is searched for and anastomosed with the peripheral end of the facial nerve in front of the stylomastoid foramen.

In 1958, Dott reported on four cases. He had achieved satisfactory results in two cases and in two others the results were excellent. After performing the operation on five patients, Drake (1960) was able to achieve good findings in four. In 1962, Loew published one case he had operated on with Miehlke, the result of which was good. In 1967, Miehlke and Bushe also achieved a good result with this technique.

It seems somewhat surprising after Dott's publication in 1958, that despite the good results achieved with this method for the last 20 years, to the best of our knowledge, only seven cases have been reported. This is probably due to the fact that the exposure of the facial nerve at the brain stem without the use of an operating microscope and microsurgical technique is too difficult. Now that microsurgical operations have become somewhat routine, one can expect that in the future the surgical treatment of cerebellopontine angle lesions should include reconstruction of the facial nerve. Since the introduction of the operating microscope, we have tried to reconstruct the facial nerve in those cases in which the nerve could not be preserved and an end-to-end anastomosis was not practicable. Instead of Dott's surgical method, a new technique could be developed in cooperation with E.N.T. surgeons (I herewith extend sincerest thanks to Professor Wigand, E.N.T. Department University Erlangen and Professor Draf, E.N.T. Department University Mainz).

If the facial nerve cannot be preserved during extirpation of the tumor, we strive to prepare the nerve at the brain stem in the region of the sulcus pontobulbaris (Fig. 32–17*A*). According to our experiences it is possible to gain a stump of the facial nerve of at least 1 to 1.5 cm length in spite of large tumors (Figs. 32–16 and 32–17*B* and *C*). Subsequently an autologous nerve graft about 5 cm in length is to be taken from the sural nerve and anastomosed with the central stump of the facial nerve at the brain stem (Fig. 32–17*D*). We place the second end of the graft into or dorsal from the internal auditory meatus. The facial nerve is exposed in its mastoidal and tympanal course through a mastoid approach. Afterward the internal auditory canal is opened by the trans-

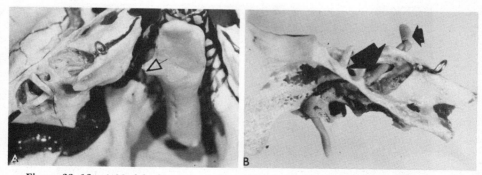

Figure 32–16   *A*, Model of a nerve defect of the facial nerve (arrow) in the cerebellopontine angle and internal auditory canal. *B*, Model of a reconstructed nerve in the cerebellopontine angle and internal auditory canal by means of nerve grafting (large arrow) between the central stump (small arrow) at the brain stem and the distal stump of the mastoidal course.

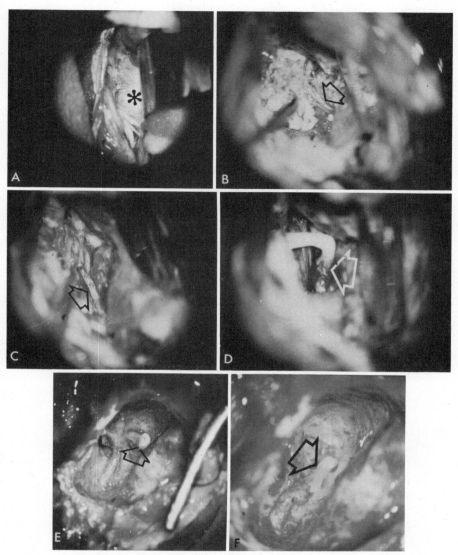

Figure 32-17 *A*, Suboccipital exposure of a left-sided acoustic neuroma (asterisk). The caudal cranial nerves are visible in the region of the lower tumor pole. *B*, After partial resection of the tumor. Exposure of the facial nerve at the brain stem (arrow). *C*, Total removal of the large tumor along with a part of the facial nerve. Exposure of the central stump of the facial nerve at the brain stem (arrow). *D*, Anastomosis between the central nerve stump of the facial nerve at the brain stem with a sural nerve graft (arrow). *E*, Mastoidectomy and translabyrinthine exposure of the internal auditory canal. Exposure of the facial nerve in the mastoidal and tympanal course. The rolled up second end of the nerve graft in the internal auditory canal is visible (arrow). *F*, The facial nerve is transected below the geniculate ganglion. The distal stump is mobilized dorsally and anastomosed with the nerve graft (arrow).

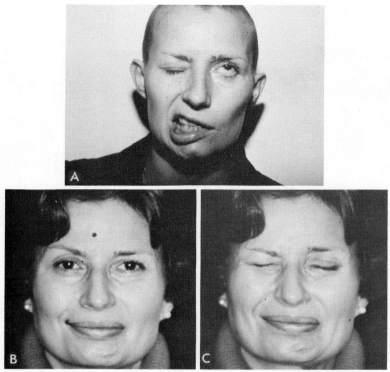

Figure 32–18   *A,* Ten days after removal of a large acoustic neuroma on the left side with reconstruction of the facial nerve by means of a 5 cm long graft between the proximal stump at the brain stem and the mastoidal segment in the petrous bone. Total paralysis of facial nerve on the left side. *B* and *C,* Functional return 13 months after nerve grafting between the intracranial and intratemporal part of the facial nerve.

labyrinthine approach at exactly the place where the graft is located (Fig. 32–17*E*). After transection of the facial nerve distal to the geniculate ganglion, the nerve stump is mobilized dorsally and anastomosed with the distal end of the graft. In this manner an intracranial–intratemporal anastomosis of the facial nerve is performed with a graft 5 cm in length (Fig. 32–17*F*). The satisfactory results in four patients operated on justify the future application of this technique (Fig. 32–18). The one and a half hours necessary for the operation means no additional strain for the patient.

The Surgical Treatment of the Facial Nerve in the Intratemporal Region

The facial nerve can be injured in the region of the petrous bone by a longitudinal or transverse fracture of the skull base, by a tumor, or the cause can be iatrogenic. In patients with craniocerebral injuries who exhibit paralysis of the facial nerve, one should ensure a possible fracture in the region of the petrous bone by use of special x-ray techniques including tomography (Figs. 32–19 and 32–20).

Sometimes it is difficult to identify a fracture line radiologically. According

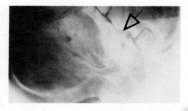

Figure 32–19 Combined longitudinal and transverse fracture (arrow) of the petrous bone.

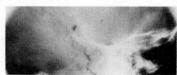

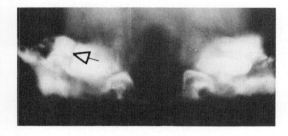

Figure 32–20 Medial pyramidal transverse fracture (arrow) on the right side reaching into the fundus of the internal auditory meatus and the vestibulum. Lateral to the fracture fissure one can recognize the upper and lateral semicircular canal.

to Fisch laterobasal fractures of the skull damage the facial nerve in the meatal–labyrinthine area. One third of the patients with early paralysis of the facial nerve after pyramidal longitudinal fractures showed a complete loss of continuity in the proximal intratemporal course of the facial nerve. Paralysis of the facial nerve due to pyramidal *longitudinal* fractures may be caused by a compression of a bony fragment or by an interruption in continuity of the nerve. In 50 per cent

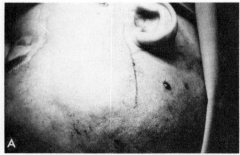

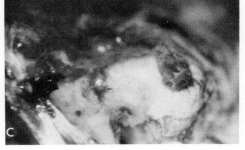

Figure 32–21 *A*, Skin incision line to the transtemporal and extradural approach to the middle fossa for the exposure of the facial nerve in the meatal and labyrinthine region. *B*, Temporal craniotomy and exposure of the dura (arrow) in the region of the middle fossa. *C*, Transtemporal decompression of the facial nerve proximal to the geniculate ganglion in a case of laterobasal skull fracture.

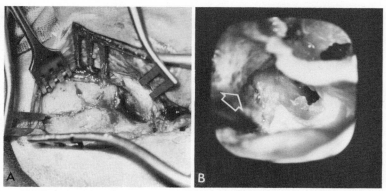

Figure 32–22   *A*, Operating feature: fracture of the mastoid and temporal bone. *B*, Operating feature: transmastoidal exposure of the facial nerve. The fracture line (arrow) is vertically crossing the facial canal at the level of the lateral semicircular canal.

of the cases a stretching of the geniculate ganglion with peri- or intraneural hemorrhage may be the cause (Fisch, 1972). Pyramidal *transverse* fractures, occurring with much less frequency (in 30 to 50 per cent of all cases), lead to early paralysis of the facial nerve. One differentiates between external transverse fractures, located distal to the internal auditory canal, and internal transverse fractures, situated proximal of the fundus meatus.

The surgical approach to the various segments of the intratemporal course of the facial nerve can differ. In the meatal and labyrinthine region, the facial nerve is reached on the transtemporal extradural approach to the middle fossa (House, 1961; Fisch, 1970). The exposure extends from the porus acusticus

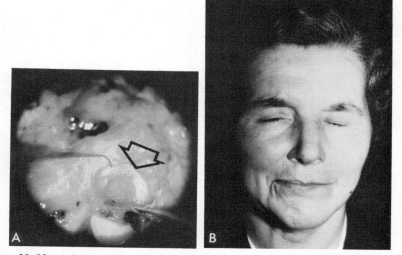

Figure 32–23   *A*, Interposition of a 2.5 cm graft (arrow) in the region of the mastoidal and tympanal segments of the facial nerve. *B*, Functional return 1½ years after the operation.

internus up to the tendon of the tensor tympani muscle without opening the internal ear space (Fig. 32–21).

The transtemporal approach renders preservation of the ear function possible. In case of deafness, the transmastoidal–translabyrinthine approach is chosen (Fig. 32–22).

If the mastoidal segment is injured, the facial nerve must be exposed by means of mastoidectomy up to the stylomastoid foramen. The nerve may be followed up to the lateral semicircular canal. In cases where the lesion is located in the tympanal segment, the preparation of the mastoidal segment can be continued in a central direction up to the geniculate ganglion without impairment of auditory function (Fig. 32–23A and B).

The Extratemporal Region

The facial nerve in the extratemporal region originates in the stylomastoid foramen and arborizes at the level of the parotid gland. After their exit from the gland the branches reach the particular face muscles.

Deep incision wounds in the face, extracranial tumors of the base of the skull in the area of the stylomastoid foramen, and tumors of the parotid gland may cause extratemporal lesions. Tumors originating in the facial nerve itself can produce an extratemporal lesion. If lacerations involve the main stem of the facial nerve directly in front of the stylomastoid foramen, complete facial paralysis will be found. An isolated transection of a peripheral branch in the region of the parotid gland must not always lead to a visible loss of function because the neighboring branches are in a position to take over the innervation of the transected branch. Should the location of the injury be more peripheral, directly at the entrance of the final spread of the particular branches into the muscle system, it may lead to an isolated, regionally limited paralysis.

For surgical treatment of lacerations in front of the stylomastoid foramen, one must begin with exposure of the central stump at the foramen. If it is impossible to obtain the distal stump outside the parotid gland, one is forced to split the gland in order to expose the peripheral stumps. One has the opportunity to perform a direct anastomosis to bridge the nerve defect. The preparation of the distal stumps in the parotid gland may be simplified by starting with the exposure of the zygomatic branch, which is located below the zygomatic bone. From there, the zygomatic nerve trunk can be followed through the parotid gland up to the injured area. Thereafter, if necessary, all other branches of the facial nerve can easily be prepared (Fig. 32–24).

Surgical treatment of transected facial nerve branches in a more peripheral region is possible, provided the surgeon can locate the distal stumps. In smooth injuries there is no difficulty in performing an end-to-end anastomosis without tension (Fig. 32–25). It is recommended that the surgeon perform the wound care, together with a nerve anastomosis or nerve grafting, if the wound is clean and the surgeon is experienced in microsurgical technique.

Very careful attention should be paid to the facial nerve during tumor surgery near the base of the skull. All surgical interventions, such as for the removal of a tumor, should concentrate on the preservation or reconstruction of

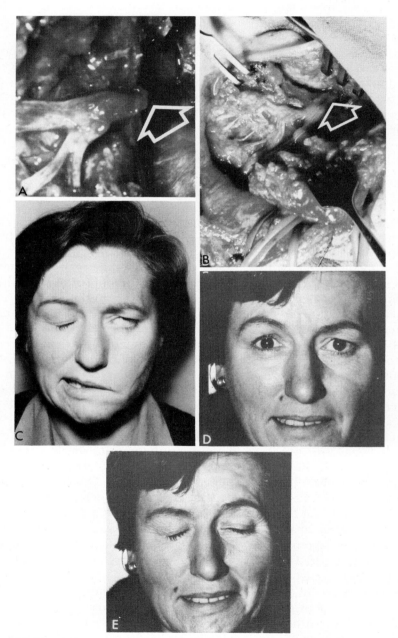

Figure 32–24   *A*, Exposure of the central and peripheral stump of the facial nerve in front of the stylomastoid foramen after a glass cut injury (arrow). *B*, The parotid gland is opened and the nerve defect is bridged by means of two nerve grafts (arrow). *C*, Complete facial palsy on the left side. *D* and *E*, Functional return after 18 months.

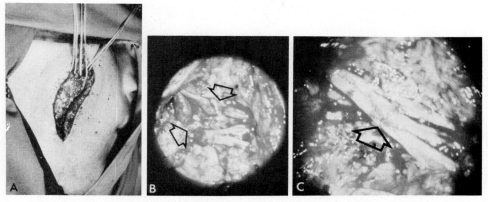

Figure 32–25   *A,* Clean-cut injury of the facial nerve in the region of the zygomatic branch and the buccal branch in the right part of the face. *B,* After microsurgical exposure of the interrupted branches of the facial nerve (between arrows). *C,* End-to-end suture without tension (arrow).

the facial nerve as part of the surgical concept. In our experience with tumor surgery of the facial nerve in its extratemporal course, we have learned that one should not sacrifice this nerve without reconstructing it at the same time. In the surgical removal of *benign tumors* the facial nerve should be preserved.

If the nerve is traumatized to a large extent without interruption of continuity, the development of scar tissues may compress the nerve and lead to persistent paralysis. In such cases, we can achieve good results with microsurgical neurolysis, even after a prolonged period of time (Fig. 32–26*A* and *B*).

Malignant parotid tumors require their total removal along with removal of the facial nerve in order to reduce the possibility of recurrence. The nerve defect should be bridged in one stage by means of a nerve graft (Fig. 32–27). *Secondary repair* of the facial nerve after parotidectomy and removal of the facial nerve followed by radiotherapy may be difficult because massive scar tissues may make

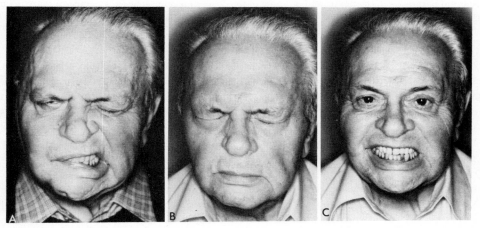

Figure 32–26   *A,* Complete peripheral facial palsy on the right side after surgery of a parotid tumor. *B* and *C,* Functional restoration six months following microsurgical neurolysis.

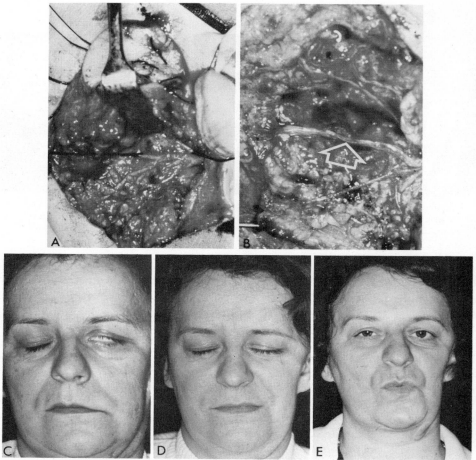

Figure 32–27 *A,* Mucoepidermoid tumor of the left parotid gland. The main stem and the individual peripheral branches of the facial nerve are exposed and marked with threads. The tumor can be removed along with the facial nerve. *B,* Total extirpation of the tumor along with the intraparotid part of the facial nerve, and bridging of the nerve defect by means of a nerve graft (arrow) at the same time. *C,* Postoperative facial palsy on the left side. *D* and *E,* Functional result 18 months after nerve grafting.

identification of the nerve trunk difficult. In a situation like this, one should try to expose the nerve outside the scar tissue field. In most cases the proximal stump in front of the stylomastoid foramen may also be damaged to such an extent as to render it impossible to gain an intact stump. Circumstances such as this make it necessary to expose the facial nerve in the bony course of the mastoid segment. After preparation of the peripheral branches in the healthy part, interposition of nerve grafts between the mastoid segment and the peripheral branches of the facial nerve is performed (Fig. 32–28*A* and *B*). Reconstruction of the facial nerve represents a special problem when the nerve is affected by neurofibromatosis. There is a difficulty that even under the microscope the local limits of the tumor extension cannot be estimated with certainty. Recurrence in many cases is most likely to occur. In one case, we were able to reconstruct the facial nerve after radical extirpation of various neurofibromas of the peripheral

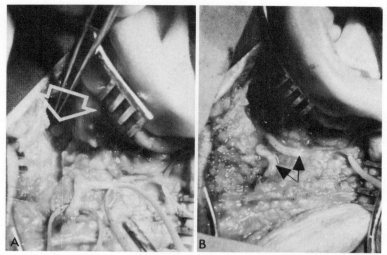

Figure 32–28 *A*, Exposure of the facial nerve in a patient following parotidectomy and radio-therapy. The central stump of the facial nerve (arrow) is exposed in its mastoidal course after opening the mastoid. The peripheral branches of the facial nerve are also exposed (tapes). *B*, After bridging the nerve defect by means of two nerve grafts (arrows).

branches of the nerve by means of several nerve grafts. However, postopera-tively we diagnosed tumor recurrence in spite of satisfactory reinnervation (Fig. 32–29*A* and *B*).

Another important aspect is the time interval between trauma and surgical treatment, which has a certain influence on functional success. According to our laboratory and clinical experience, we know that in some cases after cutting the

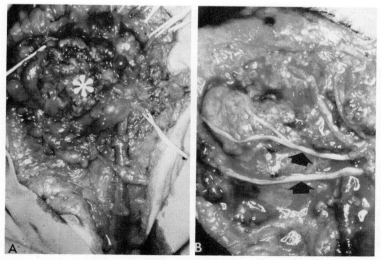

Figure 32–29 *A*, Neurofibromatosis (asterisk) in the region of the facial nerve in the left side of the face. Exposure of the central stump and the individual intact peripheral branches of the facial nerve (tapes) are seen. *B*, After total removal of the neurofibromatosis of the facial nerve with sub-sequent nerve grafting (arrows).

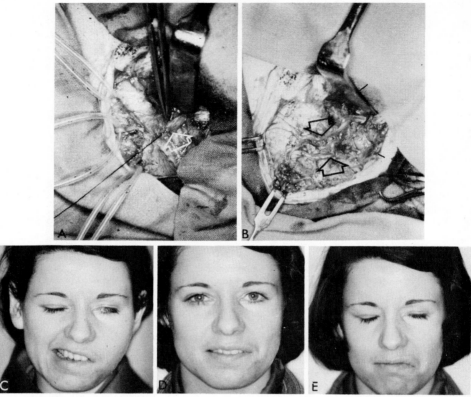

Figure 32–30   *A,* Exposure of both the central stump (arrow) and distal stumps (tapes) of the facial nerve 20 years after surgery of a hemangioma on the left side of the face. *B,* After nerve grafting (arrows). *C,* Facial palsy on the left side 20 years after surgery for a hemangioma. *D* and *E,* Functional result three years after the nerve-grafting operation.

facial nerve on one side of the face the precondition for partial innervation of the paralyzed muscles may be present because of collateral innervation (Fujita, 1934; Passerini and co-workers, 1968; Hiroko Nishimura and co-workers, 1977). This mixed innervation of the opposite facial muscles across the midline of the face may exist or be developed after transection of the nerve, owing to the sprouting of new nerve fibers from the intact side to the paralyzed muscles. Such a phenomenon must be demonstrated by electromyography, since clinical examinations still reveal a complete facial paralysis in spite of this collateral innervation. In these patients, with a paralysis lasting over many years, muscle fibers can keep on existing, so that a reconstruction of the damaged nerve can be successful. An example is the case of a 20-year-old female student who had from the fifth month of her life a complete facial paralysis on the left side. At that time she underwent an hemangioma operation, during which the facial nerve was severed. Because of the positive electromyographic findings, although there was complete clinical paralysis, we decided to reconstruct, aiming at restoring motor function to the face. During surgery we found an interruption of the facial nerve. After resecting the neuroma of the central stump and a fibrosis of the peripheral branches, we found the nerve defect to be 5 cm long; we were able to bridge this by means of an autologous nerve graft. Within 17 months reinnervation was satisfactory (Fig. 32–30). Another method for treating facial nerve lesions is to anastomose between the facial nerve and another motor nerve, thus reinnervating the paralyzed muscles. This technique is used in all cases in which direct surgical treatment of the nerve is impossible. Although the glosso-pharyngeal nerve (Ballance, 1924; Watson and Williams, 1927) and the phrenic nerve (Hardy and co-workers, 1957) are used as donors, anastomoses between the facial and hypoglossal nerve (Körte, 1903; Ballance, 1909; Bevers, 1913; Kautzky, 1956; Metelka, 1966; and others), as well as the accessory nerve, are more frequently used.

Faciofacial Anastomosis

A further development of anastomosis of the facial nerve to other cranial nerves is the faciofacial anastomosis, also known as "crossover cross face anastomosis." The advantage of this technique is that reinnervation of the paralyzed muscles can be partially achieved without sacrificing another cranial nerve and without loss of function. This technique was reported for the first time by Smith in 1971, and in the same year by Scaramella. The method was improved by Anderl (1972) and Samii (1973). The technical principle of the faciofacial anastomosis is based on the anatomical fact that the branches of the facial nerve within the face region build a kind of plexus — the pes anserinus — and that parts of these branches may be cut without risk of visible functional deficit. The central stumps of the transected branches in the healthy side of the face are anastomosed with nerve grafts crossing the face subcutaneously in the upper lip region to the damaged side. Here, they have to be sutured with the analogous branches (Fig. 32–31A and B).

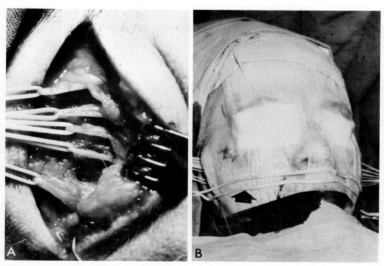

Figure 32–31 A, Exposure of the peripheral branches of the facial nerve (tapes) in the face as for a facio-facial anastomosis. B, Exposure of the peripheral branches of the facial nerve on both the intact and the damaged sides. Two grafts of sural nerve, which will be passed subcutaneously and anastomosed with both sides, are seen placed over the upper lip (arrow).

Our experience has proved the sural nerve to be the most appropriate for transplantation. However, it must be taken into consideration that the course of the peripheral branches of the facial nerve is different in each individual. Fujita (1934) found irregularities in this pattern even when comparing the two sides of the face in one person. McCormack and co-workers (1945) established eight different types of facial nerve branch distribution in the face. According to their investigations an anastomosis among the different groups of branches is lacking in only 13 per cent of all people. In general, a more or less well developed parotid plexus is to be found, whereas the mandibular branch is very seldom connected through anastomosis with the other branch groups, and the cervicalis colli branch never is.

According to Davis and co-workers (1956), this percentage varies. Intraoperative electrodiagnostic stimulation of the individual branches of the facial nerve confirms these anatomical variations. With this technique, the innervation patterns of the facial nerve of each patient can be accurately evaluated. It is our impression that the zygomatic branch is the most important of all the facial nerve branches because electrical stimulation of it produces contraction of both the orbicularis oculi and orbicularis oris muscles. Because of overlapping supply by the ocular and mandibular branches of the facial nerve, a complete transection of its zygomatic branch rarely produces a visible paralysis. In order to clarify these clinical observations, we counted the nerve fibers in the zygomatic branches in cadavers. We found that this branch makes up approximately 40 per cent of the total fibers of the facial nerve. End result studies of faciofacial anastomosis, in which each branch was anastomosed with the analogous branch of the opposite side, revealed failure of reinnervation of the frontal branch. For this reason we have now simplified the technique. We have abandoned the method of complete exposure of all peripheral branches of the facial nerve. Instead, we merely expose both zygomatic branches through two 2 cm-long incisions. These two branches are identified, transected, and anastomosed, using a sural nerve graft (Fig. 32–32*A* and *B*).

The results in 41 patients up to the present are satisfactory. In 90 per cent of the examined cases we could observe electromyographic and clinical reinnerva-

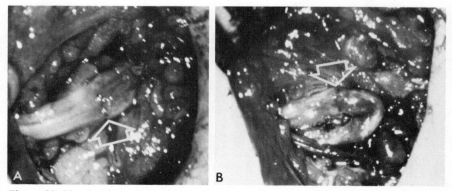

Figure 32–32   *A*, After a 2 cm skin incision below the zygomatic branch of the facial nerve on the intact side, the zygomatic branch is exposed and transected, the central stump is already anastomosed with the sural nerve (arrow). *B*, The second end of the graft is anastomosed with the distal stump of the zygomatic branch of the facial nerve on the damaged side (arrow).

tion of muscles. In 50 per cent of the patients we could ascertain symmetry of the face in a state of respose. Although in the other 40 per cent we could recognize a satisfying contraction of muscles, the paralysis of the facial nerve while in a state of repose was evident. In these cases we regularly perform a skin correction in the sulcus nasolabialis in order to achieve a symmetric position of the face in repose.

In only a few cases could we achieve an ideal symmetrical function in connection with active contraction of face muscles. The cause arises from the fact that only 50 per cent of the fibers of the facial nerve on the healthy side may be called upon for reconstruction without the risk of loss of function. In my opinion, the technique of the faciofacial anastomosis therefore constitutes only an alternative to the accessory–facial anastomosis or hypoglossal–facial anastomosis. Faciofacial anastomosis is inadequate when direct exposure and treatment of the lesion is possible.

Faciofacial anastomosis is a good additional method when direct treatment of the facial nerve lesion results only in partial reinnervation.

SURGICAL TREATMENT OF BELL'S PALSY

With regard to this idiopathic lesion of the facial nerve, the etiology of which is still uncertain, but which constitutes 58 to 88 per cent of all facial nerve lesions (according to Devriese, 58 per cent, Hosomi and Peitersen, 70 per cent, Adour, 74 per cent, Gomez, 84 per cent, and Cadena, 88 per cent), the attitude toward an operative treatment has changed very much during the past years. According to Hilger's (1949) theory of a vascular dysregulation and ischemia with following edema and compression of the nerve, principally in the fallopian canal, the only reasonable therapy seemed to be early operative decompression with neurolysis in the facial canal. Recent investigations emphasize the role of allergic factors or viral pathogenesis, with the result of a considerable decrease in the frequency of operative decompressions of the facial nerve. In about 70 to 90 per cent of all cases a return of function was possible by means of conservative therapy (Peitersen, 1977; Hosomi, 1977; Gomez, 1977). The intensity of the disease may be substantially reduced by prednisone therapy. Jongkees reported that with prednisone therapy he was able to limit the number of operative decompressions to 10 per cent.

An indication for intratemporal facial decompression, according to Esslen (1973), should be when electroneurographic examinations give the following results:

1. If more than 50 per cent of the nerve fibers show signs of degeneration four days after occurrence of the facial paralysis.
2. If about 50 per cent of the fibers are degenerated on the fourth day and a further 15 to 20 per cent are degenerating during the following two days.
3. If 90 per cent or more of the fibers have degenerated within seven days.

Owing to the fact that electroneurography is being increasingly used, several authors suggest the 90 per cent limit as the time for operative intervention. When surgical treatment is indicated, Fisch (1973) suggests exposure of the entire course of the facial nerve from the brain stem up to the stylomastoid foramen, but not only the preparation of the mastoidal and tympanal segment. In 11 of 12 such interventions he found either an exclusive or added involvement of the nerve proximal to the geniculate ganglion. About half of those cases with total decompression showed slight secondary ischemia in the mastoidal segment.

Based on experience with the decompression of the facial nerve in patients with Bell's palsy, Helms, in 1976, supported the view that an isolated transmeatal exposure of the geniculate ganglion may lead to satisfactory results. He performed decompression of the geniculate ganglion with local anesthesia. This technique, however, only applies in those cases where active muscle contraction is no longer ascertainable and electrical examinations establish a rapid decrease in muscle reaction. The period of time between onset of the paralysis and operation extends from seven days to 12 weeks. In all patients on whom transmeatal decompression of the geniculate ganglion has been done, a return of motor function in the three branches of the facial nerve could be diagnosed.

Recent studies by Jannetta on the surgical treatment of Bell's palsy show that in some patients a sudden displacement of an arterial loop in the cerebellopontine angle can lead to extensive stretching of the facial nerve. Jannetta pointed out that in some cases this mechanism may be regarded as a cause of Bell's palsy. He has found in six patients that this vascular change in the cerebellopontine angle is the cause of Bell's palsy. In five cases, he could achieve satisfactory results by decompression of the facial nerve from an arterial loop. The surgical approach and the technique of vascular decompression correspond to the findings of Jannetta (1977) regarding facial spasm.

ACOUSTIC NERVE (EIGHTH CRANIAL NERVE)

The problem of functional preservation and reconstruction of the acoustic nerve is that already after a short period of morphological interruption of this nerve, an irreversible loss of the corresponding sensory cells is unavoidable. In the past the loss of the acoustic organ and the organ of equilibrium (vestibular apparatus) as a result of tumor surgery in the cerebellopontine angle was accepted as inevitable. Efforts are now being made to preserve the acoustic nerve

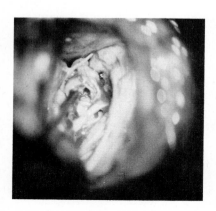

Figure 32–33 Cerebellopontine angle neuroma on the right side. After partial removal, one can clearly discern the tumor originating in the fascicle of the vestibular nerve. The facial nerve as well as the cochlear nerve in this case could be preserved. The preoperative extent of hearing remained unaltered following surgery.

in the cerebellopontine angle as well as in the internal auditory meatus by early diagnosis and with the help of microsurgical technique (Rhoton, 1976; Wigand, 1977). For the patient this is especially advantageous when the asymmetry of hearing between the two ears is not good. In two cases of cerebellopontine angle tumors (neurinoma, epidermoid) we preserved not only the continuity of the cochlear nerve but also the hearing function (Fig. 32–33).

Whether the attempt to preserve the vestibular nerve is justified seems to be open to question. On the one hand, a complete loss of this nerve may be compensated centrally, especially in younger patients, but on the other hand, partial damage may cause constant, troublesome vertigo.

GLOSSOPHARYNGEAL, VAGUS, SPINAL ACCESSORY, AND HYPOGLOSSAL NERVES (NINTH THROUGH TWELFTH CRANIAL NERVES)

It seems to be significant to classify the lesions of the cranial nerves IX-XII in three descending topographical and anatomical sections according to the possibilities of surgical approach.

1. The intracranial cerebellopontine region
2. The extradural area of the base of the skull (jugular foramen, canal of the hypoglossal nerve)
3. The neck region

The caudal cranial nerves in the first and second area lie closely together. They are often affected by pathological processes, either one after the other or at the same time, whereas each nerve in the region of the neck requires individual attention. In our experience, preservation of the glossopharyngeal and vagus nerves for the patient (particularly if their preoperative functions were intact) is almost as important as complete removal of the pathological process. While a slowly proceeding loss of these nerves (e.g., due to the growth of a tumor) is less significant with regard to swallowing, the acute interruption of continuity of the nerve leads to severe dysphagia and aspiration. In such cases only plastic reconstructive measures in the neck area, as mentioned by Denecke (1961), or partial closure of the glottis (Draf, 1977 personal communication) will allow physical rehabilitation for the patient.

In the region of the cerebellopontine angle, the protective sheath of connective tissue of the caudal cranial nerves is less thick than outside the base of the skull. Therefore, microsurgical manipulation, bipolar coagulation, and the avoidance of direct contact of the nerve are essential conditions for functional preservation. Because of the vital functions of the caudal cranial nerves, the first step after suboccipital exposure of the cerebellopontine angle during tumor operation should be the preparation and protection of the caudal cranial nerves (Figs. 32–34 and 32–35).

The *jugular foramen*, as the exit area of the cranial nerves (IX–XI), can be the place of origin of extradural space-occupying processes at the base of the skull (neurinomas, glomus tumors). Frequently, the jugular foramen is secondarily

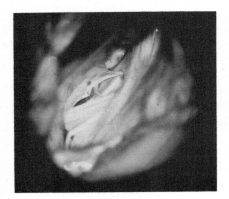

Figure 32–34 Demonstration of the normal condition of the caudal cranial nerves after suboccipital approach to the cerebellopontine angle. The dura has been opened and the cerebellum retracted.

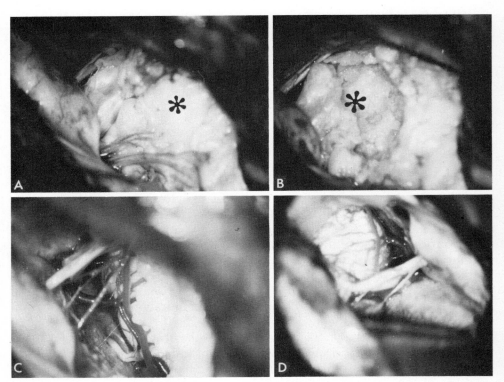

Figure 32–35 *A*, Exposure of the cerebellopontine angle on the left side with a very extensive cholesteatoma (asterisk). The tumor capsule is adherent to the caudal cranial nerves. *B*, After dissection with preservation of the caudal cranial nerves, the tumor (asterisk) is seen partially removed. *C*, Extensive removal of the tumor. The caudal cranial nerves, the facial nerves, and the acoustic nerves, as well as the vessels running to the brain stem are preserved. The hypoglossal nerve is visible. *D*, Total extirpation of the large cholesteatoma (measuring 6 × 5 cm). Preservation of the cranial nerves and the brain stem as well as the vessels. The slight depression of the pons and the anterior cerebellar artery is distinctly demonstrated.

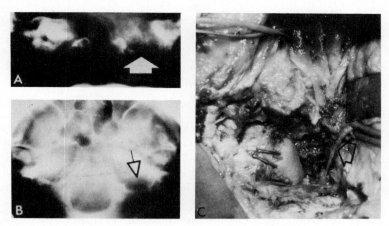

Figure 32–36 *A* and *B*, Roentgenograms of the base of the skull. Large glomus tumor with extensive destruction of the base of the skull (arrows) in the region of the jugular foramen and the petrous bone. *C* After removal of the large glomus tumor of the base of the skull, exposure of the jugular foramen. The preserved caudal cranial nerves and the internal carotid artery are visible. Bridging of a dura defect using lyophilized dura after resection because of tumor infiltration in the area of the middle and posterior fossa. The facial nerve (arrow) is exposed in the cerebellopontine angle up to its entrance into the parotid gland.

involved, as is the hypoglossal canal in processes that are located directly caudal to the base of the skull (tumors of the jugular glomus and of the tympanic glomus, as well as high lymphatic node metastases). From this point, penetration into the endocranium is also possible (Fig. 32–36). Clinical and neuroradiological examination is absolutely necessary before embarking on any surgical intervention in this region in order to estimate the exact extension of the tumor. The exposure of this area of the base of the skull was developed by Grunert (1894), Rehn (1919), Zehm (1969), Arena (1974), Conley (1975), and Fisch (1976). Among others, Denecke (1969) published essential references regarding this surgical technique.

The approach to the middle and posterior base of the skull, including the jugular foramen, is performed dorsocaudally after turning the sternocleidomastoid muscle to the side. The field of operation can be enlarged: through a temporary splitting of the lower jaw and by pulling up the neighboring part of the joint; through tangential resection of the ascending branch of the lower jaw, including the processus articularis; through resection of the styloid process and, if necessary, of the lip of the mastoid, then the internal jugular vein in the bulb or sigmoid sinus as well as the internal carotid artery and the accompanying cranial nerves can be isolated and distinctly arranged (Draf and Samii, 1977; Samii and Draf, 1978).

Processes at the jugular foramen may require the exposure or resection of the jugular bulb after ligation of the sigmoid sinus. In such a manner it is possible not only to prepare the cranial nerves IX, X and XI more distinctly in the anterior section of the jugular foramen but also to preserve them in cases of expansive tumors, provided that the tumor does not originate in one of these cranial nerves (Fig. 32–36). Injuries to the caudal cranial nerves in the neck region may be traumatic, tumorous, or iatrogenic.

Isolated *glossopharyngal nerve* lesions in the neck region are comparatively rare and are of less significance because of the mixed innervation of the pharyngoglossal area. Additionally, this nerve is located in the neck region and reaches its supply area relatively cephalad. Besides, many anastomoses exist between this nerve and the vagus nerve just caudal to the jugular foramen. Surgical interventions medial of its guide muscle (the stylopharyngeal) are performed rarely.

The clinical symptom of a *vagus nerve* disorder depends upon the location of the lesion and is characterized by dysphagia, shifting of the velum palatinum toward the healthy side, loss of the coulisse phenomenon of the pharyngeal muscles as well as paralysis of the vocal cord. Besides the disturbance of the swallowing reflex, the sensory disorder in the pharynx region, including the danger of aspiration, is especially high.

Surgical reconstruction of the glossopharyngeal nerve, because of the unimportant functional loss, is almost never considered; this nerve, therefore, is used as a donor nerve for grafting with the facial nerve (Ballance, 1924; Watson and Williams, 1927). However, all attempts are made regarding the treatment of vocal cord paralysis due to a lesion of the recurrent nerve.

The clinical disturbances due to the injury of the trunk of the vagus nerve distal to the posterior belly of the digastric muscle, with the exception of the recurrent nerve are not significant. In respect to correction of vocal cord paralysis after injury of the recurrent nerve distal to its take off from the vagus nerve (most often after thyroidectomy), Miehlke (1976) elaborated in animal experiment the recurrence decompression, an end-to-end anastomosis as well as an autograft. Hengerer and Tucker (1973) successfully performed, in animal experiments, an anastomosis of a muscle quadrant between the sternohyoid muscle still connected with a cervical branch of the hypoglossal nerve and the cricoarytenoid muscle.

The principle of this operation is, that by blunt preparation the cricoarytenoid muscle on one side, and, if necessary, at some further step on the second side, is exposed just on the plate of the cricoid cartilage. A 1×1 cm large and about 5 mm thick, cube-shaped piece of the sternohyoid muscle is prepared and kept attached to the innervating branch of the ansa hypoglossi. This piece of muscle is inserted like an inlay into the defect of the cricoarytenoid muscle.

SPINAL ACCESSORY NERVE (ELEVENTH CRANIAL NERVE)

A neurological deficit of the accessory nerve when diagnosed clinically has serious impact. Preservation of function or reconstruction of the accessory nerve is very important. Patients suffering complete loss of function of this nerve with paralysis of the trapezius muscle are no longer in a position to practice professions demanding strenuous physical activity. Damage to the accessory nerve due to accidents is relatively rare, even though the nerve lies in the lateral neck triangle close under the skin. However, the accessory nerve may frequently get damaged during extirpation of a tumor or of a lymphatic gland lateral to the posterior border of the sternocleidomastoid muscle (Fig. 32–37*A*).

Excisions of lymphatic glands and small tumors in this region must be performed very carefully. During such an intervention, the accessory nerve in

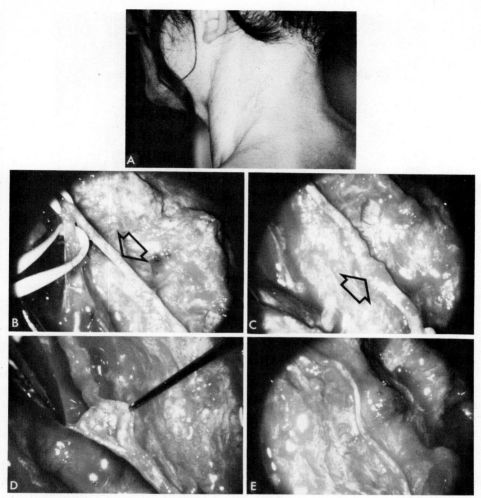

Figure 32–37 *A*, Typical scar to the lateral border of the sternocleidomastoid muscle after removal of a lymph node with injury of the accessory nerve. *B*, Exposure of the accessory nerve (arrow) at the lateral border of the sternocleidomastoid muscle. *C*, The lesion is exposed. The continuity of the nerve is preserved. One can observe a thickening of the nerve trunk (arrow). *D*, Microsurgical epineurotomy. The fascicle of the nerve is exposed. *E*, A fascicular neurolysis has been performed. The fascicle is preserved in its continuity.

this area should always be exposed at the posterior border of the sternocleido-mastoid muscle. Subsequently, the removal of a tumor or the lymphatic gland may be executed. If postoperative paralysis occurs, the accessory nerve must be operated as soon as possible, by means of neurolysis, nerve suture, or nerve grafting. When exposing the nerve, one must avoid the scar region in the area of the lesion and start with its exposure in the healthy part at the posterior margin of the sternocleidomastoid muscle. If the continuity is evident macroscopically a fascicular neurolysis can be performed under the microscope. In some cases there may be only a serious fibrosis with compression of the nerve, requiring the removal of the fibrotically changed epineurium (Fig. 32–37).

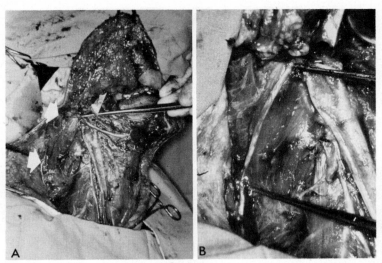

Figure 32–38 *A*, Operative field following neck dissection including the resection of the accessory nerve. Exposure of the distal and central stumps (arrows). *B*, Bridging of the nerve defect by means of a 12 cm nerve graft (between forceps).

In case of neuromatous change of the fascicles, even if the continuity is preserved, the neuroma should be resected and an end-to-end anastomosis or nerve grafting performed. If the accessory nerve is interrupted in its continuity and the neuroma of the proximal stump is located in a scar region with no relation to the distal stump, one must endeavor to trace the accessory nerve distal to the nerve lesion. Extensive damages, especially when the lesion is located at a great distance, may cause difficulties with regard to the exposure of the distal stump for the nerve at this point soon begins to branch off and ends in the anterior segment of the trapezius muscle.

Malignant tumors that involve the accessory nerve, and cases that demand radical neck dissection, require preoperative consideration of accessory nerve reconstruction. As soon as the skin flap is prepared for neck dissection, the central portion of the accessory nerve distal to the jugular foramen is marked and cut. The distal part also has to be traced and is cut before its entrance into the trapezius muscle (Figs. 32–38*A* and *B*). After neck dissection, the existing defect can be bridged by a graft approximately 12 cm long from the sural nerve.

HYPOGLOSSAL NERVE
(TWELFTH CRANIAL NERVE)

Injuries to the hypoglossal nerve in the neck region rarely occur with penetrating injuries of the soft tissues of the neck. During tumor surgery in the neck region, especially when dissecting the carotid sheath, where the hypoglossal nerve often is surrounded by a venous plexus, it may be damaged during the management of bleeding vessels. Furthermore, damage may occur during a difficult extirpation of the submandibular gland, especially when the nerve is adherent to the inflammatory mass or is infiltrated by the tumor. Tumors in the retrolingual region and on the floor of the mouth may grow around the hypo-

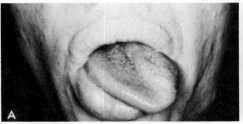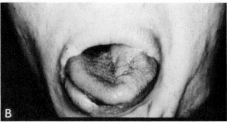

Figure 32-39 *A*, Paralysis of hypoglossal nerve on the left side after laceration of the neck in a 19-year-old patient. *B*, Functional improvement four days after a fascicular neurolysis.

glossal nerve and cause a paralysis. Paramount to the clinical symptoms there is a disturbance of articulation. Reconstruction of the hypoglossal nerve is demanded in traumatic cases and should be performed by microsurgical techniques. The spectrum of surgical treatment extends from neurolysis to nerve suture and nerve grafting, depending upon the operative findings (Fig. 32-39*A* and *B*).

REFERENCES

Adour, K.: Etiology and pathogenesis of Bell's palsy. Panel Discussion No. 10. *In* Fisch, U.: Facial Nerve Surgery. Amstelveen, The Netherlands, Kugler Medical Publ., B. V., 1977, p. 371.

Anderl, H.: A simple method for correcting the ectropion. Plast. Reconstr. Surg. *49*:156, 1972.

Arena, S.: Tumor surgery of the temporal bone. Laryngoscope (St. Louis) *84*:645, 1974.

Ballance, C. A.: A case of facial palsy treated by facio-hypoglossal anastomosis. Lancet *1*:1675, 1909.

Ballance, C. A.: An address on the results obtained in some experiments in which the facial and recurrent laryngeal nerves were anastomosed with other nerves. Brit. Med. J. *2*:349, 1924.

Ballance, C. A., and Duel, A. B.: The operative treatment of facial palsy; by the introduction of nerve grafts into the fallopian canal and by other intratemporal methods. Arch. Otolaryngol. *15*:1, 1932.

Becker, R.: Die Kontinuitätsresektion des Unterkiefers unter Erhaltung des N. mandibularis. Dtsch. Zahnärztl. Z. *22*:929, 1967.

Becker, R.: Continuity resection of the mandible with preservation of mandibular nerve. Brit. J. Oral Surg. *8*:45, 1970.

Becker, R.: Behandlung und Behandlungsergebnisse bei 38 Ameloblastomen. Fortschr. Kiefer- u. Gesichtschir. *15*:211, 1972.

Bertrand, R. A., Molina, P., and Hardy, J.: Surgical treatment of hemi-facial spasm. *In* Fisch, U.: Facial Nerve Surgery. Amstelveen, The Netherlands, Kugler Medical Publ., B. V., 1977, p. 512.

Bevers, E. C.: A case of facio-hypoglossal anastomosis. Lancet *1*:1450, 1913.

Bunnell, S.: Surgery of the nerves of the hand. Surg. Gynecol. Obstet. *44*:145, 1927.

Cadena, G.: Incidence and management of Bell's palsy according to geographic distribution. Panel Discussion No. 9. *In* Fisch, U.: Facial Nerve Surgery. Amstelveen, The Netherlands, Kugler Medical Publ., B. V., 1977, p. 328.

Campbell, E., and Keedy, C.: Hemifacial spasm: A note on the etiology in two cases. J. Neurosurg. *4*:342, 1947.

Cawthorne, T.: The pathology and surgical treatment of Bell's palsy. J. Laryngol. *65*:792, 1951.

Cawthorne, T., and Wilson, T.: Indications for intratemporal facial nerve surgery. Arch. Otolaryngol. *78*:429, 1963.

Cawthorne, T.: Geniculate ganglion facial palsy. Arch. Otolaryngol. *81*:502, 1965.

Clerc, P., and Batisse, R.: Abord des organes intra-pétreux par voi endocranienne. Ann. otolaryngol. (Paris) *71*:20, 1954.

Conley, J. J.: Facial nerve grafting in treatment of parotid gland tumors. Arch. Surg. *70*:359, 1955.

Conley, J. J.: Facial nerve grafting. Arch. Otolaryngol. *73*:322, 1961.

Conley, J. J.: Salivary Glands and the Facial Nerve. Stuttgart, George Thieme Verlag, 1975.

Davis, R. A., Anson, B. J., and Budinger, J. M., et al.: Surgical anatomy of the facial nerve and parotid gland based upon a study of 350 cervicofacial halves. Surg. Gynecol. Obstet. *102*:385, 1956.

Denecke, H. J.: Operationstechnische Probleme bei der Entfernung großer Neurinoma im Bereich von Felsenbeinpyramide. N. facialis, Pharynx, Gefäßscheide, Ösophagusmund und Zunge. H.N.O. (Berl.) *8*:343, 1959/60.

Denecke, H. J.: Korrektur des Schluckaktes bei einseitiger Pharynx- Larynxlähmung. 'HNO', Wegweiser für die fachärztl. Praxis, *9*:351, 1961.

Denecke, H. J.: Diskussionsbemerkung Nobel Symposion 10. Stockholm, Almquist and Wiksell, 1969.

Devriese, P. P.: Experimental compression of the facial nerve. *In* Fisch, U.: Facial Nerve Surgery. Amstelveen, The Netherlands, Kugler Medical Publ. B. V., 1977, p. 344.

Dott, N. M.: Facial paralysis. Restitution by extrapetrous nerve graft. Proc. Roy. Soc. Med. *51*:900, 1958.

Draf, W., and Samii, M.: Otorhinolaryngologisch-neurochirurgische Probleme an der Schädelbasis. Laryng. Rhinol. *56*:1007, 1977.

Drake, C. G.: Acoustic neuroma. Repair of facial nerve with autogenous graft. J. Neurosurg. *17*:836, 1960.

Drake, C. G.: Experiences and results with posterior approaches. *In* Schürmann, K., Brock, M., Reulen, H. J., and Voth, D., Brain Edema — Cerebellopontine Angle Tumors. Advances in Neurosurgery. New York, Springer Verlag, 1973, Vol. 1, p. 240.

Duel, A. B.: Clinical presentation of improvement in surgical repair of the facial nerve. Laryngoscope *44*:599, 1934.

Esslen, E.: Electrodiagnosis of facial palsy. *In* Miehlke, A.: Surgery of the Facial Nerve. Munich, Urban & Schwarzenberg, 1973, p. 45.

Esslen, E.: Electromyography and electroneurography. *In* Fisch, U.: Facial Nerve Surgery. Amstelveen, The Netherlands, Kugler Medical Publ. B.V., 1977, p. 93.

Fisch, U.: Operations on the facial nerve. *In* Yasargil, M. G., Microsurgery. Stuttgart, 1969, p. 208.

Fisch, U.: Transtemporal surgery of the internal auditory canal. Report of 92 cases, technique, indications and results. Adv. Otorhinolaryng. *17*:203, 1970.

Fisch, U.: Die totale Freilegung des Nervus facialis bei laterobasalen Schädelfrakturen. Arch. Klin. Exp. Ohren. Nasen. Kehlkopfheilkd. *196*:187, 1970.

Fisch, U.: Die Verletzungen des Nervus facialis bei laterobasalen Schädelfrakturen. Med. Mitteil. Braun Melsungen *46*:165, 1972.

Fisch, U.: Chirurgie im inneren Gehörgang und an benachbarten Strukturen. *In* Naumann, H. H.: Kopf- und Halschirurgie, Bd. III: Ohrregion. Stuttgart, Georg Thieme Verlag, 1976.

Fisch, U.: Facial Nerve Surgery. Amstelveen, The Netherlands, Kugler Medical Publ. B.V., 1977.

Fujita, T.: Über die periphere Ausbreitung des Nervus facialis beim Menschen. Gegenbaurs Morph. Jb. *73*:578, 1934.

Gardner, W. J., and Sava, G. A.: Hemifacial spasm: A reversible pathophysiologic state. J. Neurosurg. *19*:240, 1962.

Gardner, W. J.: Concerning the mechanism of trigeminal neuralgia and hemifacial spasm. J. Neurosurg. *19*:947, 1962.

Gomez, J. G.: Incidence and management of Bell's palsy according to geographic distribution. Panel Discussion No. 9. *In* Fisch, U.: Facial Nerve Surgery. Amstelveen, The Netherlands, Kugler Medical Publ. B.V., 1977, p. 319.

Greve, K.: Histologische Befunde bei komplizierten Kieferfrakturen mit besonderer Berücksichtigung des Mandibularkanals. Dtsch. Mschr. Zahnheilk. *45*:458, 1927.

Grunert, K. A.: Die operative Ausräumung des Bulbus venae jugularis (Bulbusoperation). Arch. Ohrenheilk. *36*:71, 1894.

Hardy, R. C., Perret, G., and Meyers, R.: Phrenicofacial nerve anastomosis for facial paralysis. J. Neurosurg. *14*:400, 1957.

Hausamen, J.-E., Samii, M., and Schmidseder, R.: Repair of the mandibular nerve by means of autologous nerve grafting after resection of the lower jaw. J. Maxillofac. Surg. *1*:74, 1973.

Helms, J.: The transmeatal approach to the geniculate ganglion. Acta Otolaryngol. Belg. *30*:84, 1976.

Hengerer, S., and Tucker, H. M.: Restoration of abduction in the paralyzed canine vocal cord. Arch. Otolaryngol. *97*:247, 1973.

Hermann, M.: Über die Verletzung der Gesichtsnerven. Zahnärztl. Praxis *9*:97, 1958.

Hilger, J. A.: The nature of Bell's palsy. Laryngoscope *59*:228, 1949.

Hitselberger, W. E. and House, W. F.: Experiences and results with the translabyrinthine approach and related techniques (Abstract). *In* Schuermann, K., et al. (eds.): Advances in Neurosurgery, Volume 1: Brain Edema: Pathophysiology and Therapy; Cerebello Pontine Angle Tumors: Diagnosis and Surgery. New York, Springer-Verlag, 1973, p. 239.

Hof, E.: Facial palsy of infectious origin in children. *In* Fisch, U.: Facial Nerve Surgery. Amstelveen, The Netherlands, Kugler Medical Publ. B.V., 1977, p. 414.

Hosomi, H.: Management of Bell's palsy. *In* Fisch, U.: Facial Nerve Surgery. Amstelveen, The Netherlands, Kugler Medical Publ. B.V., 1977, p. 382.

House, W. F.: Surgical exposure of the internal auditory canal and its contents through the middle cranial fossa. Laryngoscope (St. Louis) *71*:1363, 1961.

House, W. F.: Middle cranial fossa approach to the petrous pyramid. Arch. Otolaryngol. *78*:460, 1963.

Jacobson, J. H.: Microsurgical technique in the repair of the traumatized extremity. Clin. Orthop. *29*:132, 1963.

Jannetta, P. J.: Microsurgical exploration and decompression of the facial nerve in hemifacial spasm. Curr. Top. Surg. Res. *2*:217, 1970.

Jannetta, P. J.: Neurovascular compression of the facial nerve in hemifacial spasm: Relief by microsurgical technique. *In* Merei, F. T. (ed.): Reconstructive Surgery of Brain Arteries. Budapest, Publishing House of the Hungarian Academy of Sciences, 1974, p. 193.

Jannetta, P. J.: The cause of hemifacial spasm: Definitive microsurgical treatment at the brainstem in 31 patients. Am. Acad. Ophthalmol. Otolaryngol. *30*:319, 1975.

Jannetta, P. J.: Trigeminal neuralgia and hemifacial spasm — etiology and definitive treatment. Trans. Am. Neurol. Assoc. *100*:53, 1975.

Jannetta, P. J.: Etiology and definitive microsurgical treatment of hemifacial spasm. J. Neurosurg. *47*:321, 1977.

Jannetta, P. J.: A theory as to aetiology. Observations in six patients. Laryngoscope *89*:849, 1978.

Jongkees, L. B. W.: Die chirurgische Behandlung der intratemporalen Facialislähmung. Dtsch. Med. Wschr. *83*:865, 1958.

Jongkees, L. B. W.: Über die intratemporale Facialislähmung und ihre chirurgische Behandlung. Z. Laryng. Rhinol. *40*:319, 1961.

Jongkees, L. B. W.: Nerve excitability test. *In* Fisch, U.: Facial Nerve Surgery. Amstelveen, The Netherlands, Kugler Medical Publ. B.V., 1977, p. 83.

Kautzky, R.: Die periphere Facialislähmung und ihre Behandlung mittels Nervenpfropfung. *In* Schuchart, K., Fortschr. Kiefer- u. Gesichtschir. Bd. II, 1956, p. 119.

Kettel, K.: Repair of the facial nerve in traumatic facial palsies. Results of decompression, nerve suture and nerve grafting in one hundred twenty-seven cases. Arch. Otolaryngol. *66*:634, 1957.

Kettel, K.: Peripheral Facial Palsy, Pathology and Surgery. Copenhagen, Munksgaard, 1959.

Körte, W.: Ein Fall von Nervenpfropfung: des Nervus Facialis auf den Nervus Hypoglossus. Dtsch. Med. Wschr. *29*:293, 1903.

Koos, W. T., Böck, F. W., and Salah, S.: Experiences in microsurgery of acoustic neurinomas (Abstract). *In* Schuermann, K., et al.: Advances in Neurosurgery, Volume 1: Brain Edema: Pathophysiology and Therapy; Cerebello Pontine Angle Tumors: Diagnosis and Surgery. New York, Springer-Verlag, 1973, p. 251.

Lathrop, F. D.: The facial nerve; technique of exposure and repair. Surg. Clin. North Amer. *33*:909, 1953.

Lathrop, F. D.: Surgical repair of the facial nerve: Technique. Surg. Clin. North Amer. *36*:583, 1956.

Lathrop, F. D.: Management of the facial nerve during operations on the parotid gland. Ann. Otol. (St. Louis) *72*:780, 1962.

Loew, F.: Die kombinierte intrakranielle-extratemporale Fazialisplastik nach Dott. Langenbecks Arch. Klin. Chir. *298*:934, 1962; Saarl. Ärzteblatt *9*, 1962.

Loew, F. and Kivelitz, R.: Surgical reconstruction of intracranial lesions of cranial nerves. *In* Schuermann, K., et al. (eds.): Advances in Neurosurgery, Volume 1: Brain Edema: Pathophysiology and Therapy; Cerebello Pontine Angle Tumors; Diagnosis and Surgery. New York, Springer-Verlag, 1973, p. 242.

Martin, R. C.: Intratemporal suture of the facial nerve. Arch. Otolaryngol. *13*:259, 1931.

Martin, R. C.: Surgical repair of the facial nerve. Arch. Otolaryngol. *23*:458, 1936.

Maxwell, J. H.: Extratemporal repair of the facial nerve. Ann. Otol. (St. Louis) *60*:1114, 1951.

Maxwell, J. H.: Repair of the facial nerve after facial lacerations. Trans. Amer. Acad. Ophthal. Otolaryngol. *58*:733, 1954.

McCormack, L. J., Cauldwell, E. W., and Anson, B. J.: The surgical anatomy of the facial nerve "with special reference to the parotid gland." Surg. Gynecol. Obstet. *80*:620, 1945.

McGovern, F. H.: Etiology and pathogenesis of Bell's palsy. *In* Fisch, U.: Facial Nerve Surgery. Amstelveen, The Netherlands, Kugler Medical Publ. B.V., 1977, p. 371.

Metelka, M.: Anastomóza N. VII. A XII. lepnim plazmou. Cs. Neurol. *29*:305, 1966.

Michon, J., and Masse, P.: Le moment optimum de la suture nerveuse dans les paies du membre supérieur. Rev. Chir. Orthop. *50*:205, 1964.

Miehlke, A.: Extratemporale Gesichtsnervenplastik im Zuge der Parotischirurgie. *In* Schuchhardt, K.: Fortschr. Kiefer- u. Gesichtschir., Stuttgart, 1960, Vol. 6, p. 344.

Miehlke, A.: Extratemporale Facialischirurgie. Z. Laryngol. Rhinol. *40*:338, 1961.

Miehlke, A., and Bushe, K. A.: Die operative Freilegung der mittleren Schädelgrube und des Porus acusticus internus zur Behandlung interlabyrinthärer Läsionen des Nervus facialis. Chir. Plast. Reconstr. *3*:37, 1967.

Miehlke, A.: Functional rehabilitation of laryngoparalysis through vagus-recurrent nerve anastomosis. *In* Clinical Microneurosurgery. Stuttgart, Georg Thieme Verlag, 1976, pp. 253–272.

Miehlke, A.: Surgery of the facial nerve. Munich, Urban & Schwarzenberg, 1973.

Millesi, H., Ganglberger, J., and Berger, A.: Erfahrungen mit der Mikrochirurgie peripherer Nerven. Chir. Plast. Reconstr. *3*:47, 1967.

Millesi, H.: Operative Behandlung verletzter peripherer Nerven. Hefte Unfallheilkd. *117*:366, 1974.

Millesi, H.: Zum Problem der Überbrückung von Defekten peripherer Nerven. Wien. Med. Wschr. *118*:182, 1968.

Millesi, H., Berger, A., and Meissl, G.: Experimentelle Untersuchungen zur Heilung durchtrennter peripherer Nerven. Chir. Plast. *1*:174, 1972.

Millesi, H., and Samii, M.: Erfahrungen mit verschiedenen Wiederherstellungsoperationen am Nervus facialis. *In* Plastische Wiederherstellungschirurgie. New York, H. Köhler, 1975, p. 111.

Nishimura H., Morimoto, M. and Yanagihara, N.: Contralateral innervation of the facial nerve. *In* Fisch, U.: Facial Nerve Surgery. Amstelveen, The Netherlands, Kugler Medical Publ. B.V., 1977, p. 227.

Passerini, D., Dala, E., and Valli, G.: Contralateral reinnervation in facial palsy. Electromyography *8*:115, 1968.

Peitersen, E.: Spontaneous course of Bell's palsy. *In* Fisch, U.: Facial Nerve Surgery. Amstelveen, The Netherlands, Kugler Medical Publ. B.V., 1977, p. 337.

Rehn, E.: Die Freilegung der A. carotis interna in ihrem oberen Halsteil. Zbl. Chir. (1919) H. 17.

Rhoton, A. L.: Microsurgical removal of acoustic neuromas. Surg. Neurol. *6*(4):211, 1976.

Samii, M.: Lage und Verlauf der Sehnerven im Cisternenbild. Radiologe *10*:456, 1970.

Samii, M., Schürmann, K., Scheinpflug, W., and Wallenborn, R.: Experimental studies comparing grafting with autogenous and irradiated freeze dried homologous nerves. Excerpta Medica, Intern. Congress Series *287*:263, 1971.

Samii, M., and Wallenborn, R.: Tierexperimentelle Untersuchungen über den Einfluß der Spannung auf den Regenerationserfolg nach Nervennaht. Acta Neurochir. (Wien.) *27*:87, 1972.

Samii, M.: Die operative Versorgung peripherer Nervenverletzungen. Therapiewoche *22*:2164, 1972.

Samii, M., Schürmann, K., Wallenborn, R., and Scheinpflug, W.: Tierexperimentelle Untersuchungen über autologe und homologe Nerventransplantationen. Med. Mitt. (Melsungen) *46*:333, 1972.

Samii, M. and Kahl, R.-I.: Klinische Resultate der autologen Nerventransplantationen. Med. Mitt. (Melsungen) *46*:197, 1972.

Samii, M.: Autologe Nerventransplantation im Trigeminusbereich. Med. Mitt. (Melsungen) *46*:189, 1972.

Samii, M.: Die operative Wiederherstellung verletzter Nerven. Langenbecks Arch. Chir. *332*:355, 1972.

Samii, M.: Interfaszikuläre autologe Nerventransplantation. Indikation, Technik und Ergebnisse. Deutsches Ärzteblatt 70, *19*:1257, 1972.

Samii, M.: Visual disturbances caused by a low located optic chiasm. Excerpta Medica, Intern. Congress Series *306*:25, 1972.

Samii, M.: Sehstörungen bei tiefsitzendem Chiasma Opticum. Bericht über die 72. Zusammenkunft der Deutschen Ophthalm. Gesellsch. Heidelberg 1972. Munich, J. F. Bergmann, 1974, p. 37.

Samii, M.: Indication and operative technique of birth injuries of brachial plexus. *In* Progress in Paediatric Neurosurgery. Stuttgart, Hippokrates-Verlag, 1974, p. 243.

Samii, M., and Scheinpflug, W.: Klinische, elektromyographische und histologische Untersuchungen nach Nerventransplantation. Acta Neurochir. *30*:1, 1974.

Samii, M.: Verletzungen der Hirnnerven und des Plexus brachialis. Hefte Unfallheilkd. *117*:372, 1974.

Samii, M.: Modern aspects of peripheral and cranial nerve surgery. *In* Advances and Technical Standards in Neurosurgery. New York, Springer-Verlag, 1975, Vol. 2, p. 33.

Samii, M.: Use of microtechniques in peripheral nerve surgery — experience with over 300 cases. Microneurosurgery. Tokyo, Igaku Shoin Ltd., 1975, p. 85.

Samii, M., and Wagner, D.: Ergebnisse der autologen Nerventransplantationen bei Läsionen kranialer und peripherer Nerven. Ther. Umsch. *32*(7):453, 1975.

Samii, M.: Faziofaziale Anastomose durch Nerventransplantation. Fortschritte der Kiefer- und Gesichtschirurgie XX, (Hrsg. K. Schuchhardt) *XX*, Stuttgart, Georg Thieme Verlag, 1976, p. 115.

Samii, M.: Die Wiederherstellung peripherer Nervenverletzungen mit freien Transplantaten. *In* Hollwick, F., and Walter, C. (eds.): Plastisch-chirurgische Maßnahmen bei Spätfolgen nach Unfällen. Stuttgart, Georg Thieme Verlag, 1976, p. 174.

Samii, M.: Intraneurale Neurolyse des Nervus medianus beim Carpaltunnel-Syndrom. Handchirurgie *8*:117, 1976.

Samii, M., and Schürmann, K.: Operative treatment in relation to location and extension of pituitary adenomas. Stuttgart, Georg Thieme Verlag, 1978, p. 310.

Samii, M., and Draf, W.: Neurosurgical-ENT-treatment of processes of the base of the skull. *In* Advances in Neurosurgery, Head Injuries, Tumors of the Cerebellar Region. Berling, Springer-Verlag, vol. 5, pp. 324–330, 1978.

Scaramella, L.: L'anastomosi tra i due nervi faciali. Arch. Ital. Otol. *82*:209, 1971.

Simpson, H. E.: Injuries of the inferior dental and mental nerves. J Oral Surg. *16*:300, 1958.

Smith, J. W.: Microsurgery of peripheral nerves. Plast. Reconstr. Surg. *33*:317, 1964.

Smith, J. W.: A new technique of facial animation. Transaction Fifth International Congress Plastic and Reconstructive Surgery, Melbourne Feb. 1971, London 1971, p. 83.

Watson-Williams, E.: Glossopharyngeal facial nerve anastomosis. Proc. Roy. Soc. Med. *20*:1439, 1927.

Wigand, M. E.: Schwindel, ein Leitsymptom der Felsenbeinneurinome. Neurol. Psychiat. *2*:307, 1976.

Wullstein, H. L.: Die Methode der Dekompression des Nervus facialis vom Austritt aus dem Labyrinth bis zu dem aus dem Foramen stylomastoideum ohne Beeinträchtigung des Mittelohres. Arch. Ohren. Nasen. Kehlkopfheilkd. *172*:582, 1958.

Yasargil, M. G.: Microsurgical experience in surgery of acoustic neurinomas (Abstract). *In* Schuermann, K., et al. (eds.): Advances in Neurosurgery, Volume 1: Brain Edema: Pathophysiology and Therapy; Cerebello Pontine Angle Tumors: Diagnosis and Surgery. New York, Springer-Verlag, 1973, p. 250.

Yasargil, M. G.: Management of facial nerve in intracranial tumors. *In* Fisch, U., Facial Nerve Surgery. Amstelveen, The Netherlands, Kugler Medical Publ. B.V., 1977, p. 474.

Zehm, S.: The surgical approach to the external part of the base of the skull related to the anterior and medial cranial fossa. Nobel Symposium 10. Stockholm, Almquist and Wiksell, 1969.

33

TRAUMA INVOLVING THE BRACHIAL PLEXUS

HANNO MILLESI

BASIC CONSIDERATIONS

The severe loss of function suffered in brachial plexus injuries leads to serious consequences to the patient's family and professional life and expectations. A short time ago the chances of significant improvement by surgery of root lesions were regarded as minimal (Seddon, 1972). Today some improvement can be achieved, but expectations must not be too high. Return of function is far from satisfactory from an objective point of view; however, for the patient it means a significant improvement, and helps him to resume a somewhat normal social life. The great expenditure that is necessary for such an improvement is therefore highly justified.

Brachial plexus injuries can be caused by direct trauma causing an open injury or by foreign bodies being thrust into the neck area during an accident. These injuries are typically suffered by young people, usually consequent to motorcycle accidents. Gunshot wounds are infrequent causes during peace time. Most often the lesion is caused by traction in a longitudinal direction or by compression, or by a combination of both. The distance between the intervertebral canal and the upper arm is increased and the brachial plexus elongated if the head is moved and turned to the contralateral side while the shoulder joint and the thorax are depressed. The distance is further increased if the arm is moved away from the body by luxation of the shoulder joint or by a fractured humerus. The scalenus muscles and the connective tissue of the infraclavicular area act to prevent the elongation. Under sufficient force the scalenus medius muscle itself is elongated and the protection is lost. As a result of this damage this muscle may undergo fibrotic changes. Sometimes there are fractures of the transverse processes of the corresponding cervical vertebra. The elongation leads to ruptures within the parts of the brachial plexus until continuity is lost either partially or completely.

Compression of a brachial plexus occurs between the first rib and the clavicle. This compression is caused by an external force which presses the clavicle on the first rib. The compression occurs at the distal parts of the trunks and the proximal parts of the cords. It can cause various degrees of damage.

If the brachial plexus is compressed and the arm is moved in a caudal or lateral direction, the greatest damage will occur within the cords (fourth degree lesion).

If the compression is between the clavicle and first rib, and the head is moved to the contralateral side, the trunks and roots will be under stress and will suffer a traction lesion (second or third degree lesion).

If trauma causes movement of the head mainly to the lateral side, and there is compression of the brachial plexus, a root avulsion is likely to occur (first degree lesion).

Roots are exposed to traction in various degrees according to the position of the arm at the moment of the accident. If the arm is in a pendulous position, the greatest traction will occur in roots C5 and C6. If the arm is in lateral abduction all roots are under great stress with the greatest stress being on C7. If the arm is in an elevated position, the greatest traction is exerted on C8 and T1. If the traction force is limited, then only these specific roots are avulsed while the others remain intact or are minimally damaged. If, of course, the traction force is severe and excessive, all roots can be damaged, regardless of the position of the arm.

THE BRACHIAL PLEXUS PATIENT

The first treatment that a person with brachial plexus injury usually receives is at an emergency facility, where the saving of his life is probably the first concern. The patient has suffered a major accident with cerebral concussion, shock, and other injuries. The brachial plexus lesion is noted but not much has been done to correct it. After the patient's other problems have been attended and he is no longer in imminent danger, he is presented for consultation in relation to the brachial plexus lesion.

The average patient is a young man in a very depressed psychological state. He has begun to understand the ways in which the injury and its sequelae will influence his life. The arm is completely paralyzed; it hangs flail from the shoulder. It is in slight internal rotation. The dependent arm is cyanotic in its peripheral parts. Sensibility is completely lost, with the exception of a strip on the inner side of the upper arm supplied by the intercostobrachial nerves, coming from T2. Very often the patient suffers from severe pain, and complains of phantom limb symptoms.

At this stage the first treatment the patient needs is psychological guidance to prepare him to accept the situation, and to encourage his cooperation. It is evident that an individual approach has to be found for each patient. This support is necessary throughout the whole period of reconstruction.

Physiotherapy must be started with passive joint motion to prevent stiffness. Electrophysiologic treatment is initiated. The value of stimulation with triangular impulses having exponential slope to avoid or retard the occurrence of muscle atrophy has not been proved scientifically effective yet, but it is a fact that patients who have undergone such therapy regularly do much better for various reasons, some of which might be psychological.

By use of various examinations, a diagnosis regarding severity level and extent of the injury must be established. It is very difficult to achieve an exact diagnosis, but this is not really necessary. We must determine at this time the prognosis for spontaneous recovery.

A plan of treatment is established which includes the activities of different teams. It is necessary that somebody supervise the treatment and control its exact execution. The plan of treatment includes the following:
— Conservative treatment of patients for whom the possibility of spontaneous recovery is good.
— Conservative treatment of patients in whom surgery is indicated to cover the preoperative phase.
— Direct surgery on the brachial plexus in cases without spontaneous recovery and in patients in whom spontaneous recovery has come to a standstill.
— Conservative treatment after the operative phase.
— Evaluation of the degree of recovery during the second year, when spontaneous recovery or postoperative recovery comes to an end.
— Selection of palliative methods to get optimal use of the returned function.

It is evident that the patient needs social support during this period of time. He must have financial help to support himself and his family. He should receive training in another profession which he can carry out with one arm and one hand only. It is absolutely necessary to prevent long periods of professional inactivity.

If there is a pain syndrome everything possible to control this situation should be attempted.

The therapeutic approach does not differ much if the patient is admitted to hospital within two to five months after the accident, but after six months the optimal time for direct repair has passed and special considerations are necessary.

For closed brachial plexus injuries, the optimal time for direct surgery at the brachial plexus is between two and five months. After six months the chances for recovery become poor. Nevertheless, this does not mean that the patient should not be operated at all beyond this deadline, especially with partial lesions or with lesions of third or fourth degree. It is possible that recovery can occur even after a longer period of time. Therefore, one must consider all these facts and discuss the problems with the patient. If the patient, for instance, says that he wants to exploit any chance whatsoever, I would not hesitate to operate after six months. But the patient must know that the chances for functional improvement are reduced.

INDICATION FOR SURGERY

Surgery is indicated if spontaneous recovery cannot be expected within a reasonable time. The prospect of spontaneous recovery depends on the severity of the lesion and other factors.

Severity, Level, and Longitudinal and Lateral Extent of the Lesion

Sir Sidney Sunderland (1951) has provided a scheme to describe the different degrees of peripheral nerve damage. This scheme fits very well with some inclusions to the evaluation of brachial plexus lesions.

First Degree

First degree lesions are those in which conduction is blocked without morphologic changes. There is no wallerian degeneration peripheral to the lesion and, therefore, conduction within the motor and sensory fibers is preserved. Full spontaneous recovery should recur within some weeks. External pressure can prevent this natural development.

Second Degree

In second degree lesions there is axon damage with wallerian regeneration distal to the lesion; therefore, conduction within the motor and sensory fibers is lost a few days after the accident. There is no damage to endoneural and perineural tissues. Full spontaneous recovery can be expected within some months. Two to three weeks after the accident a Tinel–Hoffmann sign can be elicited by percussion at the site of the lesion. In the following weeks the Tinel–Hoffmann sign advances toward the periphery; after some months regeneration potentials can be detected in the proximal muscles by EMG. Spontaneous recovery can be prevented by external pressure.

Third Degree

In the third degree lesion there is damage to the axons and the endoneural tissue. The perineural tissue and the fascicular pattern remain intact. There is no motor or sensory conduction distal to the lesion. The Tinel–Hoffman sign is positive at the site of injury and starts to advance slowly to the periphery. Spontaneous recovery is possible but there will always be a deficit because not all axon sprouts reach a corresponding distal endoneural tube. Spontaneous recovery can be prevented by external pressure. Because of the traction the epineural and interfascicular tissue may suffer to such a degree that epineural fibrosis with constriction of the fascicular tissue occurs. In more severe cases the interfascicular tissue can also develop fibrosis. Third degree lesions present the best indication to perform a neurolysis and, if necessary, epineurectomy plus interfascicular neurolysis, to make spontaneous recovery possible or to speed it up.

Fourth Degree

In this type of lesion there is damage to axons and endoneural and perineural tissue. The fascicular pattern is lost. The continuity is preserved by the epineurium only, which may have developed severe fibrotic changes. There is wallerian degeneration and there is no motor or sensory conduction distal to the lesion. A Tinel–Hoffman sign develops at the site of injury and shows no significant movement in a peripheral direction. Spontaneous recovery in reasonable time and to a significant degree cannot be expected. The best method of treatment is resection of this segment and restoration of continuity by nerve grafts.

First to fourth degree lesions can be present in different parts of the brachial plexus in the same patient.

Fifth Degree

By definition, fifth degree lesions occur in all parts of the brachial plexus that have lost continuity. As far as surgery is concerned, the consequences depend very much on the level of the injury.

PREGANGLIONIC (SUPRAGANGLIONIC) LESIONS (AVULSION OF ROOTS, LEVEL I). In these lesions there is a complete loss of motor and sensory function. Motor conduction has been lost. The motor fibers undergo wallerian degeneration, but there is no wallerian degeneration in the sensory fibers because they are still in continuity with their ganglion cells in the spinal ganglion. Therefore, sensory conduction is preserved; this can be proved by electroneurography. The paralysis extends also to the very proximal muscles, including the deep muscles of the neck, supplied by the dorsal branch of the root, the serratus anterior muscle, supplied by the long thoracic nerve, and the rhomboideus muscles, supplied by the dorsal scapular nerve. The denervation of these muscles can be proved by electromyography. There is no Tinel–Hoffman sign with radiation of paraesthesias to the arm and the hand because the sensory fibers are not separated from their ganglion cells. One must avoid misinterpretation of a Tinel–Hoffman sign due to a lesion of one of the branches of the cervical plexus. The presence of a Horner syndrome, of spinal cord symptoms, and of fractures of transverse processes supports the assumption that a supraganglionic lesion is present.

If by myelography a meningocele is proven this speaks strongly for an avulsion of this root, but, there are well documented cases with a positive myelogram and no avulsion. If the myelogram is negative and does not show a meningocele, the presence of a root avulsion, a supraganglionic lesion, cannot be excluded. It is not uncommon to have a combined lesion with some roots avulsed and others ruptured.

In a case of supraganglionic lesion sympathetic functions such as sweat production and vascular response should be normal. But this is true only in very well defined lesions. The symptoms can be difficult to interpret if there is combined rupture and avulsion of different roots or if a lesion extends in a longitudinal direction involving both the supra- and infraganglionic areas (LEVELS I and II).

POSTGANGLIONIC (INFRAGANGLIONIC) LESIONS (LEVEL II).   In these lesions there is a complete loss of continuity peripherally tb the spinal ganglion, with complete loss of motor and sensory function and loss of conductivity of motor and sensory fibers, which are completely separated from their ganglion cells and undergo wallerian degeneration. The dorsal branches of the spinal nerve are not involved, and the deep muscles of the neck are fully innervated. The Tinel–Hoffman sign is positive, with radiation to the hand and fingers.

TRUNK LESIONS (LEVEL III).   The symptoms are similar to an infraganglionic lesion but the very proximal muscles such as the serratus anterior are spared.

CORD LESIONS (LEVEL IV).   There is a complete loss of motor and sensory function with loss of conductivity. The Tinel–Hoffman sign is positive in the infraclavicular area, the supra- and infraspinatus muscles, supplied by the suprascapular nerve, are not involved.

COMBINED TRUNK AND CORD LESIONS.   A combined lesion of cords and trunks is possible (III/IV). Fracture of the clavicle can cause a brachial plexus lesion at this level by direct pressure of a bony fragment.

Lateral Extension

A complete brachial plexus lesion means that all parts of the brachial plexus are involved: in a root lesion, all five roots; in a lesion of the supraclavicular fossa, all three trunks; and in a lesion of the infraclavicular fossa, all three cords. Frequently, the roots do not all suffer the same amount of damage.

Upper Brachial Plexus Lesion.   The C5 and C6 roots can be involved only; when this occurs the muscles of the shoulder and the biceps will not function. If the C7 root is included there is also a varying degree of paralysis of radial nerve supplied muscles.

Lower Brachial Plexus Lesion.   The lesion involves the C8 and T1 roots. In this case the intrinsic muscles of the hand are paralyzed but the muscles of the forearm, the upper arm, and the shoulder remain active.

Plan of Treatment

Phase One

During the first three to four months conservative treatment is performed in all cases. During this period one tries to exclude all first and second degree lesions. First degree lesions are easy to recognize because motor and sensory conduction is continuously preserved and there are early signs of recovery. In second degree lesions the return of regeneration potentials in proximal muscles can be observed. In these cases conservative treatment is continued until full recovery occurs or spontaneous regeneration stops, in which event the indications for surgery are reconsidered. Neurolysis to free the nerve from external pressure might be indicated. The presence of a mixed second and third degree lesion might cause delayed and incomplete recovery.

Phase Two

Between the fourth and the sixth month direct surgery on the brachial plexus to achieve neurotization must be considered for all patients in whom no signs of recovery can be detected and no advancement of a Tinel–Hoffman sign observed. If the operation reveals a third degree lesion and external neurolysis is performed, the epineurium is resected and, if necessary, an internal neurolysis is carried out. The surgeon must be very careful to avoid any damage to fascicular structures that might lessen the chances of spontaneous recovery within these fascicles. If a fourth degree lesion is encountered, the involved part is resected and the continuity restored by nerve grafts.

In any case of fifth degree lesion with loss of continuity below the spinal ganglion, the neuroma and the glioma are resected and the continuity restored by nerve grafting. If a lesion of the fifth degree above the spinal ganglion is present, neurotization by intercostal nerve transfer is indicated.

It should be remembered that spontaneous recovery is possible in third degree lesions but is very often delayed or prevented by extrinsic causes; however, if one waits long enough, useful recovery can occur (Alnot et al., 1975). Regeneration can be induced or speeded up by means of surgery. Delicate microsurgical technique is necessary to prevent damage to fascicular tissue. One tries to transform fourth or fifth degree lesions into something similar to third degree lesions by reestablishing the continuity by means of nerve grafts.

Phase Three

After the postoperative treatment is finished and the wounds are healed, conservative treatment is resumed, and is continued until recovery occurs. Recovery cannot be expected sooner than about one year after the operation.

Phase Four

In the second half of the second year and in the third year the amount of recovery after surgery is evaluated. By means of palliative surgery an attempt is made to achieve maximal usefulness of returned motor and sensory functions.

Phase Five

A final evaluation is done after all possibilities of palliative surgery are exhausted. If there is significant functional return a final decision regarding the patient's professional activities is made. If no improvement has occurred, amputation at the upper arm level might be considered. If the patient has good elbow flexion but no sensibility and no motility in the hand, forearm amputation and fitting of a prosthesis might be an acceptable solution.

SPECIAL PROBLEMS

Primary Treatment

When the brachial plexus injury is due to an open wound, repair of skin, bone, and subclavian vessels, which are often involved, is the aim of the primary treatment. Nerve repair is performed as an early secondary procedure some weeks after the injury.

In any case of closed injury it is extremely important to recognize the presence of continuous compression of the brachial plexus by a bone fragment, hematoma, or edema. If this occurs, emergency surgery to achieve decompression is indicated.

Delayed Admission

The chances of direct repair are significantly reduced if the patient is admitted more than six months after the injury. However, improvement is possible if a first, second, or third degree lesion is present and spontaneous recovery has been prevented by external or internal pressure.

Partial Lesions

When the lesion is partial and the remaining parts of the brachial plexus are intact, the surgeon must decide whether direct repair or immediate reconstructive surgery is indicated. In any upper brachial plexus lesion one might decide to immediately perform a pectoralis or latissimus transfer to replace the biceps muscle function. My personal view is that one should also attempt to restore the continuity in order to achieve neurotization of a paralyzed muscle; if this fails, reconstructive surgery offers a second chance.

Age

It is evident that the chances of recovery decrease with age. There might be an age limit beyond which the chances are nil. However, it is very difficult to determine this limit for individual cases. Our attitude is to actively treat the lesion in order to gain even small functional improvements if there is no general contraindication to a long operation and general anesthesia.

Pain Syndromes

Some patients suffer from a severe pain syndrome. One has the impression that the syndrome is more likely to occur in lesions in which continuity is preserved. Chordotomy is indicated in severe cases. The frequency of pain syndromes in operated patients is lower than in unoperated cases.

DIRECT REPAIR

Neurotization of the denervated part càn be achieved by direct repair, making spontaneous recovery possible if continuity is restored; continuity can be by nerve grafting or by bringing in new axons from other nerves.

Preparation

A brachial plexus repair takes six to eight hours or longer. The patient must be carefully prepared for such a long procedure. If there is a strong probability that there is a fourth or fifth degree lesion and that nerve grafts will be needed, it is wise to provide some nerve grafts as a first step. For this, the patient is placed in a prone position (remaining in this position during this part of the operation) while the two sural nerves are excised. After skin closure and dressing, the patient is turned on his back, and the operative field in the brachial plexus area is prepared. In the meantime the two nerve grafts are stored in Ringer's solution.

For exposure of the brachial plexus the patient is lying on his back with a thin pillow underneath the scapula area, so that the shoulder and thoracic wall of the paralyzed side are slightly raised. This gives sufficient access to the thoracic wall if intercostal nerve transfer is indicated. The involved side — neck, mandible, the ventral and lateral side of the thorax, the shoulder, arm, forearm and hand are cleaned. This is necessary to enable the operator to obtain additional nerve grafts by excising the medical cutaneous nerves of the arm and forearm, the superficial branch of the radial nerve, and parts of the ulnar nerve, if necessary.

Exposure

The incision follows the posterior border of the sternocleidomastoid muscle. It turns at the area of the sternoclavicular joint and follows the clavicle. At the middle of the peripheral half of the clavicle, it turns again and crosses the pectoral area by an additional zig-zag incision. The exposure is extended to the proximal part of the upper arm on its medial surface. It is not always necessary to use the whole incision, but the incision must be planned in a way that will allow it to be lengthened, as outlined above. Two skin flaps are raised, one dorsally based flap of supraclavicular area skin and one medially based flap of infraclavicular area skin (Fig. 33–1).

Precise hemostasis is necessary during all stages of this operation. The external jugular vein is exposed and ligated at its proximal end on the neck and on its distal end where it leaves the lateral neck triangle. By blunt dissection in the ventral part of the field, dorsal to the sternocleidomastoid muscle, the scalenus anterior muscle is exposed, as is the phrenic nerve, which runs on top of this

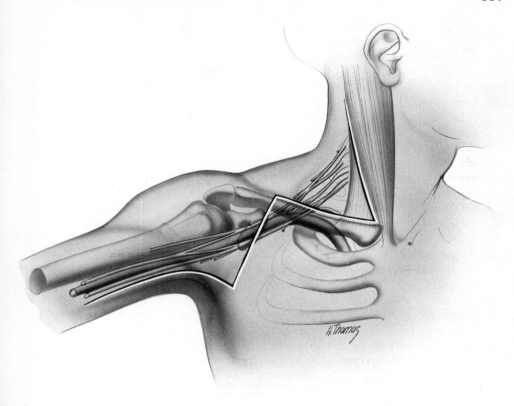

Figure 33-1   Incision recommended for complete exposure of the brachial plexus.

muscle in a slight curve from lateral cranial to caudal medial. The phrenic nerve is followed in a central direction and in this way the C4 root is easily defined. This root is usually not involved in a brachial plexus lesion; it can contribute a thick branch to the upper trunk. If the C4 root is incorporated into the brachial plexus, the plexus then contains the C4 to C8 roots; this is called prefixation. Having exposed the C4 root, the operator follows the same layer of the scalenus medius muscle in a caudal direction to expose the C5 root. In a root or trunk lesion (I, II, III) the scalenus medius muscle becomes very fibrotic, and dissection can be extremely difficult. If no root is encountered the transverse process is defined and the entrance into the intervertebral canal exposed. One must be careful to avoid damage to the vertebral artery. If no stump is met in the intervertebral canal, the root has been avulsed (I). In contrast to prefixation, the C5 root can be excluded from the brachial plexus. Then the brachial plexus will contain the C6 to T2 roots (postfixation).

The C6 root is defined by dissecting in the caudal direction. It is difficult to dissect to the remaining roots without lifting the clavicle. Therefore, at this stage, the exposure of the infraclavicular part of the brachial plexus is performed. At this stage, the operator enters between the deltoid and major pectoralis. The cephalic vein is defined. The pectoralis is detached at its origin from the clavicle. The pectoralis minor muscle is defined and put on a sling.

Depending on the situation, the operator can expose the cords below or above the pectoralis minor muscle. The first structure met is the lateral cord. Posterior to the lateral cord one can easily define the dorsal cord. Medial to the lateral cord one finds the axillary artery, and still farther medially, the axillary vein. The medial cord is exposed by entering between the axillary artery and the lateral cord; it is the deepest structure. As it is much easier to define the individual structure in normal tissue, the dissection always starts as far distally as necessary to be within healthy tissue.

After definition of the structures the dissection proceeds in a central direction. It is rather easy to proceed along the lateral and dorsal cords, exposing the interconnections between these two structures and reaching the trunk level underneath the clavicle. To follow the medial aspects of the lateral and medial cords is much more difficult because it is necessary to preserve the vessels and the nerve branches supplying the pectoralis muscles.

At this stage of the dissection, a connection is achieved between the infra- and supraclavicular fields of dissection. The clavicle is lifted. The lateral part of the sternocleidomastoid muscle is detached from the clavicle. The omohyoid muscle is transected. The subclavius muscle is also transected, and the vessels to it are carefully ligated. Now the clavicle can be lifted in a cranial direction. From the infraclavicular area the surgeon proceeds with the exposure along the dorsal and lateral cords to reach the upper and middle trunk. At this level the suprascapular nerve is seen leaving the brachial plexus and going in a lateral direction. Along the medial border of the medial cord the brachial plexus is separated from the subclavian artery. This part of the operation can be extremely difficult because at times the brachial plexus is fixed by scar tissue in the depth of the infraclavicular fossa, in the angle between the clavicle and the first rib.

Further dissection can be facilitated by transecting the clavicle, using an oblique osteotomy. This procedure is recommended by Narakas (1972). In the majority of our cases osteotomy of the clavicle has not been necessary. Sufficient exposure can be achieved by operating from above and below, lifting the clavicle in either a caudal or cranial direction. The advantage of avoiding the osteotomy is evident — no complication such as retarded bone healing or callus formation can occur. After separation of the brachial plexus from the subclavian artery, the inferior trunk can be isolated from below the clavicle. After its isolation the dissection continues in the supraclavicular fossa, lifting the clavicle in a caudal direction until the C8 and T1 roots are exposed. The C7 root is defined in a similar way.

Selection of Technique

Having completed the exposure the following questions must be answered:

1. Is the continuity of all roots, trunks, and cords preserved?
2. If continuity is interrupted, are there proximal stumps with neuromas available for all roots?
3. Do the proximal stumps have normal nerve tissue, so that regeneration can occur after restoration of continuity?

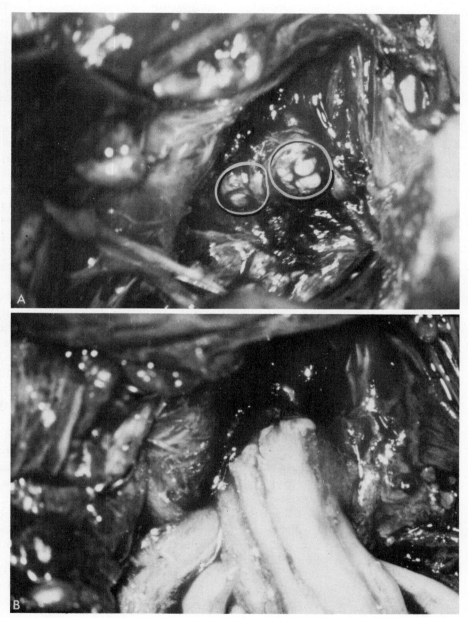

Figure 33–2 *A,* Exploration of a left brachial plexus. Close-up view of C5 and C6 roots after resection of the neuromas. *B,* The nerve grafts are in place. The grafts cover the cross sections of C5 and C6. They were united with the superior and middle trunks and with the peripheral stump of the suprascapular nerve.

(A) If continuity is preserved an external neurolysis is performed and everything removed that might compress or constrict the brachial plexus at any level. The epineurium is exposed and incised proximal and distal to the lesion. After reflection of the epineurium, the dissection proceeds toward the site of the lesion within a gap between the epineurium and the fascicular tissue. As the surgeon approaches the lesion, epineurium becomes more and more fibrotic and thickened. Very often the epineurium constricts the fascicular tissue like a tight stocking, and after its incision the fascicles can be seen to expand. This is a good prognostic sign, and in this case the operation can be finished. If the interfascicular tissue has become fibrotic, it has to be excised by interfascicular dissection, in order to relieve compression on the fascicles. If the fibrosis also involves the perineural and endoneural tissue, the damage is too great to allow spontaneous regeneration, and resection and restoring the continuity of the involved parts by nerve grafting are indicated.

(B) If continuity is interrupted at a peripheral level (II, III, IV), a neuroma will develop at the proximal stump. After proper resection until normal fascicular tissue is encountered, the continuity can be restored by nerve grafting (Figs. 33–2A and 33–2B). In certain cases the proximal stumps end within an unorganized mass of scar tissue. A complete exposure is then not necessary. After resection of the proximal stumps the fibrotic area is bypassed by nerve grafts.

If the lesion is situated at root levels and no proximal stump can be detected (I), the root has been avulsed. In combined lesions (I/II) with one or two avulsed roots (I) but three or four good-looking stumps of the remaining roots (II), the avulsion is ignored and the continuity is restored between the three or four remaining roots and the peripheral parts of the brachial plexus. If three or four roots are avulsed, a neurotization of the corresponding peripheral parts of the brachial plexus by intercostal nerve transfer is indicated, along with restoration of continuity of the stumps of the remaining ruptured roots by nerve grafts.

(C) In complete loss of continuity, if the root stumps can be exposed a resection is performed to judge a cross section. The resection is repeated until the cross section looks normal with good fascicular structures and without scar tissue. There are roots that consist of one big fascicle (monofascicular) and others that consist of small fascicles (polyfascicular). If the stump consists more or less of scar tissue, and no normal fascicular tissue can be exposed by such resections, the presence of a supraganglionic lesion is suspected. In this case the root cannot be used as a proximal stump and neurotization by intercostal nerve transfer must be performed.

Restoration of Continuity

If a proximal stump can be exposed and by resection normal looking fascicular tissue can be exposed, continuity with the corresponding peripheral part can be restored. Very rarely an end to end neurorrhaphy is possible. In the vast majority of cases the defects are too large to be overcome by mobilization and lifting of the upper arm and the shoulder girdle. Therefore, nerve grafting is the routine procedure to restore continuity. The nerve grafts are cut into pieces about 20 per cent longer than the defect to be bridged. The proximal ends of the grafts are approximated to the proximal stumps by one single 10-0 nylon stitch. In case of a big monofascicular root a fascicular nerve repair 1:4 or 1:5 is performed. If the root is polyfascicular, the nerve grafts are distributed to sectors of the root cross section (sectoral nerve grafting). Coaptation with the peripheral stumps is achieved in a similar way. If only one root stump is present, it is united with the dorsal cord to get nerve fibers into the shoulder and the radial nerve innervated muscles. If two root stumps are present, one is united with the dorsal cord and the other with the lateral cord. If three roots are available the upper one is united with the dorsal cord, the second with the lateral cord, the third with the medial cord. If four roots are present, two of them are united with the lateral cord, the third one with the dorsal cord, and the fourth one with the medial cord. If five roots are present, two of them are united with the lateral cord, two with the dorsal cord, and the remaining one with the medial cord. If there are short defects at trunk level, each trunk is restored by nerve grafts, as close to the normal anatomy as possible.

Intercostal Nerve Transfer

If only one or two roots are avulsed, intercostal nerve transfer is not worthwhile. But if at least three roots are avulsed, intercostal nerve transfer is indicated. There are three basic ways to achieve intercostal nerve transfer:

1. The whole length of the intercostal nerves is exposed, and the nerve is transposed to permit end to end coaptation with the peripheral stumps of the brachial plexus. An advantage is that only one coaptation need be performed. However, in the peripheral parts of the intercostal nerves the relation between motor and sensory fibers is changing in favor of sensory fibers.
2. If there is a root avulsion without much damage to the intraganglionic part (I) the whole root and trunk can be transposed down to get it close to the intercostal nerve. An end to end nerve repair is possible. A disadvantage is that the avulsed part might have suffered damage and neurotization be difficult.
3. A third possibility consists of exposure of the intercostal nerves in the midaxillary line, transecting them and uniting the proximal stump with a nerve graft, the peripheral end of which is coapted with the peripheral stumps of individual peripheral nerves. Up to seven intercostal nerves have been transferred in a single patient. The following peripheral nerves have been used to receive axons by intercostal nerve transfer in the following sequence of preference: musculocutaneous, median, radial, axillary, thoracodorsal and pectoral.

Wound Closure

After careful hemostasis and reattachment of the detached parts of the pectoralis major and the sternocleidomastoid muscles, the skin wound is closed carefully, avoiding translocation of the grafts by shearing forces. Small drains are inserted into the wound edges, but no suction drainage is used.

Immobilization

The head, neck, thorax, and involved arm are immobilized in plaster of Paris for 10 days, after which passive exercises to prevent joint stiffness are started.

RECONSTRUCTIVE SURGERY

The treatment of patients with brachial plexus lesions must be complete. After the results of the direct repair of the brachial plexus are fully evaluated, palliative surgery to achieve optimal use of the returned functions must be planned. The following procedures can be considered.

Arthrodesis of the Shoulder Joint. Denervation of the shoulder muscles causes a lack of soft tissue support to the shoulder joint, and subluxation of the shoulder joint develops. Subluxation of the shoulder joint is a constant feature of a long-standing brachial plexus lesion. This may indicate the need for an arthrodesis. Even in cases with rather poor regeneration after direct repair, the shoulder muscles regained sufficient tone to prevent this subluxation. In these instances there was no reason to perform an arthrodesis. As the scapula retains good active motion an arthrodesis in slightly abducted and elevated position could improve the motility of the arm. This was suggested in the past in connection with an amputation and fitting of a prosthesis at an upper arm level. According to our experience patients are not pleased with such an arthrodesis because of the fixed position of the upper arm.

Transfer of a Portion of the Trapezius Muscle to Obtain Some Abduction of the Shoulder Joint. This procedure was done in several cases, the results were encouraging if the trapezius muscle was transposed with the acromion and fixed to the humerus.

Transfer of the Pectoralis Major Muscle to Achieve Abduction of the Shoulder Joint. Wide abduction of the shoulder joint is really not necessary but some patients need only a small amount of abduction in order to lift the elbow when writing. This abduction can be achieved by transferring the pectoralis major muscle after detachment of its origin and its insertion to the level of the midportion of the deltoid muscle. This operation has to be performed in two stages because the neurovascular pedicles are not long enough to allow the transfer in a single stage.

Transfer of a Portion of the Pectoralis Major Muscle to Obtain Elbow Flexion (Clark, 1946). This is a very good operation that has proved its usefulness. However, it evidently can be performed only if a strong pectoralis muscle is present.

Transfer of the Latissimus Dorsi Muscle to Achieve Flexion (Axer, Segal, and Elkon, 1973; Zancolli and Mitre, 1973). This transposition has been performed in rare cases with good success.

Transfer of the Pectoralis Major or Latissimus Dorsi Muscle to Achieve External

Rotation. Good results can be expected if the muscle to be transposed is strong enough.

Transfer of the Triceps Muscle to Achieve Elbow Flexion. If the biceps muscle is paralyzed and the triceps muscle still functions, a transfer of the triceps tendon to the biceps tendon can provide some elbow flexion. We have no experience with this operation, but there are cases after regeneration of the biceps and triceps muscles as a result of a direct brachial plexus repair with simultaneous reinnervation of these antagonistic muscles occurs. On occasion, the patient is unable to flex his elbow because both the biceps and the triceps mucles contract simultaneously. In this instance, transfer of the triceps tendon to the biceps tendon has resulted in good flexion of the elbow joint.

Transposition of the Common Head of the Forearm Flexors to the Humerus Shaft to Achieve Elbow Flexion. Good results have been achieved by this operation in patients with upper brachial plexus lesions who had strong forearm muscles (Steindler, 1918).

Arthrodesis of the Wrist Joint. In a high percentage of cases some forearm muscle function returns, as does good elbow flexion by the biceps muscle. In these situations, arthrodesis of the wrist joint offers a possibility that the wrist flexors or extensors may be utilized to achieve the return of other functions. Arthrodesis, using a plate between the radius and the third metacarpal bones, is performed, preserving the motion in the distal radioulnar joint to preserve pronation and supination.

An individual reconstructive procedure, similar to the one used in radial and median nerve palsy, must be developed for each patient (depending on the return of function in each specific case).

Palliative Surgery at Finger Levels. When continuity has been lost function of intrinsic muscles does not return. Therefore, normal hand function is never achieved. However, it is possible in many cases to obtain primitive grip function by fixing the thumb in opposition to the fingers by a bone graft between the first and second metacarpal bone, performing an arthrodesis of the interphalangeal joint of the thumb and the proximal interphalangeal and distal interphalangeal joints of the fingers, concentrating the available muscles on the metacarpal joint of the thumb and the metacarpophalangeal joint of the fingers to achieve pinch and hook functions.

If no muscle has recovered, a tenodesis is performed to obtain pinch when the forearm is supinated by biceps muscle function.

CONSERVATIVE TREATMENT

Conservative treatment is performed before, between, and after operation. Three goals should be achieved by this treatment:

1. Preservation of joint mobility by passive motion of all joints. Soft tissue contractures are treated by active splinting.
2. Prevention of elongation of muscles and tendons and support of regenerating muscles against stronger antagonists or gravity. Elongation of the biceps muscle or the wrist extensors can be prevented by splinting the elbow joint in flexion and the wrist joint in neutral position. If regenera-

tion commences in the biceps muscle, the regenerating muscle should be protected against elongation by splinting the elbow joint in a flexed position. If the regenerating muscle is strong enough to maintain the elbow joint in flexed position against gravity, a slowly increasing amount of extension is allowed. In a similar way, transposed muscles, such as the pectoralis major or the latissimus dorsi, are protected against elongation until the transfer insertion site has regained full strength.

3. Stimulation of the denervated muscles by triangular impulses with exponential slope. Faradic stimulation is used in muscles paralyzed because of a first degree lesion only. The regular treatment before, between, and after the operations has a very important psychological effect; this is an additional reason to insist on such treatment.

RESULTS

The results are evaluated by clinical examination. We have adopted the scale developed by Wright (1912), as it is extensively described by Daniels, Williams and Worthingham (1961). Six degrees of motor function are differentiated:

> M O — complete palsy
> M 1 — muscle contraction without effect
> M 2 — muscle contraction with visible effect if gravity is excluded
> M 3 — active motion against gravity
> M 4 — active motion against gravity and resistance
> M 5 — active motion against strong resistance

M3 recovery was regarded as a useful recovery. Useful recovery for the shoulder joint was assumed if the patient could lift the arm against gravity to achieve positions of functional value, regardless of the range of motion. However, we should remember that a much lesser degree of recovery is beneficial for the patient, because subluxation in the shoulder joint is prevented. Recovery of the elbow joint was considered useful if the patient could flex the elbow joint to more than 90 degrees against gravity and simultaneously achieve supination. Recovery was regarded as useful (M3) if the patient could move a wrist joint against gravity, flex the fingers to reach the palm, and grasp an object.

As far as sensibility is concerned the return of tactilegnosis cannot be expected. Return of protective sensibility (pain, touch and temperature) could be observed in all cases.

There was also significant improvement in sympathetic functions in all patients.

Recovery of Motor Function

The following data on motor recovery are based on a series of 54 cases, operated as a continuous series between 1964 and 1972. During this period two additional patients have been observed who have suffered avulsion of all five roots. These two patients were not operated upon.

Complete Brachial Plexus Palsy due to Root Lesion

There were 18 cases within this group. Four patients had avulsion of four roots, five patients avulsion of three roots, one patient avulsion of two roots, and eight patients avulsion of one root only. All these patients had combined avulsion and rupture lesions (I/II). If we include the two cases with avulsion of all five roots who were not operated, we can state that in a group of 20 patients with root avulsion only two had avulsion of all five roots. The remaining 18 patients had, in addition to avulsion of some roots, infraganglionic lesions with nerve stumps suitable to be used to restore continuity. In 12 patients all the roots had suffered a fifth degree lesion (loss of continuity) but six patients had, in addition to root avulsion and ruptures, some roots with preserved continuity (third degree). In all six cases the upper roots were ruptured or avulsed but in the lower roots continuity was preserved.

The following useful recovery was achieved:

Shoulder	5 of 18 cases
Elbow flexion	9 of 18 cases
Elbow triceps muscle alone	1 of 18 cases
Wrist and fingers	2 of 18 cases

The results given in the above scale are a result of motor recovery after the operation. Some of these results could be improved by reconstructive surgery; as happened, for example, in a case of recovery of the triceps muscle only wherein a transfer of this tendon to the biceps tendon brought about active elbow flexion.

In four of the six patients mentioned above, who suffered rupture and avulsion of the upper roots but in whom continuity of the lower roots was preserved, useful recovery occurred in the upper root innervated muscles, which were restored by nerve grafts only, but not in the muscles supplied by the lower roots, which had only neurolysis. Alnot et al. (1975) reported similar results in a series of patients following conservative treatment without operation, with a followup of many years. It is evident that spontaneous recovery can occur only when continuity is preserved. In this series of 18 patients, continuity was lost in all roots with the exception of the lower roots of six patients who did not show any spontaneous recovery. Therefore, this series of 18 cases cannot be compared in any way with the series of Alnot et al. On the contrary, one can assume that Alnot's cases had sustained partial third degree lesions with spontaneous recovery. In our series the fifth degree lesion of the roots was transformed into a third degree lesion by restoring the continuity via nerve grafts. This assumption explains very well the similarity of the results (Fig. 33–3).

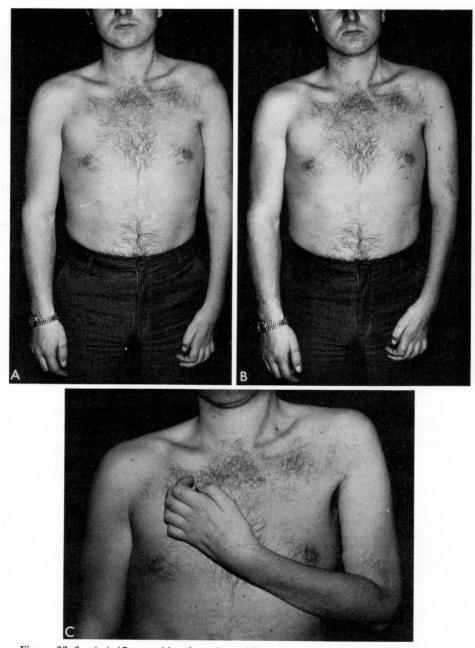

Figure 33–3 *A*, A 17-year-old male patient with a complete brachial plexus palsy following a traffic accident. There was no evidence of spontaneous recovery. Note the atrophy of the shoulder muscle and the subluxation of the humerus. *B*, Two years after restoration of continuity by interfunicular nerve grafts there is return of function in the shoulder muscles. There is less atrophy and no subluxation of the shoulder. *C*, The biceps is functioning and there is strong elbow flexion. Some of the forearm flexors recovered but no functional return of the intrinsic muscles was observed. Protective sensibility was present and there was no trophic problem. This case represents an average result.

Complete Palsy due to a Peripheral Lesion

The following useful recovery was achieved:

Shoulder	6 of 13 cases
Elbow	7 of 13 cases
Wrist	5 of 13 cases
Fingers	5 of 13 cases

In the majority of these cases continuity was preserved and neurolysis was performed to encourage spontaneous recovery.

Partial Palsy due to a Root Lesion

There were 11 cases in this group. The following useful recovery was achieved:

Shoulder	3 of 10 cases with loss of shoulder function
Elbow	7 of 9 cases with loss of elbow function
Wrist	3 of 7 cases with loss of wrist function
Fingers	3 of 7 cases with loss of finger function

In the majority of these cases nerve grafting and neurolysis had to be performed.

Partial Palsy due to Peripheral Lesions

There were 12 patients in this group. The following useful function was achieved:

Shoulder	7 of 10 cases with loss of shoulder function
Elbow	8 of 9 cases with loss of elbow function
Wrist	3 of 6 cases with loss of wrist function
Fingers	3 of 8 cases with loss of finger function

It should be noted in the partial root and peripheral nerve lesion that not all joints were equally affected. Some joints were spared.

Complications

Pseudarthrosis of the clavicle occurred in two of that group of patients in whom osteotomy of the clavicle was performed.

A hematoma developed in two patients, and this resulted in delayed healing and local infection. The cases become complete failures.

No pneumothorax or lesion of a major vessel occurred in this series.

Three of the patients with partial palsy showed temporary increased weakness after neurolysis. All three had full recovery. This indicates that none of the patients who had partial lesions and who had microsurgical neurolysis permanently lost any of their function.

One patient developed a severe pain syndrome which could not be controlled by neurosurgical intervention. Because of the persisting pain, the patient requested amputation, in spite of the fact that the biceps muscle had recovered well.

REFERENCES

Alnot, J. Y., Cadre, N., Frot, D. and Sedel, L.: Etude clinique et paraclinique plus evolution spontanée de paralysie plexus brachial. 50ème Réunion Annuelle de Soc. Francaise de Chirurgie Orthopédique et Traumatologique, Paris, Nov., 1975, p. 4.

Axer, A., Segal, D., and Elkon, A.: Partial transposition of the latissimus dorsi. J. Bone Joint Surg. *55A*:1259, 1073.

Clark, J. M. P.: Reconstruction of biceps brachii by pectoral muscle transplantation. Brit. J. Surg. *34*:180, 1946.

Daniels, S., Williams, M., and Worthingham, C.: Muscle Testing. 2nd Ed., Philadelphia, W. B. Saunders Co., 1961.

Narakas, A.: Plexo brachial Rev. Ortop. Traumatol. *16*:855, 1972.

Seddon, H. J.: Surgical disorders of the peripheral nerves. London, Churchill Livingstone, 1972.

Steindler, A.: A muscle plasty for relief of flail in infantile paralysis. Interstate Med. J., *25*:235, 1918.

Sunderland, A.: A classification of peripheral nerve injuries producing loss of function. Brain 74: 491, 1951.

Wright, N. G.: Muscle training in the treatment of infantile paralysis. Boston Med. Sci. J.: *167*:567, 1912.

Zancolli, E., and Mitre, H.: Latissimus dorsi transfer to restore elbow flexion. J. Bone Joint Surg. *55A*:1265, 1973.

34

MANAGEMENT OF NERVE COMPRESSION LESIONS OF THE UPPER EXTREMITY

MORTON SPINNER

PRINCIPLES

In the management of a neural compression lesion, early recognition of the etiology is an essential requirement. A mechanical lesion of a specific peripheral nerve, or one of its major branches, is reflected in a disturbance of specific motor and/or sensory function within the extremity. It is essential that the precise level of the lesion be identified in order to accurately plan effective treatment. This can be accomplished by careful clinical examinations and by electroneuromyographic techniques. The physician who directs his attention to the wrong pathological process or to the wrong neural localization, or to both, leaves the patient essentially untreated.

Assessment of a neural lesion may require several quantitative tests, which are repeated at regular intervals for comparison and prognosis (Omer and Spinner, 1975). Both motor and sensory function must be evaluated. The choice of therapy and the timing of necessary surgical intervention must be individualized, and a thorough evaluation of the injured nerve and its peripheral end organs, muscle fibers and sensory organelles will dictate the optimal therapeutic approach. At times, conservative care, consisting of proper immobilization, diuretics, and local steroids when indicated, may reverse the process. If the symptoms do not subside, or if they recur, then prompt surgical intervention is indicated. Complete spontaneous paralysis due to an en-

569

trapment lesion should not be left untreated surgically for more than three months because the degree of injury to the nerve worsens with the passage of time. If the total paralysis is permitted to exist without relief for 18 months, the pathological process often becomes irreversible, since internal fibrosis occurs within the nerve. The final pathological event is a fourth-degree neural lesion, a neuroma in continuity.

Advanced age in a patient is not a factor affecting recovery following neural compression because older patients do recover well following appropriate neurolysis. However, in this age group, when the neural lesion is of the fourth-degree type (neuroma in continuity), the results of nerve repair are unpredictable and often poor.

CLASSIFICATION OF NEURAL COMPRESSION LESIONS

There are two recognized methods of classifying neural injuries (Seddon, 1943; Sunderland, 1968), each of which represents an attempt to correlate the degree of injury with the characteristic symptomatology and localized neural pathology. Sir Herbert Seddon's classification employs three terms to describe the degree of the severity of the injury — neurapraxia, axonotmesis, and neurotmesis. Sir Sidney Sunderland has a five-fold system of classifying nerve injuries. They can be compared in the following manner:

Correlation of Seddon and Sunderland Classification of Nerve Injuries

		Sunderland					
		First	Second	Third	Fourth	Fifth	(Degree)
	Neurapraxia	////////					
Seddon	Axonotmesis		////////	////////			
	Neurotmesis				////////	////////	////////	

Shaded areas indicate equivalent terms.

Seddon's neurapraxia is analogous to Sunderland's first degree of injury. Neurapraxia is characterized by complete motor paralysis with little sensory or autonomic involvement, and is a transient syndrome. A classical example of neurapraxia may be seen in a limb following the passage of a bullet close to a major nerve (Mitchell, 1872). Recovery from an episode of neurapraxia is often rapid and excellent.

The next level of severity is called axonotmesis by Seddon and includes all second-degree and some mild third-degree injuries in the Sunderland classification. In this type of nerve injury, motor, sensory, and autonomic nerve dysfunction are complete. Muscle atrophy is progressive. The nerve fibers are separated into proximal and distal sections, but the continuity of their Schwann tubes is maintained (Thomas, 1964, 1966). The distal fibers are phagocytized. Restoration of muscle-nerve continuity by the regenerating proximal axons determines the motor and sensory recovery. However, while there is a good prognosis with this degree of injury, the interval of recovery depends on the distance between the muscle to be reinnervated and the site of axonotmesis.

The third-degree lesion of Sunderland may correspond, in Seddon's classification, to either axonotmesis, or to neurotmesis, depending on the extent of the neural injury. In a third-degree injury, the nerve fibers, along with their Schwann tubes, are damaged within intact nerve fascicles. Some of these lesions are reversible, and these fall into the axonotmetic group. However, in the more severely involved group of third degree neural lesions, the process may be irreversible because of the number of axons damaged and the extent of the irreversible fibrotic process within the funiculi.

The fourth-degree lesion is a neuroma in continuity. There is no gross separation of the nerve and no retraction of nerve ends but, microscopically, the axons are in complete disarray and are not structurally in continuity. Loss of continuity of the nerve trunk is designated as a fifth-degree injury. This neural lesion occurs when the nerve is actually severed and the ends retract. This degree of injury is not seen with compression lesions.

It is important to note that, while classification of nerve injury is useful to the clinician, each of the methods yields only an approximation of the true degree of nerve injury. A lesion, even in experimentally controlled situations, will seldom produce a single pattern of nerve fiber damage. In one fascicle, different fibers may suffer neurapraxia, axonotmesis, or neurotmesis. In general, the extent of the nerve fiber damage will increase in severity with time as the mechanical forces continue to influence the site of the lesion (Spinner and Spencer, 1974).

CLINICAL CORRELATION OF THE DEGREE OF NERVE INJURY

The Lesions of Neurapraxia

There appear to be three lesions of neurapraxia. The first is probably ionic and is related to electrolyte imbalance (Kuczynski, 1974). The second is vascular. Classically, it has been described as an ischemia (Denny-Brown and Brenner, 1944), but in recent years this type of neurapraxia has been thought to be due to anoxia at the capillary level within the funiculi, caused by venous obstruction in the epineurium (Lundborg, 1970; Sunderland, 1976). The third neurapractic lesion is mechanical, with structural changes of the myelin sheath in a short segment of the nerve fibers due to compression-shear forces (Gilliatt et al., 1974; Ochoa, 1974).

Clinically, the speed of return of function suggests the type of neurapractic lesion. A rapid recovery, within hours of neurolysis, suggests the ionic or anoxic type, while if thirty or sixty days passes before recovery, then a structural neurapractic lesion is most likely.

Most neurapractic lesions that respond to nonoperative treatment will do so within three months. If the patient has a neural compression persisting for more than three months, surgical exploration of the nerve at the level of the lesion is indicated. The length of the time for recovery after surgery for a neurapractic lesions depends upon whether the nerve must undergo a process of segmental demyelination and remyelination. If such a process is necessary, recovery usually takes one to two months rather than hours or days, as observed with nonstructural neurapractic lesions. If a neurapractic lesion is left untreated, it can increase in severity.

Axonotmetic Lesions

This classification of Seddon includes all of the second-degree lesions and the mild third-degree lesions of Sunderland. In a pure axonotmetic lesion the nerve fiber is damaged at the point of compression. However, the basement membrane of the axon is maintained. There is complete wallerian degeneration distal to the level of the compression. As the nerve heals, new axonal sprouting and growth from the point of disruption occurs, along with the formation of a new myelin sheath. The time for recovery depends on the distance of the motor end-plates and sensory end-organs from the lesion. The closer the end-plates, the faster the recovery. Following neurolysis of an axonotmetic neural lesion, it may take five to six months or more, because recovery depends upon the level of the lesion and the location of the closest motor end-plate to be reinnervated.

Neurotmetic Lesions

This category consists of all fourth-degree lesions and advanced third-degree lesions of Sunderland. A fourth-degree lesion is characterized by complete fibrosis of a segment of the nerve. With a complete neurotmetic lesion, a nonfunctioning, nonconductive neuroma in continuity exists. Excision of the neuroma and epineural repair is indicated. If the gap is too great for direct approximation, then interfunicular grafting is necessary. The prognosis depends upon the specific nerve involved, the duration of the paralysis, the age of the patient, and the level of the complete neurotmetic lesion. Sensory repair may be successful long after motor repair is impossible because of fibrosis of the muscle fibers and because of continued viability of the sensory organelles and of the thinly myelinated axons, which are capable of late regeneration (provided the distal endoneural tubes are patent).

When a nerve is lacerated and the ends retract, this lesion too is neurotmetic and falls into a lesion of the fifth degree, according to Sunderland's classification.

EVALUATION OF NEURAL LESIONS IN CONTINUITY

At times neural lesions in continuity can be evaluated accurately with ease but at other times may be baffling clinical dilemmas. When preoperative evaluation indicates that surgical intervention is indicated, be sure that the expo-

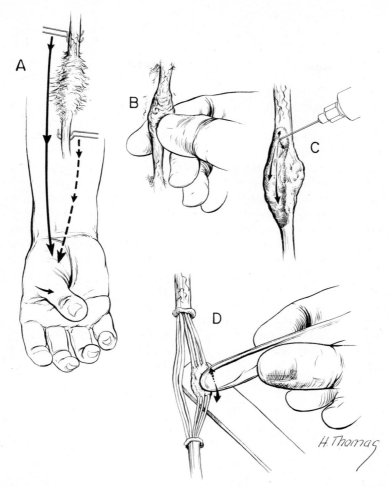

Figure 34–1   Intraoperative evaluation of a neuroma in continuity. *A*, Electrical stimulation of the nerve proximal and distal to the site of injury before the neuroma is separated from its bed. *B*, Palpation of the entire neural lesion. *C*, Saline injection followed by internal neurolysis if indicated. *D*, Palpation of several funiculi using a scalpel handle.

sure is adequate. The actual physical extent of this surgery is always much greater than the lesion itself. It is necessary to identify the normal proximal and distal regions of the nerve adjacent to the pathology, through anatomical planes. By dissecting toward the lesion from both directions, the neural lesion is exposed. One must be certain, during this phase of the external neurolysis, to avoid conversion of a first- or second-degree neural lesion to one of more advanced degree.

  Before separating the involved nerve segment from its scarred bed, electrical stimulation proximal and distal to the lesion is performed. The response to this bipolar stimulation is evaluated by observing the muscle reaction distally, or by recording the distal evoked nerve action potential (Fig. 34–1*A*). Axons of sufficient maturity to conduct nerve action potentials must extend well into the distal segment of the nerve weeks before electroneuromyographic evidence of recovery can be recorded (Kline, 1969, 1972). The extent of the axon population recovery can be correlated with the amplitude of the potential, proximal and distal to the lesion. The greater the number of conducting mature axons, the greater the amplitude of the nerve action potential that is recorded (Fig. 34–2*A* and *C*).

Palpation of the lesion may be helpful in the evaluation. A stony-hard neuroma in continuity has a poor prognosis for recovery by neurolysis, whereas a soft enlargement of the nerve is a favorable sign (Fig. 34–1*B*).

Intraneural injection of saline (Fig. 34–1*C*), followed by neurolysis — external and internal — utilizing the operating microscope or ocular magnification, is a helpful technique in dealing with some of these lesions (Brown, 1972).

The nerve can be evaluated on a funicular level. The gross appearance of the funiculi under magnification and the intraoperative firmness of the funicular neuromata can be evaluated with the aid of the scalpel handle (Fig. 34–1*D*). Single fascicular electrical recordings (Williams et al., 1976) offer a most critical intraoperative technique for evaluation of partial neural lesions (Fig. 34–2*B*).

Frequently, when dissecting the proximal and distal portions of the normal component of the nerve to the area of the compression, the nerve may be suddenly liberated. A fibrotic band or thrombosed blood vessel is released; the nerve is freed and is found to have a narrow area of indentation. There is no visible neuroma. The recovery pattern follows an axonotmetic course; the time for the first sign of motor recovery is related to the closeness to its first motor end-plate.

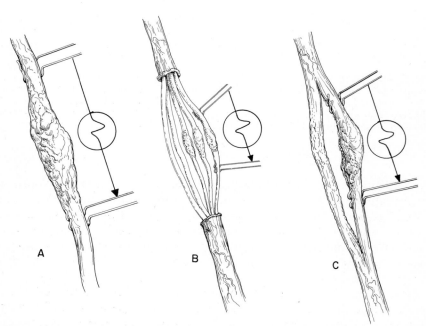

A   B   C

Figure 34–2 Intraoperative nerve action potentials can aid in the determination of the viability of the neuroma in continuity. This can be performed on the whole nerve (*A*), at the funicular level (*B*), and with the entire partial lesion (*C*).

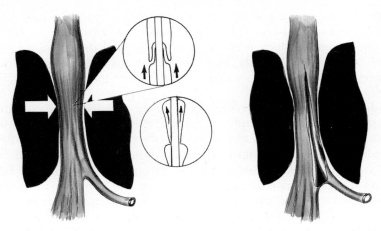

Figure 34–3 Internal neurolysis, when indicated, during the operative procedure should be limited to those funiculi which are clinically involved. This is correlated with the preoperative observations and the intraoperative findings, as well as with knowledge of the internal topography of the nerve. Even the neurapractic structural lesions (inserts), consisting of myelin intussusception or bulbous myelin formation, can heal following release of the neural compression.

With the neurapraxia group, recovery following neurolysis recovery may be prompt — hours to weeks. The neurapractic nerve lesion that responds following surgical release in this manner may reveal only locally increased or decreased vascular markings. In the carpal tunnel region, the neural injection is due to increased venous markings characteristic of the neurapractic lesion of the carpal tunnel syndrome (Sunderland, 1976). Lysis of the flexor retinaculum alone is sufficient to relieve symptoms and to restore function in this first-degree group of cases.

With elderly patients, the carpal compression symptomatology often has been permitted to exist for a prolonged period. In this group, second- and third-degree lesions are common. Depending upon the patient's predominant symptomatology, such as dysesthesia in the long finger or thumb, specific internal neurolysis, liberating only those fasciculi involved clinically, is performed (Fig. 34–3). Indiscriminate internal neurolysis can result in excessive local interfunicular fibrosis (Rydevik, 1976). Even in the severest of carpal tunnel syndromes with marked median nerve pathology (with advanced third-degree lesions), I have not as yet needed to resect, perform a neurorrhaphy, or nerve graft the lesion to relieve the patient's major complaints.

CLINICAL MANIFESTATIONS OF NEURAL ENTRAPMENT LESIONS IN THE UPPER EXTREMITY

Knowledge of the different types of clinical patterns of nerve entrapment lesions observed in practice makes it easier to diagnose the entity. Basically, the clinical presentation is relatively easy to recognize when the lesion is complete. Partial lesions, and complete lesions in upper limbs in which significant anatomical variations exist, can present diagnostic problems.

The neurological deficit follows a well-recognized distribution for each of the peripheral nerves. Basically, each nerve lesion can be clinically described as a high or low neural lesion — that is, a high or low median, radial, or ulnar lesion.

In addition, there are further refinements and localizations within this gross classification. For example, a complete low ulnar lesion at the pisiform should bring to mind a mixed lesion with a clawed ring and little finger, with sensory loss of these digits. However, when the ulnar lesion is at the hook of the hamate, sensation is normal throughout the hand. The motor intrinsic muscle paralysis is usually complete, or the hypothenar muscles may be spared. There can be many subtleties to intrinsic paralysis. For example, the intrinsic muscles of the first web space alone may be atrophic when an anatomical neural variant with a split deep motor branch exists which traverses about the hook of the hamate (Fenning, 1965; Lanz, 1974; Lassa and Shrewsbury, 1975). Similar localized atrophy of the first web space intrinsic musculature has been described as being caused by a ganglion in juxtaposition to the deep branch of the ulnar nerve at the level of the third metacarpal (McDowell, 1977). Therefore, atrophy of the muscles of the first web space can occur without ulnar nerve sensory disturbance, or other intrinsic muscle involvement can be observed when entrapment of the deep branch of the ulnar nerve occurs at a specific location. There need not be concern that the pathology must be at the spinal cord (anterior horn) cell level with purely intrinsic muscle involvement.

Pain in a particular area of the limb associated with a positive Tinel sign in the region is a valuable confirmatory physical finding, and is helpful in localizing the entrapment. Unfortunately, this combination is not always present.

Median Nerve Syndromes

Carpal Tunnel Syndrome (Paget, 1854; Marie and Foix, 1913; Phalen, 1951, 1966)

This syndrome is the result of median nerve compression at the volar aspect of the wrist. Extrinsic and intrinsic factors predispose to and can result in this condition. There is a relatively narrowed passage for the median nerve through the carpal tunnel, or the nerve is enlarged. It is a common entrapment syndrome, seen most frequently in females between the ages of 40 and 60.

Pain and paresthesias in the median nerve distribution of the hand are the usual complaints. Nocturnal burning pain, relieved by shaking the hand, is frequently reported. There are many symptoms of a carpal tunnel syndrome. All need not be present in any one case. The signs and symptoms include sensory disturbance of the radial 3-1/2 digits, atrophy of the thenar muscles, a positive Tinel sign at the wrist, a positive Phalen sign, and motor and sensory electroneuromyographic abnormalities. Frequently, however, numbness may be restricted to the long finger. There may be no thenar muscle atrophy and Tinel and Phalen signs may be negative. Twenty-five per cent of patients with this syndrome have a normal EMG, utilizing standard methods. However, with newer segmental digital-to-palm and palm-to-wrist comparative conduction studies, the correlation between clinical assessment and electrical confirmation is markedly improved (Buchthal et al., 1974).

When the recurrent motor branch of the median nerve alone is entrapped in the flexor retinaculum, there is just weakness of abduction of the thumb and thenar atrophy — no sensory disturbance in the hand (Papathanassiou, 1968). Here, neurolysis of this motor branch is essential. Sensitivity to cold may be a major presenting symptom. Sympathetic overflow, associated with carpal tunnel syndrome, has been observed (Linscheid, et al., 1967).

Median and ulnar nerve entrapment following fractures and dislocations of the wrist can be a cause of reflex dystrophy of the hand (Stein, 1962). It may be necessary to release one or both of these nerves in order to prevent or relieve the stiffness of the digits characteristic of reflex dystrophy. In this instance, early diagnosis of the neural entrapment can be confirmed by electromyographic studies and, with appropriate surgical intervention, the reflex dystrophic process can be aborted.

According to personal observations 50 per cent of patients with carpal tunnel syndrome respond to conservative treatment measures. The combined treatment of splinting the wrist in a neutral position and administering a diuretic is effective in these patients. Any underlying systemic disease should be brought under control. If conservative methods do not provide relief, it may be necessary to release the transverse carpal ligament. External neurolysis and, on occasion, internal neurolysis may be necessary (Curtis and Eversmann, 1973). Care must be taken to avoid injury to the median palmar cutaneous branch of the median nerve, as postoperative painful neuromata are a disturbing complication of this surgery (Carroll and Green, 1972; Inglis, Straub, and Williams, 1972.).

Anterior Interosseous Nerve Syndrome

This syndrome is caused by compression of the anterior interosseous branch of the median nerve, usually at a site close to its origin from this nerve. It is characterized by inability to flex the terminal phalanges of the thumb, index, and long fingers. Paralysis of the pronator quadratus muscle is also observed. There is a typical pinch attitude (Spinner, 1969) seen with this paralysis (Fig. 34–4). The remaining muscles innervated by the median nerve in the hand and forearm are intact. Sensation is undisturbed in the hand. With this localized paralysis, the patient still can oppose his thumb and can flex the proximal interphalangeal joints of the index and long fingers because the flexor digitorum superficialis is unaffected. Furthermore, there can be partial lesions of this major nerve branch, in which case there is an isolated paralysis of the flexor pollicis longus or flexor digitorum profundus of the index or long fingers. Pain in the proximal forearm frequently is a harbinger of these localized paralyses.

If a Martin–Gruber connection is present, there are variations in the clini-

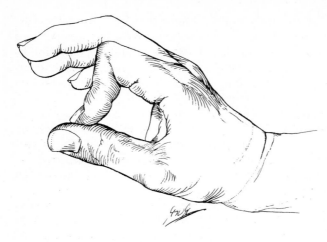

Figure 34–4 Typical pinch attitude seen with an anterior interosseous nerve paralysis.

cal pattern. This neural variant, occurring in approximately 15 per cent of limbs, transports ulnar fibers via the median nerve to the ulnar nerve in the proximal forearm. It connects frequently via the anterior interosseous branch of the median nerve and the ulnar nerve. With this anomaly, entrapment of the anterior interosseous nerve may produce some intrinsic muscle paralysis in the hand. Furthermore, through a connection within the substance of the flexor digitorum profundus muscle between the anterior interosseous branch of the median nerve and a motor branch of the ulnar nerve, the flexor digitorum profundus muscle is innervated to a variable degree by the median and ulnar nerves. Thus, flexion of the terminal phalanges may be variably disturbed in an anterior interosseous nerve syndrome (Spinner, 1970, 1978).

Exploration of this branch of the median nerve is indicated if the paralysis does not subside spontaneously within six to eight weeks. The median nerve should be identified proximal to the lacertus fibrosus and traced distally through the region of the pronator teres. The anterior interosseous nerve usually arises from the median nerve approximately 7 cm distal to the lateral epicondyle.

The most common restraining structure is the tendinous origin of the deep head of the pronator teres, which crosses the anterior interosseous branch at its hilum from the median nerve. Other causes of anterior interosseous nerve entrapment are an enlarged bicipital bursa, other variant tendinous structures, thrombosed ulnar collateral vessels, old penetrating forearm scars, and anomalous radial artery passage.

Isolated paralysis of the flexor pollicis longus, associated with axillary pain and percussion tenderness, has been described with an entrapment lesion of the median nerve in the axilla (Spinner, 1976). This is an important differential, especially when pain is not initially present in the forearm.

Pronator Syndrome

Entrapment of the median nerve in the proximal forearm is termed the pronator syndrome. While it is true that the greatest cause for, and localization of, the compression is at the pronator level, there are two other areas of potential entrapment in close proximity — at the lacertus fibrosus and at the flexor superficialis arch. Pathological localization to these areas is not as common as to the pronator teres (Johnson et al., 1979). Usually, the patient has a 9 to 24 month history of non-localized forearm pain. A frequent clinical finding is reproduction of the proximal forearm pain when forearm pronation is resisted. The pain is intensified when the flexed, pronated forearm is extended. This test is reliable for localizing the lesion to the pronator teres (Fig. 34–5A). Patients may report numbness in some digits innervated by the median nerve. While the

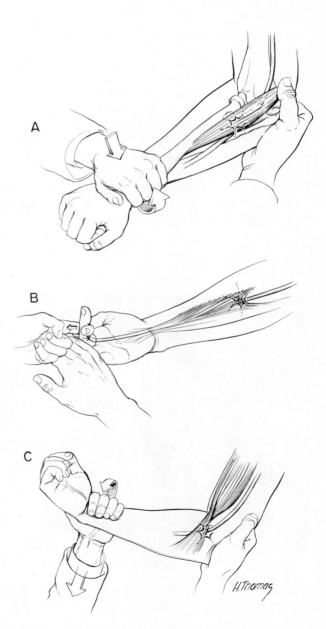

Figure 34–5 Tests for the site of compression in a pronator syndrome. *A,* When the forearm pain is reproduced by resistance to pronation of the forearm, and is aggravated by extending the elbow, the localization is to the pronator teres. *B,* When the pain occurs upon resistance to flexion of the flexor digitorum superficialis of the long finger, the examiner's fingers keep the patient's remaining fingers in extension, and resistance to flexion of the proximal interphalangeal joint of the long finger evaluates the flexor superficialis of this finger alone. This test localizes the compression to the flexor superficialis arch. *C,* When the forearm pain is reproduced by resistance to flexion of the elbow and supination of the forearm, the lacertus fibrosus is the offending fibrous structure.

Tinel sign can localize the level of the pathology, it may not appear for four to five months after the initial examination. Electromyographic evaluation can aid in the diagnosis, particularly when several serial studies are compared. It would be extremely helpful if a conduction delay were found. However, frequently, all that can be found electrically is the appearance of some positive sharp waves or fibrillations in some of the forearm median nerve-innervated muscles (Buchthal et al., 1974). It is important that these muscles be the ones innervated distal to the pronator teres to be of confirmatory value. If more proximal median innervated muscles, pronator teres, flexor carpi radialis, and palmaris longus have these findings, then a more proximal median nerve problem must be considered.

Pain in the proximal forearm, reproduced by resistance to flexion of the flexor digitorum superficialis of the long finger, helps to localize the pathology to the flexor superficialis arch (Fig. 35–5B). Consider the site of entrapment at the lacertus fibrosus when resistance to flexion of the elbow and supination of the forearm reproduce the pain (Fig. 34–5C). The Tinel sign is more proximally positive in the forearm when the lacertus fibrosus is the site of median nerve compression when compared with the other two localizations.

Conservative management should be utilized, initially. This consists of physical therapeutic measures, local steroid injections, immobilization, transcutaneous nerve stimulation, and anti-inflammatory medication. When surgical release is necessary, the median nerve is identified, first, proximal to the lacertus fibrosus and, then, as it passes through the flexor superficialis bridge. To accomplish the latter, it is necessary to develop the plane between the

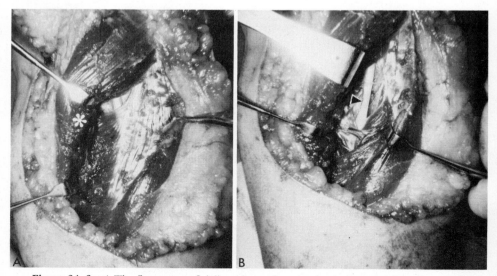

Figure 34–6   *A,* The flexor superficialis arch was found to be the compressing structure in this patient with a pronator syndrome of the right forearm. The inferior margin of the pronator teres(*) is retracted radially. The median nerve is seen passing posterior to the flexor superficialis arch. *B,* Upon release and excision of a portion of the flexor superficialis arch, the median nerve was found to be narrowed and devoid of vascular markings in the region.

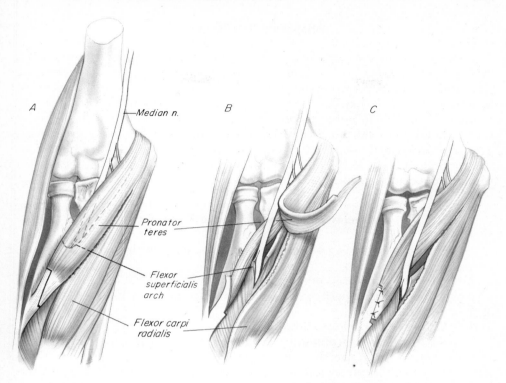

A ─Median n. *B* *C*

Pronator
teres

Flexor
superficialis
arch

Flexor carpi
radialis

Figure 34–7 *A*, When the median nerve is to be translocated into a subcutaneous bed in the proximal forearm, the median nerve is identified proximally and is traced through the two heads of the pronator teres (*A*). After opening the plane between the pronator teres and the flexor carpi radialis the median nerve is identified at its entrance to the flexor superficialis bridge (Fig. 34–6). The tendon of the pronator teres is then detached in a step-cut manner. Upon elevating the pronator teres, the median nerve is traced through the region and its numerous branches preserved. The flexor superficialis arch is incised (*B*). *C*. The median nerve is elevated. When necessary, its motor branches are liberated by opening the epineurium. The superficial head of the pronator teres is then passed posterior to the median nerve and is resutured.

lower border of the pronator teres and the proximal margin of the flexor carpi radialis. Then, the median nerve is traced between these two sites proximally and distally in the forearm, releasing all restraints upon it. These consist of the lacertus fibrosus, bands within the pronator teres, the deep tendinous origin of the pronator teres, hypertrophied pronator teres, thickened flexor superficialis arch, and accessory tendinous origin of the flexor carpi radialis from the ulna (Fig. 34–6*A* and *B*).

On occasion, with recurrent cases or with specific anomalies, such as a hypertrophied superficial head of the pronator teres, the median is translocated subcutaneously. This is accomplished by lengthening the pronator teres at its musculotendinous junction and by bringing it posterior to the median nerve. The flexor superficialis bridge is released. Branches of the median nerve are preserved and usually require mobilization in order to permit easy passage through its new subcutaneous course (Fig. 34–7).

Supracondylar Process

An anomalous spur, found 3 to 5 cm proximal to the medial epicondyle, can be another cause for median nerve entrapment in the upper extremity. The connection between these two bony prominences is the ligament of Struthers. This fibro-osseous tunnel, in the distal arm, is found in 1 per cent of limbs. The median nerve passes through this tunnel usually with the ulnar artery. Commonly, the brachial artery divides proximal to this bony process. This anomaly usually does not produce symptoms. However, after local trauma, high median nerve symptomatology may appear. On occasion, it can even result in ulnar nerve disturbance.

Infraclavicular Median Nerve Entrapment

The median nerve can be compressed at the level of the axilla. There are several causative factors:
1. Anomalous axillary arch muscles.
2. Anomalous vascular perforations of the median nerve or its roots.
3. The pectoralis minor.
4. Thickening of the deltopectoral fascia.

All of these have a common mechanism for the production of paralysis, which is abduction of the shoulder. Compression of the median nerve is aggravated by this repeated motion because the offending anatomical structures cross anteriorly or penetrate the nerve.

Langer's muscle is an example of an axillary arch muscle. It is a flat muscle which arises from the tendon of insertion of the latissimus dorsi and crosses anterior to the axillary neurovascular bundle to insert into the tendon of the pectoralis major in the region of the bicipital groove (Kaplan, 1945). According to Langer, this muscle has a 3 per cent occurrence rate. The sternalis muscle, another anomalous pectoral muscle, can be associated with an axillary arch muscle (Hollinshead, 1969). It is capable, similarly, of producing median nerve symptomatology.

I have treated six patients who have had either partial or complete median nerve paralysis caused by anomalous vascular perforations or vascular arches which compressed or tethered the median nerve in the axilla. The associated vascular anomalies were either arterial or venous in origin. When the lesion was partial, sensation was unaffected, while groups of forearm median-innervated muscles were paralyzed. On occasion, an isolated muscle, such as the flexor pollicis longus, may alone be paralyzed. More commonly, the flexor pollicis longus, pronator teres, pronator quadratus, flexor carpi radialis, and palmaris longus were nonfunctioning, while the remaining median-innervated intrinsic and extrinsic musculature was uninvolved clinically or electrically. When the flexor pollicis longus alone is paralyzed, the diagnosis must be differentiated from a partial anterior interosseous nerve paralysis or an isolated rupture of the tendon of the pollicis longus.

Subclavian arteriography, with the arm at the side and repeated with the arm abducted, is helpful in making the diagnosis of vascular penetration of the median nerve. With the arm at the side, the arterial tree is visualized, while in abduction the vessel which had an aberrant course does not fill (Fig.

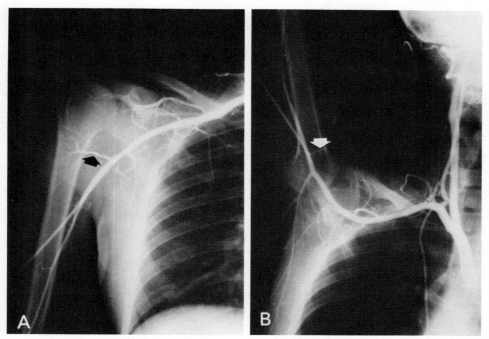

Figure 34–8 *A*, The posterior humeral circumflex artery (arrow) is seen to be wavy. *B*, The second subclavian arteriogram, with the arm abducted, reveals only the anterior humeral circumflex artery (arrow). The posterior humeral circumflex is not visualized with the arm in this position. At surgery, the posterior humeral circumflex artery was found to penetrate the median nerve.

34–8*A* and *B*). Brachial venography, with similar positioning of the arm, may reveal the pathology when a major vein penetrates the nerve. Venography should be performed utilizing the basilic vein rather than the cephalic system in order to visualize details of the venous system of the region. The most common variant perforation of the median nerve that is correlated with symptomatology is found with abnormalities of the posterior humeral circumflex artery or vein. The subscapular and anterior thoracic vessels have also been reported to follow anomalous paths. In a study of 480 human extremities, an 8 per cent aberrant relationship between the axillary artery, its major branches, and elements of the brachial plexus has been described (Miller, 1939).

Thus, some cases of high median nerve compression may be due to perforation of the median nerve by anomalous branches of the axillary vessels. It has been proposed that with repeated abduction of the arm median nerve compression is produced (Spinner, 1976). Furthermore, some cases of brachial plexus neuritis which have been previously considered to be idiopathic or viral may be caused by this mechanism.

The pectoralis minor, with the coracoid process, can cause compression of the neurovascular bundle when the arm is hyperabducted (Mayfield, 1970). Sleeping in a normal position or working continuously with the arm fully abducted in a cramped position can produce neural symptomatology in the limb. With abduction of the arm, the radial pulse is frequently obliterated in this hyperabduction syndrome. Conservative management is preferred but, on occasion, surgical release is necessary.

The deltopectoral fascia becomes thickened and its distal edge becomes fibrotic after trauma to the shoulder or brachial plexus. I have seen lesions of the brachial plexus and arm in which the distal fibrotic edge of the thickened deltopectoral fascia produced a compression of the median nerve. At the level of the compression a positive Tinel sign was present.

Radial Nerve Syndromes

Superficial Radial Nerve Entrapment

This syndrome is characterized by pain in the course of the superficial radial nerve, usually in the proximal forearm (Wartenberg, 1932), but the compression can occur at varying levels along its course in the forearm, depending upon the etiology. A tight watchband, operating room gloves, or a cast can produce symptoms of pain in the forearm and hypesthesia of the dorsum of the thumb. There is no associated muscle weakness or paralysis, and no motor conduction abnormality is noted with electroneuromyography.

Posterior Interosseous Nerve Syndrome

There are two ways in which this syndrome may present itself. In neither instance is there a sensory deficit.

In the first pattern, all of the muscles supplied by the posterior interosseous nerve are not functioning. The patient cannot extend the thumb, long, index, ring, and little fingers at their metacarpophalangeal joints. The wrist can dorsiflex and does so in a dorsoradial direction. This occurs as a result of a muscular imbalance of the wrist extensors due to paralysis of the extensor carpi ulnaris and the extensor digitorum communis.

The second pattern is characterized by a lack of extension of one or more of the digits at the metacarpophalangeal level. Paralysis of the remaining digits often develops. Finally, there is a fullblown posterior interosseous nerve syndrome. Frequently, posterior interosseous nerve entrapment occurs proximally where the nerve enters the two heads of the supinator muscle. This area, the arcade of Frohse, is fibrotendinous in 30 per cent of limbs (Spinner, 1968). Entrapment can occur spontaneously as a result of compression within the supinator or even at its distal margin (Fig. 34–9). Other causes of entrapment of the posterior interosseous nerve may be compression by a soft tissue tumor, synovial proliferations of rheumatoid disease, the Volkmann's disease process, dislocations of the radial head, or fractures of the proximal radius (Figs. 34–10 and 34–11).

The symptom complex known as lateral epicondylitis, or resistant tennis elbow, is now recognized frequently to be due to posterior interosseous nerve compression in the region of the arcade of Frohse (Capener, 1966; Roles and Maudsley, 1972). This syndrome is characterized by pain about the lateral aspect of the elbow. A significant number of patients who have not responded to conservative treatment, to release of the lateral epicondylar soft tissues, or

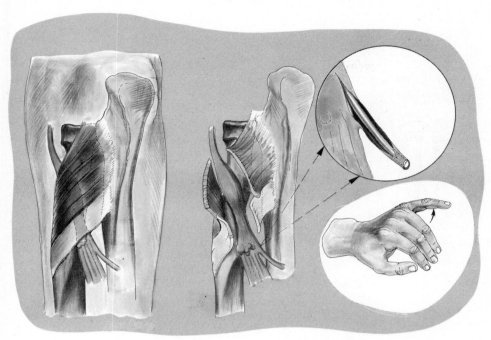

Figure 34–9   A patient had a partial posterior interosseous nerve paralysis of three years' duration. He could extend only the little finger of his left hand. The extensor carpi ulnaris was also functioning. A fibrotic band compressing the nerve was found at the distal end of the supinator. All but the most medial funiculus of the posterior interosseous nerve were severely compressed. Following both external and internal neurolysis, there was complete recovery.

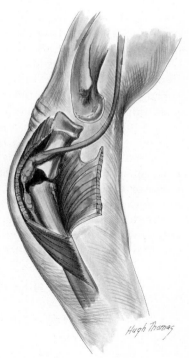

Figure 34–10   Fracture of the proximal radius can be associated with posterior interosseous nerve paralysis, especially if there is posterior angulation of the fracture site.

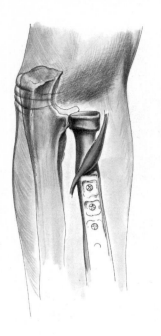

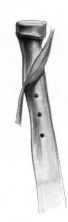

Figure 34–11 Open reduction with plate-and-screw fixation of a fracture of the proximal half of the radius can be complicated by a posterior interosseous nerve paralysis. Early removal of the plate and replacement with a shorter plate or, if the fracture is healed, neurolysis alone can restore neuromuscular function.

to excision of a portion of the orbicular ligament have been relieved by neurolysis of the posterior interosseous nerve. If pain persists following the customary surgery for tennis elbow, posterior interosseous nerve compression should be considered as a possible etiology.

There are several surgical approaches that are available to expose the entrapped posterior interosseous nerve. The approach chosen depends on the presence of muscle fusions or other anomalies in the region and on the extent of the nerve that is to be traced. Either the radial nerve is identified above the elbow, proximal to its site of division, or the superficial radial nerve is identified posterior to the brachioradialis in the forearm and traced proximally through the area of the muscular anomaly to the main radial nerve trunk. The posterior interosseous nerve is then identified and traced through the two heads of the supinator. A direct anterior approach, splitting the brachioradialis, has also been recommended (Lister, Belsole, and Kleinert, 1979).

An alternate approach is to open the internervous plane on the dorsoradial aspect of the forearm between the flexor digitorum communis and the extensor carpi radialis brevis. After detaching the tendinous origin of the extensor carpi radialis brevis from the medial epicondyle and flexing the elbow, the posterior interosseous nerve is identified proximal to its entry between the two heads of the supinator — the arcade of Frohse (Spinner, 1978). This nerve can then be traced through its entire course.

High Radial Nerve Compression

In the Arm or Axilla: Spontaneous high radial nerve paralysis can occur in the arm, usually at the level of the lateral head of the triceps (Wilhelm, 1970; Lotem et al., 1971; Manske, 1977).

As a result of an analysis of six patients with this entity that I have managed, the following conclusions are made:

1. If a patient has a spontaneous paralysis of the radial nerve in the arm that does not reveal clinical or electrical evidence of recovery by three to four months following onset, then exploration is necessary.

2. If the paralytic lesion is complete for 18 months, the procedure of choice is primary tendon transfers. If, in addition to the paralysis, pain is a persistent complaint, neurolysis of the radial nerve to relieve the chronic pain is indicated.

3. It is vital to localize the radial nerve lesion to the proper level early for optimal recovery. With a lesion at the proximal forearm, the wrist can dorsiflex in a radial direction, the thumb and fingers cannot extend at the metacarpophalangeal joints, and sensation is intact. A lesion at the midarm level produces complete drop of the wrist, fingers, and thumb. There is anesthesia of the dorsal basilar aspect of the thumb; elbow extension is normal.

4. If, in addition to a drop of the wrist, fingers, and thumb, there is partial or complete paralysis of the triceps, a higher lesion is probably present. To demonstrate the location and the etiology of this axillary lesion of the radial nerve, subclavian arteriography and basilic venography, with the arm at the side and abducted, can be helpful. An aberrant subscapular artery can penetrate the radial nerve, and with repeated abduction can produce radial nerve dysfunction. On the posterior axillary wall, an aberrant muscle, the accessory subscapularis-teres-latissimus, may cross a portion of, or all of, the radial nerve (Kameda, 1976). This anomalous muscle can involve both the radial nerve and the axillary nerve.

Ulnar Nerve Syndromes

Guyon's Tunnel

At the wrist, the ulnar nerve can be compressed at the pisiform, at the hook of the hamate, or in Guyon's tunnel. A pure motor or pure sensory deficit, or a combination of the two, may result. The main ulnar nerve or one of its terminal branches may be entrapped, depending upon the localization (Hayes et al., 1969; Shea and McClain, 1969).

Cubital Tunnel

This syndrome has been described in detail by Osborne (1957, 1970) and by Vanderpool et al. (1968). The ulnar nerve may be compressed just distal to the medial epicondyle through the two heads of the flexor carpi ulnaris. These findings have been confirmed by Apfelberg and Larson (1973).

The choice of surgical procedure varies between release of the cubital tunnel, medial epicondylectomy, and anterior translocation of the ulnar nerve. When the ulnar nerve is translocated anteriorly, it is unwise to place it in a groove in the pronator-flexor group of muscles. Traction ulnar neuritis fre-

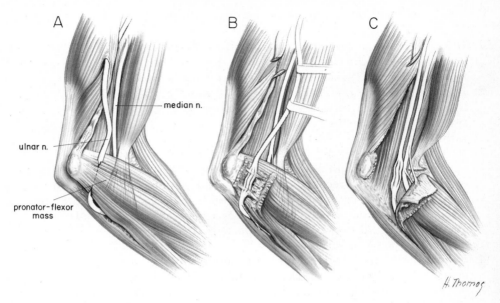

Figure 34-12 *A,* A left ulnar nerve which had been translocated anteriorly and placed in a groove in the pronator-flexor muscles by the initial treating physician. The patient developed recurrent severe ulnar neuritic symptoms one year postoperatively. *B,* At the second surgical procedure, a traction neuritis was found. *C,* The nerve was translocated deep to the pronator-flexor mass. In addition, the arcarde of Struthers was released.

quently complicates this technique (Seddon, 1972). When this problem exists, it is best to liberate the nerve and to translocate it deep to the entire pronator-flexor muscle mass. The traumatized ulnar nerve is placed in the bed adjacent to the median nerve (Fig. 34–12).

Arcade of Struthers

This is the region where the ulnar nerve passes into the posterior compartment of the distal arm (Kane et al., 1973; Spinner and Kaplan, 1976). Release of the arcade of Struthers and excision of the adjacent medial intermuscular septum prevent a secondary potential entrapment of the ulnar nerve 8 cm proximal to the medial epicondyle (Figs. 34–12 and 34–13).

Cervical Syndromes

With the thoracic outlet syndromes, the ulnar nerve is most frequently compressed at the level of the first rib or at the costoclavicular level. If appropriate studies are positive, and conservative treatment is unsuccessful, removal of the first rib is indicated.

Cervical arthritis can cause symptoms of numbness in ring and little fingers with weakness of these digits. There is pain on rotation of the neck associated with reproduction of radicular complaints and restriction of cervical motion; such symptoms can help to localize the cause of the syndrome.

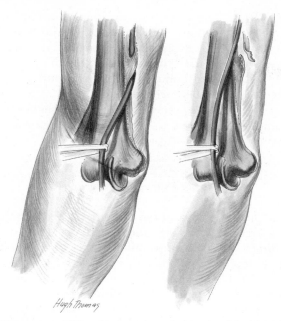

Hugh Thomas

Figure 34–13   Entrapment of the ulnar nerve at the arcade of Struthers 8 cm proximal to the medial epicondyle can be a cause for a secondary ulnar neuritis following incomplete anterior translocation of this nerve.

Pain on direct pressure or percussion along the course of the nerve can also help to locate the level of the pathology.

Musculocutaneous Nerve Entrapment

This terminal branch of the lateral cord is specifically vulnerable to entrapment where it penetrates the coracobrachialis. There are many variations both in the number of muscular components of the coracobrachialis and in the levels where the musculocutaneous nerve penetrates this muscle. A complete lesion of this nerve results in paralysis of the biceps and brachialis muscles, and there is a sensory loss on the lateral aspect of the forearm (the lateral cutaneous nerve of the forearm). I have seen this lesion occurring spontaneously with a recurring pattern in a professional athlete, in a patient who had a transfer of the coracoid process for repair of a recurrent dislocation of the shoulder, and in a patient who had plate-and-screw fixation of a fracture of the humerus through a medial approach. Surgical exploration is necessary if there is no recovery by three to four months.

Bowler's Thumb

This entity is characterized by pain in the thumb, numbness (most marked on its ulnar aspect), a palpable mass at the base of the thumb, a positive Tinel sign on percussion of this mass, and a history of habitual bowling (Dobyns et al., 1972). The use of a protective thumb-guard, redrilling of the bowling ball so it is scythed, and cessation of bowling for four to six weeks are helpful conservative measures. Surgery is indicated when conservative measures do not relieve the symptoms. In this instance, neurolysis, excision of the markedly thickened epineurium, and rerouting the involved digital nerve into a new soft tissue bed are indicated.

Similar localized digital compression neuropathy has been seen in baseball batters. The management of this condition is identical in principle — avoidance of repetitive external compression.

Multiple Entrapment Lesions

It is important to note that a nerve can be trapped simultaneously at two levels (Upton and McComas, 1973), and that more than one nerve can be entrapped in a limb. Electromyographic studies are not always sensitive enough to localize a double lesion. It may be necessary to explore a peripheral nerve at two sites. In this instance, an hereditary etiology with familial factors that can predispose the patient to multiple compression sites and to repeated episodes must be considered (Earl et al., 1964; Behse, 1972; Karparti et al., 1973). Remember also that a patient can have two completely separate neurological conditions such as syringomyelia of the cervical cord and a compressed peripheral nerve (Spinner and Spencer, 1974). Avoid the wrong diagnosis of a localized process when a diffuse peripheral neuropathy is the cause of a conduction delay. A sampling of other peripheral nerves will prevent this error.

In conclusion the following points should be emphasized:
1. Early accurate diagnosis and treatment are essential for the most favorable results in compression lesions.
2. Age is no factor in prognosis, and to deny surgical relief to the older age group is unjustified.
3. If the diagnosis is unclear, repeated clinical examinations and electroneuromyography at monthly intervals are indicated until the diagnosis is clear.
4. Pure first-, second-, third-, or fourth-degree neural lesions are unusual; one lesion-type frequently predominates. Clinical studies will usually define the variable nature of the neural pathology.
5. Surgery is indicated if there is not progressive improvement in function within three to four months.

REFERENCES

Apfelberg, D. B., and Larson, S. J.: Dynamic anatomy of the ulnar nerve at the elbow. Plast. Reconstruct. Surg. *51*:76, 1973.

Behse, F., Buchthal, F., Carlsen, F., and Knappeis, G. G.: Hereditary neuropathy with liability to pressure palsies: Electrophysiological and histopathological aspects. Brain *95*:777, 1972.

Brown, B. A.: Internal neurolysis in traumatic peripheral nerve lesions in continuity. Surg. Clin. North Am. *52*:1167, 1972.

Buchthal, F., Rosenfalck, A., and Trojaborg, W.: Electrophysical findings in entrapment of the median nerve at wrist and elbow. J. Neurol. Neurosurg. Psychiatry *37*:340, 1974.

Capener, N.: The vulnerability of the posterior interosseous nerve of the forearm. J. Bone Joint Surg. *48B*:770, 1966.

Carroll, R. E., and Green, D. P.: The significance of the palmar cutaneous nerve at the wrist. Clin. Orthop. *83*:24, 1972.

Curtis, R. M., and Eversmann, W. W.: Internal neurolysis as an adjunct to the treatment of the carpal tunnel syndrome. J. Bone Joint Surg. *55A*:733, 1973.

Denny-Brown, D., and Brenner, C.: Paralysis of nerve induced by direct pressure and by tourniquet. Arch. Neurol. Psychiatry *51*:1, 1944.

Dobyns, J. H., O'Brien, E. T., Linscheid, R. L., and Farrow, G. M.: Bowler's thumb. Diagnosis and treatment. A review of seventeen cases. J. Bone Joint Surg. *54A*:751, 1972.

Earl, C. J., Fullerton, P. M., Wakefield, G. S., and Schutta, H. S.: Hereditary neuropathy with liability to pressure palsies. A clinical and electrophysiological study of four families. Quart. J. Med. *33*:481, 1964.

Fenning, J. B.: Deep ulnar-nerve paralysis from an anatomical abnormality. J. Bone Joint Surg. *47A*:1381, 1965.

Gilliatt, B. W., Ochoa, J., Rudge, P., and Neary, D.: The cause of nerve damage in acute compression. Trans. Am. Neurol. Assoc. *99*:71, 1974.

Hayes, J. R., Mulholland, R. C., and O'Connor, B. T.: Compression of the deep palmar branch of the ulnar nerve. J. Bone Joint Surg. *51B*:469, 1969.

Hollinshead, W. H.: Anatomy for Surgeons. The Back and Limbs. 2nd ed., New York, Hoeber, 1969, Vol. 3, p. 286.

Inglis, A. E., Straub, L. R., and Williams, C. S.: Median nerve neuropathy at the wrist. Clin. Orthop. *83*:48, 1972.

Johnson, R. K., Spinner, M., and Shrewsbury, M. M.: Median nerve entrapment syndrome in the proximal forearm. J. Hand Surg. *4*:48, 1979.

Kameda, Y.: An anomalous muscle (accessory scapularis-teres-latissimus muscle) in the axilla penetrating the brachial plexus in man. Acta Anat. *96*:513, 1976.

Kane, E., Kaplan, E. B., and Spinner, M.: Observations on the course of the ulnar nerve in the arm. Ann. Chir. *27*:487, 1973.

Kaplan, E. B.: Surgical anatomy — Langer's muscle of the axilla. Bull. Hosp. Joint Dis. *6*:78, 1945.

Karpati, G., Carpenters, S., Eisen, A. A., and Feindel, W.: Familial multiple peripheral nerve entrapments — an unusual manifestation of a peripheral neuropathy. Trans. Am. Neurol. Assoc. *98*:267, 1973.

Kline, D. G., Hackett, E. R., and May, P. R.: Evaluation of nerve injuries by evoked potentials and electromyography. J. Neurosurg. *31*:128, 1969.

Kline, D. G., and Nulsen, F. E.: The neuroma in continuity. Its preoperative and operative management. Surg. Clin. North Am. *52*:1189, 1972.

Kuszynski, K.: Functional micro-anatomy of the peripheral nerve trunks. Hand *6*:1, 1974.

Lanz, U.: Lahmung des tiefen Hohlhandastes des Nervus ulnaris, bedingt durch eine anatomische Variante. Handchirurgie *6*:83, 1974.

Lassa, R., and Shrewsburg, M. M.: A variation in the path of the deep motor branch of the ulnar nerve at the wrist. J. Bone Joint Surg., *57A*:990, 1975.

Levine, J., and Spinner, M.: Neurolysis in the elderly. Clin. Orthop. *80*:13, 1971.

Linscheid, R. L., Peterson, L. F. A., and Juergens, J. L.: Carpal tunnel syndrome associated with vasospasm. J. Bone Joint Surg. *49A*:1141, 1967.

Lister, G. D., Belsole, R. B., and Kleinert, H. E.: The Radial Tunnel Syndrome. J. Hand Surg. *4*:52, 1979.

Lotem, N., Fried, A., Levy, M., Solzi, P., Najenson, T., and Nathan, H.: Radial palsy following muscular effort. A nerve compression syndrome possibly related to a fibrous arch of the lateral head of the triceps. J. Bone Joint Surg. *53B*:500, 1971.

Lundborg, G.: Ischemic nervy injury. Experimental studies on intraneural microvascular pathophysiology and nerve function in a limb subjected to temporary circulatory arrest. Scand. J. Plast. Reconstr. Surg. (Suppl.) *6*:1, 1970.

Manske, P. R.: Compression of the radial nerve by the triceps muscle. A case report. J. Bone Joint Surg. *59A*:835, 1977.

Marie, P., and Foix, C.: Atrophie isolée de l'eminence thénar d'origine névritique, rôle du ligament annulaire antérieur du carpal dans la pathogénie de la lésion. Rev. Neurol. *26*:647, 1913.

Mayfield, F. H.: Compression syndromes of the shoulder girdles and arms. *In* Vinken, P. J., and Bruyn, G. W. (eds.): Handbook of Clinical Neurology. Diseases of Nerves. New York, American Elsevier, 1970, Vol. 7, p. 441.

McDowell, C. L., and Henceroth, W. D.: Compression of the ulnar nerve in the hand by a ganglion. J. Bone Joint Surg. *59A*:980, 1977.

Miller, R.: Observations upon the arrangement of the axillary artery and brachial plexus. Am. J. Anat. *64*:143, 1939.

Mitchell, S. W.: Injuries of Nerves and Their Consequences. London, Smith Elder, 1872.

Ochoa, J.: Schwann cell and myelin changes caused by some toxic agents and trauma. Proc. Roy. Soc. Med. *67*:3, 1974.

Omer, G., and Spinner, M.: Peripheral nerve testing and suture techniques. *In* Instructional Course Lectures of the American Academy of Orthopedic Surgeons. St. Louis, C. V. Mosby Company, 1975, Vol. 24, p. 122.

Osborne, G.: The surgical treatment of tardy ulnar neuritis. J. Bone Joint Surg. *39B*:782, 1957.

Osborne, G.: Compression neuritis of the ulnar nerve at the elbow. Hand *2*:10, 1970.

Paget, J.: Lectures on Surgical Pathology. Philadelphia, Lindsay & Blakiston, 1854.

Papathanassiou, B. T.: A variant of the motor branch of the median nerve in the hand. J. Bone Joint Surg. *50B*:156, 1968.

Phalen, G. S.: Spontaneous compression of the median nerve at the wrist. J.A.M.A. *145*:1128, 1951.

Phalen, G. S.: The carpel-tunnel syndrome. Seventeen years experience in diagnosis and treatment of six-hundred forty-four hands. J. Bone Joint Surg. *48A*:211, 1966.

Roles, N. C., and Maudsley, R. H.: Radial tunnel syndrome. Resistant tennis elbow as a nerve entrapment. J. Bone Joint Surg. *54B*:499, 1972.

Rydevik, B., Lundborg, G., and Nordberg, G.: Intraneural tissue reactions induced by internal neurolysis. Scand. J. Plast. Reconstr. Surg. *10*:3, 1976.

Seddon, H.: Surgical Disorders of the Peripheral Nerves. Edinburgh, Churchill, 1972.

Seddon, H. J.: Three types of nerve injury. Brain *66*:237, 1943.

Shea, J. D., and McClain, E. J.: Ulnar nerve compression syndromes at and below the wrist. J. Bone Joint Surg. *51A*:1095, 1969.

Spinner, M.: The arcade of Frohse and its relationship to posterior interosseous nerve paralysis. J. Bone Joint Surg. *50B*:809, 1968.

Spinner, M.: The anterior interosseous nerve syndrome, with special attention to its variations. J. Bone Joint Surg. *52A*:84, 1970.

Spinner, M.: Injuries to the Major Branches of the Forearm. 2nd ed., Philadelphia, W. B. Saunders, 1978.

Spinner, M., and Kaplan, M.: The relationship of the ulnar nerve to the medial intermuscular septum in the arm and its clinical significance. Hand *8*:239, 1976.

Spinner, M., and Spencer, P. S.: Nerve compression of lesions of the upper extremity. A clinical and experimental review. Clin. Orthop. *104*:46, 1974.

Spinner, M.: The functional attitude of the hand afflicted with an anterior interosseous nerve paralysis. Bull. Hosp. Joint Dis. *30*:21, 1969.

Spinner, M.: Cryptogenic infraclavicular brachial plexus neuritis (preliminary report). Bull. Hosp. Joint Dis. *37*:98, 1976.

Sunderland, S.: Nerves and Nerve Injuries. Baltimore, Williams & Wilkins, 1968.

Sunderland, S.: Nerve lesions in the carpal tunnel syndrome. J. Neurol. Neurosurg. Psychiatry *39*:615, 1976.

Thomas, P. K.: Changes in the endoneurial sheaths of peripheral myelinated nerve fibers during Wallerian degeneration. J. Anat. *98*:175, 1964.

Thomas, P. K.: The cellular response to nerve injury. I.: The cellular outgrowth from the distal stump of transected nerve. J. Anat. *100*:287, 1966.

Upton, A. R. M., and McComas, A. J.: The double crush in nerve entrapment syndromes. Lancet *2*:359, 1973.

Vanderpool, D. W., Chalmers, J., Lamb, D. W., and Whiston, T. R.: Peripheral compression lesions of the ulnar nerve. J. Bone Joint Surg. *50B*:792, 1968.

Wartenberg, R.: Chiralgia paresthetica. Zeitschr. Neurol. Psychiat. *141*:145, 1932.

Williams, N. B., and Terzis, J. K.: Single fascicular recordings. An intraoperative diagnostic tool for the management of peripheral nerve lesions. Plast. Reconstr. Surg. *57*:562, 1976.

Wilhelm, A.: Neues Überdrückschaden des Nervus ulnaris und Nervus radialis. Handchirurgie, *2*:143, 1970.

35

THORACIC
OUTLET
SYNDROME

ROBERT D. LEFFERT

The term "thoracic outlet syndrome" is used to describe the signs and symptoms resulting from proximal compression of the neurovascular structures supplying the upper limb. This can occur in the interscalene area, between the clavicle and the first rib, and further distally, beneath the conjoined tendons attaching to the coracoid process.

It is important for the surgeon to understand the varied clinical manifestations of this entity, which commonly presents with complaints referable to the hand. Failure to consider it in the differential diagnosis may deprive the patient of an opportunity for relief, or worse, subject her to unnecessary surgical procedures in the limb, to be followed by the label "neurotic" when the complaints continue.

The normal anatomy of the thoracic outlet (Lord and Rosati, 1958), which extends from the intervertebral foramina and superior mediastinum to the axilla, must be considered not only in one plane but in three dimensions to appreciate the potential mechanisms of compression. With the normal range of movement of the shoulder joint complex, the dynamic changes in space available to nerves and vessels can produce significant symptoms in susceptible individuals. Hence, the configuration of the female chest cage, along with postural descent of the shoulder girdle, or poor musculature, predispose women to this condition. If the breasts are excessively large, the situation may be markedly aggravated (Kaye, 1972). Clavicular abnormalities, both congenital and posttraumatic, may lead to compression.

The scalene muscles, which are flexors and rotators of the neck, were formerly considered major causes of compression, leading not only to the term "scalenus anticus syndrome" but also to therapy directed solely at their release (scalenotomy) (Adson, 1951), a relatively simple procedure with a high failure rate. Since the anterior and middle scalenes both insert on the first rib, and the subclavian artery and brachial plexus must pass between them, anything that alters the funnel-shaped interscalene tunnel can produce compression. Such variations as overlapping or hypertrophy of the muscles, or fusion of their insertions by a fibrous falciform band (Law, 1920; Bonney, 1965), are diagnosed only at the time of surgery. However, when there are long cervical transverse processes or rudimentary cervical ribs present, one may sometimes anticipate the presence of a fibrous band extending from the adventitious bone to the region of the scalene tubercle where it may cause compression. Although the incidence of cervical ribs in the general population is about 1 per cent, the mere presence of such a bony variation should not lead "a priori" to a diagnosis of thoracic outlet syndrome, since this may be merely an incidental finding. If a cervical rib is long enough, it may indeed directly impinge on nerves or vessels, and the incidence of concomitant vascular abnormalities such as subclavian aneurysm is well documented (Short, 1975; Blank and Connor, 1974; Mathes and Salaam, 1974). Not only will malformations of the clavicle cause the costoclavicular interval to be narrowed but also since the normal clavicle is "S-shaped" and rotates during abduction of the arm, both the "military brace position" and hyperabduction will produce symptoms in susceptible individuals. Since the nerves and vessels change course by 180 degrees from adduction to full arm elevation, there is potential for impingement beneath the coracoid process. Needless to say, any space-occupying lesion, whether it be unusual, such as hypertrophy of the subclavius muscle (Lusskin, Weiss, and Winer, 1967), or the regrettably more common expanding Pancoast tumor, has the potential for mechanical mischief, and must be considered in appropriate patients.

SYMPTOMS AND SIGNS

It is obvious that with a multiplicity of potential causes for compression, the three structures at risk — the subclavian artery, the vein, and the lower trunk of the brachial plexus — may be affected to significantly different degrees. As has been suggested, the typical patient is likely to be a woman, usually aged 20 to 40; in our experience the ratio of women to men is approximately 5 to 1. Complaints are often vague and hard to define. The patient may experience nocturnal paresthesias, leading to confusion with carpal tunnel syndrome. However, careful history taking in the thoracic outlet group will always correctly identify their locus of complaint as the medial forearm, little finger, and ring finger. Commonly, they will experience similar symptoms with abduction of the arm, such as while hanging clothes on a line, writing on a blackboard, or even grooming a tall horse. Many patients will also describe discomfort in the posterior hemithorax, anterior chest or breast, and upper arm. Some will report quite accurately that they feel as though "the blood is being shut off in the arm," which is obviously a reflection of arterial insufficiency. A most elusive complaint, that of intermittent swelling of the limb with exercise, may not be accepted as real until the venous hypertension becomes sufficiently great to produce measurable asymmetry or a pronounced superficial venous pattern due to the formation of collaterals. The least common presentation, that of Raynaud's phenomenon (Swinton et al., 1970), may be either unilateral or bilateral, and, in the latter case, the diagnosis of collagen-vascular disease must be excluded.

It is unusual for the patient to complain of motor weakness, although careful manual muscle testing will often detect hypothenar, interosseous, or adductor pollicis weakness of subtle degree. The profundi to the little and ring fingers may be weak, and, less commonly, the median motor nerve distribution of the lower trunk may be affected. However, I have not observed this in the absence of weak ulnar innervated musculature. The sensory deficit is appropriate to the ulnar distribution plus the medial cutaneous nerve of the forearm, thus aiding in differential diagnosis of ulnar neuropathy.

The vascular signs have already been alluded to; these may be spontaneous and noted by the patient or provoked by the examiner in a series of diagnostic positions of the arm and neck. The classical Adson maneuver is performed, with the patient seated, by palpating the radial pulse with the arm dependent. The head is turned toward the side of the lesion and extended while a deep breath is taken. If the test is positive, the pulse will markedly diminish or disappear. In addition, since some normal and asymptomatic individuals will exhibit this phenomenon, the patient should at the same time reproduce her symptoms. The remaining provocative maneuvers have the same end point and consist of "the military brace," or costoclavicular maneuver, and the abduction–external rotation position of the shoulder. Finally, the patient elevates both arms fully and rapidly opens and closes the hands. In susceptible individuals this exercise will cause cramping or a fatigued sensation very quickly. Startling color changes of pallor or cyanosis and suffusion may result, depending on whether the compression is predominantly arterial or venous. Rarely, vascular compromise because of a sudden catastrophic occlusion of artery or veins may be the presenting complaint, and thus the cause may be quite obvious. In all patients being screened for thoracic outlet syndrome, it is wise to palpate and auscultate the supraclavicular fossa for the presence of a mass or bruit.

LABORATORY AND X-RAY TESTING

Plain films of the cervical spine and chest are taken to assist in the differential diagnosis. Since a significant percentage of unselected patients have some evidence of cervical spondylosis, this entity must be considered. It should be remembered that although cervical radiculopathy is a major cause of brachialgia, it is unusual for it to affect the C8–T1 outflow and produce the corresponding sensory loss and intrinsic atrophy in the hand. The AP cervical spine film should be scrutinized for the presence of cervical ribs or other osseous abnormalities, such as long transverse processes at C7. The incidence of cervical ribs in the general population is about 1 per cent, and only about 20 per cent of our operative cases have such osseous abnormalities.

The measurement of the conduction velocity of the ulnar nerve through the thoracic outlet and successively down the arm has proved to be an extremely useful and reproducible test. In order to avoid false negatives, the arm should be positioned to provoke the symptoms, usually in full abduction and external rotation. The expected normal velocity through the thoracic outlet under these circumstances is 72 meters per second, while speeds of less than 65 meters per second are considered abnormal. When the velocity in the remainder of the limb is otherwise normal, this is strong presumptive evidence for thoracic outlet syndrome (Urschel, 1968).

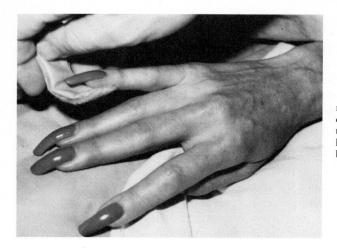

Figure 35–1 The pneumatic cuff applied to the fingers of a patient with a cyanotic hand thought to be due to thoracic outlet syndrome but actually caused by reflex sympathetic dystrophy.

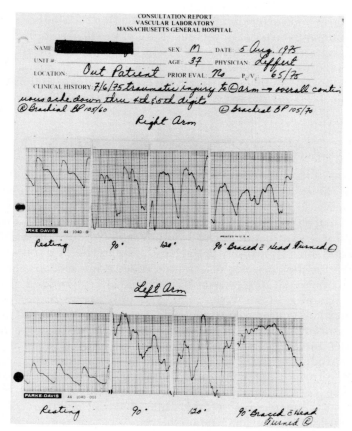

Figure 35–2 The recorded digital pulsations of a patient who had thoracic outlet syndrome. The tracing on the bottom of the figure should be compared with the top to see the damping of pulse when the left shoulder is braced. The right side is normal.

Although both arteriography and venography have been recommended for the study of these patients, we find that in most cases they are unnecessary and that noninvasive testing not only suffices but is highly reliable. Digital plethysmography (Roos, 1969) is done by means of pneumatic cuffs applied to the fingertips (Fig. 35–1). The arm is put through the standard provocative positions, thus producing a running pulse tracing that can be correlated with the clinical findings (Fig. 35–2). It is considerably more reliable than palpating the radial pulse. At the same session, an assessment of the degree of digital vascular tone can be made.

Angiography is ordinarily reserved for those patients who have significant cervical ribs, and in whom the possibility of subclavian aneurysm must be ruled out (Blank and Connor, 1974). In addition, patients who have had multiple unsuccessful previous operations in the area and who are potential operative candidates may be examined in this manner.

The place of venography in the diagnostic workup is still undecided, since a number of asymptomatic individuals will exhibit temporary occlusion of the subclavian vein with the arm in full abduction. Of course, demonstration of extensive collateralization in this situation would indicate pathology.

CONSERVATIVE THERAPY

Once the patient learns that her symptoms have an anatomic basis that can be alleviated, it is not unusual for her to want something dramatic done immediately. However, unless there is significant vascular compromise or motor loss, most patients are best treated initially by conservative methods (Britt, 1967; Peet et al., 1956). A thorough explanation of the problem is useful in enlisting the patient's cooperation in a therapeutic exercise program. Local heat, analgesics, and muscle relaxants will help to lessen the spasm of the cervical musculature. The exercises are done gently and progressively twice a day as the shoulders and neck gain strength. The patient stands erect, holding a 1 or 2 pound weight in each hand; she intermittently shrugs and relaxes the shoulders forward and upward, then backward and upward, then upward 10 times each. The second exercise is done with the weights held at the sides then raised with the elbows extended overhead until the backs of the hands meet. In the third set, the patient faces a corner of the room with one palm on each wall. With the elbows bent, she inhales as she leans into the corner, and then exhales as she pushes out. A series of neck range of motion exercises combined with breathing exercises completes the program. This course of treatment should be pursued faithfully for two to three months unless symptoms are worsened (which sometimes happens) or until it is readily apparent that there has been no improvement. In our experience, if there is significant compression, conservative therapy will not suffice and operation is indicated.

OPERATIVE THERAPY

Owing to the interest of surgeons of different specialty orientations in the treatment of thoracic outlet syndrome, there are divergent preferences for anatomical approach. However, it has become increasingly accepted that in all cases the scalene muscles should be sectioned and the first rib removed as totally as possible (Falconer and Li, 1962), since it serves as an anatomical "common denominator" for the majority of the compression syndromes (Urschel et al., 1968). Many thoracic surgeons prefer the posterior approach, as for high thoracoplasty (Clagett, 1962), but, since this approach involves a transmuscular route, we reserve it for those patients who have had previous surgery through the axilla. With either a supraclavicular or subclavicular route, I believe it is technically more difficult to do an adequate rib resection, and the neurovascular structures must be constantly retracted to avoid damage by instruments or bone fragments. The transclavicular route, or treatment by total claviculectomy is, in my opinion, excessive unless there is preoperative documentation of significant vascular abnormality, such as an aneurysm.

The transaxillary route, as originally described by Roos (1966 and 1971), has become increasingly popular because it involves trivial blood loss and transects no important muscles. The patient is in the lateral decubitus position with the affected arm held by a scrubbed assistant who can raise and lower it as the surgeon requires (Fig. 35–3). An 8 cm transverse skin incision is made in the axilla just beneath and parallel to the lower border of the axillary hairline (Fig. 35–4), from the pectoralis major to the latissimus dorsi muscle. The intercostobrachial nerve is preserved and retracted. Heney vaginal retractors are used for separating the muscular walls of the incision. Full muscular relaxation and a proper line of pull on the arm open the thoracic outlet. Blunt dissection is carried out along the rib cage until the first rib can be palpated. Ligation and division of the intercostal branches of the subclavian artery and vein allow their full mobilization to the most cephalic part of the field. They are constantly kept under direct

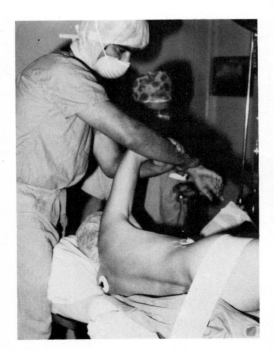

Figure 35–3 The correct position of the assistant holding the arm using a "wrist lock."

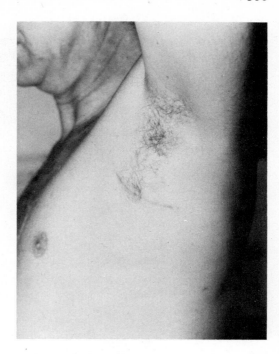

Figure 35–4 A healed transaxillary incision.

vision to avoid injury. Since the field is actually shaped like an inverted pyramid, 10 to 12 centimeters deep, it is necessary to use either lighted retractors or an operating headlight for illumination.

The areolar tissue surrounding the upper surface of the first rib and neurovascular structures is gently cleared by blunt dissection, and the scalenus anticus is identified as it attaches to the scalene tubercle between the artery and vein. Using a right-angled clamp, the muscle is pulled forward off the pleura just above the surface of the rib and sectioned with a scissors. Although the phrenic nerve is not at risk at this level, the pleura is, and a pneumothorax will result if the muscle is not separated from it prior to section. The outermost edge of the first rib may be cleared with a first rib elevator, proceeding anteriorly and then posteriorly to free the attachments of the scalenus medius. Anterior to this muscle an incision in the periosteum may be used, but only blunt dissection with a first rib elevator and a rounded periosteal elevator, such as a Matson, is permitted posteriorly to avoid injury to the long thoracic nerve. When working on the undersurface of the rib to separate it from the pleura, it is helpful to have the anesthetist hypoventilate the patient. Pressure on the instruments should be made only against the bone. If a pneumothorax results, it may not be obvious until the wound is flooded with irrigating solution, which will bubble because of the air leak. This occurs in 15 to 20 per cent of our cases, and is easily managed by inserting a chest tube through the rent in the pleura and leading it out through a stab wound to underwater suction. When the rib has been sufficiently cleared, the proposed line of section should lie at least 2 cm behind the lower trunk of the brachial plexus, and less than 2 cm from its vertebral articulation. Then, with all structures under direct vision, the Roos rib cutter is placed around

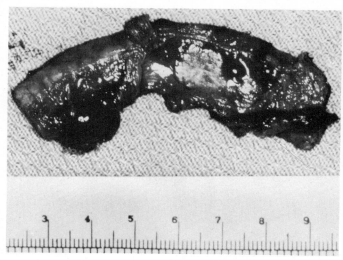

Figure 35–5   A typical resected first rib. Note the soft tissues included with the specimen. (Scale in cm.)

the rib and pushed posteriorly. After a final safety check, the jaws are closed and the rib is cut. This instrument has an angled cutting surface so that the rib is sectioned transversely, which would not be possible using other cutters. A sharply oblique bone end would pose a hazard to the adjacent structures. Attempts to substitute a ronguer are similarly unsatisfactory.

If a fibrous band from a cervical rib or a cervical rib itself is present, it can be removed at this stage if it constitutes a cause for compression as determined by inspection and palpation. Usually a short rib (less than 2 cm) need not be removed, although any bands coming from it should be sectioned. The first rib is then cut anteriorly from the sternum, and the subclavius muscle attachment can be divided then as well. As much of the rib periosteum as possible must be removed to prevent recurrence (Fig. 35–5).

The thoracic outlet is then gently digitally explored with the arm and shoulder in all positions to determine if adequate decompression has been achieved. If not, a portion of the second rib can be removed to provide more space. The wound is then irrigated to test for air leaks, and the muscles are allowed to fall back into place. The subcutaneous tissues are approximated, and the skin is closed without a drain, usually by means of a subcuticular suture.

COMPLICATIONS

Some of the potential complications of the procedure and their management have already been described. Obviously, the ultimate disaster would be a laceration of the vessels or of the brachial plexus. We have, fortunately, never had this occur, but one should be prepared to perform a modified median sternotomy to gain proximal vascular control if necessary. Laceration of the brachial plexus at this level would be irrevocable, and it should be remembered that the plexus has little excursion here. Hence, rough retraction directly on it might cause many months of neurologic deficit. Some patients will experience transient aching about the shoulder and winging of the scapula due to the stretch of the nerve to the serratus anterior, but unless the nerve has actually been cut, this will usually recover within a few weeks. The numbness of the axilla caused by traction on the intercostal brachial nerve will gradually fade over a few months if continuity has been preserved.

POSTOPERATIVE MANAGEMENT

Morbidity from transaxillary first rib resection is usually negligible, since no major muscles are cut and blood loss is often less than 50 cubic centimeters. A sling is used for the first few days, as comfort dictates, and the dressing may be removed at four or five days. Patients must be cautioned against resumption of normal activities involving heavy lifting for three or four weeks, since it is not unusual for dramatic relief of symptoms to occur in the immediate postoperative period. Even intrinsic hand muscle weakness may be reversed, although significant atrophy may be permanent. The overall results of the operation in properly selected patients who have objective signs and positive laboratory findings have been very gratifying, and in a number of cases the "functional overlay" has completely disappeared.

REFERENCES

Adson, A. W.: Cervical ribs: symptoms, differential diagnosis for section of the insertion of the scalenus anticus muscle. J. Int. Coll. Surg. *16*:546, 1951.

Blank, R. H., and Conner, R. G.: Arterial complications associated with thoracic outlet compression syndrome. Ann. Thorac. Surg. *17*:4, 1974.

Bonney, G.: The scalenus medium band: A contribution to the study of the thoracic outlet syndrome. J. Bone Joint Surg. (Brit.) *47*:268–272, 1965.

Britt, L. P.: Nonoperative treatment of thoracic outlet syndrome symptoms. Clin. Orthop. *51*:45–48, 1967.

Clagett, O. T.: Presidential Address: Research and Prosearch. J. Thorac. Cardiovasc. Surg. *44*:153, 1962.

Falconer, M. A., and Li, F. W. P.: Resection of first rib in costoclavicular compression of the brachial plexus. Lancet *1*:59, 1962.

Kaye, B. L.: Neurologic changes with excessively large breasts. South. Med. J. *65(2)*:177, 1972.

Law, A. A.: Adventitious ligaments simulating cervical ribs. Ann. Surg. *72*:497, 1920.

Lord, J. W., and Rosati, L.: Neurovascular compression syndrome of the upper extremity. Clin. Symp. *10*:35, 1958.

Lusskin, R., Weiss, C. A., and Winer, J.: The role of the subclavius muscle in the subclavian vein syndrome (costoclavicular syndrome) following fracture of the clavicle. Clin. Orthop. *54*:75, Sept–Oct., 1967.

Mathes, S. J., and Salaam, A.: Subclavian artery aneurysm; sequela of thoracic outlet syndrome. Surgery *76(3)*:506, 1974.

Peet, R. M., Henriksen, J. D., Anderson, T. P., and Martin, G. M.: Thoracic outlet syndrome: Evaluation of a therapeutic exercise program. Staff Meet. Mayo Clin. *31*:281, 1956.

Roos, D. B.: Transaxillary approach for first rib resection to relieve thoracic outlet syndrome. Ann. Surg. *163*:354, 1966.

Roos, D.: Plethysmography, a simple method of studying and following peripheral vascular disease. Surg. Clin. North Am. *49(6)*–1333, Dec. 1969.

Roos, D. B.: Experience with first rib resection for thoracic outlet syndrome. Arch. Surg. *173*:429, 1971.

Short, D. W.: The subclavian artery in 16 patients with complete cervical ribs. J. Cardiovasc. Surg. *16*:135, 1975.

Swinton, N. W., Hall, R. J., Baugh, J. H., and Blake, H. A.: Unilateral Raynaud's phenomenon caused by first rib anomalies. Am. J. Med. *48*:404, 1970.

Urschel, H. C., Paulson, M. D., and McNamara, J. J.: Thoracic outlet syndrome. Ann. Thorac. Surg. *6(1)*:1, 1968.

36

QUADRILATERAL SPACE SYNDROME

BERNARD R. CAHILL

This unusual syndrome, which has been recognized for the past nine years, is caused by a compression of the posterior humeral circumflex artery and axillary nerve in the quadrilateral space. It affects active young people of both sexes. The youngest case in a series of 134, was 22 years of age and the oldest, 43. The average duration of symptoms before seeking medical attention was 18 months.

Symptoms begin with slow, intermittent onset of pain and paresthesias in the upper extremity, usually not associated with shoulder trauma. Forward flexion and/or abduction and external rotation of the humerous aggravates the symptoms. In some cases night symptoms awaken the victims.

The pain component of this syndrome is poorly localized to the anterior aspect of the shoulder, and the paresthesias have a nondermatomal distribution in the arm, forearm, and hand. The paresthesias are described with the same adjectives used for other neurovascular compression syndromes and are also usually not dermatomal in distribution. Like other peripheral entrapment neuropathies, the atypical distribution of the pain and paresthesia makes the diagnosis difficult when relying on the history and physical examination alone (Thompson, 1959; Kopell, 1960).

Most patients, after obtaining medical consultation, have had numerous oral anti-inflammatory agents, local injection of hydrocortisone and local anesthesia into various sites in the shoulder, exercises, and physical therapy. None of these measures gives complete relief, and when partial relief occurs it is not lasting.

After entertaining a diagnosis of neurosis, the frustrated physician eventually orders a subclavian arteriogram to rule out thoracic outlet syndrome. Unfortunately, most radiologists do not follow the dye far enough peripherally to make a diagnosis of compression of the posterior humeral circumflex artery. If the subclavian artery is radiographically normal, most of these patients are

602

dismissed as neurotics, or a questionably abnormal subclavian artery is surgically decompressed without success.

Diffuse anterior and lateral shoulder tenderness may be present; however, discrete point tenderness is always found posteriorly in the quadrilateral space. This is often missed or not looked for. The tenderness tends to be lateral in the quadrilateral space, almost at the insertion of the teres minor. Abduction and external rotation (AER) of the humerus for approximately one minute will reproduce the symptoms in some patients. There may be some difference in the quality of the radial pulse in the AER position, or in other maneuvers used in the diagnosis of the thoracic outlet syndrome, and this often leads to the tentative diagnosis of thoracic outlet syndrome and a subclavian arteriogram. The neurologic examination is normal and there is no muscular atrophy, although five cases of the quadrilateral space syndrome had an associated carpal tunnel syndrome.

Electromyographic studies of the deltoid muscle are normal, as are ulnar and median nerve conduction times if this is a pure quadrilateral space syndrome.

Patients with histories and physical findings such as these should have a subclavian arteriogram, done according to the Seldinger technique (Seldinger, 1953). The dye is injected with the humerus at the side and in AER. The dye is followed distally so that the posterior humeral circumflex artery may be evaluat-

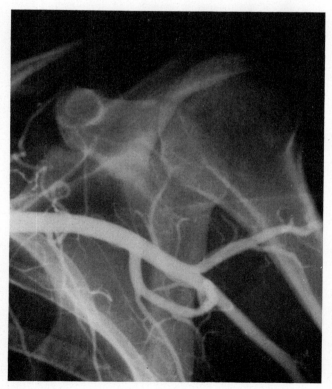

Figure 36–1   The subclavian arteriogram of the 28-year-old male with the symptomatic left arm at the side.

ed. In positive arteriograms, this artery will be patent with the humerus at the side, but may occlude with as little as 60 degrees of abduction. Other cases require full AER. The asymptomatic shoulder has a normal subclavian arteriogram, and I no longer feel it necessary to perform bilateral procedures (Figs. 36–1 thru 36–3).

Many patients have been referred after a normal subclavian arteriogram but with a compressed posterior humeral circumflex artery. Approximately 70 per cent of these do not have symptoms sufficient to justify surgery. Reassurance that they are not neurotic seems to enable these patients to live with their disability. Long-term followup on these nonoperated patients confirms this. It also confirms that the symptoms of the quadrilateral space syndrome do not cease entirely with the passage of time.

If the patient has sufficient symptoms, a positive subclavian arteriogram indicating occlusion of the posterior humeral circumflex artery, and local tenderness posteriorly over the quadrilateral space, surgical decompression of the quadrilateral space should be considered.

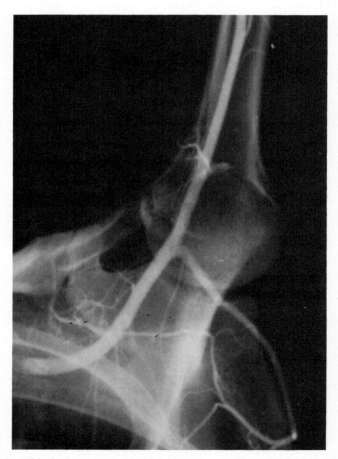

Figure 36–2   With the humerus in the AER position, arteriogram shows occlusion of the posterior humeral circumflex artery just distal to its origin.

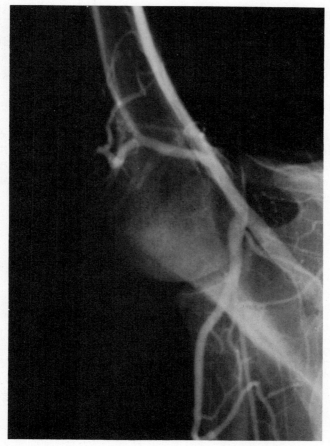

Figure 36-3 The asymptomatic right arm is shown in the AER position with the posterior humeral circumflex artery patent. The subclavian artery was bilaterally normal.

The posterior approach to the shoulder is used (Bennett, 1941). The arm is draped free. Hemostasis is essential, since bleeding into the areolar tissue of the quadrilateral space, even in minute quantities, makes visualization of the posterior humeral circumflex artery and axillary nerve extremely difficult. After the deltoid muscle is reflected laterally, the interval between the infraspinous and teres minor muscles is developed. The teres minor is then detached from its insertion into the posterior capsule, usually leaving a defect. The teres minor and its nerve are reflected medially, after dividing the nerve. Medial reflection of the teres minor aids exposure and removes a superior obstruction of the quadrilateral space. By blunt dissection the neurovascular bundle containing the axillary nerve and the posterior humeral circumflex artery are followed anteriorly for 1 to 2 cm. Prior to this dissection, on inserting an index finger into the quadrilateral space, one encounters randomly oriented tethering bands. These bands must be divided and, with the index finger on the pulse of the posterior humeral circumflex artery, the arm is taken into AER until it remains palpable to at least 110 degrees of abduction and 45 degrees of external rotation of the humerus. The axillary nerve must not be stretched over retractors while manipulating the humerus.

The quadrilateral space is consistently tethered by these fibrous bands, which have not been found on cadaver dissections. They seem to be responsible for the constriction of the neurovascular bundle. Fusiform swelling of the nerve to the teres minor may be encountered (Daniell, 1944; Getlin, 1957). The symptom complex is probably due to compression of nervous tissue and not to vascular compromise.

The teres minor muscle is not reattached but if there is a defect in the posterior capsule it is repaired. Routine closure is then carried out.

The patient is placed on active range of motion as soon as comfortable and begins shoulder girdle strengthening exercises at three weeks. Most patients are able to return to their employment within six weeks.

REFERENCES

Bennett, G. E.: Shoulder and elbow lesions of the professional baseball pitcher. J.A.M.A. *117*:510, 1941.

Daniell, H. W.: Fusiform swelling on the terminal portions of peripheral nerves. J. Neuropathol. Exp. Neurol. *13*:467, 1954.

Getlin, G.: Concerning the gangliform enlargement on the nerve to the teres minor muscle. J. Anat. *91*:466, 1957.

Kopell, H. P., and Thompson, W. A. L.: Peripheral entrapment neuropathies of the lower extremities. New Engl. J. Med. *262*:56, 1960.

Seldinger, S. I.: Catheter replacement of the needle in percutaneous arteriography; a new technique. Acta Radiol. *39*:368, 1953.

37

OPERATIVE EXPERIENCE WITH MAJOR LOWER EXTREMITY NERVE LESIONS, INCLUDING THE LUMBOSACRAL PLEXUS AND THE SCIATIC NERVE

DAVID G. KLINE

The incidence of major injury to the nerves of the lower extremity is infrequent when compared to that of the upper extremity (Seddon, 1972; Woodhall and Beebe, 1957). However, when serious injury occurs, it is often devastating, even if circumstances for regeneration are optimal. New axons must

607

travel great distances to reach effective functional end-inputs. With all pelvic plexus lesions and most sciatic nerve lesions, such regeneration may require many months to several years. By the time axons reach such distant inputs, not only are they frequently fine in caliber and poorly myelinated but also the muscle awaiting reinnervation is severely atrophic or may even be replaced by fibrosis or fat (Gutman and Young, 1944; Woodhall and Beebe, 1957). These considerations make early diagnosis, relatively early decision for or against operation and, most importantly, the correct intraoperative decision regarding need for resection and suture mandatory.

In addition to the restrictions imposed by great regenerative distances, pelvic plexus injuries, although fortunately rare, are by definition complex and difficult to correct should spontaneous recovery not occur. One of the outflows from the plexus, the peroneal or anterior tibial division of the sciatic nerve, is not only especially prone to injury but also regenerates poorly. Various explanations have been proposed for the poor results seen with peroneal injury and repair, and are nicely summarized by Sunderland (1968). The peroneal nerve has less cross-sectional perineurium than does the tibial, and this may also contribute to its relative propensity for injury, as may its lateral position at the buttocks level, which may lead to more frequent injury with fractures or dislocations of the head of the femur and hip. Its oblique course through the thigh and its relative tethering at the head of the fibula may also predispose the peroneal to more severe stretch than that encountered with the tibial nerve. In addition, the peroneal nerve also innervates muscle bundles in the anterior lower leg compartment, which are, when compared to the tibial innervated gastrocnemius–achilles, not only more distal but also smaller in volume, requiring presumably more accurate and therefore closer point-to-point reinnervation than does the tibial innervated musculature.

SPECIFIC LOWER EXTREMITY NERVE INJURIES

Table 37–1 shows that the sciatic has been the most frequently injured lower extremity nerve in our experience. This table also shows that gunshot wound was the most common mechanism of injury of the sciatic nerve, followed by transection or laceration, tumor, and injection injury. A variety of mechanisms were responsible in a small series of femoral nerve injuries cared for (seven) while laceration was the mechanism usually responsible for sural injury (four).

Sciatic Nerve

The sciatic nerve is formed from the anterior and posterior divisions of the L4, L5, S1, and S2 roots, as well as the anterior division of S3. In general, the anterior divisions make up the tibial nerve as well as the large nerve to the hamstring musculature, whereas the posterior divisions make up the peroneal nerve (Seddon, 1972). Divisions combine after the posterior elements give rise to the superior and inferior gluteal nerves in the pelvis and then emerge as the sciatic nerve from the pelvis via the sciatic notch, where they lie beneath the gluteus maximus. Gluteal nerves, the major hamstring nerve, and the gluteal

Table 37–1. Lower Extremity Nerve Lesions Operated Upon 1966–1977

	TRANS	LAC	GSW	INJ	F(x)	TUMOR	CONT	STRETCH	PRIOR OP	OTHER	TOTAL
Sciatic (Buttocks)	2	0	3	6	0	1	1	0	2	2	17
Sciatic (Thigh)	4	3	17	2	1	2	2	0	1	3	35
Tibial (Knee)	0	1	2	0	0	2	0	0	0	0	5
Peroneal (Knee)	1	0	4	0	1	3	2	2	2	1	16
Tibial (Lower leg)	0	2	0	0	0	1	1	0	4	0	8
Peroneal (Lower leg)	0	0	0	0	1	1	0	0	2	0	4
Femoral (Pelvic)	1	0	1	0	0	0	0	0	2	0	4
Femoral (Thigh)	0	1	2	0	0	0	0	0	0	0	3
Pelvic Plexus	0	0	0	0	0	3	0	0	0	0	3
Sural	0	3	1	0	0	0	0	0	0	0	4
Totals	8	10	30	8	3	13	6	2	13	6	99

Key: TRANS = transection; LAC = laceration; GSW = gunshot wound; INJ = injection injury; F(x) = fracture; CONT = contusion; PRIOR OP = Prior operation.

vessels leave the notch with the sciatic nerve. The sciatic nerve usually exits the pelvis to lie below the lower margin of the piriformis but occasionally may penetrate it or even lie above it. In some cases, the two divisions of the sciatic nerve remain discrete after their exit from the pelvis, and in this case the peroneal may penetrate the piriformis itself (Sunderland, 1968). At this level, the major nerve to the hamstrings is medial to the sciatic, while the nerve to the short head of the biceps is lateral. The contiguous nature of these structures, as well as the vasculature to the nerves and the gluteal vessels themselves, makes dissection at the level of the notch difficult but not impossible. The major branch to the hamstrings travels close to the medial or tibial division of the nerve through the buttocks, and on reaching the upper thigh it branches to supply the long head of the biceps, the semitendinosus, and the semimembranosus, as well as the ischial portion of the adductor magnus. The sciatic divisions lie on top or dorsal to the gemelli and quadratus in the midportion of the buttocks and enter the thigh somewhat deep and between medial and lateral masses of the hamstring muscles.

Sciatic Lesions — Buttock Level

The skin incision for the buttock level exposure is curvilinear and is placed around the lateral aspect of the buttock mass (Seletz, 1951). If the sciatic nerve in the proximal thigh as well as beneath the buttock needs to be exposed, the incision is swung into the buttocks crease and then down the posterior midline of the thigh. The incision extends deep between the hamstring muscles for thigh level exposure of the sciatic nerve, whereas the gluteus maximus and a portion of the medius are separated close to the lateral pelvic brim and mobilized medially to expose the nerve up to the sciatic notch. There is a somewhat avascular plane beneath the gluteal musculature and posterior to the neural structures. Enough of a rim of gluteal attachment should be left laterally to facilitate later closure.

Injection injuries and fracture dislocations are responsible for most sciatic lesions at the level of the buttocks. Gunshot wounds, rare tumors, and injury from prior operation are other sources of buttock level involvement. Owing to massive and blunt buttock contusion from falls, subgluteal clot can acutely compress the sciatic nerve. Treatment of one such case included acute evacuation of the clot and neurolysis of the sciatic nerve, which resulted in early reversal of a complete but presumably neurapractic sciatic injury.

Patients with injection injuries are often either constitutionally thin or chronically ill and thus debilitated. Poor gluteal covering predisposes to this type of injury, particularly if the injection is given with a long needle in other than the upper, outer quadrant of the buttocks. There appear to be two patterns of onset of pain and disability following such injury to the sciatic nerve. The first, and by far the most frequent, is radicular pain and paresthesias with some degree of distal deficit of almost immediate onset (Clark et al., 1970). The second, and much less frequent, pattern is delayed onset of pain, paresthesias, and deficit appearing minutes to several hours after the injection, which may or may not have produced severe local pain shortly after it was administered. These historical differences suggest the possibility that noxious drugs need not be injected directly into the nerve to damage it but rather may be deposited subepineurially or perhaps even adjacent to the nerve and with time may diffuse into or penetrate the intrafascicular structure.

To date, only a quarter of the injection injuries seen have warranted operation. Partial injuries sparing some function in both the tibial and peroneal divisions can usually be treated with vigorous physical therapy and time, although such injuries may on occasion require exploration and internal neurolysis that may or may not relieve the pain. More complete lesions to either the sciatic as a whole or to all of one division may benefit from relatively early exploration, intraoperative recording of nerve action potentials (NAP's), and differential neurolysis of each division if NAP's are present, or resection and suture if they are absent. Time for such exploration is best three to five months after the injection injury occurs. Results are poor if resection and suture are indicated for the peroneal division but better with tibial repair. Even resection of a division if it is felt to be non-repairable may not help the pain associated with some injection injuries. One of our patients who had resection of a segment of the peroneal division at the buttock level eventually had a sympathectomy with some relief even though the pain was not of a classic, causalgic nature.

The sciatic nerve is not infrequently injured at the buttock level in conjunction with posterior fractures alone or in conjunction with dislocations of the hip and acetabulum (Patterson, 1972). Treatment has usually been expectant (Seddon, 1972) rather than operative, although there are exceptions where relatively early exploration and suture may be indicated (Johnson, 1969; Spiegel, 1974). Even if the nerve is not operated on directly, every attempt should be made to reduce the dislocation and stabilize the fracture as soon as possible. One patient with a complete sciatic palsy following dislocation of the hip without fracture had complete reversal of his palsy after reduction of his hip within a few hours of injury, so that some of these patients will have recovery of function although, unfortunately, the peroneal portion of the paralysis is more likely to persist, requiring the use of a drop foot brace. If the fracture or dislocation requires operative exposure for reduction, the nerve should be inspected and freed of scar or penetrating bone fragments at the same time (Johnson, 1969; Seddon, 1972).

Sciatic Lesions — Thigh Level

At the thigh level, gunshot wounds to either the whole sciatic nerve or to predominantly one division are not uncommon (Clawson and Seddon, 1960; Kline, 1972). Such gunshot wounds produce lesions in continuity which may or may not improve with time. Hamstring function is usually spared, since these branches originate high and take a somewhat different course from the sciatic itself. Tibial division loss will be manifested by inversion weakness of the foot, plantar flexion loss, and inability to flex or spread the toes. Sensory loss will be on the sole of the foot as well as the volar surface of the toes, particularly the large toe. Peroneal division loss gives "foot drop" or "slap foot." Eversion and dorsiflexion of the foot as well as extension of the big toe by the extensor hallucis longus are lost. Sensory loss, if present, is over the dorsum of the foot. The peroneal nerve does not have as autonomous a zone for sensation as does the tibial. Overlap from the saphenous and sural nerves makes such sensory loss less definite.

Fractures and sometimes extensive soft tissue loss may accompany gunshot injury to the sciatic but should not delay exploration too long. Distances to distal inputs, should suture be necessary for regeneration, are lengthy. If the distal deficit in a suspected lesion in continuity is complete to one or both divisions of the sciatic and does not improve, the injury should be explored at two to four months. A longer wait in the face of complete loss to one or both divisions militates against recovery should resection and suture be necessary. By two to four months after injury, stimulation and recording studies should show NAP evidence of regeneration if axonal regrowth has been effective in the interim. Absence of an NAP indicates the need for resection and suture (Kline, 1977). The value of thorough preoperative and intraoperative workup can be seen in Table 37–2.

Even in the proximal thigh the sciatic nerve may travel as two distinct divisions of nerve or may cover a portion of the proximal thigh as a single nerve and then split somewhat prematurely into two nerves. As a result, even proximal thigh injury may occur to one division, sparing or minimally involving the other. Thus, loss of tibial function with peroneal sparing even with a proximal thigh level wound does not insure partial injury to the sciatic as a whole but may rather reflect complete injury to one division and partial or no injury to the other. In the usual case, if an NAP is recorded from the whole nerve despite distal functional loss of any significance, then the nerve should be split into its two divisions and each evaluated and treated separately (Kline, 1972). For example, if an NAP can be recorded from one division and not the other, neurolysis of the first and resection and suture of the second are indicated. Unfortunately, it is

Table 37–3.   Importance of Multiple Electrical Studies of Sciatic Elements in Continuity After Serious Injury*

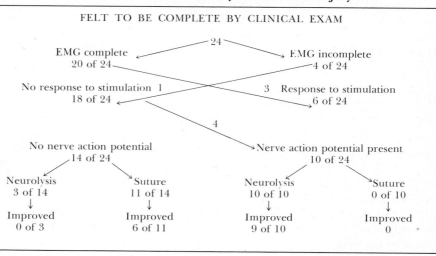

FELT TO BE COMPLETE BY CLINICAL EXAM

EMG complete 20 of 24 — 24 → EMG incomplete 4 of 24

No response to stimulation 18 of 24   1   3   Response to stimulation 6 of 24

No nerve action potential 14 of 24   4   Nerve action potential present 10 of 24

Neurolysis 3 of 14   Suture 11 of 14   Neurolysis 10 of 10   Suture 0 of 10

Improved 0 of 3   Improved 6 of 11   Improved 9 of 10   Improved 0

Key: Most of these cases were explored two or more months post-injury because of a clinically complete deficit despite suspected gross continuity. Injuries were due to gunshot wound, injections, contusion, and stretch, and in one instance, fracture. (See Table 1). EMG suggested early regeneration in four, while stimulation at operating table gave distal function in six and nerve action potentials could be recorded across and distal to the lesion in 10, indicating acceptable regeneration. Nine of these 10 cases improved with neurolysis alone.

*Follow-up of one year or more.

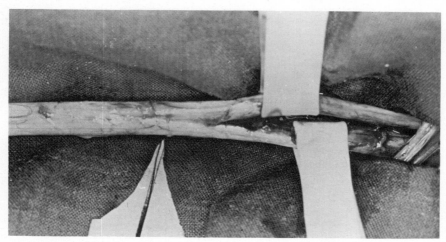

Figure 37–1 Method of splitting sciatic nerve. Tibial and peroneal nerves have been identified and are gently retracted to either side with one-half inch rubber Penrose drains. A small cleft or crease is usually discernable and/or palpable between the two divisions, and this is developed further by sharp dissection using magnification and microinstruments. Saline irrigation and microtipped bipolar forceps are used to identify and cauterize bleeding points.

frequently the peroneal division that requires resection and repair while the tibial has evidence of regeneration and can be treated by neurolysis. Occasionally, however, the reverse is true and then the prognosis for more complete return of function is more favorable, since the tibial may respond to suture even at a proximal thigh level.

The sciatic nerve may be readily split both above and below the level of the lesion. One can usually see or palpate a plane between the two divisions and, if not, the sciatic can be traced to the tibial and peroneal nerves in the lower thigh. These two nerves are then dissected in a retrograde fashion, splitting one from the other within the sciatic itself. Some magnification, such as is provided by eye loupes, is helpful as well as use of microsurgical scissors, forceps, and spatulas. A bipolar coagulator is necessary to treat the intraneural bleeding.

Loss of length in the sciatic nerve can be made up by a number of maneuvers, including complete mobilization of the complex tracing the tibial or posterior tibial division into and beneath the triceps surae. Removing the head of the fibula and tracing the peroneal and anterior tibial branches of the peroneal nerve, proximal mobilization of the nerve to the buttocks, and flexion of the lower leg on the upper leg also make up length. Hamstring branches can sometimes tether either stump, and these need to be traced into muscle as far as possible without damaging them. These methods can make up 10 to 11 cm in length as has been the case in our own as well as Clawson and Seddon's experience (Clawson and Seddon, 1960b). We prefer not to flex the lower leg on the upper beyond 60 degrees from the fully extended position. If flexion beyond this is required for end-to-end repair, one should consider the interposition of short interfascicular grafts, which have supplanted most other techniques of correcting large sciatic gaps (MacCarty, 1951). It has been rare in our experience to need hip extension or immobilization of the hip joint by spica cast.

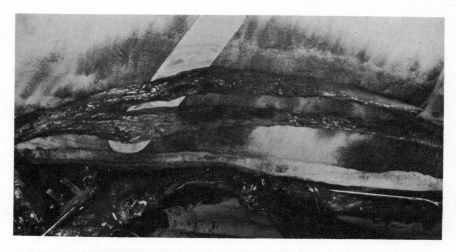

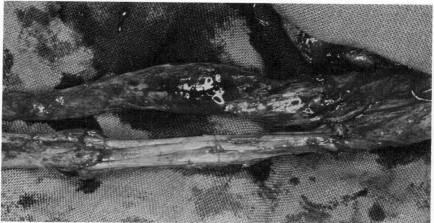

Figure 37–2   GSW to mid-thigh sciatic nerve. Since an NAP could be recorded across this lesion it was split into tibial and peroneal divisions and re-evaluated electrically (top). A small NAP could be recorded across the peroneal but not the tibial division, so the tibial neuroma was resected and a sural interfascicular graft done (bottom).

Experience with an unusual injury in five patients, complete section of the sciatic nerve at the level of buttocks crease or thigh, has suggested that primary repair, if possible, is preferable in this setting. These guillotine-like injuries usually transect hamstring musculature as well as nerve, since the transection extends to the posterior aspect of the femur (Kline, 1972). If explored secondarily, the acutely transected sciatic nerve ends will have retracted, making up length is difficult, and tension on the repair and subsequent distraction is possible. Significant retraction of one or both stumps may make even primary repair difficult.

A teenage girl tried to break out of a shower by bracing her feet on the tile wall and pushing with her buttocks against the shower door. The door broke and the glass transected both nerves at the gluteal crease. The referring neurosurgeon knew to attempt primary repair and did so successfully on one limb but

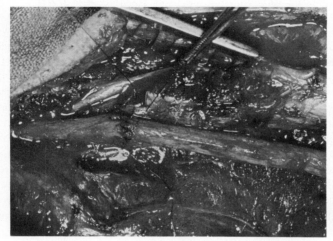

Figure 37–3 Completed epineurial suture of whole sciatic nerve at mid-thigh level following resection of a neurotmetic lesion due to GSW. Distal deficit was complete and remained so both clinically and electrically for three months preoperatively.

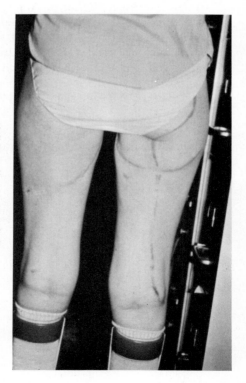

Figure 37–4 Postoperative view of patient with total transection of both sciatic nerves. Sciatic and transected muscle on the left side were repaired primarily through the original laceration. The referring surgeon tried to locate the right sciatic stumps through the original laceration but could not locate the proximal stump. Upon secondary exploration in our institution, the proximal stump had retracted well beneath the gluteus maximus. Extensive mobilization of both stumps, flexion of the lower leg, and casting were necessary to achieve satisfactory end-to-end repair.

could not locate the proximal stump in the other. After transfer to this center several days later, the proximal stump was found at the mid-buttock level, just distal to the sciatic notch, and a secondary repair was possible but only after extensive mobilization of the nerve, flexion at the knee, and casting. Four patients with a sufficient period of followup who have had primary repair have fared well compared to those having secondary repair. Tibial nerve recovery is more complete and in one instance peroneal nerve function has returned sufficiently so that the patient does not require the use of a drop foot brace.

Tumors involving the sciatic nerve or its branches at thigh or popliteal level have included neurofibromas (3), Schwannomas (2), neural ganglion (1), venous malformation (1), and desmoid tumor (1), all operated upon because of severe pain or progressive neurologic deficit, or both. The neurofibromas were removed in a gross, total fashion by splitting fascicles both proximal and distal to the tumor under magnification, tracing them into the tumor, and sparing as many as possible. One neurofibroma measuring 8 cm in diameter was successfully removed using this approach. The two other neurofibromas were not as large, and thus function was more readily preserved. One Schwannoma was readily enucleated without any deficit by removing the contents of the tumor and then teasing away the capsule from the fascicles.

Sciatic Branches — Popliteal Level

In the popliteal region, injury involving nerve usually affects one nerve, either the tibial or the peroneal, rather than both, although exceptions certainly can occur, particularly with gunshot wounds or with other penetrating lesions which may lead to a clot. One such patient in our series developed an acute clot secondary to a gunshot wound that compressed both tibial and peroneal nerves and whose functional loss was reversed by evacuation of the clot as well as neurolysis of the nerves (Kline, 1977). On rare occasions, similar injury can produce a popliteal aneurysm that can compress otherwise intact or mildly injured tibial nerve, which is closely applied to the artery through most of the popliteal fossa and then deviates slightly laterally to innervate the triceps surae

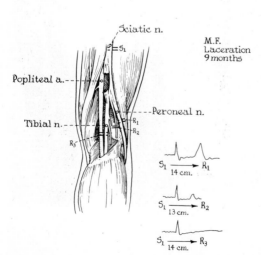

Figure 37–5 Drawing of lower thigh level partial transection of sciatic nerve explored at nine months post injury following late referral. NAP studies showed good peroneal activity (S1→R1), some sural nerve conduction (S2→R3), but no tibial activity. After splitting the sciatic into its two divisions to mid-thigh level and trimming the neuromatous proximal and gliomatous distal stumps, a three inch gap resulted, and this required sural interfascicular graft repair.

musculature. Discrete injuries to the tibial nerve in the popliteal region without vascular involvement have been rare in our experience although we have treated one patient with laceration of the tibial nerve without arterial injury.

Stretch or avulsion of the peroneal nerve associated with dislocation and/or fracture of the knee is not uncommon. These injuries are, in our experience as well as that of others (Highet and Holmes, 1943; White, 1968), difficult to treat successfully. If the lesion is complete and does not recover in the early months, wide resection and repair, usually by grafts, is the only alternative to conservative therapy. The results of either are extremely poor. Proper bracing, usually with a spring loaded dropfoot brace, and proper skin care are very effective (Stayman, 1972). Occasionally, posterior tibial tendon transfer is indicated in young and lightweight patients. Unfortunately, the peroneal nerve can be injured readily, not only by contusion or laceration at the level of the head of the fibula but also by surgical procedures in this area. Efforts to reconstruct the knee, to remove Baker's cysts, or to excise the fibular head or soft tissue tumors have resulted in tibial or peroneal nerve palsy in a number of patients subsequently referred to our service. These patients required secondary repair of the injured nerve. Usually nerve graft reconstruction is necessary.

Sciatic Branches — Lower Leg and Ankle

In the lower leg, the tibial nerve runs beneath the triceps surae and angles toward the medial malleolus, which it passes inferior to, to enter the plantar canal or tarsal tunnel.The need for exposure of the tibial nerve at the mid-calf level is infrequent, since the nerve is deep to and protected by the triceps surae. Exposure for this as well as peroneal branches, which at this level are usually sensory and therefore not of great functional importance, can be seen in the text by Seletz (1951). At the ankle level, the lateral, posterior, and medial plantar branches supply sensation to the heel and sole of the foot. This is a site for the tarsal tunnel entrapment syndrome. Although not included in Table 1, such patients present with burning paresthesias in the sole of the foot, aggravated by weight-bearing, have a Tinel's sign below the medial malleolus usually over the instep of the foot, and have poor or absent sensory conduction on stimulation of toes and attempted NAP recording proximal to the medial malleolus. All or a portion of the tarsal tunnel syndrome symptoms may also be seen with injury to the tibial nerve or its branches at the ankle.

The ankle region is, unfortunately, not an infrequent site for lacerating and contusive injury, especially those associated with fractures. Occasionally, reconstruction of such a fracture and of the collateral ligaments can secondarily entrap or compress the tibial nerve or plantar branches at this level, as was seen in three of our cases. Each case had a prior operation, usually neurolysis, but had to have a repeat neurolysis or suture with variable functional results. Usually, acceptable relief of pain was obtained.

On the lateral side of the ankle, the peroneal sensory branches as well as the sural nerve can be involved by laceration, contusion, and fracture. Fracture of the later malleolus was accompanied by peroneal nerve injury in three of our cases. Two of these had had prior operative attempts made to reduce the neural pain.

At secondary surgery the following causes for persistent symptoms were

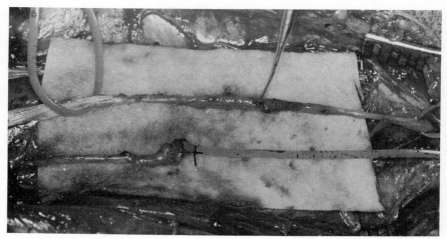

Figure 37–6   Distal lower leg tibial nerve branch mistakenly sewn to tendon. Vasaloop is around tendon, double ended instrument points to tendon to nerve suture site while second vasaloop is attached, for illustrative purposes, to neuromatous proximal stump of the nerve. Patient presented because of painful paresthesias in tibial distribution whenever posterior calf was compressed or bumped.

found: the tibial or peroneal nerve was found sutured to a tendon; the tarsal tunnel was released insufficiently to relieve the entrapment of injured plantar branches and/or tibial nerve; and, with reconstruction of the collateral ligaments of the ankle, neural entrapment occurred.

Tumors at the ankle level involving nerve are unusual (Das Gupta and Brasfield, 1970) but they can occur. For example, a neurofibroma was the diagnosis in a 37-year-old black male with painful paresthesias located in the sole of the foot on weight-bearing. Percussion over the malleolus reproduced these paresthesias but there were no masses palpable in the lower extremity and no cutaneous manifestations of von Recklinghausen's disease. At exploration, a serpiginous neurofibroma was found extending from foot to buttocks level with alternate areas of cystic and firm tumor. Function was preserved and some help was given for the painful paresthesias by decompression of the cysts without removal of the more solid portions of the tumor. One interesting case was that of a teenager who had an exquisitely tender area over the lower anterior tibial or "shin" region associated with an old contusion to this area caused by a ski boot. Tapping in the region gave exquisitely severe pain and paresthesias on the dorsum of the foot, and a neuroma although not palpable was suspected. However, at exploration, a glomus tumor was found instead. This tumor measured only a centimeter in diameter but was attached to the tibial periosteum. This is an unusual but not unreported locus for this tumor. Recurrence is a possibility, since some two years after resection she has had a few paresthetic pains and has a mild Tinel's sign in that region.

Femoral Nerve

Femoral nerve injuries fall into two categories — those distal to the inguinal ligament and thus in the femoral triangle and those proximal and by definition intrapelvic. Theoretically, injury to the pelvic portion of the femoral nerve should give, in addition to quadriceps paralysis and hypesthesia over the anteromedial thigh, loss of sartorius or "tailor muscle" function. Unfortunately, the branch to the sartorius is somewhat variable in origin and course, and thus one of our clearly intrapelvic femoral nerve lesions appeared to spare this muscle while several thigh level lesions had sartorius loss. Preservation or loss of this muscle's function does not necessarily localize the level of femoral nerve involvement.

In the thigh, the nerve branches "pes-like" one to two inches distal to the inguinal ligament to supply the quadriceps. These branches make dissection and identification of elements that need repair difficult unless the thigh injury is

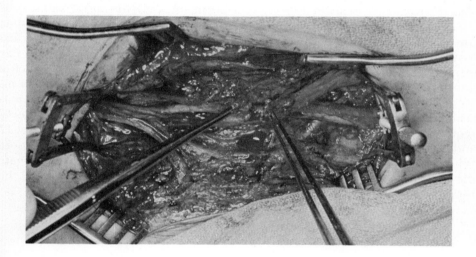

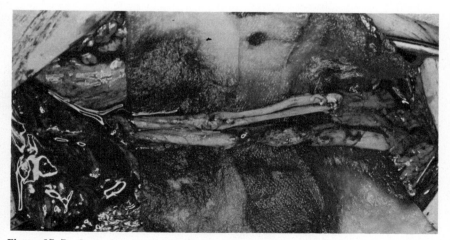

Figure 37–7 Operative site of prior femoral popliteal bypass graft which resulted in injury to femoral nerve (top). Deficit was complete and remained so for five months. At exploration, one of the branches had an NAP but the others did not. As a result, partial repair was done using interfascicular grafts for a portion and neurolysis for the rest (bottom).

immediately distal to the ligament. Four of the thigh level injuries seen had exploration and some type of repair attempted. Neurolysis sufficed in one injury due to gunshot wound (Kline and DeJong, 1968) as well as in another where a knife wound involved the femoral branches. Another thigh level nerve injury was due to a femoral–popliteal bypass procedure, which at exploration required graft repair of some branches and neurolysis of others. At the pelvic level, injury was due to herniorrhaphy in one instance, a hip replacement procedure in another and gunshot wound in a third. Surprisingly enough, a lacerating injury caused by glass that penetrated the lower abdominal wall at inguinal ligament level spared the intra-abdominal contents but transected the femoral nerve at the edge of the pelvis. This last case is worth noting, since a primary nerve repair had been attempted elsewhere. Since signs of clinical as well as electromyographic recovery failed to materialize by six months post-repair, the wound was re-explored. The distal femoral nerve was identified in the femoral triangle and traced proximally beneath the inguinal ligament, and the distal stump was attached by scar to the femoral vein. The proximal stump with a large neuroma present on it was found on the brim of the pelvis, a good distance from its usual location. After the stumps were trimmed back to healthy tissue, sural grafts (six in number) were necessary to make up a 9 cm gap. Another case in which a gunshot wound had injured the pelvic portion of the femoral nerve, also involved the bladder and large bowel. Repair of the nerve within the pelvis was achieved secondarily after the other pelvic injuries were healed. The nerve required five 7.5 cm sural grafts. Both of these patients were relatively young, 12 and 27 years of age, respectively. Both had some return of quadriceps function. When evaluating recovery following femoral nerve repair one must eliminate the mimicking action of the uninvolved tensor fascia latae, which can extend the leg as a trick movement.

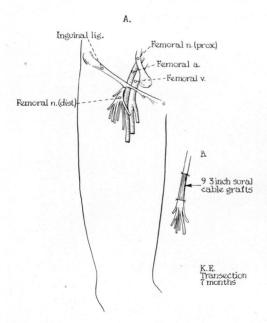

Figure 37–8 Femoral nerve transected at inguinal level by a glass injury. Initial attempt at repair elsewhere failed. At secondary exploration the neuromatous proximal stump was displaced in the distal pelvis. The distal stump was adherent to the femoral vessels. Repair was done with interfascicular grafts. At nine months post repair, quadriceps function began to recover and has progressively improved over the next six months.

Sural Nerve

The sural nerve takes its origin from both the peroneal and tibial nerves in the popliteal fossa and penetrates the gastrocnemius fascia to run beneath it until it reaches the approximate junction of the upper and middle third of the lower leg, where it leaves the fascia to lie subcutaneously in the midline posterior calf. The nerve then takes a slightly oblique course across the lower calf to lie along the lateral side of the gastrocnemius–achilles tendon. As the sural approaches the lateral malleolus it branches to innervate the nonweight-bearing surface of the heel and the lateral aspect of the foot. Laceration of the nerve can give a painful neuroma much as is seen with injury to the superficial radial sensory branch in the upper extremity. In three cases in our series the nerve was lacerated by glass, in two instances from exploded soda "pop" bottles. These patients developed painful paresthesias in the heel and on the lateral aspect of the foot. The cause of these paresthesias was initially unsuspected. Once the diagnosis was made, the neuroma was widely excised in a sharp fashion and the proximal stump was buried deep beneath the gastrocnemius fascia to minimize the symptoms brought upon by recurrence of the neuroma.

Pain due to injury of the sural nerve is less common at the level of the popliteal fossa than at the calf. Nonetheless, one patient in our series sustained a gunshot wound to the popliteal fossa producing not only partial injury and peroneal loss but also severe paresthesias and pain in the distribution of the sural nerve. Significant improvement was gained after a lengthy resection of the sural nerve that extended from the popliteal level to the middle third of the posterior calf.

As with injury to the superficial radial sensory nerve in the forearm, no attempt should be made to repair the sural nerve, for suture will lead to a neuroma and recurrence of pain. Moreover, the sural nerve innervates a functionally unimportant portion of the foot, and thus its sensory distribution can be sacrificed without detriment to the patient. For this reason, as well as because the sural nerve is relatively accessible and usually of relatively good caliber, the nerve is an excellent source for autogenous grafts. The nerve can be exposed by a linear, vertical incision placed lateral to the gastrocnemius–achilles tendon and extending up the posterior calf. Vessels, especially veins in this area, should not be mistaken for the nerve nor for superficial peroneal branches if the dissection is carried too far lateral. If identification of the nerve is in question, extend the excision toward the lateral malleolus, and, if need be, to the popliteal region to identify either the termination or the origin of the nerve. Stimulation of the sural nerve should, of course, not produce muscular function. The nerve should be sharply resected, placed in sterile, normal saline, and excess soft tissue trimmed before use for interfascicular grafts.

Pelvic Plexus

The pelvic plexus is formed by the anterior and posterior divisions of L2 to L5 as well as S1 and S2, along with the anterior division of S3 (Seddon, 1972; White, 1968). The anterior divisions form the tibial division, and the posterior the peroneal division of the sciatic nerve. Posterior divisions of L2, L3, and L4 form the femoral nerve, and branches from the posterior division of L2 and L3 from the lateral femoral cutaneous nerve. The obturator nerve is formed by the anterior divisions of L2, L3, and L4. The plexus roots are located in the posterior portion of the psoas major in front of the transverse processes of the vertebrae. The largest branch of the lumbar portion of the plexus is the femoral nerve, which descends through the fibers of the psoas major, emerging from that muscle along its lateral border, and passing between the psoas and iliacus muscles. The femoral nerve then travels beneath the inguinal ligament into the thigh, where it splits into anterior and posterior divisions. The obturator nerve lies in the pelvis medial to the femoral nerve, while even more medial is the lumbosacral trunk (L4 and L5 roots), which, along with sacral input, make up the sciatic nerve. The lumbosacral trunk appears at the medial margin of the psoas major and runs downward over the pelvic brim to join the sacral nerves and plexus, which lies at the back of the lower pelvis.

Pelvic plexus injuries are rare, and most appear in the literature as a small series of case reports or solitary cases (Patterson, 1972). In addition to gunshot wounds and other penetrating injuries to the pelvic region, fractures of the pelvis as well as of the sacrum (Byrnes et al., 1977), and rare primary tumors of the pelvic plexus provide the usual etiology. However, the pelvic plexus has been reported to be involved secondary to hematomas caused by anticoagulation, usually heparinization for thrombosis, phlebitis, or pulmonary embolus, and even in patients with disseminated intravascular coagulation (Gilden and Eisner, 1977). Our personal experience has been with gunshot wounds, and three patients with fortunately incomplete pelvic plexus losses have been treated expectantly with acceptable results. We have followed several patients who had

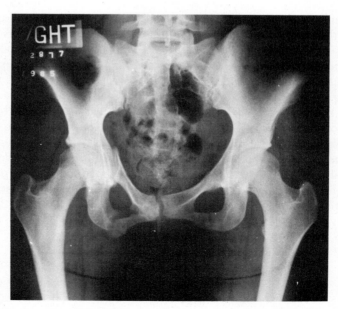

Figure 37–9   Fractures of the pelvic rami on the right associated with partial but improving pelvic plexus palsy.

pelvic, usually sacral, plexus involvement secondary to pelvic brim fractures, and these have improved without operation. The hallmark of pelvic plexus involvement is combined femoral and/or obturator as well as sciatic involvement. Branches leading to ilioinguinal, genitofemoral, saphenous, and lateral femoral cutaneous nerves can be involved but usually are not. Injury and entrapment are more likely to occur with distortion of the lower abdominal, inguinal, or upper thigh anatomy (Cox, 1974; Ecker and Woltman, 1938; Keegan and Holyoke, 1965). One of our patients had a large, recurrent intraspinal neurofibroma with extension through the L3 vertebral body as well as a greatly dilated intervertebral foramen at that level. Its origin was believed to be from a root in the pelvis with extension into the spinal canal. Because of extensive intraspinal recurrence, an attempt at total excision was elected. After subtotal removal of the intraspinal portion of the tumor to the level of the intervertebral foramen, the pelvic portion was resected using a transabdominal approach in conjunction with general surgery. The psoas muscle was split to locate the tumor, which was enucleated, sparing most but unfortunately not all of the root input to the femoral nerve.

Several sacral plexus neurofibromas have been operated on and successfully removed. One patient, a female, presented with dyspareunia; a mass was not palpable by vaginal or rectal examination; however, digital percussion of the lateral vaginal wall gave paresthesias into the medial thigh and vagina. This finding combined with a history of the patient having had a mediastinal neurofibroma removed some years earlier led to exploration of the sacral portion of the plexus, where a solitary neurofibroma was found and successfully excised. Several other unsuspected neurofibromas were found attached to the intestinal mesentery and omentum, presumably arising from autonomic fibers.

It should be mentioned that secondary attempts at repair of plexus element injury after resection of intrapelvic tumors, often unsuspected neurofibromas in the subrenal region, have usually met with frustration brought about by inability to find a proximal end for repair (Hudson, 1977).

Pelvic plexus palsies associated with lumbar, sacral, or pelvic fractures should be evaluated by myelography, since the presence of a meningocele usually impedes successful repair at this level just as it does with brachial plexus injury (Harris, 1974). If the plexus is to be explored, a transabdominal approach is favored by the author even though a lateral muscle splitting approach similar to that used for lumbar sympathectomy is also available.

PAIN SYNDROMES

A description of lower extremity nerve lesions would be incomplete without addressing at least briefly the management of the pain syndromes that accompany about 50 per cent of these injuries (Clawson and Seddon, 1960b). True causalgia is best treated by repetitive lumbar sympathetic block. If intermittent but non-sustained relief is gained from adequate sympathetic blocks, lumbar sympathectomy is done, taking care to resect all of the lumbar chain. True causalgia is usually associated with partial injury to the tibial division of the sciatic nerve. Our own experience with true causalgia in the lower extremity has for the most part been with that due to gunshot wounds to that component of the sciatic nerve. These patients have not tolerated even gentle movement or manipulation of the foot. They have had good response to both sympathetic block and surgical sympathectomy. Sympathetic dystrophy may mimic true causalgia and is accompanied by demineralization of digits and bones of the foot and ankle. This syndrome is often secondary to mild nerve injury or even to soft tissue injury alone, such as in recurrent sprain of the ankle. Two personal cases of sympathetic dystrophy of the foot were both benefited by sympathectomy.

Unfortunately, the all too common "neuralgia-like" pain associated with partial injury of the lower extremity nerves is not helped by manipulation of the sympathetic nervous system and usually requires vigorous and sustained physical therapy as well as continuous use of analgesic medications. In some cases, exploration and neurolysis will benefit and in others it will not, as is the case with the injection palsies (see sciatic section). If an area of potential entrapment is complicating a primary injury to nerve, then neurolysis, which by definition releases the surrounding tissues as well as the nerve, may be of help. If the lesion appears incomplete on clinical exam and yet is found to be complete by electrical studies at the operating table, resection and suture can be of help in the lower extremity, as it is in the upper extremity. If an NAP can be recorded and yet pain is a predominant feature, internal neurolysis may be tried, although once again the result of this procedure in our hands is 50 per cent relief of the pain caused by lower extremity neural lesions.

If the sural or saphenous nerves are injured, resection without repair may be helpful in relieving or reducing pain, particularly the dysesthesias and paresthesias associated with involvement of these elements (Cox, 1974). In our experience, the saphenous nerve is less frequently implicated in leg pain syndromes than the sural. Unfortunately, in an occasional lower abdominal operation the ilioinguinal, genitofemoral, or lateral femoral cutaneous (Ecker and Woltman, 1938; Keegan and Holyoke, 1965) nerve can be injured or secondarily entrapped by scar or suture, or both. Exploration and identification of these elements after prior operation is difficult. However, involvement of these elements is best treated by wide resection despite attendant hypesthesia which, in some cases, involves the mons pubis and the vaginal vault.

On rare occasions, a gunshot wound, particularly a shotgun blast, can lodge a pellet or shell fragment in the sciatic nerve. A hunting accident due to shotgun blast left one patient in our series with severe paresthesias in the sole of the foot and some burning pain but no true causalgia, because the extremity could be readily manipulated when the patient's attention was distracted. This patient's pain was helped considerably by removal of a pellet embedded within the tibial portion of the sciatic nerve.

Other surgeons have had favorable experience with implantation of proximal or distal nerve stimulators after a suitable trial with peripheral nerve stimulation for lower extremity pain syndromes due to nerve injury (Long, 1973). We have had no experience with the implanting of such electrodes but have had to do a neurolysis on one sciatic nerve at the buttock level because of scar and painful paresthesias due to an implant inserted at another institution. Nielson, Watts, and Clark (1976) have reported a similar situation. Hopefully, the incidence of such complications will remain low.

REFERENCES

Byrnes, O., Russo, G. L., Ducker, T. B., and Cowley, R. A.: Sacrum fractures and neurological damage. J. Neurosurg. *47*:459, 1977.

Clark, K., Williams, P., Willis, W., and McGavran, W.: Injection injury to the sciatic nerve. Clin. Neurosurg. *17*:111, 1970.

Clawson, D. K., and Seddon, H. J.: The results of repair of the sciatic nerve. J. Bone Joint Surg. *42B*:205, 1960a.

Clawson, D. K., and Seddon, H. J.: The late consequences of sciatic nerve injury. J. Bone Joint Surg. *42B*, 213, 1960b.

Cox, S. J.: Saphenous nerve injury caused by stripping of long saphenous vein. Br. Med. J. *1*:415, 1974.

Das Gupta, T., and Brasfield, R.: Tumors of peripheral nerve origin: benign and malignant solitary schwannomas. Cancer *20*:228, 1970.

Ecker, A. D., and Woltman, H. W.: Meralgia paresthetica: A report of 150 cases. J.A.M.A. *110*:1650, 1938.

Gilden, D. H., and Eisner, J.: Lumbar plexopathy caused by disseminated intravascular coagulation. J.A.M.A. *237*:2846, 1977.

Gutman, E., and Young, J. Z.: Reinnervation of muscle after various periods of atrophy. J. Anat. *78*:15, 1944.

Harris, W. R.: Avulsion of lumbar roots complicating fracture of the pelvis. J. Bone Joint Surg. *55A*:1436, 1973.

Highet, W. B., and Holmes, W.: Traction injuries to the lateral popliteal and traction injuries to peripheral nerves after suture. Br. J. Surg. *30*:212, 1943.

Hudson, A. R.: Personal communication, Toronto, Canada, 1977.

Johnson, E. W.: Nerve injuries in fractures to the lower extremity. Minn. Med. *52*:627, 1969.

Keegan, J. J., and Holyoke, E. A.: Meralgia paresthetica. J. Neurosurg. *19*:341, 1965.

Kline, D. G., and DeJong, B. R.: Evoked potentials to evaluate peripheral nerve injuries. Surg., Gynecol. Obstet. *127*:1239, 1968.

Kline, D. G.: Physiological and clinical factors contributing to the timing of nerve repair. *In* Keener, E. (Ed.): Clinical Neurosurgery, Baltimore, Williams & Wilkins Co., 1977, Vol. 24, Ch. 31, p. 425.

Kline, D. G.: Operative management of major nerve lesions of the lower extremity. Surg. Clin. North Am. *52*:1247, 1972.

Long, D. L.: Electrical stimulation for relief of pain from chronic nerve injury. J. Neurosurg. *39*:718, 1973.

MacCarty, C. S.: Two stage autograph for repair of extensive damage to the sciatic nerve. J. Neurosurg. *8*:319, 1951.

Nielson, K. D., Watts, C., and Clark, W. K.: Peripheral nerve injury from implantation of chronic stimulating electrodes for pain control. Surg. Neurol. *5*:51, 1976.

Patterson, F. P.: Neurological complications of fractures and dislocations of the pelvis. J. Trauma *12*:1013, 1972.

Seddon, H. J.: Surgical Disorders of the Peripheral Nerves. Baltimore, Williams & Wilkins Co., 1972.

Seletz, E.: Surgery of Peripheral Nerves, Springfield, Ill., Charles C Thomas, 1951, p. 119.

Spiegel, P. G.: Complete sciatic nerve laceration in a closed femoral shaft fracture. J. Trauma *14*:617, 1974.

Stayman, J. W.: Care of the nerve-injured extremity. Surg. Clin. North Am. *52*:1337, 1972.

Sunderland, S.: Nerves and Nerve Injuries, Baltimore, Williams & Wilkins Co., 1968, p. 1012.

White, J.: The results of traction injuries to the common peroneal nerve. J. Bone Joint Surg. *40B*:346, 1968.

Woodhall, B., and Beebe, G. W. (eds.): Peripheral Nerve Regeneration, VA Medical Monograph. Washington, D.C., U.S. Government Printing Office, 1957.

38

LOWER
EXTREMITY
LESIONS

HARVEY P. KOPELL

INTRODUCTION

The key to the management of peripheral nerve lesions of the lower extremities is the establishment of an accurate diagnosis. Arriving at the diagnosis is often a function of an awareness of the condition and an appropriate examination, taking into account both historical and physical factors. The history of a possible lower extremity problem reveals more information if taken first hand than if obtained from an intermediate historian or from a form. For increased effectiveness the examination should contravene the usual bias of the traditional method of inspection, which compels the examiner to start proximally and proceed distally. If, instead, the examiner starts at the periphery and works centrally, he may often be rewarded by fresher, more useful clues to the patient's condition. In keeping with this viewpoint, the organization of the following section is directed centripetally, starting with the interdigital nerves in the foot and working up.

Electrodiagnostic evaluation is a major tool for confirmation of the diagnosis in the majority of these neuropathies. The parameters of some have not yet been adequately established, as, for example, interdigital neuropathy. Another diagnostic aid, and possible treatment aid, is the use of paraneural infiltration with a locally acting steroid.

While a localized neuropathy may occur at any region of a nerve, there are certain points at which anatomical features tend to cause compression or maintain mechanical irritation. The features of some of these points will be discussed below. The most frequent compression points are emphasized because of their diagnostic importance.

A patient with a peripheral nerve lesion and a coexisting, non-related low back derangement is in jeopardy of having an unwarranted diagnosis of a compressive radiculopathy.

The nerves of the lower extremity are not exempt from primary neoplasms. No rules can be laid down for their diagnosis or site frequency. Some can be palpated, while others can be localized by careful electrical survey. Space occupying extraneural lesions may cause a neuropathy at an entrapment point but generalizations are not warranted as to frequency or location.

Similarly, it is difficult to make suggestions about the effects of missiles. Wounding in the lower extremities, with accompanying nerve injury, is usually a product of wartime activity; ordinarily, peacetime occupations lead to more upper extremity nerve lesions. The questions of type and timing of nerve repair will not be discussed in this section.

INTERDIGITAL NERVES

Anatomy

The interdigital nerves lie between the metatarsal heads. They are derived from either the medial or lateral plantar nerves via the posterior tibial nerve, and they contain fibers from the L4 to S2 nerve roots. The major function of these nerves is sensory to the skin of the toes. The 3-4 interdigital nerve is unusual in that it is formed from the junction of branches derived from both plantar nerves. Each interdigital nerve then divides into digital branches that convey sensation from the adjacent sides and palmar surfaces of the toes. The course of the nerves is from the plantar region of the foot to a more dorsal position for its final innervation.

The alteration in course from plantar to dorsal is accomplished by angulation of the nerve against the edge of the deep metatarsal ligament (Fig. 38–1). It is this relationship that offers the potential of trauma to the nerve.

Mechanism

The interdigital nerve (3-4) is most often affected. It is probably related to the more secure proximal fixation of the nerve because of its derivation. It must be remembered, that the same pathological process can occur to the adjacent second web space nerve.

Impingement of the ligament against the nerve can occur in a variety of ways. A heavy weight dropped on the dorsum of the foot can drive the ligament into the nerve. Forceful lateral deviation or extreme hyperextension can stretch the nerve tight over the ligament. The hyperextended position may be a single occurence at the time of fracturing a toe, or it may be a continuing posture induced by the wearing of high heels.

The involved nerve may present a small region of inflammation, or sufficient trauma may have occurred to cause internal scarring. The latter is a cicatricial neuroma in continuity, and is called a Morton's neuroma. It is not a true neoplasm, being the end result of repeated mechanical injury to the nerve (compression, traction, or friction).

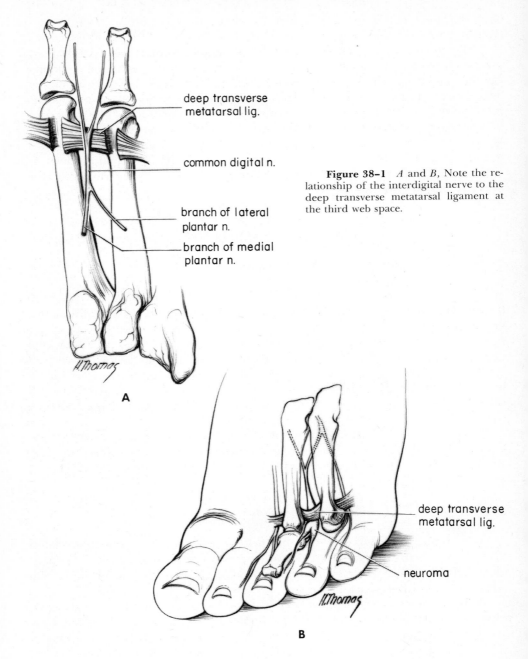

deep transverse
metatarsal lig.

common digital n.

branch of lateral
plantar n.

branch of medial
plantar n.

Figure 38–1   *A* and *B*, Note the relationship of the interdigital nerve to the deep transverse metatarsal ligament at the third web space.

A

deep transverse
metatarsal lig.

neuroma

B

Diagnosis

The patient complains of pain in the affected toes. The pain may be dull or it may be sharp and lancinating. The facts that continued walking may aggravate the pain and that rest gives relief may at times mislead the examiner into making a diagnosis of intermittent claudication on a vascular basis. This is more likely to happen from a second web space neuroma, which tends to produce upward radiation of pain. The pain is often relieved by removing the shoe and letting the toes assume a protective easy plantar flexion. On examination it is possible to pick up hypalgesia to pin prick of the involved area of skin. If a neuroma is present, it is possible to move it across the ligament by finger pressure against the sole between and just beyond the metatarsal heads. This should reproduce the pain pattern. Electrodiagnostic measurement values have not been satisfactorily established for these nerves. A paraneural infiltration with a steroid is useful. It should be performed with a fine needle and a small amount of solution, so that the possible distress caused by the injection will not cloud the issue.

Treatment

The extent of treatment for an interdigital neuropathy is determined by the relief afforded by the measures used. Since the nerves have no motor function, the major effect of the neuropathy is pain.

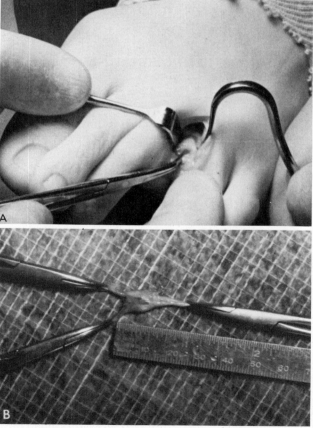

Figure 38–2 *A,* Operative exposure of the third web space neuroma. *B,* Interdigital neuroma specimen.

The first measure to be tried is to reduce the tension of the nerve against the ligament. The shoe has to have adequate room to permit flexion at the metatarsophalangeal joints and easy toe motion. A metatarsal bar or pad is prescribed. The placement of the correction is critical — if too far forward it will aggrevate the pain, if too far backward it will be ineffective.

A paraneural infiltration with a steroid will help to localize the lesion and permit some of the inflammation to subside so that the shoe correction can work more effectively.

If after an adequate trial of these measures relief is inadequate, surgical excision of the offending nerve segment is indicated. The usual approach to the lesion is through the dorsum of the foot in the region of the third web interspace (Fig. 38–2A). A neuroma, when present, is found near the bifurcation of the nerve into its digital branches (Fig. 38–2B). The lesion should be excised sufficiently proximal to prevent possible cicatricial adhesion of the remaining nerve end to the intermetatarsal ligament. Some surgeons prefer an exposure through the plantar aspect of the foot near the metatarsophalangeal crease. It would appear that this incision leads to more operative bleeding and puts the vascular supply of the toes into jeopardy. The denervation that results from the nerve section has seemed of little consequence to the patient's normal function.

POSTERIOR TIBIAL NERVE

Anatomy

The posterior tibial nerve is particularly vulnerable to compression in its course behind and below the medial malleolus on its way to the foot. As it changes its direction, in company with the artery, vein and long flexor tendons of the foot, it lies in a tunnel (tarsal tunnel) which is roofed over by the laciniate ligament The posterior tibial nerve splits up into three main branches either within or just beyond the tunnel. They are the calcaneal (sensory), medial plantar (mixed), and lateral plantar (mixed). The plantar nerves supply the small muscles of the foot and carry sensory information from the medial and lateral portions of the sole and toes distal to the region supplied by the calcaneal nerve (Fig. 38–3). The posterior tibial nerve has its root origin from L4 through S2.

Mechanism

Nerve compression within the tarsal tunnel can occur from enlargement or distortion of any of the extraneural structures in the region. The mechanism can be brought about by a flexor tenosynovitis — produced either by stress or by an infection process. Varicose engorgement of the posterior tibial vein can compress the nerve and augment the symptoms caused by the varicosities. The structural distortion produced by a fracture or dislocation of the

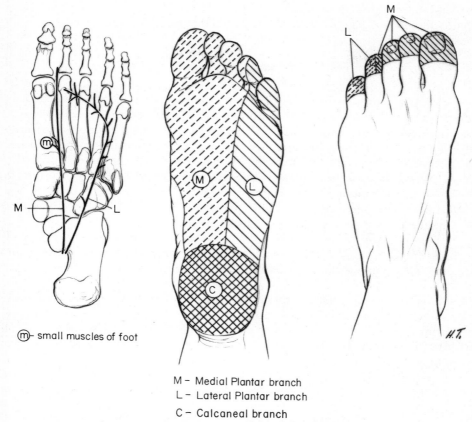

m̶ - small muscles of foot

M – Medial Plantar branch
L – Lateral Plantar branch
C – Calcaneal branch

Figure 38-3 Cutaneous distribution of the posterior tibial nerve.

calcaneus or malleolus can cause compression of the nerve either by direct pressure or by causing it to be compromised within the tarsal tunnel.

Diagnosis

A major complaint in this neuropathy is pain involving the foot and sometimes radiating upward. The patient may also complain of numbness of the foot. Skin sensation of the heel may remain intact under two circumstances: 1) if the calcaneal nerve arises above the tunnel and descends to the heel superficial to the flexor retinaculum; 2) when the compression is actually distal to the tarsal tunnel. The second instance occurs at the place where the plantar nerves enter the sole of the foot between the medial border of the abductor hallucis and the calcaneus. It is frequently difficult to distinguish between a compression neuropathy and a diabetic neuropathy. (It should be borne in mind that the peripheral nerves in a diabetic are more easily affected by compression force than are "normal" nerves and are more prone to the development of a mechanical neuropathy.) If there is reason to suspect a neuropathy, an electrodiagnostic survey is invaluable in establishing a diagnosis.

Treatment

From the standpoint of frequency of occurrence, a reactive neuropathy within the tarsal tunnel is the condition most often encountered. When a post-traumatic flexor tenosynovitis is the cause of a tarsal tunnel syndrome, anti-inflammatory medication and rest are the initial measures to be utilized. The ligament can be relaxed and the tunnel widened to some extent if the heel is placed in a varus posture. This can be accomplished by the use of a Thomas heel or a medial arch support. If the neuropathy chiefly involves the plantar nerves at their entrance into the foot, the use of an arch support could aggravate symptoms because of local pressure.

If nonoperative measures fail to bring adequate relief, surgical release of the pressure is indicated. When surgery is performed, it is best to carry the exposure sufficiently distal to visualize the entrance of the plantar nerves into the foot.

The decision on whether to decompress the nerve after trauma to the ankle–foot region involves sorting out the signs and symptoms of the neuropathy from the rest of the post-traumatic complex, and requires both clinical and electrical evaluation. If a neurolysis is elected, it should follow the course of the nerves into the foot.

COMMON PERONEAL NERVE

Anatomy

The common peroneal nerve is one of the two major branches of the sciatic nerve. Its root supply is from L4 to S2. The nerve comes to lie against the fibular head after first occupying a position in the lateral aspect of the popliteal fossa. It then passes forward through an opening in the attachment of the long peroneal muscle to the fibula. The nerve divides into three branches—the superficial peroneal, deep peroneal and recurrent peroneal nerves. The superficial and deep peroneal nerves angulate over the fascial edge of the opening. The nerves then pass down the leg to innervate the extensors and evertors of the ankle and foot, the skin of the distal anterior portion of the leg, and the dorsum of the foot.

Mechanism

The common peroneal nerve and its branches may be affected in some particular locations. This nerve is vulnerable to the effects of direct pressure as it lies on the lateral surface of the fibular neck. The pressure can compress the nerve against the unyielding bone. The condition may result from the external stress that causes a fractured fibula, from the top of a boot, from a relatively tight cast or traction tape binding, or from a leg lying in helpless eversion against a firm surface for a prolonged period. Just beyond the fibular neck where the common peroneal nerve branches, the superficial and deep peroneal nerves change their course over the fibrous edge of the long peroneal muscle another region of vulnerability. A forced strong inversion twist of the foot and ankle can pull the tight nerve against the fibrous edge to initiate a neuropathy. Further down in their course the nerves can be compressed in a compartment syndrome.

The superficial peroneal nerve pierces the deep fascia in the distal portion of the leg. The opening may provide the opportunity for a muscle hernia. The symptomatology attributed to the hernia may be the result of nerve compression rather than muscle compression. If the hernia is treated by fascial closure the resulting fascial tightness can aggravate the nerve compression. The superficial peroneal nerve ends in a gangliform expansion on the dorsum of the tarsal bones. This entity should be borne in mind when the foot is the recipient of direct trauma. Irritation of a peripheral nerve may at times evoke a disproportionately large autonomic outflow. The circumstance is sometimes seen in compression of the median nerve in the carpal tunnel. In the foot an overflow of autonomic innervation can arise from stimulation of either the posterior tibial or the peroneal branches, and this can lead to a diagnosis of an early Sudeck's atrophy. The distal portion of the deep peroneal nerve surfaces between the first and second rays. Direct pressure in this region can traumatize the branch.

Diagnosis

When there are persistent pressures on the common peroneal nerve or its branches, the patient will usually complain of pain. If the pressure has produced irreversible nerve damage, pain may disappear, leaving numbness and weakness or paralysis in the innervated region. The peroneal nerve is accessible to an electrodiagnostic survey, which should be able to localize the involved segment. Normally a diabetic neuropathy does not present the diagnostic problem that occurs with a peroneal nerve lesion.

When the neuropathy is kept active by the stretching of the nerve over a fascial edge, it is often possible to aggravate the symptoms by passively inverting the foot. Eversion should bring some relief. As in other entrapment neuropathies, firm digital pressure at the entrapment point should cause local and radiating pain. It must be kept in mind that a forced inversion twist of the foot can also cause pain from a peroneal tenosynovitis or an inflamed subastragalar joint.

Treatment

If it is has been determined that the condition is a localized neuropathy influenced by fascial and nerve tension, a trial of conservative therapy is in order. Besides the use of anti-inflammatory medication, either systematically or locally, some relief of the tension can be obtained by the use of a lateral sole wedge, which will force the foot into eversion.

The surgical treatment for a peroneal neuropathy is determined by the suspected diagnosis. When the neuropathy has been caused by pressure against the fibular neck, external and internal neurolysis with nerve mobilization are indicated if the condition has stabilized and no return is evident. Neurolysis at other sites can be achieved by fascial release. This is the operative treatment that is performed when the nerve is compressed through its course in a compartment syndrome.

SCIATIC NERVE

Anatomy

The sciatic nerve is derived from the L4, L5, S1, S2, and S3 nerve roots. The nerve passes over the sciatic notch, then descends through the gluteal region and becomes more superficial (posterior), usually under, but sometimes over and occasionally through, the piriform muscle. Below the piriform muscle the nerve trunk lies posteromedial to the hip joint and lateral to the ischial tubercle. Here the nerve is ensheathed in a layer of protective fatty tissue. The sciatic nerve carries sensation from a portion of the leg and foot, and innervates the knee flexors and all the muscles below the knee.

Mechanism

The sciatic nerve is particularly vulnerable to injury following hip dislocation or·as a complication of hip surgery performed through the posterior approach. A sciatic neuropathy is no longer considered to be a fashionable basis for a sciatica, but cases do occur. Though the nerve is seemingly well protected by the gluteal muscle mass, an external force can compress the trunk against the ischial tuberosity. A fall on the buttocks can traumatize the sciatic trunk, besides causing lower spine problems. Unfortunately, so much attention and treatment are directed to the back injury that little consideration is given to a possible peripheral sciatic trunk problem. A sciatic neuropathy can also be seen after an intramuscular injection that has been placed too low and too medial in the buttock.

Diagnosis

A sciatic neuropathy will usually signal its presence on clinical examination. Most patients complain of buttock pain with radiation down the posterior aspect of the lower extremity. If the condition is severe enough, there will be sensory alterations and motor losses in the anatomical distribution of the sciatic nerve. Pressure over the proximal portion of the trunk causes radiation of pain down the course of the sciatic nerve. The piriformis syndrome (entrapment of the sciatic nerve by the piriformis muscle), once popular, is now seldom diagnosed. In a true case, internal rotation of the hip should accentuate the sciatic pain, external rotation should relieve it. Electrodiagnostic studies are valuable not only for the diagnosis of a lesion but also as a guide to management. Repeated studies can show the direction of change more accurately than can a clinical examination.

Treatment

Treatment for a sciatic neuropathy is necessarily a function of the manner of origin and nature of the lesion. In the majority of instances, a chemically induced neuropathy will resolve under a conservative program of rest, anti-inflammatory medication, and local physiotherapy. If the clinical course is not clear, electrodiagnostic studies at appropriate intervals can monitor whether the condition is resolving or secondary cicatricization has taken place. In the latter instance, neurolysis would be an indicated procedure.

When a sciatic lesion is diagnosed after hip trauma or after a surgical exposure, the form of the lesion requires evaluation (i.e. whether the involved segment is showing the effects of a contusion, section, or cicatricial compression). It usually requires repeated evaluations to characterize the lesion. If the lesion shows progressive improvement, conservative management should be continued.

The lesions that should benefit from neurolysis are those in which nerve function is degraded by a cicatricial process.

FEMORAL NERVE

Anatomy

The femoral nerve is formed from L2, L3, and L4 nerve roots that have traversed the lumbar plexus. The nerve goes through the psoas muscle, down behind the iliac fascia, and under the inguinal ligament. After passing beneath the ligament it lies anterior to the femoral head. It is separated from the bone by a slip of the iliacus, the psoas tendon, and the hip joint capsule. Anteriorly there is only the full thickness of the skin. The nerve is held down in position over the femoral head prominence by fascia derived from the iliacus and psoas. Just past this point the nerve divides into its main branches. The nerve supplies the iliacus, psoas, pectineus, sartorius, and quadriceps muscles. It also innervates the skin of the medial and anterior surface of the thigh and the medial surface of the leg, including the medial aspect of the foot down to the metatarsophalangeal joint of the big toe.

Mechanism

The femoral nerve can be affected by the same diabetic process that causes a neuropathy elsewhere. Because of its passage through the psoas and through the retroperitoneal region, conditions that can cause psoas spasm, such as kidney pathology, or hemorrhage into the psoas fascial envelope, may affect the nerve.

The relationship of the nerve to the femoral head, the scant cushioning that intervenes between the two, and the lack of anterior protection make the nerve vulnerable to direct trauma at this point. The tethering of the nerve to its position also makes it vulnerable to pressure from an abnormal anteversion of the head or an implanted prosthesis. A large femoral hernia may irritate the nerve by lateral compression.

Diagnosis

Usually the patient with an active femoral neuropathy will complain of pain in the distribution of the femoral nerve. At one time I was of the impression that pain in the distribution of this nerve was not a frequent complaint in a diabetic neuropathy but subsequent experience has changed this view. A femoral neuropathy will cause sensory alteration and muscular weakness along with loss of the knee jerk. The electrical parameters for the femoral nerve are available so that confirmation of a diagnosis is possible.

Treatment

As of this writing there is no specific treatment for any of the diabetic neuropathies. Probably the only systemic neuropathies that respond to any degree of treatment are those based on vitamin deficiencies. Even those induced by a heavy metal or other toxic chemical intake do not respond rapidly to removal of the offending substance.

If a compressive force can be identified as the source of the neuropathy, an attempt should be made to relieve it surgically. The nerve should be released from the fascial bindings that maintain its relationship to the femoral head. Direct trauma to the nerve can cause an intraneural hematoma that has a clinical course similar to a subdural hemotoma; that is, an immediate response to trauma, a period of quiescence, and then increasing pressure effects. Release of the hematoma will usually bring about resolution of the condition.

LATERAL FEMORAL CUTANEOUS NERVE

Anatomy

The lateral femoral cutaneous nerve is formed from the roots of L2 and L3. It travels down to make a wide sweep around the pelvis under the iliacus fascia and then emerges through an opening in the lateral attachment of the inguinal ligament at the anterior superior spins. Beyond the ligament it splits into two branches, which pierce the deep subcutaneous fascia on their way to the skin (Fig. 38–4). The branches carry sensation from the anterior and lateral aspects of the thigh (Fig. 38–5). There are no skeletal muscle branches; the function of the nerve is purely sensory.

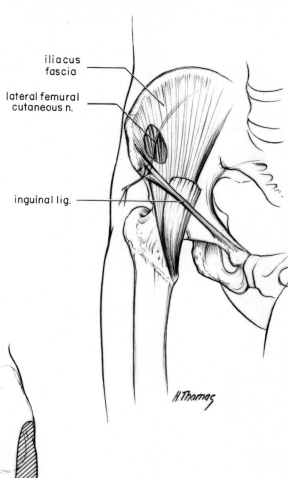

Figure 38–4 Anatomical scheme of the lateral femoral cutaneous nerve.

iliacus fascia

lateral femoral cutaneous n.

inguinal lig.

H.Thomas

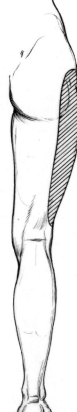

Figure 38–5 Distribution of the lateral femoral cutaneous nerve.

Mechanism

The lateral femoral cutaneous nerve is not often injured by direct trauma, although it may occasionally be injured during a full anterolateral hip exposure. Ordinarily the neuropathy presents without antecedent trauma. The fascial attachments in the thigh pull the nerve tight against the opening at the lateral end of the inguinal ligament. Thigh obesity and lateral shift in trunk posture can cause pressure against the fascial edge.

Diagnosis

The clinical manifestation of a neuropathy of the lateral femoral cutaneous nerve is known as meralgia paresthetica. In this entity there is a burning pain in the skin of the anterior and lateral surfaces of the thigh, accompanied by hypesthesia in the area. At times a low back derangement may cause pain in the trochanteric region or in the tensor fascia lata that can be distinguished from meralgia by the absence of sensory alteration in the skin. It is often possible to reproduce the pain distribution by deep digital pressure just beneath the anterior superior spine, for when a neuropathy is present the region is exquisitely tender to deep palpation. Electrodiagnosis is a useful tool for confirmation of a suspected diagnosis.

Treatment

A patient with a visible trunk shift can sometimes be relieved of pain by use of a contralateral heel lift. It is wise to accompany this with adjunctive measures such anti-inflammatory medication and physiotherapy. If the diagnosis is confirmed and the patient is not helped by conservative measures, surgical neurolysis is indicated. The nerve should be freed by section of the lateral end of the inguinal ligament and also by liberating it from the iliacus fascia for two or three inches posterior to the anterior superior spine. There have not been any untoward effects seen as yet from section of the lateral end of the inguinal ligament. Previously some surgeons have sectioned the nerve, but this can produce annoying numbness in the region of sensory innervation, and still leave a painful entrapment proximal to the end of the inguinal ligament.

REFERENCES

Goodgold, J.: Anatomical Correlates of Clinical Electromyography. Baltimore, Williams & Wilkins Co., 1972.

Kopell, H. P. and Thompson, W. A. L.: Peripheral Entrapment Neuropathies. Huntington, NY, R. E. Krieger, 1976.

39

PERIPHERAL NERVE INJECTION INJURY

ALAN HUDSON, DAVID KLINE,
AND FRED GENTILI

INTRODUCTION

The management of injection nerve injury remains a controversial subject (Linder and Gurdjian, 1970). The iatrogenically-produced drug injection injury of a peripheral nerve is of particular concern, because of both its clinical and medicolegal implications. With the numerous agents administered by intramuscular injection, this accident has come to be recognized as a not infrequent cause of pain and disability in adults (Linder and Gurdjian, 1970; Clark et al., 1970; Combes et al., 1960; Tuvo and Bouquet, 1971). Nerve injection injury in children may be responsible for permanent, severe paralytic deformities.

Peripheral nerve injury resulting from the deep injection of therapeutic and prophylactic agents has been recognized for half a century. Turner (1920) was among the first to report sciatic nerve palsy due to quinine injection. Kolb and Gray (1946) describe a "localized peripheral neuritis" in seven patients who had received multiple intramuscular injections of various penicillin preparations. The paralysis, involving motor more than sensory function, had its onset one to three weeks after the initial injection of the drug. Complete recovery was seen within four months in five of the seven patients. Subsequently, Broadbent et al. (1949), reporting on four cases, delineated the clinical syndrome of penicillin-induced peripheral nerve paralysis. All the patients experienced immediate pain radiating distally along the course of the affected nerve segment following injection of penicillin into, or adjacent to, a major extremity nerve. A transient sensory loss and early motor paralysis

639

were noted. Two patients were left with severe deficits, and two with motor palsy.

Further reports of peripheral nerve injury after the injection of agents other than penicillin soon followed (Combes et al., 1960; Hudson et al., 1950, Matson, 1950). Combes et al. (1960) reported 12 cases of sciatic nerve injection injury due to a variety of therapeutic and prophylactic agents. In contrast to earlier reports, these authors found recovery of neurological function to be disappointing in all but one case. They suggested that the site and the volume and type of injected material were important in determining the degree of injury. Curtis and Tucker (1960) stressed the relative increased frequency of sciatic nerve lesions in premature infants. This was partially related to the relatively small area of the infant buttock and the relative paucity of muscle covering the sciatic nerve. These authors reported good functional recovery in all but one patient, occurring within 45 days to seven months. Gilles and French (1961) reviewed 21 cases of sciatic palsy associated with intragluteal injections in pediatric patients. They noted that sciatic nerve palsy occurred after both single and multiple injections of antibiotic medications, either alone or in combination. The clinical presentation was most commonly that of immediate pain and disability following injection. Follow-up in 18 patients revealed that 30 per cent had complete recovery within a period of one hour to one year. Twenty-two per cent had no improvement in an interval of seven to 36 months. The remainder had partial improvement of neurological function.

Clark et al. reviewed their own experience in 26 patients, and a further 25 patients from the literature, with injury to a peripheral nerve (Clark, 1972; Lindnen and Grudjian, 1970). They noted that the neurological deficit, often associated with pain, had its onset immediately or within minutes of injection. The degree of injury was often profound, motor function being more severely involved. Residual deficit was found to be present in the majority of cases, only two of 51 recovering completely. Early onset of return of function appeared to be the only favourable prognostic factor noted.

Although the sciatic nerve is by far the most commonly affected nerve, because of its size and the frequency of intramuscular injections in the buttock, injection injury of a number of other peripheral nerves has been reported, including the radial, ulnar, axillary, posterior interosseus, and lateral femoral cutaneous (Broadbent et al., 1949; Ling and Loong, 1976; Holbrook and Pilcher, 1950).

There is a great deal of controversy regarding the treatment of postinjection nerve palsies. If the complication is noted immediately, some authors have advocated immediate open operative irrigation (Elkington, 1942). Others have recommended early exploration at three to four weeks, with thorough external neurolysis (Matson, 1950). In contrast, some authors, citing the experimental work of Tarlov, which implicated intraneurial pathology in this lesion, favor conservative management for at least a year in children, before resorting to surgical neurolysis. Other workers have felt that exploration of the nerve should be carried out if there is complete loss of nerve function of sufficient duration that spontaneous return can be considered unlikely, and that the absence of a nerve action potential through the injury is an indication for resection and suture (Nulsen and Kline, 1973; Clark, 1972).

There have been few experimental studies on drug injection injuries in animals. Tarlov et al. (1951) were among the first to study the experimental pathology of injection injuries in animals. They injected the sciatic nerves of rabbits with penicillin in various forms and with streptomycin. Light microscopy studies revealed that injection of these substances around the nerve produced no effect, and that epineurial injections resulted in mild inflammatory changes with no, or minimal, axonal degeneration. On the other hand, intraneural injection produced an intense inflammatory reaction with axonal and myelin degeneration and connective tissue scarring within the nerve. Control injection with normal saline and autologous blood resulted in no abnormality. These authors concluded that drug injection injury of the peripheral nerve was predominantly an intraneural lesion attributable to the introduction of the material directly into the parenchyma of the nerve. The delayed impairment seen in a few animals was felt to be attributable to progressive inflammatory and fibrotic changes. Holbrook and Pilcher (1950) studied the effects of various penicillin preparations and their vehicles which were injected into the sciatic nerves of dogs. They reported immediate marked axonal degeneration and necrosis, with prompt polymorphonuclear leukocyte infiltration, followed by an infiltration of mononuclear cells and fibroplasia with formation of granuloma. Of the various drugs injected, they noted that calcium penicillin produced the most severe degree of damage.

The studies of Woodhall et al. (1950) in cats confirmed the above and extended the findings. They reported complete axonal degeneration with intrafascicular injection of both penicillin and streptomycin. Extrafascicular injection, on the other hand, resulted in an inflammatory reaction but no axonal changes. Hanson (1963) injected the sciatic nerve in rabbits and noted that the degree of injury was dependent, in part, on the vehicle of suspension. Burkel and McPhee (1970) reported wallerian degeneration, followed by nearly complete regeneration, in rat sciatic nerve after the injection of phenol.

Combes and Clark (1960) examined the effect of intragluteal injection of a wide variety of drugs in rat and dog, and reported that intraneurial injection of tetracycline, erythromycin and gantrisin produced sciatic nerve damage. In contrast, extraneural injections had no effect. Similarly, no abnormality was noted after repeated injections of saline, or after direct needling. They concluded that nerve injury following intragluteal injection in the sciatic nerve resulted from a combination of chemical irritation and constriction by scar tissue.

Clark et al. (1970, 1972) have studied the effects of injections of various preparations in the sciatic nerves of cats, using neurophysiological criteria. They noted a prompt decrease in the size of both afferent and motor action potentials following the injection of paraldehyde and promazine. Normal saline and autologous blood produced no changes in the conduction time. They concluded that the two most important factors in determining the degree of nerve injury were the nature of injected material and the location within the nerve.

More recently, Sun and White (1974), and Chino et al. (1974) have reported regeneration of nerve fibers following the injection of alcohol and propylene glycol, respectively, in rat sciatic nerve.

Gentili et al. (1978) conducted a light and electron microscopic study of nerve injection injury in rats. They concluded that the main target of the

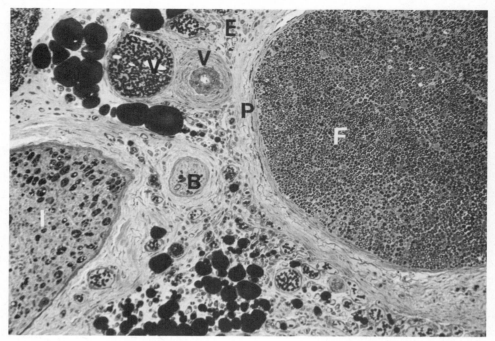

Figure 39–1 Rat sciatic nerve—injection injury site. E = epineurium; P = perineurium; V = epineurial blood vessels; F = normal fascicle; I = fascicle injected with diazepam; B = branch of damaged fascicle. Note that the nerve fiber damage is confined to the fascicle which received the direct injection (I). Damaged fibers in the small branch (B) are presumably derived from that damaged fascicle. Slight thickening of the perineurium is apparent, but the target is primarily the nerve fibers within the injected fascicle. Epineurial blood vessels, of varying calibre, are not affected by the injection. (×550.)

assault on the peripheral nerve was the nerve fiber itself, and that the perineurium and endoneurial microvessels were relatively spared. The site of injection was found to be the major defining factor. Direct intrafascicular injection always gave rise to a more severe injury when compared to an identical extrafascicular injection (Fig. 39–1). Certain drugs proved to be relatively innocuous, but other injectibles injured all nerve fibers at the point of injection. Diazepam and penicillin were found to evoke the most severe injury in this particular study. Alteration in dosage of the injected drug gave rise to the anticipated alteration in severity of injury. One of the most striking findings, however, was the finding of excellent regeneration which occurred even in the most severely affected nerves.

MANAGEMENT OF PATIENTS WITH INJECTION INJURIES

The available experimental and clinical data suggest that it is extremely unlikely that the course of events following nerve injection injury can be altered by any immediate surgical manoeuver. The exact date of nerve injury is available. The patient is managed along the well established lines for patients suffering from lesions in continuity (Nulsen and Kline, 1973; Kline and Hudson, 1976; Kline, 1975; Hudson and Kline, 1975). It is reasonable to anticipate regeneration at approximately one inch per month, and it is appropriate to examine the first target muscle clinically and with electrophysiological studies to see if there is evidence of recovery after the appropriate duration of waiting. Percussion of the nerve at the injured site will almost always cause abnormal sensory symptoms and is of no prognostic value. The clinician may record an advancing Tinel's sign along the anatomical course of the nerve. This indicates that at least some fine fibers have traversed the injured area. This, unfortunately, is no guarantee of a successful outcome, which requires more numerous fibers to reach end-organs and subsequently mature so that they can transmit action potentials. The lack of an advancing Tinel's sign is probably much more significant and suggests that very little regeneration is occurring. During the period of waiting, the patient should maintain all joints through a full range of passive movement so that contractures do not develop.

Case Report 1

A 55-year-old right-handed male experienced extreme pain when he received an injection of meperidine hydrochloride in his right arm. The injection site was on the lateral aspect of the arm, just distal to the spiral groove. The severe pain radiated down his forearm to the dorsal aspect of his thumb. The patient immediately experienced a complete wrist drop. Examination at the University of Toronto revealed a complete radial nerve palsy. The patient was managed expectantly, and, 20 weeks after the incident, electrical and clinical evidence of reinnervation of the first target muscle, the brachioradialis, was evident. Subsequent visits revealed serial reinnervation of the forearm muscles supplied by the radial nerve, and eventual reinnervation of the muscles supplied by the posterior interosseus nerve.

COMMENT. The pathology in this instance was presumably akin to that observed by Gentili et al. (1978) following intrafascicular injection of meperidine hydrochloride; that is, axonal disintegration with associated myelin digestion leading to wallerian degeneration of all elements distal to the point of injury. Subsequent reinnervation of the bands of Büngner led to restoration of function.

Unfortunately, a group of patients exists in whom this desired course of events does not take place. *It is essential that surgical intervention not be unduly postponed in these patients.* The limiting factor in the eventual successful outcome in these patients is the ability of the end-organs to receive regenerating axon sprouts and resume full function. In an adult, it is unlikely that muscle will make a good recovery following denervation intervals in excess of 18 months.

Case Report 2

A 32-year-old patient received an injection of tetanus toxoid into the lateral aspect of his right arm following a minor surgical procedure on his left hand. The pain on injection was severe and extreme, and he immediately developed a wrist drop. The patient was told that he had probably suffered a compression palsy from resting his

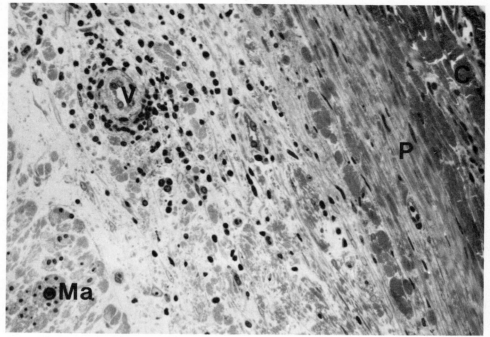

Figure 39–2   Human radial nerve—injection injury site. C = collagen; P = perineurium; V = endoneurial blood vessel with surrounding inflammatory infiltration; Ma = macrophage in endoneurial tissue. Note the absence of any viable nerve fibers in the endoneurial tissues. (× 1375.)

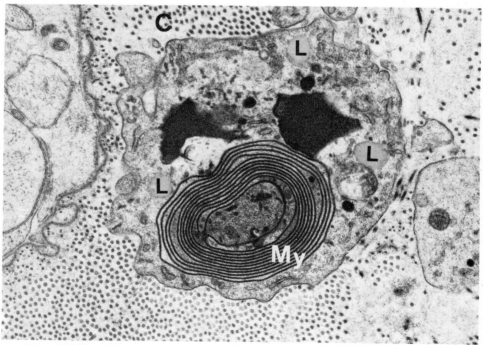

Figure 39–3   Human radial nerve—injection injury site. (detail of a macrophage in Fig. 39–2). L = lipid inclusions within macrophage; C = collagen; My = Myelin figures which have assumed a physical relationship of true myelin around an intracytoplasmic structure which is not an axon. (× 24,200.)

644

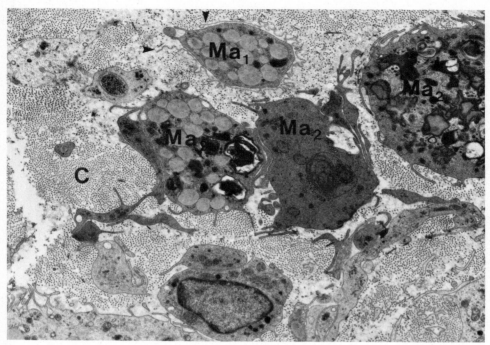

Figure 39–4 Human radial nerve—injection injury site. (Details of another area from Fig. 39–2). C = collagen; Ma_1 = macrophage containing lipid inclusion, either entering or leaving a ruptured basement tube; (►) = points of rupture of basement membrane tube; Ma_2' = macrophage containing myelin remnants free in endoneurium. Surface membrane finger processes are interpreted as evidence of cell mobility. (× 13,100.)

arm against the side of the stretcher. He was subsequently told that he had probably suffered a stroke. Examination 21 weeks after this incident revealed no evidence of reinnervation of the brachioradialis. The radial nerve was promptly explored at the University of Toronto. Stimulation of the radial nerve proximal to the injury site did not result in any brachioradialis contraction. Recording below the injection site failed to reveal any evidence of axonal transmission, and no satisfactory nerve action potential (N.A.P.) could be recorded. The nerve was divided and the ends inspected under an operating microscope. No fascicular pattern could be seen. Frozen section revealed an absence of fascicular pattern. Serial resections were made on both stumps until examination under the operating microscope and quick section confirmed the presence of a fascicular pattern. An 8 cm. gap was reconstituted using sural nerve for interfascicular grafts. The patient made a partial recovery and subsequently required tendon transfers to obtain satisfactory wrist and digit extension.

COMMENT. The pathology in this case was clearly quite different from that of the first case report (Figs. 39–2 through 39–8). Just what the factor is that causes the blocking of regenerating axons by inflammatory and fibrous tissue is as yet unclear. It is possibly related to an admixture of blood with the offending drug.

The two cases quoted represent extremes of the pathological and clinical spectrum. Surgeons will see cases in intermediate grades. Injudicious resection of nerves with normal fascicular pattern will result in a disservice to the patient, and, contrariwise, external neurolysis in a situation that requires resec-

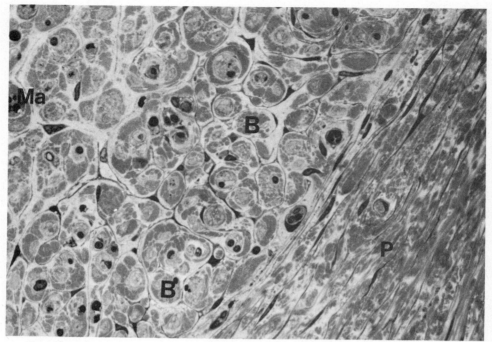

Figure 39–5   Human radial nerve distal to injection site. Ma = macrophage; P = perineurium; B = bands of Büngner. Note the total absence of axons. Myelin remnants are visible, but no normal myelin is present. This is the end state of wallerian degeneration at a level distal to the injury point. (× 2200.)

tion and suture or grafting is the result of equally bad judgment. Surface inspection of the nerve alone will not reveal the critical factor of the fascicular pattern, and the authors favor the various electrical techniques that are used to resolve this dilemma (Nulsen and Kline, 1973; Kline and Hudson, 1976).

Pain is frequently a major symptom. The surgeon should content himself with an external neurolysis that will free the nerve of any surrounding muscle contraction, if the injury has already transmitted a significant number of axons.

LOUISIANA STATE UNIVERSITY SURGICAL SERIES

Radial nerve

Table 39–1 summarizes the courses of patients who received radial nerve injury as a result of nerve injection. Triceps function is preserved, as the branches to that muscle are derived from the nerve proximal to the point of injury. The patients experience wrist drop. They cannot extend the thumb after it has been flexed into the palm and can only achieve limited extension of the fingers by the intrinsic hand muscles. The sensory loss is variable and is seldom a practical problem.

(Text continued on page 650)

Table 39 –1 Injection Injuries – Radial

PATIENT	AGE	AGENT	LOSS	EMG	LESION AGE	STIMU- LATION	N.A.P.	OPERATION	RESULT	FOLLOW- UP
E.H.	55	Terramycin	C	C.D.	5 mos.	Ab	Ab	Suture	4	12 yrs.
C.J.	7	DPT	C	C.D.	2 mos.	Ab	–	Suture	5	7 yrs.
G.R.	48	Tetanus Toxoid	I	I.D.	2 mos.	P	P	Neurolysis	5	6 yrs.
A.R.	39	Vistaril	C	C.D.	3 mos.	Ab	Ab	Suture	4	1 yr.
D.T.	41	Vistaril	C	C.D.	20 mos.	Ab	Ab	Suture	1–2	9 mos.

C = complete, I = incomplete, D = denervation, Ab = absent, P = present.

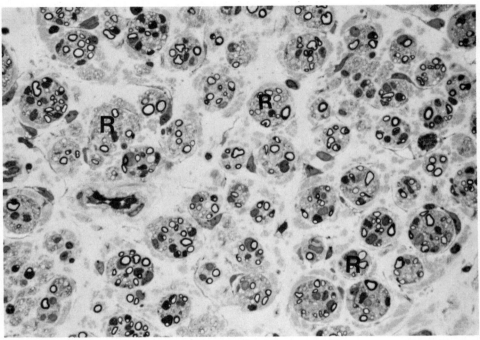

Figure 39–6 Human radial nerve proximal to injection injury site. R = regenerative units within a single fascicle. Note the intense regenerative activity at the level of most proximal sections made prior to reconstitution of the nerve with interfascicular grafts. Compare the microtopography of the fascicle with Figure 39–1. The grouping of fibers in this figure is an expression of axonal sprouting within basement membrane tubes. It is essential that all damaged tissue be trimmed back to this level before a graft is inserted. The surgeon receives indirect evidence that he has reached this point when he observes definition of the fascicular pattern of the nerve on the proximal stump. (× 2200.)

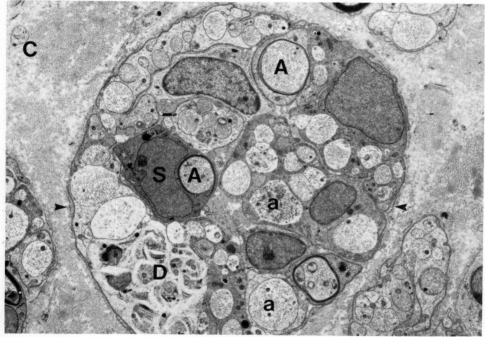

Figure 39–7 Human radial nerve proximal to injection injury site. S = Schwann cell nucleus: A = axons showing early remyelination; a = unmyelinated axons; C = collagen; D = debris; (▶) points to basement membrane. (This is a high-power view of one of the regenerative units in Fig. 39–6). Note intense regenerative axon sprouting. All these sprouts are contained within the original basement membrane system of the fibre, which was injured at the time of the injection. Remnants of Schwann cell and macrophage components are noted in the lower left corner. (× 7752.)

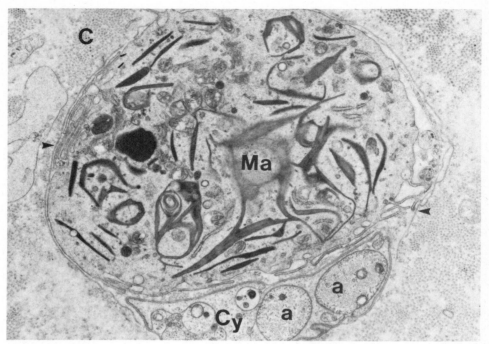

Figure 39–8 Human radial nerve proximal to injection injury site. Ma = macrophage; a = unmyelinated axon sprouts; C = collagen; Cy = Schwann cell cytoplasm; (►) points to basement membrane. This macrophage either has invaded the basement membrane tube at another plane of section, or, alternatively, is a transformed Schwann cell. It contains numerous cytoplasmic organelles indicative of its function of phagocytosis and digestion of cell remnants. Regenerating unmyelinated axon sprouts, presumably derived from the nodes of Ranvier further proximally along this fiber, are included within the original basement membrane tube. This section is taken distal to Figures 39–4 and 39–5 and shows the transition zone between the zone of degeneration and the zone of regeneration. (× 13,680.)

A radial nerve is easily found at operation by separating the brachialis from the brachioradialis. The nerve lies at the bottom of the trough (Sunderland, 1968). It is followed back to the injury site. The nerve is stimulated proximal to the lesion and N.A.P. recordings are made. If the lesion is resected, the proximal and distal stumps are freed up and the nerve is sutured. If the ends cannot be opposed, interfascicular grafts are sewn in, using the sural nerve (Kline et al., 1972).

Recovery is heralded by the return of function to the brachioradialis. Wrist extension is initially performed with radial deviation, as the extensor carpi radialis is supplied by the radial nerve. Subsequently, the extensor mass supplied by the posterior interosseus nerve resumes function and the digits extend through a normal range.

Sciatic nerve

The sciatic nerve is managed as two nerves. The function of the tibial and peroneal divisions is assessed separately. The nerve is exposed at the gluteal fold-line and followed proximally. The gluteus maximus is divided at its attachments to the iliotibial tract and femur. If this does not give good access,

Table 39–2 Injection Injuries—Sciatic*

PATIENT AGE	AGENT	LESION AGE	LOSS	OPERATION** Tibial	OPERATION** Peroneal	RESULT Tibial	RESULT Peroneal	FOLLOWUP
60	Demerol Atropine	6 wks.	Inc.	N	N	4	0	9 yrs.
22	Demerol Phenergan	6 wks.	Compl.	N	S	4	2	7 yrs.
3	Demerol Scopolamine	5½ mos.	Inc.	N	S	5	2	5 yrs.
60	Demerol	10 mos.	Inc.	N	N	4	4	5 yrs.
46	Demerol Phenergan	4 mos.	Inc.	N	R	4	0	2 yrs. Subsequent sympathectomy
39	Castor oil	2 yrs.	Inc.	N	N	5	5	1½ yrs.
56	Unknown	6 mos.	Inc.	N	N	4	4	½ yr.

*Operative stimulation and N.A.P. recording done on each nerve.
**N = neurolysis, S = suture, R = resection.

Table 39–3 Injection Injuries—Median

PATIENT	AGE	AGENT	LOSS	LESION AGE	EMG	STIMULATION	N.A.P.	OPERATION	RESULT	FOLLOW-UP
V.B.	28	Contrast	I	2 mos.	I.D.	P	P	Neurolysis	5	3 yrs.
J.D.	18	Demerol	C	6 wks.	C.D.	Ab	P	Neurolysis	3	4 yrs.

C = complete, I = incomplete, D = denervation, P = present, Ab = absent.

the dissection is carried up to the iliac crest so that the injured nerve can be thoroughly exposed. The nerve is split into its two components, and stimulation and recording studies are carried out on the tibial and peroneal components (Table 39–2).

The patient must protect the heel of the foot from blisters until the calcaneal branches of the posterior tibial nerves are reinnervated. A temporary drop-foot splint allows the patient good mobility, as the superior gluteal, femoral and obturator nerves give sufficient lower limb control.

Median nerve

The median nerve supplies sensation to the terminal phalanges of the thumb and index finger. This function is critical both to the recognition of objects and to the coordinated action of the hand. Note that in the case of J.D. there was no response to stimulation. This indicates that axons have not made functioning connections with the muscles of the thenar mass. Nerve action potentials were recorded, however, indicating that axons had traversed the lesion, so that the surgeon performed a neurolysis and did not resect the nerve (Table 39–3).

CONCLUSION

The authors believe that an aggressive attitude should be taken toward all cases that do not exhibit recovery in an appropriate period following nerve injection injury. It is essential that these patients not be managed conservatively in the vain hope of some future magical recovery. The lesion should be assessed by intraoperative study, and, where appropriate, resection of the lesion with suturing and grafting should be accomplished.

REFERENCES

Bischoff, A., and Thomas, P. K.: Microscopic anatomy of myelinated nerve fibres. *In* P. J. Dyck, P. K. Thomas, E H. Lambert (eds.): Peripheral Neuropathy. Philadelphia, W. B. Saunders Co., 1975, p. 104.
Broadbent, T. R., Odom, G. L., and Woodall, B.: Peripheral nerve injuries from administration of penicillin. J.A.M.A.*140*:1008, 1949.
Burkel, W. E., and McPhee, M.: Effect of phenol injection into peripheral nerve of rat. Arch. Phys. Med. Rehab. *51*:391, 1970.
Chino, N., Award, E. A., and Kottke, F. J.: Pathology of propylene glycol administered by perineural and extramuscular injection in rats. Arch. Phys. Med. Rehab. *55*:33, 1974.
Clark, K., Williams, P. E., Jr., Willis, W., and McGravan, W.: Injection injury of the sciatic nerve. Clin. Neurosurg. *17*:111, 1970.
Clark, W. K.: Surgery for injection injuries of peripheral nerves. Surg. Clin. North Am. *52*:1325, 1972.
Combes, M. S., Clark, W. K., Gregory, C. F., and James, J. A.: Sciatic nerve injury in infants: Recognition and prevention of impairment resulting from intragluteal injection. J.A.M.A. *173*:1330, 1960.
Curtis, P. A., Jr., and Tucker, H. J.: Sciatic palsy in premature infants: A report and follow-up study of 10 cases. J.A.M.A. *174*:1586, 1960.
Elkington, J. St. C.: Peripheral nerve palsies following intramuscular injections of sulphonamides. Lancet *2*:425, 1942.

Gentili, F., Hudson, A., Kline, D. G., and Hunter, D.: Peripheral nerve injection injury — an experimental study. Read at Annual Meeting A.A.N.S., New Orleans. April, 1978.

Gilles, F. H., and French, J. H.: Post-injection sciatic nerve palsies in infants and children. J. Pediat. *58*:195, 1961.

Hanson, D. J.: Intramuscular injection injuries and complications. Gen. Pract. *27*:109, 1963.

Holbrook. T. J., and Pilcher, C.: The effects of injection of penicillin, peanut oil and beeswax, separately and in combination upon nerve and muscle. Surg. Gynecol. Obstet. *90*:39, 1950.

Hudson, A. R., and Kline, D.: Progression of partial experimental injury to peripheral nerve. Part 2: Light and electron microscopic studies. J. Neurosurg. *42*:15, 1975.

Hudson, A. R., Morris, J., Weddell, G., et al.: Peripheral nerve autografts. J. Surg. Res. *12*:267, 1972.

Hudson, F. P., McCandless, A., and O'Malley, A.: Sciatic paralysis in newborn infants. Br. Med. J. *1*:223, 1950.

Kline, D. G., and Hudson, A. R.: Early management of peripheral nerve injury. *In* Morley T. (ed.): Current Controversies in Neurosurgery. Philadelphia, W. B. Saunders Co., 1976, p. 181.

Kline, D. G., Hackett, E. R., Davis, G. D., et al.: Effect of mobilization on the blood supply and regeneration of injured nerves. J. Surg. Res., *12*:254, 1972.

Kline, D. G., Hudson, A. R., Hackett, E. R., et al.: Progression of partial experimental injury to peripheral nerve. Part 1: Periodic measurements of muscle contraction strength. J. Neurosurg. *42*:1, 1975.

Kolb, L. C., and Gray, S. J.: Peripheral neuritis as a complication of penicillin therapy. J.A.M.A. *132*:323, 1946.

Linder, D. W., and Gurdjian, E. S.: Injuries of nerves: clinical aspects. *In* Vinken, E. P. T., and G. W. Bruyn (eds.): Handbook of Clinical Neurology. New York, American Elsevier, 1970, pp. 257.

Ling, C. M., and Loong, S. C.: Injection injury of the radial nerve. Injury *8*:60, 1976.

Matson, D. D.: Early neurolysis in the treatment of injury of the peripheral nerves due to faulty injection of antibiotics. New Engl. J. Med. *242*:973, 1950.

Morris, J., Hudson, A. R., and Weddell, G.: A study of degeneration and regeneration in the divided rat sciatic nerve based on electron microscopy. Z. Zellforsch Mikrosk Anat. *124*:76, 1972.

Nulsen, F. E., and Kline, D. G.: Acute injuries of peripheral nerves. *In* Youmans, J. R. (ed.): Neurological Surgery. Philadelphia, W. B. Saunders Co., 1973, p. 1094.

Ochoa, J.: Microscopic anatomy of unmyelinated nerve fibres. *In* Dyck, P. J. Thomas, P. K., and Lambert, E. H. (eds.): Peripheral Neuropathy. Philadelphia, W. B. Saunders Co., 1975, p. 131.

Olsson, Y., and Reese, T.: Permeability of vasa nervorum and perineurium in mouse sciatic nerve studied by fluorescence and electron microscopy. J. Neuropath. Exper. Neurol. *30*:105, 1971.

Ranvier, L. A.: Lecons Sur L'Histologie du Systeme Nerveaux. Paris, F. Savy, 1878.

Sun, C. N., and White, H. J.: Dysfunction and remyelination of peripheral nerve after alcohol injury. Exp. Path. *9*:169, 1974.

Sunderland, S.: Nerves and Nerve Injuries. Edinburgh, Livingstone, 1968.

Tarlov, I. M., Perlmutler, I., and Berman, A. N.: Paralysis caused by penicillin injection: Mechanism of complication — a warning. J. Neuropath. Exper. Neurol. *10*:158, 1951.

Thomas, P. K., and Jones, D. G.: The cellular response to nerve injury. 2: Regeneration of the perineurium after nerve section. J. Anat. *101*:45, 1967.

Turner, G. G.: The site for intramuscular injections. Lancet *2*:819, 1920.

Tuvo, F., and Bouquet, F.: Clinical and instrumental contribution to the knowledge of painful iatrogenic paralysing sciatica in the adult and pediatric age. Minerva Med. *62*:784, 1971.

Woodhall, B., Broadbent, T. R., and Taver, J.: The neuropathology of antibiotic-induced peripheral nerve paralysis. Surg. Forum, *1*:394, 1950.

Special Problems

VI

40

DIFFERENTIAL DIAGNOSIS OF PERIPHERAL NERVE TUMORS

JAMES C. HARKIN

Most peripheral nerve neoplasms are derived from Schwann cells. In other, less differentiated neoplasms it may not be possible to identify the cell of origin. Neoplastic neurons are not found in primary peripheral nerve neoplasms except in the neuroblastoma–ganglioneuroma–pheochromocytoma group, members of which are almost never seen in the extremities (Table 40–1).

The nomenclature of the tumors is that generally accepted (Stout, 1949; Harkin and Reed, 1969; Kramer, 1970; Urich, 1975; Russell and Rubinstein, 1977). Neurofibromas of the skin and those in other parts of the body have been considered separately because of their different behavior.

Von Recklinghausen's disease of nerves (VRD) modifies the location and character of nerve tumors (Harkin and Reed, 1969; Canale and Bebin, 1972). At the end of the description of each tumor the effect of VRD on the neoplasm is described.

Von Recklinghausen's disease is inherited as an autosomal dominant, and is characterized by a wide variety of lesions, only some of which will be present in one patient. Marked difference in expressivity is usual. A common pattern is the formes fruste (incomplete expression), in which only a few lesions are found and the diagnosis may be readily overlooked. The characteristic lesions of VRD are a) *abnormal cell growths and hamartomatous lesions:* cafe-au-lait cutaneous spots formed by increased melanin in the basal layer of the epidermis, localized gigantism, scoliosis (Rezain, 1976), and fibrous cortical defect of bone; and b)

Table 40–1   Classification of Peripheral Nerve Neoplasms

I. Benign primary nerve sheath cell tumors
    A. Schwannoma (neurilemoma)
        Variants: ancient schwannoma, cystic schwannoma
            and plexiform schwannoma
    B. Neurofibroma, cutaneous
    C. Neurofibroma of a peripheral nerve, neither
        cutaneous nor plexiform
II. Locally aggressive primary nerve sheath cell tumors
    that tend to undergo malignant transformation
        Plexiform neurofibroma
III. Malignant primary nerve sheath cell tumors
    A. Malignant schwannoma
    B. Nerve sheath cell sarcoma (neurogenic sarcoma)
IV. Neuroectodermal tumors of primitive type and tumors
    with nerve cell differentiation
    A. Neuroblastoma
    B. Ganglioneuroma
    C. Pheochromocytoma
V. Tumors metastatic to peripheral nerves

neoplasms: benign schwannomas and neurofibromas (sometimes of enormous size), locally aggressive tumors, and malignant tumors, as well as some lesions that could be called either hamartomas or neoplasms. Almost all of the separate lesions seen with VRD can be found in patients who do not have the disorder.

SCHWANNOMA

Schwannoma is a benign, slowly growing, encapsulated neoplasm that originates in a nerve and is composed of Schwann cells and a collagenous matrix.

The tumor usually grows by expanding within the nerve of origin, pushing the axons aside and then projecting to one side of the nerve, allowing the lesion to be removed without sacrificing the nerve (Fig. 40–1). However, a schwannoma on the acoustic nerve and dorsal spinal nerve roots invariably involves the nerve to the extent that separation of tumor and nerve is impossible.

Grossly the schwannoma is pale gray, smooth surfaced, and rubbery. When cut across, it is either pale gray and homogeneous or may contain cysts filled with clear fluid. Rarely the tumor presents as a cyst, and only after microscopic examination is the true nature of the lesion identified. In older schwannomas

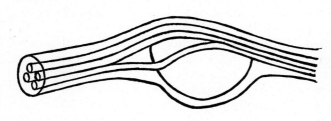

Figure 40–1 Diagram of schwannoma of peripheral nerve. At the left the structure of a normal nerve is illustrated: four nerve fascicles are seen (each fascicle contains a number of myelinated and nonmyelinated axons sheathed by Schwann cells and each fascicle is surrounded by a perineurium containing cells and collagen). The oval mass is a schwannoma. The nerve fascicles are stretched across the tumor. The epineurial sheath and the nerve fascicles lie over the tumor.

there may be yellow and reddish-brown zones representing collections of fat-filled and hemosiderin-laden macrophages.

Common sites for schwannomas are along the peripheral nerves and major nerve plexuses, but not in the small cutaneous nerves. Schwannomas in the acoustic nerve (acoustic neuroma) and on the dorsal nerve roots of the spinal cord are common. The nerve root lesions may grow on both sides of the intervertebral foramen, creating a dumbbell tumor. Mediastinal schwannomas are also common. Intraosseous schwannomas are not common but may occur in many sites and must be considered in the differential diagnosis of a lytic bone lesion (Wirth and Bray, 1977).

Microscopically, the schwannoma is a cellular tumor with oval nuclei, often oriented in parallel array with indistinct cell boundaries (Fig. 40–2). In some tumors the cells form palisades; however, it should be noted that this feature is generally overemphasized. Palisading of cells is a much more prominent feature of leiomyomas than of schwannomas. Sometimes the cells are clumped in little structures resembling nerve end organs; these are called Verocay bodies. In schwannomas the cells are closely packed with relatively little extracellular space (Antoni type A pattern) except in some foci with abundant extracellular space (Antoni type B pattern). Electron microscopy shows the tumor cells to have convoluted plasma membranes (similar to hyperplastic Schwann cells) and an encasing basement membrane. Most of the collagen has a normal pattern, but in some tumors the collagen is aggregated extracellularly into long spacing collagen — a mass of banded material that does not form true fibrils. Long spacing collagen can occur in other tissues but has been seen most frequently in schwannomas (Harkin and Reed, 1969; Urich, 1975).

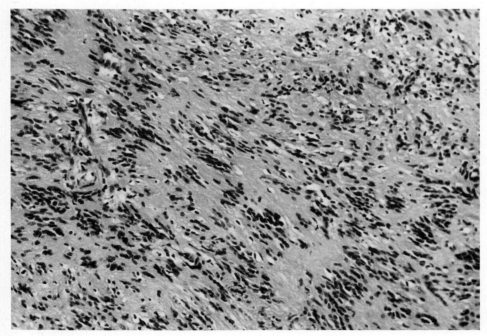

Figure 40–2   Schwannoma, photomicrograph. Oval, relatively regular nuclei are arranged in streams and palisades. Most of the tissue between nuclei is cytoplasm of the tumor cells. Some extracellular collagen is present. (×124.)

Variants include the ancient schwannoma with increased cellularity and marked nuclear variation. Ancient schwannomas are benign tumors, and the cellular atypia should not lure the observer into an erroneous diagnosis of malignant tumor. Some schwannomas are cystic. A rare form is the plexiform schwannoma, a lesion that grossly somewhat resembles a plexiform neurofibroma but microscopically is a typical benign schwannoma with the same good prognosis as other benign schwannomas. We believe this lesion to be the one briefly noted by Masson as a plexiform tumor that had features of schwannoma and one that we have recently studied (Masson, 1956).

Differential Diagnosis

The site of some lesions (acoustic nerve, dorsal spinal nerve roots) is so characteristic that the diagnosis is not in doubt. In the mediastinum, thymic tumors and cysts may resemble schwannomas. Along peripheral nerves a nodule of metastatic carcinoma can resemble grossly a schwannoma. Soft tissue tumors other than schwannomas are common around joints, whereas in the soft tissue between joints the schwannomas comprise a larger share of the tumors. Hemangiomas involving peripheral nerves usually extend for some distance along the nerve rather than forming discretely localized tumors.

Relationship to VRD

Von Recklinghausen's disease modifies the sites where schwannomas are found. Schwannoma is only one of many lesions that can be found in VRD. Multiple schwannomas can be found in this condition. Bilateral acoustic schwannomas have not been reported in the absence of VRD, and intestinal schwannomas are virtually unknown except with VRD. Schwannomas that grow into the substance of the brain and spinal cord are found only with VRD. However, single schwannomas located on peripheral nerves are not usually associated with VRD, and there is no relationship between plexiform schwannoma and VRD insofar as is known.

Schwannomas do not undergo malignant transformation even in patients with VRD. An unusual malignant schwannoma may resemble an ancient schwannoma, but the mitotic figures and evidence of invasion should allow the correct diagnosis of malignant schwannoma. The most common error is to call an ancient schwannoma a malignant tumor. When examining an individual schwannoma there is no way to determine if the patient has VRD.

CUTANEOUS NEUROFIBROMA

Neurofibroma is a benign, slowly growing, localized but nonencapsulated neoplasm that contains Schwann cells and a massive extracellular collagenous matrix. Scattered fibrocyte-like cells may sometimes be found within the lesion but these are probably not neoplastic cells. In the skin the nerve of origin is rarely seen.

Externally the lesion is seen as a smooth elevation of the skin that is rubbery

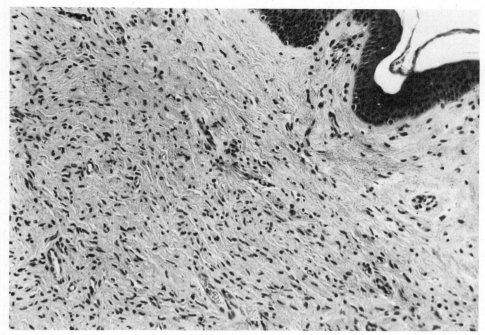

Figure 40-3 Cutaneous neurofibroma, photomicrograph. A thin layer of dermis lies between the epidermis and the tumor, which is not sharply outlined. The somewhat irregularly arranged tumor cells are separated by a considerable amount of collagen. (×124.)

or soft. Pain is not a prominent feature. On section the tumor is pale gray and glistening, localized but not encapsulated. Skin appendages may be embedded within the lesion. Grossly and microscopically the overlying epidermis may be flattened. The large lesions may be gelatinous. Microscopically the lesion is not very cellular, containing nuclei that are oval and somewhat irregularly arranged (Fig. 40-3). Sometimes cell borders are seen and the cells are stellate or fusiform. Electron microscopy shows that the vast majority of the tumor is made up of extracellular collagen, and the scattered Schwann cells have little infolding of the plasma membrane.

Differential Diagnosis

The dermal lesions grossly resemble dermatofibromas, dermal nevi, lipomas, or granular cell tumors (myoblastoma) but histologically these lesions are readily separated.

Relationship of VRD to Cutaneous Neurofibromas

The neurofibroma is the characteristic lesion of VRD. On the other hand, having one or a few cutaneous neurofibromas does not automatically indicate that the patient has VRD. The majority of surgically excised cutaneous neurofibromas come from patients who do not have VRD, insofar as can be determined. The massive cutaneous neurofibromas so frequently illustrated in reviews yet so infrequently seen clinically are found only with VRD.

Patients with VRD may also have dermal fibromas. The cafe-au-lait pigmented zones may or may not be associated with sites of neurofibromas.

Malignant lesions may develop in the skin or subcutaneous tissue of patients with VRD. Some of the malignancies arise de novo, others from malignant transformation of a *plexiform* neurofibroma. In general, cutaneous neurofibromas (other than plexiform) do not become malignant.

NEUROFIBROMA OF A PERIPHERAL NERVE, NEITHER CUTANEOUS NOR PLEXIFORM

The neurofibroma of a larger peripheral nerve is a neoplasm of Schwann cells with a massive extracellular collagenous matrix that often contains a considerable amount of mucoid material.

The tumor may be sharply demarcated and grow out from a nerve, or the nerve may pass through the tumor and be lost, at least in part. On section the lesion is very pale gray, soft, somewhat rubbery, and gelatinous. Microscopically the lesion is similar to the dermal neurofibroma but with a much looser extracellular matrix (Fix. 40–4). Axons may be trapped within the tumor. Identifica-

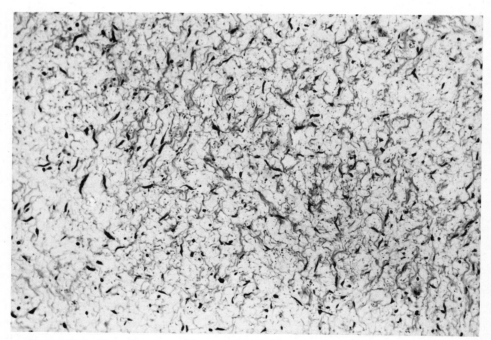

Figure 40–4 Neurofibroma, neither cutaneous nor plexiform, of a large nerve, photomicrograph. The loose hypocellular pattern of the tumor is seen. Irregularly arranged cells have long cytoplasmic processes. Grossly the lesion was gelatinous. (×124.)

tion of axons within the tumor is not necessary for classification of the lesion as a neurofibroma.

Differential Diagnosis

The tumor must be distinguished from a lipoma and lipofibromatous hamartoma of nerve (Seddon, 1972). Clinically, cysts around joints may resemble neurofibromas.

Relationship to VRD

In the majority of cases of neurofibromas involving larger nerves there is definite evidence of VRD. In some cases no evidence can be found of a relationship.

PLEXIFORM NEUROFIBROMA

Plexiform neurofibroma is a distinct lesion that should be separated from other neurofibromas. It is invariably associated with von Recklinghausen's disease (VRD). The neoplasm arises within a nerve and distorts the nerve structure (Fig. 40–5).

Grossly the lesion resembles a tangle of worms of varying sizes. When cut across, it is soft and gelatinous. The tangled nerve fascicles can fade into adjacent soft tissue or into more solid masses of tumor. In the early stage of development the lesion may be difficult to identify because the swollen neoplastically overgrown nerve fascicles may appear to be nodular swellings of the nerve.

Microscopically the abnormal nerve fascicles are swollen and hypocellular, containing Schwann cells, endoneurial cells, and relatively few axons. As the lesion develops, the grossly enlarged nerve fascicles contain increased numbers of Schwann cells, endoneurial cells and primitive cells that cannot be identified as to origin (Fig. 40–6). When examined by electron microscopy the lesions resemble cutaneous neurofibromas. The plexiform neurofibroma may continue in a relatively hypocellular pattern for long periods of time with slow growth, or the lesion may become increasingly cellular and transform into a malignant neo-

Figure 40–5 Diagram of plexiform neurofibroma. The normal nerve is to the left. Four nerve fascicles (each containing many axons sheathed by Schwann cells and the fascicles each sheathed by perineurium) are surrounded by an epineurial sheath. Moving to the right the progressive expansion and distortion of nerve fascicles can be seen as they are transformed into a plexiform neurofibroma.

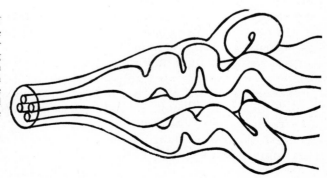

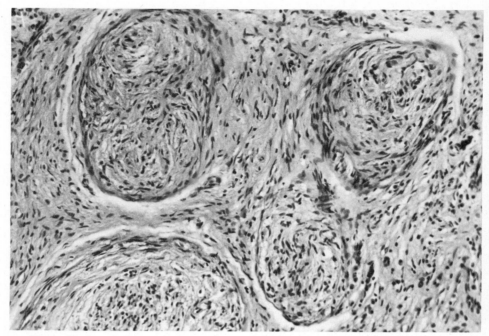

Figure 40-6. Plexiform neurofibroma, photomicrograph. Four enlarged distorted nerve fascicles are seen filled with neoplastic Schwann cells arranged in an irregular pattern. Many axons would have been displaced by this stage. (×132.)

plasm. Accurate documentation of the complete natural history of the lesion remains incomplete.

Plexiform neurofibromas may occur in any of the major nerve plexuses (e.g., brachial, lumbosacral), in the major nerves, particularly·those in the legs and the neck, and occasionally in small peripheral nerves, such as those of the eyelids. Lesions can also be found in the tongue and the viscera.

Differential Diagnosis

The principal differential diagnosis is between a simple plexiform neurofibroma and a malignant nerve sheath cell tumor that has developed in a plexiform neurofibroma. On microscopic examination, traumatic neuromas in the early stage of development, before the characteristic miniature nerve fascicles are well formed, may resemble plexiform neurofibromas. The history, location, and symptoms may be helpful to the pathologist in such cases (and in some others as well). The rare tumor plexiform schwannoma may grossly resemble a plexiform neurofibroma, but not microscopically.

The prognosis for plexiform neurofibroma must be guarded. The lesions are difficult to excise completely without massive nerve destruction. The lesions often recur, possibly because the proximal limit of the tumor could not be identified, or because the neoplasm was already developing in other sites where it was unrecognizable. The tumor tends to grow toward the central nervous system and can even progress into the spinal cord and cause severe damage there. The gravest danger faced by a patient with a plexiform neurofibroma is that it might develop into a malignant nerve sheath cell tumor; many of these malignant tumors start as plexiform neurofibromas.

A consideration of the relationship of VRD to plexiform neurofibroma is irrelevant, since all cases are associated with VRD. Other lesions that can be associated with plexiform neurofibroma in the VRD patient are local gigantism of the involved part; for example, the tongue or leg.

MALIGNANT PRIMARY PERIPHERAL NERVE SHEATH CELL TUMORS (MALIGNANT) SCHWANNOMA AND NERVE SHEATH CELL SARCOMA; RELATED TERM–NEUROGENIC SARCOMA

Malignant primary peripheral nerve sheath cell tumors derive from Schwann cells or cells insufficiently differentiated to allow identification. Approximately one fourth of such tumors can be definitely identified as malignant schwannomas by light and electron microscopy.

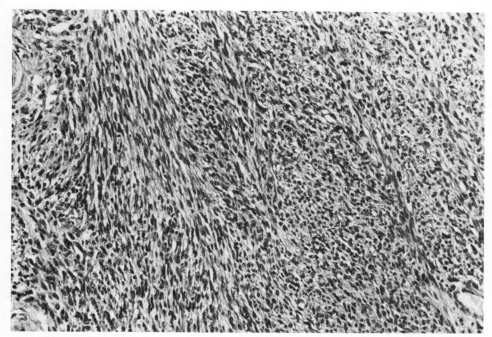

Figure 40–7. Malignant schwannoma, photomicrograph. The malignant nerve sheath cell tumor is very cellular and has streams of cells. Mitotic figures were present. An objective diagnosis wound not be possible on the basis of this illustration alone, although the histologic pattern is characteristic of the tumor. (×124.)

On gross examination primary malignant peripheral nerve neoplasms are moderately firm and reddish-gray. The tumor extends into the adjacent tissue without a sharp line of demarcation. The malignant tumor either arises in a plexiform neurofibroma or de novo in a peripheral nerve. The normal or abnormal nerve is trapped within the malignant tumor.

Microscopically, the *malignant schwannoma* is a cellular tumor with some variation in nuclear size and shape (Fig. 40–7). Scattered mitotic figures are seen. There may be clumps of lymphocyte-like cells. Sometimes there is an epithelioid pattern, with cells having a distinct cell margin. Electron microscope examination shows that the tumor cells have a basement membrane surrounding the cells, a feature that helps identify the cells as Schwann cells.

The *nerve sheath cell sarcoma* (neurogenic sarcoma) resembles a fibrosarcoma or spindle cell sarcoma, with occasional clumps of cells arranged in streams. Some of the tumors differentiate into typical malignant mesenchymoma.

Differential Diagnosis

Differentiation of primary malignant nerve sheath cell tumors from other soft tissue sarcomas rests principally on identifying a lesion extending from a nerve and having a histologic pattern consistent with a primary nerve tumor. If the tumor has arisen in a plexiform neurofibroma it may be possible to observe a transition from the locally aggressive lesion into the frankly malignant one, making it possible to identify the malignant tumor as being of nerve origin.

Frozen section diagnosis is not very satisfactory. Probably half the tumors can be recognized as being malignant, but almost never can the tumor be identified as being a nerve tumor without knowledge of its relationship to a nerve as well as other pertinent clinical data. It is important to have all the information possible (clinical, gross, family history, etc.) in order to make the diagnosis.

Relationship to VRD

The majority of malignant nerve sheath cell tumors arise in patients with VRD. The most common origin is in a plexiform neurofibroma. Some of the tumors arise in apparently normal nerves in patients with or without VRD. A VRD patient may have more than one malignant tumor of nerve origin. It is uncommon to find a malignant primary peripheral nerve tumor. The frequency is not known. Probably fewer than 13 per cent (the most used figure) of VRD patients will develop malignant tumor (Seddon, 1972). It is known that malignant primary peripheral nerve tumors occur about 15 to 20 times more often in VRD patients than in the general population. Although it has been alleged that surgical interference with a neurofibroma can precipitate malignant change, the evidence is inconclusive; more likely, the usual condition is that partial resection of a tumor failed to include the tumor that had become malignant (Seddon, 1972).

A number of the patients with malignant primary peripheral nerve sheath cell tumors are recognized as having VRD only after the tumor has been biopsied or removed.

NEUROECTODERMAL TUMORS OF PRIMITIVE TYPE AND TUMORS WITH NERVE CELL DIFFERENTIATION: NEUROBLASTOMA, GANGLIONEUROMA, AND PHEOCHROMOCYTOMA

Tumors in this group rarely involve nerves of the extremities. They can involve the spine by extension from lesions in sympathetic ganglia, particularly the ganglioneuromas in the neck and thorax (mediastinum).

Differential Diagnosis

Ganglion cells (neurons) can be found in ganglioneuromas and in neurofibromas infiltrating normal nerve ganglia. The histologic pattern may be similar. The differentiating feature is the presence of cap cells surrounding the ganglion cell — in the infiltrating neurofibroma the normal ganglion cells are surrounded by cap cells, whereas the neoplastic ganglion cells of the ganglioneuroma, with rare exceptions, are not.

Pheochromocytoma and neuroblastoma are found in the autonomic part of the peripheral nervous system, most often in the adrenal.

Relationship to VRD

All tumors in this group can occasionally be found associated with VRD.

NEOPLASMS PRIMARY IN OTHER SITES SECONDARILY INVOLVING PERIPHERAL NERVES

Malignant neoplasms that arise outside the nervous system occasionally metastasize to peripheral nerves. A complete history and physical examination together with x-rays and suitable laboratory tests will usually establish the nature of these growths. In practice, unsuspected metastatic tumors in peripheral nerves occur more often than might be anticipated. The reason is that a comprehensive workup of the patient may not have been considered necessary before excising what appeared to be a ganglion cyst on the wrist or a focus of nodular synovitis on the foot. One should suspect that the nerve lesion may be metastatic if the patient has had a previous malignant neoplasm elsewhere, even though the primary tumor was apparently treated successfully. Carcinomas of the breast, lung, and thyroid have been the common tumors metastatic to peripheral nerves. The most unusual lesion we have seen was what was thought to be a "clear cell adenoma" of uncertain origin, apparently primary in the ulnar nerve. Finally, it was found that the patient had had a parathyroid tumor which was of equivocal malignancy histologically. The nerve tumor was apparently a solitary metastasis from the parathyroid carcinoma.

Lymphomas may involve peripheral nerves and nerve roots, but usually the diagnosis is not in doubt by the time masses are recognizable in the peripheral nerves.

Malignant melanoma metastatic to a peripheral nerve is sometimes not recognized microscopically because of the lack of pigmentation of the tumor cells. Almost all cases referred to us as malignant melanocytic schwannomas have proved to be metastatic malignant melanomas. Melanomas are notorious for reappearing years after the original tumor was excised.

As to *sites* where metastatic tumors are found in nerves, the nerve roots of the spinal cord are common sites, with or without involvement of the adjacent bone.

In *von Recklinghausen's neurofibromatosis,* tumors may be found invading or metastasizing to peripheral nerves. Sometimes the lesion is a metastasis from a previously recognized malignant nerve sheath cell tumor. At other times the tumor may be one that is not of nerve origin, since patients with VRD can have a variety of different tumors.

REFERENCES

Canale, D. J., and Bebin, J.: Von Recklinghausen's disease of the nervous system. *In* Vinken, P. J., and Bruyn, G. W.: Handbook of Clinical Neurology, Volume 14: The Phakomatoses. Amsterdam, North-Holland Publishing Company, 1972.

Harkin, J. C., and Reed, R. J.: Tumors of the Peripheral Nervous System. Fascicle 3, Atlas of Tumor Pathology. Second Series. Washington, Armed Forces Institute of Pathology, 1969.

Kramer, W.: Tumours of nerves. *In* Vinken, P. J., and Bruyn, G. W., Handbook of Clinical Neurology, Volume 8: Diseases of Nerves, Part II. Amsterdam, North-Holland Publishing Company, 1970.

Masson, P.: Human Tumors. 2nd ed., English translation (published originally as P. Masson: Tumeurs Humaines, 2ème édition, Paris, France. Librarie Maloine, 1956), Detroit, Wayne State University Press, 1970.

Rezain, S. M.: The incidence of scoliosis due to neurofibromatosis. Acta Orthop. Scand. *47*:534, 1976.

Russell, D. S., and Rubinstein, L. J.: Pathology of Tumors of the Nervous System, 4th ed., Baltimore, Williams & Wilkins, 1977.

Seddon, H.: Surgical Disorders of the Peripheral Nerves. Baltimore, Williams & Wilkins, 1972.

Stout, A. P.: Tumors of the Peripheral Nervous System. Section II, Fascicle 6, Atlas of Tumor Pathology. Washington, Armed Forces Institute of Pathology, 1949.

Urich, H.: Pathology of tumors of cranial nerves, spinal nerve roots, and peripheral nerves. *In* Dyck, P. J., Thomas, P. K., and Lambert, E. H.: Peripheral Neuropathy. Philadelphia, W. B. Saunders Company, 1975, Chap 68.

Wirth, W. A., and Bray, C. B.: Intra-osseous neurilemoma. J. Bone Joint Surg. *59A*: 252, 1977.

41

CURRENT CONCEPTS IN THE MANAGEMENT OF PERIPHERAL NERVE TUMORS

IRVING M. ARIEL

Any tumefaction of the soft somatic tissue demands critical evaluation of all factors related to the tumor and the patient before a therapeutic regime can be embarked upon. On simple clinical evaluation a benign neuroma cannot be separated from the most malignant neurilemoma. This presentation reviews the basic factors upon which one plans the therapeutic regime that will be instituted. In a previous chapter, a histologic classification was presented, defining the various sub-varieties of tumors of the peripheral nerves. This presentation is devoted to the clinical approach, establishing the diagnoses, and the therapeutic procedures to be instituted based upon the natural history of the various sub-types of tumors inflicted on the peripheral nervous system.

Tumors of soft somatic tissues involve nearly all the tissues of the human body. In clinical treatment, however, certain of these malignant tumors are differentiated into subspecialty groups. Thus neuroblastomas of the adrenal glands would be treated by pediatric oncologists and surgeons, whereas malignant retinoblastomas would be treated by ophthalmologic surgeons and oncologists. The general surgeon, including the orthopedic surgeon is called upon to treat those tumors afflicting the torso and extremities; the greatest emphasis in this chapter shall be devoted to these structures.

The soft somatic tissues constitute over 50 per cent of the body weight and the greatest amount of tissue in the human organism. They consist of that mass of flesh situated between the epidermis and the parenchymal organs, and are composed of connective tissue, blood and lymphatic vessels, smooth and striated muscle, fat, fascia, synovial structures, and nerves. They are present in every organ of the human body. As mentioned above, this discussion will include only neoplasms in what are usually considered the organs of locomotion and support. Neoplasms of parenchymal organs and bone structures are excluded, as are those of lymph nodes, which neoplastic practice has placed in separate categories.

The following discussion is based on personal experience with over 1000 patients treated for various tumors of the soft somatic tissues.

The overall plan of treatment is based on four major considerations: 1) an overall evaluation of the patient, 2) the histology of the neoplasm, 3) the local anatomic setting, and 4) whether the tumor is primary or recurrent.

EVALUATION OF THE PATIENT

Age

The average age of patients suffering malignant neurilemomas with von Recklinghausen's disease is 32 years; without von Recklinghausen's disease it is about 42 years. Patients with other forms of sarcomas usually fit into the same age patterns. For example, those with Kaposi's sarcoma averaged 40 years of age, and those with giant cell tumors of the tendon sheaths also averaged 40 years of age. Synovial sarcomas appeared more often in slightly younger adults, averaging 36 years of age, although they have been seen in every age, from two weeks to 70 years. The rhabdomyosarcomas are seen in patients between 40 and 70 years of age, and patients with sarcomas of undetermined histogenesis averaged 36 years of age. The tremendous age overlap of the patients offers no assistance in evaluating the type of lesion from the standpoint of developing treatment principles.

Sex

Of the 70 patients with tumors of nerve tissues treated by the author, 55 per cent were male and 45 per cent were female. Thus, the difference is not statistically significant. A similar, almost equal distribution was found in other sarcomas; for example, rhabdomyosarcomas occurred in 61 per cent of male patients, and sarcomas of undetermined histogenesis occurred slightly more frequently in female patients (54 per cent). Kaposi's hemorrhagic sarcoma, however, is notorious for occurring in the male, being observed in males in 92 per cent of the cases. Giant cell tumors of the tendon sheaths were observed more often in females (70 per cent). The overall conclusion would be that most

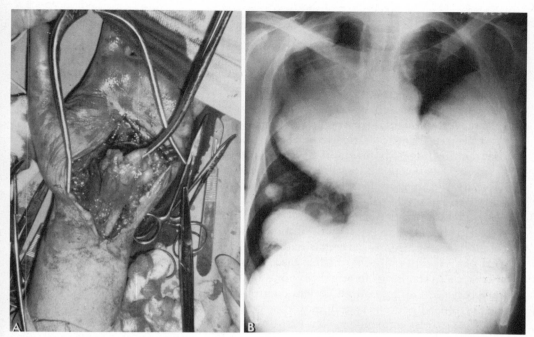

Figure 41-1 *A*, Recurrent malignant neurilemoma of the median nerve in the wrist, treated by wide resection. A recurrence developed associated with pulmonary metastases. *B*, Extensive pulmonary metastases from which the patient expired. Cells left behind when the initial operation was performed were probably the ones which produced the recurrence and the metastases.

tumors of the soft somatic tissues cannot be identified on the basis of sexual predilection except for Kaposi's sarcoma.

It is not wrong to mention here that neither age nor sex should influence the surgeon in deciding treatment policies. Old age should never be a deterrent to major amputation where indicated. The anatomic and physiologic age of the patient is more important than the chronologic age.

As loathsome as it may be to perform a major amputation on a young child or a lovely young girl in her teens, it must be realized that a live cured patient, even minus a limb, is preferable to a dead patient. *One can be most conservative at times by being radical at the onset.*

Etiologic Factors

Nothing is known concerning the formation of these neoplasms in humans, therefore, very little can be said about etiology. Heredity does play a role in certain of these tumors. There are several neurocutaneous syndromes associated with congenital angiomas which are further associated with tumors of nervous tissue origin. These consists of von Recklinghausen's neurofibromatosis and angiomas of the skin, Bourneville's syndrome with tuberous sclerosis, and others. The most severe underlying etiologic factor in tumors of the peripheral nervous system is von Recklinghausen's disease, which will be discussed in further detail.

HISTOLOGY OF NEOPLASM OF SOFT SOMATIC
TISSUES

There are approximately 56 classifications of tumors afflicting the soft somatic tissues, of which 35 are considered benign and 21 malignant. Each of these tumors represents a separate entity with its own natural history, methods of dissemination, and principles of growth, and, accordingly, each demands specific and individual treatment. Included in the overall group are some of the most bizarre forms of cancers that affect the human, and some of the largest, such as the huge lipomas and liposarcomas (a liposarcoma weighing 32 kilograms has been reportedly removed). Some of the smallest and yet most painful neoplasms, the glomus tumors, are included. Some of the growths remain limited to the site of origin, where they grow to huge proportions and practically never metastasize (a dermatofibrosarcoma protuberance). Others have metastasized throughout the body by the time of the initial diagnosis (Kaposi's hemorrhagic sarcoma). Many sarcomas extend imperceptibly along muscular and fascial planes, especially the diffuse fascial fibrosarcomas. The high incidence of metastasis to the lungs in angiosarcomas that are encountered demands pulmonary roentgenograms on all patients with this disease. The fact that tumors of the peripheral nervous system may arise de novo from different nerve segments demands careful neurologic examination and other diagnostic aids to determine whether the entire dermatome may be doomed; hence, local resection of a solitary tumor would be an incomplete treatment. Furthermore, other cancers may extend along the nerve sheath for varying distances producing different signs and symptoms. Accordingly, the surgeon must be familiar with the natural history of each of these lesions; therefore the emphasis of this presentation is on the natural history of the different tumors arising from the peripheral nervous system.

THE LOCAL ANATOMIC SETTING OF THE
NEOPLASM

The local anatomic setting is one of the most important factors in determining the type and extent of resection. After the histology has been determined and the knowledge of the natural history of that particular type of tumor evaluated, the manner in which the tumor exists within its own anatomic setting is an important factor in determining treatment policy. *No sarcoma is encapsulated; hence simple enucleation is never indicated for any malignant tumor of the soft somatic tissue.*

For example, if the neoplasm involves a single muscle, the preferred treatment is excision of the entire muscle from origin to insertion. Wide excision may on occasion be performed, removing a large block of the involved muscle, but this is associated with recurrence in approximately one half of the cases. If major nerves or blood vessels are involved, removal of which would render an extremely frail extremity, an amputation should be performed. On occasion a blood vessel may be excised and a defect repaired with a graft, and even a nerve may be resected with the resultant damages being understood and explained to the patient preoperatively. When the sarcoma involves a joint, with extensive infiltration throughout all the surrounding tissue, nothing short of an amputation can be performed.

TREATMENT POLICY FOR TUMORS OF THE PERIPHERAL NERVOUS SYSTEM. The degree of surgical extirpation is often one of the first things this author evaluates in the initial procedure. If one suspects a malignant tumor, then an initial operation is performed, preferably under general anesthesia, to expose the tumor, a formal biopsy is taken, and an evaluation of the extent of the lesion is made. Previously, our policy was simply to get a report of a malignant tumor from the pathologist. In view of the headway being made in the multimodality treatment of certain sarcomas, with better results for some (such as embryonal rhabdomyosarcomas) when treated by combined surgery, radiation therapy, and chemotherapy, we now prefer to get a formal biopsy and await the results of a paraffin section in order to determine treatment policy. When the exact histologic variety has been diagnosed, and the anatomic setting has been determined, the treatment policy can be planned as to the degree of excision, whether one must resort to an amputation or whether it is possible to avoid this extreme measure.

PRIMARY OR RECURRENT SARCOMAS

Most recurrent sarcomas are more malignant than the ones excised at the primary operation. The anatomic setting is often distorted, and amputations are more frequently indicated for recurrent sarcomas.

Biopsy

Biopsy must be meticulously performed in a setting geared for immediate and proper treatment. Certain tumors which are obviously benign, such as lipomas or benign neuromas, can be locally excised. If the tumor is fungating through the skin, a conventional biopsy may be taken with a biopsy forceps or a scalpel. If the tumor is situated in the depths of the extremity and the skin is intact, an exposure of the tumor is indicated. It must be borne in mind that incisional biopsy can be a dangerous procedure and may often penetrate a dense pseudocapsule, permitting expansive growth of the cancer unless therapy can be instituted with dispatch. Certain sarcomas are extremely vascular, so that intractable hemorrhage may result.

NOSOLOGY OF TUMORS OF THE PERIPHERAL NERVOUS SYSTEM

Most tumors of the peripheral nervous system, surprisingly, do not arise in the nerve elements themselves, but, rather, in the tissues that sheath the nerves (Schwann cells, neurilemma). Previous concepts were that these tumors were of nervous tissue origin, and they were thus labeled neurogenic. Because of the large amounts of fibrous tissue intermingled througout the malignant tumors, the sarcoma suffix was affixed. The term "neurogenic sarcoma" has now been largely abandoned, because it has been demonstrated that the tumors arise from the cells of Schwann, which, although apparently ectodermal in origin, have a propensity for producing connective tissue fibers and other mesodermal structures. Tumors arising from these cells if benign are termed benign neurilemoma, encapsulated or diffuse (plexiform) if malignant, malignant neurilemoma or malignant schwannoma. If the tissue is composed of a combination of nerve tissue and fibrous tissue, it is termed a neurifibroma. Von Recklinghausen's disease consists of multiple neurifibromatoses, representing an error of metabolism with a proclivity toward the formation of neuroectodermal tumors.

THE ANATOMY OF THE NERVES

The peripheral nervous system is that part of the nervous system wherein the neurons and their processes (axons) are encased by Schwann cells. In the central nervous system the axons are sheathed by glial cells. "In most cranial and all spinal nerves, the Schwann cell sheath starts at the site where the nerve is recognizable grossly emerging from the brain or the cord" (Harkin and Reed, 1969). The Schwann cell is defined by Harkin and Reed as: "A neuroectodermal cell which sheaths an axon of the peripheral nervous system, and is surrounded by an extracellular basement membrane. Nonmyelinated axons are encased in a tunnel within Schwann cells, and a number of axons share a common Schwann cell. In myelinated nerves, axons are sheathed by a spiral wrap, formed by the Schwann cell itself, each Schwann cell surrounding only one axon for a longitudinal segment. Other Schwann cells do not intimately encase axons, but form the perineural sheath." It thus becomes obvious that tumors may arise from the nerve elements themselves, and would thus be true neurogenic sarcomas. However, most of the tumors arise from the Schwann cells and are thus termed schwannomas or malignant neurilemomas.

BENIGN NERVE SHEATH TUMORS

Included in this group are solitary, benign, slowly growing, usually encapsulated tumors arising in the nerve and composed of Schwann cells within a framework of collagen, enveloping the peripheral, cranial, and autonomic nerves. Related terms or synonyms, are neurinoma, neurilemoma, schwannoma, encapsulated neurilemoma, perineurial fibroblastoma, and acoustic neuroma.

Inasmuch as acoustic neuromas are the specialty of neurosurgeons or head and neck surgeons they will not be discussed in this chapter. Schwann cells apparently can synthesize collagen, but differ from collagen-producing fibrocytes of mesodermal origin by the presence of a basement membrane (Harkin and Reed, 1969). The histologic studies of Masson and Nageotte and the tissue culture studies of Murray and Stout seem to demonstrate that the neuroectodermal Schwann cells can form reticulin fibers in vitro. Because of the similarity of the reticulin produced by the Schwann cells and the fibrils produced by fibroblasts, the difficulty in separating malignant neurilemomas from ordinary fibrosarcomas by histologic methods is evident. In addition to the neuroectodermal derivatives and fibrous tissues, blood vessels, lymphatics, and fat cells are frequently found in the nerve trunk.

Etiology

No known etiologic factor exists. These benign tumors have been described in every country on earth, and there is no racial predilection for them. They are extremely rare in animals. Certain of these tumors of goldfish were previously described as schwannomas, but on electron microscopy no recognizable Schwann cells appear (Harkin and Reed, 1969).

Clinical Data

These tumors are usually asymptomatic when small, but as they grow, and pressure to the nerve develops, pain will occur, and often paraesthesias may develop. The pain may radiate throughout the entire nerve. Usually on physical examination the tumor can be moved from side to side, but rarely in a longitudinal manner. They are occasionally tender, but this is no distinguishing characteristic. They usually arise from posterior spinal roots and thus produce symptoms which are sensory, but motor symptoms develop when compression of the spinal cord or anterior nerve roots occurs. On inspection, the tumor will be found growing out of the nerve, especially in peripheral lesions. They are usually thick walled, and large vessels may be seen within the tumor. In retroperitoneal and thoracic schwannomas, the nerve of origin often can not be identified. The solitary, benign, encapsulated neurilemomas occur most commonly in the neck, the mediastinum, and the flexor surface of the extremities. They are found frequently in patients with von Recklinghausen's disease, and often in normal people. They are encapsulated, solid or cystic, slow growing, and rarely recur after complete surgical excision. It is fundamental to know that these tumors grow by expansion in such a manner that they push the nerve of origin aside or expand it. The literature reports very few authentic examples of locally infiltrating or recurrent types of benign encapsulated neurilemomas.

A variant of benign neurilemoma is reported by de Santo (1940), who described a primary benign, encapsulated neurilemoma arising in the midshaft of the ulna which was cured by resection of the bone, and in another case arising from the fifth lumbar nerve and locally invading the right sacral wing and ligamentum flavum. In the benign encapsulated neurilemoma, wide local excision is necessary. In the author's experience of 50 benign encapsulated neurilemomas, not one malignant neurilemoma was encountered.

Treatment

If the tumor arises from the surface of the major nerve trunk, the encapsulated tumor is readily separated from the nerve with little or no disability resulting, as there are no funiculi in the tumor. They are splayed in the tumor capsule, where they have been displaced by the expanding tumor. When the tumor originates in a large trunk, such as the sciatic, the functional fibers of the nerve are expanded around the neoplasm. Dissection or separation of the fibers parallel to the nerve and meticulous dissection make it possible to remove the encapsulated neoplasm intact. Sacrifice of the nerve is not necessary. As benign encapsulated neurilemomas may occur along any somatic or sympathetic nerve, procedures for their extirpation are the same as described above. They may occur in the neck and the spine as a so-called hourglass tumor, where a combination of peripheral resection plus the neurosurgical attack on the spinal portion of the tumor is necessary. They occur in the cerebellopontine angle and also arise from the acoustic nerve.

A variant is the so-called cellular schwannoma, in which nuclear atypism and hypercellularity exist. Ackerman introduced this term under the broader term of "ancient schwannoma"; that is, schwannomas that show extensive hyalinization with loosely arranged cells in a dense fibrous matrix. The overall prognosis for these variants is the same as that for the usual schwannomas.

Solitary Neurofibroma

These tumors are benign, circumscribed, nonencapsulated lesions, arising in a nerve, and composed principally of Schwann cells. The intercellular matrix of the solitary neurofibroma contains collagen fibrils and a myxomatous extracellular component. There may be a variation in the proportion of tissue fibrils and matrix. Because of the intermingling of the two cell types, they are called neurofibromas. Although this tumor is the one most frequently seen in generalized neurofibromatoses, local lesions have been described in patients without a generalized disorder. Treatment is by simple surgical excision, and the prognosis is extremely good. When encountered, however, a careful examination for von Recklinghausen's neurofibromatosis should be made.

Multiple Neurofibromatoses (von Recklinghausen's Disease)

Definition

Neurofibromatosis is a developmental diathesis of the neuroectodermal system with a strong tendency toward neoplastic proliferation (neurofibromas). The condition is most frequently inherited. It may manifest itself in a variety of ways, from a simple tendency to epidermal pigmentation to a generalized widespread pathologic involvement of many portions of the nervous system (both central and peripheral). Other ectodermal structures (such as the skin), various mesodermal structures (e.g., bones and connective tissue), and even certain endodermal structures (e.g., certain portions of the intestine and appendix) may be involved. With the exception of a terratoid tumor, which consists of a localized abnormal growth involving the three germ layers, there is no other disease process by which the human organism can be afflicted that produces abnormalities of the tissue derivatives of the three germ layers than does neurofibromatosis, so-called von Recklinghausen's disease. Von Recklinghausen first described the entity in 1882. Associated pathologic involvement of neurofibromatosis, in addition to the classic stigmata mentioned below, are certain neoplasms of the

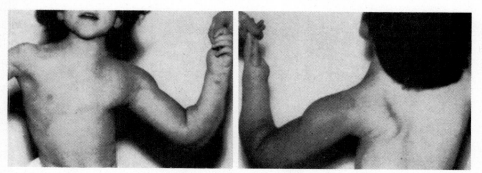

Figure 41-2 Diffuse Neurilemomatosis in a young girl. Note gigantism of arm, a result of both the plexiform neurilemomas and overgrowth of bone.

central nervous system, such as meningiomas, acoustic neuromas, and optic nerve gliomas. The classic stigmata involve other entities, such as tuberous sclerosis, Lindau–von Hippel disease, Sturge–Weber syndrome, mental retardation from unknown pathology, abnormal non-neoplastic hypertrophy of the skin and bones, hirsutism, mesodermal tumors (lipomas, fibromas, and others), and congenital malformations, such as hypospadias, spina bifida, cerebral meningocele, and congenital defects of the fingers and toes. These may all be expressions of the broad nosologic developmental defect designated by the term "von Recklinghausen's disease."

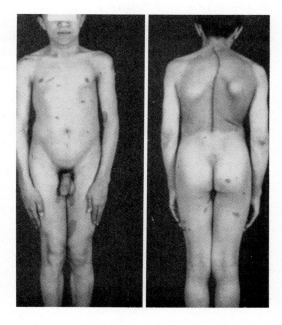

Figure 41-3 A patient with generalized neurofibromatosis showing bone deformities and café au lait spots.

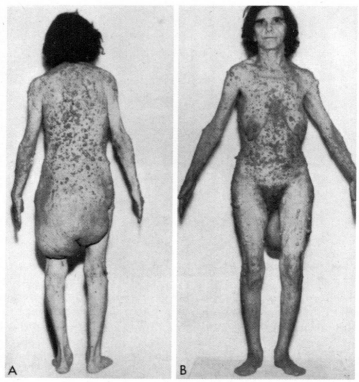

Figure 41–4 Von Recklinghausen's disease. An advanced stage of neurofibromatosis with elephantiasis nervosum.

Incidence: Genetic Features

It has been estimated that neurofibromatosis occurs in about 0.05 per cent of the population. It has been reported in all races, as well as in some animals, and it has been shown that about half of the offspring of a parent with neurofibromatosis will present certain stigmata.

Thirty families with von Recklinghausen's disease demonstrated some evidence of multiple neurofibromatosis in 43.5 per cent of the offspring. According to mendelian laws, this would accord von Recklinghausen's disease a dominant genetic characteristic. The offspring may present the same type and location of lesions as do the parents.

Neurofibromatosis

Neurofibromatosis consists of multiple nerve sheath tumors which may either be schwannomas or neurofibromas, and in some of these (plexiform) malignant transformation takes place producing malignant neurilemomas. The majority may be so mild as to go unrecognized, and those with a simple, single lesion are referred to formes frustes. Harkin and Reed (1969) consider that any

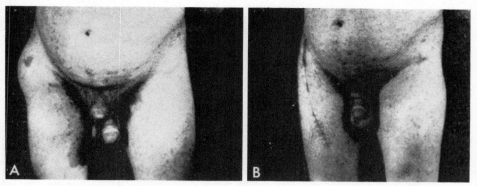

Figure 41-5 Multiple malignant neurilemomas in a patient with neurofibromatosis. *A*, Malignant neurilemomas of the right upper thigh. *B*, The patient two months after surgical excisions. He has now been cured of the neurilemoma for over 20 years. Previously, a malignant neurilemoma of the right upper arm had been excised. The patient has remained well for 26 years.

patient who has a plexiform neurofibroma also has neurofibromatosis, even if it is the only manifestation of the disease. The age of onset is variable, and the disease may not present its full characteristics until adulthood. There has been described an accentuation of disease with pregnancy, suggesting an endocrine relationship. The course of neurofibromatosis is often one of dynamic progression, sometimes infuenced by heredity, physiologic stresses (manifested in adolescence by growth), and the probable unknown specific factors engendered by puberty, pregnancy, and menopause. Any one patient may present with lesions of complex morphology, the individual variations of which are unlimited. The variability in location of neurofibromas or benign plexiform neurilemomas of the skin associated with café au lait spots, and the elephantoid derangements and tortuous conglomerate masses occurring in the deeper nerves, both somatic and sympathetic, are well known. The osseous changes associated with elephantiasis neuromatosa and the isolated subperiosteal cyst present rather interesting phenomena in this disease.

Treatment

Patients with the classic, generalized form of the disease have little to gain from operative treatment, but they should be kept under observation to note excessive growth of certain tumors or other complicating features that may be amenable to surgical intervention. Pregnancy may provoke dramatic changes. Whereas before pregnancy the patient may exhibit only the abortive type of disease, with pregnancy many new lesions may appear, and those already present may increase markedly in size. Succeeding pregnancies will bring about a similar response. Sterilization may be considered when progression of disease causes serious changes.

Complications of the generalized type of disease that call for surgical intervention are: (1) increased size of the tumor that causes pain or interference with activity; (2) cosmetic disfigurements; (3) hemorrhage into or infection of the large pachydermatocele; and (4) rapid progression in size with the danger of

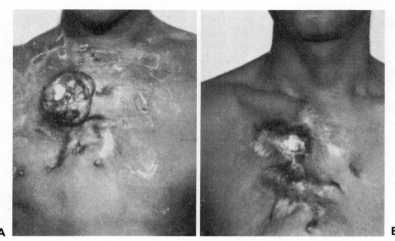

A   **B**

Figure 41–6 *A*, Malignant neurilemoma of the chest wall treated by surgical excision and irradiation. *B*, Appearance 11 years later. This patient is living and well 25 years after treatment.

transformation to malignant neurilemoma. When the disease appears in its abortive type, complete eradication of the presenting lesion is possible by surgical treatment. Many large or isolated plexiform masses will appear to be infiltrated because of their tendency toward diffuse distribution. Surgical removal of small tumors for microscopic study or cosmetic effect has not been followed by increased growth phenomena. Whenever conglomerate, irregular masses of plexiform neurilemomas within the subcutaneous tissue require extirpation, they can be readily dissected, and no nerve repair is necessary; however, when similar masses occur in which the involvement of major nerve trunks would necessitate their sacrifice and repair by nerve suture, the surgical procedure should not involve sacrifice of these nerves unless an accurate diagnosis of malignant change is obtained. Whenever the overlying skin is pigmented or takes the form of pachydermatocele, portions of it must be excised along with the underlying neuromatous process to obtain a good cosmetic result. *In principle, therefore, no major nerve trunk should be sacrificed in the treatment of benign plexiform neurilemomas of von Recklinghausen's disease.* Occasionally, owing to pressure necrosis of the skin over a saculated plexiform neurilemoma, infection of a gelatinous-appearing tumor tissue content will result. With infection, the mass will continue to discharge necrotic material, and the chronic inflammatory process can be eradicated only by radical resection of the mass after suitable preparation with antibiotics.

It has been estimated that approximately 10 per cent of plexiform neurilemomas in von Recklinghausen's disease will undergo malignant transformation. Patients should be watched, for any massive growth so that these may be eradicated. It has been the author's policy to observe patients with plexiform neurofibromas as part of von Recklinghausen's syndrome, and not to treat them unless specific indications develop. At times the tumors may grow to huge dimensions, and major amputation may be necessary as a palliative procedure. This should not be done with any patient unless there are clinical indications. The results of our treatment of malignant neurilemomas as part of the von Recklinghausen's disease syndrome are presented later in this chapter.

Other Neuromatous Syndromes

Multiple Mucosal Neuromas

A syndrome recently described (and similar to von Recklinghausen's disease) under the heading of multiple mucosal neuromas, contained lesions that have been classified in the past as true neuromas. Harkin and Reed (1969) state that, in contrast to neurofibromatosis, the lesions in this syndrome are true neuromas that resemble traumatic neuromas rather than neurofibromas. The syndrome is considered familial and has been associated with carcinoma of the thyroid gland, usually of the medullary or amyloid producing type. Pheochromocytomas have occurred in association with medullary tumors of the thyroid, and have also occurred in a multiple mucosal neuroma syndrome. These are probably manifestations of the APUD syndrome.

Neurocutaneous Melanosis Syndrome

This disorder, which is not familial, presents giant pigmented nevi of the skin and melanosis of the meninges. Malignant tumors develop in either the skin or the central nervous system that are either melanomas and neurilemomas, tend to be very extensive and tend to be localized over the posterior surface of the tunk, and usually are multiple. Histologically, the benign cutaneous lesions are either typical blue nevi of Jadasshan, cellular nevi, or neurofibromas.

The malignant tumors that develop in the skin often show a typical melanoma, but some have been reported which resemble a malignant schwannoma in certain parts, and in others there are distributed throughout the specimen immature ganglion cells. Not enough is known about these entities to warrant any discussion regarding clinical treatment of such patients, but they do demonstrate the close relationship between the various histologic types of oncologic expression.

Malignant Tumors of Peripheral Nerves

Malignant tumors of the peripheral nervous system are, as mentioned before, tumors that arise from cells of Schwann. Various terms have been applied to these neoplasms; malignant neurilemoma, malignant schwannoma, malignant nerve sheath tumor, perineural fibrosarcoma, neurogenic sarcoma, neurofibrosarcoma, fibromyxosarcoma of nerve, fibrosarcoma, myxomatodes, fibrosarcoma of nerve sheath, malignant peripheral glioma, myosarcoma of nerve sheath, neurilemosarcoma, sarcoma of peripheral nerves, and secondary malignant neuroma. The definitions of these tumors follow.

A malignant Schwannoma is a malignant neoplasm of nerve sheath origin that infiltrates locally and widely, and metastasizes. It contains an intercellular component which may be either collagenous or mucinous. They may develop in an apparently normal nerve or in a neurofibroma. The cell of origin is considered to be the Schwann cell. They may occur in isolated instances in patients without von Recklinghausen's disease, or in patients with the forme-fruste state of von Recklinghausen's disease. They occur in approximately 10 per cent of patients with von Recklinghausen's disease. It is essential that the pathologist make a complete distinction between a benign solitary or plexiform benign neurilemoma and a malignant schwannoma. Several authoritative pathologists in the field of soft tissue sarcomas have advised that the term neurilemoma be used for benign tumors of nerve sheath origin and the term malignant schwannoma be used for malignant tumors. However, in view of the fact that various terminologies are utilized, it is necessary that the surgeon be familiar with the description his pathologist offers.

The various components that exist within these tumors are responsible for the bizarre and different classifications. The reason for these different components is unknown. We have called attention previously to the fact that various sarcomas can develop different features depending upon their particular environment, and have presented a patient who had a wide resection of a chondosarcoma. When a recurrence developed years later in the shoulder region, it presented the features of fibrosarcoma, for which an interscapular thoracic amputation was done. We hypothesized that the change in environment caused the basic mesodermal cell to undergo change in cell type. It may be recalled that the matrix of a chondrosarcoma, which is cartilaginous in nature contains chondroitin sulphuric acid, whereas the matrix of fibrosarcoma is devoid of chondroitin sulphuric acid. Accordingly, the various manifestations of these nerve sheath tumors possibly represent different expressions of one underlying cell type. Although the cells of Schwann are considered ectodermal in origin, there are many mesodermal potentialities within the nerve sheath that may enter into the formation of the tumorous entity.

Harkin and Reed (1969) have divided the malignant tumors of the peripheral nervous system into the following categories:
1. Nerve sheath tumors
   a. Malignant schwannomas
   b. Malignant epithelioid schwannomas.
   c. Malignant melanocytic schwannomas
   d. Nerve sheath fibrosarcoma and malignant mesenchymoma of nerve sheath origin
2. Neurectodermal tumors of primitive type and with nerve cell differentiation

They further state: "Included in Group 'a' are those neoplasms arising in plexiform neurofibromas that show local infiltration but little propensity for metastasis. Groups 'b' and 'd' are usually highly malignant. Behavior of tumors in group 'c' is not known due to lack of followup and their rare occurrence. Tumors in groups 'a' and 'd' often overlap histologically. An assignment of a given tumor to one or the other category is therefore arbitrary. Rarely, the pattern seen in tumors in group 'b' is found as a regional variation in tumors in groups 'a' and 'd'."

The clinical diagnosis of benign and malignant nerve tumors may not be possible before actual operative exposure. In patients with von Recklinghausen's disease, the recent, more rapid growth of a small mass which may have begun to cause pain or inconvenience should be suspected of being malignant. A nerve will withstand much abuse by stretching or pressure from a benign tumor, but infiltration by malignant cells may soon destroy some degree of function of a peripheral nerve.

When neurologic signs are present, they may offer a clue that a given tumor may arise in a peripheral nerve, but the fact that a nerve is incorporated in a tumor mass is not sufficient proof that the tumor arose from that nerve. Sarcomas may surround and destroy major nerves. The final diagnosis of malignant nerve tumor then depends on gross anatomical–pathologic dissection plus the careful interpretation of tissue sections. When there is a possibility of resection of a major nerve trunk, or amputation, biopsy alone is the indicated procedure, and definitive therapy is deferred until permanent microscopic sections have been confirmed by authoritative pathologists.

In order to plan adequate treatment, certain pathologic characteristics of malignant neurilemomas must be stressed. In the solitary form, the growth may remain encapsulated or confined within the nerve sheath, expanding it, or forming a round or fusiform mass whose shape is determined by the denseness of the surrounding tissue in which the nerve tissue is expanding. These solitary tumors may reach large proportions without showing any noticeable gross infiltration of surrounding tissues, and they tend to grow along the nerve trunk more than into the tumor bed. However, at the points where the "capsule" adheres to the muscle fascia or vessels, viable tumor cells are present. These tumors thus grow by continuity along the nerve trunk and also by embolization along the lymphatics coursing with the nerve well beyond the fusiform swelling produced where the tumor appears to be limited. Nodular swelling along the nerve of origin or its branch are common. Satellite nodules of malignant neurilemomas may be interspersed with fusiform enlargements of contiguous nerves that on microscopic section will depict only benign plexiform neurilemomas. Thus, the various

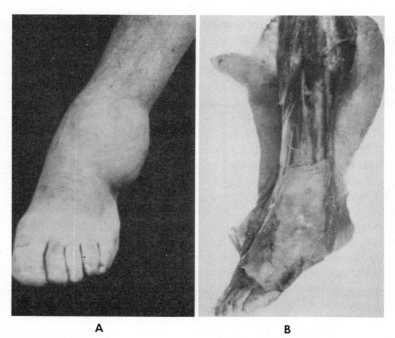

A **B**

Figure 41-7 *A,* Diffuse malignant neurilemoma of the lower leg. *B,* Dissection specimen after amputation demonstrating the intimate attachment of the neoplasm to all the contiguous structures.

nodules noted proximal or distal to the main mass acutally demonstrate a multicentricity of origin for some of the malignant neurilemomas. These growth characteristics are especially evident in those malignant neurilemomas associated with von Recklinghausen's disease. Thus, the multicentricity of origin, growth by continuity along the nerve, tumor embolization along the lymphatics, and seeding of the operative area with neoplastic cells may all be factors concerned in the local persistence or recurrence after attempted resection.

Recurrences of the tumor due to inadequate removal are, in the main, more anaplastic than the original neoplasm, thus setting the stage for fatal blood-borne metastases. Furthermore, the malignant neurilemomas that arise in major nerve trunk plexuses are clinically more malignant.

Treatment

Successful treatment of malignant tumors of peripheral nerves demands radical surgery at the earliest opportunity. In our experience, the various subvarieties often designated by the pathologist have not influenced the course of therapy. Once the diagnosis of malignant tumor of nerve sheath origin has been established, it behooves the surgeon to treat the lesion by radical surgery at the earliest opportunity. These tumors must be treated by either radical local resection or amputation. Each case must be considered on an individual basis. The type of therapy must be determined whether the procedure is for extirpation of a primary neoplasm or for a recurrence, and whether the tumor is high or low grade malignancy when a primary radical local excision cannot adequately eradicate the local disease. By "radical local excision" is meant that the tumor plus its bed and any attached nerve, bone, muscle, or blood vessels must be extirpated en bloc. Thus, any "shelling" out of the neoplasm can only lead to local recurrence. Of necessity, the resulting operative defect must be through normal tissue on all surfaces. The nerve of origin must be dissected proximally and distally from the tumor. Frozen section at the time of excision is helpful, to be certain that the line of nerve sections is outside the area of intraneural spread of the neoplasm. If radical local excision cannot be performed adequately, an amputation must be carried out.

When, at surgical exploration, it is noted that in addition to the original tumor mass there are nodular enlargements or tortuosity and thickness of branches of the involved nerve trunk or adjacent nerve trunks — even though a biopsy reveals only a plexiform neurilemoma in these satellite foci — it is a safer procedure to radically sacrifice the limb by amputation at the highest level, by interscapular–thoracic amputation or conservative hemipelvectomy. There have been instances when we have performed wide radical excisions or minor amputations only to have some of the above-described fusiform nodules undergo malignant changes and present themselves with malignant neurilemomas. When a malignant neurilemoma occurs in an extremity whose nerves are the site of multiple plexiform neurilemomas, although the malignant tumor may be removed by radical dissection the other nerves in the area have a tendency toward the same type of malignant transformation. This observation is especially noteworthy in the malignant neurilemomas that appear on the bases of multiple neurofibromatoses of von

Recklinghausen. Thus, one must deal in these instances not with local recurrence but with multicentricity of origin in condemned segments of nerve tissue that may give rise to various histologic grades of malignant neurilemoma. This important pathologic concept makes the most radical type of local excision or amputation mandatory.

One exception is in the treatment of the smaller group of malignant nerve tumors classified as Grade 1 malignant neurofibromas or neurilemomas. These grossly resemble the benign encapsulated neurilemoma, but are not completely encapsulated. Histologically, there may be typical areas of palisading of nuclei, the Antoni type A architecture, but for the most part the neoplasm is made up of the tissue of the reticulated structure designated as Antoni Type B. An occasional large hyperchromatic nucleus will be seen interspersed with this particular pattern. This observation is often the earliest recognized manifestation of malignant neurilemoma. These changes have been noted, for the most part, in the plexiform neurilemoma.

Local excision of this rare group need not be as radical, but the nerve of origin must be excised. It may also be possible to adequately excise the neoplasm and restore continuity to the nerve of origin by nerve suture. From a practical standpoint, however, this fortuitous circumstance is not often encountered.

In isolated instances, in order to radically excise a malignant nerve tumor through normal tissue on all sides, the main blood vessels to an extremity may of necessity be sacrificed. Repair of the vascular structures by vein graft has avoided amputation in these instances.

If a wide local resection can be accomplished with sacrifice of the nerve, this should be done. Cases have been recorded of resection of malignant neurilemomas of the sciatic nerve, with the foot and lower extremity being placed in a brace, after which a triple arthrodesis permitted satisfactory function for the patient.

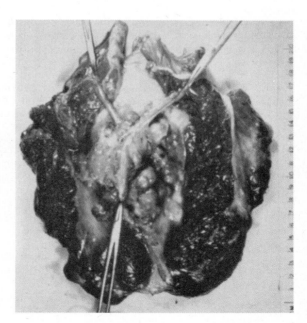

Figure 41-8 Malignant neurilemoma of the right radial nerve. This patient was treated by wide local resection encompassing a satisfactory margin of normal soft tissue about the tumor. The patient remained alive and well 20 years after this resection.

Repair of Sacrificed Nerves

When the nerve has been sacrificed and can be repaired by end-to-end suture, there must be no rotation of the cut ends when the approximation is effected. Sling sutures of any material that pierces the entire nerve trunk are traumatic, increase intraneural fibrosis, and should not be used.

Nerve grafts have been used with success. Homografts are uniformly unsuccessful, although autogenous nerve grafts have been used successfully.

Radiation Therapy

Peripheral nerve tumors, both benign and malignant, are notoriously radioresistant. Occasionally, however, the size can be diminished with radiation therapy. The shrinkage may be the result of either the effect on the tumor itself or, more plausibly, the effect of the therapy on the anatomic structures of the tumor bed. In some cases treated by radical local resection, we have administered postoperative radiation therapy with the idea of preventing local recurrence. But nothing from a curative standpoint can be said regarding these results.

Our observation in treating a large number of patients with radiation therapy would indicate that this does not destroy the tendency of a new tumor to develop, or prevent the recurrence of an original tumor if cells have been left behind. We know of no malignant neurilemomas that have been cured by radiation therapy. Its use for palliation can be great, as evidenced by the following case reports.

CASE I

MALIGNANT NEURILEMOMA OF PELVIS RENDERED OPERABLE BY RADIATION THERAPY
W.W. is a 27-year-old machinist who had a left nephrectomy performed in 1954, on his third birthday, for a Wilms' tumor of the kidney, followed by x-ray treatments. In 1970, an osteochondroma of the thoracic spine was removed. In 1975, because of lower abdominal pain, he was admitted to a local hospital where a mass the size of a golf ball was found in the pelvis and removed through a posterior incision. It was diagnosed as a benign neuroma. This was a presacral lesion. A recurrent mass appeared about one year later. Following a wide sacral excision the mass was found to infiltrate into the abdomen. At this time, an abdominal incision was performed, and a tumor was removed from the left prostatic region. This was diagnosed as a malignant neurilemoma. The mass recurred and gradually filled the entire pelvis. When first seen by me on January 18, 1977, the tumor was found fixed to the pelvis, and, accordingly, it was decided to give the patient a course of radiation therapy. He received approximately 3000 rads to the pelvis over a period of six weeks. On May 19, 1977, a pelvic exenteration was performed. The liver was free of tumor and there was no tumor involving the upper abdomen. The cancer was found to invade the entire pelvis, adhering to the left iliac bone and involving the prostate, the bladder, the rectum, and a loop of small bowel. These were all removed, and a Bricker type of ileoconduit was performed. The tumor was dissected off the iliac and pubic bone, to which it was intimately attached. The final diagnosis at this time was neurofibrosarcoma of the pelvis invading rectal tissue, left periseminal fascicular tissue, striated muscle, and fat. Post-radiation therapy fibrosis was noted. The tumor had shown increased anaplasia since 1975.

The patient had postoperative infection which was drained; numerous sinuses later developed throughout the entire pelvis, demonstrating residual cancer throughout. He died from local sepsis six months later.

Comment. This case represents an instance of what was originally diagnosed as a benign ganglioma of the presacral region undergoing progressive anaplasia into a malignant neurilemoma which invaded the entire pelvis, necessitating a palliative pelvic exenteration. Although neurilemomas are notoriously radioresistant, it is believed that radiation therapy here had the beneficial effect of making an inoperable cancer operable from a gross standpoint.

Case II

MALIGNANT NEURILEMOMA OF LOWER LEG WITH METASTASES TO CHEST WALL

M.A.P. is a 45-year-old female who had a malignant neurilemoma involving the lower leg. She was treated in 1976 by a mid-thigh amputation, which she tolerated well, but recovery was slow. About one year later she developed a large, hard mass involving most of the lateral aspect of the left chest. Accordingly, a resection of the eighth and ninth ribs and the chest wall including the underlying pleura was performed, which revealed metastatic malignant neurilemoma. Three months later she developed severe pain involving the stump, and x rays revealed an osteoblastic lesion and a gallium scan demonstrated increased pickup at the head of the femur. In view of the fact that this represented metastases, she was treated by cobalt irradiation with complete relief of all bone pain. She was then treated systemically with chemotherapy utilizing combined actinomycin D and Alkeran, following which she received a modified Maxfield course of therapy consisting of large doses of testosterone plus fractionated radioactive phosphorus given intravenously for a total dose of 8.5 millicuries. She tolerated this therapy well and at the time of this writing, she is asymptomatic.

Comment. A malignant neurilemoma of the lower extremity treated by a mid-thigh amputation resulted in bizarre metastases involving the left chest wall which were treated surgically. Subsequently, metastases developed at the head of the femur which were treated with radiation therapy, producing remarkable relief of excruciating pain in that area. This demonstrates the value of radiation therapy in such instances. Incidentally, she also received postoperative radiation to the chest wall following surgical resection. One cannot state the effects of the combined ^{32}P and testosterone, which has been shown to be beneficial for metastatic cancer to the bone, particularly of the prostate, and also of the breast. The patient is currently well but, of course, she has an extremely guarded prognosis.

Case III

MALIGNANT NEURILEMOMA OF RIGHT HAND

A.M., a 50-year-old male, presented with a history of having received an injury while working; a swelling that developed was removed and a diagnosis of benign neurilemoma was made. It recurred six months later, was operated upon, and a diagnosis of malignant neurilemoma was made. An additional recurrence took place 18 months later, and a wide excision was performed, sacrificing the median nerve, which left surprisingly good function. Postoperative examination revealed complete anesthesia in the entire left median nerve distribution of the left hand. This included numbness of the thumb, index and middle fingers, and part of the ring finger. Motor function was fairly good, in that he was able to flex the involved fingers. There was no noticeable atrophy of the thenar eminence.

The patient remained well for 13 months, when another recurrence took place for which a local resection was done. An axillary lymph node was also removed and was reported to be hyperplastic adenopathy. Thirteen months later, another recurrence developed; this required resection and removal of a carpal bone. The patient was given chemotherapy in a combination of adriamycin, methotrexate, and Alkeran. He was continued on this regimen postoperatively on an outpatient basis.

One year later, there was metastasis to his lung for which he received a course of chemotherapy. There was a large recurrence of the neurilemoma of his left hand, but, because of the metastasis to the lung, an amputation was considered unjustified. Accordingly, he was given radiation therapy (3000 rads at mid-plane in three weeks), with tremendous relief of all symptoms and a marked reduction in the degree of swelling. Although he was continued on a course of Cosmegen and actinomycin D, the lung metastasis continued to increase in extent. The metastasis to the lung was a contraindication to radical amputation, which would be done only for palliation, and this was not indicated at the time. The patient died in respiratory failure four years after the initial surgery.

Comment. This case demonstrates: (1) the apparent benignity of the neurilemoma at its first onset; (2) that wide local excision was unsuccessful; (3) that metastases to the lung were extensive and resistant to any form of therapy; (4) that chemotherapy had an uncertain effect; but that (5) there was an almost dramatic, although transient, effect from the radiation therapy to the hand recurrence.

Other Treatment Methods

We have used various chemotherapeutic agents both systemically and interarterially in the form of infusion, with questionable results. Continued exploration of cancer chemotherapy and immunologic therapy is greatly needed for this form of tumor. Efforts to treat some of these tumors by isolation infusion plus heating of the injected material to high temperatures have met with practically no success.

Results of Treatment

Seventy patients suffering malignant tumors of the nerve sheath were treated at the Pack Medical Group between 1940 and 1970. A review of these patients indicates certain principles of surgery that must be followed in order to effect favorable results. Of the 70 patients, 25 were considered indeterminable, the reason being that eight died from other causes without evidence of recurrence, nine were lost to followup without evidence of recurrence, and eight have been followed for less than a five-year span. There were, accordingly, 45 patients who

Table 41–1   Five-Year End Results of Treating 70 Patients with Malignant Neurilemoma

Total number of patients			70
Indeterminable group		25	
Died from other causes without evidence of recurrence	8		
Lost track of without recurrence	9		
Patients followed for less than 5 years	8		
Determinable group		45	
(Total number minus those of the indeterminable group)			
Failures		25	
Died of tumor	17		
Lost tract of with recurrence and presumed dead	5		
Living with recurrence and/or metastases	3		
Successful results		20	
Free of cancer 5 years or longer	20		
Net 5-Year End Results			
Successful results divided by determinate group			44%

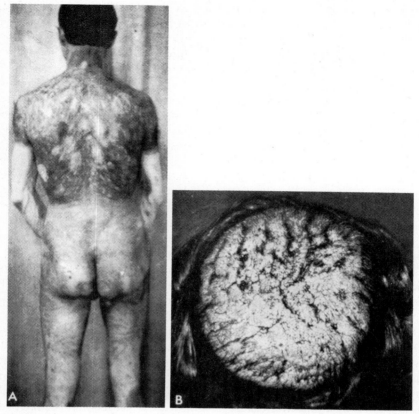

Figure 41–9 Malignant melanoma associated with von Recklinghausen's neurifibromatosis. *A,* Bathing trunk nevus in which a melanoma developed which metastasized to the axillary nodes and brain. Note the numerous cutaneous fibromas scattered throughout. *B,* Turban's tumor (bulldog scalp). A malignant melanoma developed in this lesion and metastasized to the cervical lymph nodes. Both patients died of the metastatic malignant melanoma.

composed the determinable group. Of these, 25 are considered failures. Seventeen died from the cancer, five with recurrences were lost to followup and are presumed dead, and although three are living with recurrences and/or metastases, a successful result is not anticipated. Twenty patients survived five years or longer after treatment. The five-year end result, which equals the successful result divided by the determinable group, is thus 44 per cent. An examination of the histories of all the patients to note if any indices could be obtained regarding the causes for failure revealed that 30 of the 70 were treated surgically before being referred here for therapy. Surgical exploration of the site of the cancer had been performed, and some had had repeated resections for recurrences. One patient had had three such excisions. Of these patients, 20 had had a previous "wide excision and 18 revealed evidence of cancer on re-exploration, or had clinical evidence of recurrence. In only two patients was the resection adequate, and those patients were followed by us. Ten patients were treated by radiation therapy, in some instances before a diagnosis had been adequately established. Of these 10, four demonstrated evidence of shrinkage of tumor size from the radiation therapy, which was given most frequently by orthovoltage techniques. No person was cured by radiation, but recurrences appear to have been slowed by the therapy inasmuch as they did not appear in some patients from six months to 15 months after the irradiation. One patient, an orthodontist, had a huge sarcoma intimately bound to the sciatic nerve that was diagnosed histologically as a synovial sarcoma, but its intermingling with the nerve tissue was so intimate that dissection could not be performed, and it was believed that it represented a mesodermal modification of the tumors involving the nerve sheath. A hemipelvectomy was suggested, but the patient refused it. He was then treated by an energetic radiotherapist, receiving 9000 rads to the tumor site over a period of six weeks. The radiation therapy caused severe clinical symptoms to the rectum and excruciating pain to the site of the tumor, for which the patient begged for a hemipelvectomy. This was performed through heavily irradiated tissue and was the only instance in over 125 hemipelvectomies performed at the Pack Medical Group when a prolapse occurred. Examination of the tumor after the 9000 rads revealed no histologic effect from the irradiation upon this particular tumor.

These examples of failure after local resection illustrate two factors: 1) Preoperative irradiation does not usually make certain tumors resectable. Postoperative irradiation cannot produce a cure and is not a substitute for adequate surgery. Nevertheless, several impressive examples of the effects of irradiation have been observed. 2) Tumors in nerves proximal to the site of excision became manifest, or spread of the tumor along the nerve trunk or nerve lymphatics occurred. One such patient was treated first by a wide resection of the malignant neurilemoma of the forearm, followed by an amputation of the forearm for recurrences, after which another neurilemoma occurred just above the elbow. This was treated by a mid-humeral resection; for the subsequent recurrence she received an interscapulothoracic amputation. She, nevertheless, developed an interspinal lesion and expired one year after the amputation. This case demonstrates the proclivity of certain nerves to form tumors.

The two major sites for the failures from wide local excision occurred in the hands and the feet where the excisions were not adequate enough because the anatomic structure surrounding the tumor limited the degree of resection. In two patients with malignant neurilemoma of the arm, new tumors kept forming proximally, necessitating more proximal resections until tumors appeared as the nerves emerged from the spinal cord in the cervical region. Wide excision was the only procedure available for the cervical neoplasms.

Eleven of 20 amputations were performed after a recurrence had occurred following a wide local resection. Of this group, five failed. Two patients lived less than five years after the amputation. Six patients survived five years or longer, but died of pulmonary metastases. Nine patients of the series survived five years or longer and are apparently cured. Of the 50 patients who were treated by wide local resection, 14 are alive and well five years or longer, and 36 have died. Twelve patients were inoperable when first seen, thus treatment was palliative, consisting of either radiation therapy, local excision of a painful or ulcerated lesion, or amputation. Five patients had palliative amputations performed at their insistence.

A previous report from this clinic demonstrated that the classification of the tumor grading utilizing Broder's classifications of Grades 1, 2, 3, and 4 evidenced

Table 41–2 Relationship of Neurofibromatosis to End Results in Malignant Neurilemoma 5-Year Followup

Number of patients with neurofibromatosis	30	100%
Number dying	16	53%
Number living	14	47%
Number of patients without neurofibromatosis	40	100%
Number dying	24	60%
Number living	16	40%

that the more anaplastic the lesion, the more likely a poor prognosis. Two patients were classified as Grade 1, Broder's classification, and each of these later developed pulmonary metastases and died. Thus, a low grade on Broder's scale is no assurance of a favorable prognosis.

The relationship of neurofibromatosis to malignant neurilemoma is summarized in Table 41–2. Many authors believe that patients with malignant neurilemoma occurring with von Recklinghausen's neurofibromatoses are infrequently cured. Our data do not agree with this statement. Thirty patients presented evidence of generalized neurofibromatoses, and 40 either did not have neurofibromatosis or had it in an undetectable manner and are to be considered

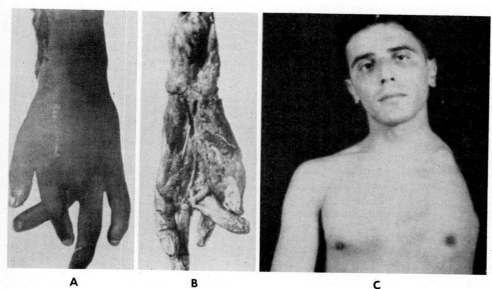

A　　　　　　**B**　　　　　　　　**C**

Figure 41–10 A malignant neurilemoma of the hand treated by interscapulothoracic amputation. *A*, Amputated specimen showing the malignant neurilemoma. Note the congenital deformed middle finger. *B*, Dissected specimen demonstrating the extent of the malignant neurilemoma and congenital deformity. *C*, Postoperative photograph subject to interscapulothoracic amputation which was necessitated by repeated proximal recurrences, the last of which was in the base of the neck. The patient was living and well 25 years after the last operation. He was then lost to follow-up. This patient had been treated first by local resection, followed by an amputation at the level of the forearm. He developed a recurrence about a year later necessitating a mid-humeral amputation. A more proximal recurrence occurred, which necessitated the interscapulothoracic amputation. His last recurrence was a mass in the neck which was excised. This case demonstrates a nerve plexus doomed to the formation of multicentric malignant neurilemomas.

free of generalized neurofibromatoses in this presentation. The explanation for the better result in patients with generalized fibromatoses may be that these patients are under more careful clinical surveillance and hence are treated sooner, as soon as tumors increase in size or produce any disability.

SUMMARY AND CONCLUSIONS

1. Most tumors (benign and malignant) do not arise from the nerves per se but arise from the supporting cells, the cells of Schwann or neurilemma, and are termed schwannoma or neurilemoma, benign or malignant.
2. Surgical extirpation is the only way to treat these neoplasms. Radiation therapy can offer significant palliation and prolongation of life but no cures have been observed. Other forms of therapy, such as chemotherapy, and immunotherapy, have little to offer at this time.
3. Benign tumors can be treated by local surgical extirpation; malignant tumors must be radically resected, including major amputation.
4. Certain dermatomes have a proclivity to produce tumors, and new growths (benign and malignant) proximal to the one clinically manifest can be expected in certain patients.
5. Neurofibromatosis (von Recklinghausen's disease) is a genetic error of metabolism with a proclivity to produce multiple neurofibrosarcomas and, in about 10 per cent of the patients, malignant neurilemomas.
6. Of 70 patients with malignant neurilemomas treated by the author, 45 were considered determinable; in these a 44 per cent five year "cure" rate was obtained.
7. Patients with von Recklinghausen's disease had a better prognosis (47 per cent living) than those without evidence of von Recklinghausen's disease (40 per cent living). This may be due to the greater awareness and earlier treatment of von Recklinghausen's disease.

REFERENCES

Ackerman, L. V., and Taylor, F. H.: Neurogenous tumors within the thorax. Cancer 4:699, 1951.

Brasfield, R. D., and Das Gupta, T. K.: Von Recklinghausen's disease: A clinicopathological study. Ann. Surg. 175:86, 1972.

Brewer, D. B.: Differences in the fine structure of collagen and reticulin as revealed by the polarizing microscope. J. Path. Bact. 74:371, 1957.

Bull, J. W. D.: Spinal meningiomas and neurofibromas. Acta Radiol. 40:283, 1952.

Carey, L. S., Ellis, F. H. Jr., Good, C. A., and Woolner, L. B.: Neurogenic tumors of the mediastinum; A clinicopathologic study. Am. J. Roentgenol. 84:189, 1960.

Carpenter, W. B., and Kernohan, J. W.: Retroperitoneal ganglioneuromas and neurofibromas. Cancer 16:788, 1963.

Chapman, R. C., Kemp, V. E., and Taliaferro, I.: Pheochromocytoma associated with multiple neurofibromatosis and intracranial hemangioma. Am. J. Med. 26:883, 1959.

Cohn, I.: Epithelial neoplasms of peripheral and cranial nerves: Report of three cases, review of the literature. A.M.A. Arch. Surg. 17:117, 1928.

Crowe, F. W., Schull, W. J., and Neel, J. V.: A Clinical, Pathological, and Genetic Study of Multiple Neurofibromatosis. Springfield, Ill., Charles C Thomas, 1956.

D'Agostino, A. N., Soule, E. H., and Miller, R. H.: Primary malignant neoplasms of nerves (malignant neurilemomas) in patients without manifestations of multiple neurofibromatosis (von Recklinghausen's disease). Cancer 16:1003, 1963.

D'Agostino, A. N., Soule, E. H., and Miller, R. H.: Sarcomas of the peripheral nerves and somatic soft tissues associated with multiple neurofibromatosis (von Recklinghausen's disease). Cancer *16*:1015, 1963.

Dart, L. H. Jr., MacCarty, C. S., Love, J. G., and Dockerty, M. B.: Neoplasms of the brachial plexus. Minn. Med. *53*:959, 1970.

DeSanto, D. A., and Burgess, E.: Primary and secondary neurilemoma of bone. Surg. Gynecol Obst. *71*:454, 1940.

Duncan, T. E., and Harkin, J. C.: Ultrastructure of spontaneous goldfish tumors previously classified as neurofibromas. (Abstract) Am. J. Pathol. *52*:33, 1968.

Fawcett, K. J., and Dahlin, D. C.: Neurilemoma of bone. Amer. J. Clin. Path. *47*:759, 1967.

Fox, H., Emery, J. L., Goodbody, R. A., and Yates, P. O.: Neurocutaneous melanosis. Arch. Dis. Child. *39*:508, 1964.

Harkin, J. C., and Reed, R. J.: Tumors of the Peripheral Nervous System. Washington, D.C., Armed Forces Institute of Pathology, 1969.

Herrmann, J.: Sarcomatous transformation in multiple neurofibromatosis (von Recklinghausen's disease). Ann. Surg. *131*:206, 1950.

Hosoi, K.: Multiple neurofibromatosis (von Recklinghausen's disease), with special reference to malignant transformation. Arch. Surg. *22*:258, 1931.

Jones, H. M.: Neurilemoma of bone (metacarpus). Brit. J. Surg. *41*:63, 1953.

Langford, J. A., and Cohn, I.: Expendymal neoplasm of the median nerve. South Med. J. *20*:273, 1927.

Lichtenstein, B. W.: Neurofibromatosis (von Recklinghausen's disease of the nervous system): Analysis of the total pathologic picture. Arch. Neurol. *62*:822, 1949.

Lukash, W. M., Morgan, R. I., Sennett, C. O., and Nielson, O. F.: Gastrointestinal neoplasms in von Recklinghausen's disease. Arch. Surg. *92*:905, 1966.

Masson, P.: Experimental and spontaneous schwannomas (peripheral gliomas). Am. J. Pathol. *8*:367, 1932.

Masson, P.: Tumeurs encapsulées et bénignes des nerfs. Rev. Canad. Biol. *1*:209, 1942.

Murray, M. R., and Stout, A. P.: Characteristics of human Schwann cells in vitro. Anat. Rec. *84*:275, 1942.

Murray, M. R., and Stout, A. P.: Schwann cell versus fibroblast as the origin of the specific nerve sheath tumor. Am. J. Pathol. *16*:41, 1940.

Murray, M. R., and Stout, A. P.: Demonstration of the formation of reticulin by schwannian tumor cells in vitro. Am. J. Pathol. *18*:585, 1942.

Nageotte, J.: Sheaths of the peripheral nerves. *In* Penfield, W.: Cytology and Cellular Pathology of the Nervous System. New York, Paul B. Hoeber, Inc., 1932, Vol. 1, p. 191.

Randall, J. T., and Jackson, S. F.: Nature and Structure of Collagen. New York: Academic Press, Inc., 1953.

Reed, W. B., Becker, S. W. Sr., Becker, S. W. Jr., and Nickel, W. R.: Giant pigmented nevi, melanoma, and leptomeningeal melanocytosis. Arch. Derm. *91*:100, 1965.

Ruppert, R. D., Buerger, L. F., and Chang, W. W.: Pheochromocytoma, neurofibromatosis and thyroid carcinoma. Metabolism *15*:537, 1966.

Shuangshoti, S., Tangchai, P., and Netsky, M. G.: Neoplasms of the nervous system in Thailand. Cancer *23*:493, 1969.

Stout, A. P.: Malignant tumors of the peripheral nerves. Amer. J. Cancer *25*:1, 1935.

Stout, A. P.: Neurofibroma and neurilemoma. Clin. Proc. *5*:1, 1946.

Stout, A. P.: Tumors of the Peripheral Nervous System. Fascicle 6, Atlas of Tumor Pathology. Washington, D.C.: Armed Forces Institute of Pathology, 1949.

Tarlov, I. M.: Structure of the nerve root. I. Nature of the junction between the central and the peripheral nervous system. Arch. Neurol. *37*:555, 1937.

Vieta, J. O., and Pack, G. T.: Malignant neurilemomas of peripheral nerves. Am. J. Surg. *82*:416, 1951.

Williams, E. D., and Pollack, D. J.: Multiple mucosal neuromata endocrine tumours: a syndrome allied to von Recklinghausen's disease. J. Path. Bact. *91*:71, 1966.

Willis, R. A.: The hamartomatous syndromes; their clinical, pathological and fundamental aspects. Med. J. Aust. *1*:827, 1965.

Wilson, J. S., and Anderson, A. A.: Cutaneous and intestinal neurofibromatosis. Am. J. Surg. *100*:761, 1960.

Woodruff, J. M., Chernik, N. L., Smith, M. C., Millett, W. B., and Foote, F. W., Jr.: Peripheral nerve tumors with rhabdomyosarcomatous differentiation (malignant "triton" tumors). Cancer *32*:426, 1973.

42

SURGICAL TREATMENT OF PERIPHERAL NERVE TUMORS OF THE UPPER LIMB

RICHARD J. SMITH and
ROBERT W. LIPKE

Tumors of the peripheral nerves of the upper limb are infrequent. Most are neither suspected nor diagnosed preoperatively (Posch, 1956, Strickland and Steichen, 1977). The hand surgeon may have had only limited experience in treating these tumors. Therefore, it is important that he become familiar with the clinical findings, gross appearance, and accepted methods of treating these lesions in order that he may be able to deal with them appropriately.

Tumors of the peripheral nerves may involve the axons, the Schwann cells, or the connective tissue cells of the perineurium or epineurium. In neurofibromatosis, tumors will usually involve both the axon and its supporting tissues. Rarely, primary nerve tumors may consist of cartilage, bone, and muscle or adipose tissue. Malignant tumors of the peripheral nerves are uncommon and most frequently originate from the Schwann cells. Although a traumatic neuroma may be considered a peripheral nerve tumor, as there is proliferation of axons and supporting tissue following nerve transection, the neuroma is not a primary neoplasm, and will not be considered in this chapter.

SCHWANNOMA OR NEURILEMOMA

The most common solitary peripheral nerve tumor originates from the Schwann cells that surround the axon. There had been controversy for many years regarding the origin of this tumor. Careful clinical and laboratory investigation, including tissue cultures, has now established rather conclusively that these lesions do not arise from the fibrous tissue of the perineurium and epineurium, but rather from the Schwann cells which are formed from the neuroectodermal crest (Stout, 1935a, 1953; Harkin and Reed, 1969; Geschickter, 1935; Byrne, 1966). The schwannoma most commonly is located in a major nerve trunk or one of its branches and is not found in the intradermal nerve ends (Penfield, 1927; Biggart, 1958). The tumor usually is solitary, but multiple schwannomas have been found within the same nerve (Heard, 1962). As many as six isolated schwannomas have been described in one patient (White, 1967). The tumor occurs with equal frequency in both sexes. It is more frequently located on the flexor than the extensor surfaces of the upper limb, particularly in the region of the wrist and elbow (Stout, 1935a). On rare occasions, schwannomas have been found within bone (Seth et al., 1963; Hart and Basom, 1958). In 18 per cent of cases, schwannomas are associated with von Recklinghausen's disease (Stout, 1935a). Twenty per cent of all schwannomas are found in the upper limbs, 15 per cent in the lower limbs. In 45 per cent they are located in the head or neck region (Dasgupta, 1969).

The typical schwannoma develops gradually, and the patient is first aware of a slowly growing mass deep to the skin. Although paresthesia may occur, motor weakness is unusual (Seddon, 1972). About 40 per cent of patients complain of some pain and tenderness in the region of the mass. Clinically, the tumor is well defined and can be moved from side to side but not longitudinally. On occasion, there may be cystic degenerative changes within the larger schwannomas that will allow them to be transilluminated. A mistaken diagnosis of ganglion cyst may be made preoperatively (Stout, 1935a).

At surgery, the appearance of the tumor is typical. A shiny, white, oval, encapsulated mass measuring up to 2 to 4 centimeters in diameter is seen within the substance of the peripheral nerve. Although the tumor usually has a firm consistency, there may be areas of cystic degeneration. The nerve both proximal and distal to the tumor will appear normal and the adjacent tissues are uninvolved (Stout, 1946).

The tumor should be explored utilizing magnification. As the schwannoma is a tumor of the tissues surrounding the axons, nerve fascicles are compressed and spread by the tumor but do not enter it. Careful sharp dissection should allow each fascicle to be freed of the tumor and the schwannoma enucleated without damage to the axon bundles (Cutler and Gross, 1936; Jenkins, 1952; Marmor, 1965; Barrett and Cramer, 1963). If the axons are intimately entwined within the tumor, or if the tumor does not appear encapsulated and is adherent to the surrounding soft tissues, the diagnosis should be in doubt and incisional biopsy performed (Phalen, 1976).

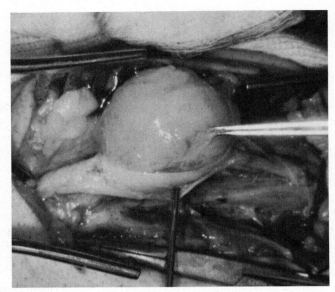

Figure 42–1 *Benign schwannoma (neurilemoma).* This benign schwannoma is sharply dissected from the nerve fascicles which surround it. The tumor can be excised from the peripheral nerve under magnification by sharp dissection without sacrificing the nerve fascicles. The benign schwannoma does not become malignant.

Histological examination of the schwannoma is discussed in detail in Chapter 40 by Harkin. If no malignant change or atypical cells are noted, recurrence after enucleation is rare. Malignant degeneration of a benign schwannoma has not been documented (Stout, 1935*a*). Full recovery can usually be anticipated postoperatively (Fig. 42–1).

MALIGNANT SCHWANNOMA WITH SCHWANN CELL DIFFERENTIATION

Some authors suggest that the term "malignant schwannoma" be restricted only to those nerve sheath tumors that show distinctive features of Schwann cell differentiation histologically. Such tumors appear to arise principally from the Schwann cells of the axon sheath.

The malignant schwannoma does not develop from malignant degeneration of a benign schwannoma, but is thought to originate by malignant degeneration of normal Schwann cells (Gore, 1952). As with the benign schwannoma, the tumor is most frequently observed on the flexor aspect of the wrist and elbow. Typically, it begins as a painless mass that slowly grows in size and ultimately may cause paraesthesia, hypaesthesia, and muscle weakness. The tumors occur equally in males and females and are most prevalent in patients 30 to 60 years of age. Grossly, the tumor is white and appears as a fusiform enlargement within the nerve, or as a globular infiltrative mass of nerve surrounded by a pseudocapsule (Fig. 42–2). The tumor may involve several centimeters of the nerve trunk. Unlike the benign schwannoma, a malignant schwannoma usually consists of axon

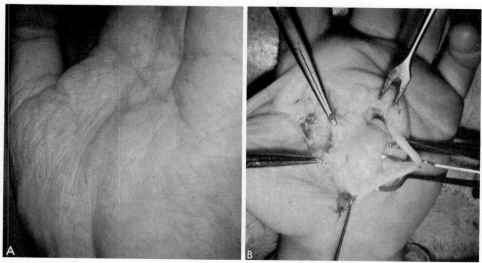

Figure 42–2 *Malignant schwannoma (well differentiated). A,* This 32 year old man complained of pain in the palm radiating to the middle finger. He had noted a slowly growing mass just distal to the carpal canal for several months. There was no antecedent trauma. There was mild hypesthesia in the index, middle and ring fingers. *B,* Exploration of the palm revealed a tumor approximately 4 cm in length. It involved the digital branches of the median nerve to the ring and middle fingers. Fascicles entering the tumor could not be separated from it. Incisional biopsy revealed malignant schwannoma. As this tumor had well differentiated Schwann cells histologically, local en bloc resection was indicated. If the histological appearance were similar to that of fibrosarcoma, wide en bloc excision or amputation would be considered.

filaments intimately intertwined within the tumor mass. Some authors have referred to "skip areas" where malignant schwannoma will be found in more than one location along a nerve trunk with normal nerve between the tumors. Such "skip tumors", however, are rare.

A malignant schwannoma may develop within a plexiform neurofibroma of von Recklinghausen's disease. In these cases, there will usually be a history of increased growth in the plexiform neurofibroma, or recurrence of a tumor mass after a plexiform neurofibroma has been removed. Grossly, the malignant schwannoma is somewhat larger than a plexiform neurofibroma and when incised, it is more homogeneous, reflecting its increased cellularity. Although malignant schwannomas with well differentiated Schwann cells are locally infiltrative, they rarely metastasize. Thus, if a malignant schwannoma that arises de novo or from a plexiform neurofibroma reveals Schwann cell differentiation on microscopic examination, the tumor may be treated by local en bloc excision. If the borders of the excised tissue are free of tumor, surgical reconstruction with a nerve graft may be considered. Neurorrhaphy should be delayed if there is uncertainty as to whether the tumor is completely removed.

About 10 per cent of these tumors contain epithelial elements with acinar and rosette patterns characteristic of neuroepithelial origins (Michael, 1967). Occasionally, metaplasia of the malignant Schwann cells may form bone, striated muscle, cartilage, or fatty tumors. If rhabdomyosarcoma is found in the metaplastic elements of the malignant schwannoma, the prognosis is exceedingly poor (Woodruff, et al., 1973).

MALIGNANT SCHWANNOMA — UNDIFFERENTIATED TYPE

Many malignant tumors of the peripheral nerve sheath appear undifferentiated when examined microscopically. Some authors believe that these tumors are of fibroblastic origin; others consider them to be either partly or totally of Schwann cell origin. They have been called fibrosarcomas, neurogenic fibrosarcomas, and malignant schwannomas. Histologically the lesions may appear similar to fibrosarcomas of non-neurogenic soft tissue. The differentiation often can be made best at operation. The nerve sheath tumor is intimately associated with the nerve, and only secondarily invades the surrounding soft tissues, whereas the gross appearance of a fibrosarcoma arising from surrounding tissues is the reverse. Compared with fibrosarcomas of adjacent soft tissues, the nerve sheath fibrosarcoma or malignant schwannoma is usually more aggressive, more likely to recur, and more likely to infiltrate along the nerve trunk.

The results of treatment of the more undifferentiated malignant schwannomas (as contrasted with those with Schwann cell differentiation) is poor. Five year survival rates have ranged from 10 to 50 per cent (White, 1971). The prognosis is particularly poor if the tumor is treated by incomplete local resection.

With recurrence, the tumor shows a tendency toward anaplasia, with increasingly poor prognosis (Vieta and Pack, 1951). The tumor may spread proximally along the nerve trunk and may involve the brain and spinal cord. Metastases occur in 20 per cent of cases and are most common to the lung and pleura (Stout, 1935b).

Most important in the treatment of the malignant schwannoma is its prompt diagnosis. Malignant schwannomas occur in approximately 10 per cent of patients with von Recklinghausen's disease and usually arise from deep plexiform neurofibromata (Hosoi, 1931). Thus, surgical exploration is indicated in any patient with von Recklinghausen's disease who notes a rapid enlargement of a tumor mass. The value of xerography, computerized axial tomography, and angiography in diagnosing the size and location of any deep soft tissue tumor is well known. If the surgeon suspects a benign nerve or soft tissue tumor and finds a lesion of a peripheral nerve which is poorly encapsulated, adherent to the surrounding soft tissues, or intricately entwined in peripheral nerve fascicles, malignant schwannoma should be suspected. Incisional biopsy should be performed and further treatment should await histological diagnosis.

Once a diagnosis of malignant schwannoma of the fibrosarcomatous type is established, radical resection is indicated (D'Agostino et al., 1963). Chest roentgenograms and tomograms should be studied for possible metastases. The limb should be palpated meticulously for more proximal lesions in the involved nerve trunk. As with any soft tissue sarcoma, either amputation or en bloc radical excision is indicated if the tumor is to be completely removed. As this type of malignant schwannoma is a most aggressive lesion with a high mortality rate, the surgeon's primary concern should not be reconstruction or hand function. Local resection and nerve graft jeopardizes not only the entire limb but also the life of the patient. If the lesion appears relatively localized at the time of initial exploration and incisional biopsy, radical en bloc excision may permit safe extirpation without amputation. The involved nerve should be resected for several centimeters proximal to the level of resection. The tumor and the soft tissues adjacent to it should not be exposed during the dissection. The borders of the excised soft tissue mass and nerve ends should be examined, and if tumor tissue is found, amputation must be considered. If skin is excised, the defect must not be covered by remote pedicle flaps. Remote flaps increase the risk of seeding malignant cells to distant areas. Secondary reconstructive procedures should be delayed for several months until there is satisfactory healing and no evidence of local recurrence. Recurrence usually requires amputation (Smith, 1977).

In dealing with malignant schwannomas of the fibrosarcomatous type, the hand surgeon should consider total extirpation of the lesions as his primary role. Reconstruction, if possible, is secondary to saving the life of the patient. As malignant schwannomas are not radiosensitive and do not appear to be affected by chemotherapeutics, total surgical excision is the only chance for cure (D'Agostino et al., 1963; Dasgupta and Brasfield, 1970).

NEUROFIBROMA

A neurofibroma is an unencapsulated proliferation of Schwann cells, fibrous connective tissue, and axons. When a neurofibroma occurs at the distal end of a peripheral nerve, a subcutaneous or intradermal neurofibroma develops. A more deeply located neurofibroma that produces a tortuous mass of Schwann cells, fibrous tissue, and axon is called a plexiform neurofibroma (Stout, 1946). Although a neurofibroma may occur as a solitary lesion, they are seen most frequently with von Recklinghausen's disease.

The *solitary neurofibroma* is a benign, slowly growing neoplasm often found in patients with von Recklinghausen's disease. It may be located in the skin or subcutaneous tissues; it is moderately firm, circumscribed, and usually not tender. Those that occur in the skin are well localized but not encapsulated. The nerve of origin is rarely seen. Deeper solitary neurofibromata usually are well encapsulated. The nerve of origin enters the substance of the tumor where it becomes part of the tumor mass and cannot be separated from it. The solitary neurofibroma is composed of axon cylinders, Schwann cells, collagen, and a myxomatous matrix. It is rarely cystic. Excision of the solitary neurofibroma is usually curative as recurrence is infrequent.

Von Recklinghausen's disease (VRD), or neurofibromatosis, is an inherited disorder which typically consists of multiple neurofibromata of the spinal, cranial, and peripheral nerves. Both cutaneous and plexiform neurofibromata may be formed. The majority of cases of von Recklinghausen's disease are mild and may be unrecognized. Abnormalities associated with von Recklinghausen's disease include (McCarroll, 1956):

1. Cutaneous café-au-lait spots and verrucous skin hypertrophy ("fibroma molluscum").
2. Multiple skeletal changes, such as scoliosis, congenital pseudarthrosis of the tibia, bone cysts, bone resorption, and bone hypertrophy.
3. Cutaneous vascular changes, consisting of diffuse, flat hemangiomata or plexiform venous dilatation.
4. Lymphatic edema.

Local gigantism of the digits, with soft tissue and bony hypertrophy is often

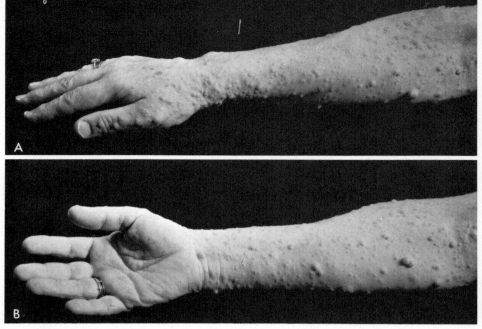

Figure 42–3 Multiple cutaneous neurofibromata or "fibroma molluscum". This woman has hundreds of intracutaneous neurofibromatous cutaneous lesions throughout her body. She also has large areas of skin hyperpigmentation. She has no other stigmata of neurofibromatosis. Several of the lesions were excised when they became extremely pruritic or painful. She has no motor nor sensory abnormality. Unfortunately, there is no successful treatment available to control these unsightly lesions.

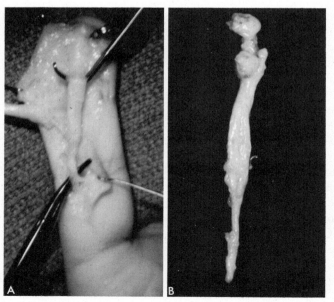

Figure 42–4 Solitary benign plexiform neurofibroma. *A,* This 45 year old woman noted a rapidly enlarging mass to the radial and dorsal sides of her left index finger. Exploration reveals marked enlargement of the dorsal and volar branches of the radial digital nerve of the index finger. The tumor could not be separated from the fascicles of the digital nerve. *B,* The dorsal and volar branches of the digital nerve were removed. Biopsy had revealed the tumor to be a plexiform neurofibroma.

considered a variant of von Recklinghausen's disease. This lesion will be considered separately.

Multiple cutaneous neurofibromata, "fibroma molluscum," presents a most striking appearance. This feature of neurofibromatosis occurs in less than 10 per cent of patients with von Recklinghausen's disease (McCarroll, 1956). The intracutaneous neurofibromata cause multiple sessile or pedunculated skin lesions that are often associated with the café-au-lait spots (Fig. 42–3). They develop early in life and may remain unchanged for many years (Preston et al., 1951). Frequently, they enlarge at puberty or with pregnancy (Sharpe and Young, 1936). They cause unsightly skin lesions which may be pruritic or painful. Rarely, if ever, do they undergo malignant transformation (McCarroll, 1956).

In *plexiform neurofibromata,* axons are intimately intertwined with proliferating Schwann cell and fibrous tissue from the perineurium. If an asymptomatic plexiform neurofibroma is discovered in a patient with neurofibromatosis, the tumor should be carefully observed. These tumors may remain dormant for many years and suddenly begin to grow rapidly. If a more central plexiform neurofibroma grows proximally along the nerve trunk towards the spinal cord and brain, paralysis or death may result. As the tumor is unencapsulated, surgical excision is difficult and the lesion may recur locally if it is incompletely excised. Fifty per cent of malignant schwannomas develop in the plexiform neurofibromas of patients with neurofibromatosis. In these patients, the mortality rate is greater than 50 per cent if the tumor is not well differentiated histologically (D'Agostino et al., 1963).

Any patient with neurofibromatosis who has a rapidly enlarging or suddenly painful nerve tumor should be suspected of having a plexiform neurofibroma with malignant degeneration that demands immediate attention. If there is no evidence of local invasion, and if biopsy reveals no evidence of malignant degeneration, the tumor is excised. If there is malignant change, radical en bloc excision is required.

Unlike the schwannoma, the plexiform neurofibroma cannot be enucleated leaving axons intact. Thus, with a benign enlarging neurofibroma, an entire segment of the nerve must be removed, including axons, Schwann cells, and supportive connective tissues (Fig. 42–4). The gap may be bridged by nerve graft, although the recovery of nerve function is often indifferent (Seddon, 1972; Barfred and Zachariae, 1975). If neurofibromatosis has caused bone or joint deformity, appropriate reconstructive procedures may be performed to restore function to the hand without necessarily excising the nerve lesions (Fig. 42–5).

LOCAL GIGANTISM DUE TO NEUROFIBROMATOSIS

Although local bone and soft tissue hypertrophy are frequently associated with neurofibromatosis of von Recklinghausen's disease, local gigantism, or macrodactyly, may occur as an isolated abnormality unassociated with the other stigmata of hereditary neurofibromatosis.

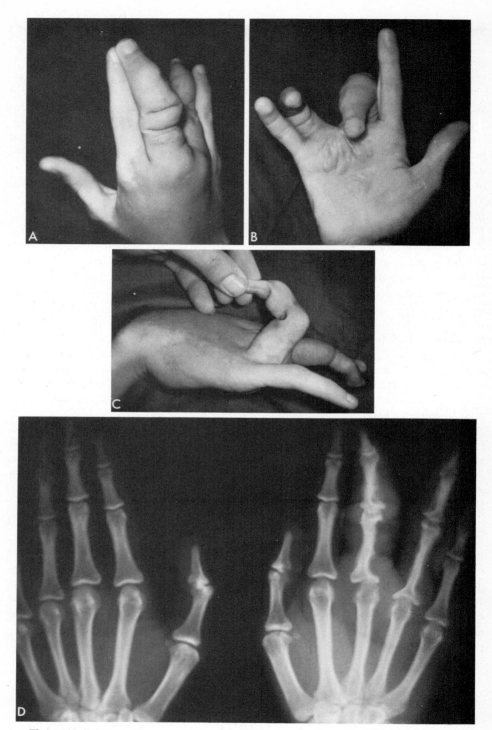

Figure 42–5 Neurofibromatosis, ("von Recklinghausen's disease"). This patient has many of the stigmata of neurofibromatosis. *A*, The café-au-lait hyperpigmentation on the dorsum of the hand extending to the middle and ring fingers is seen. There is extensive soft tissue swelling about these fingers but no true "gigantism." *B*, Thumb, index, and little fingers are uninvolved. In the palm proximal to the middle and ring fingers there is a soft tissue tumor which is soft and nontender. *C*, There is gross instability of all three joints of the involved fingers. With loss of stability, the fingers were not used for grasp. *D*, Roentgenograms of the right hand revealed narrowing of the proximal and middle phalanges of the involved central fingers. The scalloped appearance is suggestive of a defect caused by extrinsic pressure.

Legend continued on the opposite page

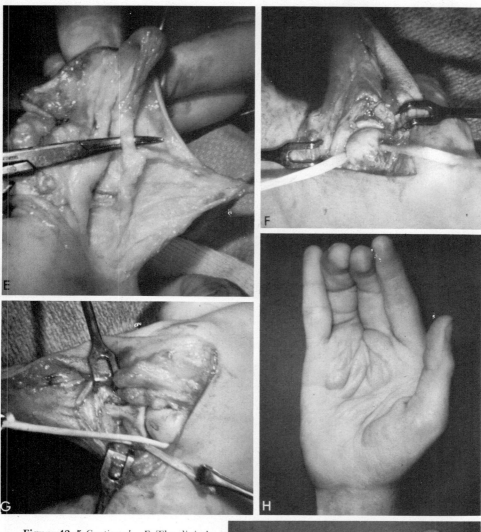

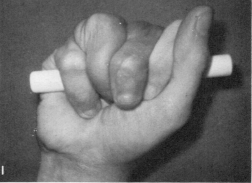

Figure 42–5 *Continued.* *E*, The digital nerves to the involved fingers are thick, yellow, and fatty. Generous amounts of subcutaneous tissues have the characteristics of abdominal fat and appear coarse and globular. *F* and *G*, Surgical reconstruction included resection of redundant skin and excessive fatty tissue in each finger, reconstruction of collateral ligaments using free tendon grafts and arthrodesis of the distal interphalangeal joint, *H* and *I*, Postoperatively, the function of the hand was much improved and he was able to grasp objects using the involved central fingers.

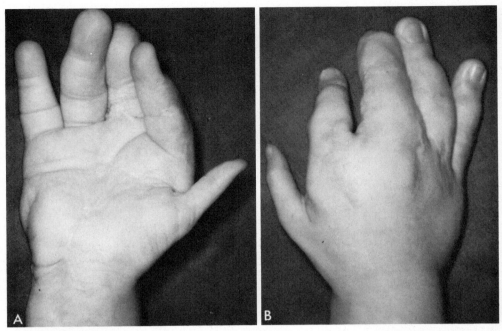

Figure 42–6 Neurofibromatosis with "elephantiac hypertrophy." This patient with von Recklinghausen's neurofibromatosis has café-au-lait spots and massive soft tissue swelling of all four fingers.

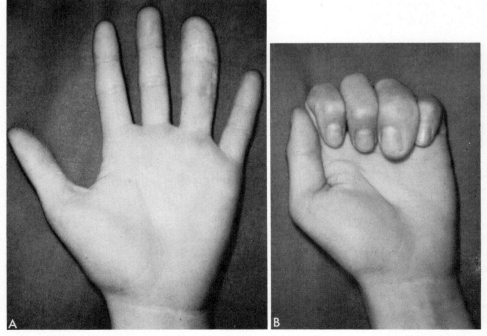

Figure 42–7 Macrodactyly. This woman with moderate enlargement of the left ring finger has no other stigma of neurofibromatosis. There are no café-au-lait spots. The soft tissue swelling does not extend into the palm. She has a "static primary" type of macrodactyly.

Macrodactyly, or gigantism of the digits, may be primary or it may be secondary to tumor or exogenous factors. With primary macrodactyly, there is enlargement of all tissues of the involved finger (Fig. 42–6). Finger enlargement may be seen at birth or may develop within the first two years of life. Disproportionate enlargement of the involved fingers may continue through puberty. With *static macrodactyly,* there is enlargement of only one finger or toe and no involvement of the contiguous palm or sole (Fig. 42–7). With *progressive macrodactyly,* more than one digit is usually involved, and the palm or sole adjacent to it is thickened (Fig. 42–8). The phalanges of the involved digit are increased in length and breadth, and growth centers show advanced maturation. Asymmetric growth of the phalanges causes deviation of the fingers toward the less involved side. There may be diminution of sensibility, but trophic changes are uncommon (Barsky, 1967).

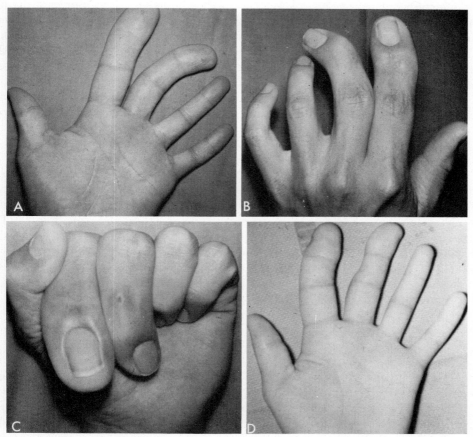

Figure 42–8 *Macrodactyly-progressive type. A, B,* and *C,* This patient had no stigma of neurofibromatosis. There was enlargement of bone, nails, and all soft tissues of the index and middle fingers. The middle finger deviated ulnarly toward the relatively uninvolved side. *D,* Surgery can shorten and straighten markedly deviated fingers of macrodactyly. A normal appearing finger should not be anticipated.

Blood vessels in the involved digits are elongated, and angiography has revealed hypertrophy which usually affects only one vessel of the finger. Subcutaneous fat is hypertrophic and has the appearance of adult abdominal fat. Large fat globules are found throughout the finger, intimately associated with nerve fibrils. The most consistent and distinctive pathological changes are found in the digital nerves. They are broad, tortuous, and covered by a rather thick epineurium that lacks the luster and sheen normally seen in the digital nerve of a child. Nerve branches are intimately adherent to the fat globules they appear to envelop. Histological section reveals proliferation of fibrous endoneurium and perineurium, coarse nerve fascicles, narrow myelin sheaths, and compression of the axons. Fatty and bony enlargement of the finger is restricted to the areas in which nerve changes are found. Proliferation of fibroblastic tissue has been found between the bone cortex and the periosteum, in the region of peripheral nerve fibrosis (Ben-Bassat et al., 1966; Khanna et al., 1975; Moore, 1942).

The close association between peripheral nerve abnormality and macrodactyly, as well as the occasional association of neurofibromatosis with enlarged digits, has led many to question whether primary macrodactyly is a *forme fruste* of neurofibromatosis. This association appears unlikely. Neurofibromatosis is usually an inherited disorder, with many members of a family showing various stigma of the disease in the skin, spine, and peripheral nerves. Such is not found with primary macrodactyly. In addition, fibrolipomatous changes found about the branches of the median nerve with primary macrodactyly are not similar to those found with neurofibromatosis (Inglis, 1950).

The possibility of a neurogenic cause of macrodactyly remains. Some authors have suggested a neuro-intrinsic factor which may cause finger hypertrophy; others have suggested disturbance in "growth limiting factors."

Secondary macrodactyly may be associated with neurofibromatosis. These patients have other stigma of neurofibromatosis.

Usually a macrodactylous digit is unsightly and stiff and has poor function. The goals of surgery are to decrease its size, prevent its continued growth, correct its angular deformity, and, if possible, increase motion at its stiffened joints. If only one finger is involved and if it is unsightly, deformed, and stiff, serious consideration should be given to amputation. Digital nerve transection has been suggested by some to slow the growth of a macrodactylous digit. However, nerve division to prevent formation of "neuro-intrinsic factor" interferes with the sensibility of the finger and has met with disappointing results in the control of finger growth (Tsuge, 1967; Jones, 1964).

LIPOFIBROMATOSIS OF THE MEDIAN NERVE

Fatty and fibrous enlargement of the supporting structures of the median nerve were described in the 1960's (Watson-Jones, 1962; Pulvertaft, 1964; Mikhail, 1964; Emmett, 1965; Johnson and Bonfiglio, 1969). These lesions have been found principally in the median nerve at the distal forearm, palm, and fingers (Fig. 42–9). The lesion begins as a slowly growing, painless, soft mass that develops in early childhood and often continues to enlarge through adolescence (Bergman et al., 1970). Although there may be local soft tissue swelling,

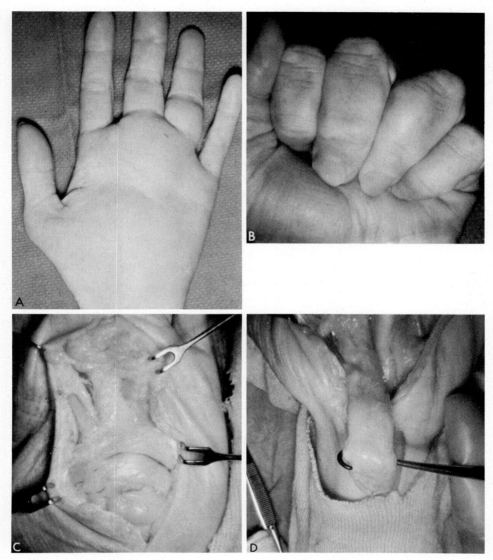

Figure 42–9 Lipofibromatosis of the median nerve. *A* and *B*, This 25 year old woman had noted progressive enlargement of a palmar mass extending into the middle and ring fingers since the age of six. She had no other abnormalities. In recent years, she had symptoms suggestive of a carpal tunnel syndrome with hypesthesia to the median nerve distribution. The swelling was non-tender and extended to the contiguous sides of the dorsum of the middle and ring fingers. *C*, Exploration of the palm revealed marked swelling of the digital branches of the median nerve to the middle and ring fingers. The nerve appeared yellow and fatty. Fascicles could be defined among the supporting tissues of the nerve. *D*, More proximal dissection revealed the median nerve to have been broadened several centimeters proximal to the wrist. No attempt was made to remove the tumor. The transverse carpal ligament was not repaired and the symptoms of carpal tunnel syndrome subsided. The mass has remained but is relatively asymptomatic.

the lesion is not associated with gigantism of the digits. Frequently, the patient will develop median nerve paraesthesia and thenar weakness suggestive of carpal tunnel syndrome. This lesion is not associated with the stigma of neuro-fibromatosis.

The median nerve may be enlarged to five or six times its normal diameter. This enormous swelling is symmetrical and may extend for several centimeters, involving the common or proper digital nerves. The involved nerve is slightly yellow in color but has a sheen and glistening appearance of a normal nerve. It is not adherent to surrounding tissues. Longitudinal dissection of the nerve will reveal large quantities of fibrous and fatty tissue surrounding the nerve fascicles. Histologically, fatty and fibrous infiltration of the epineurium and perineurium is seen to extend between the fascicles, engulfing and intimately associated with the axons. At no time has this lesion become malignant. Symptoms appear to be those of a carpal tunnel syndrome associated with painless palmar and digital swelling. The preoperative neurological deficit is usually due to compression of the median nerve at the carpal canal. Carpal tunnel release should result in relief of the pain and paraesthesia. Return of motor function is variable (Johnson and Bonfiglio, 1969). Although there have been published reports of extensive dissection of these tumors to free the fibrous and fatty tissues from about the axons, this treatment may jeopardize median nerve function by inadvertent axon damage (Friedlander et al., 1969). Such dissection would appear warranted only in cases of excessive enlargement that interferes with hand function (Callison et al., 1968; Rudolph, 1975; Paletta and Rybka, 1972; Rowland, 1967).

Lipofibromatous infiltration of the median nerve is a localized tumor of the supporting fatty and fibrous tissues of the nerve with little or no malignant potential. It is unclear why this lesion is restricted to the median nerve in the distal forearm and palm.

OTHER TUMORS OF PERIPHERAL NERVES

There are many other tumors of the peripheral nerves which very rarely will be encountered by the hand surgeon. They include variants of the malignant schwannoma, such as malignant epithelioid schwannoma and melanocytic schwannoma, and other soft tissue sarcomas and carcinomas, such as malignant mesenchymomas, neuroblastomas, and metastatic lesions to the nerve sheath. These lesions require histological diagnosis by a neuropathologist. Once the lesion has been diagnosed, treatment may best be determined by those most familiar with their histological behavior.

CONCLUSIONS

The hand surgeon will infrequently be called upon to diagnose and treat neoplasms of the peripheral nerves. Even less frequently will the diagnosis of peripheral nerve tumor be made preoperatively on a patient not previously treated. For this reason the surgeon must be prepared for the unexpected. A few basic rules should be remembered:

1. If a small (less than 4 cm), well encapsulated, fusiform or globular lesion is found within the substance of a peripheral nerve, and if under magnification the axons are found to be splayed around the lesion but do not penetrate it, the surgeon may be reasonably certain that he or she is dealing with a benign schwannoma. The tumor should be enucleated and the nerve preserved.

2. If the surgeon encounters a larger lesion (2 to 6 cm in diameter) which is adherent to surrounding soft tissues, and through which the axons run, he or she may be dealing with a malignant schwannoma. This is a dangerous tumor, which has up to a 50 per cent five year mortality rate if not totally excised. An incisional biopsy should be performed. If the diagnosis is confirmed, the surgeon and the patient should be prepared for major extirpative surgery consisting either of radical en bloc excision or amputation if the lesion appears fibrosarcomatous, or en bloc excision with later reconstruction if Schwann cell differentiation is seen histologically.

3. At operation, a solitary neurofibroma of the skin may appear to be a fibroma. Excision is usually curative. When the correct diagnosis is made histologically, the surgeon should carefully re-examine the patient for stigma of von Recklinghausen's disease. If none are found, no further treatment is indicated. The solitary deep neurofibroma is usually well encapsulated and rarely recurs after excision. If the nerve trunk requires transection in order to remove the tumor, secondary neurorrhaphy or nerve grafting may be indicated.

4. In cases of neurofibromatosis or von Recklinghausen's disease, cutaneous lesions should be removed only if symptomatic. They will not become malignant. The deeper neurofibromata should be removed if they rapidly enlarge or cause local symptoms. As these tumors may become malignant, they should be biopsied if they enlarge. Histological evaluation of the lesion is important in determining the extent of resection. If the tumor is not malignant, it may be locally resected and the nerve reconstructed.

5. A lipofibroma of the median nerve should be treated by carpal tunnel release. These lesions rarely, if ever, become malignant. As the axons are intimately entwined in fibrous and fatty tissue, extensive dissection to remove the tumor is usually unwarranted.

REFERENCES

Barfred, T., and Zachariae, L.: Neurofibroma in the median nerve treated with resection and free nerve transplantation. Scand. J. Plast. Reconstr. Surg. 9:245, 1975.

Barrett, R., and Cramer, F.: Tumors of the peripheral nerves and so-called "ganglia" of the peroneal nerve. Clin. Orthop. 27:135, 1963.

Barsky, A. J.: Macrodactyly. J. Bone Joint Surg. 49A:1255, 1967.

Ben-Bassat, M., Casper, J., Kaplan, I., and Laran, Z.: Congenital macrodactyly. A case report with three years follow-up. J. Bone Joint Surg. 48B:359, 1966.

Bergman, F. O. et al.: Radical excision of a fibrofatty proliferation of the median nerve with no neurological loss symptoms. Plast. Reconstr. Surg. 46:375, 1970.

Biggart, J. H.: Peripheral nerve tumors. J. Bone Joint Surg. 31B:134, 1958.

Bryne, J. J.: Nerve tumors. In Flynn, J. E. (ed.): Hand Surgery. Baltimore, Williams & Wilkins Co., 1966.

Callison, J. R., Oliver, J. T., and White, W. C.: Fibrofatty proliferation of the median nerve. Plast. Reconstr. Surg. 42:403, 1968.

Cutler, E. C., and Gross, R. E.: Surgical treatment of the peripheral nerves. Ann. Surg. 104:436, 1936.

D'Agostino, A. N., Soule, E. H., and Miller, R. H.: Primary malignant neoplasms of nerves (malignant neurilemomas) in patients without manifestations of multiple neurofibromatosis (von Recklinghausen's disease). Cancer *16*:1003, 1963.

D'Agostino, A. N., Soule, E. H., and Miller, R. H.: Sarcomas of the peripheral nerves and somatic soft tissues associated with multiple neurofibromatosis (von Recklinghausen's disease). Cancer *16*:1015, 1963.

DasGupta, T. K., and Brasfield, R. D.: Solitary malignant schwannoma. Ann. Surg., 419, 1970.

DasGupta, T. K., Brasfield, R. D., et al.: Benign solitary schwannomas (neurilemomas). Cancer *24*:355, 1969.

Emmett, A. J. J.: Lipomatous hamartoma of the median nerve in the palm. Br. J. Plast. Surg. *18*:208, 1965.

Friedlander, H. L., Rosenberg, N. S., and Grabbard, D. J.: Intraneural lipoma of the median nerve. J. Bone Joint Surg. *51A*:352, 1969.

Geschickter, C. F.: Tumors of peripheral nerves. Am. J. Cancer *25*:377, 1935.

Gore, I.: Primary malignant tumors of nerve: a report of eight cases. Cancer *5*:278, 1952.

Harkin, J. C., and Reed, R. J.: Tumors of the Peripheral Nervous System. Washington, D.C., Armed Forces Institute of Pathology, 1969.

Hart, M. S., Basom, W. C.: Neurilemoma involving bone. J. Bone Joint Surg. *40A*:465, 1958.

Heard, H. G.: Nerve sheath tumours and von Recklinghausen's disease of the central nervous system. Ann. R. Coll. Surg. *31*:229, 1962.

Hosoi, K.: Multiple neurofibromatosis (von Recklinghausen's disease) Arch. Surg. *22*:258, 1931.

Inglis, K.: Local gigantism (a manifestation of neurofibromatosis): Its relation to general gigantism and to acromegaly illustrating the influence of intrinsic factors in disease when development of the body is abnormal. Am. J. Path. *26*:1059, 1950.

Jenkins, S. A.: Solitary tumours of peripheral nerve trunks. J. Bone Joint Surg. *34B*:401, 1952.

Johnson, R. J., and Bonfiglio, M.: Lipofibromatous hamartoma of the median nerve. J. Bone Joint Surg. *51A*:984, 1969.

Jones, K. G.: Megalodactylism. A case report treated by epiphyseal resection. J. Bone Joint Surg. *45A*:1704, 1963.

Khanna, N., Gupta, S., Khanna, S., and Tripathi, F.: Macrodactyly. Hand *7*:215, 1975.

Marmor, L.: Solitary peripheral nerve tumors. Clin. Orthop. *43*:183, 1965.

McCarroll, H. R.: Clinical manifestations of congenital neurofibromatosis. J. Bone Joint Surg. *32A*:601, 1950.

McCarroll, H. R.: Soft tissue neoplasms associated with congenital neurofibromatosis. J. Bone Joint Surg. *38A*:717, 1956.

Michel, S. L.: Epithelioid elements in a malignant neurogenic tumor. Am. J. Surg. *113*:404, 1967.

Mikhail, I. K.: Median nerve lipoma in the hand. J. Bone Joint Surg. *46B*:726, 1964.

Moore, B. H.: Macrodactyly and associated peripheral nerve changes. J. Bone Joint Surg. *24*:617, 1942.

Paletta, F. X., and Rybka, F. J.: Treatment of hamartomas of the median nerve. Ann. Surg. *176*:217, 1972.

Penfield, W.: The encapsulated tumor of the nervous system. Surg. Gynecol. Obstet. *45*:178, 1927.

Phalen, G. S.: Neurilemomas of the forearm and hand. Clin. Orthop. *114*:219, 1976.

Posch, J. L.: Tumors of the hand. J. Bone Joint Surg. *38A*:517, 1956.

Preston, F. W., Walsh, W. S., and Clarke, T.: Cutaneous neurofibromatosis (von Recklinghausen's disease). Arch. Surg. *68*:813, 1951.

Pulvertaft, R. G.: Unusual tumors of the median nerve. J. Bone Joint Surg. *46B*:731, 1964.

Rowland, S.: Lipofibroma of the median nerve in the palm. J. Bone Joint Surg. *49A*:1309, 1967.

Rudolph, R.: Painless fibrofatty hamartoma of the median nerve. Br. J. Plast. Surg. *28*:301, 1975.

Seddon, H. J.: Surgical Disorders of Peripheral Nerves. Baltimore, Williams & Wilkins, 1972.

Seth, H. N., Rao, B. D., et al.: Neurilemoma of bone. J. Bone Joint Surg. *45B*:382, 1963.

Sharpe, J. C., and Young, R. H.: Neurofibromatosis: The effect of pregnancy on skin manifestations. J.A.M.A. *106*:1682, 1936.

Smith, R. J.: Who is best qualified to treat tumors of the hand? J. Hand Surg. *2*:251, 1977.

Stout, A. P.: Peripheral manifestations of specific nerve sheath tumor (neurilemoma). Am. J. Cancer *24*:751, 1935a.

Stout, A. P.: The malignant tumors of the peripheral nerves. Am. J. Cancer *25*:1, 1935b.

Stout, A. P.: Neurofibroma and neurilomoma. Clin. Proc. *5*:1, 1946.

Stout, A. P.: Tumors of peripheral nerves. J. Bone Joint Surg. *40A*:959, 1958.

Stout, A. P.: Tumors of the peripheral nervous system, A.F.I.P. In Atlas of Tumor Pathology, Section II: Fascicle 6. Washington, D.C., U.S. Armed Forces Institute of Pathology, 1953.

Strickland, J. W., and Steichen, J. B.: Nerve tumors of the hand and forearm. J. Hand Surg. *2*:285, 1977.

Tsuge, K.: Treatment of macrodactyly. Plast. Reconstr. Surg. *39*:590, 1967.

Vieta, J. O., and Pack, G. T.: Malignant neurilomomas of peripheral nerves. Am. J. Surg. *82*:416, 1951.
Watson-Jones, R.: Encapsulated lipoma of the median nerve at the wrist. J. Bone Joint Surg. *44A*: 1353, 1962.
White, N. B.: Neurilemomas of the extremities. J. Bone Joint Surg. *49A*:1605, 1967.
White, H. R.: Survival in malignant schwannoma. Cancer *27*:720, 1971.
Woodruff, J. M., Chernik, N. L., et al.: Peripheral nerve tumors with rhabdomyosarcomatous differentiation (malignant "Triton" tumors). Cancer *32*:426, 1973.
Yeoman, P. M.: Fatty infiltration of the median nerve. J. Bone Joint Surg. *46B*:737, 1964.

43

DIFFERENTIAL DIAGNOSIS OF PERIPHERAL NEUROPATHIES

PETER TSAIRIS

DEFINITIONS AND SYMPTOMATOLOGY

A peripheral neuropathy is a disorder affecting, to a variable degree, the peripheral motor, sensory, or autonomic nerves. If only one nerve is affected, it is considered a mononeuropathy. If several nerves are involved in a distal symmetrical or asymmetrical fashion, then this pattern is characterized as a polyneuropathy. If there are multiple single peripheral nerves or their branches involved, then this pattern is referred to as a mononeuritis multiplex.

Patients who suffer from any form of peripheral neuropathy will often describe their symptoms by characteristic expressions, using such words as prickling, burning, or jabbing sensations, which will often indicate to the knowledgeable physician whether or not there is disease in the peripheral nerves. Similarly, patients who present with muscle weakness will talk about their functional disability; for example, the difficulty they might have with their hands in fastening buttons or safety pins, or with their feet, such as an inability to pick up their feet or toes without stumbling. It should be emphasized that a patient's statement that some part of his extremity is "numb" may not indicate disease of the peripheral nervous system. The term "numbness" may be used loosely by patients to mean tiredness, fatigue, or heaviness of a limb or limbs. Patients with arthralgias and myalgias, especially if they are poorly localized, frequently do not have a neuropathy and, thus, the misinterpretation to mean a neuritis can be misleading. In addition to analyzing the symptoms, several lines of inquiries should be followed in every suspected case of peripheral neuropathy. The patient who presents with symptoms suggesting an isolated mononeuropathy should also be asked about symptoms suggesting systemic disease, since some diseases such as diabetes mellitus, nutritional deficiency states, or renal failure may first manifest as a mononeuropathy. Inquiries should be made regarding recent infectious illnesses. A knowledge that the patient has had a recent infectious disease (for example, infectious mononucleosis) may lead to a correct diagnosis. Exposure to toxic substances at home or at work, and whether a patient is taking alcohol or drugs excessively should be determined. A history of travel abroad, or past habitation in Asia, Africa, or the southwestern United States could lead to a correct diagnosis of leprosy. In rare situations, arsenic or thallium poisoning should be suspected if the patient is depressed or if there is any knowledge of marital infidelity. The family history is equally important. There may be relatives with systemic diseases such as diabetes mellitus or acute intermittent porphyria or several relatives with signs suggesting a hereditary neuropathy. Occasionally, patients may have a hereditary neuropathy but be unaware of the similarity of their disorder to that of others within the same kinship. Furthermore, patients will often attribute neuromuscular dysfunction in other members of their families to other, unrelated diseases when they are actually all afflicted by the identical disease process. Dietary histories are important, especially in alcoholic or elderly patients who may be malnourished. Careful detective work may also uncover conditions such as diabetes mellitus or chronic renal failure in patients who are neurologically asymptomatic but exhibit significant sensory or motor abnormalities on examination.

Once the diagnosis of a peripheral neuropathy is established, either by examination or electrophysiological studies, other laboratory tests are necessary to determine the cause of the neuropathy. The tests most frequently ordered (Table 43–1) obviously depend on what diagnostic possibilities are suggested by the history and examination. Even with these tests, an etiology can be found in no more than 50 per cent of the patients who are admitted to hospital for evaluation. When the cause is determined, therapy can be direct and affective. If an etiological diagnosis is not established, various forms of therapy are available to ameliorate the disabilities which these patients experience.

CLASSIFICATION SYSTEMS

We now recognize that clinical neurophysiological techniques, biochemical studies, and morphological analyses of nerve biopsies have contributed immensely to the classification of the systemic and hereditary polyneuropathies. However, since the definition of a neuropathy may be based on a variety of clinical features, and since the definition is somewhat arbitrary, several classification systems have been proposed. These systems have been based on etiological factors, clinical features, results of nerve electrophysiology, nerve pathology, and associated chemical disturbances; for example, changes in spinal fluid protein. Miller's classification (Miller, 1966) appeals to most neurologists

Table 43–1   Evaluation of Peripheral Neuropathy

TEST	DISEASE STATE
Glucose metabolism	Diabetes mellitus
Blood urea metabolism	Uremia
Serological/antibody studies	Collagen vascular diseases
Thyroid function	Myxedema, acromegaly
Hematological studies, Schilling test	Pernicious anemia — coagulation disorders
Stool fat, blood carotene	Malabsorption syndrome
Protein electrophoresis, ±bone marrow	Multiple myeloma, Waldenstrom's dysglobinemia
Porphyrins (Watson-Schwartz Test)	Acute intermittent porphyria
Heavy metal determinations (Pb, As, Hg, thallium)	Toxic neuropathies
Heterophil	Infectious mononucleosis
Special malignancy studies	Carcinomatous neuropathy
Infectious disease studies	Herpes zoster, leprosy
OTHER LESS COMMON TESTS	
Phytanic acid (urine)	Refsum's disease
Urinary sulfatides (aryl sulfatase A)	Metachromatic leukodystrophy (MLD)
α Lipoproteins	Tangier's disease
β Lipoproteins	Bassen-Kornzweig's syndrome
Rectal or gingival biopsy	Amyloidosis
Nerve biopsy (selected cases)	Leprosy, MLD, amyloidosis, vasculitis or periarteritis, peroneal muscular atrophies

because of its simplicity. In this classification, he divides neuropathy into four categories:

1. Loss of neurons in anterior horn or dorsal ganglia or both.
2. Proximal demyelinization with nerve root involvement.
3. Dying-back neuropathies due to toxic poisoning or systemic diseases.
4. Lesions affecting the supporting tissues of peripheral nerves.

Table 43–2 lists these different categories and gives some examples. In some instances, the disease, either genetic or systemic, may affect both central and peripheral nerve tissues. This creates some difficulty in classification (for example, in disorders of a dorsal sensory root); there may also be degeneration of axons in the peripheral nerve and in the dorsal columns of the spinal cord. Additional confusion may arise as to the site of involvement and the cause of a peripheral neuropathy. For example, some disorders of motor or

Table 43–2   Classification of Peripheral Neuropathies (Miller)

1. Disease of motor or sensory neurons or both — peroneal muscular atrophy (CMT), hereditary sensory neuropathy, carcinomatous neuropathy
2. Proximal demyelination with spinal root damage — Landry-Guillain-Barré syndrome, diphtheritic neuritis
3. Dying-back neuropathies due to toxins or systemic illnesses — heavy metals, isoniazid, nutritional deficiencies, acute intermittent porphyria
4. Lesions affecting supporting tissues, including vasculature — collagen vascular diseases, leprosy, amyloidosis

sensory neurons whose cell bodies lay near or in the central nervous system are first revealed by symptoms and signs in the most distal portions of their axons, or the so called dying-back phenomenon (Spencer and Schaumburg, 1976). Spinal muscular atrophies in which anterior horn cells undergo degeneration, thus leading to a loss of the motor axons in peripheral nerves, are not customarily considered peripheral neuropathy. Nevertheless, it must be remembered that in many neuropathies in which there is primary degeneration of motor axons, the disturbance may lie within the cell body, and thus distinction between an anterior horn cell disorder (spinal muscular atrophy) and a peripheral motor neuropathy may well be artificial. Diabetic neuropathy defies clearcut classification because its pathogenesis is multifactorial, e.g., there may be a disturbance of lipid metabolism in the myelin sheath and/or ischemia due to arterial sclerosis or vasculitis of the vasa nervorum.

Focal nerve involvement by trauma, compression, traction, and tumors is, by convention, not included in an outline of medical mononeuropathies and polyneuropathies. However, it is important to remember that a few genetic, metabolic, and inflammatory conditions of peripheral nerves or roots may masquerade as isolated mononeuropathies. These mononeuropathies may be misdiagnosed as entrapment neuropathies and thus lead to unnecessary surgery. At the end of this section, I will discuss those medical and neurological disorders that increase a patient's susceptibility to focal compression of nerves.

There have been many advances in our understanding of the pathogenesis and pathophysiology of peripheral nerve disease. For those who would like a fuller explanation of this subject, excellent reviews can be found in recently published monographs by Dyck, Thomas, and Lambert, 1975; Vinken and Bruyn, 1970; and Bradley, 1975.

CLINICAL DIAGNOSTIC ASPECTS

In most patients with polyneuropathy, distal weakness is more prominent than proximal weakness, and usually there is an accompanying sensory abnormality. In a mononeuropathy, muscles innervated by a single peripheral nerve are weak and/or atrophic. This pattern must be differentiated from that in a patient with a radiculopathy in which only the muscles supplied by a single root are affected, or that in a patient with a plexopathy in which the pattern of motor and sensory dysfunction is in a multiple root or peripheral nerve distribution. Ascertaining the anatomical distribution of a nerve lesion is probably the most important aspect of the examination. In most cases, the mapping of the motor and sensory loss will quickly point to one of the several patterns of involvement previously defined. Differentiation, however, is not always easy. The detection of sensory abnormalities can be quite difficult at times, and thus tests with greater degrees of sophistication have been designed. Dyck (1972) states that much of the reason for lack of sensory findings is due to the crude testing that is generally done, or to unreliable or uncooperative patients. A more quantitative evaluation of touch can be gained by using von Frey hairs. Other methods have been devised for quantitative evaluation of touch and the thermal sensations (Dyck et al, 1972; Dyck et al., 1974). The loss of sensation in peripheral neuropathies may involve all sensory modalities, or the impairment may be restricted to particular forms of sensation. Two patterns of selective sensory loss have been recognized; in one form there is a selective loss of pain and temperature sensation which correlates with loss of small myelinated fibers. In the other there may be a loss of touch-pressure, tactile two-point discrimination, and joint position sense, which correlates with disease and/or loss of large myelinated fibers. It should be remembered that in testing position sense of the finger joints, the normal patient should be able to perceive the smallest movement of the joint that can be made by the examiner. The examiner's proprioceptive mechanisms are used to rate those of the patient. In testing joint position of the toes, larger movements must be made. The testing of vibration sense requires the use of a good tuning fork, preferably at 128 Hz. Hysterical abnormalities of vibration sense are best detected by demonstrating differences on two sides of a bony structure; for example, at the forehead or on the sternum. If there is splitting of the midline (one side normal and the other abnormal) of such a bony structure, then this should be a clue that there is no real defect in sensory appreciation.

When there is a pattern of dissociated sensory loss, the sensory dysfunction may be limited to pain and temperature appreciation and there is preservation of proprioception and touch-pressure modalities. In this pattern one finds a diffuse but selective loss of small myelinated axons and also a substantial loss of unmyelinated axons. Cases of this pattern of sensory disturbance have been recognized for over 50 years, and may be seen as the primary manifestation in patients with syringomyelia, hereditary sensory neuropathy, and hereditary primary amyloidosis of the peripheral nervous system.

In Friedreich's ataxia there is a selective loss of proprioception and vibratory sensation and impairment of touch-pressure sensibility, whereas pain and temperature is preserved. This is due to degeneration of the primary afferent neurons with a concomitant selective disappearance of larger myelinated fibers (Dyck, 1972).

When patients complain of tingling, prickling or abnormal thermal sensations, these symptoms fall into the category of *paresthesias*. This sensory disturbance is the most frequent manifestation of a purely sensory or a mixed sensorimotor neuropathy. Paresthesias may be felt in the territory of a single nerve. In a symmetrical polyneuropathy they exhibit a distal glove and stocking distribution. Their origin is not clear. The terms hyperesthesia and hyperpathia have been employed in a variety of ways but in general refer to an unpleasant quality that a patient experiences following a light cutaneous stimulation. With painful stimuli such as following a pin prick the threshold for appreciation of the sensation is usually elevated but if one repeats application of the pin sensation at the same site, this may lead to a steadily increasing unpleasant stinging or burning pain that radiates diffusely from the site of stimulation. When this reaction occurs, the term hyperalgesia may be used. All of these phenomona are usually encountered following peripheral nerve injury or recovery from such injury. Such sensations may also be primary manifestations of alcoholic or diabetic sensory neuropathies and may be localized manifestations of postherpetic neuralgia.

One cannot adequately discuss the nature of peripheral neuropathies without mentioning pain, which may constitute the most troublesome symptom in many types of neuropathies. In mononeuropathy, pain can occur within a territory of distribution of a nerve; for example, the burning pain of meralgia paresthetica. At other times, involvement of single nerves may result in widely radiating pain which may create diagnostic problems. Some polyneuropathies are uniformly painless whereas others have pain of varying severity. Patients with diabetic neuropathy or ischemic neuropathy frequently have nocturnal pains in the lower leg or thighs, or lancinating pain similar to the "lightning" pains of tabes dorsalis. The neuropathy of multiple myeloma or dysglobulinemia is frequently painful. In general the mechanisms of pain in these and other neuropathies are as yet unknown. A discussion of causalgia is covered in other sections of this book (see Chapters 12 and 17).

Ataxic limb movements and tremor of outstretched hands are sometimes observed in neuropathies in the absence of any detectable central nervous system disturbance. When there is a primary sensory ataxia, resulting from proprioceptive deafferentation of the upper extremities, this may be reflected in the occurrence of peculiar movements of the fingers when the hands are outstretched with the eyes closed (pseudoathetosis). These movements and associated limb ataxia may occur in certain types of diabetic neuropathy affecting large myelinated fibers (diabetic pseudotabes).

Autonomic nervous system dysfunction or dysautonomias should alert the physician to the possibility of a generalized neuropathy. Disturbances of the sympathetic system and of the sacral parasympathetic outflow may occur in a number of polyneuropathies (Table 43–3); however, the differential diagnosis should include the systems degenerations and spinal cord diseases which affect the preganglionic neuron. Disturbances of pupillary function, orthostatic hypotension, anhidrosis, disturbances of genitourinary or alimentary tract functions are the most commonly seen manifestations of dysautonomia. Pupillary disturbances (that is, sluggish responses to light) are common in diabetic autonomic neuropathy. Although Horner's syndrome is seen with localized lesions affecting the first thoracic nerve root or cervical sympathetic chain, by and large, ocular sympathetic involvement is not a frequent accompaniment of generalized neuropathies. Defects of vasomotor function have been demonstrated in a variety of conditions associated with peripheral neuropathy; namely, acute intermittent porphyria, carcinomatous neuropathy, the Guillain-Barré syndrome, amyloidosis, and sometimes alcoholic neuropathy. Orthostatic hypotension may be the presenting symptom in amyloid neuropathy. Diabetic patients with autonomic neuropathy may also have excessive heat

**Table 43–3   Causes of Dysautonomia in Peripheral
Neuropathies**

1. Diabetes mellitus (diabetic dysautonomia)
2. Amyloidosis
3. Inflammation of nerves and roots (infectious and post-infectious polyradiculoneuropathy)
4. Porphyria
5. Alcoholism (toxic-nutritional neuropathy)
6. Uremia
7. Paraneoplastic syndromes
8. Multiple endocrine adenomata
9. Familial and genetic disorders

intolerance or excessive sweating in the upper parts of the body. This sweating abnormality is due to a deficiency in pseudomotor innervation and may occur in a cutaneous territory of a peripheral nerve. Patients with diabetic and amyloid neuropathy may also have profound disturbances of genitourinary function; for example, they may have voiding difficulties or retention with overflow incontinence, owing to a motor disturbance or lack of awareness of bladder fullness as a result of a disturbance in the sensory arc of the bladder reflex. Some patients may be impotent as a result of failure of erection or ejaculation, or both, due to interference with parasympathetic innervation. Retrograde ejaculation may sometimes be encountered in diabetic subjects. Most of the symptoms related to dysfunction of the gastrointestinal tract are seen in diabetic autonomic neuropathy; for example, the occurrence of megacolon is not uncommon.

Palpation of peripheral nerves is an integral part of the examination and should be carried out in normal patients as well as those suspected of having a peripheral neuropathy. Only after repeated testing does it become possible to decide whether a nerve has become hypertrophic. The ulnar nerve in the cubital fossa, the median nerve at the elbow, the superficial cutaneous nerves of the neck above the clavicle, and the peroneal nerve at the head of the fibula are common sites for palpation. Hypertrophic nerves are commonly seen in genetic polyneuropathy, namely those that come under the category of peroneal muscular atrophy. Nerve enlargement may also be found in lepromatous neuropathy, especially of the ulnar nerve. In leprosy, the enlargement of the nerve usually extends for a greater distance up the arm or may be maximal at some distance proximal to the elbow. In contrast, a simple entrapment of the ulnar nerve at the elbow produces enlargement usually restricted to a few cemtimeters in and above the groove. Less commonly, nerve enlargement may be found in acute Guillain-Barré syndrome, chronic relapsing polyneuritis, amyloid neuropathy, and the neuropathy sometimes seen in acromegaly. Schwann cell proliferation is the hallmark of both the genetic and acquired forms of hypertrophic neuropathy. Although the enlargement in acromegaly has been referred to as hypertrophic neuropathy, the nerves become larger as a result of connective tissue overgrowth. When one sees a localized swelling subcutaneously in relation to nerve trunks, one should also consider the possibility of neurofibromatosis or some other solitary peripheral nerve tumor, such as a schwannoma.

Chronic neuropathies frequently give rise to foot, hand, and spinal deformities. If there is significant denervation then trophic changes may become quite profound. Clawing of the toes and fingers may develop in any type of chronic neuropathy but the presence of this deformity or pes cavus or spinal deformity usually indicates onset in childhood, and this may be of diagnostic importance. Hand and foot deformities can, in most cases, be attributed to muscle weakness. In the hereditary hypertrophic neuropathies these deformities are usually seen in the legs; for example, equinovarus positions of the foot, cavus deformity of the foot, and clawing of the toes. Kyphoscoliosis is more commonly seen in the spinocerebellar degenerations rather than in the pure forms of hereditary polyneuropathy.

When we refer to trophic changes we are talking about the alterations in the skin, nails, and subcutaneous tissues that follow denervation in a longstanding neuropathy. This does not mean that there is a loss of specific trophic function by nerve fibers. In addition to their occurrence in diabetic neuropathy, trophic changes are also encountered in hereditary neuropathy, lepromatous neuropathy, the various types of peroneal muscular atrophy with sensory loss, and hereditary amyloid neuropathy. The term acrodystrophic neuropathy (Spillane and Wells, 1969) describes cases of a mixed sensorimotor neuropathy in which there are distal trophic alterations and bony changes, or what we may call a "neuropathic arthropathy." Osteomyelitis can occur in this setting.

The diagnosis, localization, and prognosis of any neuropathic process is facilitated by using various methods of electrodiagnosis. While diagnosis and localization can often be determined by a simple examination, prognosis requires repeated testing and sometimes specific biochemical and pharmacological studies. Generally speaking polyneuropathies can be subdivided into those in which there is widespread segmental demyelination and those in which the primary disturbance is axonal degeneration. When there is a substantial reduction in nerve conduction velocity, this usually implies extensive or widespread segmental demyelination. Conduction velocities tend to be within normal limits or slightly reduced when there is primary involvement of the axons. In the latter case, the evaluation of motor conduction velocities may not be helpful in distinguishing these diseases from anterior horn-cell involvement in which motor conduction may be similarly affected. In most peripheral neuropathies, sensory nerve conduction studies are abnormal, even in situations when no sensory dysfunction can be determined by examination. It must be remembered, however, that in lesions affecting the sensory roots proximal to the dorsal root ganglia, the sensory conduction in the limbs will be preserved even if there is evidence of total sensory loss. In some patients, when there is difficulty in distinguishing between a motor neuropathy and a myopathic process, needle electromyography recordings are usually decisive.

Nerve biopsy is rarely necessary to substantiate a diagnosis of peripheral neuropathy. It may be helpful in some instances in confirming or defining the nature of the pathological process; for example, in amyloidosis, leprosy, and metachromatic leukodystrophy. The indications, however, are highly individualized; furthermore, all biopsies should be done in a center where there are adequate technical facilities, especially electron microscopy.

DIFFERENTIAL DIAGNOSIS

When the etiology of a peripheral neuropathy is not apparent, several other clinical features must be used to construct a differential diagnosis. The neuropathies beginning in infancy or childhood are usually genetic or inflammatory. Those beginning in adulthood are either metabolic, toxic, or inflammatory. Determining the distribution of neural involvement, or a pattern of a neuropathy, may suggest a diagnosis or even limit the diagnostic possibilities. In severe symmetrical polyneuropathies, a mixed motor and sensory loss in a distal distribution is usually the case. This pattern is associated with a loss of tendon reflexes at the ankles or wrists but not at the knees or elbows. A variety of factors may be involved in determining this type of selective distal

**Table 43–4   Some Commonly Used Drugs that Cause
Peripheral Neuropathy**

Chloramphenicol	Gold salt
cis-dichloramineplatinum (II): DDP	Hydralazine (Apresoline)
Citrated calcium carbimide (Abstem)	Isoniazid (INH)
Dapsone (Avlosulfon)	Methaqualone (Quaalude)
Diphenylhydantoin	Metronidazole (Flagyl)
Disopyramide phospate (Norpace)	Nitrofurantoin (Furadantin)
Disulfiram (Antabuse)	Nitrofurazone
Ethionamide	Vinblastine (Velban)
Glutethemide (Doriden)	Vincristine (Oncovin)

distribution. Some of these neuropathies may be of the "dying-back" type; i.e., there is degeneration of the distal axons, suggesting that the neurons that have the longest axons to maintain may be the first to suffer. Neuropathies due to drug toxicity fit into this category (Table 43–4). The first indications of these types of polyneuropathy are usually in the legs, but occasionally the initial symptoms and signs may be in the upper extremities. Lead neuropathy may begin with a bilateral wrist drop before symptoms appear in the lower extremities. Symptoms of a distal sensory neuropathy, beginning in the hands, should suggest a vitamin deficiency disorder, especially vitamin B_{12}. Some of these distal sensory neuropathies, which may mimic carpal tunnel syndrome, can be the initial manifestation for a dominantly inherited amyloid neuropathy. Symptoms of compression of the median nerve in the carpal tunnel by amyloid deposits in the synovium and even in the transverse carpal ligament have been reported (Mahloudji et al., 1969). In some symmetrical polyneuropathies, a proximal distribution of muscle weakness may be seen, and this is sometimes confused with a primary muscle disorder such as muscular dystrophy or polymyositis. Electrophysiological studies are helpful in pinpointing a neurogenic process. When one is found, one should consider a Guillain-Barré syndrome or a polyneuritis related to infectious mononucleosis. Occasionally, this type of proximal weakness is seen in acute intermittent porphyria where there also may be an associated proximal distribution of sensory loss. Several explanations have been given for this selective type of proximal involvement; some clinicians attribute this to an underlying polyradiculopathy because of an associated elevation of spinal fluid protein. Others attribute it to the fact that proximal portions of limbs are supplied by myelinated fibers larger than those innervating more distal areas and the trunk, suggesting that there may be a difference in susceptibility to immunological insults or metabolic changes. Lepromatous neuropathy, still a very common cause through the world, should be considered in any patient with a distal sensory neuropathy or a hypertrophic mononeuropathy. There may be depigmented and atrophic skin lesions in the tuberculoid type. In the lepromatous type there is usually a pattern of sensory deficit where there is sparing of some skin areas in the forearms or hands and involvement of some proximal areas, such as the ears. This type of deficit is felt to be related to tissue temperature gradients, i.e. the manifestations are due to infiltration by bacilli of the cooler body tissues (Hastings et al., 1968).

The clinical course of a neuropathy, that is the length of its progressive phase, may be of some diagnostic importance. Neuropathies with an abrupt onset and often associated with pain are usually of an ischemic origin, as in rheumatoid arthritis and polyarteritis nodosa (this disease may affect multiple nerves, leading to a mononeuritis multiplex), or in some mononeuropathies of diabetes mellitus, such as the cranial nerve palsies or femoral neuropathy (Raff, Sangalang, and Asbury, 1968). This presentation, of course, should be differentiated from nerve compression resulting from hemorrhage into or around a nerve trunk, or some direct external compression due to thermal injury, or to inadvertent injection into the nerve trunk. Neuropathies that evolve over a few days may be due to industrial intoxications, such as are seen with thallium or tri-ortho-cresyl phosphate. Diphtheria, which is now relatively uncommon and presents predominantly as a motor neuropathy, or some types of the Guillain-Barré syndrome may present with an abrupt onset. A neuropathy evolving over many weeks or months is commonly seen and should suggest several possibilities: exposure to toxic agents or drugs, nutritional deficiencies, a chronically abnormal metabolic state or a remote effect of a malignant disease, or even a genetic polyneuropathy which may have an insidious onset at any age. Despite the type of presentation, we are left with a large group of chronic progressive neuropathies of uncertain etiology which often leaves the neurologist perplexed (Prineas, 1970).

Disorders Which Can Simulate a Peripheral Neuropathy

Primary diseases of muscle are not usually confused with peripheral neuropathies, but in some cases electrophysiological studies are required for differentiation. If the neuromuscular dysfunction, mainly motor weakness, is gradual in onset and proximal in distribution, one must differentiate between polymyositis or one of the other dystrophic or biochemical diseases of muscle and an acute or subacute form of the Guillain-Barré syndrome. In some patients with polymyositis who have no muscle tenderness or involvement of other organ systems the disorder can be confused with the Guillain-Barré syndrome. Rarely, chronic polymyositis may present with a distal pattern of muscle weakness and wasting and, thus, may resemble a chronic motor neuropathy or a chronic distal spinal muscular atrophy (Prineas, 1970). Myotonic dystrophy will usually affect the distal muscles. In some of these patients there may be clinically undetectable myotonic phenomena, and thus the pattern may look like a peripheral motor neuropathy. However, other features of this disorder are usually evident, such as selective atrophy of the sterno-mastoid muscles, ptosis, atrophy and weakness of the temporalis muscles, frontal baldness, and cataracts. There are rare cases of muscular dystrophy beginning in adulthood which present as distal motor weakness, but these usually commence in the upper extremities. In children or adolescents who present with acute or subacute proximal weakness in the limbs, the diagnosis of myasthenia gravis should be considered even if there is little or no oculobulbar involvement. These patients will fatigue easily during repetitive exercise of the limbs, and this may be a significant differentiating feature. In adults, the Eaton-Lambert-Rooke syndrome (Lambert and Rooke, 1965) may be confused with a peripheral neuropathy. These patients have weakness mainly in the proximal distribution of their lower extremities with no ocular, facial, or bulbar weakness. The confusion lies in that they have a generalized depression of their tendon reflexes, and occasionally there is associated autonomic dysfunction. Electrophysiological studies are usually necessary to differentiate this syndrome from a peripheral neuropathy. In brief, these patients will show a post-tetanic facilitation either on examination or during repetitive nerve stimulation.

Spinal muscular atrophies and progressive motor neuron disease, (amyotrophic lateral sclerosis) may present with distal weakness (bilateral foot-drop and absence of ankle jerks), and thus may simulate a predominantly peripheral motor neuropathy. Initially, signs of spasticity may be absent, making diagnosis difficult, but may appear later on in the course of the disease. The spinal muscular atrophy patient will not develop signs of spasticity and will continue to have progressive weakness with no sensory change. Obviously, careful sensory testing and electrophysiological examinations of sensory nerve action potentials are required to differentiate these cases from peripheral mixed motor sensory neuropathy.

Distal sensory neuropathies may be confused with several disorders. The distal sensory neuropathy of diabetes may be clinically similar to that seen in tabes dorsalis, but differentiation between tabes and a distal sensory neuropathy is usually not difficult, mainly because there is no impairment of tactile sensation in the former, and also because a serological test for syphilis will give the answer. Distal symmetrical or asymmetrical paresthesias in the extremities without a significant component of muscle weakness should be differentiated from the spinal cord disorder seen with multiple sclerosis, cervical spondylytic myelopathy, or occasionally from extradural tumors of the cervical cord. Constant severe pain in the neck or pain with flexion of the neck (Lhermitte's sign) usually indicates cervical cord disease. Sometimes, symptoms or signs of spasticity may occur later in these myelopathies, and this creates problems in diagnosis, but electrophysiological testing usually resolves the issue.

In some patients, hysterical sensory loss may simulate a peripheral neuropathy. These patients usually have a glove-stocking distribution, but inconsistencies revealed by sensory testing along with the preservation of reflexes and sensory nerve action potentials on electrodiagnostic tests will indicate the nature of the problem. Patients with chronic tension and anxiety who have paresthesias in their limbs are frequently suspected of having a sensory neuropathy, but appropriate testing will reveal otherwise. Furthermore, the hyperventilation syndrome will sometimes present in this fashion and may not always be noticed or admitted by the patient.

Neuropathies Simulating Other Disorders

Although relatively uncommon, certain mononeuropathies or polyneuropathies may masquerade as other degenerative muscle diseases or other systemic illnesses. As indicated, acute or subacute neuropathies with proximal muscle weakness, normal tendon reflexes, and no sensory loss can be mistaken for acute or indolent polymyositis. It must be emphasized that patients who have proximal weakness without sensory changes must be looked at very carefully for the simple reason that several neuropathic diseases will give the appearance of primary disease of muscle or a disorder of neuromuscular transmission. Some systemic diseases (e.g., sarcoidosis) may present with cranial nerve involvement initially and be confused with myasthenia gravis. Similarly, other neuropathies may simulate spinal cord disease. Tangier's disease may present with muscle weakness and wasting, areflexia, and associated pain and temperature loss, which may be on a central basis, in addition to their peripheral neuropathy (Kocen et al., 1973). Lastly, patients who present with acute or subacute weakness, but who have intact reflexes and no sensory loss, and who on examination exhibit bizarre personality or psychotic disturbances, will sometimes be diagnosed as hysterical when, in fact, a positive Watson–Schwartz test will indicate that they have porphyria.

DISORDERS AFFECTING LIABILITY TO PRESSURE NEUROPATHY

There are several medical disorders and polyneuropathies which may be complicated by superimposed isolated nerve lesions as a consequence of a patient's abnormal susceptibility to focal compression of peripheral nerves:

1. Diabetes mellitus

We know that patients with longstanding or poorly controlled diabetes are more prone to neuropathies but, in addition, there is also an increased incidence of focal pressure neuropathies in these patients (Mulder et al., 1961). The metabolic disturbance in diabetes mellitus may reduce the safety factor of nerve conduction and produce abnormalities in excitability of the nodal membrane, all of which may predispose the diseased nerve to be excited by the slightest degree of traction or compression. Involvement of most peripheral nerves has been reported, but the most often affected are the ulnar, median, radial, femoral, lateral cutaneous of the thigh, and peroneal nerves. A case of selected involvement of the deep palmar branch of the ulnar nerve has been described in a diabetic woman (Finelli, 1975). This patient experienced trauma to the palmar surface of the hand and then noticed progressive weakness and wasting of her hand without associated pain or sensory loss. The significance of this case is that the disorder was misdiagnosed as motor neuron disease, based on an electromyographic study which was limited to the affected extremity. An incomplete interpretation or misinterpretation of an EMG study may be a key source of such errors. Motor neuron disease is not an uncommon misdiagnosis when there is involvement of the deep palmar branch of the ulnar nerve. This case illustrates two points: that metabolic peripheral nerve disorders may masquerade as isolated mononeuropathies and that it is extremely important to accurately diagnose diseases that cause intrinsic muscle weakness and wasting of the hand.

Other commonly reported sites for external pressure palsies in diabetics are the radial nerve in the upper arm (Mulder et al., 1961), the common peroneal nerve at the neck of the fibula (Shohani and Spalding, 1969), and common entrapment sites such as the median nerve in the carpal tunnel or the ulnar nerve in the cubital tunnel (Gilliatt and Willison, 1962).

2. Hereditary Neuropathies

In addition to systemic diseases, genetic factors also predispose to the development of pressure neuropathies. Most of these neuropathies are transient; however, some have resulted in persistent deficits. Davies (1954) described a familial form of multiple mononeuropathy which was precipitated by minor pressure or traction. Members of the afflicted family gave a history of recurrent weakness and sensory symptoms in the distribution of one peripheral nerve that was exposed to minor compression or traction. In some families with similar predispositions to the development of pressure neuropathies, electrophysiological abnormalities were also found in non-symptomatic members (Earl et al., 1964: Behse et al., 1972). In addition, sural nerve biopsies on some affected members of these families have shown irregular thickening of the myelin sheath and demyelination (Behse et al., 1972). The cause for increased susceptibility of isolated peripheral nerves in the genetic polyneuropathies remains unknown.

3. Guillain-Barré Syndrome

Patients recovering from this type of inflammatory polyradiculoneuropathy sometimes develop external pressure palsies; for example, of the median nerve at the wrist, the ulnar nerve at the elbow, or the peroneal nerve at the knee (Lambert and Mulder, 1964). These patients usually do not complain of the classical symptoms of these isolated neuropathies at these various sites.

Pressure neuropathies are also frequent complications in patients suffering from malnutrition (Denny-Brown, 1947), alcoholism, and renal failure (Preswick and Jeremy, 1964). The cause for this increased susceptibility in these systemic illnesses also remains unknown, but it is clear that peripheral nerves are more sensitive to the effects of minor trauma or compression when there is underlying systemic or genetic disease, and this should be kept in mind with every patient who presents with a mononeuropathy.

SOME ASPECTS OF TREATMENT

Successful treatment or rehabilitation of a patient with a peripheral neuropathy requires a multi-disciplined approach. Obviously, an accurate diagnosis, an assessment of the extent of the disease, prognostic indicators for recovery, and quantitative methods of documenting improvement are prerequisites to successful treatment. Electrodiagnostic techniques may be helpful in documenting improvement. Prevention of complications resulting from disuse (immobility) and recumbency is of paramount importance. For example, some patients with a severe sensory deficit must be warned against burning themselves. In elderly patients with vascular insufficiency the diseased peripheral nerve tissues cannot meet the demands of increased local metabolism that may be induced by excessive temperature. To prevent the breakdown of dry skin, and other trophic changes, the skin, especially in those patients with diabetic neuropathy, should be protected with a thin coat of lanolin cream. It is also important to retrain patients with muscle weakness so that they may achieve maximal independence. In addition, a number of therapeutic measures may be directed at the musculoskeletal system. Passive and active physiotherapy may prevent contractures across weakened joints and disuse atrophy at larger, more proximal joints. Hand or foot splints, and other ingenious devices in the hands of skilled occupational therapists, may allow performance of fine motor skills that otherwise would be impossible. These and other rehabilitative measures are more extensively covered in another part of this book (see Section VII).

Neuropathic pain can be a most troublesome feature of a peripheral neuropathy, even if there is associated anesthesia. The origin of neuropathic pain is speculative and will not be discussed here. When drug therapy is utilized for treatment of pain, we usually try to manage this symptom with mild analgesics alone or with codeine. However, the disabling aching pain that complicates chronic neuropathies may require long-term therapy with narcotics. The episodic or lancinating pains of diabetic neuropathy may respond to diphenylhydantoin (Dilantin); 300 to 500 mg per day has proved effective in some cases (Ellenberg, 1968). Some patients who fail to respond to Dilantin have a good chance of responding to Tegretol, 200 to 800 mg per day (Wilton, 1974). The tricyclic antidepressant drugs in combination with phenothiazines have been used effectively for relief of chronic intractable pain; they also have a mood-elevating action. It must be remembered, however, that chronic administration of Dilantin or the tricyclic antidepressants can cause neuropathy in itself (Table 43–4).

Nerve blocks or surgical section of a nerve or root or percutaneous cervical tractotomy have been variably ineffective for pain relief. Cutaneous electrical stimulation applied over injured isolated nerves or multiple diseased nerves has been reported to relieve intractable pain but to a variable degree and only for short time periods. Acupuncture therapy for the treatment for neurogenic pain has been a controversial issue. Basically, the usually transient improvement with acupuncture seems to reflect an alteration in the subject's acceptance of pain, but not in his threshold for noxious stimuli (Mann et al., 1973; Clark and Yang, 1974).

In many cases of peripheral neuropathy, an etiology can be found and a specific treatment instituted. However, where the cause is not known, several different types of therapies are available to lessen the disabilities of these patients. Achievement of treatment goals and demands by the patient require a close cooperation between physicians and other health professionals who are sufficiently aware of the complications to prevent them, and who also possess the skills for rehabilitation of patients who desire to become more functional.

REFERENCES

Behse, F., Buchthal, F., Carlsen, F., and Knappeis, G. G.: Conduction and histopathology of the sural nerve in hereditary neuropathy with liability to pressure palsies. Brain 95:777, 1972.

Bradley, W. G.: Disorders of Peripheral Nerves. Oxford, Churchill Livingstone, 1975.

Clark, W. C. and Yang, J. C.: Acupuncture analgesia? Evaluation by signal detection theory. Science 184:1096, 1974.

Davies, D. M.: Recurrent peripheral nerve palsies in a family. Lancet 2:266, 1954.

Denny-Brown, D.: Neurological conditions resulting from prolonged and severe dietary restriction. Medicine 26:41, 1947.

Dyck, P. J., Curtis, D. J., Bushek, W., and Offord, K.: Description of "Minnesota thermal disks" and normal values of cutaneous thermal discrimination in man. Neurology 24:325, 1974.

Dyck, P. J., Lambert, E. H., and Nichols, P. C.: Quantitative measurement of sensation related to compound action potential and number and sizes of myelinated and unmyelinated fibers of sural nerve in health, Friedreich's ataxia, hereditary sensory neuropathy, and tabes dorsalis. In Cobb, W. A. (ed.): Handbook of Electroencephalography and Clinical Neurophysiology. Amsterdam, Elsevier, 1972, Vol. 9, p. 83.

Dyck, P. J., Schultz, P. W. and O'Brien, P. C.: Quantitation of touch–pressure sensation. Arch. Neurol. 26:465, 1972.

Dyck, P. J., Thomas, P., and Lambert, E. H. (eds.): Peripheral Neuropathy. W. B. Saunders Co., Philadelphia, 1975.

Earl, C. J., Fullerton, P. M., Wakefield, A. S., and Schutta, H. S.: Hereditary neuropathy, with liability to pressure palsies. Quart. J. Med. 33:481, 1964.

Ellenberg, M.: Treatment of diabetic neuropathy with diphenylhydantoin. N.Y. State Med. J. 68:2653, 1968.

Finelli, P. F.: Mononeuropathy of the deep palmar branch of the ulnar nerve, a case occurring in a diabetic woman. Arch. Neurol. 32:564, 1975.

Gilliatt, R. W., and Willison, R. G.: Peripheral nerve conduction in diabetic neuropathy. J. Neurol. Neurosurg. Psychiatry 25:11, 1962.

Hastings, R. C., Brand, P. W., Mansfield, R. E., and Ebner, J. D.: Bacterial density in the skin in lepromatous leprosy as related to temperature. Lepr. Rev., 39:71, 1968.

Hollinrake, K.: Polymyositis presenting as distal muscle weakness: A case report. J. Neurol. Sci. 8:479, 1969.

Kocen, R. S., Thomas, P. K., Kind, R. H. M., and Haas, L. F.: Nerve biopsy in two cases of Tangier's disease, Acta Neuropath. 26:317, 1973.

Lambert, E. H., and Mulder, D. W.: Nerve junction studies in experimental polyneuritis electroencephalography. Clin. Neurophysiol. Suppl. 22:29, 1964.

Lambert, E. H., and Rooke, E. D.: Myasthenic state and lung cancer. In Brain, R. L., and Norris, F. H., Jr. (eds.): The Remote Effects of Cancer on the Nervous System. New York, Grune & Stratton, 1965, p. 67.

Mahloudji, M., et al.: The genetic amyloidoses, with particular reference to hereditary neuropathic amyloidosis, type II. Medicine 48:1, 1969.

Mann, F., Bowsher, D., Mumford, J., Lipton, S., and Miles, J.: Treatment of intractable pain by acupuncture. Lancet 2:57, 1973.

Melzack, R.: Prolonged relief of pain by brief, intense transcutaneous somatic stimulation. Pain 1:357, 1975.

Miller, H.: Polyneuritis. Brit. Med. J. 2:1219, 1966.

Mulder, D. W., Lambert, E. H., Bastron, J. A., and Sprague, R. G.: The neuropathies associated with diabetes mellitus. A clinical and electromyographic study of 103 unselected diabetic patients. Neurology 11:275, 1961.

Preswick, G., and Jeremy, D.: Subclinical polyneuropathy in renal insufficiency. Lancet 2:731, 1964.

Prineas, J. Polyneuropathies of undetermined cause. Acta Neurol. Scand. 46 (Suppl 44):1, 1970.

Raff, M. C., Sangalang, V., and Asbury, A. K.: Ischemic mononeuropathy multiplex associated with diabetes mellitus. Arch. Neurol. 18:487, 1968.

Shahani, B., and Spalding, J. M.: Diabetes mellitus presenting with bilateral foot drop. Lancet 2:930, 1969.

Spencer, P. S., and Schaumburg, H. H.: Central-peripheral axonapathy: The pathology of dying-back polyneuropathies. In Zimmerman, H. (ed.): Progress in Neuropathology. New York, Grune & Stratton, 1976, p. 253.

Spillane, J. D., and Wells, C. E. C.: Acrodystrophic Neuropathy. London, Oxford Medical Publications, 1969.

Thomas, P. K., Lascelles, R. G., Hallpike, J. F., and Hewer, R. L.: Recurrent and chronic relapsing Guillain-Barré polyneuritis. Brain 92:589, 1969.

Vinkin, P. J., and Bruyn, G. W. (eds.): Handbook of Clinical Neurology. Elsevier (North Holland), 1970, Vols. 7 and 8.

Wilton, T. D.: Tegretol in the treatment of diabetic neuropathy. S. Afr. Med. J. 48:869, 1974.

44

NEUROLOGICAL INVOLVEMENT OF THE EXTREMITIES ASSOCIATED WITH RHEUMATOID ARTHRITIS

LEWIS H. MILLENDER and MARK HALLETT

Pain, weakness, and sensory loss are prominent symptoms in patients with rheumatoid arthritis and can be caused by neuropathy, but the diagnosis can be difficult. The most frequent cause of pain, of course, is the arthritis itself, which can affect virtually all of the synovial joints in the body. Additionally, the inflammatory process can affect tendon sheaths and can lead to a painful tenosynovitis, such as flexor tenosynovitis associated with carpal tunnel syndrome. Destruction of the joints can lead to deformity, restriction of range of motion, and disuse, all of which produce weakness. Tendon rupture is another cause of weakness without neurologic involvement. The clinical assessment of true muscle weakness may be impossible in the face of significant joint pain and deformity. Since sensory symptoms can be experienced as a kind of pain, it is not surprising that, in this setting, they may be ascribed initially to the arthritis. When weakness is out of proportion to the joint disease, and when numbness and paresthesias are recognized, neurological involvement is clear, but even then one is faced with the differential diagnosis of myopathy, radiculopathy, and myelopathy as well as neuropathy. We will discuss the details of the several varieties of neuropathy encountered in patients with rheumatoid arthritis and then touch on the major features of the principal differential diagnostic entities.

727

NEUROPATHIES

There are three main classes of neuropathies in rheumatoid arthritis: (1) entrapment neuropathies, (2) a typically severe mononeuropathy multiplex, and (3) a mild, distal, mainly sensory polyneuropathy. The relative incidence of each type is not well established. Neuropathy seems not to be an inevitable concomitant of the disease, as it is, for example, in diabetes mellitus or uremia. On the other hand, nerve biopsies or electromyographic studies of asymptomatic patients may be abnormal (Beckett and Dinn, 1972).

Entrapment Neuropathies

Compression neuropathies are a frequent manifestation of rheumatoid arthritis, being seen mainly in the upper, but also in the lower, extremity. Their incidence has been reported to be as high as 45 per cent (Nakano, 1975). The most frequent cause of the compression is a proliferative rheumatoid tenosynovitis or synovitis which causes local compression over a segment of the nerve as it passes through a fibrous or fibro-osseous canal. In addition to this, bony protrusion, joint subluxations, and joint deformities can cause the syndrome. Two complete chapters in this text (35 and 37) are devoted to the compression neuropathies; therefore, in this section we will discuss only the specific characteristics that the rheumatoid patient presents.

Upper Extremity Compression Neuropathies

Median Nerve

Carpal tunnel syndrome is the most common rheumatoid compression neuropathy, being seen in approximately 23 per cent of rheumatoid patients (Chamberlain and Corbett, 1970) (Fig. 44–1). It may be the initial manifestation of the disease, and it is not uncommon to have the diagnosis of rheumatoid arthritis made by the pathologist after carpal tunnel release for what was thought to be an idiopathic carpal tunnel syndrome.

The early signs and symptoms of rheumatoid carpal tunnel syndrome are identical to those of carpal tunnel syndrome of other causes and include nocturnal symptoms, paresthesias in the median nerve distribution, and pain which extends both proximally and distally. As with idiopathic carpal tunnel syndrome, a high percentage may present bilaterally. As the condition progresses, involvement of the flexor tendons plus thenar atrophy can significantly affect hand function.

Wrist flexor tenosynovitis initially causes only symptoms of median nerve compression. However, as the proliferation continues, flexor tendon function becomes affected (Millender and Nalebuff, 1975). The early effects of this proliferation are minimal loss of active digital flexion, with passive flexion preserved. However, as the disease progresses, severe limitation of digital flexion may be seen. In addition to the wrist flexor tenosynovitis, the tenosynovium may extend into the palm and digits, and one should evaluate these areas

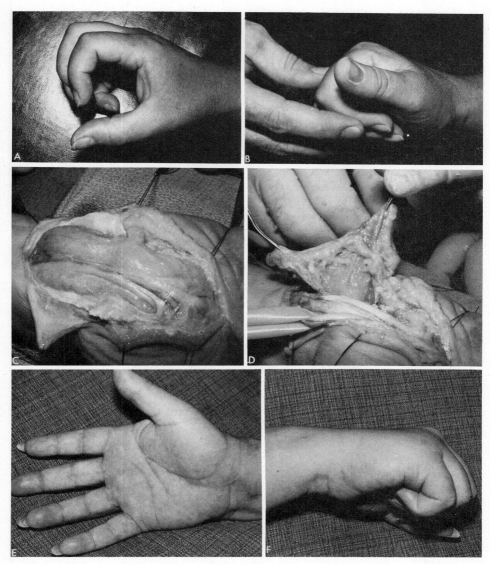

Figure 44–1   *A*, Patient complains of numbness in median nerve distribution and limited active digital flexion. *B*, Passive digital flexion preserved. *C*, Carpal tunnel exposed and median nerve seen surrounded by large amount of flexor tenosynovitis. *D*, Median nerve retracted with Penrose drain. Flexor tenosynovium plus large bursa exposed prior to tenosynovectomy. *E* and *F*, Full digital motion restored.

(Nalebuff and Potter, 1968). Digital fullness, palpable tendon nodules, and triggering are the common signs of palmar and digital flexor tenosynovitis.

Another complication of wrist flexor tenosynovitis is tendon rupture (Nalebuff, 1969). Although not common, tenosynovium can infiltrate into the flexor tendons, resulting in their rupture. When a tendon rupture is diagnosed, one must differentiate whether the rupture occurred at the wrist, palm, or digital level.

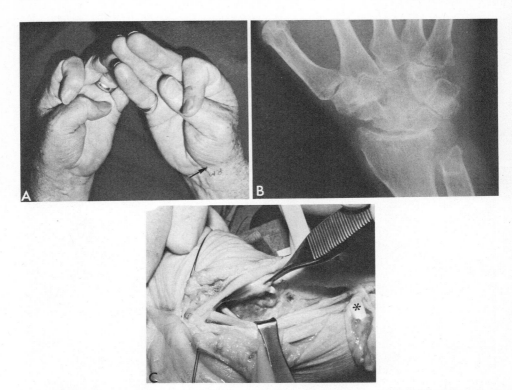

Figure 44-2 *A*, Patient with inability to actively flex interphalangeal joint of thumb or distal interphalangeal joint of index finger. Anterior interosseous nerve palsy suspected. Note arrow pointing to localized area of tenderness. *B*, Roentgenogram of the wrist demonstrates punched out lesion in the scaphoid often seen with ruptured flexor pollicis longus. *C*, Carpal tunnel exposed. Ruptured flexor pollicis longus held with forceps. The synovium from the wrist joint can be seen bulging through the capsule. The proximal end of the flexor pollicis longus has also been identified (asterisk).

An interesting manifestation of tendon rupture which must be differentiated from anterior interosseous nerve paralysis is the Mannerfelt syndrome (Fig. 44-2). In this condition there may be rupture of the flexor pollicis longus alone, or of the flexor pollicis longus plus the flexor digitorum profundus to the index and long digits from a sharp spur which develops on the anterior aspect of the scaphoid (Nalebuff, 1969). When a patient presents with inability to flex the interphalangeal joint of the thumb and the distal interphalangeal joint of the index finger, anterior interosseous nerve paralysis must be suspected (Spinner, 1972). Although anterior interosseous nerve paralysis is no more common in the rheumatoid patient than in the general population, the condition must be considered in differential diagnosis and ruled out. Oblique films of the wrist sometimes will show an erosion of the scaphoid. Additionally, electromyography can help confirm the diagnosis of anterior interosseous nerve paralysis.

The other serious complication of wrist flexor tenosynovitis is involvement of the thenar muscles. Generalized intrinsic muscle atrophy is commonly seen in the rheumatoid patient and is associated with cervical spine disease, median and ulnar nerve involvement, and disuse atrophy secondary to pain and joint involvement. Thenar atrophy can significantly affect the rheumatoid thumb, especially if there is associated joint involvement (Millender and Nalebuff, 1975). As thenar atrophy progresses, there is loss of active opposition which will lead to a fixed supination contracture with loss of effective pulp or key pinch. The end result of this ineffective side pinch is destruction of the interphalangeal joint or the metacarpophalangeal joint, or both.

The diagnosis of rheumatoid carpal tunnel syndrome can usually be established clinically, especially if there are wrist fullness and limited active digital flexion. One must be careful not to attribute all thenar atrophy to carpal tunnel syndrome, because of the multiple factors which can cause its appearance. When the clinical diagnosis is in doubt, electromyography and nerve conduction velocity studies should be obtained to confirm the diagnosis.

In addition to tenosynovitis, carpal tunnel syndrome can be associated with both wrist joint subluxation and lateral or fixed flexion contractures. One manifestation of rheumatoid arthritis is volar wrist dislocation associated with wrist destruction. This can cause symptoms of both median and ulnar nerve compression. Correction of the deformity by wrist arthrodesis or arthroplasty will usually alleviate the symptoms, although carpal tunnel release may be necessary (Millender and Nalebuff, 1975).

For early carpal tunnel syndrome associated with flexor tenosynovitis, steroid injection plus wrist splinting may give temporary or long-term remission, depending on the general condition of the disease. However, for persistent symptoms, especially if tendon function or thenar atrophy is associated, early carpal tunnel release with flexor tenosynovectomy is indicated. In addition to the wrist flexor tenosynovectomy, palmar or digital flexor tenosynovectomy, or both, should be carried out if indicated (Millender and Nalebuff, 1975). If flexor tendon ruptures are present, tendon transfers or intercalary tendon grafts may be necessary.

Ulnar Nerve

Ulnar nerve compression at the elbow is not especially common in rheumatoid arthritis (Nakano, 1975). It can be seen secondary to elbow synovitis, which bulges medially and compresses the nerve as it passes through the tunnel behind the medial epicondyle (Fig. 44–3). It can also be associated with scarring and narrowing of the ulnar tunnel secondary to the inflammatory process and destruction of the elbow joint. A less frequent cause is bony deformity. Rarely, ulnar nerve compression has been seen in association with a large olecranon bursa that has extended medially. Although many rheumatoid patients have elbow flexion contractures and cubitus valgus, few of them manifest symptoms of ulnar nerve compression. Even in cases of elbow instability due to joint destruction with ligamentous laxity, ulnar nerve involvement is not especially common.

Two additional causes of ulnar nerve compression are seen after lower extremity surgery and after total elbow replacement. Following major lower extremity surgery, such as total hip or total knee replacement, patients with weak hands sometimes will tend to push themselves up on their elbows. If done excessively, this can result in symptoms of ulnar nerve irritation. Also, patients using platform crutches can develop ulnar nerve symptoms if the crutches are inadequately padded or do not fit properly.

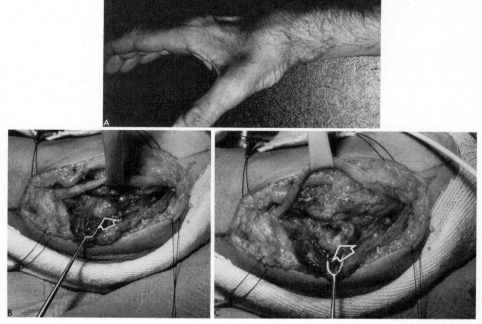

Figure 44–3 Ulnar nerve palsy associated with elbow joint synovitis. *A*, Interosseous muscle atrophy. *B*, The ulnar nerve is retracted and the synovium (arrow) is demonstrated bulging from medial aspect of the elbow joint. *C*, The capsule of the elbow joint is opened, demonstrating the proliferative synovitis (arrow).

A postoperative complication of total elbow replacement is the presence of ulnar nerve irritation symptoms. These symptoms are especially seen when the nerve is not completely mobilized and retracted prior to the joint resection or introduction of the methyl methacrylate. The symptoms are usually transient, and are probably related to traction on the nerve during surgery. They also may be associated with the heat of the methyl methacrylate. Permanent symptoms of ulnar nerve compression may be related to postoperative compression of the nerve, especially if it was not completely mobilized at the time of total joint replacement.

When ulnar nerve symptoms are associated with elbow joint synovitis, steroid injections into the joint and immobilization will often alleviate the condition. If elbow synovectomy is indicated, a separate medial incision should be made to release the ulnar nerve. In cases of ulnar nerve involvement associated with severe elbow destruction, total joint replacement is indicated. The nerve should be completely mobilized at the time of total elbow replacement.

Ulnar nerve entrapment at the wrist in Guyon's canal is seen much less frequently than median nerve compression associated with carpal tunnel syndrome (Shea and McClain, 1969; Spinner, 1972). This is understandable, since there are no tendons, and therefore no tenosynovium, within Guyon's canal. Rarely, ulnar nerve compression at the wrist level can be associated with large amounts of wrist flexor tenosynovitis. Swanson (1973) has stated that he has seen several cases of ulnar nerve motor impingement within Guyon's canal associated with flexor tenosynovitis. Ulnar nerve involvement at the wrist can also be associated with wrist dislocation and wrist joint deformities similar to median nerve involvement (Millender and Nalebuff, 1973).

When patients present with symptoms of ulnar nerve compression, the diagnosis may not be easily established. Many of these patients have multiple joint involvements and can have, in addition to wrist and elbow involvement, evidence of cervical spine disease (Nakano, 1975). As with the median nerve, the ulnar nerve may become entrapped concomitantly with lower cervical spine disease or also with thoracic outlet syndrome.

Posterior Interosseous Nerve Paralysis

Posterior interosseous nerve paralysis is a rare but well-documented complication of rheumatoid arthritis (Millender, Nalebuff, and Holdsworth, 1973) (Fig. 44–4). It results from elbow synovitis bulging anteriorly and compressing the posterior interosseous nerve as it enters into the supinator muscle. Depending upon the degree of nerve compression, either a partial or complete paralysis of the muscles innervated by the posterior interosseous nerve will be seen. The clinical appearance of the compression neuropathy, especially when it is partial, is quite similar to extensor tendon ruptures, and in two cases reported in the literature, patients were initially explored for extensor tendon ruptures (Marmor, Lawrence, and Dubois, 1967; Millender, Nalebuff, and Holdsworth, 1973).

The presenting manifestation will be inability to extend either all or some of the digits and thumb. In two of the three cases we have seen there was inability to extend the ulnar three digits at the metacarpophalangeal joint, with extension preserved in the index finger and extension and abduction preserved in the thumb (Millender, Nalebuff, and Holdsworth, 1973).

The proper diagnosis is readily established by careful clinical examination. The patient will show evidence of elbow synovitis with pain, limitation of digital extension, and tenderness over the anterior aspect of the elbow joint. There is usually absence of dorsal tenosynovitis, which would tend to rule out extensor tendon rupture. When the wrist is passively flexed the metacarpophalangeal joints will extend, demonstrating that the extensor tendons are intact (Fig. 4B and D). In tendon rupture, the distal ends usually retract distal to the wrist joint, thereby giving a negative tenodesis effect when the wrist is flexed. The most important physical findings are radial deviation of the wrist on active extension due to paralysis of the extensor carpi ulnaris with preservation of the extensor carpi radialis longus and brevis. In addition, any digital extensor tendons that are functioning will show definite weakness. Electromyography can be used to confirm the diagnosis.

The treatment will depend upon the degree of involvement and the length of time the compression has existed. In one of the cases that we treated with a steroid injection into the elbow joint the patient showed partial recovery of extensor tendon function in two weeks and full recovery with full strength in six weeks. In another case, anterior exploration of the posterior interosseous nerve with elbow synovectomy was carried. out. The patient showed return of extensor tendon function within 24 hours and full return of function within four days. In

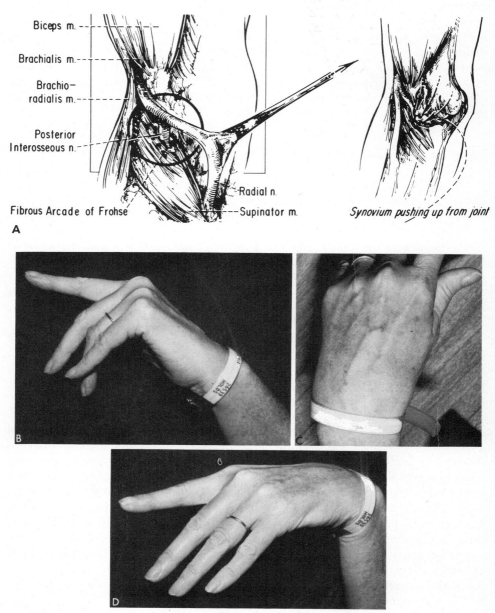

Figure 44–4 Posterior interosseous nerve paralysis associated with rheumatoid arthritis. *A*, Diagram demonstrates the elbow synovitis bulging anteriorly and compressing the posterior interosseous nerve as it penetrates the two heads of the supinator muscle. *B*, Partial posterior interosseous nerve paralysis with inability to extend lateral three digits. *C*, Wrist extension is associated with radial deviation due to paralysis of extensor carpi ulnaris. *D*, Positive tenodesis effect demonstrating that the extensor tendons are intact.

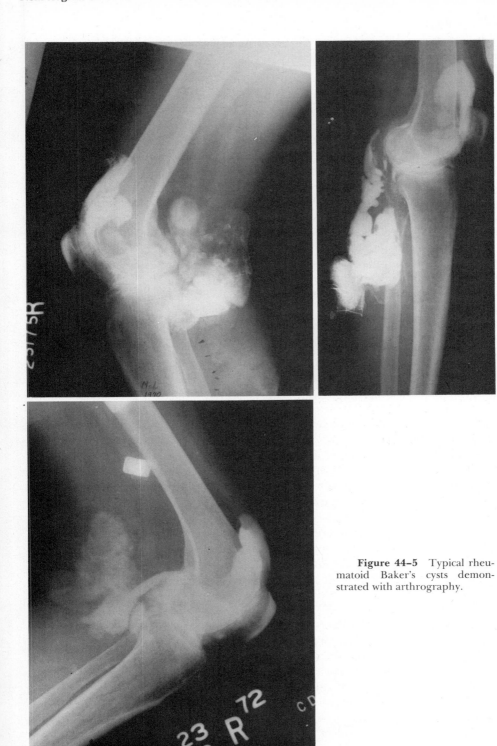

Figure 44–5 Typical rheumatoid Baker's cysts demonstrated with arthrography.

a case which was explored for ruptured extensor tendons, tendon transfer was carried out because the patient had shown inability to extend the digits for approximately two years (Millender, Nalebuff, and Holdsworth, 1973).

Lower Extremity Compression Neuropathies

Lower extremity compression neuropathies associated with rheumatoid arthritis are basically confined to the tibial and peroneal nerves, owing to compression from popliteal cysts plus tarsal tunnel syndrome and lateral and medial plantar nerve syndrome (Nakano, 1975). Sciatic nerve palsies can be seen as a complication of hip surgery or following improperly administered intramuscular injections, but are not directly associated with rheumatoid arthritis. Additionally, bed-ridden patients or patients with cast immobilization can develop common peroneal nerve palsies secondary to external pressure over the vulnerable area at the proximal fibula. Although these neuropathies are seen with rheumatoid arthritis and the latter must be differentiated from popliteal cysts, they are not a direct complication of rheumatoid arthritis.

Popliteal (Baker) Cyst

Rheumatoid synovitis of the knee joint may cause popliteal cyst resulting in entrapment syndrome of the posterior tibial or peroneal nerve (Gardner, 1972) (Fig. 44–5). It has been suggested etiologically that elevated intra-articular pressure within the knee joint may lead either to a herniation of rheumatoid synovial tissue posteriorly or to distention into normally communicating bursas, thereby resulting in the so-called Baker's cyst (Good, 1964; Jayson and Dixon, 1970; Weissman and Sosman, 1975). Although these cysts are a frequent manifestation of rheumatoid arthritis, they rarely cause compression neuropathies. However, they can become extremely large and exhibit symptoms suggestive of thrombophlebitis or they can rupture into the posterior knee compartment (Hollingsworth, 1968). Additionally, entrapment of either the tibial or peroneal nerve, or both, can result.

When the common peroneal nerve is involved, patients will demonstrate partial or total paresis of the peroneal muscles, tibialis anterior, extensor hallucis longus, extensor digitorum longus, and extensor digitorum brevis (Nakano, 1975). Additionally, sensory loss will be noted over the lateral aspect of the leg and dorsum of the foot, including the web interspaces of the second and third toes. When the tibial nerve is compressed, patients will show weakness of the gastrocnemius, soleus, tibialis posterior, flexor digitorum longus, flexor hallucis longus, and intrinsic muscles of the foot, plus sensory loss over the plantar aspect of the foot and the posterior lateral aspect of the calf.

The diagnosis of this should be relatively easy, as the compression symptoms are generally associated with a large cyst and pain in the posterior aspect of the knee. Sometimes the patients will have symptoms quite suggestive of thrombophlebitis. Routine x-rays will demonstrate the soft tissue swelling, and knee arthrography will demonstrate the extent of the popliteal cyst.

Treatment of these cysts, especially when large, is posterior exploration with decompression of the nerve and knee joint synovectomy. Decompression, if carried out early, is generally successful in restoring function.

Tarsal Tunnel Syndrome

Tarsal tunnel syndrome results from compression of the posterior tibial nerve as it passes through the tarsal tunnel along with the posterior tibial tendon, flexor hallucis longus, and flexor digitorum longus tendons. The tunnel is bounded by the bony structures of the foot and ankle and the flexor retinaculum, which extends from the medial malleolus to the bony structures of the foot. Although the tarsal tunnel syndrome is uncommon in rheumatoid arthritis, it can be seen secondary to tenosynovitis of the involved tendons or entrapment of the posterior tibial nerve secondary to various foot and ankle deformities (Aita, 1972; Dixon, 1971).

The symptoms are those of painful dysesthesias and intrinsic muscle weakness. Early symptoms are those of burning feet, especially at night. As the neuropathy progresses, patients lose more feeling in the feet and show progressive intrinsic muscle paralysis.

The diagnosis is made by careful physical examination. Intrinsic muscle weakness is demonstrated, as is diminished sensation over the sole of the foot. Sometimes tenosynovitis can be demonstrated medially and tenderness elicited behind the medial malleolus. When the compression is associated with foot and ankle deformities, these are evident. The diagnosis is confirmed by electromyography and nerve conduction velocity studies. If the compression is associated with tenosynovitis, local steroid injections will sometimes alleviate the condition. For progressive symptoms, release of the flexor retinaculum, decompression of the posterior tibial nerve, and tenosynovectomy are indicated.

Medial and Lateral Plantar Nerve Syndrome

In addition to entrapment of the posterior tibial nerve, entrapment of either the medial or lateral plantar nerve can cause symptoms similar to those of posterior tibial nerve entrapment (Nakano, 1975). Distal to the tarsal tunnel, the posterior tibial nerve branches into the calcaneal and lateral and medial plantar nerves. When either the lateral or medial plantar nerve becomes entrapped, symptoms similar to tarsal tunnel syndrome will be seen. However, on physical examination one will find that the decreased sensation is only along one side of the foot, with heel sensation preserved. Again, electromyography and nerve conduction studies have been helpful in establishing the diagnosis. After appropriate diagnosis has been established, steroid injections have been helpful in alleviation of the symptoms.

Mononeuropathy Multiplex

In this disorder, individual large nerves are involved asymmetrically at slightly different times. The onset is acute, in days or at most weeks. The legs tend to be involved more often than the arms, and motor function can be impaired significantly. Foot drop, for example, is common. The patient is usually suffering with severe chronic rheumatoid arthritis. Rheumatoid nodules are present; the patients are all seropositive, and there is a clear tendency to have a decreased complement and increased immunoglobulins in the serum. Often there are signs of a disseminated vasculitis including fever, weight loss, and skin lesions. The clinical picture of the vasculitis is similar to that of polyarteritis nodosa, but renal involvement in rheumatoid vasculitis is rare. Most series show a strong male preponderance, which is unusual, since rheumatoid arthritis in general has a female predominance. The etiology is an arteritis that leads to an ischemic injury of the nerve. The mortality of patients with this kind of neuropathy is high (Pallis and Scott, 1965; Chamberlain and Bruckner, 1970; Conn and McDuffie, 1976).

Individual nerves are involved, just as in entrapment neuropathies. An important point in differential diagnosis is that in the mononeuropathy multiplex the onset of the deficit is rapid. Nerve conduction studies show a reduction in action potential amplitudes (or absence of action potentials) with preserved conduction velocities in mononeuropathy multiplex, whereas there is segmental slowing of conduction velocity in an entrapment neuropathy at the site of the entrapment.

There are no good studies of methods of therapy. There was an early impression that steroids, especially with rapid increases or decreases in dose, were a predisposing feature to the development of the mononeuropathy multiplex, but this has not been convincingly demonstrated in subsequent series. At this time, high dose steroid therapy is often used, especially when the progression of the disease is rapid. The mainstay of therapy is penicillamine, but the response takes several months (Jaffe, 1970). In aggressive cases, cytotoxic therapy with a drug such as cyclophosphamide would be recommended.

SENSORY POLYNEUROPATHY

This syndrome is characterized by symmetrical sensory loss in the feet with little motor involvement. The rheumatoid arthritis can be milder and the sex ratio is more heavily female; most patients with this disorder have longstanding disease, seropositivity, and nodules. Typically, ankle jerks will be absent. Pathology of nerve biopsies reveals demyelination of large fibers and occasional blood vessels which show an arteritis. Some investigators feel that there is probably some toxic effect directly on myelin, while others feel that the demyelination is an ischemic change due to the vasculitis. Those who subscribe to the latter viewpoint feel that the difference between the mononeuropathy multiplex and the polyneuropathy is in the severity of the vasculitis and possibly the size of the involved blood vessel (Pallis and Scott, 1965; Chamberlain and Bruckner, 1970; Conn and McDuffie, 1976).

In general, prognosis in this disorder is good. Many patients seem to improve spontaneously, and no change in therapy is necessary. Occasional patients, however, have progressed to mononeuropathy multiplex from this state.

DIFFERENTIAL DIAGNOSIS

Myopathy

Muscle disease, common in rheumatoid arthritis, can be responsible for weakness without sensory loss. Nodular interstitial myositis seems to be an extension of the rheumatoid process in muscle and is associated with muscle cell necrosis. Most commonly it produces an asymptomatic periarticular atrophy, but it can cause a severe proximal muscle atrophy having the appearance of limb girdle dystrophy. Nodular interstitial myositis has been found to be present in 70 to 80 per cent of muscle biopsies of unselected patients with rheumatoid arthritis (Williams, 1974).

Polymyositis, which occurs in 4 to 6 per cent of patients with rheumatoid arthritis, presents as the subacute development of proximal muscle weakness. Patients' early complaints usually relate to inability to rise from a chair or to climb stairs. Involvement of the neck flexors is very common. Muscle pain and tenderness are present in about half of the cases, and skin lesions characteristic of dermatomyositis may occur. Muscle enzymes (CPK and aldolase) are almost always elevated. Electromyography shows a myopathic pattern rather than the neurogenic pattern of all the other entities considered in this section (Nakano, 1975).

Radiculopathy

Pressure on the nerve roots as they exit from the vertebral column can occur in rheumatoid arthritis secondary to bony changes at the foramina or ruptured discs. It is not known if there is an increased incidence of radiculopathy in rheumatoid arthritis. Symptoms of radiculopathy include: (1) local pain in the neck or low back; (2) radicular pain radiating into the arm, back of head, or leg; and (3) neurologic deficit, with motor and sensory symptoms and signs in a root pattern. It is not uncommon for a peripheral nerve entrapment to occur simultaneously with a radiculopathy of a root of the entrapped nerve. An example would be a carpal tunnel syndrome and a C6 radiculopathy. This is the so-called "double-crush" syndrome and might be the underlying cause of the failure of peripheral entrapment surgery to remedy the patient's syndrome.

Myelopathy

The rheumatoid process often affects the articulations of the cervical spine and can lead to subluxation. The incidence of subluxation is in the range of 30 per cent and is more common in severe disease, but can be a relatively early manifestation. The most common subluxation is at C1–2 with separation of the odontoid from the atlas. The next most common is the "staircase" subluxation, with multiple successive subluxations in the mid-cervical spine. Other varieties include lateral, anterior, or upward movement of C2 with respect to C1. Subluxation can lead to brain stem signs or a myelopathy (Stevens et al., 1971; Nakano et al., 1978).

Brain stem signs are usually transient, similar to those in transient ischemic attacks. The mechanism of this may relate to upward movement of the odontoid or to vertebral artery compression, or both.

A mild asymptomatic myelopathy characterized by an increase in tendon reflexes and possibly Babinski's signs is very common with subluxation and in fact is occasionally seen in patients with rheumatoid arthritis who do not have subluxation. The more severe symptomatic myelopathy is less common. Patients complain of numbness of either the hands or feet, or of both. Spastic quadriparesis is characteristic and can develop very rapidly. A radiating pain into the occiput is common, presumably from C2 root compression, but there are no radiating pains into the arms. Patients have neck pain, crepitus, Lhermitte's sign (electrical sensation radiating down spine and into the limbs with neck flexion), and a feeling that the head may "slip off." A common complaint is that there is difficulty in using the hands for fine tasks. The upper motor neuron signs are the keystone to the clinical diagnosis; for example, active ankle jerks in the presence of numbness and sensory loss in the feet. The pathophysiology of the myelopathy relates to direct compression of the cord or to vascular compression, or both.

CONCLUSION

Separation of the surgically remediable entrapment neuropathies from the other entities discussed is difficult but valuable because operation can be an effective means of reversing symptoms. Electromyography and nerve conduction studies are extremely useful in sifting through the differential diagnosis.

REFERENCES

Aita, J. A.: Neurologic manifestations of rheumatoid arthritis, 1972. Nebraska Med. J. 57:439, 1972.

Beckett, V. L., and Dinn, J. J.: Segmental demyelination in rheumatoid arthritis. J. Med. 41:71, 1972.

Chamberlain, M. A., and Bruckner, F. F.: Rheumatoid neuropathy: Clinical and electrophysiological features. Ann. Rheum. Dis. 29:609, 1970.

Chamberlain, M. A., and Corbett, M.: Carpal tunnel syndrome in early rheumatoid arthritis. Ann. Rheum. Dis. 29:149, 1970.

Conn, D. L., and McDuffie, F. C.: Neuropathy: the pathogenesis of rheumatoid neuropathy. In: Organic Manifestations and Complications in Rheumatoid Arthritis. Stuttgart, F. K. Schattaner Verlag, 1976.

Dixon, A. S.: The rheumatoid foot. In Hill, A. G. S.: Modern Trends in Rheumatology. London, Butterworths, 1971.

Gardner, D. L.: Pathology of Rheumatoid Arthritis. Baltimore, The Williams & Wilkins Co., 1972.

Good, A. E.: Rheumatoid arthritis, Baker's cyst, and "thrombophelebitis." Arth. Rheum. 7:56, 1964.

Hollingsworth, J. W.: Local and Systemic Complications of Rheumatoid Arthritis. Philadelphia, W. B. Saunders Co., 1968.

Jaffe, I. A.: The treatment of rheumatoid arthritis and necrotizing vasculitis with penicillamine. Arth. Rheum. 13:436, 1970.

Jayson, M. I. V., and Dixon, A. St. J.: Valvular mechanisms in juxta-articular cysts. Ann. Rheum. Dis. 29:415, 1970.

Marmor, L., Lawrence, J. F., and Dubois, E. L.: Posterior interosseous nerve palsy due to rheumatoid arthritis. J. Bone Joint Surg. 49A:381, 1967.

Millender, L. H., and Nalebuff, E. A.: Arthrodesis of the rheumatoid wrist. An evaluation of sixty patients and a description of a different surgical technique. J. Bone Joint Surg., 55A:1026, 1973.

Millender, L. H., and Nalebuff, E. A.: Reconstructive surgery in the rheumatoid hand. Orthop. Clin. North. Am. 6(3):709, 1975.

Millender, L. H., and Nalebuff, E. A.: Preventive surgery — tenosynovectomy and synovectomy. Orthop. Clin. North. Am. 6(3):765, 1975.

Millender, L. H., Nalebuff, E. A., and Holdsworth, D. E.: Posterior interosseous nerve syndrome secondary to rheumatoid synovitis. J. Bone Joint Surg. 55A:753, 1973.

Nakano, K. K.: The entrapment neuropathies of rheumatoid arthritis. Orthop. Clin. North. Am. 6(3):837, 1975.

Nakano, K. K.: Neurologic complications of rheumatoid arthritis. Orthop. Clin. North. Am. 6(3):861, 1975.

Nakano, K. K., Schoene, W. C., Baker, R. A., and Dawson, D. M.: The cervical myelopathy associated with rheumatoid arthritis. Ann. Neurol. 3:144, 1978.

Nalebuff, E. A.,: Surgical treatment of tendon rupture in the rheumatoid hand. Surg. Clin. North. Amer. 49:811, 1969.

Nalebuff, E. A., and Potter, T. A.: Rheumatoid involvement of tendons and tendon sheaths in the hand. Clin. Orthop. 59:147, 1968.

Pallis, C. A., and Scott, J. T.: Peripheral neuropathy in rheumatoid arthritis. Brit. Med. J. 1:1141, 1965.

Shea, J. D. and McClain, E. J.: Ulnar-nerve compression syndromes at and below the wrist. J. Bone Joint Surg. 51A:1095, 1969.

Spinner, M.: Injuries to the Major Branches of Peripheral Nerves of the Forearm. 2nd ed., Philadelphia, W. B. Saunders Co., 1978.

Stevens, J. C., Cartlidge, N. E. F., Saunders, M., Appleby, A., Hall, M., and Shaw, D. A.: Atlanto-axial subluxation and cervical myelopathy in rheumatoid arthritis. J. Med. 40:391, 1971.

Swanson, A. B.: Flexible Implant Resection Arthroplasty in the Hand and Extremities. St. Louis, The C. V. Mosby Co., 1973.

Weissman, B. N. W., and Sosman, J. L.: The radiology of rheumatoid arthritis. Orthop. Clin. North. Am. 6(3):653, 1975.

Williams, R. C.: Rheumatoid Arthritis as a Systemic Disease. Philadelphia, W. B. Saunders Co., 1974.

45

THE
MANAGEMENT
OF LEPROUS
NEURITIS

CARL D. ENNA

INTRODUCTION

The management of leprous neuritis requires knowledge of the pathogenesis of leprosy and of the histopathology of neural involvement. Three etiological factors related to leprous neuritis are (1) the *Mycobacterium leprae*, which is the causative organism, and the host response to its invasion; (2) auto antigens that sensitize and damage nerves without the presence of *M. leprae*, and (3) the anatomical physiological factors responsible for predisposing peripheral nerves to trauma besides providing a temperature related environment optimal for the growth of *M. leprae* (Brand, 1959).

The primary objectives of treatment are to halt the disease activity and prevent the development of insensitivity and deformity caused by the destruction of peripheral nerves. Thus the "sine qua non" of treatment is specific anti-leprosy therapy to control, inactivate, and cure the disease. Certain features related to involvement of peripheral nerves in leprosy must be considered in evaluating the efficacy of the specific drugs.

Early paralysis may sometimes be reversed and recovery enhanced by specific therapy. Also, the increase in size of the affected nerve does not necessarily correlate with the degree of neuropathy. The nerve is not infrequently enlarged in lepromatous leprosy, yet it is without deformity. Numerous organisms may be present as a result of inadequate cell mediated immune response, which allows widespread dissemination and growth of *M. leprae*. Edema and progressive increase in the neural connective tissue are mainly responsible for destruction, which occurs slowly by compression. In the tuberculoid type of leprosy there is a granulomatous cellular infiltration that destroys fasciculi by caseation necrosis. Involvement of fasciculi may be focal or

742

extensive to the point of transecting the nerve (Fig. 45–1). There is the problem, however, of differentiating the disease-causing peripheral neuropathy from the various drugs commonly used in treatment (Sabin, 1974; Valden, 1976; Vivier and Fowler, 1974).

In tuberculoid leprosy neuritis there is an ascending centripetal infection that begins with the entry of *M. leprae* into fine sensory nerves and progresses to larger trunks of mixed nerves. The bacilli infect the Schwann cells, being confined intially within the endoneurium and spread centrally along the length of the nerve before the perineurium is penetrated at any point to produce a localized involvement (Sunderland, 1973). In both lepromatous and tuberculoid leprosy it is characteristic for the *M. leprae* to localize and multiply at sites of predilection; these are the primary areas of nerves to which surgery is directed. The most common affected nerves and their sites of predilection are as follows, in order of frequency.

1. The ulnar nerve is affected at the medial aspect of the elbow proximal to the cubital tunnel (Fig. 45–2). Involvement occurs later at, or proximal to, the pisohamate tunnel in the wrist (Enna et al., 1974).
2. The median nerve is clinically affected only if there is ulnar nerve involvement. It is affected at the wrist as it emerges from under the flexor digitorum superficialis to course superficially before entering the carpal tunnel.
3. The common peroneal nerve is affected at the lateral aspect of the knee as it winds around the neck of the fibula.
4. The tibial nerve is usually affected at the medial aspect of the ankle, proximal to the tarsal tunnel. However, the terminal plantar branches are liable

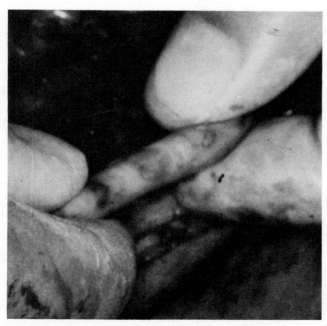

Figure 45–1   Focal deposits of caseation in ulnar nerve.

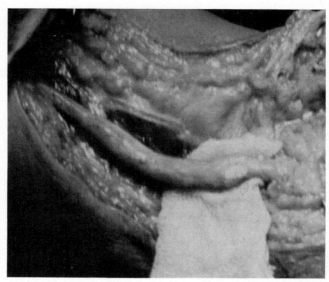

Figure 45–2   Fusiform enlargement of ulnar nerve in distal forearm, with swelling terminating abruptly before entering cubital tunnel.

to entrapment at the "portis pedis" as they pass into the plantar aspect of the foot.

5. The zygomatic branch of the facial nerve that innervates the orbicularis oculi, the paralysis of which causes lagophthalmos, is superficial and thus is subject to compression as it passes over the zygomatic arch (Antia, 1974).

6. The radial nerve is less frequently affected. It is usually involved distal to the musculospiral groove of the humerus, but it is also sometimes affected at the elbow where it bifurcates proximal to the arcade of Frohse. Infrequent paralysis is probably due in great part to the nerve assuming a deep position within muscles, which provide a warm environment.

Certain features common to sites of predilection are considered to contribute to local aggravation of the disease. Their superficial position makes them liable to injury from extrinsic forces besides providing the optimum temperature of 27 to 30° C for the growth of *M. leprae* (Shepard, 1975). Also, the proximity of the nerves to bone and joints makes them vulnerable to injury from compression against unyielding bone or to stretch with joint movement to produce deformation with increased intraneural pressure (Pandey and Singh, 1974). Grooves, tunnels, fibrous bands, and anomalous structures contribute to entrapment, which aggravates the disease process by increasing intraneural tension with increasing ischemia.

TREATMENT OF LEPROUS NEURITIS

Acute manifestations of leprous neuritis develop suddenly and progress rapidly, with intense pain and tenderness affecting the peripheral nerve. Occasionally there is fever, and loss of function may develop within 24 to 48 hours. The initial treatment is usually with steroids. We have found prednisone to be effective, with minimal side effects, in halting the process, often with reversal of sensory and motor changes. Unsuccessful therapy with steroids is usually due to delayed and inadequate treatment. Patients are given 60 mg of prednisone daily. Response is immediate in terms of fever, neuritic pain, and tenderness; these usually resolve within 24 to 48 hours. This dosage is continued for an additional two to three days, after which it is gradually decreased over a period varying from 10 days to several months, depending upon the patient's reaction to withdrawal. If symptoms recur, it is necessary to resume the higher dosage for a slightly longer period. Subsequent withdrawal attempts are made until it is accomplished without recurrence of symptoms.

Mild to moderate manifestations usually respond to prednisone within 10 days to three weeks; however, a number of patients will require a maintenance dosage of prednisone for many months. In such chronic cases, drug therapy is usually changed to either thalidomide for lepromatous cases, or clofazimine (B663), which is effective in both lepromatous and dimorphous (borderline) types of leprosy.

The dosage of thalidomide and also clofazimine is 100 to 200 mg daily, which is gradually decreased over several months to two to three years until it can be discontinued without recurrence of neuritis. Specific anti-leprosy therapy (DDS), however, is continued during the administration of steroids, thalidomide, or clofazamine and for the lifetime of patients with dimorphous and lepromatous disease. Each drug is given concomitantly with prednisone as the dosage of the steroid is tapered to be discontinued. This is necessary in order to avoid the recurrence of neuritis, which may happen if the steroids are suddenly withdrawn. Clofazimine is slower acting than thalidomide; therefore, a slightly longer period is required before the prednisone can be discontinued. Thalidomide and clofazimine are classified as investigational drugs requiring approval by the Food and Drug Administration (FDA), thus the drugs are now available only from the U.S. Public Health Service Hospital, Carville, Louisiana.

Supplemental measures are applied directly to the affected extremity as the patient is receiving medical therapy. These include the following methods.

Splinting. Extremities with acute neuritis are splinted in optimum position to decrease neural tension and relieve pain. A molded splint or light plaster of paris cast is worn for four to six weeks, but may be reapplied for a longer period if necessary.

Physical Therapy. Several measures have been tried at Carville but without remarkable benefit (Shipley, 1964). The various methods employed were for the purpose of relieving pain, increasing the warmth of the extremity to discourage multiplication of the *M. leprae* or to improve nerve function (Abramson et al., 1966; Riordan, 1960). The more frequent methods employed were the wearing of an insulated sleeve and the use of diathermy, microthermy, ultrasound therapy, and hot paraffin baths.

Intraneural Injections. Steroids, hyaluronidase, and tolazoline (Priscol) have been injected into and around nerves (Garrett, 1956; Joplin and Cochrane, 1957; Ramanujan, 1964; Sepaha and Sharma, 1964; Tio, 1966). Relief of pain is obtained with injection of the steroids. Hydrocortisone acetate, 12.5 to 25 mg, is recommended, although repeated injections at weekly intervals may be required to obtain complete and permanent relief. Benefits from the other drugs are supplemental, as they are given to enhance the effect of the steroids.

This method is not without harmful effects. The injection may increase the intraneural pressure to augment ischemia and add to existing damage; there is also the possibility of an iatrogenic abscess as a complication (Enna et al., 1974). For these reasons, and because relief is generally obtained from appropriate anti-reaction therapy, intraneural injection with steroids is reserved for chronic leprous neuritis associated with advanced deformities where additional nerve damage is unlikely or inconsequential.

Surgical Procedures

Various surgical procedures have been suggested. for those cases that do not respond to medical and conservative treatment. The surgical management remains controversial; this is reflected in the variety and number of procedures employed, (Basombrio and Malbran, 1941; Carayon and Giraudeau, 1976; Childress, 1975; Enna et al., 1974; Joplin and Cochrane, 1957; McLeod et al., 1975; Pandey and Singh, 1974; Riordan, 1960; Vaidyanathan and Vaidyanathan, 1968). The objectives of surgery are primarily to provide a warmer environment that is adverse to the multiplication of *M. leprae,* and to obviate the effects of anatomical and physiological features responsible for trauma of either extrinsic or intrinsic origin that may aggravate the neural pathology. Our preoperative assessment includes subjective and objective manifestations, nerve conduction velocity studies, and thermograms, which are used as a baseline for postoperative evaluation of the surgical procedure. Our indications for surgery are:

1. Failure to relieve pain after 48 to 72 hours of anti-inflammatory treatment
2. Development of progressive signs of denervation in spite of apparent control of the disease with specific anti-leprosy therapy
3. Persistence of a tender localized swelling due to an abscess
4. Recurrent episodes of neuritis requiring frequent prolonged periods of hospitalization that interfere with normal life.

The following procedures are employed where applicable, depending upon the pathology encountered.

External Neurolysis

This method involves mobilization of the nerve to free it from inflammatory adhesions; in the case of ulnar nerve, it precedes transposition. This measure has been recommended as the sole measure for treating leprous neuritis (Vaidyanathan and Vaidyanathan, 1968). However, it is more often done as the first of multiple measures performed in coping with the various problems encountered, such as the elimination of various causes involved in entrapment

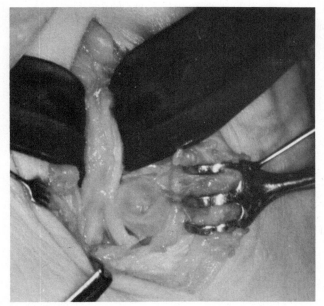

Figure 45-3   Tendon sheath ganglion compressing tibial nerve within tarsal tunnel.

(Basombrio and Malbran, 1941; Enna and Callaway, 1964). Common non-leprosy extrinsic causes of neural pressure include hypertrophic and rheumatoid arthritis, deformity due to trauma (Harrison and Nurick, 1970), and the presence of tendon sheath ganglion (Fig. 45-3).

Transposition and Burial of the Nerve

This measure was recommended for ulnar leprous neuritis by Riordan (1960). It avoids replacement of the nerve into the original bed, where adhesions are prone to redevelop, and it places the nerve in a warm environment that is unfavorable to the growth of *M. leprae*. Also, it obviates the elongation and deformation that produce ischemia when the nerve is stretched upon flexing the elbow.

The performance of certain steps of this procedure is essential to accomplish an effective transposition as recommended. As considerable variations have been observed from clinical examinations and during secondary surgical procedures, re-emphasis of these features is indicated.

1. The nerve is mobilized from the upper arm distally into the proximal forearm. This is facilitated because the ulnar nerve does not innervate any muscle in the arm.
2. Increased mobilization is obtained by sacrificing the articular branch to the elbow and by dissecting the nerve a short distance into the flexor carpi ulnaris muscle, which it innervates. The extensive mobilization permits a gradual alteration in the course of the nerve that obviates an abrupt an-

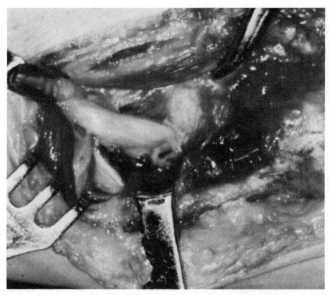

Figure 45–4   Acute angulation of ulnar nerve resulting from inadequate mobilization prior to transposition.

gulation, which is especially likely to occur at the distal end (Fig. 45–4). Inadequate surgery is a cause for performing secondary procedures (Lluch, 1975). In our experience, the extent of mobilization has not resulted in harm to the nerve.

3. The medial intermuscular septum is excised to eliminate the taut fibrous ridge that the nerve would cross with transposition.

4. Dissection is carried out between the biceps and the brachialis muscles, exposing the median nerve, along the side of which the ulnar nerve is placed.

5. Distally, an incision is made below the epicondyle through the common origin of the forearm flexors. The fibrous septa are divided to provide a soft muscle bed into which the transposed nerve will be placed.

6. The nerve is retained in the new location by suturing the marginal fibers of the brachialis to the triceps in the upper arm and the biceps to the brachialis in the lower arm, and by resuturing the superficial fascial layer of the common forearm flexors.

7. The extremity is immobilized postoperatively, with the elbow extended 165 to 180 degrees. This position takes up most of the redundancy of the nerve, which results from transposition, and is necessary to prevent excessive adaptive shortening.

Neurolysis continues to be controversial for several reasons. The procedure is not always beneficial and one is not certain that the natural course of the lesion has been affected, also it is difficult to obtain either a large series with a 10 year followup for an adequate evaulation or a valid control group for comparison. In a review of 103 procedures done at Carville between 1960 and 1972, immediate results appeared to be good, as evidenced by the relief of pain in the majority of patients. Long term results, however, were not as satisfactory, with pain recurring in most cases albeit less severe than the original pain. Other reasons for the recurrence of symptoms include progressive active disease, recurrent erythema nodosum leprosum (ENL), the development of a nerve abscess, and inadequate surgery during the primary procedure, of which 13 cases (12 per cent) required secondary surgical intervention (Enna and Jacobson, 1974).

Medial Epicondylectomy

This procedure is recommended as an independent method for the treatment of ulnar neuritis (Carayon and Giraudeau, 1976). It is indicated for the relief of increased pressure on the nerve within the cubital tunnel, especially when the elbow is flexed. The increased pressure interferes with the neural circulation to produce pain due to intraneural hypertension besides directly injuring the nerve.

The question is raised as to the indication for epicondylectomy versus neurolysis with transposition. Experience with this procedure is limited because it has only recently been applied as a method of treating leprous neuritis. It appears that the mobility of the nerve may be used as a means of selecting one procedure over the other (Childress, 1975; Gore and Larson, 1966). If the nerve remains within the cubital tunnel when the elbow is flexed, and the increased pressure results in pain from intraneural tension, the unyielding epicondyle is considered to be causative, and its removal is recommended. However, in a small number of cases the mobility of a recurrent luxating nerve subjects it to friction as it moves over the epicondyle, suggesting that greater benefit would be obtained with neurolysis and transposition. The decrease in pressure obtainable from epicondylectomy is evident during surgery, and when it is apparent that the increased pressure persists with flexion of the elbow after the epicondyle is excised, one may proceed with transposition. Based upon the principle of changing the location of the ulnar nerve to a warmer domicile in which *M. leprae* can less readily multiply, there are advocates who recommend prophylactic transposition of the nerve when it is thickened and enlarged, with or without localized tenderness. Epicondylectomy, however, is not recommended as a prophylactic procedure.

Internal Neurolysis

This method requires incision into the epineurium and possibly extended into the perineurium to isolate fasciculi. A simple incision into the epineurium is done for the relief of edema and for evacuation of abscesses. Edema of the nerve is an early manifestation of inflammation and is only rarely encountered during surgery because of its transient nature. Immediate results with relief of pain are dramatic. However, there are two types of peripheral nerve abscess, the caseous abscess usually seen in tuberculoid leprosy and the liquefied abscess seen more often in lepromatous leprosy. Both types, however, are uncommon.

Histologically, there is destruction of nerve with axonal degeneration and an increase of endoneurial collagen (Fig. 45–5). Although there is a loss of structure, the affected fasciculus remains adherent and is removable by excision, which may be undertaken upon determining that the affected segment is electrically inactive. If the process is allowed to continue, caseation will develop, leaving a "cheesy" material that is easily removed by "spooning it out" with a

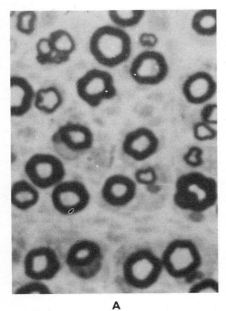

A

Figure 45–5 *A*, Microscopic cross section of a normal nerve. *B*, Intraneural fibrosis due to chronic leprous neuritis with destruction of the axons.

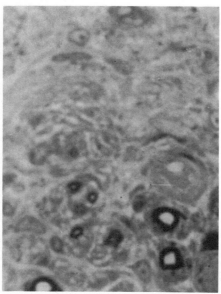

B

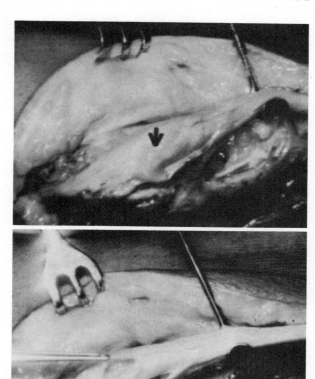

Figure 45–6 Abscess of ulnar nerve associated with erythema nodosum leprosum and a liquefied abscess.

blunt instrument. Liquefied abscesses are evacuated (Fig. 45–6). It is necessary to remove all caseous material immediate to the abscess wall, or else the abscess will recur or a sinus tract will develop that will require a secondary surgical procedure. In any case, the incisional wound is closed primarily (Enna and Brand, 1970).

Decapsulation

This method consists of stripping a segment of thickened epineurium (Gramberg, 1955). The difficulty is in determining the extent of the segment and the inability to differentiate paraneural scarring from epineural and endoneural fibrosis. The procedure is reserved for releasing cicatricial constriction from previous surgery.

Fascicular Neurolysis

This procedure is recommended by Carayon (1974); however, it has not been generally accepted. It is considered a radical procedure because there is a danger of injuring the plexus of diverging fasciculi during dissection, and possibly damaging the fasciculi further by deprivation of circulation. Furthermore, one can never be certain that it will in any way alter the course of the lesion (Enna and Jacobson, 1970).

Partial Neurectomy

A fasciculus or a segment of a nerve may be excised for biopsy. They are preferably obtained from sensory nerves or from fasciculi that are to be destroyed. The sural nerve has been used for differentiating peripheral neuropathy and is commonly used in leprosy to ascertain activity of the disease when there is a progressive neural deficit, although inactive disease is demonstrated by skin biopsy (Enna et al., 1970). Cutaneous nerves, which are also involved in leprosy, are also available for biopsy.

Segmental excision of a totally destroyed nerve is done for relief of pain in patients with chronic leprous neuritis who have multiple deformities, as relief is obtainable without augmenting existing disabilities.

Nerve Graft

Although this procedure is not recommended in leprosy, a small number of cases have been undertaken (McLeod et al., 1975). There were no harmful effects; however, the benefits were limited to recovery of "useful protective sensation" in only a few patients. Nerve grafting is discouraged, since it is impossible to determine the length of nerve that should be grafted because the extent of infiltration of the nerve by *M. leprae* may not be determined accurately at surgery and it is uncertain whether the remaining axons will bridge the graft.

SUMMARY

1. The management of leprous neuritis poses a greater challenge than does that of peripheral neuritis due to other causes because the primary treatment is directed to the disease proper, and the timing, location, and severity of the episodes of neuritis that may result are unpredictable.
2. Surgery consists of secondary procedures to alleviate or remove the factors that contribute to injury of the nerve.
3. The indications for surgery of leprous neuritis are established; however, the actual procedure performed is determined only upon viewing the pathology.
4. Indications for surgical intervention in cases of leprous neuritis are limited by the fact that most cases respond to appropriate anti-reaction therapy. Therefore, the liberal utilization of these methods for prophylactic or de-

finitive treatment remains controversial in the absence of an adequate evaluation of the procedures compared with a valid control group.

REFERENCES

Abramson, D. L., Chu, L. S. W., Tuck, S., Lee, S. W., Richardson, G., and Levin, M.: The effect of time, temperature and blood flow on motor nerve conduction velocity. J.A.M.A. *198*:1082, 1966.

Antia, N. H.: Surgery of the nerves. *In* McDowell, F., and Enna, C. D. (Eds.): Surgical Rehabilitation in Leprosy. Baltimore, The Williams & Wilkins Co., 1974. Chap. 4, p. 31.

Basombrio, G., and Malbran, C.: Pseudoleprous neuritis of the cubital nerve with osteoarthritis of the elbow. Rev. Argentina Dermatosif *25*:87, 1941.

Brand, P. W.: Temperature variation and leprosy deformity. Int. J. Leprosy *27*:1, 1959.

Brand, P. W.: The practical management of neuritis. *In* McDowell, F., and Enna, C. D.: Surgical Rehabilitation in Leprosy. Baltimore, The Williams & Wilkins Co., 1974. Chap. 6, p. 50.

Carayon, A. and Giraudeau, P.: Valeur de la resection de l'epitroclee dans la decompression et le deroutement de 87 Nevrites cubitales Hanseniennes. Med. Trop. 36:163, 1976.

Carayon, A. E., and Huet, R.: The value of peripheral neurosurgical procedures in neuritis. *In* McDowell, F., and Enna. C. D.: Surgical Rehabilitation in Leprosy. Baltimore, The Williams & Wilkins Co., 1974, Chap. 5, p. 37.

Childress, H. M.: Recurrent ulnar nerve dislocation at the elbow. Clin. Orthop. Rel. Res. *108*:168, 1975.

Enna, C. D.: Neurolysis and transposition of the ulnar nerve in leprosy. J. Neurosurg. *40*:734, 1974.

Enna, C. D., Berghtholdt, H. T., and Stockwell, F.: A study of surface and deep temperatures along the course of the ulnar nerve in the pisohamate tunnel. Int. J. Leprosy *42*:43, 1974.

Enna, C. D., and Brand, P. W.: Peripheral nerve abscess in leprosy. Leprosy Review *41*:175, 1970.

Enna, C. D. and Callaway, J. C.: Tarsal tunnel syndrome. Case report tibial leprous neuritis associated with tendon sheath ganglion. Int. J. Leprosy *32*:279, 1964.

Enna, C. D., and Jacobson, R. R.: A clinical assessment of neurolysis for leprous involvement of the ulnar nerve. Int. J. Leprosy *42*:162, 1974.

Enna, C. D., Jacobson, R. R., and Mansfield, R. E.: An evaluation of sural nerve biopsy in leprosy. Int. J. Leprosy *38*:278, 1970.

Garrett, A. S.: Hyalaze injection for lepromatous nerve reaction. Leprosy Review *27*:61, 1956.

Gore, D., and Larson, S.: Medial epicondylectomy for subluxing ulnar nerve. Am. J. Surg. *111*:851, 1966.

Gramberg, K. P. C. A.: Nerve decapsulation in the leprosy patient. Int. J. Leprosy *23*:115, 1955.

Harrison, M. J. G. and Nurick, S.: Results of anterior transposition of the ulnar nerve for ulnar neuritis. Brit. Med. J. *1*:27, 1970.

Joplin, W. H., and Cochrane, R. G.: The place of cortisone and corticotropin in the treatment of certain acute phases in leprosy. Leprosy Review *28*:5, 1957.

Lluch, A. L.: Ulnar nerve entrapment after anterior transposition at elbow. N.Y. State J. Med., *75*:75, 1975.

McLeod, J. G., Hargrave, J. C., Gye, R. S., Pollard, J. D., Walsh, J. C., Little, J. M., and Booth, G. C.: Nerve grafting in leprosy. Brain *98*:203, 1975.

Pandey, S., and Singh, A. K.: Treatment of neural involvement in leprosy. Leprosy in India *46*:83, 1974.

Pechan, J., and Julio, I.: The pressure measurement in the ulnar nerve. A contribution to the pathophysiology of the cubital tunnel syndrome. J. Biomechanics *8*:75, 1975.

Ramanujan, K.: The use of intraneural corticosteroids in acute leprosy neuritis. Leprosy in India *36*:261, 1964.

Riordan, D. C.: The hand in leprosy. A seven year clinical study. J. Bone Joint Surg. *42A*:661, 1960.

Sabin, T. D.: Thalidomide neuropathy and leprous neuritis. Lancet *1*:165, 1974.

Sepaha, G. C., and Sharma, D. R.: Intraneural cortisone and Priscol in treament of leprosy. Leprosy in India *36*:264, 1964.

Shepard, C. C.: Temperature optimum for Mycobacterium Leprae in mice. J. Bact. *90*:1271, 1975.

Shipley, D.: Personal communication. 1964.

Sunderland, S.: The internal anatomy of nerve trunks in relation to the neural lesions of leprosy. Observations on pathology, symptomatology and treatment. Brain *96*:865, 1973.

Tio, T. H.: Neural involvement in leprosy. Treatment with intraneural injection of prednisolone. Leprosy Review *37*:93, 1966.

Vaidyanathan, E. P. and Vaidyanathan, S. I.: Treatment of ulnar neuritis and early ulnar paralysis. Leprosy Review *39*:217, 1968.

Valden, G.: Neurotoxicity — a side effect of sulfones. Acta Derm. Venereol. (Stockh.) *56*:77, 1976.

Vivier, A. du and Fowler, T.: Possible dapsone induced peripheral neuropathy in dermatitis herpetiformis. Proc. Roy. Soc. Med. *67*:439, 1974.

46

BURN INDUCED PERIPHERAL NERVE INJURY

ROGER E. SALISBURY and
A. GRISWOLD BEVIN

One does not often relate nerve damage to burn injury, since the latter is usually considered a purely cutaneous injury. However, the extremely variable etiology of a burn, thermal, chemical, electrical, or radiation, may result in transient neurapraxia or large masses of necrotic tissue, requiring extirpation of muscle groups and peripheral nerves, perhaps even amputation. The purpose of this chapter is to define the peripheral nerve problems that result from burn injury and how to manage them.

THERMAL INJURY

Fire, hot liquids, or steam heat may result in peripheral nerve loss on the basis of: (1) ischemic necrosis secondary to undiagnosed vascular insufficiency after a circumferential burn; (2) the heat itself causing coagulation necrosis. For instance, the patient in Figure 1 had a circumferential deep second and third degree burn to his arm and was transferred to our Burn Unit four days after the injury. Diminished radial sensation, wrist drop (Fig. 46–1*C*), and a questionable pulse at the wrist made it obvious that a compression injury had occurred. Exploration and debridement revealed deep second and third degree burns of the skin; in addition, ischemic necrosis of the whole extensor muscle compartment including the radial nerve was noted.

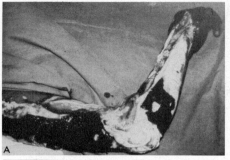

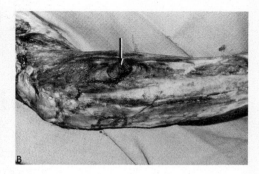

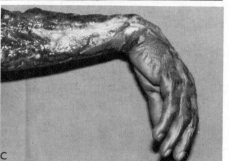

Figure 46–1 Delayed escharotomy (*A*) following a circumferential burn of the upper extremity revealed ischemic muscle; excision of necrotic extensor muscle (*B*) and radial nerve secondary to ischemia resulted in a drop wrist (*C*).

The mechanism of this injury is the tourniquet effect of the nondistensible, unyielding burn eschar. As edema increases following loss of capillary integrity, first venous and then arterial flow is compromised, resulting in a vascular emergency. The ensuing gangrene, or Volkmann's contracture of the upper extremity, or anterior tibial compartment syndrome of the lower extremity can be prevented by the physician who considers this compression phenomenon when seeing a patient with a circumferential burn. Immediate elevation of the extremity and frequent exercise of the hand or foot may help to decrease edema (Moylan, 1971) and maintain circulation. If the palpating finger cannot detect a pulse, however, the examiner should use a Doppler Flowmeter, which is extremely sensitive in detecting blood flow. If no arterial flow is heard, the physician must first be sure intravenous resuscitation is adequate. If urine output is 30 to 50 cc per hour in an adult or proportionately less in a child, the state of hydration is satisfactory and an absent pulse means vascular compression secondary to burn edema. The treatment is immediate escharotomy. This procedure can be done at the bedside or in the emergency room with a scalpel or electrocautery. The incision should be made laterally (Fig. 46–2) or medially through the constricting eschar into unburned soft tissue along the entire length of the wound (Pruitt, 1968). After waiting several minutes to allow resumption of blood flow, Doppler evaluation is repeated. If arterial flow is still unsatisfactory, escharotomy along the other side should be done. The extremity should be elevated to aid venous flow. No anatomical structures are at risk during the escharotomy as long as the incisions are lateral and extended only into the interface between eschar and viable tissue. Care should be taken at the elbow, however, to make the incision anterior to the medial epicondyle, as the ulnar nerve lies in the soft tissue posteriorly. Burn wound invasion is not a complica-

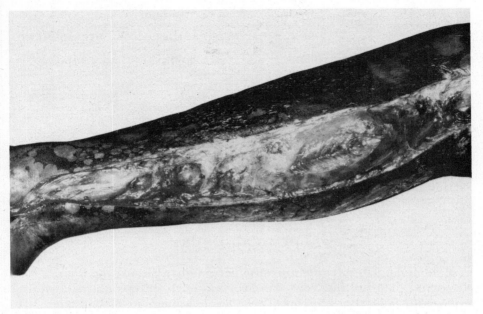

Figure 46–2   A single lateral incision may be enough to fully decompress the edematous extremity. In electrical burns, fasciotomy may be one way to decompress injured muscle.

tion of the procedure if the wounds are treated regularly, with a topical chemotherapeutic agent being used on the rest of the burns.

Direct thermal injury of peripheral nerves is not rare and is seen in patients who have had prolonged contact with hot objects, such as occurs with an unconscious driver following an automobile or motorcycle wreck, or an inebriate who is found in a burning house. The ulnar nerve at the elbow, the radial nerve at the distal humerus, and the peroneal nerve at the fibular head are especially at risk. The ulnar nerve, shielded by the flexor carpi ulnaris in the arm, and the median nerve (except at the wrist where it is superficial) are well protected. While diagnosis of sensory loss may be masked initially because of the generalized pain of the deep burn, motor loss is obvious.

Treatment of the nerve lesion must be delayed until the burn wound has healed. Necrotic tissue, high bacterial counts, and the necessity for early and aggressive splinting and exercise make immediate nerve reconstruction impossible. The physician may elect to treat the wounds with topical antibiotics, daily debridement of eschar, and, finally, skin grafting of the granulating wound. In selected cases he may opt for the more rapid course of primary excision and grafting of the burn wound. Significantly, a good wound bed for future nerve reconstruction is not characteristic of either treatment. Unfortunately, whether nerve injury is secondary to compression or direct heat, the length of nerve damage is usually too great for excision and direct repair. Nerve grafts require an excellent soft tissue bed, which might have to be provided by a large flap. Unquestionably, early tendon transfer in appropriate cases is the best solution for the patient with a motor deformity because it is the fastest and least expensive path to rehabilitation (Bevin, 1976).

	46–1	Treatment of Acid Injury	
AGENTS	**NSING**	**NEUTRALIZATION**	**DEBRIDEMENT**
Phenol	ohol	Sodium bicarbonate solution	Loose, nonviable tissue and blebs
Hydrofluoric acid		Zepharin or Hyamine chloride soaks	Nonviable tissue and blebs
(Consider primary excision of full thickness injuries)			
Sulfuric acid Nitric acid Hydrochloric acid Trichloroacetic acid	Water	Sodium bicarbonate solution	Loose, nonviable tissue and blebs

CHEMICAL INJURY

Chemical burns infrequently cause nerve injury because the wounds rarely cause more than full thickness skin loss. Although different acids and alkalis have specific neutralizing agents (Tables 46–1 through 46–3) (Salisbury, 1976), valuable time is often lost until they can be obtained. Copious lavage with water remains the single best immediate treatment for most chemical burns. Phosphorus burns are an exception in that the particles continue to destroy tissue as they erode below the skin and into soft tissue (Curreri, 1970). White phosphorus ignites on exposure to air and is oxidized to phosphorus pentoxide. The heat of reaction is more destructive than the inorganic acids of phosphorus formed, and the particles should be removed immediately in the operating room to prevent further damage. The particles may be located easily if they are smoking, or by washing the wounds with 1 per cent copper sulfate, which colors the particles black and permits easy identification. It is emphasized that the copper wash is not definitive treatment but removal of the particles is. The phosphorus creates ulcers of variable thickness, which, if debrided and treated with topical antibiotics so no infection results, usually heal by contraction.

ELECTRICAL INJURY

Electrical burns cause the highest incidence of nerve injury. In a recent review of electrical burns of the upper extremity in 84 patients (Salisbury, 1973),

Table 46–2   Treatment of Alkali Injury

AGENTS	**CLEANSING**	**NEUTRALIZATION**	**DEBRIDEMENT**
Lime	Brush off powder, then wash with water	0.5–5.0% Acetic acid	Loose nonviable tissue
Potassium hydroxide Sodium hydroxide Ammonia	Water	0.5–5.0% Acetic acid 0.5–5.0% Acetic acid 0.5–5.0% Acetic acid	Loose nonviable tissue

Table 46–3 Treatment of Other Chemical Injuries

AGENTS	CLEANSING	NEUTRALIZATION	DEBRIDEMENT
Mustard gas	Water	M-5 Ointment	Aspirate; then excise blebs while flushing with water
Tear gas	Water	Sodium bicarbonate solution	Debride loose tissue
Phosphorus	Water	1% Copper sulfate rinse	Debride and remove particles; keep particles moist

there were 17 different peripheral nerve lesions. Electricity follows the path of least resistance (Table 46–4), and thus often destroys neurovascular bundles. The resulting defect is frequently permanent and is secondary to irreversible destruction of the nerve. Diagnosis may be initially obscured if the patient has a markedly edematous extremity and decreased sensation secondary to ischemia. Since edema most frequently involves the muscle and is therefore subfascial, escharotomy is not sufficient and fasciotomy must be performed to achieve adequate decompression (Pruitt, 1968).

A cornerstone of early management is timely excision of nonviable musculature so gas gangrene does not occur. This debridement may leave exposed nerve of questionable viability. The clinician is confronted with finding a technique to cover the nerve or it will desiccate. Biologic dressings (Levine, 1976) such as cadaver allograft or porcine xenograft will maintain nerve viability because both simulate a normal internal environment. The wound should then be covered with dressings soaked in lactated Ringer's solution and changed daily. Within several days it will often become apparent by visual inspection that the nerve is nonviable and should be debrided. A wire suture placed through the epineurium of the cut ends of the nerve to tack it to the surrounding soft tissue will prevent retraction. The necessity for a longer nerve graft is obviated and future identification is simplified. Once all necrotic tissue is removed, a split thickness skin graft should be used to cover the whole wound if it is very large. For a more localized injury, a flap is obviously preferable, as it replaces the necrotic soft tissue, protects the nerve, and provides a reasonable bed through which future reconstruction may be undertaken.

Although the techniques of nerve repair are beyond the scope of this chapter, preparation of the patient for reconstruction is of paramount importance. As in other extremity problems, all viable tissue should be conserved initially. The importance of this principle cannot be overemphasized. In electri-

Table 46–4 Tissue Resistance to Electricity

Resistance ↑
Bone
Fat
Tendon
Skin
Muscle
Blood vessels
Nerves

cal injury involving large muscle masses, such as the trunk or the thigh, the demand for rapid and complete excision is high because of the risk of gas gangrene.

In the hand (where muscle mass is minimal) and even in the forearm, however, the concern is for future function, and, if necessary, dressing changes and debridement are done daily to evaluate the status of the wound. In an isolated finger injury, it is often stated that it is better to amputate if any three tissues are permanently damaged (skin, nerve, tendon, or bone; however, it is more common to have involvement of multiple fingers following electrical trauma. Thus, only obviously nonviable fingers should be amputated before the plan for the patient's reconstruction is formulated. For example, the patient in Figure 46–3 lost the index fingers of both hands and sustained damage to other fingers as well. The radial neurovascular bundle of the long finger was coagulated, and thus effective pinch was impaired. The proximal interphalangeal (PIP) joint of the long finger was exposed and the radial collateral ligament destroyed. The flexor tendons, however, were perfect, as was the ulnar digital bundle. The obvious necrotic tissue was debrided, the PIP joint pinned in moderate flexion, and the bone rongeured to stimulate granulation tissue. The finger was then grafted to achieve wound closure. Moderate radial instability of the PIP joint caused overriding on the ring finger which could be corrected by arthrodesis, and neurovascular island transfer from the ulnar to the radial portion of the long finger should render satisfactory pinch sensation. If the outcome of these combined procedures is unsuccessful, amputation is still a viable alternative. The point is that the reconstructive surgeon and the patient have a choice that would not exist if early, thoughtless debridement had been performed.

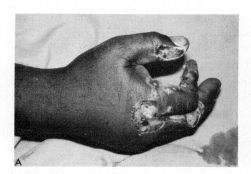
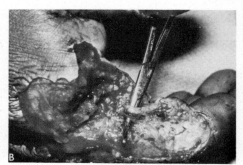

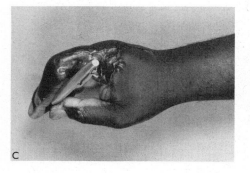

Figure 46–3 An obviously devitalized index finger (*A*) and the radial aspect of the long finger were debrided, including the neurovascular bundle (*B*). Satisfactory range of motion and strength could be complemented with a neurovascular island transfer to provide sensation.

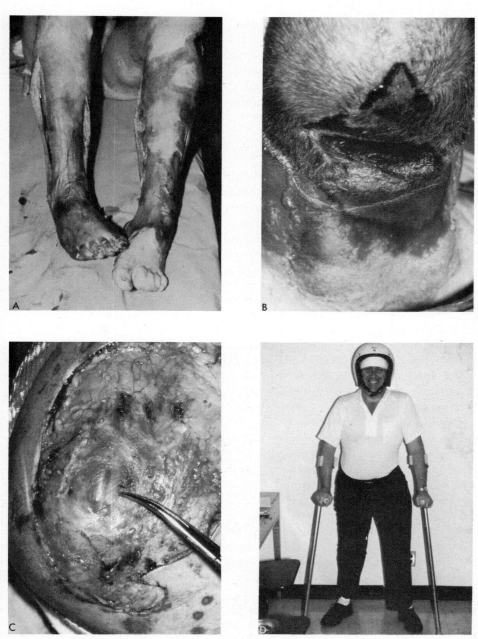

Figure 46–4   In the severe electrical burn, nerve repair may not be the top priority. Entrance (*A*) and exit (*B*) wounds resulted in bilateral AK amputations and the loss of posterior skull in addition to the ulnar nerve (*C*). Mobilizing the patient on crutches to help prevent recurrent deep vein thrombosis took precedence over early ulnar neurorrhaphy (*D*).

Nerve reconstruction may have to be delayed if the patient's general condition presents other priorities. For example, the current entered through the feet and exited through the arm and posterior skull of the patient shown in Figure 46–4. Debridement revealed a nonviable ulnar nerve at the condyle for a distance of 6.0 cm. Early nerve grafting would have been desirable except that bilateral above-knee amputations were followed by deep vein phlebitis. The patient requires crutches to walk presently, and upper extremity surgery would confine him to a bed or wheelchair, making him a prime risk for recurrent phlebitis or pulmonary embolus. Thus, nerve reconstruction will be delayed until the patient is independent on crutches.

RADIATION INJURY

The increased use of various radiation sources in the twentieth century led initially to large numbers of injuries, frequently with hand and peripheral nerve involvement. X-ray and radium were the common agents. As newer and more powerful radiation sources were developed, they were treated with extreme care, and only a few peripheral injuries in the arms, hands, and feet have been recorded. The damage from these various sources is similar, varying only in degree, and may be acute, subacute, chronic, or degenerative, leading to malignant change.

Biologically, electromagnetic radiations follow the laws of quantum mechanics, and injury is the result of the application of excessive energy into the normal biochemical systems of cells. Longer-wave-length sources, such as electricity, various radio waves, and light, promote an excitation phenomenon in which the high energy causes electrons to become displaced from inner to outer orbits in the affected atoms. The shorter-wave-length radiation sources, such as certain x-rays and atomic particles, deliver their energy by causing atoms to yield an electron, forming negative–positive ion pairs, or by striking an atom and producing various secondary radiations. The result of these mechanisms may be disorganization of nucleic acid synthesis, prevention of enzyme synthesis, interference with normal cellular division, or alterations in membrane permeability. These injuries may be reversible or irreversible, causing temporary or permanent changes in cellular function.

Low energy radiations, such as alpha and beta particles, ultraviolet light, and others, injure the superficial tissues most, the injurious effect being reduced as the depth increases. Sources with high energy, such as supervoltage x-ray and products of linear-type accelerators, cause secondary radiant energy primarily; thus the deeper tissues are most affected. This principle, which allows relative sparing of the normal, more superficial tissues, forms the basis for modern solid tumor therapy.

Tissues that have a high metabolic rate, or that have high reproductive capability, are vulnerable to radiation injury because of the effects upon mitosis. The extremities, particularly the hand, are relatively radiosensitive because of their small size and variety of functional tissues, including sweat and sebaceous glands, fingernails, marrow-containing bones, blood vessels, nerves, and soft tissues. Generally, hematopoietic tissues are most sensitive to higher energy radiation, followed by the skin and its appendages, the vascular endothelium, connective tissue, fat, bone, and, finally, nerve and muscle.

Nerve tissue is rather resistant to radiant injury because of its depth, its low cellular reproduction, and its metabolic characteristics. Nerve injury may ensue, however, because of proximity to affected structures that yield or transmit heat. As a corollary, in denervated tissues the vulnerability to radiant energy increases because of cellular turnover, changes in vascularity, and diminution of sensory feedback to the patient. Although infrared, visible, and ultraviolet light sources cause no unique injury to nerve tissue itself, they often cause pronounced injury to denervated tissues. In the hands and feet, for example, peripheral nerve injury frequently results in soft tissue changes. Because of exposure and impaired sensory feedback, protective measures and patient education are necessary to prevent further injury by these energy sources. Very high energy sources such as x-ray and gamma radiation may injure some or all of the tissues in the extremities, and, because of the smaller bulk of these structures, considerable damage may ensure.

The partially damaged cells constitute the major clinical radiation problem, as lethally injured tissues quickly become necrotic and separate. In damaged tissue, the initial hyperemia or early response to injury gradually diminishes after three to four weeks, and is due to arteritis characterized by thrombosis and obstructive endothelial proliferation with unyielding diminution of fibroplasia and capillary proliferation. Even if such wounds eventually epithelialize, they are atrophic, ischemic, and vulnerable to further mechanical injury. These cellular injuries are similar to those caused by certain biochemical material often called "radiomimetic" drugs.

Significantly, in acute radiation injury there may only be erythema of the skin and little or no pain, with resolution in a few days, although skin pigment changes may remain for months to years. In more severe acute exposure, necrosis and painful ulceration may ensue. Usually the ulcerations do not heal and the likelihood of malignant degeneration in the skin and soft tissues is high over a long period of time. There have been two reported instances (Andrews, 1968) of fatal massive exposure to the hands alone with destruction of all soft tissue, but usually massive exposure is to the whole body. Malignant degeneration commonly occurs in the skin, but no instances of selective malignant peripheral nerve degeneration have been noted.

In the treatment of radiation injured tissues, the general principles of wound management including excision, dressing, resurfacing, antisepsis, and revascularization must be practiced. Radiation wounds of significance rarely heal primarily, and are subject to chronic degenerative changes. Wound excision, usually with wide margins to include all injured tissues, is indicated. Repeated debridement is often required, much as with electrical burns, as inadequate excision with graft coverage alone commonly fails. The injury is more diffuse than may be appreciated initially, and a recipient area must be appropriately vascularized or have the capability for vascularity before definitive wound coverage can be successful. Adherent dressings for debridement, and, later, non-adherent dressings are applicable. Split or full thickness skin graft coverage may be useful at this point if evidence of vascularization of the recipient site is present. Often, however, local cutaneous skin flaps may be required for coverage. Direct or free muscle flaps with skin graft coverage, or myocutaneous flaps may be required in the extensive injury, especially where neovascularization or reinnervation of a particular area is critical. Pain caused by wound ischemia and

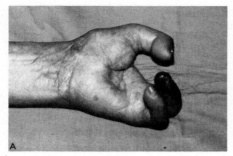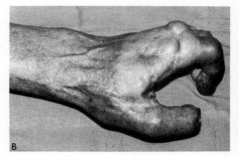

Figure 46–5 Chronic repetitive debridement, grafting, and serial amputations (*A* and *B*) reveal why nerve reconstruction is rarely a viable option following radiation injury.

neuritis or exposure of nerve tissue is common, and peripheral neuritis is associated with the more severe injuries. Since denervation from any cause renders the tissues more vulnerable to injury of all types, consideration must be given to reinnervation techniques such as neurorrhaphy, nerve grafts, or neurovascular pedicle methods. If these are not possible, protection of the reconstructed but denervated area by means of patient education and mechanical assistance, as in paraplegic patients, is required.

The handling of hazardous radioactive materials is becoming increasingly common; therefore caution and prevention must be stressed. Our patients with implanted materials in the form of sutures or prosthetic devices must be educated to avoid energy sources such as diathermy. If basic wound management principles are practiced by responsible clinicians, chronic changes, such as malignant degeneration, and susceptibility to further injury in the patient with previously denervated extremities may be reduced. Clinicians must be increasingly aware of the causes, time factors involved, and certain special characteristics of radiation injuries so that prevention and efficient rehabilitation can be achieved.

CONCLUSION

Under the general heading of burn injury reside several different etiologic agents. Although total nerve destruction may be immediate, as in some electrical injuries, and thus defy therapeutic intervention, many patients may be helped. An awareness of the specific biologic result rendered by radiation, electricity, fire, or chemical, a concern for early diagnosis, and a knowledge of specific treatments may lessen the incidence of crippling deformities (Fig. 46–5).

REFERENCES

Andrews, J. R.: The Radiobiology of Human Cancer Radiotherapy. Philadelphia, W. B. Saunders Company, 1968.
Bevin, A. G.: Early tendon transfer for radial nerve transection. Hand *8*:134, 1976.
Curreri, W. P., Morris, J., and Pruitt, B. A. Jr.: The treatment of chemical burns: Specialized diagnostic therapeutic, and prognostic considerations. J. Trauma *10*:634, 1970.

Levine, N. S., and Salisbury, R. E.: Early removal of the eschar in upper extremity burns. *In* Salisbury, R. E., and Pruitt, B. A. Jr.: Burns of the Upper Extremity. Philadelphia, W. B. Saunders Company, 1976.

Moncrief, J. A., and Pruitt, B. A. Jr.: Electric Injury. Postgrad. Med. *48*:189, 1970.

Moylan, J. A., Inge, W. W., and Pruitt, B. A. Jr.: Circulatory changes following circumferential extremity burns evaluated by the ultrasound flowmeter. J. Trauma *11*:763, 1971.

Pruitt, B. A. Jr., Dowling, J. A., and Moncrief, J. A.: Excharotomy in early burn care. Arch. Surg. *96*:502, 1968.

Salisbury, R. E., Hunt, J. L., Warden, G. D., and Pruitt, B. A. Jr.: Management of electrical burns of the upper extremity. Plast. Reconstr. Surg. *51*:648, 1976.

Salisbury, R. E., Pruitt, B. A. Jr.: Burns of the Upper Extremity. Philadelphia, W.B. Saunders Company, 1976.

Report of the U.N. Scientific Committee on the Effects of Atomic Radiation, Supplement No. 16 (A/5216).

Rehabilitation

VII

47

SENSORY RE-EDUCATION AFTER PERIPHERAL NERVE INJURY

RAYMOND M. CURTIS and
A. LEE DELLON

   The hand is unable to function without sensibility. Moberg (1962, 1966) was one of the first to emphasize that hand function was dependent upon the degree of sensibility obtained following nerve repair. In adults with median and ulnar nerve laceration at the wrist, Önne (1962) described poor recovery of two-point discrimination following repair. In reports by other authors (McEwan, 1964; Nicholson and Seddon, 1957; Nielsen and Torup, 1964; Stromberg et al., 1961) only 2 per cent of adults obtained two-point discrimination of 3 to 5 mm following repair of the median and ulnar nerves. Önne (1962) reported excellent recovery of two-point discrimination in children. This could be based on the fact that the child has better nerve regeneration; however, it is undoubtedly due in part to the fact that the child has the ability to achieve a more perfect sensory re-education pattern in the cerebral cortex following peripheral nerve repair.

   Mitchell (1895) described the phenomenon of false localization following nerve regeneration. This he refers to as the inability to accurately localize a point of stimulation on the skin despite good return of function of the basic modalities of sensation following nerve severance and regeneration. He cites, for example, that following the repair of a lacerated median nerve, a point stimulus to the index finger will be clearly localized to another point in the distribution of this nerve. Increasing the intensity of the stimulation only makes the patient more convinced that it has occurred on the falsely localized area.

Mountcastle and coworkers (1957) first proposed the unit column theory of cortical organization based on his electrophysiologic recordings and the previous work of Sperry (Sperry, 1947). This experimental work was done by stimulating a single nerve fiber distally in the cutaneous nerve of the paw of the cat and recording with microelectrodes from the somatic sensory cerebral cortex (Brodmann's areas 3 and 1 of the postcentral gyrus of the brain). Mountcastle demonstrated that there was a discrete area of the brain that received the distal signal. This could be mapped as a specific localized area (such as the tip of the thumb or the tip of the index finger) on the cerebral cortex using a microelectrode.

Paul and associates (1972), using adult rhesus monkeys, sectioned the median nerve and resutured it. Mapping experiments were carried out on both hemispheres of six operated monkeys six and a half or seven and a half months following operations. The right hemisphere served as the control; the left hemisphere (contralateral to the denervated hand) served as the experimental model. Nerves of both hands were dissected out and photographed. Short sections of the digital nerve distal to the anastomotic site and sections from the anastomotic site were removed and stained with special myelin stains for histologic examination. In all six experiments following nerve section and repair there was a significant disorganization of the somatotopic representation of the skin of the monkey's paw in the cortex. This somatotopic experimental model demonstrated that the input to the cortical columns in the brain is radically altered following peripheral nerve severance repair and regeneration.

In 1962 Vinograd and associates described the use of common objects, such as blocks, cubes, and triangles, to re-educate sensibility in the hemiplegic hand (Vinogrod, Taylor, and Grossman, 1962). In 1966 Wynn Parry demonstrated the usefulness of sensory re-education using a similar technique (Wynn Parry, 1966a, 1966b). In 1970 Fragiadakis and coworkers observed that the results of nerve suture were better in patients who were dextrous rather than in those who were not, such as heavy manual laborers. Dellon and associates reported on a sensory re-education program in which the patient was assigned a specific sensory exercise at the appropriate time in his recovery; that is, when specific clinical tests indicated he had reached the degree of recovery that would allow for re-education of deep touch, light touch, movement, two-point discrimination, and the use of objects normally used in activities of daily living (Dellon, Curtis, and Edgerton, 1971, 1972).

The blind have no greater capacity for touch than do the sighted, but their intensive training of tactile discriminating capacity reaches very high levels. In Braille printing each dot is 1 mm above the surface, and the dots are separated by 2.5 mm. This is just above the two-point discrimination threshold for the fingertips. An experienced blind reader can read 100 words (approximately 600 letters) per minute. This is about the rate we read aloud. If the blind person presses his finger against the letter and prevents the scanning movements (moving two-point), his reading capacity is almost abolished. The practiced braillist uses the left index finger even when he is right-handed. In 1969 Heinrichs and Moorhouse recorded two-point discrimination of 1.5 mm in blind diabetic patients (Heinrichs and Moorhouse, 1969). Bach-y-Rita (1972) trained blind subjects to "see" by using a multipoint stimulator against the skin receptors of the back. The blind subject was taught to interpret the stimuli and thereby to recognize objects, and to operate an oscilloscope.

NEUROPHYSIOLOGY OF CUTANEOUS SENSIBILITY

It has been estimated that there are as many as 2000 nerve endings in 9 sq. mm of the tip of the finger. These nerve endings are supplied by myelinated or nonmyelinated fibers. These nerve fibers may terminate free or in a specific structure, such as a Meissner corpuscle, Merkel disk, or pacinian corpuscle. The sensory endings possess a threshold; that is, there exists a physically definable stimulus of appropriate quality to which they respond with the discharge of a nerve impulse (Mountcastle, La Motte, and Giancarlo, 1972). The large, myelinated fibers (group A-beta fibers) mediate the perception of touch and have been divided by Mountcastle and associates into two populations, based on the way in which they respond to a constant touch stimulus (Mountcastle et al., 1967). These are the quickly adapting fibers and the slowly adapting fibers. The quickly adapting fibers are further divided into two groups, one of which responds

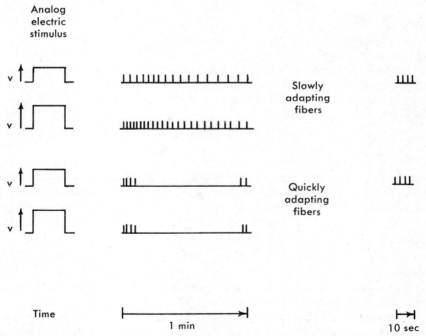

Figure 47–1   The response patterns of slowly adapting and quickly adapting fibers to mechanical stimuli of constant duration. Both the stimulus and response are illustrated by an electrical analog; a square-wave stimulus and a spike-potential response from single fiber recordings. Each type of fiber is stimulated first with a low intensity (voltage, v), and then with a higher intensity, which is analogous to the depth to which the mechanical stimulus penetrated, and which corresponds to a human experience of a constant-touch stimulus of two different pressures. Stimuli of both short- and long-time duration are used.

maximally to a vibratory frequency in the range of 2 to 40 Hz, and one of which responds best in the range of 60 to 300 Hz (Fig. 47–1). The large, myelinated sensory fibers end in mechanoreceptors (Merkel disks, Meissner corpuscles, and pacinian corpuscles). These latter structures transform the external stimulus into a conductible action potential that moves along the afferent neuron and is conducted, after relays in the brain stem and thalamus, to the postcentral gyrus of the sensory cortex.

After nerve laceration the sensory endings begin a progressive degeneration (Dellon, Witebsky, and Terrill, 1975). Following nerve repair, axons regrow down the endoneurial tube to its termination, reinnervate the degenerating end-organ, and, providing too long a time interval has not elapsed, reverse the process of degeneration (Dellon, 1976).

It is the group A-beta nerve fiber system that gives man the precision his hands possess. Each nerve fiber has a small peripheral receptive field. The fields of different fibers partially overlap. In the hand we have the greatest number of receptive fields per body area. There is, therefore, a very high peripheral innervation density. The perception of form and the direction of movement of a stimulus is not explained as an activation of isolated nerve fibers but rather as the cortical interpretation of profiles of the activities of these partially overlapping peripheral receptive fields (Mountcastle, 1974).

METHOD OF RE-EDUCATION

The object of sensory re-education is to improve sensation. The program should be introduced as soon as possible in the recovery period, and this is determined by the patient's pattern of recovery of sensation. The pattern of sensory recovery is mapped at regular intervals, and the following are charted: Tinel sign, constant- and moving-touch perception, perception of vibration at 30 and 256 Hz by tuning fork and two-point discrimination (Dellon, Curtis, and Edgerton, 1972). Two-point discrimination is not tested until perception of constant touch returns (Fig. 47–2).

The retraining session lasts 10 to 15 minutes and is carried out by the patient three to five times a day at home in a room with as few distractions as possible. During this session the patient observes what he is doing, thinks about how it feels, turns his head, closes his eyes, and verbalizes aloud what he is doing (Fig. 47–3).

The therapist re-evaluates the patient at regular intervals, introduces the appropriate exercise based on the degree of recovery, and reinforces the learning process by the interest shown in the improvement. When possible, the therapist should encourage the patient to use the forearm and hand muscles in the exercise. This enhances the learning process.

Early phase re-education is begun over the areas in which constant and moving touch are perceived but in which no two-point discrimination has returned. If a 256 Hz stimulus is perceived before touch stimuli, the patient also is ready for early phase re-education. Early phase re-education can be started in the palm and proximal phalanx. The object can be a pencil eraser or even another finger (Fig. 47–4). Once constant touch is perceived at the fingertip, late phase re-education is begun. The patient is instructed to move an object

Text continued on page 776

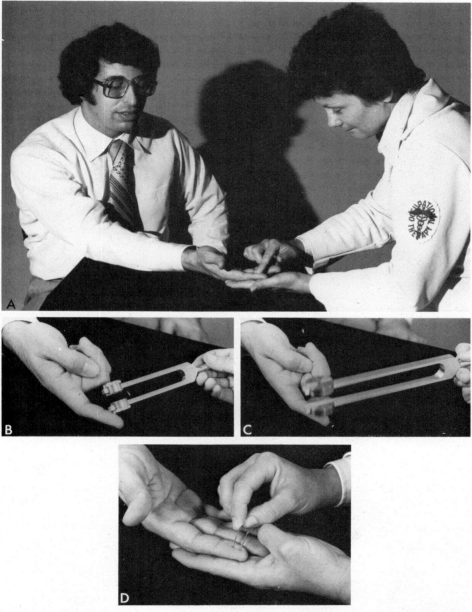

Figure 47–2   Evaluation of sensibility: *A*, With the examiner and patient arranged comfortably, and the tested digit supported fully, perception of constant and moving touch are tested using the examiner's fingertip. Evaluation of the quickly adapting fiber/receptor system is then detailed with the 256 cycle per second (pacinian corpuscle) (*B*) and the 30 cycle per second (Meissner corpuscle) (*C*) tuning forks. Applying the vibrating prong's edge gives a maximum stimulus amplitude. *D*, A paper clip serves to test two-point discrimination.

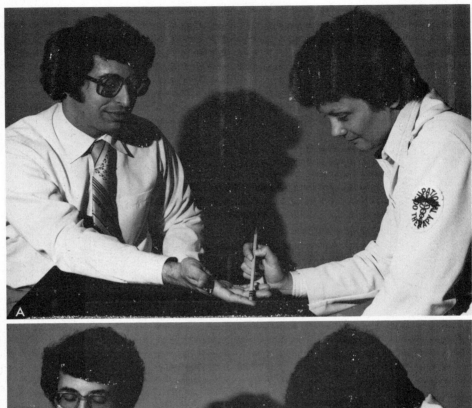

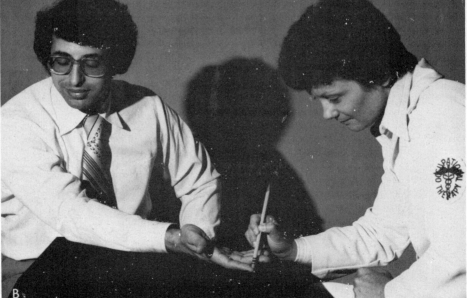

Figure 47–3 Basic technique in sensory re-education involves the patient's direct observation of the sensory stimulus (*A*). Then, with head turned and eyes closed (*B*), the patient concentrates on this same, repeated stimulus. He must learn to associate the new, altered profile of peripheral nerve impulses his brain is receiving with the old, once-familiar stimulus.

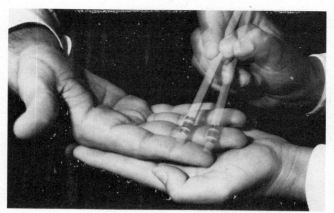

Figure 47–4 Early phase sensory re-education is begun when sensory evaluation indicates that a constant and/or moving touch, or a 256-cycle-per-second stimulus is perceived in the palm. In this phase, touch stimuli are delivered to the reinnervated area to re-educate gross tactile discrimination and localization. Any blunt-tipped object is suitable to use.

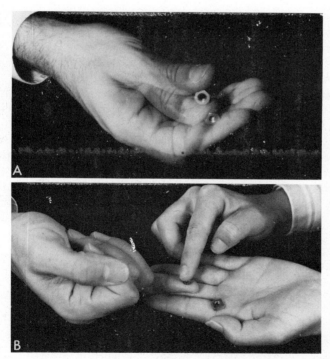

Figure 47–5 Late phase sensory re-education is begun when touch stimuli are perceived at the fingertip. For median nerve recovery, varying sized metal hex or square nuts are compressed or rolled between index and thumb, concomitantly helping motor function (*A*). For ulnar nerve recovery, these objects must be pressed on to the little finger (*B*). Again, the patient observes the action, then with eyes closed concentrates on making the new sensory associations.

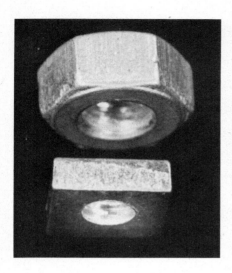

Figure 47-6 As sensory recovery proceeds, gradually smaller nuts may be used, and objects of daily living and work introduced into the routine. Here the difference in edge length between a square and a hex nut illustrates how fine discrimination can be trained simply and inexpensively.

back and forth between the thumb and the fingers in the normal hand, to shift the object to the injured hand, and to try to identify it with his eyes open and closed (Fig. 47–5).

These objects are used for retraining:

Early phase re-education

1. Fingertip of normal hand
2. Soft object, such as the eraser on a pencil

Late phase re-education

3. Various sizes of square, hexagonal, and round objects, starting with an object about 3 cm in diameter (such as square or hexagonal metal nuts and washers) (Fig. 47–6)

4. Objects used in daily living, such as keys, coins, safety pins, screwdrivers, writing instruments, buttons on clothing, typewriters, nuts threaded on bolts, and tools used in work

Where there is hypesthesia or pain over the distribution of the regenerating nerve, a procedure for desensitization must be carried out prior to sensory re-education. It will not be possible to re-educate the hypersensitive hand. The technique consists of stroking the hypersensitive area with the finest piece of cotton that can be tolerated, progressing to wool fiber and felt (Maynard, 1977). In some instances, treatment with a transcutaneous stimulator may be necessary.

DISCUSSION

Dellon and associates (1974) reported recovery of normal or near-normal sensation in four adults following sensory re-education after nerve repair. Wynn Parry and Salter (1976) reported on sensory re-education in 23 patients following median nerve repair. They were followed from one to three years, and an improvement in the time it took the patients to identify test objects and texture was noted. In almost all patients point localization returned to normal. The occupational therapist and workshop technicians reported a marked improvement in function once training began. Reid (1977) reviewed the testing of 150 adult patients with median nerve injury one to five years after injury and found that these patients had nothing more than protective sensation. To retrain sensation he used the Weber two-point test using a Boley gauge. The re-education was begun after a preliminary battery of clinical tests had been carried out and when 256 Hz could be detected at the fingertip. There was an improvement in sensation in all patients re-educated, as evidenced by improved two-point discrimination, point localization, Moberg object identification, Moberg picking-up test, and Porter letter test. In addition, the patients used the area of the hand supplied by the repaired median nerve.

The patients studied by Reid (1977) maintained the improvement in two-point discrimination even after many years. One adult from the series, with a primary repair of a median nerve that had been lacerated 12 cm proximal to the wrist crease, had two-point discrimination greater than 45 mm when tested at six months following repair. Following six weeks of sensory re-education, he had two-point discrimination of 11 to 15 mm. When he was examined seven years later, the two-point discrimination was 7 mm over the thumb and index finger. The patient used the area of the hand innervated by the median nerve for all functions without visual help.

SUMMARY

The nervous system faces the external world not directly but by an afferent input through a system of mechanoreceptors in the hand. When stimulated, these produce an impulse that travels by way of the nerve fibers to a specific area of the cerebral cortex. This area for the hand is massive, and consequently tactile acuity is very highly developed in the fingers.

Following repair of a lacerated peripheral nerve, axons regrow down an endoneurial tube to reinnervate the mechanoreceptors. This regrowth generally results in less than 100 per cent of the distal endoneurial tubes being filled, in axons misdirected into other than their former endoneurial tube, and often in improperly reinnervated mechanoreceptors at the periphery. This produces an altered profile of neural impulses in the cerebral cortex compared to the pre-injury profile when the repaired nerve is stimulated.

A sensory re-education program introduced at the appropriate time in the patient's clinical recovery leads to measurable improvement in sensation and, ultimately, to improved hand function.

REFERENCES

Bach-y-Rita, P.: Brain mechanisms in sensory substitution. New York, Academic Press, 1972.
Dellon, A. L., Curtis, R. M., and Edgerton, M. T.: Evaluating recovery of sensation in the hand following nerve injury. J. Johns Hopkins Hosp. *130*:235, 1972.
Dellon, A. L., Curtis, R. M., and Edgerton, M. T.: Re-education of sensation in the hand following nerve injury. J. Bone Joint Surg. *53A*:813, 1971.
Dellon, A. L., Curtis, R. M., and Edgerton, M. T.: Reeducation of sensation in the hand after nerve injury and repair. J. Plast. Reconstr. Surg. *53*:297, 1974.

Dellon, A. L., Witebsky, F. G., and Terrill, R. E.: The denervated Meissner corpuscle: a sequential histologic study following nerve division in the Rhesus monkey. J. Plast. Reconstr. Surg. *56*:182, 1975.

Dellon, A. L.: Reinnervation of denervated Meissner corpuscles: A sequential histologic study in the monkey following fascicular nerve repair. J. Hand Surg. *1*:98, 1976.

Fragiadakis, D. G., Lamb, D. W., and Honner, R.: An investigation of factors affecting the results of nerve division. Hand *2*:21, 1970.

Heinrichs, R. W., and Moorhouse, J. A.: Touch perception in blind diabetic subjects in relation to the reading of Braille type. N. Engl. J. Med. *280*:72, 1969.

Maynard, J.: Sensory reeducation after peripheral nerve injury. American Society for Surgery of the Hand. Symposium on Rehabilitation of the Hand, Philadelphia, 1977.

McEwan, L. E.: Median and ulnar nerve injuries. Aust. N. Zeal. J. Surg. *32*:89–104, 1964.

Mitchell, J. K., Jr.: Remote consequences of injuries of nerves and their treatment. Examination of the present condition of wounds received 1863–65 with illustrative cases. Philadelphia, Lea Bros. and Co., 1895, p. 255.

Moberg, E.: Criticism and study of methods for examining sensibility in the hand. Neurology (Minneap.), *12*:1, 1962.

Moberg, E.: Methods of examing sensibility of the hand. *In* Flynn, J. E. (ed.): Hand Surgery. Baltimore, Williams & Wilkins Co., 1966.

Mountcastle, V. B.: Sensory receptors and neural encoding: introduction to sensory processes. In Mountcastle, V. D., (ed.): Medical Physiology, 13th ed. St. Louis, C. V. Mosby Co., 1974, Vol. 2, p. 285.

Mountcastle, V. B., Talbot, W. H., and Kornhuber, H. H.: The neural transformation of mechanical stimuli, delivered to the monkey's hand. In de Reuck, A. V. S., and Knight, J., (eds.): Ciba Foundation Symposium. Boston, Little, Brown & Co., 1966, p. 325.

Mountcastle, V. B., Talbot, W. H., Darian-Smith, I., and Kornhuber, H. H.: A neural base for the sense of flutter-vibration. Science *155*:597, 1967.

Mountcastle, V. B.: Modality and topographic properties of single neurons of cat's somatic sensory cortex. J. Neurophys. *20*:408, 1957.

Mountcastle, V. B., LaMotte, R. H., and Giancarlo, C.: Detection thresholds for stimuli in humans and monkeys: Comparison with threshold events in mechanoreceptive afferent nerve fibers innervating the monkey hand. J. Neurophys. *35*:122, 1972.

Nicholson, O. R., and Seddon, H. J.: Nerve repairs in civil practice: Results of therapy of median and ulnar nerve lesions. Br. Med. J. *2*:1065, 1957.

Nielsen, J. B., and Torup, D.: Nerve injuries in the upper extremities. Dan. Med. Bull. *11*:92, 1964.

Önne, L.: Recovery of sensibility and sudomotor function in the hand after nerve suture. Acta Chir. Scand. (Suppl.) *300*:1, 1962.

Paul, R. L., Goodman, H., and Merzenich, M.: Alterations in mechanoreceptor input to Brodmann's areas 1 and 3 of the postcentral hand area of *Macaca mulatta* after nerve section and regeneration. Brain Res. *39*:1, 1972.

Reid, R. L.: Preliminary results of sensibility reeducation following repair of the median nerve. Am. Soc. Surg. Hand Newsletter 15, 1977.

Sperry, R. W.: Cerebral regulation of motor coordination following multiple transection of sensorimotor cortex. J. Neurophysiol. *10*:275, 1947.

Stromberg, W. B., McFarlane, R. M., Bell, J. L., Koch, S. L., and Mason, M. L.: Injuries of the median and ulnar nerves. J. Bone Joint Surg. *43A*:717, 1961.

Vinograd, A., Taylor, E., and Grossman, S.: Sensory retaining of the hemiplegic hand. Am. J. Occup. Ther. *16*:246, 1962.

Wynn Parry, C. B.: Diagnosis and aftercare of peripheral nerve lesions in the upper limb. Founders Lecture, American Society for Surgery of the Hand. J. Bone Joint Surg. *48A*:607, 1966*a*.

Wynn Parry, C. B.: Rehabilitation of the hand, London, Butterworth & Co., 1966*b*.

Wynn Parry, C. B., and Salter, M.: Sensory reeducation after median nerve lesions. Hand *8*:250, 1976.

48

NEUROVASCULAR CUTANEOUS ISLAND PEDICLE FLAPS

GEORGE E. OMER, Jr.

Surgical procedures to restore sensibility following irreparable nerve loss have been utilized primarily for the hand. In 1955, during a discussion of tactile-sense restoration, Moberg (1955) suggested the digital neurovascular pedicle sensory island. Littler (1956) developed the technique for transfer, incorporating a digital nerve and artery as the pedicle. Intact sensibility, peripheral circulation, and corniferous skin are all restored by this method. (Littler, 1976) Subsequent techniques were developed to utilize double islands from two digits (McGregor, 1969; Omer et al., 1970) and a radial-innervated island for the thumb. (Holevich, 1963). Since the operations are elective and are performed for irreparable nerve loss, they should be delayed until all indicated tendon transfers have been accomplished and the patient has supple tissues with an established range of motion.

Three general uses for the neurovascular cutaneous island pedicle flap have been developed: (1) reconstruction of the thumb distal to the level of the metacarpophalangeal joint, (2) islands of sensibility over the radial half of the hand that has total median nerve loss distal to the volar carpal ligament, and (3) islands of sensibility over weight-bearing areas of the foot.

THUMB PULP DEFECT

Many techniques have been devised for reconstruction following total thumb loss, such as pollicization of an available finger (Bunnell, 1952; Littler, (1953), free toe transfers (Buncke, 1976), or the osteoplastic composite flap

779

(McGregor and Simonetta, 1964). Several experienced surgeons (Chase, 1969; Littler, 1956; Tubiana and Duparc, 1961) advocate osteoplastic reconstruction, including a delayed neurovascular cutaneous island, when all other fingers are normal in the presence of a mobile first metacarpal with distal avulsion. The neurovascular cutaneous island pedicle is even more useful in providing a sensible, nonslip, durable surface for the volar pulp of the thumb with an avulsion injury.

Surgical Considerations

The volar sensory supply of the digits of the hand is primarily from the median and ulnar nerves. These nerves terminate as common digital nerves which bifurcate into proper digital nerves, each supplying sensation to one hemidigit. The most common arrangement is for the median nerve to supply sensation on both sides of the thumb, index finger, and long finger, and on the radial half of the ring finger. The ulnar nerve usually supplies both sides of the little finger and the ulnar half of the ring finger. The superficial radial nerve is important in the dorsal sensory supply of the fingers. The nerve is distributed to the radial–dorsal aspect of the hand, with one nerve branch tending to pass to each side of the dorsum of each digit. The superficial radial nerve fibers terminate over the proximal two thirds of the proximal phalanx.

The superficial palmar vascular arch of the hand is a continuation of the ulnar artery, and from this arch three common volar digital arteries arise and then bifurcate into the proper digital arteries on the ulnar side of the index finger, both sides of the long and ring fingers, and the radial side of the little finger. The superficial palmar vascular arch underlies a transverse palmar line extending along the ulnar side of the widely abducted thumb. An Allen test should be done at the carpal level to evaluate the arterial supply of the hand. The superficial vascular arch may have to be interrupted and the radial portion freed to swing with the neurovascular pedicle attached to the cutaneous island. In patients over 40 years of age, circulatory problems should be carefully investigated before surgery is attempted.

Technique Using the Median Nerve for Sensibility

A paper pattern is made of the avulsed pulp area of the thumb or the new area of sensibility desired on the ulnar–volar aspect of the reconstructed thumb. The completed pattern is outlined in sterile ink. It is then laid on the skin of the ulnar–volar aspect of the long finger or the radial–volar aspect of the ring finger. A large pattern includes more of the donor nerve and is not a disadvantage (Hueston, 1965). The distance from the proximal edge of the pattern on the finger to the "swing-point" on the superficial vascular arch is measured, compared, and adjusted to the distance from the "swing-point" to the proximal edge of the original drawing on the thumb. These measurements should be made with the thumb widely abducted from the palm on a flat surface. Uneven distances indicate the superficial volar vascular arch will have to be interrupted and the radial portion freed to swing with the cutaneous island.

A zigzag longitudinal palmar incision avoiding the pads over the metacarpal heads is made along the course of the common digital nerve and vessels between the long and ring fingers. The incision extends proximally from the distal edge of the palm to the level of the superficial volar vascular arch. If there is abnormal vessel or nerve distribution, the palmar incision should be closed without further injury to the hand. If the anatomy is normal, the neurovascular pedicle distances should be measured again under direct visualization of the "swing-point" where the common digital artery leaves the superficial arch.

Liberation of the neurovascular pedicle requires cleavage of the common digital nerve in the palm into its two proper digital nerve components. This must be a meticulous procedure if loss of sensation is to be avoided. The nerve is dissected from its distal end to its proximal end, beginning at the bifurcation in the web space. The proper digital arterial branch to the cutaneous island is freed, while the proper digital artery to the remaining finger is ligated. Perforating branches of the digital artery are tied. Ligation of the branch too close to the major trunk can distort the patent vessel and cause eddy currents with subsequent thrombosis (Peacock, 1971). Optical magnification is required for an optimal result.

The cutaneous island is carefully dissected in a proximal to distal direction. The nerve branches should be superficial to the dissection. Sufficient subcutaneous tissue is removed to expose the flexor tendon sheath and perhaps the extensor mechanism, but a very thin transparent layer of tissue is left behind over the tendon structures. Small vessels are carefully ligated. A zigzag transverse palmar incision from the proximal portion of the initial palmar incision to the thumb recipient site is made through the palmar fascia just distal to the superficial volar arch, thus creating a fascial trough. The neurovascular pedicle is then placed in the fascial trough without tension, acute angulation, or constriction. The tourniquet is released to prove the viability of circulation to the cutaneous island and to obtain meticulous hemostasis.

If the procedure is an osteoplastic reconstruction, and if there is no avulsion of the thumb pulp, a full thickness skin graft is removed from within the ink pattern outlined as the recipient site. This skin graft fits exactly in the island donor site on the long finger. It is sutured into place, with the ends of some of the sutures left long enough to tie around a glycerin and mineral oil soaked cotton wedge compression dressing. If the thumb pulp is avulsed, the full thickness skin graft can be obtained from the nonweight-bearing portion of the sole of the foot or from the hypothenar area of the hand.

The neurovascular island is then fitted into the recipient site on the thumb. The glycerin and mineral oil soaked cotton wedge dressing is tied in place for even compression. The hand is immobilized for three weeks after surgery, but the extremity is free for an exercise program.

Technique Using the Ulnar Nerve for Sensibility

The procedure for the ulnar nerve is the same as for the median nerve, except the common digital nerve and vessels are exposed between the ring and little fingers, and the neurovascular cutaneous island is obtained from the ulnar–volar aspect of the ring finger (Fig. 48–1).

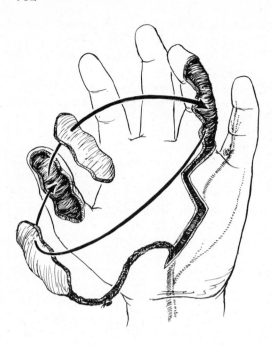

Figure 48–1 Neurovascular cutaneous island from the ulnar-innervated aspect of the ring finger to the thumb to restore volar pulp sensibility.

Technique Using the Superficial Radial Nerve for Sensibility

When the superficial radial nerve is used, it is advisable to carry out preoperative evaluation by digital block of the proper volar digital nerves to the index finger. Occasionally the dorsal surface of the proximal phalanx of the index will

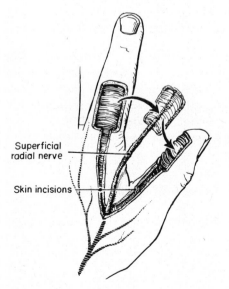

Superficial
radial nerve

Skin incisions

Figure 48–2 Radial innervated island flap from the index finger to the thumb pulp. This procedure is precarious because there is no constant vascular supply to the island. The technique is usually modified so that instead of an island pedicle, a cross-finger flap is created from the index finger to the thumb.

be supplied by the median nerve (Adamson, Horton, and Crawford, 1967). Careful study with light touch and two-point discrimination distance is indicated after the appropriate nerve blocks.

If the preoperative evaluation proves favorable, a V-shaped skin incision is made, with one limb of the "V" at the level of the midlateral line on the radial side of the index finger and the other limb at the midlateral line on the ulnar side of the thumb. The point of the incision is near the first dorsal metacarpal branch of the radial artery. Gentle dissection will expose the longitudinal branches of the superficial radial nerve and vascular structures dorsal to the second metacarpal. If the vessels can be followed distally to the area of the proximal phalanx, a racquet-shaped cutaneous island with a neurovascular pedicle is dissected from the dorsal–radial surface of the index finger. This neurovascular island is then fitted into the volar–ulnar aspect of the thumb pulp (Fig. 48–2). This procedure is precarious, because the arterial supply to the cutaneous island is not constant. Consequently, the procedure is usually modified in one or two ways: (1) a narrow dorsal strip of skin may be retained proximally from the index cutaneous island (Holevich, 1963), or (2) a cross-finger flap from the index finger to the thumb may be used instead of the free cutaneous island (Adamson, Horton, and Crawford, 1967; Bralliar and Horner, 1969; Gaul, 1969).

Results

Moberg (1964) has indicated that all neurovascular sensory island transplants will have three negative aspects: (1) a loss of sensibility at the donor site, (2) a margin of hyperesthesia around the edges of the cutaneous island, and (3) a loss of the quality of sensibility secondary to cortical disorientation.

Murray and associates (1967) reported their results in 16 patients who were followed one to 10 years after surgery. Based on two-point discrimination distance and light touch, the sensibility in the neurovascular island was less than normal. Twelve patients had continued intolerance to cold and seven had significant hyperesthesia at all times. Reorientation of sensation, so that stimuli on the cutaneous island were referred to the thumb and not to the donor finger, occurred in four patients only after long periods ranging from 18 months to eight years. Reid (1966) reported deficient two-point discrimination in the neurovascular cutaneous islands of fourteen patients. In contrast, Tubiana and Duparc (1961) noted the gradual spread of protective sensibility into the tissue surrounding the transplanted cutaneous island, which may be related to the transferred nerve.

MEDIAN NERVE LOSS

The median nerve supplies the sensibility required for the precise prehension normally performed with the radial side of the hand. If there is an associated loss of motor function from a high (proximal) median nerve injury, the normal pattern of activity is reversed; the radial side of the hand is used for gross grip, while the ulnar side, with its intact muscles and ulnar nerve, is used for precise prehension. A neurovascular island transfer should not be considered in such cases until all possible tendon transfers have been accomplished (Omer, 1975).

Surgical Consideration

Only the common digital nerve between the ring and little fingers is available for a neurovascular cutaneous island, since sensibility along the ulnar aspect of the little finger is essential in total median nerve loss. The usual technique is to transfer a neurovascular cutaneous island from the ulnar aspect of the ring finger to the ulnar–volar aspect of the thumb pulp. To obtain a greater area of sensation, a larger island can be dissected by using half of the volar skin of the donor finger rather than only the distal volar skin from the tip of the donor finger (Hueston, 1965). This technique requires less dissection of the neurovascular bundle but also results in a shorter neurovascular pedicle. The superficial vascular arch may have to be interrupted and the radial portion freed to swing with the cutaneous island.

Technique Using Double Cutaneous Island

The outline of the double island is drawn with a sterile skin marker along the ulnar aspect of the ring finger and the radial aspect of the little finger. The island on the ring finger extends to the distal interphalangeal joint level. This preserves the distal pulp tip of the little finger for precise tactile activity. Both islands extend proximally to the distal edge of the palm. A narrow skin bridge is drawn on the web, dorsal to its palmar edge. A pattern of the double island is made and traced on the skin at the selected recipient area along the ulnar–volar aspect of the thumb and the thumb–index web and proximal radial–volar aspect of the index finger.

A zigzag longitudinal palmar incision is made, avoiding the nonslip pads over the metacarpal heads and following the course of the common digital nerve and vessels between the ring and little fingers. If there is abnormal vascular or nerve distribution, the incision is closed without further surgery. The neurovascular pedicle distances are measured in the same way as is done for a single island transplant, and a decision is made concerning interruption of the superficial vascular arch. Interruption and extensive dissection of the vascular arch increases the danger of an ischemic flap, while the more proximal release of the common digital nerve threatens the sensibility of the cutaneous island.

The two islands are dissected free at the donor sites and full thickness skin grafts are developed at the recipient site. The skin graft from the thumb–index finger area fits exactly in the neurovascular cutaneous island site at the ring–little finger area. The free full thickness graft is sutured into place with the ends of some sutures left long enough so that later a glycerin and mineral oil soaked cotton wedge compression dressing can be tied between the ring and little fingers.

A transverse palmar incision from the proximal point of the initial incision to the midpoint of the selected thumb–index finger recipient site is made through the palmar fascia just distal to the position of the superficial volar

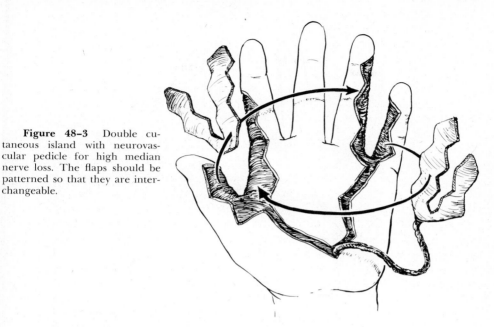

Figure 48–3 Double cutaneous island with neurovascular pedicle for high median nerve loss. The flaps should be patterned so that they are interchangeable.

vascular arch. The neurovascular pedicle is placed in this fascial trough without tension, acute angulation, or constriction (Fig. 48–3). If the narrow skin bridge between the wide double islands does not fit without uneven skin tension, a small, free, split thickness skin graft can be added in the center of the thumb–index web along the dorsal margin of the neurovascular cutaneous islands. A bulky dressing without tie-over compression is used in the web space between the thumb and index finger. The hand is immobilized for three weeks after surgery.

Results

There is disorientation of sensitivity in all neurovascular sensory island transplants. For several months after transplant the patient recognizes stimulation in the island as coming from the original donor digit. Later, sensation is localized in both the recipient and donor sites. Finally, some patients learn to interpret the sensibility to the recipient digit. If the hand is immobilized and nonfunctional for any period of time, however, the interpretation process must be repeated. Also, in an emergency, such as a flame burn, the patient loses his interpretation ability and moves the original donor digit.

Omer and associates (1970) reported their findings in 15 patients with high (proximal) median nerve loss who were followed with evaluation tests at eight week intervals for 14 to 43 months after surgery. The two point discrimination distance recognition and the von Frey light touch pressure tests demonstrated a gradual reduction from normal sensation to merely protective sensation. It was believed that this gradual loss of sensibility was directly related to the associated motor loss for the radial side of the hand; and without adequate motion and power for precise prehension, the sensibility for precise prehension must be lost

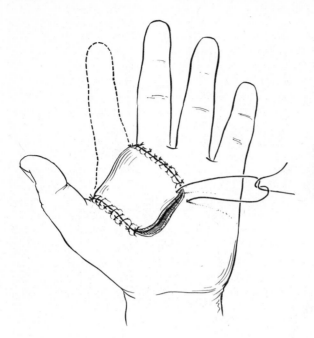

Figure 48–4 Radial innervated dorsal skin flap for combined high median–high ulnar palsy. The insensitive palmar skin is excised to create space for the flap. (From Orthop. Clin. N. Amer. 5:377, 1974.)

(Omer, 1975). Murray, Ord and Gavelin (1967) believed the sensibility loss to be caused by repeated traction on the transferred nerve pedicle.

Combined high median and ulnar nerve loss is a major functional impairment. Sensibility can be restored only to the radial–volar aspect of the hand. The skeleton of the index finger is removed distal to the carpometacarpal joint of this ray. All index tendons except the extensor digitorum communis are then available for tenodesis or active tendon transfers. The insensitive skin distal to the level of the index proximal phalanx is discarded. The fillet of finger is then fitted into a defect created for it in the insensitive palmar skin (Omer, 1974). This broad-based flap is innervated by the superficial radial nerve and will provide protective sensibility for grasp (Fig. 48–4).

WEIGHT-BEARING AREAS OF THE FOOT

In the patient with a neurotrophic ulcer of the foot, a neurovascular cutaneous island transplant will enhance the circulation and stability of the weight-bearing area and afford protective sensation. Moberg (1964) first utilized a cutaneous island transplant in the foot when he moved the pulp of a filleted great toe on a neurovascular pedicle to fill a neurotrophic ulcer of the heel.

Surgical Conditions

The dorsalis pedis artery is the terminal branch of the anterior tibial artery. In midfoot the artery has two named branches, the medial and lateral tarsal arteries. Further distally, the deep branch penetrates the second dorsal interosseous muscle to communicate with the deep plantar arch. The dorsal vein of the foot and the deep peroneal sensory nerve accompany the proper dorsalis pedis artery and the lateral plantar artery, which is the larger of the terminal branches of the posterior tibial artery. The plantar metatarsal arteries run on the surface of the interosseous muscles and may pass dorsal or volar to the transverse metatarsal ligament. The medial plantar nerve divides into digital branches to the great toe, the second and third toe, and the tibial aspect of the fourth toe. The foot is more variable in its blood supply than the hand, and arteriography or a Doppler probe is most helpful in previewing the anatomic variations.

Technique Using Toe for Heel Coverage

The neurotrophic ulcer on the heel is excised to the periosteum of the os calcis. A zigzag longitudinal incision is then made on the nonweight-bearing medial aspect of the sole, extending from the medial aspect of the heel pad to the metatarsophalangeal joint level of the great toe. A flap is dissected, and the medial plantar neurovascular bundle is identified in the interval between the abductor hallucis and flexor digitorum brevis muscles. This dissection is continued to isolate the neurovascular bundle to the medial side of the great toe. Further dissection will identify the plantar metatarsal neurovascular bundle to the adjacent sides of the big toe and the second toe. The digital nerve to the tibial aspect of the second toe is dissected from the common digital nerve from the trunk of the medial plantar nerve, and the vascular branch to the tibial aspect of the second toe from the first metatarsal artery is ligated. If the first metatarsal artery is primarily supplied by the dorsalis pedis artery, then a long vascular pedicle is easily developed. If the major contributor to the first metatarsal artery is the lateral plantar artery, the dissection must be carried proximally into the sole of the foot between the first and second metatarsals to obtain an adequate vascular pedicle. The cutaneous island is developed from the volar skin and subcutaneous tissue overlying the phalanges and the metatarsophalangeal joint. The neurovascular cutaneous island is then rotated into the heel defect and sutured into position. The big toe is disarticulated through the metatarsophalangeal joint, and remaining dorsal skin provides the necessary flap to cover the donor defect.

Results

Toe to heel transplants of sensory cutaneous islands on neurovascular pedicles have been reported by Moberg (1964), Snyder and Edgerton (1965), and Kaplan (1969). No detailed evaluations were recorded by all these surgeons, but the follow-up to two years demonstrated that the cutaneous islands were well vascularized, and the patients appreciated sensation in the cutaneous islands. Sensibility was referred to the donor toe.

Technique Using the Dorsum of the Foot

The entire dorsum of the foot can be safely elevated as an island flap, provided that the deep branch of the dorsalis pedis artery is ligated and the distal

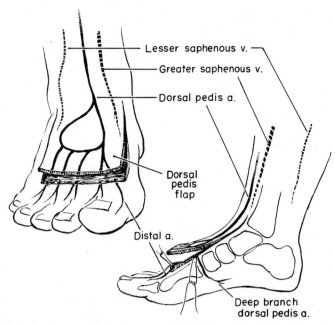

Figure 48–5   The dorsum of the foot as an island flap. If possible, the entire dorsal venous arch should be included in the island.

dorsalis pedis artery is retained with the flap (Fig. 48–5). McGraw and Furlow (1975) state that the island elevation is begun medially, and only after identifying the deep dorsalis pedis branch, the proper dorsalis pedis artery, and the distal dorsalis pedis branch, should the deep branch be ligated. The dissection is then carried distally just superficial to the extensor tendons. Proximal to the deep branch of the dorsalis pedis artery, the proper dorsalis pedis artery is densely adherent to the tarsal bones, and one must dissect precisely on the surface of the tarsal bones. The cutaneous island cannot survive if it is separated from the vascular pedicle at this point. Further proximal, the lateral tarsal branch of the dorsalis pedis artery is ligated where it passes beneath the short toe extensors. The extensor retinaculum can be divided, but the island cannot be extended more proximally, as the dorsalis pedis artery enters the island just distal to the extensor retinaculum. If possible, the entire dorsal venous arch should be included in the island. The dorsal venous arch has numerous intercommunications above the superficial fascia, and the arch communicates distally with the dorsalis pedis vein. The venous valves direct drainage into the greater saphenous vein from the distal venous arch.

Results

The full range of this island transplant has not been determined, since it has usually been used as a flap. The flap has been used to resurface defects of the dorsum of the foot, both malleoli, the Achilles tendon, and the sole. Employed as a cutaneous island, coverage of portions of the weight-bearing area of the heel and the pretibial areas should also be practicable (McGraw and Furlow, 1975). McGraw and Furlow reported no complications at the donor site after nine cases, but the donor site has potential for shear pressure problems.

COMMENTS

The advent of the microsurgically transferred free neurovascular cutaneous island flap promises the restoration of protective sensibility in weight-bearing areas of the lower extremity and perhaps tactile gnosis for sensory depleted hands. Survival of the free island is dependent on re-establishment of a functional circulation and reinnervation of the sensory end-organs through the microneural anastomosis. Cortical localization of sensation may prove to be superior to the neurovascular cutaneous island pedicle, since the proximal connections are the original tracts for impulse transmission.

REFERENCES

Adamson, J. E., Horton, C. E., and Crawford, H. H.: Sensory rehabilitation of the injured thumb. Plast. Reconstr. Surg. *40*:53, 1967.

Bralliar, F., and Horner, R. L.: Sensory cross-finger pedicle graft. J. Bone Joint Surg. *51A*:1264, 1969.

Buncke, H. J.: Free toe-to-hand transfers. *In* Daniller, A. I., and Strauch, B. (eds.): Symposium on Microsurgery. Educational Foundation of the American Society of Plastic and Reconstructive Surgeons, St. Louis, C. V. Mosby Co., 1976, p. 216.

Bunnell, S.: Digit transfer by neurovascular pedicle. J. Bone Joint Surg. *34A*:772, 1952.

Chase, R. A.: An alternate to pollicization in subtotal thumb reconstruction. Plast. Reconstr. Surg. *44*:421, 1969.

Gaul, J. S., Jr.: Radial-innervated cross finger flap from index to provide sensory pulp to injured thumb. J. Bone Joint Surg. *51A*:1257, 1969.

Holevich, J.: A new method of restoring sensibility to the thumb. J. Bone Joint Surg. *45B*:496, 1963.

Hueston, J.: The extended neurovascular island flap. Br. J. Plast. Surg. *18*:304, 1965.

Kaplan, I.: Neurovascular island flap in the treatment of trophic ulceration of the heel. Br. J. Plast. Surg. *22*:143, 1969.

Littler, J. W.: The neurovascular pedicle method of digital transposition for reconstruction of the thumb. Plast. Reconstr. Surg. *12*:303, 1953.

Littler, J. W.: Neurovascular pedicle transfer of tissue in reconstructive surgery of the hand. J. Bone Joint Surg. *38A*:917, 1956.

Littler, J. W.: On making a thumb: One-hundred years of surgical effort. J. Hand Surg. *1*:35, 1976.

McGraw, J. B., and Furlow, L. T.: The dorsalis pedis arterialized flap. A clinical study. Plast. Reconstr. Surg. *55*:177, 1975.

McGregor, I. A., and Simonetta, C.: Reconstruction of the thumb by composite bone-skin flap. Br. J. Plast. Surg. *17*:37, 1964.

McGregor, I. A.: Less than satisfactory experiences with neurovascular island flaps. Hand *1*:21, 1969.

Moberg, E.: In Discussion of "The place of nerve-grafting in orthopaedic surgery" by Donal Brooks. J. Bone Joint Surg. *37A*:305, 1955.

Moberg, E.: Evaluation and management of nerve injuries in the hand. Surg. Clin. North Am. *44*:1019, 1964.

Murray, J. F., Ord, J. V. R., and Gavelin, G. E.: The neurovascular island pedicle flap. J. Bone Joint Surg. *49A*:1285, 1967.

Omer, G. E., Jr., Day, D. J., Ratliff, H., and Lambert, P.: Neurovascular cutaneous island pedicles for deficient median-nerve sensibility. J. Bone Joint Surg. *52A*:1181, 1970.

Omer, G. E., Jr.: Tendon transfers in combined nerve lesions. Orthop. Clin. N. Amer. *5*:377, 1974.

Omer, G. E., Jr.: Neurovascular island flaps and fillet of finger *In* Grabb, W. C., and Myers, M. B.: Skin Flaps. Boston, Little, Brown and Company, 1975, p. 471.

Peacock, E. E., Jr.: Island pedicle gymnastics. *In* Cramer, L. M., and Chase, R. A.: Symposium on the Hand. Educational Foundation of the American Society of Plastic and Reconstructive Surgeons, St. Louis, C. V. Mosby Company, 1971, p. 209.

Reid, D. A. C.: The neurovascular island flap in thumb reconstruction. Br. J. Plast. Surg. *19*:234, 1966.

Snyder, G. B., and Edgerton, M. T.: The principle of the island neurovascular flap in the management of ulcerated anesthetic weightbearing areas of the lower extremity. Plast. Reconstr. Surg. *36*:518, 1965.

Tubiana, R., and Duparc, J.: Restoration of sensibility in the hand by neurovascular skin island transfer. J. Bone Joint Surg. *43B*:474, 1961.

49

SENSORY REHABILITATION OF THE HAND UTILIZING FREE MICRONEUROVASCULAR FLAPS FROM THE FOOT

HARRY J. BUNCKE, JR.
and BERISH STRAUCH

Restoration of sensibility to the hand and fingers when the skin coverage lacks the normal neural pathways or terminal sensory receptors was until recently an insurmountable problem for the reconstructive hand surgeon. Small defects of the fingertips may be adequately covered with local sensory flaps, and slightly larger defects of the thumb may be resurfaced and reinnervated with island vascular flaps. These flaps, however, are limited in size, are dependent on the length of the intact neurovascular leash, require a cortical relearning process, and impose an area of decreased sensibility at the long finger donor site.

Only with advancing microsurgical capabilities in the past few years has it been possible to replace insensible areas of the hand and fingers with microneurovascular free flaps (Fig. 49–1). The ideal characteristics of such flaps should

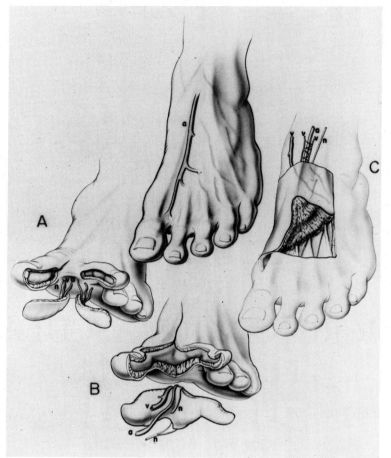

Figure 49–1 Composite drawing of the various neurovascular free flaps from the foot. *A,* Island vascular flaps from the lateral aspect of the big toe and the medial aspect of the second toe. In each of these flaps the respective digital nerve is utilized, as is the digital artery. A dorsal vein is utilized for venous drainage. *B,* Entire first web space. This is a relatively large flap of glabrous skin measuring 14 cm long by 7.5 cm wide. Three nerves innervate this flap. The common digital nerve may be split into its two components. The deep peroneal nerve also provides sensory input into this flap. The dorsalis pedis artery extended by the first dorsal metatarsal artery is utilized as the donor vessel. The dorsal draining veins are dissected proximally over the dorsum of the foot and utilized as the donor veins. *C,* The dorsum of the foot flap is innervated by the superficial peroneal nerve. The donor vessel is the dorsalis pedis artery. The venae commitantes of the dorsalis pedis artery are used for venous drainage. This flap has the characteristics of hairy skin.

include the following: the possibility of achieving critical sensibility; that the sensory pattern of the flap be reasonably predictable; and that the donor skin approximate the quality of the skin of the hand and fingers.

Daniel, Terzis, and Midgley in 1976 described the use of the dorsum of the foot, a hair-bearing area, as a free microneurovascular flap. Gilbert (1975*a,* 1975*b;* 1976) performed the initial first web speace neurovascular flap in 1975. This flap utilizes the glabrous skin of the first web space of the foot.

DORSUM OF THE FOOT FREE
NEUROVASCULAR FLAP

The skin on the dorsum of the foot has a relatively sparse adipose layer, making it an ideal donor site for use in selected locations requiring reinnervation. Skin from the entire dorsum of the foot may be used, an area 14 cm × 12 cm in size in most adults. The superficial peroneal nerve provides sensation to this skin. The flap has the characteristics of hair-bearing skin, with an initial two-point discrimination of 20 to 30 mm.

The main arterial supply to this flap is the dorsalis pedis artery, arising from the terminal branch of the anterior tibial artery. As the dorsalis pedis artery runs distally, it gives off many small branches to the skin. It is these cutaneous branches that provide the main arterial supply to the flap. The venae comitantes of the dorsalis pedis artery provide the major draining system of the flap. The greater and lesser saphenous systems are of lesser importance.

If the distal extension of the dorsalis pedis artery, the first dorsal metatarsal artery, is not superficial, then the distal portion of the flap must be considered to have a random blood supply and this part of the flap should be delayed seven to 10 days prior to transfer.

When the first dorsal metatarsal artery is more deeply situated (as is found in 20–30% of feet), the likelihood of its sending direct arterial vessels to the overlying skin is more remote. In these patients the skin distal to the base of the metatarsals is considered to have a random blood supply as opposed to being truly an arterialized flap. Therefore, initial delay of this random segment is indicated.

The dissection of the flap is begun medially, and the dorsalis pedis artery is identified lateral to the extensor hallucis longus tendon. The plane of dissection is deepened and the first dorsal metatarsal artery identified. The penetrating portion of the dorsalis pedis artery is ligated as it dips between the base of the first and second metatarsals. The dorsalis pedis artery and the first dorsal metatarsal artery must be left attached to the flap. The superficial peroneal nerve is identified proximally and taken with the flap. The donor site is resurfaced with a split thickness skin graft.

At the recipient site, the flap is attached distally to stabilize it. Utilizing the operating microscope, the venous repairs are accomplished with an interrupted repair using 10-0 nylon with a 100 micron needle. The arterial anastomosis is similarly performed and the flap perfused with blood. The nerve repair is done under magnification, again using 10-0 nylon.

NEUROVASCULAR FLAPS FROM THE FIRST
WEB SPACE OF THE FOOT

Reconstruction of the insensible volar surface of the hand and fingers requires composite skin of comparable sensitivity and texture. The glabrous skin found in the first web space, richly supplied with three peripheral nerves, makes an ideal choice for replacement of these areas. Two-point discrimination of this skin in the intact web space is 11 to 12 mm. Depending on the size of the defect to be resurfaced and reinnervated, a portion of the first web space, either the lateral surface of the big toe or the medial surface of the second toe, or the entire web space, may be utilized for transfer. When the skin of the entire web space is utilized, the flap measures 14 cm in length and 7.5 cm in width.

The arterial supply to the adjacent sides of the web space is via the digital arteries extending from the dorsal and plantar metatarsal arteries. When a smaller defect, such as the volar surface of a finger or a thumb, needs to be resurfaced, then the outline is drawn on the toe, with a dart extending to the base of the web (Figs. 49–2 and 49–3). In elevating the flap, the digital nerve, digital artery, and a dorsal vein are identified and divided at the web space. The artery at this level measures 1 mm in external diameter. The flap is transferred to the digit where appropriate vascular anastomosis and nerve repairs are accomplished under magnification.

Alternatively, if the entire web space tissue is required for transfer, then the dorsal circulation is utilized as the donor vessel (Fig. 49–4). The dorsalis pedis artery at the level of the base of the first and second metatarsals continues plantarward to join the plantar circulation. At this point, the first dorsal metatarsal artery arises and proceeds toward the web space, joining the digital arteries on adjacent sides of the first and second toes. If the penetrating portion of the dorsalis pedis artery is ligated, then the web space tissue will be perfused directly through the dorsalis pedis artery–first dorsal metatarsal system. The dorsalis

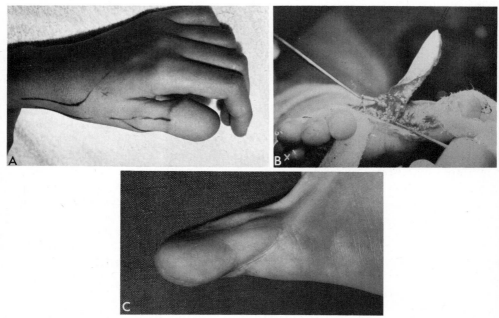

Figure 49–2   A 13 year old female had sustained a traumatic amputation of the left thumb through the proximal phalanx seven months previously. *A,* Initial treatment was by a tube pedicle flap, which developed only protective sensibility. *B,* A free neurovascular island flap was transferred from the lateral surface of the great toe to the thumb. The digital artery of the thumb was anastomosed to the metatarsal artery of the great toe, a superficial vein to a vein in the first web space of the hand, and the radial digital nerve of the thumb was sewn to the lateral digital nerve of the great toe. *C,* At 10 months, two-point discrimination was 5 mm.

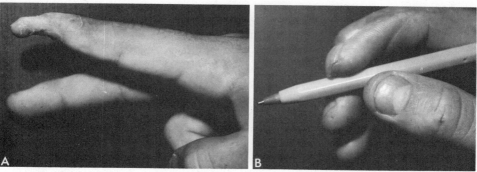

Figure 49–3 A 20 year old male had been bitten by a cottonmouth snake six months previously, with soft tissue loss of the distal phalanx of the right index finger. *A,* The scar was adherent to the bone and the tip was anesthetic. A free neurovascular island flap was transferred from the left second toe to the right index finger. The radial digital artery and nerve of the right index finger were attached to the medial digital artery and nerve, respectively, of the second toe. A superficial toe vein was anastomosed to the dorsal vein of the index finger. *B,* At 16 months, two point discrimination was 5 mm.

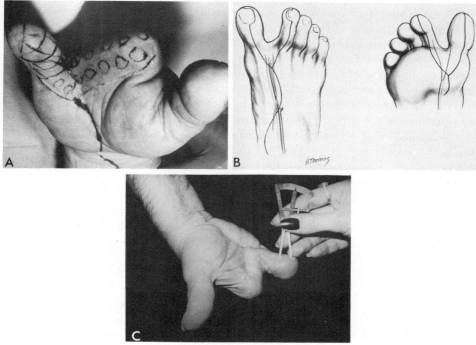

Figure 49–4 A 47 year old male sustained amputation of all the fingers of his right hand. Five years prior to his present surgery he had undergone an ulnar post reconstruction and resurfacing with an abdominal pedicle flap. *A,* The abdominal flap covering the post was totally anesthetic and the more proximal portion of the flap (marked with circles) had only protective sensibility. *B,* A free neurovascular flap of the entire first web space was used to replace the abdominal skin. Microneurorrhaphies were done between the deep peroneal nerve and the common digital nerve to the third web space, as well as between the common plantar nerve and the common digital nerve to the second web space. The dorsalis pedis artery was sewn to the ulnar artery at the wrist, and a common dorsal draining vein was anastomosed to a superficial vein on the radial side of the wrist. *C,* At 24 months post surgery, two point discrimination varied between 3 and 7 mm, depending on the site of the flap tested.

pedis artery on the dorsum of the foot measures 2.0 to 2.5 mm in external diameter, making the microvascular anastomosis relatively much easier. The added length of the vascular leash allows the anastomosis to be accomplished at the level of the wrist. The venous drainage is by way of the dorsal veins draining the web space. These are dissected proximally over the dorsum of the foot until they converge into one or two large veins. The added length also allows the venous anastomosis to be done at the level of the wrist.

The first web space is innervated by the common plantar nerve, which bifurcates and supplies the adjacent sides of the first web space. In addition, the deep peroneal nerve innervates the dorsal skin in the same manner that the superficial radial nerve supplies sensation to the dorsum of the first web space in the hand. All of these nerves are dissected with the web space. The common plantar nerve may be separated into its two component parts so that three microneurorrhaphies are possible if there is an adequate supply of recipient nerves in the hand.

DISCUSSION

Free transfer of composite skin on a neurovascular pedicle has been described experimentally (Daniel et al., 1975) and clinically to restore tactile gnosis in the hypesthetic hand (Robinson, 1976; Ohmori and Harii, 1976; May et al., 1977; Strauch and Tsur, 1978). The neurovascular flap from the first web space, however, most closely resembles the quality of tissue normally present on the palmar aspect of the hand and the volar aspect of the fingers. Of initial benefit to the patient is the enriched vascular supply delivered to the resurfaced area that was previously suboptimally vascularized.

The quality of reinnervation in a neurovascular flap would be expected to be far superior than is generally achieved with a conventional flap, for in a conventional flap reinnervation depends on random penetration of the flap by cutaneous fibers present in the surrounding skin and in the recipient bed. In the authors' series of eight free neurovascular flaps from the first web space, not only has reinnervation occurred but final sensibility after a period of two years has approached normal. The quality of two-point sensibility in the transferred skin was better than that present prior to transfer. Final two-point discrimination in the transferred flaps ranged from 3 to 8 mm.

Tactile acuity varies as a function of position on the body surface (Weinstein, 1969). The most sensitive areas are on the tips of the fingers and the least sensitive areas are usually on the back. It is assumed that this difference in sensory capability is related to differences in the density of cutaneous innervation; the density of innervation is thought to be greatest in those areas that have the best tactile acuity, and least in those areas for which cutaneous sensory performance is the poorest. Furthermore, it is assumed that innervation density is directly correlated with receptor density (Boring, 1942; Sinclair, 1967).

The presence of a normal or close to normal two-point test in the reinnervated first web space skin is difficult to reconcile with existing concepts. The modern concept of two-point discrimination requires that two discriminably different populations of receptors activate different populations of cortical neurons which have specific spatial and functional connections among themselves (Weber, 1852; Ruch, 1955; von Bekésy, 1959). That it is possible for a transferred skin region once having a 10 mm two-point threshold to acquire a 3 mm two-point threshold is an observation that cannot be accounted for. Our observations suggest that either the reinnervation density in the transferred flap is greater than was the original innervation density or that innervation density is less important and the more important factor is the functional characteristics of that portion of the central somatosensory cortex which serves the hand.

REFERENCES

Boring, E. G.: Sensation and Perception in the History of Experimental Psychology, New York, Appleton-Century Crofts, 1942.

Daniel, R. K., Terzis, J., and Midgley, R. D.: Restoration of sensation to an anesthetic hand by a free neurovascular flap from the foot. Plast. Reconstr. Surg. 57:275, 1976.

Daniel, R. K., Terzis, J., and Schwartz, G.: Neurovascular free flaps. Plast. Reconstr. Surg. 56:13, 1975.

Gilbert, A. L.: Composite tissue transfers from the foot: Anatomic basis and surgical technique. In Daniller, A. I., and Strauch, B. (eds.): Symposium on Microsurgery. St. Louis, The C. V. Mosby Co., 1976.

Gilbert, A., and Melka, J.: Bases anatomique et technique du transfert de gros orteil, reunion d'automme du group–Etude de la Main. Paris. 1975.

Gilbert, A., Morrison, W. A., and Tubiana, R.: Transfert sur la main d'un lambeau libre sensible. Chirurgie. 101:691, 1975.

May, J. W., Chait, L. A., Cohen, B. E., and O'Brien, B. M.: Free neurovascular flap from the first web of the foot in hand reconstruction. J. Hand Surg. 2:387, 1977.

Ohmori, K., and Harii, K.: Free dorsalis pedis sensory flap to the hand with microvascular anastomosis. Plast. Reconstr. Surg. 58:546, 1976.

Robinson, D. W.: Microsurgical transfer of the dorsalis pedis neurovascular island flap. Brit. J. Plast. Surg. 29:209, 1976.

Ruch, T. C.: In Fulton, J. F. (ed.): Textbook of Physiology. Philadelphia, W. B. Saunders Co., 1955, p. 302.

Sinclair, D.: Cutaneous Sensation. London, Oxford University Press, 1967.

Strauch, B., and Tsur, H.: Sensory restoration of the hand and fingers with a microvascular transfer of a glabrous skin flap from the first web space of the foot. Plast. Reconstr. Surg. 62:361, 1978.

von Bekésy, G.: J. Acoust. Soc. Am., 21:1236, 1959.

Weber, E. H.: Ber. Sach. Ges. Wiss., Math-phys. Cl., 85–164, 1852.

Weinstein, S.: In Kenshale, D. R. (ed.): The Skin Senses. Springfield, Ill., C C Thomas, 1969, pp. 195.

50

TENDON TRANSFERS AS INTERNAL SPLINTS

WILLIAM E. BURKHALTER

The basic goal of the treatment of upper extremity peripheral nerve injury is to restore maximum function as rapidly as possible following the initial injury. This may be difficult in the more proximal nerve injuries because of the time involved with axon regrowth to the distal muscle and sensory end organs. The modalities available to us include neurorrhaphy or nerve graft, or both, external splintage to prevent deformity, and tendon transfer. This discussion will mostly be about tendon transfers in upper extremity peripheral nerve injuries.

The timing of tendon transfers in peripheral nerve injuries is of interest to all who deal with nerve trauma (Brown, 1970). A tendon transfer should be utilized when functional recovery does not occur following neurorrhaphy or when the lesion is irreparable. In certain cases, however, such as in radial nerve injury, it has been said that tendon transfer should be performed to the exclusion of nerve repair. The use of appropriate early tendon transfers following a peripheral nerve injury and repair may make the overall goal of early return to function of the limb more possible (Burkhalter, 1974). We feel that the major reason for thinking in terms of early tendon transfer in peripheral nerve injury is predicated on three major problem areas. In a peripheral nerve injury some type of splinting is usually required in order to avoid poor patterns of motion and poor habit patterns. In the more proximal nerve injuries, splinting may be difficult to maintain during axon regrowth because of the time involved. Without splinting, however, stiffness and deformity may result. Prolonged and very frequently cumbersome splinting interferes with overall hand function, and so, in our enthusiasm to prevent stiffness and deformity, we actually compromise the overall function of the hand by use of an external device. Since our goal is to promote recovery of the hand as rapidly as possible following the injury, if we could temporarily substitute for motor loss by tendon transfer in the form of an internal splint we might very well be able to return the patient to function relatively early without the use of an external device. This early tendon transfer might take three distinct forms. Early following the injury, the transfer may work as a complete substitute during regrowth of the nerve and allow the patient to be splint-free, with nearly full use of the part during axon regrowth. This is an internal functional splint. Secondly, if following axon regrowth there has been less than optimum reinnervation of the musculature, then the transfer might act as a helper, aiding the muscular recovery from neurorrhaphy. Very frequently, the results of transfer plus those of nerve repair are better than those of either one separately. Obviously, if there is no functional recovery from the neurorrhaphy, or if the lesion is irreparable by exploration, then the transfer may be a complete substitute on a permanent basis for muscle function.

If we elect to perform an early tendon transfer to avoid some of the problems that we have already mentioned, we should not create a new deformity if significant functional recovery occurs following the neurorrhaphy. Some of us have seen patients with radial nerve transfers done at the time of radial nerve suture who have had a good deal of difficulty with finger flexion. Secondly, the tendon unit should be transferred so as not to significantly decrease the remaining hand function, and, thirdly, the transfer should allow rapid retraining so that prolonged rehabilitative efforts for the patient are not necessary in order to gain control of the transfer. With these indications and prerequisites let us examine the individual nerve problems and see how the transfers in these individual groups might act as internal splints and allow the patient to be free of external devices. In injury to the median nerve, loss of abduction and pronation of the thumb is obvious. In higher lesions there is also loss of extrinsic flexor power in the forearm. The use of an opponens splint or a C-bar to maintain thumb opposition during axon regrowth may position the thumb satisfactorily but may interfere with overall use of the extremity. If there is going to be a wait of several months or several years before the reinnervation of the abductor pollicis brevis becomes functional, then the use of an internal splint will allow the patient a mobile opposable thumb without the use of external devices. Whether or not this transfer is required will depend upon the action of the remaining portion of the flexor pollicis brevis. The radial portion may be sufficiently functional to allow maximum thumb mobility and prevent external rotation adduction contractures. If it is not, however, we feel that the functional deficit associated with median nerve injury is so disabling that all reasonable attempts to improve motor function should be carried out early in order to make the patient as functional as possible. If the radial head of the flexor pollicis brevis is not functioning, the extensor pollicis longus, the extensor pollicis brevis, the adductor pollicis, and the deep head of the flexor pollicis brevis plus the abductor pollicis longus will all be supinating forces with a tendency to create a fixed supination deformity of the first metacarpal even without significant adduction contracture. In a patient with a high median nerve injury or combined median and ulnar nerve injury, or in a patient with an isolated median nerve injury with significant muscle damage in the forearm, the list of available motors for transfer that would satisfy our criteria is somewhat limited. We feel that the use of the positioning muscles, such as the extensor indicis proprius, as described by Burkhalter et al. (1973), or the extensor digiti quinti, as described initially by

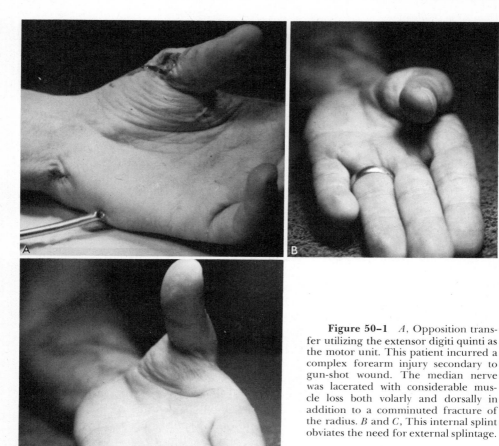

Figure 50–1   *A*, Opposition transfer utilizing the extensor digiti quinti as the motor unit. This patient incurred a complex forearm injury secondary to gun-shot wound. The median nerve was lacerated with considerable muscle loss both volarly and dorsally in addition to a comminuted fracture of the radius. *B* and *C*, This internal splint obviates the need for external splintage.

Cook (Taylor, 1921) and later by Schneider (1969), are probably the best transfers for this purpose. They are phasic with the function of the abductor pollicis brevis, they do not create a significant disability when removed, and they are of adequate strength to restore opposition to the thumb (Fig. 50–1).

The radial nerve is the most suitable nerve in the upper extremity for neurorrhaphy, yet poor functional results are common. What is the cause for the functional disability associated with radial nerve paralysis? Certainly, the major function of the radial nerve musculature may be to extend the fingers and thumb, but perhaps its most important function from the standpoint of the hand is to act as an antagonist to all finger flexors. That is, if the radial nerve musculature is able to stabilize the wrist so that power grip is possible, then there is very little functional disability referrable to the hand in the case of the radial nerve injury. The greatest functional loss in radial nerve injury then is not in finger or thumb extension but in strength of power grip because the patient is unable to stabilize the wrist in extension. Power grip is actually impossible even though there is no volar injury. The classic transfer of the pronator teres to the extensor carpi radialis brevis fulfills all the criteria we have pointed out for early transfer. No disability is created by transferring the pronator teres. While assisting in dorsiflexion of the wrist, it is also able to function as a pronator of the forearm. If functional return occurs following the neurorrhaphy to the extensor carpi radialis brevis, the pronator teres, which has been sutured end-to-side to the wrist extensor, may at that point function as a helper to improve dorsiflexor strength and thereby power grip. During muscle reinnervation following the transfer, however, the patient may very well be able to be splint-free because of the control of wrist dorsiflexion by the transfer. This dorsiflexor wrist control allows full mobility of the fingers and thumb and allows power grip activities. Passive volar flexion of the wrist by relaxation of the transfer allows extension of the fingers and thumb. We feel that a complete transfer, that is, a transfer to bring about finger extension plus thumb extension abduction, is not necessary as an internal splint and that even weak finger extension can be regained if neurorrhaphy or a nerve graft to the radial nerve is possible. We feel that the greatest functional disability in radial nerve injury is the inability to stabilize the wrist. Early transfer should be performed to bring about this stabilization (Fig. 50–2).

In ulnar nerve or combined median and ulnar nerve lesions there are deficits of intrinsic muscle control in the hand because there is no prime metacarpophalangeal joint flexor. A poor flexor pattern develops, there is weakness of power grip, and a claw deformity with the development of PIP joint contractures occurs. Functionally, if the metacarpophalangeal joints can be given some type of passive assist in avoiding hyperextension, difficulties with claw deformity can be eliminated. However, the splints that do this frequently interfere with overall hand function. We feel that by giving the patient the prime metacarpophalangeal flexor we can avoid the problems associated with metacarpophalangeal joint hyperextension — that is, poor pattern and the development of the claw deformity. Likewise, we feel that if the patient has been given a metacar-

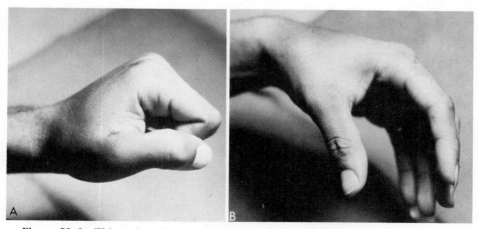

Figure 50–2 This patient incurred complete radial nerve laceration at the mid-arm level. At the time of neurorrhaphy a transfer of the pronater teres to the extensor carpi radialis brevis was performed. The pronator teres was sutured end-to-side to the wrist extensor carpi radialis brevis. This transfer allows functional use of the hand without external splintage during axon regrowth.

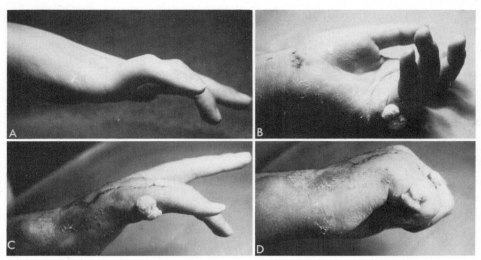

Figure 50–3 *A*, Claw deformity of ring and small fingers secondary to ulnar nerve injury in mid-forearm. Following neurorrhaphy the patient underwent transfer of the prolonged extensor carpi radialis longus to the proximal phalanx of the ring and small fingers. *B–D*, At the time of removal of the plaster immobilization four weeks after the operation, note the flexed position of the metacarpophalangeal joints and the lack of proximal interphalangeal joint stiffness.

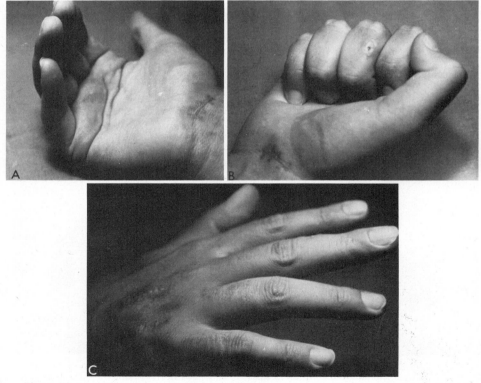

Figure 50–4 *A*, The above patient at three months post-op has the ability to achieve the intrinsic plus position. *B* and *C*, He has good control of the claw deformity with no proximal interphalangeal joint stiffness.

pophalangeal joint flexor replacement he can gain a considerable increase in power grip. Regardless of the method of transfer available, as long as one is able to control the metacarpophalangeal joint through the action of the transfer, none of the residuals associated with intrinsic muscle paralysis will result. It is important to do this transfer, however, prior to the development of a flexor habitus of the wrist. In volar transfer, such as in using the flexor superficialis or any other motor that passes volar to the axis of the wrist, the flexor habitus reduces the effectiveness of the tendon transfer. This flexor habitus normally accompanies a longstanding intrinsic paralysis of the hand. Once the pattern develops it will be very difficult to rehabilitate the patient following any type of transfer because the patient becomes accustomed to working with the wrist in varying degrees of flexion, from perhaps 45 to 90 degrees rather than 30 degrees of flexion to 45 degrees of dorsiflexion. If the patient develops this flexor position of the wrist the best way to avoid the problem of loss of usefulness of the transfer is to bring the transferred motor unit dorsal to the axis of the wrist joint, as initially described by Brand. In this manner wrist flexion actually passively tightens the transfer and brings about metacarpophalangeal joint flexion (Figs. 50–3 and 50–4).

The procedures developed by Stiles (1922) and popularized by Bunnell (1942), and later by Brand (1958, 1961) and Riordan (1959, 1964), all attempt to substitute directly for loss of intrinsic function. That is, they all attempt to

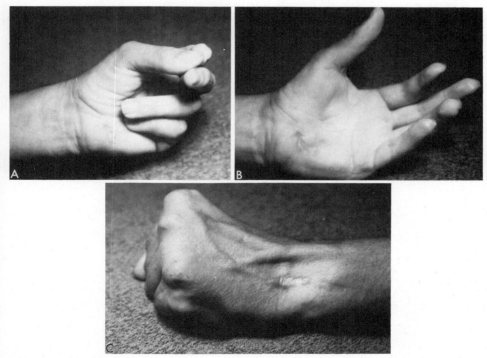

Figure 50–5 *A*, This patient incurred lacerations of the median and ulnar nerves proximal to the elbow three years prior to this photograph. *B*, and *C*, Two and one-half years earlier, he had undergone extensor indicis proprius opponensplasty and four-tailed metacarpophalangeal replacement. He has been splint free during the period of reinnervation and is free of contractures.

improve simultaneously both interphalangeal joint extension and metacarpophalangeal joint flexor function. The procedures mentioned by de Carvalho et al. (1970), Burkhalter and Strait (1973), and Brooks and Jones (1975), however, all concentrate on metacarpophalangeal joint flexor control. We feel that concentrating on a single motion gives an easily learned pattern of use that does not require extensive retraining. The transfer controls the major difficulty associated with intrinsic muscle paralysis in the fingers and does not significantly reduce overall hand function. In conclusion, we feel that maximum functional rehabilitative effort in upper extremity peripheral nerve injury will come when maximum function is instituted in the limb as soon as possible after injury and neurorrhaphy. In order to achieve a state of active function as early as possible, we think that certain selected tendon transfers for these injuries are indicated. It must be pointed out that the criteria of not reducing overall hand function, not creating opposing deformities, and making sure that the transfer can be learned quickly by the patient must be followed. The transfers outlined may work at various times during the overall rehabilitative effort as an internal splint and a complete substitute, as a helper, and, in certain places, as a complete permanent substitute for denervated musculature (Fig. 50–5).

REFERENCES

Brand, P. W.: Paralytic claw hand. With special reference to paralysis in leprosy and treatment by the sublimus transfer of Stiles and Bunnell. J. Bone Joint Surg. *40–B*:618, 1958.

Brand, P. W.: Tendon grafting. Illustrated by a new operation for intrinsic paralysis of the fingers. J. Bone Joint Surg. *43–B*:444, 1961.

Brooks, A., and Jones, D.: A new intrinsic tendon transfer for the paralytic hand. J. Bone Joint Surg. *57–A*:730, July 1975.

Brown, P. W.: The time factor in surgery of upper-extremity peripheral nerve injury. Clin. Orthop. *68*:14, 1970.

Bunnell, S.: Surgery of the intrinsic muscles of the hand other than those producing opposition of the thumb. J. Bone Joint Surg., *24*:1, 1942.

Burkhalter, W. E., and Strait, J.: Metacarpophalangeal flexor replacement for extrinsic muscle paralysis. J. Bone Joint Surg. *55–A*:1667, 1973.

Burkhalter, W. E., Christensen, R., and Brown, P.: Extensor indicis proprius opponensplasty. J. Bone Joint Surg. *55–A*:725, 1973.

Burkhalter, W. E.: Early tendon transfer in upper extremity peripheral nerve injury. Clin. Orthop. *104*:68, 1974.

De Carvalho, M. I. and Coura, Z.: Restoration of the functional balance of the hand in the paralysis of the lumbrical and interosseous muscles. The American Digest of Foreign Orthopaedic Literature, Fourth quarter, p. 18, 1970.

Riordan, D.: Surgery of the paralytic hand. *In* Instructional Course Lectures. The American Academy of Orthopaedic Surgeons. St. Louis, The C. V. Mosby Co., 1959, Vol. 16, p. 79.

Riordan, D.: Tendon transfer for nerve paralysis of the hand and wrist. Curr. Prac. Ortho. Surg. *2*:17, 1964.

Schneider, L.: Opponensplasty using the extensor digiti minimi. J. Bone Joint Surg. *51–A*:1297, 1969.

Stiles, H. J., and Forrester-Brown, M. F.: Treatment of injuries of the peripheral spinal nerves. London, H. Frowde, 1922, p. 166.

Taylor, T.: Reconstruction of the hand. A new technique in tenoplasty. Surg. Gynecol. Obstet. *32*:237, 1921.

51

RECONSTRUCTION OF THE SHOULDER AND ELBOW FOLLOWING BRACHIAL PLEXUS INJURY

ROBERT D. LEFFERT

The shoulder and elbow provide the "reach" without which man's "grasp" is impossible. When loss of power or control of these joints due to a nerve lesion occurs, the individual's ability to manipulate his environment is severely compromised. The surgical literature devoted to reconstruction under such circumstances is large and varied. Until recently the most common cause of such incapacity was poliomyelitis, and many of the indications and techniques used to treat polio are directly transferable to patients with nerve injuries. However, because there are important differences in the two groups, further consideration of the treatment alternatives for the brachial plexus injury is necessary. The functional loss in patients with brachial plexus injury will usually be considerably greater than in those with polio because of the lack of sensation and proprioceptive feedback in the former. Although both lesions may produce profound paralysis, the closed traction injury of the plexus will tend to conform to one or two patterns in an "all-or-nothing" distribution. In general, the shoulder and elbow are paralyzed by postganglionic lesions of C5 and C6. If the C7 root is in-

cluded, a functional radial palsy also results. The trapezius, being largely crani-
ally innervated, is almost always spared, even in severe traction injuries to the
brachial plexus, and the serratus anterior, since it comes from root collaterals of
C5, C6, and C7, is usually preserved unless the patient has sustained an unusual
series of preganglionic avulsions of the upper roots.

Although a number of ingenious procedures have been described for the
treatment of the paralytic shoulder due to polio, many of them are not applicable to the adult traumatic brachial plexus patient; therefore, we have most
frequently used arthrodesis for this group. However, it must be pointed out that
the patient with a birth palsy who is not seen until adolescence or adulthood has
had the factor of growth to modify his deformity. Thus, important considerations of static and dynamic nature must be entertained. These will be enlarged
upon in the section on techniques. Finally, the birth palsy patient may have the
additional and troublesome factor of dyskinesia, especially about the elbow,
which probably results from a combination of spinal injury and imperfect or
confused regeneration, and which can totally frustrate attempts to restore active
control (Milgram, 1962). This phenomenon may also be seen in adult traction
injuries after imperfect spontaneous recovery as well as following grafting
operations upon the plexus.

TIMING OF RECONSTRUCTION

Patients who have acquired brachial plexus injuries in adulthood have
usually lost function of a limb that is crucial to their established way of life. The
timing of their reconstruction takes on an urgency usually not present in those
with congenital palsies.

Following initial assessment in an adult brachial injury, an accurate prognosis for functional recovery must be made. In closed traction injuries it is unusual
for preganglionic root avulsion of C5 and C6 to occur; although avulsion may
happen here, it is more common in the lower roots. Myelography will clarify this
issue, whereupon peripheral reconstruction can begin immediately if the roots
are avulsed. Since the neurological reconstruction of these lesions has been
discussed elsewhere in this volume, we will assume either that neural continuity
cannot be restored surgically or that sufficient time has elapsed so that spontaneous recovery is unlikely to occur. This judgment is based on carefully documented recovery statistics (Barnes, 1949; Bonney, 1959; Leffert and Seddon, 1965)
compared with regular clinical and electromyographic examination of the particular patient under consideration. In general, if functional shoulder control is
not present by one year after the injury, it is not likely to improve. For the elbow,
and especially after nerve suture or graft in the supraclavicular fossa, the onset
of useful recovery may not be appreciated for one and a half to two years. With
these time periods in mind, one may proceed with reconstruction according to
the needs of the individual patient.

In the case of the growing child, not only must the possibility of evolving
bone and joint deformity be anticipated but also whatever normal growth is
possible must not be thwarted by ill-conceived or poorly executed surgery. A
neonate with a typical traction lesion of the Erb's type usually has greater deficit
in shoulder control than in elbow function. If injudicious abduction splinting is

avoided and a conscious effort is made to encourage use of the limb, continued recovery and improvement may be seen in a high percentage of children. Consideration of these patients' management will be given separately from the adult traumatic injuries. Patients who sustain their injuries at birth, but who are seen for reconstruction either in adolescence or adult life, will be considered with the first group.

TECHNIQUE

The adult patient who has a flail or paretic shoulder due to a lesion at C5–C6 usually has weakness of the lateral rotators of the humerus and the deltoid, as well as of the clavicular pectoralis major and elbow flexors. If this were not so, more aggressive attempts to maintain the mobility of the glenohumeral joint by means of tendon transfers would be indicated. An extensive experience with these is described in the literature and is especially documented by Saha (1967). In order for significant functional improvement to result from tendon transfers about the shoulder, the complex kinesiology of the normal shoulder must be recalled, and an attempt made to approximate it. In most cases this will simply not be possible because of the lack of available adjacent motors. However, in some few selected adult patients with traction lesions, and others with partial lesions due to open wounds, surprisingly good results may be achieved. In all cases, multiple transfers must be performed. The following muscles may be transferred: the latissimus and teres major posteriorly, the long head of biceps and triceps to the acromion, and the posterior or medial deltoid anteriorly (Fig. 51–1). The isolated transfer of the trapezius to replace the function of the deltoid has not proved to be effective. Because of the predictable results of shoulder fusion in this group with few alternate motors and shoulder instability, arthrodesis remains the technique of choice at this time in our clinic. Obviously, unless there is good scapular control, especially intact trapezius and serratus anterior, the ultimate function of the scapulohumeral complex will be deficient. Fortunately, this is unusual in uncomplicated cases.

It is helpful, when discussing this operation with a patient, to have someone available who has already had the procedure done and with whom the patient can talk. Since this is an irrevocable step, it is vital that all questions regarding postoperative function be completely answered preoperatively. A successful fusion should eliminate pain from local "drag" or subluxation but obviously will not influence pain due to more central nerve injury. The patient should be able to reach the midline in front as well as the back pocket and anal area. In the sagittal plane he ought to be able to bring the arm almost to the horizontal and thereby allow the hand to reach the head and mouth. At rest the arm should lie in a natural-appearing position at the side, without causing undue strain on the scapulothoracic musculature or winging of the scapula. Assuming normal scapular control and sound fusion, then, all of these functions should depend on the proper choice of position for the fusion. However, this is not a simple matter to determine, as is indicated by the significant differences of opinion in the literature (Rowe, 1974). Not only is the final position in three planes debated, even the reference points cannot be agreed upon. One can use the appearance of the "arm-at-the-side" (a rather arbitrary guideline) or the relationship of the axis of

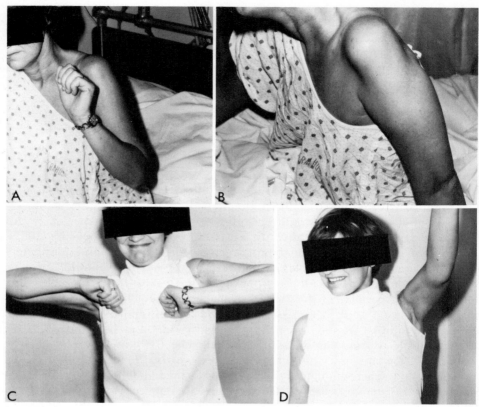

Figure 51–1 Shoulder paralysis due to a partial laceration of the upper trunk of the left brachial plexus. *A*, Elbow flexion is possible but no abduction. *B*, Only the posterior deltoid is intact. The middle and anterior portions are atrophic. *C* and *D*, Function following extensive tendon transfer which included: (1) posterior deltoid rotated anteriorly to the position of the middle deltoid; (2) posterolateral transfer of the latissimus dorsi and teres major; (3) transfer of the long head of the biceps to the anterior acromion; and (4) transfer of the origin of the clavicular head of the pectoralis major laterally to the acromion.

the humeral shaft with each of three bony landmarks: the spine or the scapula, its lateral (axillary) border, or the vertebral border. If internal fixation is used at the time of the procedure, the position at operation is permanent, so the landmarks used for angular measurements should be definitely accessible to the surgeon. I find that the vertebral border of the scapula is easily palpable using either posterior or lateral approaches. Since I rarely employ an anterior approach, this landmark has proved to be the most convenient.

It should be appreciated that the position recommended by the Research Committee of the American Orthopaedic Association in 1942 (45 to 50 degrees of abduction from the vertebral border, forward flexion of 15 to 25 degrees from the plane of the scapula, and 25 to 30 degrees of external rotation) should be considered in light of the fact that this study was done on children and adolescents with polio. In most cases, no internal fixation was used. With time, fortunately, much of the abduction was lost. Rowe (1974) has published a re-evaluation of this position and pointed out the disadvantages of excessive abduction as well as the fallacy of external rather than internal rotation. He recommends (using the same landmarks) 15 to 20 degrees of abduction, 25 to 30 degrees of forward flexion, and 40 to 50 degrees of internal rotation. Although I am substantially in agreement with these recommendations, they must be individualized. For patients who are to have Clark's pectoral transfers in the future, as much as 30 degrees of abduction may be permissible to attempt to improve the line of pull of the transfer. For patients with flexion contracture of the elbow, either congenital, posttraumatic, or postsurgical reconstruction, a lessening of both forward flexion and medial rotation should avoid a potentially embarrassing standing and resting position with the hand positioned at the crotch.

Numerous techniques and their rationales have been shown to be successful in achieving solid arthrodesis of the shoulder (Gill, 1931; Charnley and Houston, 1964; Watson-Jones, 1933; Brooks, 1959; Milgram, 1963). Although extra-articular fusion and avoidance of internal fixation were mandated by the presence of tuberculous arthritis, these are not a consideration for brachial plexus injury. With the caveat that the bone is usually porotic and the position chosen must be correct, internal fixation is a significant factor in lessening the incidence of non-union. No supplementary bony grafts are necessary if the articular surfaces of the glenoid, humerus, and inferior surface of the acromial process are decorticated and properly prepared.

Two techniques for shoulder fusion are presently in use in our clinic. In both, the patient is placed on the operating table in the lateral decubitus position with the arm draped free. The first utilizes a lateral approach, proceeding with cautery through the deltoid in the line of the incision to remove the rotator cuff attachments as well as the glenoidal ligaments and labrum. Care must be taken to avoid the circumflex humeral vessels on the medial side of the humerus, since these are difficult to control from this approach. The head of the humerus is decorticated after the glenoid, since to do the reverse would cause obscured vision due to bleeding. With the undersurface of the acromial process bared, and the head translocated cephalad, two firm points for fusion are available. Depending on the desired position and the particular anatomy, it might be necessary to partially osteotomize the acromion and deflect it down to fit into a defect cut in the humeral head. The arm can rest on a padded, sterile Mayo stand during the procedure, so that fatigue of the second assistant will not result in loss of the ultimate position. Fixation is by means of AO cancellous lag screws with washers, guided by the surgeon's fingers held parallel with the scapula on each side of the humeral head. Usually it is possible to get firm fixation with three or four 75 mm screws extending at different angles between the head and the neck of the scapula (Fig. 51–2). Steel sternal wire in a figure-of-eight configuration between the acromion and humerus completes the fixation. A suction drain is usually necessary, especially if the procedure is done under hypotensive anesthesia. Postoperative immobilization is a problem, since the application of a well-fitting shoulder spica to an anesthetized patient is quite difficult. We, therefore, use an adjustable metal abduction splint in the immediate postoperative period and apply a plaster spica when the patient has recovered sufficiently and can stand to have this done. Because the cast must be worn for 10 to 12 weeks to insure fusion, techniques using multiple compression plates without spica immobilization are very appealing, and we are doing more of them (Mueller, et al., 1970; Riggins, 1976).

For the second arthrodesis procedure the patient is in the same position on

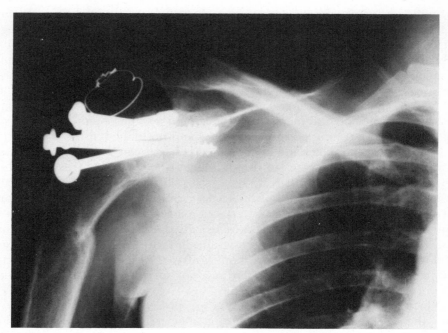

Figure 51–2   Postoperative appearance of shoulder fusion. The healed fracture of the proximal humerus was sustained a year after the fusion when the patient fell from parallel bars during gymnastics.

the operating table, but the incision is posterolateral and extends along the spine of the scapula to the lateral aspect of the humeral head. The cautery and periosteal elevators are used to bare the spine and neck of the glenoid as well as the adjacent joint and proximal humerus. A 10-hole plate is contoured to extend along the spine of the scapula to embrace the decorticated head of the humerus and glenoid. Care must be taken to insure that the proposed fusion site is not gapped as multiple screws are inserted; when this has been verified, a "T" plate is applied across the joint and fixed to the head and scapular neck. Fixation is usually quite firm, allowing the advantage of support in the postoperative period by means of just a sling. One should try to choose reasonably intelligent and cooperative patients for this technique, however. We have had two patients in the past six months loosen their fixation, one by riding his motorcycle at two weeks, and another by getting a job as a furniture mover at three weeks postoperatively. One shoulder fused spontaneously when the arm was protected in a sling, and the other after eight weeks in a plaster spica.

Since a considerable amount of hardware is present in both types of fusion, radiographic assessment of bony union is aided by tomography and stress films. These are routinely employed at about 12 weeks, by which time there is usually solid fusion. If after muscle re-education has been completed, an additional scapulothoracic range of motion, especially anteriorly and medially, is desired, the lateral end of the clavicle may be resected, but the integrity of the coracoclavicular ligaments must be preserved (Milgram, 1962).

The problem presented by the patient with a congenital palsy of the shoulder is quite different (Sever, 1916; Wickstrom, 1962). Usually the lesion is incomplete. Often there is paresis rather than complete paralysis, and the anatomic deficit is most obvious in abduction and lateral rotation. Since there are few activities of a "helper" hand (which these invariably become) that require shoulder abduction in the scapular plane, primary consideration should be given to forward flexion and the ability to bring the well-supported hand to the midline. This will permit bimanual activities or such obligatory functions as shaking hands or opening doors.

In addition to the obvious motor deficits described above, one must be aware of a number of concomitant skeletal deformities which, if ignored, can seriously prejudice the results of treatment. In the infant, one may overlook an epiphyseal separation or unreduced glenohumeral dislocation. With growth and muscle imbalance, the acromion and coracoid processes may elongate and project anteroinferiorly, thus restricting motion and contributing to posterior displacement of the humeral head. With time, the combination of a retroverted, flattened head and shallow glenoid along with persistence of the adducted and internally rotated position of the humeral head may eventually lead to posterior subluxation and even dislocation. It should not automatically be assumed, however, that this will invariably be the nature of the osseous abnormality, since occasionally one may observe anteroinferior dislocation or subluxation. In all cases under study, multiple x-ray views must be taken, and fluoroscopy performed if possible, to ensure that significant skeletal changes or subluxations are absent. In general, these must be anticipated and dealt with approximately before any further reconstruction can be considered.

I believe that no child should be considered for soft tissue correction or tendon transfer before the age of four or five unless it is for release of a significant contracture, which should not occur if proper stretching exercises are done. It will be seen that as the involved arm is raised in front of the body, the weight of the limb devoid of adequate lateral rotators will cause medial rotation of the arm, with the elbow sticking out awkwardly laterally, and the hand dropped to waist level. With time, the normally innervated medial rotators undergo contracture, so that even passive lateral rotation is impossible. For the patient with this combination of problems, it is desirable to achieve as much correction as possible so that more normal functional patterns of use will develop. Although surgical release of contracted anterior structures as described by Sever (1916) will initially result in cosmetic improvement, the continued deficit of active lateral rotators will allow recurrence of the problem with time. Therefore, transfer of muscles that are normally medial rotators posterolaterally, such as advocated by several authors (Zachary, 1957; L'Episcopo, 1939), will achieve more significant and lasting results. Through an anterior approach, the contracted pectoralis major is lengthened and the subscapularis released. Ordinarily the capsule need not be incised, but the tendons of attachments of both the latissimus dorsi and teres major are released and tagged. Then, through a posterior approach adjacent to the medial border of the deltoid, the interval between the long and lateral heads of the triceps is entered. The radial and circumflex nerves must be protected. Then the tendons of the latissimus and teres major are routed posterolaterally and then fixed to the lateral triceps head or an osteoperiosteal flap with the arm in lateral rotation and abduction. This position is maintained for three weeks by a spica or splint, after which active exercises are begun. Although it has been said that the benefit is mostly cosmetic

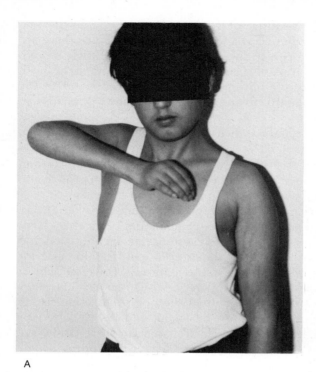

A

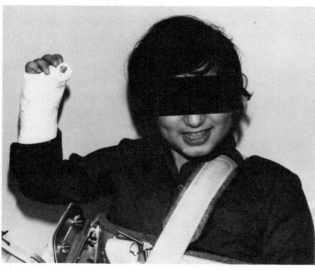

B

Figure 51–3 *A*, Preoperative appearance of abduction and attempt at lateral rotation. *B*, Following Zachary's tendon transfer of latissimus dorsi and teres major.

and that the shoulder is really no stronger postoperatively, the patients I have observed have been very gratified with the results (Fig. 51–3).

If there is significant flattening of the humeral head and a small glenoid, such that changing their rotational relationships would likely result in incongruity or subluxation, then lateral rotational osteotomy of the proximal humerus done above the level of the deltoid insertion can be a useful procedure. Not only is the arm placed in a more favorable position, but there may even be improvement in the mechanical advantage and strength of the deltoid.

It is for the patient with an established posterior subluxation or tendency to dislocation that the ingenuity of the reconstructive surgeon may be maximally taxed. Although posterior bone blocks have been advocated, one may combine anterior release with posterior capsular reefing and/or osteotomy and tendon transfer. In one notable case in which the dislocations were thought to be

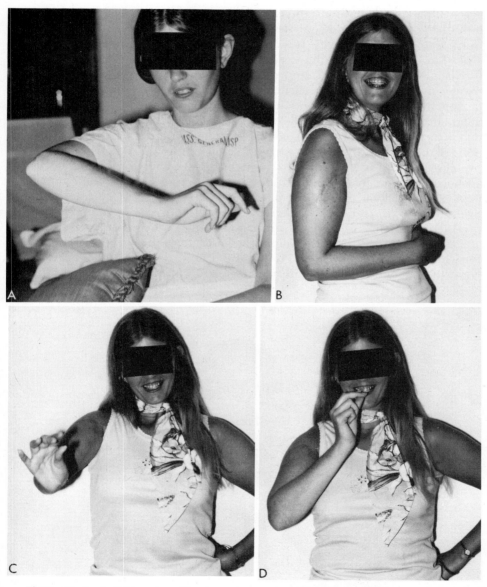

Figure 51–4   *A*, Erb's palsy with recurrent anterior dislocations requiring constant use of pillow splint to prevent dislocation. *B*, Following capsulorrhaphy and rotational osteotomy—medial rotation. *C*, Abduction. *D*, Patient now has the ability to reach her mouth.

posterior but were actually anterior, and in which the head was deformed, a conventional anterior Putti-Platt "to keep the head in," and lateral rotation osteotomy of the humerus relieved the patient's pain completely and allowed her to reach her face for the first time in her 26 years. (Fig. 51–4).

THE ELBOW

The adult patient who is afflicted with a lesion of the upper trunk of the brachial plexus will have lost the major power of active elbow flexion, although, if the arm can be raised to or above the horizontal, elbow flexion can be achieved by trick motion using gravity. It is obvious, then, that the status of the shoulder is crucial to the function of the weak or paralyzed elbow. If the flexor–pronator forearm muscles are intact, and especially with the brachium horizontal, the patient may pronate the forearm, strongly clench the fist, and achieve elbow flexion by supplementary motion (Steindler effect) (Fig. 51–5). This led Dr. Steindler in 1917 to design the flexorplasty that bears his name (Steindler, 1940), and which was performed in countless polio patients, with increased function as the result. Simply stated, the origin of the relatively normal flexor-pronator muscles was detached from the medial epicondyle of the humerus and advanced proximally to the intermuscular septum to increase the moment for flexion at the elbow. Obviously, passive elbow motion must be free preoperatively. There are two disadvantages to the procedure, however. The first is a persistent tendency to forearm pronation, which can be somewhat offset by attaching the pedicle more laterally to the midshaft of the humerus. The second, for which there is little remedy, is that the transfer is really not very powerful. Nevertheless, one should not infer that it is not a good operation, rather that it is

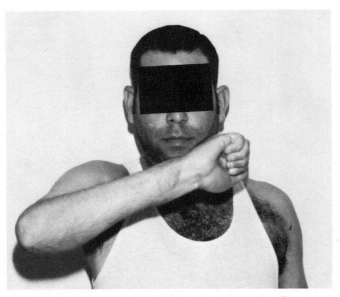

Figure 51–5   Elbow flexion using the Steindler effect.

more suited to the polio patient than to the brachial plexus patient who has more limited distribution of weakness and, therefore, often more rigorous demands for more normal strength (Kettlekamp and Larson, 1963).

It is because of this problem of strength that Clark's pectoral transfer has become my procedure of choice for the restoration of active elbow flexion (Clark, 1946). The prerequisites are, in addition to free passive elbow motion, a fused shoulder, or one under excellent control, and an essentially normal sternal head of the pectoralis major. Even though the clavicular head will be paralyzed by a lesion of C5 and C6, the sternal head will often still be functioning, and a pedicle about 5 cm wide can be raised from the chest and turned with its blood and nerve supply (lateral anterior thoracic nerve) to be rerouted down the arm. The tunnel is made subcutaneously, and attachment is to the biceps tendon in the antecubital fossa. There must be no scarring in the proposed site of transfer (hence avoid an anterior incision for shoulder fusions) and the length of the pedicle can only be adequate if additional tissue from the rectus sheath is included in continuity when the dissection is done. It is absolutely essential to identify and protect the lateral anterior thoracic nerve throughout the procedure, which can be greatly facilitated by the use of a nerve stimulator. Postoperatively, the elbow is maintained in flexion for four weeks before gentle, guarded exercises are begun. It is kept in a sling between exercise periods for three months to encourage a permanent flexion contracture of about 30 degrees, which will aid the mechanical advantage in initiation of flexion. The active power of the transfer is quite good, since the tendency to medial rotation or to adduction of the humerus is prevented by shoulder fusion. It is these mechanical points that have resulted in extremely satisfactory function in the patients we have so treated, as opposed to published evaluations of this procedure in the literature (Segal, Seddon, and Brooks, 1959).

The Brooks-Seddon technique of pectoral transfer was designed for those patients in whom the biceps and sternal pectoralis major are completely paralyzed and the clavicular pectoralis major is preserved. The biceps is surgically devascularized and used as a tendon for the clavicular head. However, this is an unusual pattern for traction injuries of the brachial plexus and, although it does work, it is not a particularly strong transfer.

A similar situation regarding availability pertains to the use of the latissimus dorsi, which can be utilized quite successfully to replace either the flexors or the extensors of the elbow (Hovnanian, 1956; Harmon, 1949; Zancolli, 1973). I have no personal experience with this transfer.

Finally, the triceps brachii may be used to replace a paralyzed biceps and brachialis. The technique of Carroll (1952), which is a modification of the procedure described by Bunnell (1951), can provide excellent elbow flexion. The entire triceps is detached from its insertion, and is prolonged by elevating several inches of the deep fascia of the proximal forearm with the pedicle. This allows the muscle to be routed subcutaneously and to be inserted directly into the biceps tendon without having to interpose a fascial graft. The transfer works particularly well when there has been confused reinnervation with simultaneous contraction of the triceps when the patient attempts to flex the elbow. Although the operation can provide very gratifying results (even though gravity extends the elbow), there are several problems that must be anticipated preoperatively. Obviously, it should not be done bilaterally, since significant disability would result in such activities as getting out of a chair or turning over in bed. Crutch walking is hindered by lack of a triceps, and pushing a revolving door or working overhead is impossible. Nonetheless, it is a very useful procedure, and phase conversion has not been a problem.

REFERENCES

Barnes, R.: Traction injuries of the brachial plexus in adults. J. Bone Joint Surg. *31B*:10, 1949.
Bonney, G.: Prognosis in traction lesions of the brachial plexus. J. Bone Joint Surg. *41B*:4, 1959.
Brooks, D. M.: Arthrodesis of the shoulder in reconstructive surgery of paralysis of the upper limb. J. Bone Joint Surg. *41B*:207, 1959.
Brooks, D. M. and Seddon, H. J.: Pectoral transplantation for paralysis of the flexors of the elbow. J. Bone Joint Surg. *41B*:36, 1959.
Bunnell, S.: Restoring flexion to the paralytic elbow. J. Bone Joint Surg. *33A*:3, 1951.
Carroll, R. E.: Restoration of flexor power to the flail elbow by transplantation of the triceps tendon. Surg. Gynecol. Obstet. *95*:685, 1952.
Charnley, J., and Houston, J. K.: Compression arthrodesis of the shoulder. J. Bone Joint Surg. *46B*:614, 1964.
Clark, J. M. P.: Reconstruction of biceps brachii by pectoral muscle transplantation. Brit. J. Surg. *34*:180, 1946.
Gill, A. B.: A new operation for arthrodesis of the shoulder. J. Bone Joint Surg. *13*:287, 1931.
Harmon, P. H.: Technique of utilizing latissimus dorsi muscle in transplantation for triceps palsy. J. Bone Joint Surg. *31A*:409, 1949.
Hovnanian, A. P.: Latissimus dorsi transplantation for loss of flexion or extension at the elbow. Ann. Surg. *143*:493, 1956.
Kettlekamp, D. B., and Larson, C. B.: Evaluation of the Steindler flexorplasty. J. Bone Joint Surg. *45A*:513, 1963.
Leffert, R. D., and Seddon, H. J.: Infraclavicular brachial plexus injuries. J. Bone Joint Surg. *47B*:9, 1965.
L'Episcopo, J. B.: Restoration of muscle balance in the treatment of obstetrical paralysis. N. Y. J. Med. *39*:357, 1939.
Milgram, J. E.: Discussion of "A Technique for Shoulder Arthrodesis." Davis, J. B., and Cottrell, G. J. Bone Joint Surg. *44A*:661, 1962.
Milgram, J. E.: (Personal communication).
Milgram, J. E.: Reconstruction of the paralytic shoulder and elbow. J. Bone Joint Surg. *45A*:1, 1963.
Mueller, M. F., Allgower, M., and Willenegger, H.: Manual of Internal Fixation. New York, Springer-Verlag, 1970, p. 278.
Report of the Research Committee of the American Orthopaedic Association: A survey of the results on stabilization of the paralytic shoulder. J. Bone Joint Surg. *24*:699, 1942.
Riggins, R.: Shoulder fusion without external fixation. J. Bone Joint Surg. *58A*:7, 1976.
Rowe, C. R.: Re-evaluation of the position of the arm in arthrodesis of the shoulder in the adult. J. Bone Joint Surg. *56A*:5, 1974.
Saha, A. K.: Surgery of the paralyzed and flail shoulder. Acta Orthop. Scand. (Suppl.) *97*:5, 1967.
Segal, A., Seddon, H. J., and Brooks, D. M.: Treatment of paralysis of the flexors of the elbow. J. Bone Joint Surg. *41B*:44, 1959.
Sever, J. W.: Obstetric paralysis: Its etiology, pathology, clinical aspects, and treatment with a repair of four hundred and seventy cases. Am. J. Dis. Child. *12*:541, 1916.
Steindler, A: Orthopedic Operations. Springfield, Ill., Charles C Thomas, 1940, p. 129.
Watson-Jones, R.: Extra-articular arthrodesis of the shoulder. J. Bone Joint Surg. *15*:862, 1933.
Wickstrom, J.: Birth injuries of the brachial plexus. Treatment of defects in the shoulder. Clin. Orthop. *23*:187, 1962.
Zachary, R. B.: Transplantation of teres major and latissimus dorsi for loss of external rotation at the shoulder. Lancet *2*:757, 1957.
Zancolli, E., and Mitre, H.: Latissimus dorsi transfer to restore elbow flexion. J. Bone Joint Surg. *55A*:1265, 1973.

52

TENDON TRANSFERS FOR RECONSTRUCTION OF THE FOREARM AND HAND FOLLOWING PERIPHERAL NERVE INJURIES

GEORGE E. OMER, Jr.

Tendon transfers restore motor balance to an extremity crippled by partial loss of muscle–tendon unit function. The successful transfer has one basic objective, to eliminate a deforming force that will produce further imbalance or to replace a single motion to assist grasp, pinch, or release. The anticipated result should be a balanced simplification of functional performance, because the surgical procedure redistributes assets rather than creating new ones.

PATIENT EVALUATION

Homeostasis of the involved extremity must be established before elective tendon surgery. There should be stable skeletal alignment with near normal joint motion. Tendon transfers performed across or distal to sites of bony non-union fail because the telescoping skeleton prevents the development of adequate tension for motion. Soft tissues should be free of scar contracture and have adequate circulation. Chronic wounds are contraindications to elective surgery. The functional performance expected after tendon transfer should be possible to effect easily by passive movement before surgery.

The involved neuromuscular mechanisms must be evaluated. Is the nerve mixed or pure? Is the injury at a proximal or distal level or injured over a considerable distance, such as following an electrical burn? The metabolic response of the nerve differs in proximal and distal injuries (Ducker and Kauffman, 1977). Return of good motor function across two joints distal to the nerve injury is rare (Omer, 1974a). Is the muscle–tendon unit disrupted, avulsed, or fibrotic? Assessment of the neuromuscular mechanisms requires multiple quantitative tests that are repeated at regular intervals for comparison and prognosis. A minimal test battery would include the following: a voluntary muscle test with a recorded range of motion, light touch two-point discrimination distance over autonomous zones or pertinent peripheral nerves, a wrinkle test for sudomotor function, gross grip and finger pinch strength tests, and a timed pick-up test (Omer and Spinner, 1975).

The etiology of the motor imbalance is important in predicting the future involvement of additional muscle-tendon units with progressive functional impairment. Tendon transfers can be done in selected progressive disease conditions, such as rheumatoid arthritis, but both the patient and the surgeon should comprehend the therapeutic limitations and potential problems posed by the surgical procedure. The extent of muscle imbalance is usually static after traumatic injury, but many developmental conditions, such as syringomyelia, involve progressive muscle–tendon impairment complicated by an unpredictable rate of involvement. Muscle imbalance related to vascular problems may be limited, as in an injection injury or Volkmann's ischemia, or may be progressive secondary to a series of cerebrovascular accidents. The prognosis for the muscle imbalance, based on knowledge of the etiology and physical homeostasis, should indicate a time frame for surgery or make it obvious that the muscle imbalance will never be static.

Patient evaluation must be factored into the clinical decision for tendon transfers. The patient must have developed the cerebral imprint for the proposed function, be able to comprehend what is to be done, and be ready to accept the postoperative discipline. One should determine whether the patient desires an increase in functional performance or cosmetic improvement.

SELECTION OF THE MOTOR MUSCLE

In the normal forearm and hand there are half a hundred muscles to activate movement. Five control supination and pronation, seven move the hand at the wrist, 18 flex and extend the digits, and 20 small muscles of the hand

Table 52-1.   Work Chart for Tendon Transfers (Radial Palsy)

NEEDED FUNCTION	AVAILABLE MOTOR MUSCLE	MOTOR MUSCLES RETAINED FOR BALANCE
Wrist extension	Pronator teres	Pronator quadratus
Finger and thumb extension	Flexor carpi ulnaris (or)	Flexor carpi radialis
	Flexor digitorum superficialis (middle/ring) (or)	Flexor digitorum profundus (middle/ring)
	Flexor carpi radialis and palmaris longus	Flexor carpi ulnaris
Proximal thumb stability	Palmaris longus tenodesis with extensor pollicis brevis	Flexor carpi radialis

contribute to precise motion (White, 1960). One should use as few transfers as necessary to meet the objective, because all tendon transfers complicate the basic problem.

The motor muscle selected must be more than strong enough for its new task, because it will have to pull itself free of the healing process after surgery and will usually lose one grade of strength on Lovett's clinical scale (Omer, 1968). The selected motor muscle–tendon unit should have amplitude adequate for the anticipated arc of motion. Normal amplitude approximates 33 mm for wrist movers, 70 mm for finger flexors, and 50 mm for finger extensors and the thumb motor muscles. A muscle's work capacity is calculated by multiplying strength times amplitude. The range of normal work capacity for forearm muscles is illustrated by the following: flexor carpi ulnaris, 2.0 kg; flexor digitorum profundis, 1.2 kg each or 4.8 kg for the entire muscle; extensor digitorum communis, 0.5 kg each, or 2.0 kg for the whole muscle (Boyes, 1954; Steindler, 1946). The motor muscle selected must have a work capacity equal to that of the antagonist of the anticipated motion. One can utilize the principle of dynamic tenodesis to enhance amplitude. Joints that are involved in the dynamic tenodesis must be mobile and stable. Arthrodesis of the wrist is rare in reconstructive surgery because wrist motion often enhances tendon transfer through dynamic tenodesis.

The present action of the selected motor muscle should be synergistic with the anticipated action or at least retrainable by conscious control (Littler, 1964). Paralyzed muscles that have regained function following nerve suture usually lack the individualized control and strength desirable for successful transfer. Even synergistic action muscles are not predictable in some conditions, such as cerebral palsy (Omer, 1974c).

The available motor muscles are then charted against needed motion to determine that secondary dysfunction will be avoided. (Table 1)

OPERATIVE TECHNIQUES

Incisions are placed so that tendon junctures are beneath skin flaps and free of subcutaneous scar. In general, incisions should be transverse to the subcutaneous path of the transferred tendon. The subcutaneous pathway must glide with the transferred tendon (Mayer, 1916).

The motor muscle should be carefully mobilized to protect its neurovascular bundle, which usually enters the proximal third of the muscle. Amplitude is related to the length of the muscle fibers, and excursion can be increased by a more complete release of the muscle from the surrounding tissue (Boyes, 1954). The texture, vascularity, and excursion of the selected motor muscle should be re-evaluated under direct vision at the operating table.

The transferred tendon should not cross raw bone. Muscle–tendon units that must move through fascial planes, such as an interosseous membrane, should have as large an opening in the fascia as possible. The muscle should be placed in the fascial window, because the exterior muscle fibers will "freeze" but the interior muscle fibers will retain motion; if the tendon is placed in the fascial window, it will bind fast and motion will be lost (Omer, 1974c).

The direction of pull for the transferred tendon should be in as near a straight line as possible. In addition, most muscles are parallel to bone, and the angle of approach between the transferred tendon and its insertion should be small. The greater the angle of approach of the tendon to its insertion point, the greater the force the muscle can exert, but this creates a bowstring. A pulley is required to increase the approach angle, and the result is actually a loss of force secondary to friction when the angle is greater than 45 degrees. Eventually a bowstrung tendon will shift to a straight line and then become too slack for effective action. The more distal to the axis of motion of a joint a tendon is anchored, the more force the muscle can exert on the joint, but also the more the excursion required of the tendon to provide a normal range of motion in the joint. If the insertion of a transferred tendon is split, the motor will act primarily on the slip under greater tension. A tendon transfer is most effective when it crosses only one joint. If a tendon bowstrings across a proximal joint, its mechanical advantage at that joint will be so great that it may force that joint into unwanted movement or use up all its amplitude so that it cannot move the distal joint. An example is the transfer of the brachioradialis into the flexor pollicis longus: when the elbow and wrist are extended, the patient can hold an object tightly, but when he flexes his elbow the muscle–tendon power is dissipated at the elbow, and the patient drops the object.

Suture material for tendon fixation should be monofilament steel or synthetic material with minimal tissue reaction. The suture material should be relatively large, 2-0 or 3-0 in most situations. To prevent tendon ischemia, the suture should be inserted through the center of the tendon and then circle only half the tendon; sutures along the length of the tendon should alternate the circle to be tied from side to side to further protect circulation. "Lacing" a transferred tendon into a group of paralyzed muscle–tendon units should be avoided because it creates bulk, twist, and friction, and increases scar. A precise insertion point should be selected, but at that point a short length of paralyzed and transfer tendon should be sutured side to side to prevent "whipsawing." One may disconnect the paralyzed tendon from its fibrosed muscle and connect it directly to the transferred muscle. However, complete excision of the paralyzed muscle belly may bring unwelcome hemorrhage and should not be done unless the paralyzed muscle mass is causing deformity.

The tension of a tendon transfer is judged best while the hand is placed in the position it will assume when the new tendon contracts. For extensor transfers, resting tendon tension should be strong enough to passively hold the extremity in functional position against gravity. Flexor tendons often cross more than one joint and should be fixed at greater than normal tension against gravity. In any case when re-education is likely to be required, it is better to attach the transferred tendon under greater than normal tension. This brings perception of the new muscle more readily into consciousness as stretch reflexes and other feedback mechanisms are stimulated when opposing muscles restore the neutral position of the extremity (Brand, 1966).

POSTOPERATIVE CARE

The extremity should be immobilized in the proper position to maintain the desired result. For example, after tendon transfers for intrinsic minus thumb and the clawed fingers of ulnar palsy, the hand should be positioned with the metacarpophalangeal joints of the fingers flexed and the interphalangeal joints straight, the so called "hoe hand." Extremity fixation is more extensive when two joint length tendons have been transferred and in children. Flexor tendon transfers should be immobilized for three to four weeks and protected with a splint for one more week, but extensor tendon transfers should be immobilized for five weeks and protected for two more weeks with a volar splint.

FUNCTIONAL RE-EDUCATION

There are many clinical observations suggesting that precise sensibility depends upon total extremity homeostasis and activity (Omer, 1974b). Sensibility re-education programs depend upon movement as an important factor in appropriate stimulation of sensory organs. The patient will alter motor patterns to obtain the best available sensory function. For example, the patient with loss of index volar pulp sensibility secondary to median palsy will adapt by "divorcing" the index finger and extending it out of the pinch pattern, which will then be altered to a chuck between the thumb and ring or middle finger. The Moberg pick-up test is a good check of functional motor patterns if one of the objects is a short length of soft chalk. The chalk will rub against the fingers and leave a visible trail of functional surfaces (Omer, 1971). The abnormal motor function that usually accompanies nerve loss enhances the distorted sensibility patterns and contributes to dysesthesia. These problems are the basis for an aggressive motor re-education program which would include visual monitoring of activity patterns and tendon transfers for improved motor function.

Surgical results should be assessed only after a minimum of six months follow-up. Many elements of function should be considered: power on the voluntary clinical scale; range of motion; balance, or the passive equilibrium between opposing myotonic forces; stability, or the positive action between antagonist muscles; synergism balance such as the action between wrist flexors and finger extensors or wrist extensors and finger flexors; and coordination, the smooth transference of force from one synergistic muscle group to another.

TIMING OF TENDON TRANSFERS

Tendon transfers to restore muscle balance should be performed 12 weeks after the time of expected recovery in traumatic nerve lesions. For clinical purposes, 1 mm per day is an acceptable rate of nerve recovery after suture. Spontaneous nerve recovery after axonotmesis carries a varied latent period from three to nine months (Omer, 1974a). However, tendon transfers undertaken to meet special requirements, such as internal splinting, should be done within 12 weeks following injury (Omer, 1974b).

EARLY TENDON TRANSFERS

Selected early tendon transfers as internal splints enhance function while awaiting the return of nerve control and total muscle activity. The objectives of early tendon transfers are to stimulate sensibility re-education and to improve the coordination of residual muscle–tendon units. The use of tendon transfers as internal splints is discussed by Burkhalter in Chapter 50.

The muscle-tendon units used for early internal support should be synergistic with the muscle–tendon unit to be replaced, such as a wrist flexor in substitution for a finger extensor. A synergistic tendon will be able to utilize spinal reflex arcs and other automatic feedback mechanisms to enhance re-education. Two principles should be followed: (1) use as few muscle–tendon transfers as possible, since any active muscle–tendon unit used to restore a useful extremity position will weaken the strength of the residual active function; and (2) the muscle–tendon transfer must not cause deformity when nerve function is recovered. For example, it would be foolish to transfer the flexor carpi ulnaris, the palmaris longus, and the flexor carpi radialis to varied wrist and digit extensors in a case of radial palsy; subsequent recovery of radial nerve function would result in an inability to actively flex the wrist.

Table 52–2.   Early Tendon Transfers as Internal Splints

PALSY	FUNCTIONAL NEED	AVAILABLE MOTOR MUSCLES
Low Median	Thumb opposition (APB)	Extensor indicis proprius (or) Flexor digitorum superficialis (ring) (or) Palmaris longus (or) Extensor digiti quinti
Radial	Wrist extension (ECRB)	Pronator teres
Low Ulnar	Thumb adduction (AP) and Finger clawing (interosseoi)	Multi-tailed flexor digitorum superficialis (ring) (or) Extensor carpi radialis longus (plus graft) (or) Brachioradialis (plus graft)

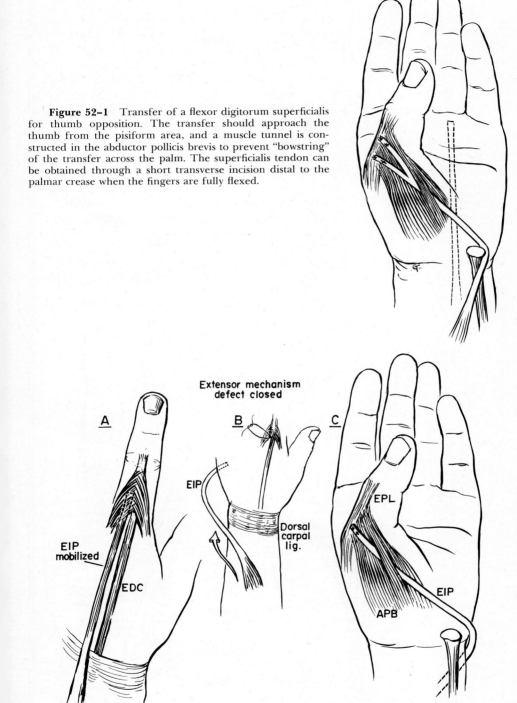

Figure 52-1 Transfer of a flexor digitorum superficialis for thumb opposition. The transfer should approach the thumb from the pisiform area, and a muscle tunnel is constructed in the abductor pollicis brevis to prevent "bowstring" of the transfer across the palm. The superficialis tendon can be obtained through a short transverse incision distal to the palmar crease when the fingers are fully flexed.

Extensor mechanism
defect closed

A

B

C

EIP

Dorsal
carpal
lig.

EIP
mobilized

EDC

EPL

EIP

APB

Figure 52-2 Transfer of the extensor indicis proprius for thumb opposition. The transfer should approach the thumb from the pisiform area. A muscle tunnel is constructed in the abductor pollicis brevis to prevent "bowstring" of the transfer across the base of the palm, and minimize a painful power grasp.

Low Median Palsy

A single tendon should be utilized to restore opposition to the thumb, and a variety of muscle-tendon units are available (Table 52–2). Transfer of the flexor digitorum superficialis tendon of the ring finger to the dorsoulnar aspect of the base of the proximal phalanx of the thumb will produce active opposition. The principles for this procedure were reported in 1890 by Codivilla (Riordan, 1974). The tendon should pass subcutaneously from the thumb insertion in the direction of the pisiform bone (Bunnell, 1938), and a pulley is created there (Fig. 52–1). Burkhalter and his associates have utilized a direct transfer of the extensor indicis proprius subcutaneously around the ulnar border of the wrist into the extensor pollicis longus across the metacarpophalangeal joint capsule (Burkhalter, Christensen, and Brown, 1973) (Fig. 52–2). Transfer of the extensor digiti minimi, as described by Schneider (1969), has the same technique and advantages as the extensor indicis proprius transfer. If the median nerve is lacerated by an oblique injury that spares the palmaris longus tendon, the tendon can be lengthened with a strip of palmar fascia and transferred to the insertion of the abductor pollicis brevis, as described by Camitz (1929) (Fig. 52–3). Both of the extensor muscle–tendon transfers have the advantage of introducing new strength into the power train for flexion, while the flexor muscle–tendon

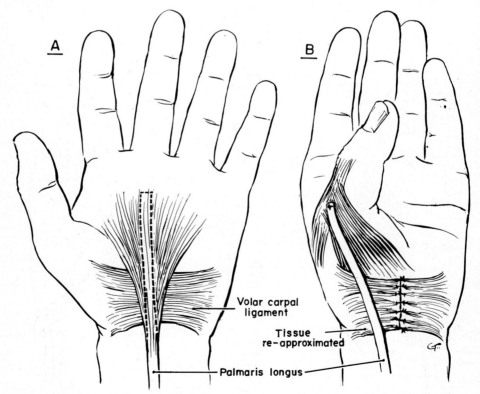

Figure 52–3 Transfer of the palmaris longus for thumb opposition. The tendon is lengthened to reach the insertion of the abductor pollicis brevis by cutting a strip from the volar carpal ligament.

transfers represent a rearrangement of volar muscle strength already involved in the power train for flexion.

Radial Palsy

The pronator teres transferred to the extensor carpi radialis brevis will produce active wrist extension and permit ulnar-innervated intrinsic muscle–finger extension. The pronator teres, while acting for dorsal extension of the wrist, still performs as a pronator of the forearm. The insertion described by Jones (1916), into both the extensor carpi radialis brevis and the extensor carpi radialis longus, often results in radiodorsal extension, and the pronator teres should be inserted only into the extensor carpi radialis brevis in the forearm (Fig. 52–4). Increasing dorsal extension power by an increment of one may increase power grip by an increment of two to four times (Burkhalter, 1974).

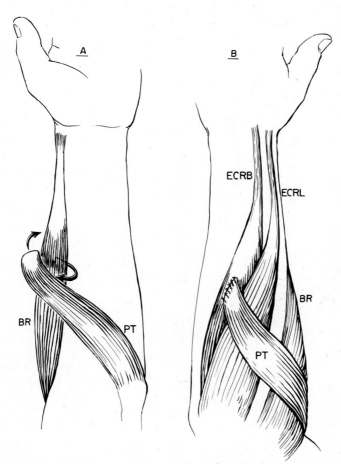

Figure 52–4   Transfer of the pronator teres for wrist extension. The transfer should pass subcutaneously over the brachioradialis and the extensor carpi radialis longus to an insertion limited to the extensor carpi radialis brevis. (From Omer, G. E., Jr.: J. Bone Joint Surg. *50(A)*: 1454. 1968.)

Low Ulnar Palsy

These patients have loss of power for thumb–index pinch and loss of intrinsic muscle power for a gross grip. There is weakness of interphalangeal joint extension, associated with hyperextension of the metacarpophalangeal joint, usually for the ring and little fingers (Table 2). One tendon transfer cannot restore the power requirements, but Omer has stabilized the clawed fingers and improved thumb–index pinch power with a single flexor digitorum superficialis tendon (Omer, 1974d). The flexor digitorum superficialis of the ring or long finger is available, but the ring finger superficialis cannot be used if the ulnar-innervated portion of the flexor digitorum profundus is paralyzed. The flexor digitorum superficialis is first split longitudinally, and the ulnar half is again split into two slips. The two slips of the ulnar half of the tendon are directed volar to the intermetacarpal ligament into the central slip of the extensor mechanism insertion on the middle phalanx in the ring and little fingers for correction of metacarpophalangeal hyperextension and to improve interphalangeal extension. The distal volar insertion of the radial half of the superficialis tendon is released proximal to the proximal interphalangeal

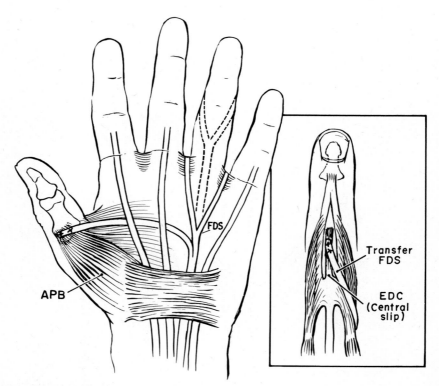

Figure 52–5 Transfer of the long or ring flexor digitorum superficialis for thumb adduction and to prevent clawing of the ring and little fingers. The two slips of the ulnar half of the tendon pass volar to the intermetacarpal ligament and insert in the central slip of the extensor digitorum communis distal to the proximal interphalangeal joint. The radial slip of the tendon passes across the adductor pollicis beneath (dorsal) to the profundi and superficialis tendons and inserts in the abductor tubercle of the thumb.

joint to prevent hyperextension of the joint after completion of the transfer. The radial half of the superficialis tendon is directed across the adductor pollicis, distal to the volar carpal ligament, and dorsal to the flexor tendons, into the insertion of the abductor pollicis brevis for improved pinch strength and to reinforce thumb pronation (Fig. 52–5).

If a power grip is a major consideration, Burkhalter extends the extensor carpi radialis longus or the brachioradialis with a multiple tailed free tendon graft through the lumbrical space, volar to the intermetacarpal ligament, to an insertion on the radial aspect of the proximal phalanx of the clawed digits (Burkhalter and Strait, 1973). This transfer does not correct thumb–index pinch patterns, but does introduce new power from extensor muscles into the flexion action.

COMPLETE NERVE LESIONS

Correction of a complete neuropathy should be designed to provide essential function. The key to success for surgical technique is simplicity; complexity invites failure. Increased power for function must be introduced from a normal power train.

Median Palsy

The requirements for restoration of forearm and hand function following median palsy are: (1) flexion of the index and long fingers (on examination, flexion of the index finger may be the obvious function defect because for the index finger there is a separate profundus muscle belly, but for the long, ring, and little fingers there is a common muscle belly partially innervated by the ulnar nerve), (2) flexion of the thumb, (3) opposition of the thumb, and (4) sensation on the volar pulp surfaces of the thumb and index and long fingers (Table 52–3). There is associated weakness of wrist flexion and forearm pronation.

Flexion of the index and long fingers is obtained by suturing (tenodesing)

Table 52–3. Median Nerve Palsy

NEEDED FUNCTION	PREFERRED MOTOR	ALTERNATE MOTORS
Index and long finger flexion (FDP – index and long)	Flexor digitorum profundus tenodesis	
Thumb flexion (FPL)	Brachioradialis	
Thumb opposition (APB)	Extensor indicis proprius	*Low*
		Palmaris longus
		(or)
		Extensor digiti quanti
		High
		Extensor carpi ulnaris
		(or)
		Abductor digiti quanti
Sensibility (thumb-index)	Neurovascular–cutaneous island pedicle from ring finger	Free neurovascular cutaneous island flap

the index and long tendons of the flexor digitorum profundus to the ring and little tendons of the flexor digitorum profundus so that the ulnar-innervated portion of the muscle will pull the tendons of the median-innervated portion of the muscle through a functional range of motion (Fig. 52–6). The flexor digitorum profundus to the index finger can be tenodesed across the distal interphalangeal joint to increase the mechanical advantage at the proximal interphalangeal joint (Omer, 1968).

Thumb flexion is obtained by releasing the brachioradialis from the radius and transferring its tendon to the flexor pollicis longus (White, 1960) (Fig. 52–7). Failure after this transfer resembles failure after transfer of the pronator teres in that the brachioradialis tends to reattach to the radius unless it has been freed completely from its attachment to the radius. In addition, releasing the brachioradialis will increase the amplitude of excursion for the transferred tendon.

Restoration of thumb opposition following a low median palsy has been discussed under early tendon transfers. Curtis has reviewed the many procedures recorded and the expected result (Curtis, 1974). The extensor indicis

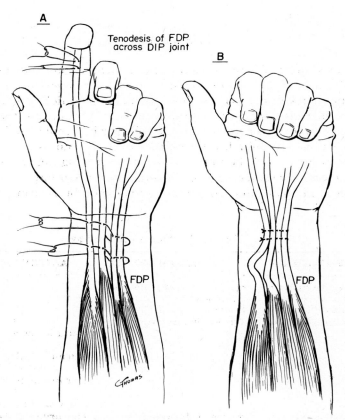

Figure 52–6   Tenodesis of the index and long tendons to the active ring and little tendons of the flexor digitorum profundus for flexion of all four fingers. A double line of sutures is important to prevent "whipsawing" of the tendons with a power grip.

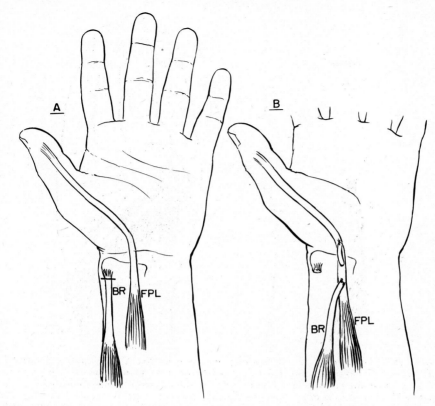

Figure 52–7   Transfer of the brachioradialis into the tendon of the flexor pollicis longus for thumb flexion. The brachioradialis should be free into the proximal third of the forearm, but avoid damage to the neurovascular bundle to the muscle. (From J. Bone Joint Surg. *50(A)*: 1454, 1968.)

proprius transfer would be preferable in a high median palsy (see Fig. 2). Active thumb opposition may be provided by transferring the extensor carpi ulnaris around the ulnar side of the forearm and prolonging its tendon with a free graft (plantaris or palmaris longus tendons) and inserting the transfer under the tendinous portion of the paralyzed abductor pollicis brevis and into the extensor pollicis longus (Henderson, 1962). The suture junction between the extensor carpi ulnaris and the graft should be proximal enough to prevent adhesions near the pisiform pulley (Fig. 52–8). An alternate method to the free tendon graft would be transfer of the extensor carpi ulnaris to the proximal tendon of the extensor pollicis brevis (Kessler, 1969; Phalen and Miller, 1947). The tendon of the adductor pollicis can be switched from the ulnar to the radial side of the proximal phalanx to reinforce pronation of the thumb (de Vicchi procedure) (Brand, 1966). The abductor digiti quinti can be folded from the hypothenar to the thenar area on its neurovascular bundle to provide active opposition (Huber procedure) (Littler and Cooley, 1963). This transfer has limited amplitude and reduces the power for gross grip by its loss from the hypothenar area.

Neurovascular island pedicle transfers and related procedures to restore

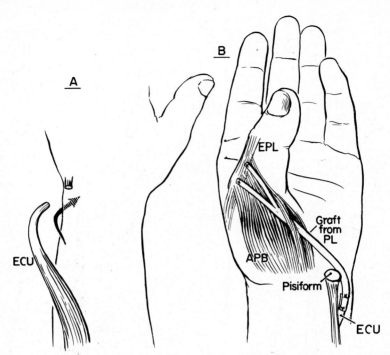

Figure 52–8   Transfer of the extensor carpi ulnaris, extended by a free graft (palmaris longus or plantaris) for thumb opposition. The suture line between the tendon and the free graft should be well proximal to the pisiform area fascia. The graft should pass through a muscle tunnel in the abductor pollicis brevis to prevent "bowstring" of the transfer across the base of the palm. (From Omer, G. E., Jr.: Amer. Acad. Orthop. Surg. Instructional Course Lectures *18*(Jl):93, 1962–1969.)

sensation following median palsy are discussed by Omer in Chapter 48, and by Buncke in Chapter 49. Procedures to restore sensibility in median lerve loss should not be considered until all possible tendon transfers have been accomplished, or the cutaneous transfer will lose precise sensibility.

If wrist flexion and forearm pronation is a special requirement, the extensor carpi radialis longus can be transferred to the flexor carpi radialis.

After operation, the patient's hand and forearm are kept in a bulky soft dressing for two to five days with a dorsal splint to prevent accidental extension of the fingers. A circular plaster cast is then applied which holds the thumb in full opposition, has a dorsal slab which extends distally to the proximal interphalangeal joints, and holds the elbow at a right angle to protect the brachioradialis transfer. After three weeks the plaster cast is shortened to below the elbow, and motion of the wrist and fingers is instituted approximately five weeks after the surgical procedure.

Radial Palsy

The requirements for restoration of forearm and hand function following radial palsy are: (1) wrist extension, (2) finger extension, (3) thumb extension, and (4) stability of the carpometacarpal joint of the thumb (Table 4).

Table 52–4.   Radial Nerve Palsy

NEEDED FUNCTION	PREFERRED MOTOR	ALTERNATE MOTORS
Wrist extension (ECRB)	Pronator teres	
Finger extension (EDC) and thumb extension (EPL)	Flexor carpi ulnaris (or) Flexor digitorum superficialis (long and ring)	
Proximal thumb stability (APL)	Palmaris longus tenodesis with extensor pollicis brevis	Split insertion–flexor carpi radialis (or) Palmaris longus to Extensor pollicis longus

Wrist extension is obtained by transferring the pronator teres to the extensor carpi radialis brevis tendon (see Fig. 52–4).

Finger and thumb extension is provided by transfer of either the flexor carpi ulnaris (Fig. 52–9) or the flexor digitorum superficialis tendons of the long and ring fingers (Fig. 52–10) (Boyes, 1954; Riordan, 1964). The flexor carpi ulnaris should be released to the proximal third of the forearm and directed subcutane-

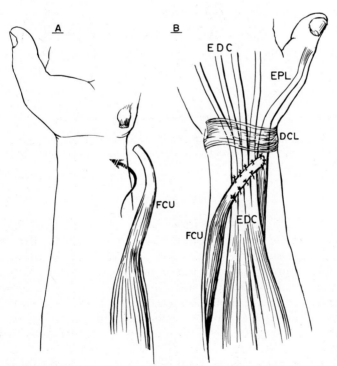

Figure 52–9   Transfer of the flexor carpi ulnaris for finger and thumb extension. The flexor carpi ulnaris should take a subcutaneous oblique route that is superficial to the tendons of the extensor digitorum communis and extensor pollicis longus. Each tendon anastomosis should have a proximal and distal suture to prevent "whipsawing" of the tendons.

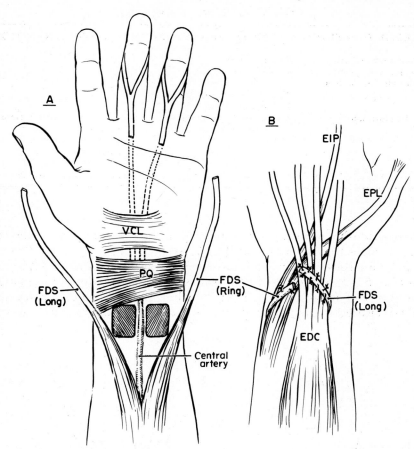

Figure 52–10　Transfer of the long and ring flexor digitorum superficialis tendons through the interosseous membrane for finger and thumb extension. The holes in the interosseous membrane must be large, but not damage the central artery on the volar side of the forearm. The long finger superficialis provides extension of the four fingers, while the ring finger superficialis provides extension of the thumb and index finger. (From Omer, G. E., Jr.: Amer. Acad. Orthop. Surg. Instructional Course Lectures *18*(Jl):93, 1962–1969.)

ously around the ulna and across the tendons of the extensor digitorum communis so that from the little finger to the index finger the transferred tendon is attached in a progressively more distal line of sutures. The tendons of the extensor digitorum communis should be left in their normal bed while the flexor carpi ulnaris is brought subcutaneously and dorsally across each tendon for the oblique anastomosis. A suture should be placed both proximally and distally at the site of attachment to each slip of the extensor digitorum communis or motion will result in "whipsawing" between the tendons. Monofilament stainless steel is a suitable suture material. Tension is increased across the wrist from the little finger to the index finger so that the fingers are held in functional position against gravity. The anastomosis should be proximal to the dorsal carpal ligament and should not be obstructed with full flexion of the wrist and fingers. After the tension has been set and suturing completed for the extensor digitorum communis tendons, the extensor pollicis longus is added as the final insertion of the flexor carpi ulnaris transfer. Failure of the transfer can be recognized because it is in a subcutaneous position. This transfer usually results in a slight radial deviation of the hand. After twenty-four months or more, the patient will be able to selectively extend one finger or all fingers at will, through selective flexor power.

Finger extension can be obtained by transfer of the flexor digitorum superficialis tendons of the long and ring fingers. The tendons are released at the level of the distal palmar crease and withdrawn into the forearm. Large windows are made in the interosseous membrane just proximal to the pronator quadratus. It is worthwhile to release the tourniquet before passing the tendons through the interosseous membrane windows to determine that there is no damage to the central vessels volar to the interosseous membrane. Each transfer should place the muscle of the superficialis within the interosseous membrane windows because the bare tendon will stick with loss of motion. The superficialis of the long finger is attached to the extensor digitorum communis tendons, while the superficialis of the ring finger is attached to the extensor pollicis longus and the extensor indicis proprius. A passive fist is formed with the wrist in 45 degrees of

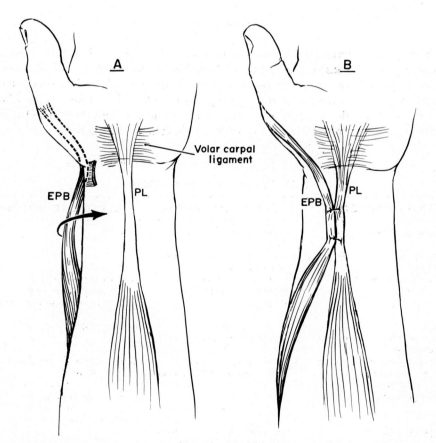

Figure 52–11   Tenodesis of the palmaris longus and the extensor pollicis brevis for proximal thumb stability. The extensor pollicis brevis is mobilized from the first dorsal compartment.

dorsiflexion, then the tendons are sutured at greater than normal tension; or a functional position against gravity can be utilized to determine the tension for transfer.

Stability of the proximal joints of the thumb is obtained by removing the intact extensor pollicis brevis from the first dorsal compartment, bringing it across the volar side of the wrist, and suturing it side-to-side under tension to the palmaris longus (Fig. 52–11). A second technique is to split the flexor carpi radialis tendon for five centimeters from its distal end and to transfer the distal end of the radial half of the split tendon into the abductor pollicis longus.

Postoperatively, the hand and forearm are kept in a bulky soft dressing for two to five days, with a "sugar tong" splint around the elbow and extending to the fingertips. The forearm is in 30 degrees pronation, the wrist in 45 degrees dorsal extension, the metacarpophalangeal joints in 0 degrees extension, and the interphalangeal joints in 15 degrees flexion. The hand and forearm are then placed in a circular cast from the elbow to the proximal interphalangeal joints to maintain the postoperative positions. Six weeks after surgery the patient is placed in a spring action cockup splint to obtain independent wrist and finger extension.

Ulnar Palsy

The requirements for restoration of forearm and hand function following ulnar palsy are: (1) stable pinch between the thumb and index, and (2) prevention of hyperextension at the metacarpophalangeal joint, with associated improved extension at the interphalangeal joints (Table 52–5). There is associated weakness of wrist flexion and an occasional persistently abducted little finger.

Restoration of power for thumb adduction has been discussed under early

Table 52–5. Ulnar Nerve Palsy

NEEDED FUNCTION	PREFERRED MOTOR	ALTERNATE MOTORS
Wrist flexion (FCU)	Palmaris longus to FCU insertion	
Finger flexion (FDP – ring and little)	Flexor digitorum profundus tenodesis	
Thumb adduction (AP)	Split insertion, flexor digitorum superficialis (Omer)	Direct insertion, flexor digitorum superficialis (Edgerton/Brand/Goldner) (or) Brachioradialis
Index abduction (first dorsal interosseous)	Extensor indicis proprius	
Metacarpophalangeal joint flexion/interphalangeal joint extension (finger clawing)	Extensor carpi radialis longus (Brand/Burkhalter)	Flexor digitorum superficialis (Stiles/Bunnell) (or) Flexor carpi radialis (or) Brachioradialis
Sensibility (ring-little)	Free neurovascular cutaneous island flap (in low ulnar palsy)	

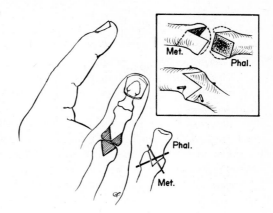

Figure 52–12 The chevron-shaped mortise cut for arthrodesis of the meta-carpophalangeal and proximal interphalangeal joints. The metacarpal bone cut is inclined proximally from the dorsal to volar surface to obtain the desired flexion of the joint. Crossed buried Kirschner wires are used for fixation.

tendon transfers (Omer, 1974d) (see Fig. 5). The thumb is more stable for pinch if there is arthrodesis of the metacarpophalangeal joint. The joint surfaces are cut back to produce a chevron-shaped mortise, with the point of the chevron directed proximally. The apex of the phalangeal half of the chevron mortise is made perpendicular to the long axis of the phalanx, while that of the metacarpal portion of the chevron is inclined palmarward to obtain the desired flexion angle for the arthrodesed joint. The mortise is then stabilized with buried crossed Kirschner wires (Omer, 1968) (Fig. 52–12).

A flexor digitorum superficialis tendon to the long or ring fingers can be utilized as an isolated adductor transfer (Brooks, 1975; Edgerton and Brand, 1965; Goldner, 1967; Tubiana, 1969). If more power for grasp is required, a dorsal muscle, such as the brachioradialis (Boyes, 1970) or one of the wrist extensors can be prolonged with a tendon graft and passed palmarward between the third and fourth metacarpals across the adductor muscle belly to the adductor tendon. The extensor indicis proprius has also been used (Brown, 1974) but often is not strong enough for this function.

Pinch of the index finger has been improved by splitting the tendon of the

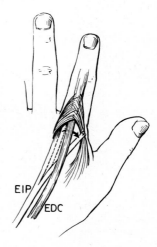

Figure 52–13 A split insertion for the extensor indicis proprius to strengthen pinch of the index finger. The insertion should remain dorsal to the axis of motion of the index metacarpophalangeal joint. (From Omer, G. E., Jr.: J. Bone Joint Surg. 50(A):1454, 1968.)

extensor indicis proprius, passing the radial half of the tendon beneath the index extensor digitorum communis and suturing it on the radial side of the extensor hood (Omer, 1968) (Fig. 52–13). This gives stability, but not active radial deviation of the finger.

A persistent abducted little finger is troublesome during any activity that requires inserting the adducted and extended fingers into a tight space. The extensor digiti quinti produces this deformity and must be transferred. If there is no associated clawing of the metacarpophalangeal joint of the little finger, the entire tendon is transferred to the phalangeal attachment of the radial collateral ligament of the metacarpophalangeal joint of the little finger. If there is clawing as well as abduction, the tendon is transferred volar to the intermetacarpal ligament into a radially based flap of the flexor tendon sheath distal to the proximal pulley (Blacker, Lister, and Kleinert, 1976) (Fig. 52–14).

Restoration of the grasp pattern for the fingers involves procedures to gain interphalangeal joint extension and metacarpophalangeal joint flexion simultaneously. The Stiles–Bunnell transfer is usually accomplished with two to four slips of a flexor digitorum superficialis (Bunnell, 1942) (Fig. 52–15). Each slip is passed down the lumbrical canal volar to the intermetacarpal ligament and then along the radial side of each finger to be inserted into the lateral band of the extensor apparatus. When four slips of a single superficialis tendon are required, the slip to the index finger can be inserted on the ulnar side of the index extensor hood to assist in opposing the index finger to the thumb. If the patient has hyperextensible proximal interphalangeal joints, one half of the superficialis is left across the volar side of the joint and sutured as a tenodesis. In addition, a Brooks insertion (Brooks, 1975) is accomplished by suturing the tendon slip into a radially based flap of the annular ligament of the flexor tendon sheath volar to

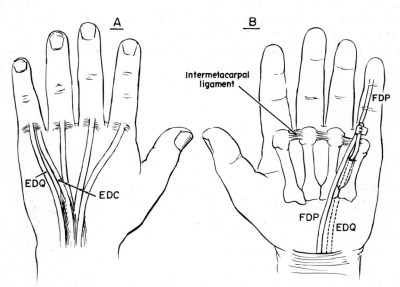

Figure 52–14 Transfer of the extensor digiti quinti for adduction of the little finger. The tendon is passed volar to the intermetacarpal ligament into a radially based flap in the flexor tendon sheath distal to the proximal pulley.

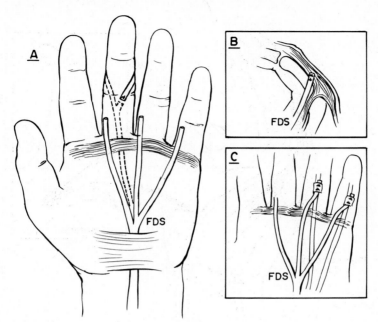

Figure 52–15 Transfer of a flexor digitorum superficialis for correction of finger clawing. The tendon is divided into two to four slips, which are passed through the lumbrical canals and volar to the intermetacarpal ligament. Each slip may be inserted into the lateral band of the extensor apparatus (Insert B) or into a radially-based flap of the flexor tendon sheath (Insert C). One-half of the donor superficialis tendon is left across the proximal interphalangeal joint and sutured to prevent hyperextension at a later date. This transfer does not add power to flexion activities.

the proximal phalanx. The transfer will not stretch and should be sutured under normal muscle tension with the wrist in 20 degrees of extension, the metacarpophalangeal joints in 45 degrees of flexion, and the proximal interphalangeal joint in 0 degrees.

Patients with marked wrist flexion contractures should have the flexor carpi radialis transferred as described by Riordan (1964). The flexor carpi radialis is passed subcutaneously around the dorsal side of the forearm and prolonged with a multiple-tailed graft, usually from the plantaris. The tails are then passed through the lumbrical canals volar to the intermetacarpal ligament and inserted into the extensor mechanism of the fingers.

The incidence of absence of the plantaris is about 8 per cent, while the incidence of absence for the palmaris longus is approximately 11 to 14 per cent. There seems to be no relationship between the absence of the palmaris longus and that of the plantaris. When the plantaris is absent, it is usually absent bilaterally. However, when the palmaris longus is absent, its absence is bilateral in about 60 per cent of cases (Kaplan, 1969).

Transfers utilizing extensor tendons will add strength to the power train for grasp. Brand's dynamic transfer is accomplished by passing the extensor carpi radialis longus around the radial side of the wrist and prolonging the tendon through the carpal tunnel with a many-tailed graft, usually taken from the plantaris tendon. Each tail is threaded down one of the lumbrical canals volar to the intermetacarpal ligament and inserted into the extensor mechanism (Brand,

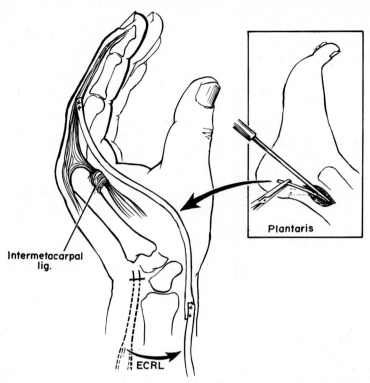

Figure 52–16   Transfer of the extensor carpi radialis longus for correction of finger clawing. The extensor carpi radialis is passed around the radial side of the forearm and extended by a graft (plantaris or palmaris longus), in two to four slips, down the carpal tunnel and out the palm through an incision at the level of the distal palmar crease. A tendon passer is then inserted retrograde from the radial lateral band of the extensor mechanism and directed volar to the intermetacarpal ligament. Each graft slip is then pulled to its insertion of the radial aspect of the extensor mechanism.

A similar technique would extend the extensor carpi radialis longus or brachioradialis. The graft would pass through the interosseous spaces between the metacarpals, then volar to the inter-metacarpal ligament. Each slip can be inserted into the extensor mechanism, the proximal phalanx, or into a flap in the flexor tendon sheath. These transfers do add power to flexion activities.

1961) (Fig. 52–16). Burkhalter has emphasized the need for a prime metacar-pophalangeal flexor (Burkhalter and Strait, 1973). The extensor carpi radialis longus or the brachioradialis is extended with a multiple-tailed graft through the lumbrical canal volar to the intermetacarpal ligament to an insertion on the radial aspect of the proximal phalanx.

Postoperatively, the patient's hand and forearm are kept in a bulky dressing for two to five days, with a "sugar tong" splint around the elbow and extending to the fingertips. The wrist is neutral, the metacarpophalangeal joints in 70 degrees of flexion and the interphalangeal joints in 15 degrees of flexion. The thumb is adducted and pronated against the second metacarpal. A circular cast is utilized to maintain this position for four weeks after surgery, when active motion is allowed, but protected for two additional weeks with dynamic traction from a wrist band to finger cuffs.

COMBINED NERVE LESIONS

When more than one nerve is injured, the problem is much more complicated. Circulation is usually impaired, resulting in increased fibrosis. Tendons are often lacerated or avulsed, complicating the neuromotor impairment. Sensibility loss is more profound in combined nerve lesions, and motor return after multiple nerve involvement is better than sensory recovery. The selected tendon transfers should be done as soon as practical in combined nerve lesions in order to increase sensory feedback and to establish more normal patterns of function.

Low Median-Ulnar Palsy

This is the most common combined nerve injury, and the complete loss of volar sensation and intrinsic motor muscles produces an almost useless claw hand. There is a flat transverse palmar arch with hyperextension at the metacarpophalangeal joints and hyperflexion at the proximal interphalangeal joints. An abducted little finger, with the flat transverse palmar arch, is troublesome, and the extensor digiti quinti tendon should be transferred as described for ulnar palsy (Blacker, Lister, and Kleinert, 1976). The patient flexes his wrist to obtain greater finger extension, a functional tenodesis, but in time a fixed flexion contracture of the wrist results. The thumb–index pinch is markedly weakened (Table 52–6).

Table 52–6.   Combined Low Median–Low Ulnar Palsy

NEEDED FUNCTION	PREFERRED MOTOR	ALTERNATE MOTORS
Thumb adduction (AP)	Split insertion, flexor digitorum superficialis (Omer)	Direct insertion, flexor digitorum superficialis (Brand/Goldner)
Thumb opposition (APB)	Extensor indicis proprius	Extensor digiti quinti (or) Extensor carpi ulnaris
Metacarpophalangeal joint flexion/interphalangeal joint extension (finger clawing)	Extensor carpi radialis longus (four-tailed graft)	Flexor carpi radialis (or) Brachioradialis (or) Flexor digitorum superficialis (Stiles/Bunnell)
Volar sensibility	Cross finger – index to thumb – neurocutaneous flap	Free neurovascular cutaneous island flap

High Median-Ulnar Palsy

The hand will rarely be used for precision work following this severe injury. Atrophy of the finger pulps will discourage both precise and power grip. Tip pinch is unstable, and it is best to direct surgical endeavor toward a key pinch and a simple grasp (Table 52–7).

The extensor carpi radialis brevis has the best mechanical advantage for wrist extension and should remain in place, but all other extrinsic muscles on the

Table 52-7. Combined High Median–High Ulnar Palsy

NEEDED FUNCTION	PREFERRED MOTOR	ALTERNATE MOTORS
Thumb flexion (FPL) Finger flexion (FDP) Thumb adduction (AP) Thumb opposition (APB)	Brachioradialis Extensor carpi radialis longus Extensor indicis proprius Extensor digiti quinti	Extensor carpi ulnaris Extensor pollicis brevis (rerouted)

Thumb stability
Metacarpophalangeal joint
  flexion/interphalangeal
  joint extension
  (finger clawing)
	M–P arthrodesis
	Extensor carpi ulnaris (four-
	  tailed graft)
		Parks tenodesis
		      (or)
		Zancolli capsulodesis
		      (or)
		Brachioradialis
		      (or)
		Extensor carpi radialis longus

Volar sensibility	Radial innervated finger fillet flap	

extensor side can be used. The extensor carpi radialis should be transferred around the radial side of the wrist into the flexor digitorum profundus for finger flexion (Fig. 52–17). The suture junction is proximal, near the musculo-tendinous junction (Omer, 1974d). The brachioradialis is transferred to the flexor pollicis longus, to obtain thumb flexion and improve forearm pronation. There is no wrist extensor muscle with enough amplitude to provide digit flexion unless the motion is reinforced by wrist extension.

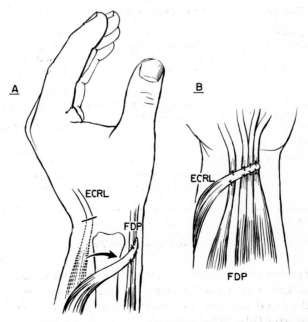

Figure 52–17 Transfer of the extensor carpi radialis longus around the forearm for finger flexion. The range of motion is less than normal. (From Amer. Acad. Orthop. Surg. Instructional Course Lectures *18*(J1):93, 1962–1969.)

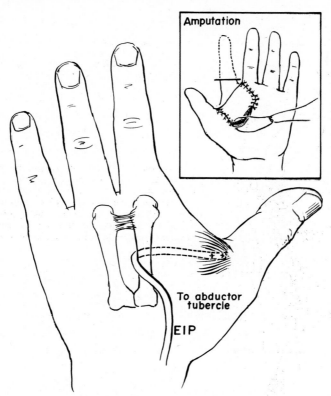

Figure 52–18   Transfer of the extensor indicis proprius for adduction of the thumb in a high median–high ulnar palsy. The index ray is excised, and a radial-innervated flap inset for palmar sensation (Insert). The extensor indicis proprius is usually not strong enough to be an effective adductor pollicis substitute.

Thumb adduction can be obtained by passing the extensor indicis proprius through the third–fourth metacarpal space and across the volar surface of the adductor pollicis. The extensor indicis proprius should be inserted into the abductor tubercle rather than the adductor tubercle (Fig. 52–18). The extensor pollicis brevis may be rerouted anteriorly to abduct the thumb while it continues to extend the metacarpophalangeal joint (Brand, 1970) (Fig. 52–19), or the abductor digiti quinti can be transferred around the wrist for thumb opposition (Schneider, 1969). If there is instability of the thumb in pinch, one should arthrodese the metacarpophalangeal joint in about 15 degrees of flexion, 10 degrees of abduction, and 10 degrees of pronation.

The extensor carpi ulnaris, the extensor carpi radialis longus, or the brachioradialis may be used for intrinsic action on the fingers. If the fingers begin to flex unduly at the distal interphalangeal joints and inadequately at the proximal interphalangeal joints, one should consider arthrodesis of the distal interphalangeal joints in neutral position (Brand, 1970).

Tenodesis procedures may be utilized in several situations but have been most effective in restoration of the grasp pattern for the fingers (Enna and Riordan, 1973; Parkes, 1973; Zancolli, 1957) (Fig. 20). The Parkes procedure,

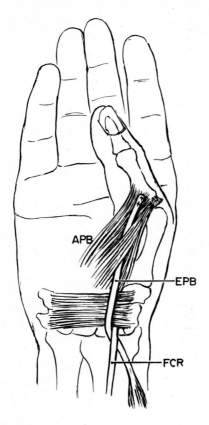

Figure 52–19 Rerouting of the extensor pollicis brevis for abduction of the thumb. The tendon is divided at its insertion and rerouted around the radius and beneath the flexor carpi radialis just proximal to the volar carpal ligament. The tendon then passes subcutaneously in the direction of the fibers of the abductor pollicis brevis to the abductor tubercle.

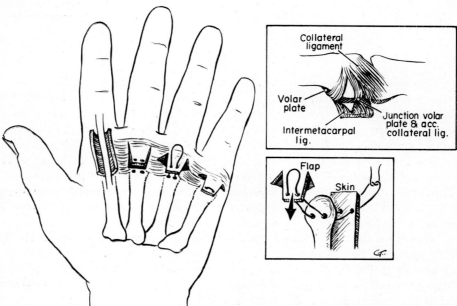

Figure 52–20 Zancolli capsulodesis of the metacarpophalangeal joint to correct finger clawing. The excised triangles extend into the intermetacarpal (deep transverse metacarpal) ligament, and into the accessory collateral ligament on each side of the flap in the volar plate. In the very mobile hand, the sutures can be tied over tubing on the dorsum of the hand.

Figure 52–21 Free graft tenodesis to correct clawing of the fingers. The distal attachment is the central slip of the extensor digitorum communis distal to the proximal interphalangeal joint. The graft passes through the lumbrical canal to the intermetacarpal ligament (deep transverse metacarpal ligament) or to the flexor retinaculum in the palm.

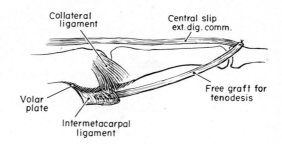

with a free graft from the flexor retinaculum through the lumbrical canal to the dorsal extensor mechanism just beyond the proximal interphalangeal joint has been very effective (Parkes, 1973) (Fig. 52–21).

Sensibility can be provided only to the radial–volar aspect of the hand (Omer, 1974d, 1975a). The skeleton of the index finger is removed distal to the carpometacarpal joint of this ray. The extensor indicis proprius is then available for transfer. The insensitive skin distal to the level of the proximal phalanx of the index finger is discarded. The fillet index finger flap is then fitted into an additional volvar defect created for it in the insensitive palmar skin (see Chapter 48). This broad based fillet finger flap is innervated by the superficial radial nerve and will provide protective sensibility (see Fig. 52–18). A free neurovascular cutaneous island flap would require extensive nerve grafts.

High Median–Radial Nerve Palsy

Tendon transfers in this combined lesion result in a wrist and hand that operate only slightly more effectively than a prosthesis (Table 52–8).

A wrist arthrodesis is one technique to free some tendons for digit motion. The flexor profundi tendons are sutured side to side for ulnar innervated motion (see Fig. 52–6). Digit extension is restored by transferring the flexor carpi ulnaris to the extensor digitorum communis and the extensor pollicis longus (see Fig. 52–9). The metacarpophalangeal joint of the thumb is arthrodesed, and the flexor pollicis longus is tenodesed across the interphalangeal

Table 52–8. Combined High Median–Radial Palsy

NEEDED FUNCTION	PREFERRED MOTOR	ALTERNATE MOTOR
Wrist flexion–extension	Wrist arthrodesis	
Index and long finger flexion (FDP–I and L)	Flexor digitorum profundus tenodesis	
Finger extension (EDC) and thumb extension (EPL)	Flexor carpi ulnaris	
Thumb opposition (APB)	Abductor digiti quinti	Adductor pollicis (abductor insertion)
Thumb flexion (FPL)	I–P tenodesis	
Thumb stability (APL)	M–P arthrodesis APL tenodesis	
Sensibility (thumb–index)	Neurovascular cutaneous island pedicle from ring finger	

joint. Thumb opposition is obtained by the Huber technique (Littler and Cooley, 1963) or the de Vecchi technique (Brand, 1970).

High Ulnar–Radial Nerve Palsy

These patients retain thumb–index sensibility, and reconstruction is a useful investment for improved function (Table 52–9).

Transfer of the pronator teres to the extensor carpi radialis brevis for wrist extension will result in radial deviation of the hand, and a double insertion into the extensor carpi ulnaris and the extensor carpi radialis longus is preferable (Brand, 1966). Proximal thumb stability may be obtained by splitting the insertion of the flexor carpi radialis and yoking it to the abductor pollicis longus insertion.

Table 52–9. Combined High Ulnar–Radial Palsy

NEEDED FUNCTION	PREFERRED MOTOR	ALTERNATE MOTORS
Wrist extension (ECRB)	Pronator teres (yoke to ECRL and ECU)	
Wrist flexion (FCU)	Palmaris longus (to FCU insertion)	
Finger extension (EDC) and thumb extension (EPL)	Flexor digitorum superficialis (long and ring)	
Finger flexion (FDP–ring and little)	Flexor digitorum profundus tenodesis	
Proximal thumb stability (APL)	Flexor carpi radialis (yoke insertion)	APL tenodesis
Thumb adduction (AP)	Flexor digitorum superficialis (index)	M–P arthrodesis
Metacarpophalangeal joint flexion/interphalangeal joint extension (finger clawing)	Parkes' tenodesis	Zancolli capsuloplasty
Sensibility (ring–little)	Free neurovascular cutaneous island flap	

COMMENT

Kaplan and White (1972) summarize the technique of tendon transfers: "In general, nothing is more unpredictable and nothing varies more with time than tendon transfers. Nevertheless, the end effect is generally more desirable than the disability for which the operation was done." The key to success for the surgical technique is simplicity, since complexity invites failure.

REFERENCES

Blacker, G. J., Lister, G. D., and Kleinert, H. E.: The abducted little finger in low ulnar nerve palsy. J. Hand Surg. *1*:190, 1976.

Boyes, J. H.: Tendon transfers for radial palsy. Bull. Hosp. Joint Dis. *15*:97, 1954.

Boyes, J. H.: Bunnell's Surgery of the Hand. 5th ed., Philadelphia, J. B. Lippincott Company, 1970.

Brand, P. W.: Tendon grafting. Illustrated by a new operation for intrinsic paralysis of the fingers. J. Bone Joint Surg. *43B*:444, 1961.

Brand, P. W.: Tendon transfers in the forearm. *In* Flynn, J. E. (ed.): Hand Surgery. Baltimore, The Williams & Wilkins Company, 1966, p. 331.

Brand, P. W.: Tendon transfers for median and ulnar nerve paralysis. Orthop. Clin. North Am. *1*:447, 1970.

Brooks, A. L.: A new intrinsic tendon transfer for the paralytic hand. J. Bone Joint Surg. *57A*:730, 1975.

Brown, P. W.: Reconstruction for pinch in ulnar intrinsic palsy. Orthop. Clin. North Am. *5*:323, 1974.

Bunnell, S.: Opposition of the thumb. J. Bone Joint Surg. *20*:269, 1938.

Bunnell, S.: Surgery of the intrinsic muscles of the hand other than those producing opposition of the thumb. J. Bone Joint Surg. *24*:1, 1942.

Burkhalter, W. E., and Strait, J. L.: Metacarpophalangeal flexor replacement for intrinsic muscle paralysis. J. Bone Joint Surg. *55A*:1667, 1973.

Burkhalter, W. E.: Early tendon transfer in upper extremity peripheral nerve injury. Clin. Orthop. *104*:68, 1974.

Burkhalter, W. E., Christensen, R. C., and Brown, P.: Extensor indicis proprius opponensplasty. J. Bone Joint Surg. *55A*:725, 1973.

Camitz, H.: Surgical treatment of paralysis of the opponens muscle of the thumb. Acta Chir. Scand. *65*:77, 1929.

Curtis, R. M.: Opposition of the thumb. Orthop. Clin. North Am. *5*:305, 1974.

Ducker, T. B., and Kauffman, F. C.: Metabolic factors in surgery of peripheral nerves. Clin. Neurosurg. *24*:406, 1977.

Edgerton, M. T., and Brand, P. W.: Restoration of abduction and adduction to the unstable thumb in median and ulnar paralysis. Plast. Reconstr. Surg. *36*:150, 1965.

Enna, C. D., and Riordan, D. C.: The Fowler procedure for correction of the paralytic claw hand. Plast. Reconstr. Surg. *52*:352, 1973.

Goldner, J. L.: Replacement of the function of the paralyzed adductor pollicis with flexor digitorum sublimis — a ten year review. J. Bone Joint Surg. *49A*:583, 1967.

Henderson, E. D.: Transfer of wrist extensors and brachioradialis to restore opposition of the thumb. J. Bone Joint Surg. *44A*:513, 1962.

Jones, R.: On suture of nerves and alternate methods of treatment by transplantation of tendon. Br. Med. J. *1*:641, 679, 1916.

Kaplan, E. B.: Personal communication, October 26, 1969.

Kaplan, I., and White, W. L.: Tendon transfer. *In* Goldwyn, R. M. (ed.): The Unfavorable Result in Plastic Surgery. Avoidance and Treatment. Boston, Little, Brown and Company, 1972.

Kessler, I.: Transfer of extensor carpi ulnaris to tendon of extensor pollicis brevis for opponensplasty. J. Bone Joint Surg. *51A*:1303, 1969.

Littler, J. W., and Cooley, S. G. E.: Opposition of the thumb and its restoration by abductor digiti quinti transfer. J. Bone Joint Surg. *45A*:1389, 1963.

Littler, J. W.: Principles of Tendon Transfer. *In* Converse, J. M. (ed.): Reconstructive Plastic Surgery. Philadelphia, W. B. Saunders Company, 1964, Vol. IV, p. 1678.

Mayer, L.: The physiological method of tendon transplantation. Surg. Gynecol. Obstet. *22*:182, 298, 1916.

Omer, G. E., Jr.: Evaluation and reconstruction of the forearm and hand after acute traumatic peripheral nerve injuries. J. Bone Joint Surg. *50A*:1454, 1968.

Omer, G. E., Jr.: Assessment of peripheral nerve injuries *In* Cramer, L. M., and Chase, R. A. (eds.): Symposium on the Hand. Educational Foundation of the American Society of Plastic and Reconstructive Surgeons, St. Louis, C. V. Mosby Company, 1971, Vol. 3, p. 1.

Omer, G. E., Jr.: Injuries to nerves of the upper extremity. J. Bone Joint Surg. *56A*:1615, 1974a.

Omer, G. E., Jr.: Sensation and sensibility in the upper extremity. Clin. Orthop. *104*:30. 1974b.

Omer, G. E., Jr.: The technique and timing of tendon transfers. Orthop. Clin. North Am. *5*:243, 1974c.

Omer, G. E., Jr.: Tendon transfers in combined nerve lesions. Orthop. Clin. North Am. *5*:377, 1974d.

Omer, G. E., Jr.: Neurovascular island flaps and fillet of fingers. *In* Grabb, W. C., and Myers, M. B. (eds.): Skin Flaps. Boston, Little, Brown and Company, 1975a, p. 471.

Omer. G. E., Jr., and Spinner, M.: Peripheral nerve testing and suture techniques. Instructional Course Lectures. Am. Acad. Orthop. Surg. *24*:122, 1975b, St. Louis, C. V. Mosby Company.

Parkes, A.: Paralytic claw fingers — a graft tenodesis operation. Hand *5*:192, 1973.

Phalen, G. S., and Miller, R. C.: The transfer of wrist extensor muscles to restore or reinforce flexion power of the fingers and opposition of the thumb. J. Bone Joint Surg. *29*:993, 1947.

Riordan, D. C.: Tendon transfers for nerve paralysis of the hand and wrist. Curr. Prac. Orthop. Surg. *2*:17, 1964.

Riordan, D. C.: Radial nerve paralysis. Orthop. Clin. North Am. 5:283, 1974.

Schneider, L. H.: Opponensplasty using the extensor digiti minimi. J. Bone Joint Surg. *51A*:1297, 1969.

Steindler, A.: The Traumatic Deformities and Disabilities of the Upper Extremity. Springfield, Charles C Thomas, 1946.

Tubiana, R.: Anatomic and physiologic basis for the surgical treatment of paralyses of the hand. J. Bone Joint Surg. *51A*:643, 1969.

White, W. L.: Restoration of function and balance of the wrist and hand by tendon transfers. Surg. Clin. North Am. *40*:427, 1960.

Zancolli, E. A.: Claw-hand caused by paralysis of the intrinsic muscles. J. Bone Joint Surg. *39A*:1076, 1957.

53

MICROSURGICAL FREE MUSCLE TRANSPLANTATION

YOSHIKAZU IKUTA

The purpose of nerve suture in the treatment of peripheral nerve damage is, as is well known, to restore sensation and mobility to the affected member. To achieve this restoration, the skin supplied by the nerves to be repaired must be healthy; similarly, the muscles must also be healthy or, if atrophied from disuse, they must at least be healthy enough to allow them to be rehabilitated.

Most damage to peripheral nerves seen in clinical practice involves only the nerve trunk; in most cases, the muscles are spared injury. However there are occasions when the motor branches of the nerve are injured at the site of entry into the muscle, rendering nerve suture impossible, and occasions when the muscle per se has been damaged.

When the extent of muscle injury is limited, it is still possible to reconstruct the hand into a fairly useful instrument by tendon transfer and tenodesis, but if the damage involves the greater part of the muscles of the forearm, such as in Volkmann's contracture, some compromises must be made in the extent of effort devoted to reconstruction; the reason being that there is a limit to the amount of muscles available for the power source. If, however, muscles for grafting are available from another site, suturing the nerve of that muscle to the motor nerve of the recipient site will be helpful in attempts to reconstruct a useful hand.

Pedicle muscle transfer is a procedure in which a muscle is removed from its site and used not to serve its original purpose but to restore the function of an injured muscle of another site. The oldest and most widely employed utilization of this technique is transfer of the gracilis muscle, which is done for a variety of purposes, such as in the treatment of incontinence (Pickrell et al., 1952; Pers and Medgyesi, 1973), and the transfer of abdominal wall muscle to cover the chest wall (Simpson and Gossage, 1971; Demos et al., 1971) and large vessels (Pers and Medgyesi, 1973).

However, the major disadvantages of pedicle muscle transfer are that the number of muscles which can be used is highly limited and that they can only be transferred to adjacent sites. These shortcomings have been studied for over a century (Zielonkos, 1874; Gluck, 1881; Salvia, 1883).

Recently, Thompson et al. (1971) have developed a method of clinical application, and a number of successful cases have been reported; however, there are still two major problems associated with free muscle graft. One is the uncertainty of achieving a successful "take." For the transfer of the muscle to be successful, it is necessary that its viability be temporarily maintained by tissue fluid, after which circulation within the transferred muscle should be provided by incoming host site vessels. Therefore, in order for the muscle to maintain viability under such conditions, its volume must not be too large.

The other problem is in restoration of motor function. After the transferred muscle has "taken," unless there is so-called neurotization of the motor nerve fibers from the surrounding muscles (Aitken, 1950, 1965), restoration of motor power in the transferred site cannot be achieved.

As a means of overcoming these two weaknesses at the same time, muscle graft experiments employing microsurgical techniques were undertaken by Tamai et al. (1970) and Kubo et al. (1975), who demonstrated its practical use. Harii et al. (1975) and the author and his colleagues have succeeded in its clinical application.

CLINICAL STUDIES

Case 1

This six-year-old boy fell from a height of about 1 meter on June 28, 1974, and his right arm was immobilized in a plaster cast for about 50 days. The diagnosis by a local doctor was supracondylar fracture of the right humerus. After removal of the cast, motor disturbance of the hand and sensory disturbance in the median and ulnar nerve regions were noticed, and the patient was referred to our department. At the time of initial examination, the case presented characteristic findings of Volkmann's contracture (Fig. 53–1).

On November 15, 1974, five months after injury, the author performed amputation of the distal phalanges of the middle and ring fingers, neurolysis of the median and ulnar nerves, and excision of the necrotic flexor muscles of the forearm (Fig. 53–2). Five months after surgery, there was some degree of sensory recovery and restoration of intrinsic function; extension of fingers was practically normal, and side pinch of thumb and index finger became possible. However, finger flexion was totally impossible except at the MP joints (Fig. 53–3).

On May 23, 1975, free muscle graft, using the right pectoralis major muscle, was performed for the purpose of obtaining flexion of the thumb and four fingers.

SURGICAL PROCEDURE. A 25 cm skin incision was made beginning at the crest of the greater tuberosity of the humerus along the outer edge of the right pectoralis major muscle to the sternum. Next, the muscular origin and insertion were released and detached from the chest wall, as shown in Figure 53–4.

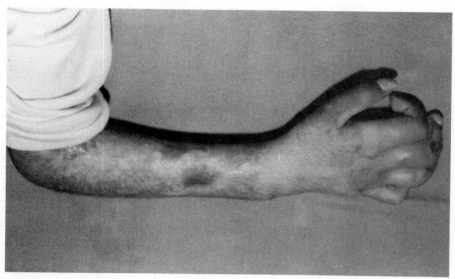

Figure 53-1   This case presented characteristic findings of Volkmann's contracture, such as pronation of forearm, flexion contracture of wrist, and claw deformity of all fingers with sensory disturbance of median and ulnar nerve regions. The tips of the middle and ring fingers were necrotic.

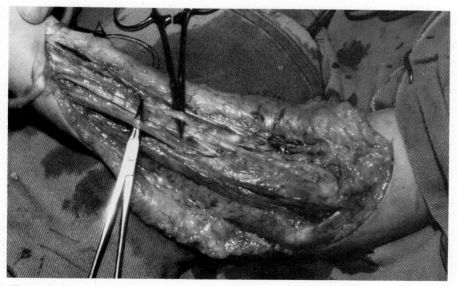

Figure 53-2   Five months after injury, ablation of the distal phalanges of the middle and ring fingers and neurolysis of the median and ulnar nerves were performed. All flexor muscles were excised. In this figure, the median and ulnar nerves are lifted with clamps.

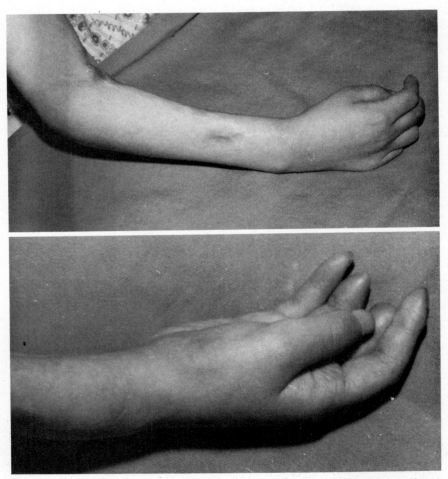

Figure 53-3   These photographs, taken five months after the initial operation, show some restoration of intrinsic function. Some sensory recovery was noted. However, finger flexion was possible only at the metacarpophalangeal joints.

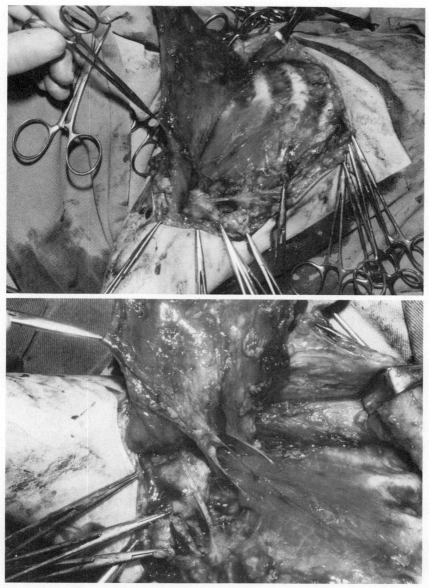

Figure 53–4 *Top,* The origin of the right pectoralis major muscle was released and detached from the chest wall. *Bottom,* The branch of the thoracoacromial artery, the accompanying veins, and the nerves from the chest wall are identified and preserved.

The branch of the thoracoacromial artery, the accompanying veins, and the nerves from the chest wall were identified.

Next, a tourniquet was applied to the right upper arm. With the skin incision used in the previous procedure, a 20 cm zigzag incision was made on the forearm, and the scarred median and ulnar nerves and the anterior interosseous nerve, which was to be used at time of nerve suture, were identified (Fig. 53–5). Search for the ulnar artery revealed that the artery, together with the two accompanying veins, disappeared at the junction of the middle and proximal thirds of the forearm. Next, the neurovascular bundle of the pectoralis major muscle, which had been confirmed earlier, was transected and the muscle was excised.

The tendinous insertion of the pectoralis major muscle was then sutured to the medial epicondyle of the humerus, and the muscular origin was sutured to the flexor tendons of the fingers and thumb at the distal portion of the forearm (Fig. 53–6).

In order to reduce the period of ischemia, the arteries were anastomosed first, and then the nerves, followed by the vein. The branch of the thoraco-acromial artery and the ulnar artery were sutured together by end-to-end anastomosis using 10-0 monofilament nylon suture under Zeiss OPMi II operating room microscope. The tourniquet was removed and good venous return was confirmed. Funicular suture of the four nerve branches of the pectoralis major and the anterior interosseous nerve was performed using 10-0 nylon, after which one of the veins was anastomosed. Figure 53–7 shows the anastomosed artery, vein, and nerves.

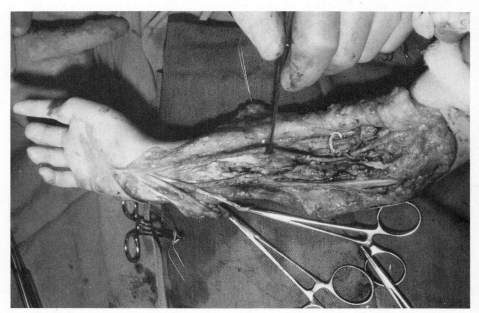

Figure 53–5 All flexor tendons, the ulnar artery and veins, the scarred median and ulnar nerves, and the anterior interosseous branch are identified.

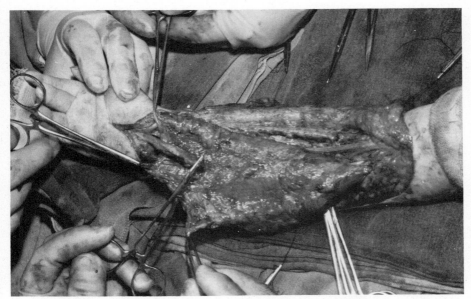

Figure 53–6 The insertion of the pectoralis major muscle was sutured to the medial epicondyle of the humerus and the muscular origin was sutured to the flexor tendons of the fingers and thumb.

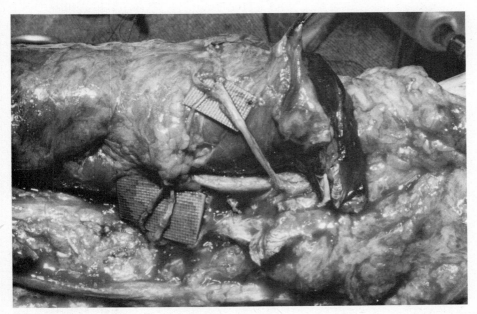

Figure 53–7 Close-up findings of the vessel and nerve anastomosis site. The diameters of the artery and vein of the muscle were about 1.2 and 1.5 mm, respectively.

To conclude the procedure, as shown in Figure 53–8, the wounds were closed with drains inserted.

Low molecular weight dextran and urokinase were administered intravenously as anticoagulants for 10 days after surgery. Heparin was not used.

POSTOPERATIVE FINDINGS.   Three months after surgery, very slight contraction of the grafted muscle could be palpated; this increased as time went by.

Five months after the operation, powerful flexion of the thumb and four fingers could be seen (Fig. 53–9). The boy could hold a pencil, write, and carry a school bag. The functional recovery of the muscle was confirmed by EMG.

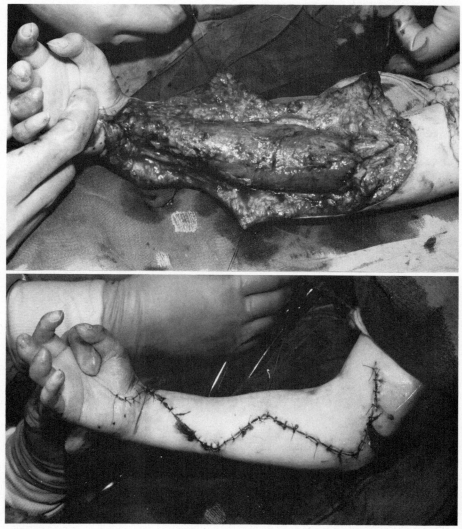

Figure 53–8 *Top,* The circulation of the muscle was confirmed by bleeding from the muscle surface. *Bottom,* The grafted muscle was covered with original skin under moderate tension.

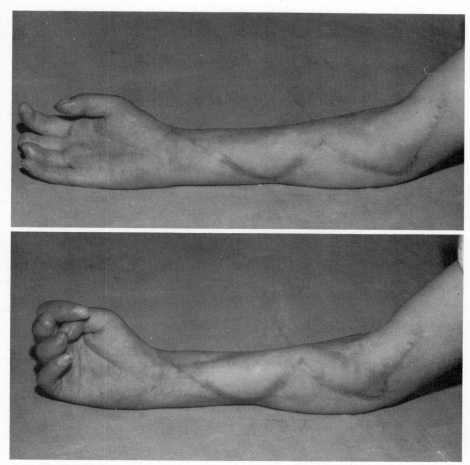

Figure 53–9 Five months after operation. Sensation of the fingers is almost normal and strong flexion of thumb and fingers is possible.

Case 2

An eight-year-old patient had had his left upper arm to palm immobilized in a cast for about one month from December 1969 by a local doctor, whose diagnosis was supracondylar fracture. After removal of the cast, the patient was referred to this department with a diagnosis of Volkmann's contracture.

Examination revealed typical findings of Volkmann's contracture, such as the wrist being in flexion, claw deformity of the fingers, adduction contracture of the thumb, and sensory disturbance in the median and ulnar nerve region. In June 1970, a zigzag incision was made on the anterior side of the left forearm and neurolysis of the ulnar and median nerves was performed. The flexor muscles, excluding those of the ring and little fingers, were practically all necrotic, and severe fibrosis was present. The fibrotic muscles were excised and the live muscles were slid distally, and attempts were made to restore flexion to the fingers. Sensation of the median and ulnar nerves was gradually regained, but

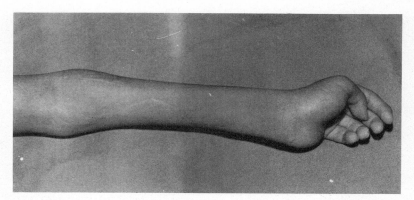

Figure 53–10 Patient had undergone neurolysis of median and ulnar nerves, and resection of fibrotic muscles. This photograph shows the arm five months after operation.

dorsiflexion of the wrist and adduction contracture of the thumb became more severe and five years after surgery, the fingers, thumb, and wrist became almost immovable (Fig. 53–10).

SURGICAL PROCEDURE. First, to correct the dorsiflexion deformity of the wrist, an L-shaped incision was made on the dorsal aspect of the left forearm; then the extensor carpi radialis brevis, extensor carpi ulnaris, and extensor digitorum communis were lengthened in a Z-shaped manner and sutured, after which the skin was closed.

Next, a zigzag incision exactly like that of the scar of the previous operation was made on the volar aspect of the forearm. The anterior interosseous branch of the median nerve, ulnar artery, and vein were isolated. All the flexor tendons were identified and preserved. The fibrotic mass was resected. Subsequently, the flexor tendons were severed in the distal forearm (Fig. 53–11).

An inverted S-shaped incision 15 cm in length was made on the inner side of

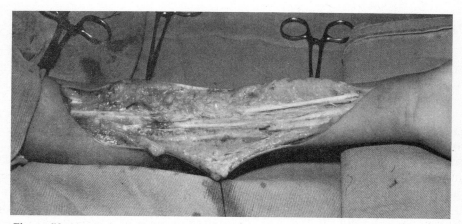

Figure 53–11 A zigzag incision was made on the flexor side of the forearm and the scar tissue was resected. This anterior interosseous branch of the median nerve and the ulnar artery and veins were isolated for the microsurgical anastomoses.

the right thigh and the gracilis muscle was exposed. The motor branch of the obturator nerve, which enters the muscle at a point one-third from the proximal end, the branch of the medial circumflex femoral artery, and two concomitant veins were isolated and severed at points as proximal as possible (Fig. 53–12). This muscle is supplied by four vascular bundles, and the other three were ligated and severed. A portion of the gracilis muscle, which measured at normal tension the length from the medial epicondyle of the left humerus to about 3 cm proximal to the wrist, was excised for transfer. The proximal end of the muscle was sutured to the medial epicondyle, and the distal end was sutured to the

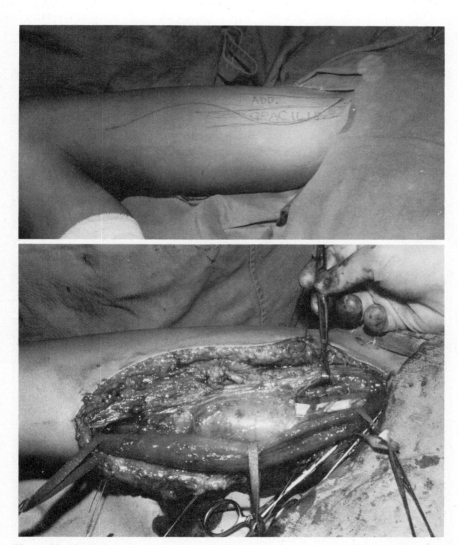

Figure 53–12 *Top,* An inverted S-shaped skin incision was made on the inner side of the right thigh, and the gracilis muscle was exposed. *Bottom,* There are four arteriovenous bundles into the gracilis muscle. The motor branch of the obturator nerve and the second arteriovenous bundle were used for anastomoses. This neurovascular pedicle enters the muscle at a point one third from the proximal end.

earlier isolated flexor tendons of the thumb and fingers, as though to wrap them into the muscle (Fig. 53–13).

The artery of the excised muscle was anastomosed to the ulnar artery of the recipient site by end-to-end suture with Crown 10-0 nylon under a Zeiss OPMi II microscope. The nerve of the muscle was severed at a point as close to the muscle as possible and sutured to the earlier isolated anterior interosseous nerve by funicular suture. Throughout this time the vein was left unsutured and the flow of blood from the anastomosed artery was observed. After neurorrhaphy, the two veins of the muscle and the concomitant veins of the ulnar artery were anastomosed by end-to-end suture.

After closing the incision, the elbow was immobilized at 90 degrees and the wrist at 40 degrees flexed position, and a moderate compression dressing and plaster slab were applied.

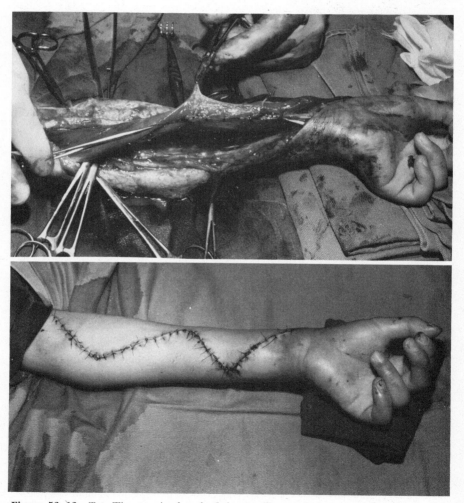

Figure 53–13 *Top,* The proximal end of the gracilis muscle was sutured to the medial epicondyle, and the distal end was sutured to the flexor tendons of the thumb, index, and middle fingers. *Bottom,* At the conclusion of the operation, there was no difficulty in covering the grafted muscle.

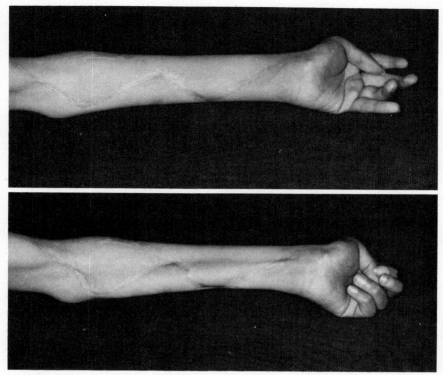

Figure 53–14 Six months after surgery. *Top,* Fingers at rest. *Bottom,* Powerful flexion of the thumb and the finger can be seen. Functional recovery of the grafted muscle was confirmed by histochemical activity and morphological findings of the end-plates.

Intravenous infusion of low molecular weight dextran, 500 cc, was administered daily for 10 days after surgery. No other medications except antibiotics were provided. At three weeks after surgery only the elbow was left immobilized and at four weeks all immobilization was discontinued.

POSTOPERATIVE FINDINGS. Four months after the surgery, slight contraction of the grafted gracilis muscle could be seen and palpated, and powerful flexion of the thumb, index, and middle fingers could be seen at six months after surgery (Fig. 53–14).

At this time, the histochemical activity and morphological findings of end-plates had returned to almost normal.

DISCUSSION

SELECTION OF MUSCLE TO BE GRAFTED

As determined from experiments, muscles supplied by a simple nutrient vessel arrangement (one artery and one vein) render good take rates, and the technical procedure is simple. However, the muscle must be selected from an area where its transplantation will not create a serious functional disorder.

The pectoralis major muscle used in the first case is supplied by a branch of the thoracoacromial artery and accompanying veins, the motor nerve arrangement is uncomplicated, and all of the above mentioned conditions have been satisfied. Further, from our experience with cadavers and clinical cases, it is felt that the extensor digitorum brevis muscle and gracilis muscle are also good donors.

In order that the grafted muscle may function normally, a certain degree of tension and excursion is necessary. If tension of the grafted muscle is excessive, ischemia will develop; contrarily, if it is too long, contraction will be inadequate. In our cases, enough tension not to cause circulatory disturbance was provided. This was considered the proper length, and it was grafted to the bed. As it is difficult to increase or decrease the length of the muscle per se, the tension of the muscle is controlled by the length of the tendon to be sutured.

CONDITIONS OF THE GRAFT BED

It is necessary that the graft bed have vessels and nerves to which the nutrient vessels and motor nerves of the muscle to be grafted may be anastomosed. Difference in vessel size does not pose a serious technical problem in vessel anastomosis. In order that the grafted muscle may have good function and almost normal volume, there must be complete recovery of the motor nerve. To accomplish this, ideally the funicular pattern of the motor nerves of the grafted muscles and the recipient sites must be almost exactly the same quantitatively. In our cases, there were slightly fewer funiculi in the donor free muscle than in the anterior interosseous nerve of the recipient site. A further good feature of the anterior interosseous branch of the median nerve is that it is basically a motor nerve.

SURGICAL TECHNIQUE

To prevent circulatory disturbance due to excessive pressure on the grafted muscle after surgery, attention should be paid to the skin incision, and a local flap and skin graft should be administered, if necessary. It is advisable not to place a skin graft directly upon the grafted muscle but to first use a local flap and administer the skin graft to the skin defect.

It is better not to irrigate the transferred muscle. In transplantation procedures, the duration of ischemia of the tissue to be transferred usually poses a problem; however, in auto-transplantation procedures, such as free flap transfer and free muscle transfer, the time required is only one hour at the longest, and thus ischemia can be disregarded. However, to shorten the period as much as possible, it is best to anastomose the artery first, as is done by the author.

REFERENCES

Aitken, J. T.: Growth of nerve implants in voluntary muscle. J. Anat. *84*:38, 1950.
Aitken, J. T.: Problems in reinnervation of muscle. Progr. Brain Res. *14*:232, 1965.
Demos, N. J., McKeon, J., and Timmes, J. J.: Free and pedicle muscle grafts in thoracic surgery. N.Y. State J. Med. *71*:1928, 1971.

Harii, K., Ohmori, K., Murakami, F., Torii, S., and Ohmori, S.: Free muscle transplantation with neurovascular anastomoses. Jap. J. Plast. Reconstr. Surg. *18*:551, 1975.

Ikuta, Y., Kubo, K., and Tsuge, K.: Free muscle transplantation by microsurgical technique to treat severe Volkmann's contracture. Plast Reconstr. Surg. *58*:407, 1976.

Kubo, K., Ikuta, Y., and Tsuge, K.: Free muscle transplantation in dogs by microneurovascular anastomoses. Plast. Reconstr. Surg. *57*:495, 1976.

Pers, M., and Medgyesi, S.: Pedicle muscle flaps and their application in the surgery of repair. Br. J. Plast. Surg. *26*:353, 1973.

Pickrell, K. L., Broadbent, T. R., Masters F. W., and Metzger, J. T.: Construction of rectal sphincter and restoration of anal continence by transplanting gracilis muscle; report of 4 cases in children. Ann. Surg. *135*:853, 1952.

Simpson, J. S., and Gossage, J. D.: Use of abdominal wall muscle flap in repair of large congenital diaphragmatic hernia. J. Pediatr. Surg. *6*:42, 1971.

Tamai, S., Komatsu, S., Sakamoto, H., Sano, S., Sasuchi, N., Hori, Y., Tatsumi, Y., and Okuda, H.: Free muscle transplants in dogs, with microsurgical neurovascular anastomoses. Plast Reconstr. Surg. *46*:219, 1970.

Thompson, N.: Autogenous free grafts of skeletal muscle. A preliminary experimental and clinical study. Plast. Reconstr. Surg. *26*:353, 1973.

54

MANAGEMENT OF SENSORY LOSS IN THE EXTREMITIES

PAUL W. BRAND

Sensory loss in the extremities rarely comes as a single problem. It may be part of a generalized medical disease, as in diabetes or leprosy; it may be accompanied by motor imbalance, as in a nerve injury; or it may be accompanied by gross paralysis, as in some cases of meningomyelocele or paraplegia.

The key to proper management of the insensitive limb is to distinguish between the various actual and immediate causes of damage and to help the patient to be aware of them. Protection of the limb is not difficult if one knows what to protect it from. For too long the word "trophic" in relation to ulcers and breakdown of denervated limbs has turned our attention inward. We have looked for weakness and inadequacy of the tissues when we should have been looking outward to ward off excessive forces or high temperatures.

In this chapter we shall consider the various factors that cause problems in the denervated limb. Each factor will be seen to be significant in some cases and not in others. Specific protective and treatment methods will be noted in the same sequence.

The factors will be discussed in the following order:

1. Loss of vasomotor control
2. Loss of sweating
3. Pressure sores from ischemia
4. Injury from mechanical and thermal energy
5. Tissue autolysis from repetitive stress
6. Spreading infection
7. Neuropathic bone and joint damage

LOSS OF VASOMOTOR CONTROL

In nerve injury as in many peripheral neuropathies, the sympathetic nerves are lost along with sensation. The immediate result is that from vasodilation the limb becomes warmer than normal, and then gradually, over a few weeks, the limb becomes cooler than normal as humeral control takes over. Vasoconstriction becomes the "normal" condition of the resting limb.

Because the limb feels cold, and the pulses and Doppler readouts are reduced, the denervated limb is often regarded as having a reduced vascular capability. In fact, such a limb responds very well to the demand for extra blood supply. In the event of infection, trauma, or stress the vessels will open up and the limb become warm. The pattern of response is different from normal, but the capability is there.

We have found that the cool baseline temperature allows us to observe the progress of inflammation very easily by thermometry. A warm limb does not get much warmer when it is inflamed, but a cold limb has a wide spectrum of temperature which can be used to alert the patient and his physician when some hidden and unfelt problem has called for extra local blood supply.

LOSS OF SWEATING

Many denervated extremities are very dry, owing to loss of sweating and diminished sebaceous secretion. The insensitive patient who has good control of his muscles may notice that objects slip out of his hands, and may complain that he is "weak." The combination of loss of sensation and very dry, slippery skin makes the hands extra clumsy. If the skin is kept moist by soaking and oiling, the hands become better able to hold and retain objects.

A more serious result of dryness is a change in the physical qualities of keratin in the cuticle of the skin. Hydrated cuticle is soft and compliant; it can be folded and stretched like a rubber membrane. Dry cuticle is hard and brittle. It will not stretch and it breaks when folded. The areas of the hands and feet that have to bend and stretch suffer damage when they are dry. This is noted in the flexures of the fingers and toes, and in the curved "shoulder" of the foot where the sole meets the sides. At every step the convexity of this shoulder increases and then decreases, and great shear stresses are absorbed by these tissues. It can be likened to the shoulder of an automobile tire that cracks after too much flexing and extending. The cuticle layer of the skin cracks and exposes the deeper layers of epidermis. Continued movement opens and closes the cuticular crack until it becomes inflamed and infected. Cuticle builds up into a thick callus along the margins of the crack, further ensuring that the skin cannot stretch; thus the crack acts as the only expansion joint between the rigid plates of cuticle. Finally the crack deepens through the skin and becomes a true ulcer and a source of infection for the whole limb.

Treatment

Loss of sweating is often permanent in cases of neuropathy such as diabetes, leprosy, some radicular neuropathies, and spina bifida. The patient must learn a routine of skin care that will have to be practiced daily for his or her lifetime. The dry limb must be soaked in water every day for 15 minutes, and then blotted lightly with a towel. The whole skin area is then rubbed with vaseline or some oil or cream, the whole purpose of which is to prevent evaporation of the water, which has now hydrated the skin. Complex and expensive "moisturizing" creams are better avoided, as they are inadequate, and over a long period some may produce allergic reactions. It is water that is needed. The purpose of the vaseline is only to keep the water in.

If cracks have already occurred, the thickened cuticle around the edges may be pared down and the floor of the crack painted with gentian violet. If the crack is in a finger flexure, the finger should be splinted in extension so that the crack may heal without causing a flexion contracture, which would otherwise tear open as soon as the finger was extended after healing.

PRESSURE SORES OR TROPHIC ULCERS

These terms have been used to lump together a variety of conditions that have three things in common: (1) they occur in denervated skin, (2) they are associated with mechanical force, and (3) they result in open infected ulcers. If a patient is to keep his limbs intact for a lifetime in spite of insensitivity, it is essential that both he and his physician understand the nature and variety of these ulcers, and learn how to prevent and to heal them.

I have found it best to divide these ulcers into four groups, each of which has a different etiology and pathology, and thus a different type of prevention. Each also is associated with a different level of mechanical force.

Pathology	Typical Force	Time Factor
Ischemic necrosis	$1/2$–5 lb/inch^2	Several hours continuously
Mechanical disruption	600 lb/inch^2 and over	Immediate
Enzymatic autolysis	25–75 lb/inch^2	Thousands of repetitions over several days
Spreading infection	Any uneven intermittent pressure	Just a few repetitions

We will consider these individually.

Pressure Sores from Ischemia

In theory, any pressure that is high enough to occlude the capillary circulation should result in ischemic necrosis if it is maintained for long enough. It is well known that a pressure of 30 to 50 mm Hg is enough to do this. However, there is a great variability both in the pressures that will actually result in necrosis and in the time that is needed to accomplish the destruction. Part of this variability is due to the texture of the supporting tissues. The sole of the foot has a thick skin and a reticulum of fibers behind it. This helps to protect the small blood vessels, so that higher external pressure is needed to flatten them. In identical tissues anywhere, higher pressures cause necrosis in a shorter time.

This may be simply because a larger depth of tissue is exsanguinated by higher external pressure so that the center of the area cannot be nourished by diffusion through tissue fluids, as might be possible if only a shallow area were ischemic. Skin maceration and shear stresses all contribute to the damage. However, the basic damage is due to ischemia, and the important fact is that necrosis in the limbs from ischemia rarely occurs in less than four or five hours. This is because it is quite exceptional for a limb to be subjected to more than three or four pounds per square inch for any continuous period of time. All the high pressures on the hand or foot are intermittent.

The only common cause of continuous pressure is a tight shoe. The damage from a tight shoe can be prevented either by making sure that all pressures inside the shoe are less than 1/2 lb per square inch or by making sure that no tight shoe is worn for more than a short time.

I have found it impractical to try to measure these small pressures inside a shoe. I have sometimes measured one spot in a shoe and found it a safe 0.2 lbs per square inch only to discover later that a half inch further distally the pressure was 2.0 lbs per square inch, and that a patch of gangrene had resulted (Fig. 54–1).

The only way to be safe is to measure time rather than pressure. The following rules work well for diabetics and others who have insensitive but otherwise normal feet. The patient has to accept responsibility for keeping these rules.

1. Take care to buy good shoes, well fitted, and with leather uppers (leather will accommodate to the foot over a period of time).
2. Never wear new shoes for more than two hours on the first day or three hours on the second. Look carefully at the foot when the shoe is first removed to see the danger signs of previous pressure, such as a red flush (or hot spot) or an area where the impression of the fabric of the sock is marked on the skin.
3. In the absence of signs of pressure, wear the shoe for longer periods of time, but aim always to change shoes at midday and on return home in the evening. An ideal is to have three five-hour shoe periods each day — morning, afternoon, and evening — with a different pair of shoes or slippers for each. To simplify the routine, one pair of shoes can be kept at the work-place, office, or factory.

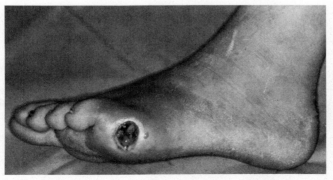

Figure 54–1   Ulcer on lateral border of foot caused by a tight shoe.

If this routine is followed there will never be an ischemic pressure sore, even if a new pair of shoes is a little tight when first purchased.

Direct Damage from Mechanical or Thermal Energy

It takes approximately a thousand times more pressure to cause mechanical disruption of the skin than it does to cause ischemic damage. Since pressure is force divided by area, the pressure can be high either because of very high force or because the force is applied through a very small area.

This type of foot damage is rare in people who wear shoes. Barefoot walkers get into trouble by stepping on objects such as thumbtacks or broken glass. All this can be prevented by a simple rule. People who have insensitive feet should not walk barefoot, and should shake out their shoes before putting them on, to remove any small sharp object that may have fallen in.

It is much more difficult to avoid mechanical damage to the hand. It is hard for people who cannot feel to learn to estimate *pressure* and *shear* stress. They can estimate force better than pressure.

To protect the hand from high pressure, the best rule is to "beware of small handles," or better, "never use small handles." Our occupational therapists will go to the workbench or home of a person with insensitive hands and remove all small handles and replace them with larger ones. Other small handles may be augmented to make them larger. The edges of the handles of small keys often cause damage, so we cover key handles in a leather sandwich (Fig. 54–2). Some of the worst offenders are the little metal knobs on drawers or cupboards, which look pretty, but have vicious edges on their rims. If the drawer sticks, a patient can tear the skin of his finger trying to open it. The little serrated knobs that are sometimes used to adjust the color on television sets may be stiff and are so small that they play havoc with the skin of patients who may have trouble using normal pinch mechanisms because of intrinsic paralysis and therefore have to use their knuckles. We sometimes provide our patients with a simple pair of general purpose pliers to use for such problems.

Because heat is a constant hazard, patients must be alert for all sorts of unexpected situations. The feet may rest on a hot floor of an automobile. The handles of steam heating coils may be too close to the heater, causing an accidental contact burn. The kitchen is full of hazards. We try to ensure that all

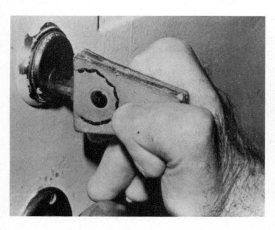

Figure 54–2 This insensitive distorted hand had been injured by the edge of a key which was stiff in a lock. A leather sandwich around the handle made it safe.

cooking implements have long wooden or plastic handles. Cigarettes are bad from every point of view; they cause vasoconstriction of the hands and feet when the patient inhales, and they burn the fingers when he forgets he is holding a cigarette. We advise the use of cigarette holders for patients who cannot quit smoking. Gloves should be advised for use in the kitchen and for some types of manual work.

Tissue Autolysis from Repetitive Stress

I believe this to be the commonest cause of damage to the active but insensitive limb. Ischemia is common in the severely paralyzed person who sits or lies still. The person who is active and works and walks becomes ulcerated at points of repetitive stress. This ulceration commonly occurs in response to a range of pressures between 25 and 75 lbs per square inch. These pressures are harmless for a few repetitions, and are painless to a normal limb. Pressures in this range are potentially harmful if there is an element of shear stress and friction with the pressure and if the tissues that receive the stress are already inflamed by previous repetitions of similar stress.

Our own extensive experiments on the footpads of rats have shown that at the pressure level of 25 lbs per square inch several thousand repetitions result in an inflammatory change in the tissues. Hyperemia develops and numbers of inflammatory cells migrate into the tissue spaces along with edema fluid. 10,000 repetitions is about equivalent to a brisk seven mile walk, and this may be the stage at which a normal individual begins to feel that his feet are sore at one or two points of pressure or friction. In response to this feeling of soreness he or she will change the length of stride or limp a little to spare one part of the foot and involve another. The person who is insensitive may have the same or a little more inflammatory change, but he does not limp because he feels no discomfort. *This failure to adapt to changes in the internal state of the tissues is probably more significant than failure to perceive external forces.* The inflammatory state of the tissues that follows the frequent repetition of quite moderate stresses can be observed by noting localized swelling and redness of the part and by noting an area of increased temperature ("hot spot") which is usually easily distinguished by the hand.

This inflammation develops slowly and persists over a few days. If the repetitive stress is continued day after day, an area of necrosis develops at the center of the inflammation. Further stress, from further walking increases the amount of necrosis, which then breaks through the skin as an ulcer.

Too Much, Too Often

When the ulcer appears, patients are often at a loss to explain it. They do not recall any gross trauma or stress, so they say, "It just happened by itself." At this time the physician must explain the whole process and point out that the presence of the ulcer proves two things: (1) that the way the patient has been walking in the shoes he wears has resulted in pressure or friction that is too high, and (2) that the patient has been walking too much during the past few days (or weeks). In most cases both these factors have been present. The pressure in the shoe might have been acceptable if there had been less walking. The amount of walking might have been acceptable if the local pressure had been less.

To prevent recurrence, both should be changed. The patient must learn to walk less, to take shorter steps, and to walk more slowly. Also, the shoe should be changed or modified to spread the stress of weight-bearing more evenly over the foot. This latter can often be accomplished by obtaining an extra-depth shoe, such as those by P. Minor (Treadeasy) or Alden or Scholls, and putting a molded insole in place of the removable insole that comes with the shoe. For insensitive feet, no shoe insert should be used that is preformed for standard feet. It must be made individually and molded on the patient's own foot or on a plaster model of the foot. There are materials now available (Plastazote, Pelite, Alimed, and other closed-cell polyethylene foams) that can be heated to 280° F and then molded directly on the patient's foot. This may be done by any good pedorthist or prescription shoemaker who is experienced in the technique. It may even be done in the office of a podiatrist or surgeon. These polyethylene foams last better if they are covered by a thin layer of microcell rubber, which is itself covered by nylon fabric, as in a Spenco insole (Fig. 54–3).

If ulceration under the metatarsal heads recurs in spite of molded insoles, then a more radical change of footwear may be needed. The forefoot is very vulnerable to breakdown both because it takes the whole thrust of body weight at the push-off phase of gait and because of the shear stresses of the rollover as the toes extend and stretch the soft tissues over the exposed ends of the metatarsal heads.

For these problem cases it is best to use a clog-type shoe with a sole that is rigid from end to end. Here the foot rolls over rather than bends and there is a minimum of shear stress and no movement of metatarsophalangeal extension. It is still better to have a "rocker shoe," which has a rigid sole that tilts or pivots on a proximal bar so that the end of the forefoot takes very little stress (Fig. 54–4). These special shoes can usually be made from an extra-depth shoe by stiffening the sole and adding the clog or rocker feature underneath. Some patients may need custom-made shoes.

The problem is that patients will accept a special pair of shoes, but then will go home and wear some more fashionable type of shoe, at least part of the time. This battle to make a patient wear sensible shoes is hopeless. The physician cannot win unless the patient fully understands the problem and takes responsibility for his own feet. The patient must learn to palpate his feet every evening

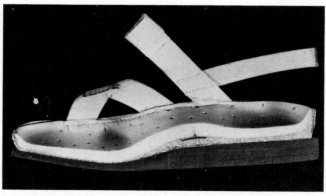

Figure 54–3   Molded Plastazote sandal. The Plastazote was molded directly on the patient's foot.

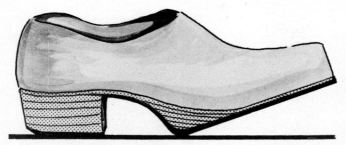

Figure 54–4 Diagram of rigid-soled rocker shoe. The toe slope is high enough so the heel can be lifted without the toe touching the ground.

when going to bed. It is the patient's own responsibility to find hot spots and know what they mean. Then he may modify his program to allow the inflammation to subside. The patient has to discover how well the special shoes keep his feet cool. Some of my patients keep a skin thermometer beside the bed and keep a graph of their metatarsal head temperature as compared to the heel temperature. They quickly learn the limits of what their feet can tolerate.

Spreading Infection

Ulceration is bad but reversible. It will heal. The real disaster for a foot is spreading infection. It starts from an ulcer that then involves bone, joint, and tendon sheath. Soon the whole foot may be hot, swollen, and septic, and bones may be destroyed. This is the sort of problem that results in amputation. This is what has given rise to the idea that insensitive feet and diabetic feet cannot deal with infection. In leprosy they used to speak of "non-healing flesh."

The Problem is Mechanical

Most neuropathic feet would heal nearly as well as normal feet if the patients did not walk on them. No person with normal sensation could put a wounded ulcerated foot to the ground and put weight on it. That is why normal feet heal. Pain forces them to rest, and the patient's own cells are able to localize the infection and heal the wound.

For insensitive feet the physician often has to force a reluctant patient to do what pain would have made him do if he had sensation. Most doctors tend to rely on medication for healing wounds and controlling infection, and forget that these are only ancilliary to the real essential of rest to the part. For most patients every acute ulcer or infection of the foot should be treated by complete rest in bed until the infection has localized. When the swelling has reduced and the fever subsided, a total-contact plaster cast may be applied and the patient allowed to walk. For very careful and cooperative patients who prefer not to have a cast, the use of crutches is permitted. However, the cast is the best method if it is properly applied.

Total-Contact Casting

The special value of a total-contact plaster cast is that it takes the weight evenly all over the foot and up the leg. Thus, no part of the foot takes more than

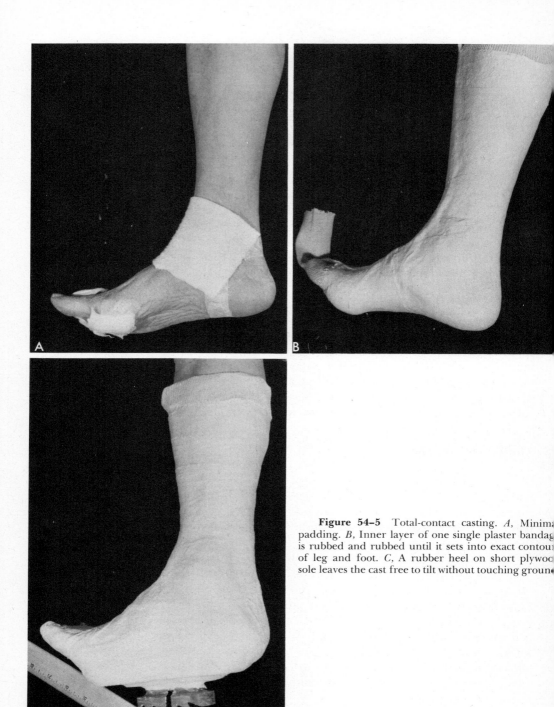

Figure 54–5 Total-contact casting. *A*, Minima padding. *B*, Inner layer of one single plaster bandag is rubbed and rubbed until it sets into exact contou of leg and foot. *C*, A rubber heel on short plywoo sole leaves the cast free to tilt without touching groun

about five pounds per square inch. A padded cast cannot take the weight from the calf, as the padding is compressible, and the cast therefore moves (piston effect) on the leg. It is unnecessary to inspect or dress a wound after it has been immobilized in a cast. It is harmful to leave a "window" in a cast, as it usually results in localized swelling of the tissues in the window and thus shear stresses take place at the edge of the opening, causing secondary wounds.

Technique is important. The inner lining must be smooth and wrinkle free. The following routine has proved safe and effective (Fig. 54–5).

1. The patient should be in bed with the foot elevated for a long enough time to allow the swelling to subside before the cast is applied.

   If a cast is applied before the swelling has subsided it must be removed within a few days and reapplied because swelling subsides rapidly in the cast and a loose cast is the commonest cause of friction blisters or secondary ulcers.

2. The patient lies face down on a plinth with the knee flexed and the foot horizontal.

3. The ulcer is dressed with cotton gauze held in place with adhesive.

4. A saddle of felt or a few thicknesses of Webril are applied to cover the malleoli and the dorsal angle between the foot and the leg. A strip of felt is laid along the anterior margin of the leg and foot and fixed with strips of adhesive. This strip is only to facilitate removal of the cast with a saw.

   The whole leg is covered with a tube of stockinette. The assistant has the responsibility of ensuring that the foot is kept at right angles to the leg, and that the toes are held slightly dorsiflexed. No change in position is allowed after the first turns of plaster are applied, even if the plaster is still soft. If the position is wrong, the turns are unwound and a fresh start is made.

5. One single plaster bandage is applied loosely, around and around the foot and leg. This will give not more than about two layers of plaster bandage. Before any more plaster is wetted, this first bandage is rubbed and rubbed around all the hollows and prominences of the limb until it has started to set. At this stage, continued firm rubbing around the contours of the foot and into the arch will ensure absolutely even pressure and absence of movement inside the case.

6. Once the first layer has set, the rest of the plaster can be applied rapidly. Slabs of plaster may be applied under the sole and up the back of the leg, and from side to side under the heel, and held in position by circular bandages. Finally, a sole plate of 4 mm plywood is applied under the sole, and plaster is tucked into the hollows between it and the cast. A rubber "heel" is placed on the plywood at about the center of the foot and fixed with a few turns of plaster bandage. The toes may be left exposed on the dorsum or may be completely enclosed. If enclosed, it is good to cover them with felt or polyurethane foam.

7. The cast should be kept fully exposed while it sets, to allow evaporation and loss of heat. No weight-bearing is allowed for the first 24 hours. After this, reasonable activity is permitted, including return to work in most cases. Patients are warned to return at once if the plaster gets soft or cracks, or if any pain or fever is experienced.

8. The first cast should be removed within a few days, because it will become

loose as the swelling subsides. The next cast may be kept on for a month or more and in most cases will be all that is needed for sound healing of the ulcer.

NEUROPATHIC BONE AND JOINT DAMAGE

In the foot most neuropathic bone and joint damage is due to infection (Hodgson, 1948). The neuropathy allows one of the various mechanisms of breakdown of the skin to result in an ulcer. The patient then goes on walking on the infected foot. Infection spreads to the bone, or the bone becomes decalcified and weak because of the chronic infection and hyperemia. Finally, the infected or decalcified bone collapses under the continued strain of uninhibited walking. This can all be prevented by attention to the wound as outlined under Total-Contact Casting (Page 869).

Sometimes neuropathic bone and joint changes may take place in the absence of infection. The process usually begins as a small crack that results from a sudden strain or twist of the foot, or it may begin as a fatigue fracture. Such small cracks are much more common in normal feet than is realized. However, in normal feet, where they are often diagnosed as a "sprain" or "strain," the pain that accompanies them forces the patient to limp until the condition settles down. In the case of fatigue fractures, the healthy foot feels the pain before the crack occurs and the patient slows down or limps, and thus may prevent the fracture. The insensitive person walks on without a limp, and the small crack extends to become a major fracture. Harris and Brand (1966) have described the typical patterns of neuropathic collapse: (1) os calcis, (2) talus, (3) navicular, (4) cuneiform, and (5) metatarsal. Common to all of them is the feature of localized heat and usually swelling. If a person presents with a "hot spot" in the absence of a wound, the surgeon should think about possible bone damage and have an x-ray done.

Early neuropathic damage will usually heal by immobilization in a plaster cast. Late cases with more extensive damage may be better treated by surgical intervention and arthrodesis. Neuropathic joints have a bad reputation for non-union after surgery. However, I have had good success by insisting upon two rules — (1) the bone must be excised back until good bleeding bone is exposed; (2) internal fixation must be reinforced by external plaster cast immobilization, and both must be maintained for 50 per cent longer than would be expected for normal bones. This may be partly because neuropathic bones heal slowly and form callus poorly. However, the main reason is that, whereas normal people spare their operated limbs and limp when first free from their plaster cast, patients with insensitive limbs will walk with full uninhibited stride as soon as restraint is removed.

REFERENCES

Harris, J. R., and Brand, P. W.: Patterns of disintegration of the tarsus in the anaesthetic foot. J. Bone Joint Surg. (Brit.) *48B*:4, 1966.
Hodgson, J. R., Pugh, D. G., and Young, H. H.: Roentgenologic aspect of certain lesions of bone: Neuropathic or infectious? Radiology *50*:65, 1948.

55

TENDON TRANSFERS AS RECONSTRUCTIVE PROCEDURES IN THE LEG AND FOOT

GEORGE E. OMER, Jr.

Tendon transfers may enhance the rehabilitation of patients with peripheral nerve injuries and paralysis of the lower extremity. The successful tendon transfer should have only one basic objective: to eliminate a deforming force that will produce further imbalance, to replace a single lost motion, or to produce stability. Stability against gravity is much more important than mobility and range of motion in the lower extremity, in contrast to the upper extremity. The best reconstructive procedure in many patients is an effective orthosis.

Tendon transfers to restore motor balance to a lower extremity were performed first by Nicoladoni of Austria (Riordan, 1974; Westin, 1965). He transferred the peroneus longus and brevis to a paralyzed gastrocnemius. The procedure failed because the suture line separated, but the principle of tendon transfer was established. The anticipated result should be a balanced simplification of function, because the tendon transfer redistributes motor assets rather than creating new ones.

TISSUE HOMEOSTASIS

Tendon transfers should not be done until the paralyzed muscle has had adequate postural support, no matter how long the interval since the onset of the paralysis. Splinting the lower extremity in a functional position is extremely important, and appropriate care should be taken to avoid pressure sores. The series of sciatic nerve injuries reported by Clawson and Seddon (1960) demonstrated that every patient with persistent skin ulceration also suffered from fixed deformity of the foot or toes. Vasomotor and trophic changes are related to painful over-response (paresthesia), which occurs in half of those patients with sciatic nerve injury, and paresthesia is more disabling for functional recovery than is inadequate neurological regeneration. Adequate sensibility depends upon total extremity homeostasis and functional activity (Brand and Ebner, 1969).

Arthrodesis is an important adjunct for improving the result of tendon transfers in the lower extremity, especially about the foot (Hoke, 1921). However, the skeleton must be stable prior to tendon transfer. Tendon transfers performed across sites of bony nonunion fail because the telescoping skeleton prevents normal tension for the muscle–tendon unit.

OPERATIVE TECHNIQUES

Tendon transfers in the lower extremity are affected by the phasic activity of the muscles (Close and Todd, 1959). The anterior muscles of the calf and the posterior muscles of the thigh are swing-phase muscles, while the posterior muscles of the calf and the anterior muscles of the thigh are stance-phase muscles. Considerable difficulty may be encountered in training the non-phasic muscle–tendon transfer, and re-education is indicated over a prolonged period.

The operated extremity should be supported in a corrected position, and a brace or splint is usually indicated for at least 8 to 12 weeks after surgery. However, splinting cannot be correlated with phasic conversion.

Femoral Palsy

The muscles innervated by the femoral nerve are not critical for an upright stature or locomotion on an even surface. A femoral palsied patient with strong hip extensor muscles and strong plantar flexor muscles of the foot can have a near normal gait unless there is a flexion contracture of the knee. Quadriceps loss is most evident while climbing stairs or an inclined plane (Rakolta and Omer, 1969).

Correction of quadriceps muscle paralysis is best done by anterior transfer of the biceps femoris muscle through a lateral approach (Herndon, 1961) (Fig. 55–1). It should be emphasized that the short head of the biceps femoris muscle must be freed from the shaft of the femur to obtain a straight-line pull to the patella. The tensor fascia and the intramuscular septum are excised for 3 to 4 inches to allow free excursion of the biceps femoris tendon and to help prevent flexion contracture of the knee. The biceps femoris tendon is passed deep to the

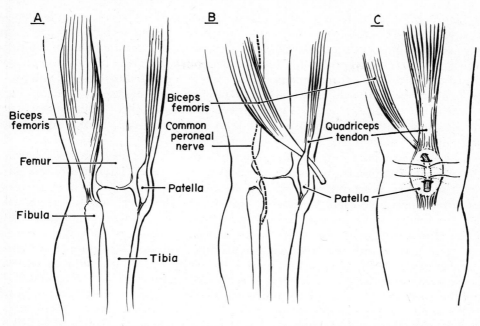

Figure 55–1 Transfer of the biceps femoris tendon to the quadriceps tendon–patellar mechanism. *A*, Biceps tendon insertion, together with an osteoperiosteal flap from the head of the fibula, is removed. *B*, The peroneal nerve is identified and protected. A section of tensor fascia and intermuscular septum is excised. The short head of the biceps is freed as far proximally as possible without injuring the neurovascular bundle to the muscle. *C*, Quadriceps tendon is split longitudinally, and the biceps tendon passed to the patella. The biceps tendon is anchored with the knee in full extension. Reinforcing sutures are placed between the tendon and the quadriceps to anchor the biceps tendon on the medial side of the patella.

quadriceps tendon, proximal to the suprapatellar pouch, and threaded through a vertical split in the quadriceps tendon to the anterior surface of the patella. A small drill hole is made transversely through the central portion of the patella and a steel 00 wire suture is passed through the hole and the transferred biceps femoris tendon. An alternate technique is the elevation of a vertical osteoperiosteal flap on the anterior surface of the patella. The biceps femoris tendon is anchored to the medial-central aspect of the patella.

The extremity is immobilized in plaster for four to six weeks and in a brace for an additional four to six weeks. Muscle re-education begins with muscle setting before surgery and active range of motion exercises 12 weeks after surgery. Supervised re-education continues until maximal strength and phase conversion have been achieved.

Common Peroneal Palsy

These patients have loss of dorsiflexion of the foot with associated loss of eversion. The result is an equinovarus deformity secondary to the mechanical advantage of the tibialis posterior muscle.

The drop foot resulting from paralysis of the common peroneal nerve demands prompt stretching of the plantar fascia and the posterior ankle structures. If a deformity is present, an attempt should be made to correct it with a series of wedging casts. Rarely, plantar fascia stripping, tendocalcaneus lengthening, or posterior capsulotomy may be necessary. External apparatus can be utilized to maintain a functional position, such as a molded orthosis of polypropylene (O'Leary, Bianchi, and Foulds, 1976). The splint must prevent dropping of the great toe as well as ankle equinus because intractable flexion contracture of the great toe will prevent using a shoe. A supple foot usually requires only a light orthosis to maintain functional position.

Operative reconstruction of equinovarus usually includes a bony stabilization as well as tendon transfers. The usual procedures are a Lambrinudi subtalar arthrodesis or a posterior bone block at the ankle joint. Triple arthrodesis leaves the foot less supple than a posterior bone block. However, residual varus deformity increases the patient's impairment, and is an expected complication of isolated posterior bone block without an associated triple arthrodesis.

The Lambrinudi operation excises a wedge of bone from the plantar and distal portion of the talus so that the talus remains in complete equinus at the ankle joint while the rest of the foot is in the desired dorsiflexion. Clawson and Seddon (1960) performed the Lambrinudi arthrodesis in twenty cases, but only five patients were pleased with the result. Following the operation, 13 patients had increased pain and 10 had a rigid varus deformity. MacKenzie (1959) studied 100 Lambrinudi procedures followed from one to 27 years: 29 patients had more than 30 degrees of equinus; 26 feet had symptomatic varus deformity, and five patients had osteoarthritis in the joints distal to the arthrodesis.

A posterior bone block procedure has been reported by Campbell, Gill and others (Ingram, 1971). The calcaneus provides the graft material for the bone block, which is placed posterior and across the tibial-talar joint. Ingram and Hundley (1951) reviewed 90 cases of posterior bone block and found a recurrence of the equinus deformity in one third of the patients, and osteoarthritic changes in 40 ankles. Ingram (1971) recommends that a triple arthrodesis be combined with a posterior bone block.

Even with stabilization of the foot, the ankle will dislocate without tendon transfers or an orthosis. In addition, unless the influence of the tibialis posterior muscle is removed, varus deformity will occur at the ankle joint.

Anterior transfer of the tibialis posterior tendon can be either through the interosseous membrane or around the medial side of the tibia (Cozen, 1969). The tibialis posterior is freed at its insertion through a longitudinal incision. A second incision is made along the medial border of the tibia, and the muscle–tendon unit is mobilized until the distal 2 or 3 inches of the muscle are free (Fig. 55–2). Another skin incision is made anteriorly over the dorsum of the foot. A large hole is made in the interosseous membrane proximal to the malleoli. The tibialis posterior muscle–tendon unit is passed through the generous opening until the muscle belly is across the interosseous membrane, because the tendon alone will fibrose to the interosseous membrane with loss of motion. The tendon is not passed beneath the cruciate ligament. A drill hole is made in the third cuneiform bone, and osteoperiosteal flaps are made. The tendon is anchored in the hole with a steel 00 wire suture loop that is tied over a button or length of tubing on the plantar surface of the foot. The osteoperiosteal flaps are sutured to the ten-

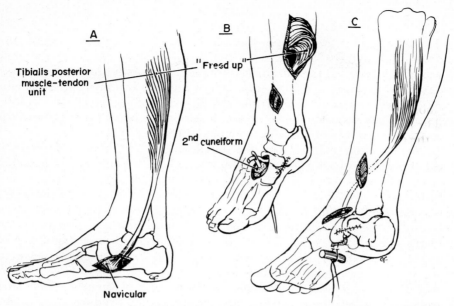

Figure 55-2 Transfer of the tibialis posterior tendon to the dorsum of the foot. *A*, The tendon of the tibialis posterior is identified and divided at its attachment, then withdrawn through a posterior incision over the muscle at the junction of the middle and distal thirds of the leg. *B*, A large window is made in the interosseous membrane, and a subcutaneous tunnel is made to the third cuneiform. The anterior tibial artery and vein should be avoided. *C*, The tibialis posterior tendon is anchored to a drill hole in the cuneiform. The tendon is anchored with a steel 00 wire loop that is tied over a gauze pad or button or length of rubber tubing on the plantar surface.

don. After six weeks, one end of the wire loop is cut, and the wire is pulled out of the foot. The extremity is immobilized in a long leg cast for three weeks, followed by a short leg cast for three more weeks. The transfer is protected for at least six months by an orthosis that maintains a dorsiflexion position. Full active dorsiflexion is rarely restored by this transfer alone.

This procedure is not a phasic transfer, but electromyograms at Brooke Army Medical Center have demonstrated normal voluntary motor unit action potentials following transfer. The tibialis posterior tendon transfer does require re-education, and it may take months to revise compensatory movements, such as lifting and flexing the leg to step forward.

Lipscomb and Sanchez (1961) had satisfactory motion when they transferred the tibialis posterior tendon medially around the tibia without passing through the interosseous membrane. Carayon and his associates (1967) transfer the flexor digitorum longus and the tibialis posterior tendons through the interosseous membrane to the tendons of the extensor digitorum longus and the extensor hallucis longus. They have obtained a total active excursion of 20 to 30 degrees in 17 of 31 feet. The tibialis anticus and the extensor digitorum communis tendons may be tenodesed to the distal tibia. Tenodesis procedures may be utilized as ancillary procedures, but are ineffective primary operations. Clawson and Seddon (1960) had failed tenodesis procedures in four of five patients.

Tibial Palsy

Talipes calcaneus is the deformity caused by paralysis of the triceps surae while the other extrinsic foot muscles remain functional. The tendo calcaneus becomes elongated, and the calcaneus is rotated into dorsiflexion by the intrinsic muscles. Gravity assists in the development of forefoot equinus, and the plantar fascia becomes contracted. Unfortunately, no external appliance will replace a paralyzed triceps surae nor prevent the development of talipes calcaneus with the secondary changes of cavus deformity and clawing of the toes.

In the skeletally mature foot, the initial surgery for talipes calcaneus is a triple arthrodesis with an associated plantar fasciotomy (Steindler, 1920) if there is a cavus deformity. Any foot stabilization procedure should displace the foot as far posteriorly as possible to lengthen the bony lever arm and lessen the muscle power required to plantar flex the foot. The Hoke procedure (Hoke, 1921), with shortening of the neck and head of the talus, is more effective than a standard triple arthrodesis. Patterson and associates (1950) reported an evaluation of 305 stabilization procedures. Pseudoarthroses occurred in 56 cases (18 per cent), with most involving the talonavicular joint.

The tibialis anterior is the strongest muscle in the foot after the triceps surae and is the only isolated tendon with sufficient strength to produce active plantar flexion (Herndon, 1961). The tibialis anterior transfer should be done through the interosseous membrane (Fig. 55–3). The tibialis anterior is divided at the base of the first metatarsal and is withdrawn proximally through a longitudinal anterior incision over the junction of the middle and distal thirds of the leg. The interosseous membrane is then exposed, and a large hole is made after visualization of the deep peroneal nerve and the anterior tibial artery and vein. The tendo Achillis is split at its insertion, and an osteoperiosteal flap is developed in the calcaneus. The tendon of the tibialis anterior is passed through the interosseous membrane and posterior to the tendo Achillis through the longitudinal split in the tendon. The tibialis anterior muscle should be across the interosseous membrane for satisfactory excursion of the muscle–tendon unit. The tibialis anterior tendon is anchored with nylon 00 suture while the foot is in full plantar flexion. Plaster immobilization is indicated for eight weeks, followed by a brace with a reverse calcaneal stop for at least six months after the operation.

An alternate transfer is the peroneus longus tendon. The tendon is placed in a longitudinal groove in the calcaneus by Bickel and Moe (1944), but should be withdrawn and anchored to the bone without extensive undermining of skin. It is a rare case that demonstrates active plantar flexion while weight-bearing.

When clawing of the great toe persists after appropriate foot stabilization and tendon transfers to restore plantar flexion of the ankle, the interphalangeal joint of the toe is arthrodesed, and the extensor hallucis longus tendon is transferred to the flexor hallucis longus tendon. The extensor tendon is passed on the medial side of the first metatarsal, proximal to the head of the bone, and anchored with interrupted 00 nylon sutures to the flexor tendon (Westin, 1965). Weight-bearing can be resumed four to six weeks after surgery. Arthrodesis of the interphalangeal joint was successful in all 13 cases done by Clawson and Seddon (1960).

Amputation is not indicated in any traumatic nerve palsy in the lower extremity unless there is severe secondary ulceration and chronic infection.

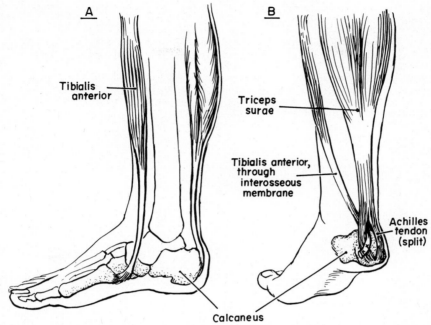

Figure 55–3 Transfer of the tibialis anterior to the heel. *A*, The tendon of the tibialis anterior is identified and divided at its attachment, then withdrawn through an anterior incision over the muscle at the junction of the middle and distal thirds of the leg. *B*, A large window is made in the interosseous membrane, and the tibialis anterior tendon is drawn through a distal split in the Achilles tendon. The deep peroneal nerve and the anterior tibial artery and vein must be protected. The tendon of the tibialis anterior is anchored into a osteoperiosteal trench-flap in the os calcis and the slit in the Achilles tendon.

REFERENCES

Bickel, W. H., and Moe, J. H.: Translocation of the peroneus longus tendon for paralytic calcaneus deformity of the foot. Surg. Gynecol. Obstet. *78*:627, 1944.

Brand, P. W., and Ebner, J. D.: Pressure sensitive devices for denervated hands and feet. J. Bone Joint Surg. *51A*:109, 1969.

Carayon, A., Bourrel, P., Bourges, M., and Touze, M.: Dual transfer of the posterior tibial and flexor digitorum longus tendons for drop foot. J. Bone Joint Surg., *49A*:144, 1967.

Clawson, D. K., and Seddon, H. J.: The late consequences of sciatic nerve injury. J. Bone Joint Surg. *42-B*:213, 1960.

Close, J. R., and Todd, F. N.: The phasic activity of the muscles of the lower extremity and the effect of tendon transfer. J. Bone Joint Surg., *41A*:189, 1959.

Cozen, L.: Management of foot drop in adults after permanent peroneal nerve loss. Clin. Orthop., *67*:151, 1969.

Dickson, F. D., and Diveley, R. L. Operation for correction of mild claw-foot, the result of infantile paralysis. J.A.M.A. *87*:1275, 1926.

Herndon, C. H.: Tendon transplantation of the knee and foot. Instructional Course Lectures. Am. Acad. Orthop. Surg., *18*:145, 1961.

Hoke, M.: An operation for stabilizing paralytic feet. J. Orthop. Surg., *3*:494, 1921.

Ingram, A. J., and Hundley, J. M.: Posterior bone block of the ankle for paralytic equinus. J. Bone Joint Surg. *33A*:679, 1951.

Ingram, A. J.: Anterior poliomyelitis. *In* Crenshaw, A. H. (ed.): Campbell's Operative Orthopaedics. 5th ed., St. Louis, C.V. Mosby Co., 1971, Chap. 21, p. 1517.

Lipscomb, P. R., and Sanchez, J. J.: Anterior transplantation of the posterior tibial tendon for persistent palsy of common peroneal nerve. J. Bone Joint Surg. *43A*:60, 1961.

MacKenzie, I. G.: Lambrinudi' arthrodesis. J. Bone Joint Surg., *41B*:738, 1959.

O'Leary, J.P.; Bianchi, B S., and Foulds, R. A.: A low cost vacuum-forming system. Orthotics Prosthetics. *30*:23–30, 1976.

Patterson, R. L., Jr., Parrish, F. F., and Hathaway, E. N.: Stabilizing operations on the foot. A study of the indications, techniques used, and end results. J. Bone Joint Surg. *32A*:1, 1950.

Rakolta, G. G., and Omer, G. E., Jr.: Combat-sustained femoral nerve injuries. Surg. Gynecol. Obstet. *128*:813, 1969.

Riordan, D. C.: Radial nerve paralysis. Orthop. Clin. North Am. 5:283, 1974.

Steindler, A.: Stripping of the os calcis. J. Orthop. Surg. *2*:8, 1920.

Westin, G. W.: Tendon transfers about the foot, ankle, and hip in the paralyzed lower extremity. J. Bone Joint Surg. *47A*:1430, 1965.

Experimental Approaches and Laboratory Methods

VIII

56

CONTEMPORARY MORPHOLOGICAL TECHNIQUES FOR EVALUATING PERIPHERAL NERVES

PETER S. SPENCER and
MONICA C. BISCHOFF

The currently available morphological techniques routinely employed in research laboratories provide sensitive methods for the evaluation of peripheral nerve structure and pathology. Since these methods are generally available in pathology laboratories, our primary purpose has been to discuss the methodological details and information yield of these techniques. The reader is referred elsewhere for the purposes of obtaining a broader review of possible morphological procedures for examination of peripheral nerves (Thomas, 1970). The following techniques are those specifically recommended for the study of biopsies and experimentally injured nerves.

NERVE BIOPSY

The surgeon's interest in appraising the structure of an excised nerve is frequently restricted to the integrity of the fascicular arrangement and vasculature, number, type, and size of nerve fibers, and the amount of collagen in the epineurial, perineurial and endoneurial compartments. This information may be readily obtained by examining the nerve in cross sections with the light microscope after appropriate fixation, dehydration, and embedding (Figs. 56–1 and 56–2) (Sunderland, 1968). Such preparations are amenable to quantitative analysis, should this be necessary, the most useful being the determination of fascicular area and the diameter distribution of the myelinated nerve fiber population (Dyck et al., 1968; O'Sullivan and Swallow, 1968). The correlation of the nerve fiber spectrum with the components of the compound nerve action potential have represented two of the more important applications of the quantitative histology of peripheral nerves (Cragg and Thomas, 1961; Dyck and Lambert, 1966). Examination of sections with the electron microscope is required to quantitate the unmyelinated nerve fiber population (Fig. 56–3) (Ochoa and Mair, 1969). Electron microscopy is also needed to identify the cellular components of an abnormal nerve and to make a detailed description of the nerve fiber pathology.

It is usually helpful to have a three-dimensional image of the structure of the nerve fibers under study. While this may be gleaned from laborious correlation of longitudinal and transverse sections, a broad overview may be rapidly obtained by examining single myelinated nerve fibers isolated by the teasing technique described below (Fig. 56–4). Such nerve fibers are also amenable to

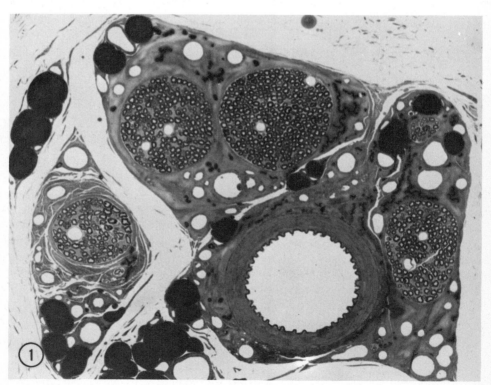

Figure 56–1   Cross section of a multifascicular nerve from a perfused animal. (This figure and Figures 56–2, 9, 10, and 11 are 1 μm epoxy sections stained with toluidine blue. Bright field light micrograph. × 200.)

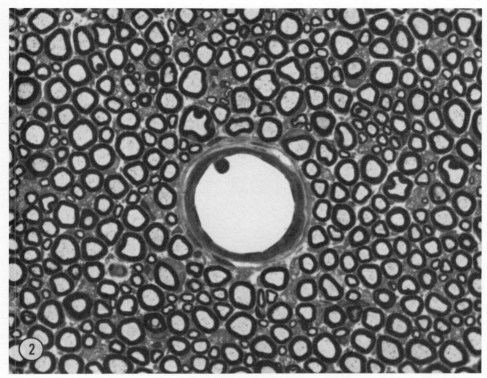

Figure 56–2 Cross section of a peroneal nerve composed of myelinated and unmyelinated fibers of various diameters. (Bright field light micrograph. × 2000.)

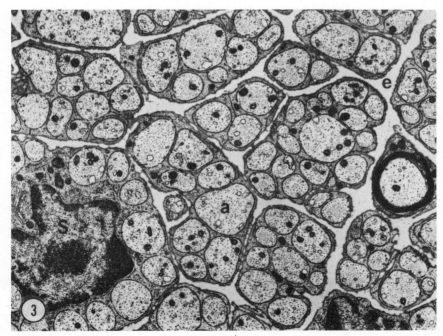

Figure 56–3 Cross section of cervical sympathetic nerve of a rat showing a large number of unmyelinated fibers and a myelinated fiber on the right. a, Axon; S, Schwann cell; e, endoneurium. (Electron micrograph of a thin epoxy section stained with uranyl acetate and lead citrate. × 10,500.)

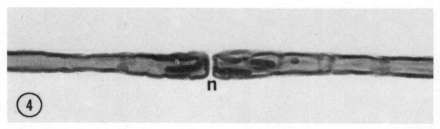

Figure 56–4 Single teased nerve fiber showing a node of Ranvier (*n*). (This and Figures 56–5, 6, and 7 were fixed in glutaraldehyde followed by osmium tetroxide and teased in Spurr® epoxy resin. Bright field light micrograph. × 400.)

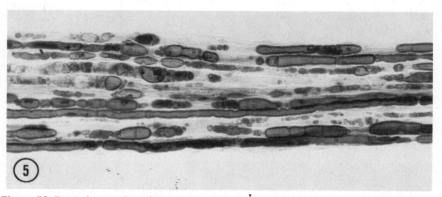

Figure 56–5 A cluster of myelinated nerve fibers undergoing wallerian degeneration. Note the formation of cylindrical ovoids of myelin. (× 200.)

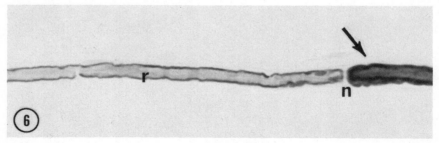

Figure 56–6 Single teased nerve fiber showing a node of Ranvier (n) separating a thickly myelinated (arrow) preserved portion and thinly remyelinated region (r). (× 300.)

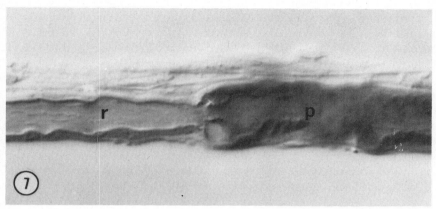

Figure 56–7   Single teased nerve fiber composed of a preserved (p) and a remyelinated (r) portion. (Nomarski micrograph. × 1800.)

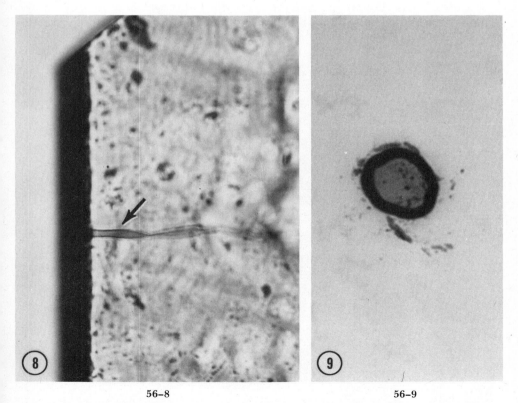

56–8   56–9

Figures 56–8 and 56–9   Single nerve fiber (arrow) embedded in an epoxy block which has been faced, ready for sectioning (left). (× 185.) Cross section of the single fiber (right). (× 1760.)

both qualitative and quantitative study with the light microscope. The presence of myelin perturbations, axonal degeneration or regeneration is readily detected by bright-field examination (Fig. 56–5), while the newer Nomarski technique may be employed to increase contrast and examine the internal structure of the fiber, including the diameter and structure of the axon (Figs. 56–6 and 56–7) (Spencer and Schaumberg, 1979). Teased fibers may also be used to determine myelinated fiber diameter, internodal length (distance between nodes of Ranvier), and nodal width (Lascelles and Thomas, 1966). Internodal length is uniformly reduced in regenerated myelinated fibers of all diameters (Vizoso and Young, 1948). Remyelinating internodes recovering from traumatically induced demyelination are also abnormally short (Lubinska, 1961; Spencer et al., 1975). Research techniques are also available for the examination of isolated single nerve fibers in the scanning electron microscope and sections of single fibers in the light and transmission electron microscope (Figs. 56–8 and 56–9) (Spencer and Thomas, 1970; Spencer and Lieberman, 1971; Ochoa, 1972).

NERVE EXCISION

Unlike many tissues, peripheral nerves are very sensitive to mechanical trauma. During excision, special care should be taken to avoid pulling, stretch-

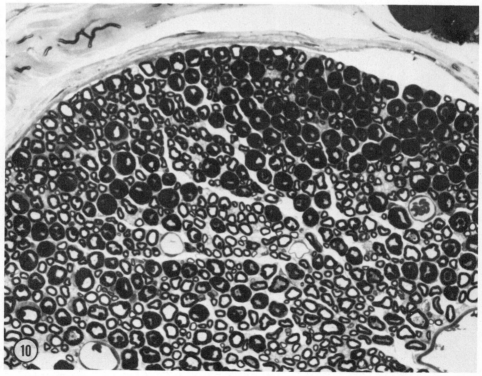

Figure 56–10   Cross section of a peroneal nerve displaying nerve fibers with greatly thickened myelin sheaths produced by trauma. (× 640.)

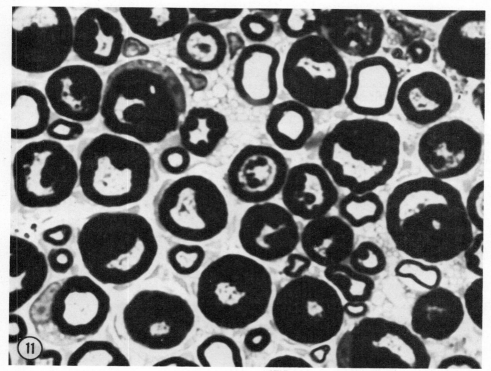

Figure 56–11 Higher magnification of traumatically altered myelinated fibers. (× 1600.)

ing, or pinching the nerve. Such treatment may cause striking changes to develop in the fibers which may easily be mistaken for pathology (Figs. 56–10 and 56–11) (Haftek and Thomas, 1968; Thomas, 1970). To avoid these changes, the nerve should always be gripped by the epineurium during excision. Cutting the nerve also introduces pronounced changes which may be eliminated by trimming away the cut ends of the specimen after fixation. Only a short length (1 to 2 cm) of nerve is required to perform a morphological examination.

CHEMICAL FIXATION

The purpose of fixation is to preserve the architecture of the nerve as closely as possible to the living state. Rapid fixation with minimal shrinkage and tissue distortion is therefore desirable. Preservation of ultrastructure is desirable, even for the purpose of light microscopy. The chemical fixative of choice is glutaraldehyde, which cross-links proteins and stabilizes lipids. Primary fixation is in glutaraldehyde, with osmium tetroxide as a secondary fixative (Sjöstrand, 1962; Dyck and Lofgren, 1968). This solution fixes and stains the lipids black, enhancing contrast for light microscopy and introducing part of the electron density needed for tissue examination in the transmission electron microscope (TEM).

Table 56–1

PHOSPHATE–BUFFERED 5% GLUTARALDEHYDE*
50 ml Sorensen's phosphate buffer
5.5 ml 50% Glutaraldehyde biological grade
0.27 ml 1% Calcium chloride
pH to 7.4
Shelf life — 2 weeks (cold)
Note: Severe allergic reactions are known

DALTON'S 2% CHROME OSMIUM TETROXIDE*
Stock solution:
4% osmium tetroxide in boiled distilled water stored in ultra-clean reagent bottle protected from
  light in refrigerator
Note: Fumes are highly toxic, especially to the cornea
Working solution: 5 ml
  2.5 ml 4% Osmium tetroxide
  1.25 ml 4% Potassium dichromate
  1.25 ml 3.4% Aqueous calcium chloride
Shelf life — 2 days (cold)

---

*Prepare under extraction hood.

Table 56–2

SORENSEN'S PHOSPHATE BUFFER
250. ml Stock
  1.9 g Sodium phosphate (dibasic) in 200 ml distilled water
  .45 g Potassium phosphate in 50 ml distilled water
  Maintain pH 7.3–7.4

Table 56–3

PARAFORMALDEHYDE*
100 ml   Distilled water
  4 g   Paraformaldehyde
50 mg   Sodium phosphate
0.5 ml   1% Calcium chloride
Heat ½ distilled water; add sodium phosphate and paraformaldehyde; stir to dissolve. Remove
  from heat. Add remaining water and calcium chloride. Filter solution into flask set in ice bucket.
  Adjust pH to 7.3–7.4. Use at room temperature.
Shelf life — 4 weeks (cold)

---

*Prepare under extraction hood.

Both fixatives are used as dilute solutions, and careful attention is given to both the hydrogen ion concentration (pH) and osmolality to minimize tissue shrinkage and distortion (Table 56–1) (Ohnishi et al., 1974, 1976).

In practice, the excised nerve is first gently stretched and adhered to a piece of firm card. This facilitates handling and prevents coiling during fixation. Proximal and distal orientation may be marked on the card, or a suture may be introduced to denote one end of the nerve. The mounted nerve segment is then immersed in the primary fixative at room temperature for a few minutes to harden the outer tissues. The nerve is then cut longitudinally, if possible without disturbing the individual nerve fascicles. Fixation in glutaraldehyde continues for three to five hours (maximum 12 hours), during which time the fixative may be replaced if desired. Tissue to be examined at a future date may be stored in a phosphate buffer solution (Table 56–2).

Optimal preservation of peripheral nerves is only achievable in animals where whole body perfusion with buffered glutaraldehyde is possible (Table 56–2) (Webster and Collins, 1964). For this purpose, the animal is anesthesized with sodium barbitone containing heparin, and secured on an autopsy table provided with an extraction hood. Once the animal is anesthetized, the thoracic cavity is cut bilaterally and retracted. The right atrium and ventricular apex are opened, and a cannula spurting fixative is rapidly introduced via the opened left ventricle and clamped into position in the aortic arch. The circulatory system is cleared of blood by perfusing for 15 seconds with phosphate-buffered 4 per cent paraformaldehyde at 100 to 160 mm of mercury (Table 56–3). This is followed without interruption by a continuous stream of buffered glutaraldehyde for 10 to 15 minutes. During this time, the animal becomes rigid and the nerves become yellow in color. Nerves removed from well-perfused animals are not subject to the types of artifacts found in tissue fixed by immersion.

Primary fixation by immersion or perfusion with glutaraldehyde is followed by secondary fixation (post-fixation) in osmium tetroxide for one to three hours. Periodic agitation of the specimen vial will ensure satisfactory fixation. Because the penetration of osmium is extremely poor, it is necessary to cut the nerve into blocks of tissue measuring no larger than $2 \times 2 \times 8$ mm. Failure of osmium to penetrate the nerve will ultimately be visible in sections as a central core of low contrast and poor preservation.

EMBEDDING

Before embedding the nerve in epoxy resin, the fixed tissue must be dehydrated stepwise in alcohol, and then immersed in a clearing agent such as propylene oxide. This solvent is miscible with both the alcohol and the liquid resin used for embedding. Resin infiltration is also a stepwise procedure, the aim in both cases being to achieve complete penetration with minimum tissue distortion. Resin infiltration is achieved by immersing tissue samples in a 1:1 ratio of propylene oxide and epoxy resin, and then into pure resin. After resin infiltration, the nerve segments are placed into flexible molds. A number written in pencil on a slip of card may be introduced into the mold at this stage. The mold is then filled with liquid resin and heated stepwise (37 to 45 to 60°C over 48 hours) in ovens to achieve controlled polymerization.

THICK SECTIONING AND LIGHT MICROSCOPY

Special microtomes or ultramicrotomes are used to cut the plastic-embedded tissue. The nerve is first exposed by trimming away the excess plastic with a razor blade and then introduced into the block holder of a microtome. Glass knives prepared with special glass knife-breakers are used to smooth the tissue face. After "facing" the block, one micrometer sections are cut with new glass knives equipped with water-baths made of electrical tape and sealed with nail varnish. The floating sections are rolled onto a fine brush and transferred to a drop of water on a glass slide.

After the sections are flattened with chloroform vapor, the slides are heated on a hot plate at 300°C for 30 minutes. During this time the plastic sections flatten and anneal to the glass surface. Basalm or epoxy-mounted sections may be examined unstained by phase-contrast microscopy or, after staining for 45 seconds with borate-buffered 1 per cent toluidine blue, with the light microscope in bright-field mode (Table 56–2).

THIN SECTIONING AND ELECTRON MICROSCOPY

Areas of interest identified in one micrometer sections are commonly studied in detail with the greater magnification and resolution of the TEM. For this purpose, the block face is trimmed to the area of interest and thin sections (approximately 50 nm) are floated onto the water bath of a glass or diamond knife. Sections are flattened with chloroform vapor and collected on clean copper grids of appropriate mesh size.

Electron density in the section is enhanced by immersing the grids in a solution of uranyl acetate followed by a solution of lead citrate (Table 56–4), taking care to wash the grid thoroughly after each stage (Venable and Coggleshall, 1965).

Finally, a carbon layer is evaporated onto the grid to provide a conducting layer to remove electrical charges produced in the section during irradiation

Table 56–4

TOLUIDINE BLUE
1 g Toluidine blue to 100 ml distilled water
+0.5 g Borax
Shelf life — 3 months
    pH to 9.0 with borax

URANYL ACETATE
  0.5 g Uranyl acetate
12.5 ml 50% Ethanol in boiled distilled water
Stir 10 minutes and filter. Store refrigerated in light-tight container.
Shelf life — 2 weeks

LEAD CITRATE
30 mg Lead citrate
10 ml 0.1N Sodium hydroxide
Solution must be clear. Make fresh for each use. When staining grids, place ultra-clean staining
    tray in Petri dish with potassium hydroxide pellets and cover while staining. This procedure pre-
    vents lead carbonate precipitate from forming.

with the electron beam. All stages of thin section preparation require special attention to cleanliness.

NERVE FIBER TEASING

A thin nerve fascicle is used for this procedure. An identical preparative procedure is employed except that it may be necessary to extend the individual steps and to use a low viscosity epoxy resin.

The nerve is dissected in liquid resin with the aid of mounted sewing needles and a stereo-binocular microscope. At first the epineurium is cleared, and the perineurium slit longitudinally and removed as a colorless sleeve from the blackened fascicular contents. The fascicle is repeatedly divided longitudinally until bundles of approximately 100 myelinated nerve fibers remain. Individual fibers are then teased apart from the bundles, picked up on the end of a sharpened wooden applicator stick, and transferred to a carefully cleaned glass slide.

After several fibers are aligned in parallel fashion, the slide is put in a covered Petri dish and placed in a 60°C oven overnight to polymerize the resin and affix the fibers to the slide. A coverslip is later positioned over the fiber using a drop of resin, which is then polymerized. No additional staining is needed. Unused nerve fibers may be stored in liquid resin at sub-zero temperatures.

SUMMARY

Formalin fixation with paraffin embedding is routinely used in pathological laboratories for the examination of nervous tissues, including peripheral nerve. The technique has been omitted here, since the procedure is totally unsatisfactory for the purposes of evaluating traumatic nerve injuries. By contrast, the techniques described here — nerve fiber teasing, light and electron microscopic analysis of epoxy sections — provide a satisfactory and uniform methodology for the contemporary evaluation of peripheral nerve structure and pathology.

REFERENCES

Cragg, B. G., and Thomas P. K.: Changes in conduction velocity and fibre size proximal to peripheral nerve lesions. J. Physiol. *157*:315, 1961.

Dyck, P. J., Gutrecht, J. A., Bastron, J. A., Karnes, W. E., and Dale, J. J. D.: Histologic and teased-fiber measurements of sural nerve in disorders of lower motor and primary sensory neurons. Proc. Mayo Clin. *43*:81, 1968.

Dyck, P. J., and Lambert, E. H.: Numbers and diameters of nerve fibers and compound action potential of sural nerve: Controls and hereditary neuromuscular disorders. Trans. Am. Neurol. Assoc., *91*:214, 1966.

Dyck, P. J., and Lofgren, E. P.: Nerve biopsy: Choice of nerve, method, symptoms and usefulness. Med. Clin. North Am. *52*:885, 1968.

Haftek, J., and Thomas, P. K.: Electron-microscope observations on the effects of localized crush injuries on the connective tissues of peripheral nerves. J. Anat. *103*:233, 1968.

Lascelles, R. G., and Thomas, P. K.: Changes due to age in internodal length in the sural nerve in man. J. Neurol. Neurosurg. Psychiatry *29*:40, 1966.

Lubińska, L.: Demyelination and remyelination in the proximal parts of regenerating nerve fibers. J. Comp. Neurol. *117*:275, 1961.

Ochoa, J.: Ultrastructural longitudinal sections of single myelinated fibers for electron microscopy. J. Neurol. Sci. *17*:103, 1972.

Ochoa, J., and Mair, W. G. P.: The normal sural nerve in man. Part 1: Ultrastructure and numbers of fibres and cells. Acta Neuropath. *13*:197, 1969.

Ohnishi, A., Offord, K., and Dyck, P. J.: Studies to improve fixation of human nerves. Part 1: Effect of duration of glutaraldehyde fixation on peripheral nerve morphometry. J. Neurol. Sci. *23*:223, 1974.

Ohnishi, A., O'Brien, C., and Dyck, P. J.: Studies to improve fixation of human nerves. Part 3: Effect of osmolality of glutaraldehyde solutions on relationship of axonal area to number of myelin lamellae. J. Neurol. Sci. *27*:193, 1976.

O'Sullivan, D. J., and Swallow, M.: The fibre size and content of the radial and sural nerves, J. Neurol. Neurosurg. Psychiatry *31*:464, 1968.

Sjöstrand, F. S.: Critical evaluation of ultrastructural patterns with respect to fixation. *In* Harris, R. J. C. (ed.): The Interpretation of Ultrastructure. New York, Academic Press, 1962, p. 47.

Spencer, P. S., and Lieberman, A. R.: Scanning electron microscopy of isolated peripheral nerve fibers. Normal surface structure and alterations proximal to neuromas. Zeit. Zellforsch. Mikroskop. Anat. *119*:534, 1971.

Spencer, P. S., and Schaumburg, H. H.: Central and peripheral distal axonopathy. The pathology of dying-back polyneuropathies. *In* Zimmerman, H.: Progress in Neuropathology. New York, Grune and Stratton, 1976, Vol. 3, p. 253.

Spencer, P. S., and Thomas, P. K.: The examination of isolated nerve fibers by light and electron microscopy, with observations on demyelination proximal to neuromas. Acta Neuropath. *16*:177, 1970.

Spencer, P. S., Weinberg, H. J., Raine, C. S., and Prineas, J. W.: The perineurial window — a new model of focal demyelination and remyelination. Brain Res. *96*:323, 1975.

Sunderland, S.: Nerves and Nerve Injuries. London, Livingstone, 1968.

Thomas, P. K.: The quantitation of nerve biopsy findings. J. Neurol. Sci. *11*:285, 1970.

Venable, J. H., and Coggeshall, R.: A simplified lead citrate stain for use in electron microscopy. J. Cell Biol. *25*:407, 1965.

Vizoso, A. D., and Young, J. Z. Internode length and fibre diameter in developing and regenerating nerve. J. Anat. *82*:110, 1948.

Webster, H. deF. and Collins, G. H.: Comparison of osmium tetroxide and glutaraldehyde perfusion fixation for the electron microscopic study of the normal rat peripheral nervous system. J. Neuropath. Exp. Neurol., *23*:109, 1964.

57

CONTEMPORARY MUSCLE MORPHOLOGY AS RELATED TO NERVE PATHOLOGY

ALFRED J. SPIRO

Denervating a muscle by any means has a profound effect on its structure. To understand these effects better and to assess their clinical usefulness, an overview of muscle morphology and of how this tissue responds to certain intrinsic and extrinsic pathological processes is needed. The following descriptions are based on analysis of muscle biopsy material acquired during the investigation of a large number of patients with a wide spectrum of neuromuscular disorders.

MUSCLE MORPHOLOGY

Routine Light Microscopy

Muscle fibers are long, thin, multinucleated cells which generally traverse the entire length of the muscle. On longitudinal sections, regular cross striations are observed, giving voluntary muscle its name. On cross sections, which are much more useful for diagnostic studies, the individual fibers are polygonal in shape in adults and children (Fig. 57–1), but appear essentially round in infants (Fig. 57–2). Fiber size, which on cross section can be measured by several methods, is dependent on several factors, including type of fixation (or lack of fixa-

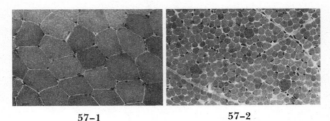

57-1   57-2

Figure 57–1   Cross section of normal adult muscle. Fibers are polygonal and of similar size. Nuclei are subsarcolemmal. (Trichrome × 200.)

Figure 57–2   Cross section of normal infant muscle. Fibers are small and round. Scattered large fibers are seen. (Trichrome × 200.)

tion), age, and sex (Dubowitz and Brooke, 1973). Generally the fibers are relatively uniform in size when compared with one another, but scattered "small" or "large" fibers may be normal. Nuclei are found in the periphery of the fiber (subsarcolemmal region).

Large numbers of fibers are observed close to one another in cross section, forming bundles or fascicles, the individual fibers being separated by small amounts of endomysial connective tissue. Bundles are surrounded by perimysial connective tissue, which is very variable in amount, and the entire muscle is surrounded by epimysial connective tissue, which is similarly variable.

In muscle biopsy specimens, in addition to the muscle fibers, intramuscular nerve twigs, blood vessels, and muscle spindles can be assessed.

Light Microscopy, Histochemical Reactions

When fresh unfixed muscle tissue is frozen rapidly in liquid nitrogen, and cross sections cut in a cryostat are subjected to a variety of histochemical reactions (two of the most useful are the adenosine triphosphatase [ATPase] reaction and the nicotinamide adenine dinucleotide [NADH] reaction, which reflects mitochondrial oxidative enzymatic activity) a typical pattern is observed (W. K. Engel, 1962). With each of the above reactions at least two types of fibers can be seen (Figs. 57–3 through 57–5) to occur *randomly* throughout the specimen, those

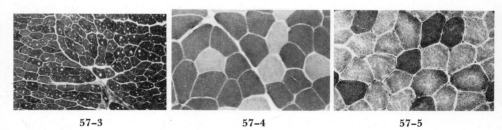

57-3   57-4   57-5

Figure 57–3   Cross section of muscle showing freezing artifact. (Trichrome × 80.)

Figure 57–4   Cross section showing mosaic with two types of fibers: dark reacting are type II and light reacting are type I. (ATPase × 200.)

Figure 57–5   Cross section showing mosaic with two types of fibers: dark reacting are type I and light reacting are type II. (NADH × 200.)

that are dark reacting and those that are light reacting. When serial sections are observed, those fibers that are light reacting with the ATPase reaction are generally dark reacting with the NADH reaction (conventionally type I fibers); those fibers reacting darkly with the ATPase reaction react lightly with the NADH reaction (type II fibers). Many other histochemical reactions can be used for special purposes, and the pH of the ATPase reaction can be altered to subdivide type II fibers into at least three subgroups, 2A, 2B, and 2C (Brooke and Kaiser, 1970). For the present purposes it is adequate to state that there are approximately equal numbers of type I and type II fibers in most human muscles biopsied for clinical purposes, but the proportion varies with individual muscles, and with such factors as age and sex. Type I fibers are roughly equivalent to "red" muscles in lower forms, and type II fibers are roughly equivalent to "white" muscles.

It is important to note that the histochemical type of muscle fiber is greatly influenced by its innervation, and is subject to alteration if its nerve supply is changed (Buller, Eccles, and Eccles, 1960).

Ultrastructure

With the electron microscope, several submicroscopic structures can be identified (Mair and Tome, 1972; Neville, 1973). Thick filaments arranged in parallel fashion extend throughout the length of the A band. Thin filaments, also arranged in parallel fashion, interdigitate with the thick filaments. The thin filaments, attached to a relatively thick Z line situated in the middle of the I band, extend through this band into part of the A band. The portion of muscle tissue between two adjacent Z lines is called a sarcomere. A myofibril is composed of a repetitive sequence of sarcomeres; a muscle fiber is composed of large numbers of parallel myofibrils. Each myofibril is separated from adjacent myofibrils by the intermyofibrillary space.

The intermyofibrillary space contains aqueous sarcoplasm in which several subcellular structures are found; these include mitochondria, glycogen granules, sarcoplasmic reticulum, and the transverse tubular system. Mitochondria are small organelles concerned with the energy supply of the muscle fiber. The transverse tubular system courses transversely across the myofibrils; in humans it is generally located near the junction of the A and I bands. The sarcoplasmic reticulum forms a discontinuous sheath surrounding individual myofibrils. Small saccular expansions of the sarcoplasmic reticulum are observed when it comes in contact with the transverse tubular system. The small transverse system tubules and two lateral sarcoplasmic reticulum sacs are known as triads, and are usually located at the junction of the A and I bands.

OBTAINING MUSCLE TISSUE FOR STUDY

Skeletal muscle is a readily accessible tissue, and biopsies can be performed whenever needed in the study of motor unit disorders. However, analysis of muscle is much less clinically useful in the study of peripheral nerve disorders, with the exception of angiopathic neuropathy and sarcoidosis (Hinterbuchner and Hinterbuchner, 1964). In nerve disorders muscle tissue is secondarily involved, and, for this reason, may not provide information that is significant in establishing an etiology.

To obtain the maximum information from the muscle biopsy, it must be performed in a manner that will provide well-oriented and virtually artifact-free tissue. The muscle to be biopsied should be one which is affected by the disorder but not too severely involved. In some instances in which a muscle that is severely wasted or that has been diseased for a prolonged period of time is biopsied, it becomes a fruitless venture, because no muscle fibers remain in the specimen to be analyzed. A muscle that has had a recent injection, electromyography, trauma, or acupuncture should also be avoided, because of the artifactual changes induced by these procedures.

Virtually all muscle biopsies can be performed under local anesthesia. The anesthetic is injected only into the tissue overlying the muscle, not into the muscle itself. Most patients experience pain (like a charleyhorse) when the muscle is being clamped. For this reason immediately before the biopsy we inject meperidine (approximately 1 mg per kg), followed by saline to clear the tubing of the butterfly needle, then up to 10 mg of diazepam all intravenously. This usually results in adequate sedation, which is of sufficient duration for the procedure.

An incision approximately 3 cm long is made over the muscle to be biopsied, in the same direction as the muscle bundles; the incision is then carried down to the superficial fascia. The wound is spread with a self-retaining retractor. The fascia is then *gently* lifted, without injuring the underlying muscle, and incised, again in the same direction as the muscle fibers, and the retractor is replaced under the fascia. With a great deal of caution, the superficial connective tissue immediately overlying the muscle can be cleared with a blunt instrument, always moving in the direction of the muscle fibers to minimize trauma. Specimens can then be taken, always *parallel* to the muscle bundles. If a muscle biopsy clamp is available (several types and sizes are commercially obtainable), a specimen approximately 2 cm long and 2 mm wide and thick can be clamped and removed by sharp dissection, and placed with the clamp into 4 per cent glutaraldehyde to be further processed for electron microscopy. If a clamp is unavailable, the specimen can be sutured to the shaft of a sterile cotton-tip applicator and then sharply cut from the muscle belly; the applicator stick with the specimen sutured to it is then placed into glutaraldehyde. Using a clamp or sutures in this manner ensures artifact-free preservation of the central portion of the specimen.

A slightly larger section (approximately 2 cm by 5 mm by 5 mm) is then removed in a similar fashion by using a special muscle clamp or by suturing to an applicator stick, being careful to orient the specimen in the direction of the muscle bundles. It is then placed, with the clamp or applicator stick, directly into 10 per cent formalin for subsequent embedding in paraffin and for utilization of routine microscopy for morphological studies.

Another specimen, similar in size to the last mentioned, is removed by using a clamp, as above, or between two hemostats. The specimen is then carefully removed from the clamps and cut in half with a razor blade. The two halves are then mounted onto cryostat chucks to which gum tragacanth has been applied. The cut ends are placed in an upright position. The specimens, thus mounted to enable cross sections to be cut, are then frozen in 2-methylbutane cooled to approximately −160 degrees C by liquid nitrogen. The specimens may then be cut in a cryostat at approximately −20 degrees C or stored in a deep freeze below that temperature. The cut sections may then be subjected to the necessary histochemical reactions. It is to be noted that *no fixation* or embedding has been used in this process.

PATHOLOGICAL REACTIONS

Myopathies

In disorders that in the conventional sense are considered to be primary diseases of muscle — myopathies — several types of alterations are observed in muscle biopsies (Walton, 1974). One of the earliest pathological changes observed in light microscopy is an increase in the variability of fiber size. Instead of the usual relative homogeneity of fiber sizes, random large and small fibers are abundant, and are best observed in cross sections (Figs. 57–6 and 57–7). In histochemical preparations it is noted that, typically, fibers of both types are affected, and that one type of fiber is not preferentially involved. Characteristically, in myopathies there is an increased amount of endomysial connective tissue. In addition, the nuclei, instead of being in their normal subsarcolemmal position, may be located in the internal portion of the cell. In myopathies, isolated, randomly occurring degenerative changes or architectural abnormalities of the fibers are commonly seen. Using the histochemical reactions, nemaline rods, central cores, and excessive glycogen or lipid can readily be detected (Spiro, 1975).

Because of the nonspecificity of changes that are seen at the ultrastructural level in human skeletal muscle diseases, it is difficult to ascribe myopathy to certain abnormalities and neuropathy to others. The morphological alterations, however, involve subcellular organelles such as mitochondria, lipid, or sacroplasmic reticulum. Reactions of the Z band and abnormalities of the nucleus, cell surface, and filaments may also be noted.

Neuropathies

Profound effects on the morphology of muscle fibers occur if the innervation is disturbed, either by a disorder of the anterior horn cells or by pathological

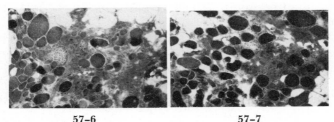

57–6   57–7

Figure 57–6 Cross section of biopsy from a child with muscular dystrophy, showing severe involvement with increase in endomysial connective tissue and fat. (Trichrome ×80.)

Figure 57–7 Same as Figure 57–6, different area. Large round dark fibers are a common feature of genetic myopathies.

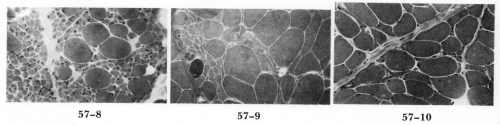

57–8   57–9   57–10

Figure 57–8   Cross section of biopsy from an infant with spinal muscular atrophy. Groups of small and very large fibers. Compare with Figure 57–2. (Trichrome × 200.)

Figure 57–9   Cross section of biopsy from a 17-year-old boy with spinal muscular atrophy showing groups of small, acutely angulated fibers. (Trichrome × 80.)

Figure 57–10   Cross section of biopsy from a patient with amyotrophic lateral sclerosis showing small groups of small, angulated fibers. (Trichrome × 200.)

changes in the peripheral nerve to that muscle. Changes in muscle structure are also associated with disturbances of the trophic effects of the nervous system on the muscle, and with disorders such as immobilization, abnormal nutritional states, and remote malignancies (Drachman, 1974; Gutmann, 1976).

In the light microscopic examination of denervated muscle, one of the most common morphological features is the presence of small fibers (Figs. 57–8 through 57–10), frequently in small or large groups (Bethlem, 1970). In cross section abnormal shrunken fibers are often acutely angular in shape instead of having the normal polygonal configuration; however, they may be otherwise structurally normal. In long-standing denervation, the nuclei of these small fibers may become pyknotic. Because of the shrunken volume of the fiber, the nuclei can appear to be increased in number. The remaining fibers are generally normal appearing; however, in chronic denervation, varying degrees of degenerative changes (so-called "myopathic" changes) may be observed. The average cross-sectional diameter of these remaining mucle fibers may be normal, but occasionally it is very much enlarged (Brooke and Engel, 1969), perhaps by compensatory hypertrophy; this feature is observed commonly in infantile and juvenile progressive spinal muscular atrophy, but can also be seen in peripheral neuropathies. In neuropathies the endomysial connective tissue is not generally increased in amount as it is in myopathies.

In histochemical studies it frequently can be demonstrated that the groups of small, acutely angulated fibers are darkly reacting with the NADH reaction (Fig. 57–11), which reflects oxidative enzymatic activity. When reacted for ATPase, it can often be shown that the groups consist of fibers of both histochemically defined types.

Target fibers (DeReuck et al., 1977) may also be observed in type I fibers in denervation, optimally with the NADH reaction. With this reaction, the absent or diminished oxidative enzymatic activity is clearly seen in the central portion of the fibers; this is surrounded by an area in which the reaction is increased. Toward the outer portion of the cell the reaction is essentially normal (Fig. 57–12).

An abnormality of fiber distribution termed fiber type grouping (Brooke and Engel, 1966) is also frequently seen in denervation (Fig. 57–13). Rather than the normal random distribution of type I and type II fibers, which produces a mosaic or checkerboard appearance on cross section, there may be clustering of

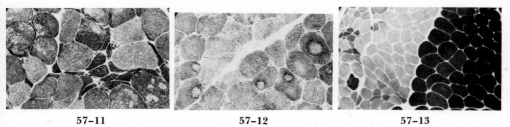

57–11   57–12   57–13

Figure 57–11 Cross section, same patient as Figure 57–10. Small fibers are dark reacting. (NADH × 200.)

Figure 57–12 Cross section of biopsy from a patient with toxic peripheral neuropathy showing several target fibers. Center of "target" is light reacting. (NADH × 200.)

Figure 57–13 Cross section of biopsy from a patient with chronic peripheral neuropathy showing grouping of both type I and type II fibers. (ATPase × 80.)

type I and type II fibers in denervation. This is probably related to coexisting denervation and reinnervation (Morris and Raybould, 1971). When fibers are reinnervated, collateral sprouting of terminal axons may occur, resulting in uniformity of histochemical type in the muscle fibers. As noted above, the histochemical typing of a muscle fiber is dependent on its innervation.

Electron microscopic studies of muscle are not routinely employed in the diagnostic study of muscle in denervating disorders. However, with experimental denervation studies performed in animals, profound changes can be demonstrated (Engel, 1974). These include myofibrillary atrophy and changes in mitochondrial mass, sarcoplasmic reticulum, and basement membrane. There is a degenerate core in the internal portion of target fibers in which there is disorganization of myofibrils, absence of mitochondria, and depletion of the sarcoplasmic reticulum. None of these changes as described in denervated muscle fibers can be regarded as entirely specific.

COMMENTS

Although the effect on muscle tissue of denervation induced by cutting the nerve or by nerve compression of various types can be studied sequentially in animal experiments, this is obviously impossible in humans. Even if it were possible to obtain repeated muscle biopsies in humans with peripheral nerve lesions, for example with a needle biopsy technique, the information obtained from such studies would be limited for several reasons. A muscle biopsy is a random sample of a much larger structure and may or may not reflect the general status of the remaining portions. We have frequently noted striking differences from one portion of a biopsy to the next when large samples are selected. In addition, only limited sequential data are available with respect to human muscles following acute and chronic peripheral nerve lesions. On the basis of limited information it is not generally possible to state with a great deal of certainty how long a muscle has been denervated or if recovery will occur. Results of animal muscle studies may prove helpful but, since many animal muscles are made up of fibers of different histochemical types from those present in human muscle, extrapolation may be imprudent (Beermann et al., 1977).

REFERENCES

Beermann, D. H., Cassens, R. G., Couch, C. C., and Nagle, F. J.: The effects of experimental denervation and reinnervation on skeletal muscle fiber type and intramuscular innervation. J. Neurol. Sci. *31*:207, 1977.

Bethlem, J.: Muscle Pathology: Introduction and Atlas. New York, American Elsevier, 1970.

Brooke, M. H., and Engel, W. K.: The histologic diagnosis of neuromuscular diseases: A review of 79 biopsies. Arch. Phys. Med. Rehab. *47*:99, 1966.

Brooke, M. H., and Engel, W. K.: The histographic analysis of human muscle biopsies with regard to fiber types. 2. Diseases of the upper and lower motor neurons. Neurology *19*:378, 1969.

Brooke, M. H., and Kaiser, K. K.: Muscle fibre types: How many and what kind? Arch. Neurol. *23*:369, 1970.

Buller, A. J., Eccles, J. C., and Eccles, R. M.: Interactions between motoneurones and muscles in respect of the characteristic speeds of their responses. J. Physiol. *150*:417, 1960.

DeReuck, J., De Coster, W., and Vander Eecken, H.: The target phenomenon in rat muscle following tenotomy and neurotomy: A comparative light microscopic and histochemical study. Acta Neuropath. *37*:49, 1977.

Drachman, D. B.: Trophic actions of the neuron: An introduction. Ann. N.Y. Acad. Sci., *228*:3, 1974.

Dubowitz, V., and Brooke, M. H.: Muscle Biopsy: A Modern Approach. Philadelphia, W.B. Saunders Co., 1973, p. 74.

Engel, A. G.: Morphological effects of denervation of muscle: A quantitative ultrastructural study. Ann. N.Y. Acad. Sci., *228*:68, 1974.

Engel, W. K.: The essentiality of histo- and cytochemical studies of skeletal muscle in the investigation of neuromuscular disease. Neurology *12*:778, 1962.

Gutmann, E.: Neurotrophic relations. Ann. Rev. Physiol. *38*:177, 1976.

Hinterbuchner, C. N., and Hinterbuchner, L. P.: Myopathic syndrome in muscular sarcoidosis. Brain *87*:335, 1964.

Mair, W. G. P., and Tome, F. M. S.: Atlas of Ultrastructure of Diseased Human Muscle. London, Churchill Livingstone, 1972.

Morris, C. J., and Raybould, J. A.: Fiber type grouping and end-plate diameter in human skeletal muscle. J. Neurol. Sci. *13*:181, 1971.

Neville, H. E.: Ultrastructural changes in muscle disease. *In* Dubowitz, V., and Brooke, M. H.: Muscle Biopsy: A Modern Approach. Philadelphia, W.B. Saunders Co., 1973, p. 383.

Sprio, A. J.: Unusual myopathies of childhood. *In* Swaiman, K. F., and Wright, F. S.: The Practice of Pediatric Neurology. St. Louis, C.V. Mosby Co., 1975, p. 1008.

Walton, J. N.: Disorders of Voluntary Muscle. London, Churchill Livingstone, 1974.

58

INTRANEURAL MICROCIRCULATION AND PERIPHERAL NERVE BARRIERS: Techniques for Evaluation — Clinical Implications

GÖRAN LUNDBORG

The normal vascularization of peripheral nerves and the vascular factor in peripheral nerve lesions have regained increasing interest among surgeons and neurologists. The membrane processes associated with impulse transmission require a continuous supply of oxygen, which is normally satisfied by the intra-neural microvessels. It is well known that ischemia is followed by rapid deterioration of nerve function (for review, see Lundborg, 1970). It has recently been demonstrated that local ischemia also blocks the fast axoplasmic transport in the corresponding segments (Ochs, 1974). Interference with intraneural blood flow may result from such surgical procedures as mobilization or stretching of a nerve, internal neurolysis and resection of the epineurium, and various opinions concerning the vascular consequences of these procedures have been reported (Bateman, 1962; Smith, 1966; Lundborg, 1970; Peacock and van Winkle, 1970; Lundborg and Rydevik, 1973; Rydevik, Lundborg, and Nordborg, 1976).

The existence of a blood–nerve barrier, corresponding to the blood–brain barrier of the central nervous system, and made up of the endothelium of the endoneurial capillaries, has been verified in experimental studies (Waksman, 1961). Nerve trauma and ischemia may deteriorate this barrier (Olsson, 1966; Lundborg, 1970). The consequent endoneurial edema might interfere with normal nerve fiber physiology, and if such an edema becomes organized, an endoneurial scar could occur. The possible role of intraneural edema formation in the etiology of the carpal tunnel syndrome has recently been extensively discussed by Sunderland (1976).

Thus, the structure and function of the intraneural microvessels have proved to be of considerable interest to anyone treating peripheral nerve injuries. The purpose of this chapter is to review the techniques used at our laboratory for studies of the intraneural microcirculation and peripheral nerve barriers of man and experimental animals under normal and experimental conditions, and to give data of relevance to the understanding and management of peripheral nerve problems.

HUMAN NERVES

Technical Procedures

These studies have all been performed on fresh human arms, amputated electively at varying levels because of malignant tumors. Within the first hour after amputation the brachial or ulnar and radial arteries were cannulated. After infusion of 5 cc 0.5 per cent lidocaine (Xylocaine) and 4 cc of heparin solution (5000 cc) the vessels were perfused with India ink at a pressure of about 100 mm Hg (13.3 kPa) for one to two hours. The specimens were then fixed in 4 per cent buffered formaldehyde for at least two weeks.

After fixation, different techniques can be used to study the surfacial as well as the intrinsic microvascular systems, respectively. The India ink perfused epineurial vessels stand out in bright contrast to the white connective tissue elements, and after resection of the superficial layers of the epineurium, deep epineurial vessels as well as perineurial vessels can be observed (Fig. 58–1). By treating the nerve according to Spalteholtz (Romeis, 1948), the tissues can be made transparent, and the intrinsic microvascular system can then be observed (Fig. 58–2).

A more detailed picture of the intraneural vascular system — especially the exact location of the vessels in relation to other intraneural tissues and cell components — can be achieved after embedding formalin-fixated nerves in paraffin. Nonstained sections 50 to 100 microns thick give an excellent microangiographic picture of the *intraneural* as well as *intrafascicular* microvascular bed when studied in a light microscope (Figs. 58–3, 58–4, and 58–5). With thinner

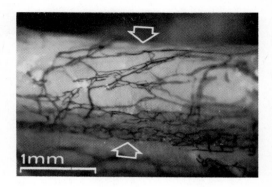

Figure 58-1 The perineurial vascular plexus as observed on the surface of a large fascicle from a non-clarified human median nerve. (India ink perfusion.) The outlines of the fascicle are indicated by arrows.

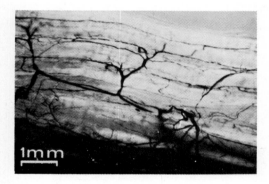

Figure 58-2 Detail of human median nerve after India ink perfusion and clarification according to Spalteholtz. The fascicular pattern of the nerve is recognized. Deep epineurial venules, each of them draining several fascicles, are seen.

Figure 58-3 Microangiogram of human median nerve. (India ink perfusion, non-stained sections of 50 microns thickness.)

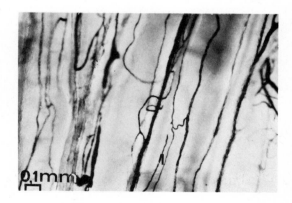

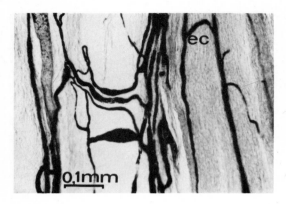

Figure 58–4 Microangiogram of human median nerve. Transverse anastomosing vessels between two adjacent fascicles (to the left and right, respectively) are seen. (India ink perfusion. Nonstained sections of 50 microns thickness.) ec indicates endoneurial capillaries.

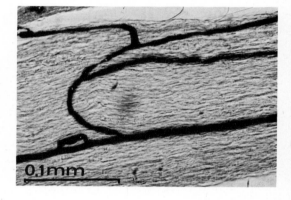

Figure 58–5 Histoangiogram of human median nerve showing typical endoneurial capillary formations. (Longitudinal nonstained section, 50 microns thick. India ink perfusion.)

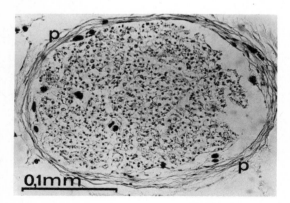

Figure 58–6 Histoangiogram of one single fascicle from a human median nerve showing numerous intrafascicular capillaries, many of them situated immediately beneath the perineurial membrane (p). (Transverse sections, 10 microns thick. India ink perfusion, hematoxylin-eosin staining.)

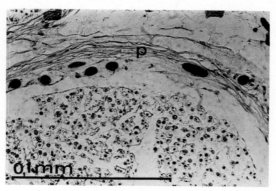

Figure 58-7 Detail of a fascicle from a human nerve, showing the distribution of vessel in various layers of the *perineurium*. (India ink perfusion, transverse section, 10 microns thick. Hematoxylin-eosin staining.)

sections, 10 to 20 microns thick, hematoxylin-eosin and van Gieson staining gives detailed "histoangiograms" with which the perfused vessels as well as intraneural tissues and cellular components can be analyzed (Figs. 58–6 and 58–7).

Results

The human peripheral nerve trunk is very well vascularized. In the epineurium, perineurium, and endoneurium there are well defined vascular plexuses, anatomically well separated but intimately anastomosing with each other.

In the epineurium a characteristic finding is large, longitudinal vessels located not only in the superficial parts of the nerve but also in the deep layers between the fascicle bundles. Numerous venules are seen, each of them collecting blood from several fascicles (see Fig. 58–2). The epineurial system is reinforced on various levels by regional arteries and veins from surrounding tissues.

If the epineurium is resected, distinct perineurial vascular plexuses are easily seen covering each single fascicle (see Fig. 58–1). The perineurial plexus constitutes a vascular network, but also exhibits numerous longitudinal vessels in continuity along the fascicle. The plexus is located in the peripheral connective tissue layers of the perineurium, but vessels are also frequently seen between the lamellae of the perineurial membrane (Fig. 58–7).

Intrafascicularly, the vessels are mainly of capillary size (Fig. 58–6). They are generally longitudinally oriented, but there are also numerous loop formations in planes perpendicular to the long axis of the nerve. Centrally, the capillaries are spread uniformly within the fascicle, but there seems to be a concentration of vessels in the area immediately beneath the perineurial membrane. Thus, capillaries can be seen running longitudinally close to the perineurial membrane for considerable distances. Frequently, anastomosing vessels are seen piercing obliquely through the perineurium or running for long distances between the lamellae of this membrane before they appear on the outside of the perineurium.

Thus, from the vascular point of view, each fascicle seems to represent a vascular unit composing a longitudinal noninterrupted vascular system separated from yet intimately anastomosing with the supporting epineurial vascular bed. The perineurial and endoneurial vascular plexuses are in immediate communication with each other. The localization of capillaries immediately beneath the strong and indistensible perineurial membrane as well as between the lamellae of this membrane might indicate that any increase in intrafascicular pressure tends to diminish or close the lumina of these vessels, thereby compromising their blood flow. Such increased intrafascicular pressure could be expected in nerve trauma and endoneurial edema formation; this is further discussed under "Comments and Conclusions."

NERVES OF EXPERIMENTAL ANIMALS

Technical Procedures

All our studies have been performed on the tibial sciatic nerve of rabbits, which can be very easily exposed in the lower limb and thigh. Anesthesia was induced by an intravenous (ear vein) injection of sodium nembutal, 30 mg per kg b.w. Supplementary doses of 12 to 15 mg were given whenever necessary to maintain adequate anesthesia.

Microangiography

For studies of the microvascular architecture we perfused the vascular system with India ink (see above) or Micropaque 25 per cent. Carefully suspended and filtered Micropaque was slowly infused at room temperature through a catheter in the abdominal aorta at a pressure slightly above the systemic arterial pressure. Before infusion the animals were heparinized and a vasodilator (Xylocaine, 0.5 per cent) was given intra-arterially before, and intermittently during the infusion in doses of 0.5 cc. As the medium was infused, blood was withdrawn from the jugular vein. This procedure resulted in a survival time of about one hour, with a fluid exchange of 200 to 300 cc corresponding to 3 to 5 cc per minute. The perfusion was continued for about 45 minutes after death to ensure a maximal filling of the vascular bed.

The tibial nerve was then removed and fixated in 5 per cent formaldehyde for at least 24 hours. Contact radiograms were produced on Kodak MR plates with a Matchless OEG-50 tube with a copper anode, operated at 12 kV and 15 mA at a focus film distance of 200 mm. The exposure time was from 5 to 10 minutes. The microangiograms were then analyzed in an ordinary light microscope (Fig. 58–8).

Fluorescence Microscopy

Fluorescence microscopic tracing of intravenously infused Evans blue-albumin was utilized to study the permeability of the intraneural microvessels under normal and various experimental conditions. Topical application of this

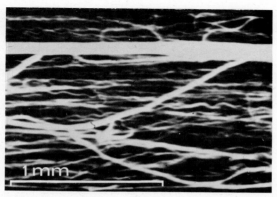

Figure 58–8 Microradiogram from the tibial nerve of rabbit. Perfusion with Micropaque. Thickness of nerve: 0.5 mm.

tracer around the nerve also enabled an analysis of the diffusion barrier constituted by the perineurium. For the vascular studies, a solution of 5 per cent bovine serum albumin* mixed with 1 per cent Evans blue** was infused intravenously. One cc of solution per 100 grams of body weight was used as a standard dose. After a half hour the nerve was removed and fixated in 5 per cent formaldehyde for at least 24 hours. For studies of the perineurial barrier the solution was applied topically around the nerve for two hours before the nerve was removed and fixated. Frozen longitudinal sections 10 microns thick were mounted in 50 per cent aqueous glycerin and were immediately studied in a Leitz fluorescence microscope equipped with a dark-field condensor. An Osram HBO 200 W mercury superpressure lamp was used as light source. The light was filtered through a Schott BG 12/3 mm filter. In the tubes the emitted light was filtered through a K 510 filter.

This technique is based on the fact that Evans-blue albumin (EBA) emits a bright-red fluorescence in formalin frozen sections (Steinwall and Klatzo, 1965; Lundborg, 1970). As the nerve tissue itself gives off a green autofluorescence, the exact location of the albumin could be easily determined (Fig. 58–9). For photographic recording a Kodak high-speed EHB 135 color film was used.

Vital Microscopy

For an analysis of the intraneural blood flow patterns in vivo, an intravital microscopic technique was used. The tibial nerve was used as experimental model. The nerve was carefully exposed in the lower limb, and by a quartz glass rod or a glass prism it could be transilluminated (Fig. 58–10). Low voltage lamps and xenon lamps were used as sources of light, and the light passed through a modified light microscopic condensor system. In recent years we have preferred a fiberoptic light system. The circulation in the nerve could then be observed in a modified Leitz intravital microscope (Lundborg, 1970). As the tibial nerve is very

---

*Nutritional Biochemical Corporation, Cleveland, Ohio.
**E. Merck AG, Darmstadt, Germany.

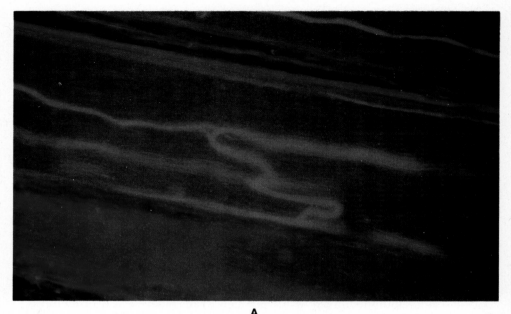

A

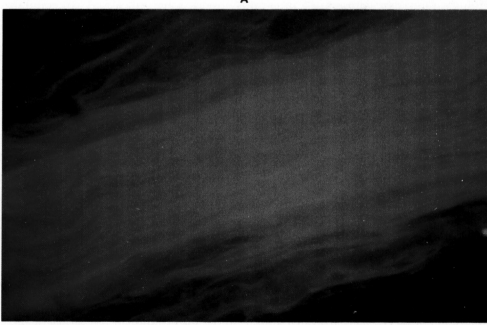

B

Figure 58–9 *A,* Fluorescence microscopic appearance of a normal tibial nerve of rabbit after perfusion with Evans-blue albumin. One fascicle passes obliquely over the field. The endoneurial capillaries are well perfused, and the red-fluorescing albumin complex is strictly confined to the capillary lumen. The nerve tissue exhibits a green autofluorescence. *B,* The same nerve after crush injury. Owing to increased capillary permeability the albumin complex is now distributed diffusely in the endoneurial space. This is the picture of an endoneurial edema.

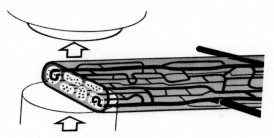

Figure 58–10　Schematic representation of the technique used for vital microscopic observation of the tibial nerve of the rabbit. Here the nerve has been cut; the end is placed on the light conductor (here a quartz glass rod). The intraneural microcirculation can be microscopically observed in vivo.

thin, the tissue appears as a living histological preparation, and the intraneural microcirculation can be studied under various experimental conditions. By this technique it is possible to achieve a very high resolution of nerve, as well as vascular structures and it is even possible to observe the endoneurial capillary circulation (Fig. 58–11).

Results

Microvascular Architecture

The intraneural vascularization of the rabbit nerves proved to be essentially the same as in human nerves. Thus, the three vascular plexuses, situated in the epi- peri- and endoneurium, respectively, were verified; the intimate anastomoses between these systems were striking. An overall view of the intraneural vascular system shows a network dominated by longitudinally oriented vessels of various calibers, intimately anastomosing with each other (see Fig. 58–8). The

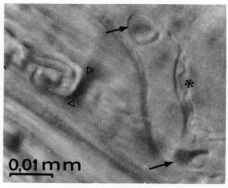

Figure 58–11　Vital microscopic appearance of nerve fibers and endoneurial capillary flow in a fascicle of rabbit tibial nerve. Δ indicates a node of Ranvier. An endoneurial capillary passes obliquely over the picture. * indicates an endothelial cell. Arrows indicate erythrocytes.

intrafascicular capillary system showed the characteristic longitudinal pattern and the typical loop formations observed also in human nerves.

Intraneural Flow Patterns

Normally the picture is dominated by numerous large, longitudinal venules situated in the superficial and deep layers of the epineurium exhibiting a well developed anastomosing system. There is no uniform direction of blood flow in the various vessels; on the contrary, the direction of flow in one such venular vessel might even be suddenly reversed if damage is induced to parts of the vascular bed. The comparatively slow blood flow in these venular vessels is in sharp contrast to the very fast flow seen in the epineurial arterioles. Also, the arterioles are longitudinally oriented, exhibiting a well developed collateral system.

Damage to regional nutrient vessels has no visible effect on the intraneural blood flow, except for the change of flow direction sometimes seen in the adjacent venules. Not even a more extensive mobilization of the nerve seems to compromise the intraneural blood flow, which remains intact because of the very well developed longitudinal intraneural collaterals. We have found it possible to mobilize the whole tibial sciatic nerve (15 cm) of the rabbit before observing any impairment of the intraneural blood flow (Lundborg, 1970, 1975).

The longitudinal collaterals seem to offer a considerable reserve capacity when the nerve is damaged. When the nerve is transected, a good capillary flow can still be observed very close to the margin of the proximal segment as well as the distal segment, even if the latter has been mobilized for several centimeters.

Even when the epineurial vascular plexus is damaged considerably, the vessels in the perineurium and endoneurium seem to be very resistant. When the nerve has been slightly traumatized during the dissection procedure, we have often observed pronounced edema formation in the epineurium and standstill of blood flow in most of the epineurial vessels, while there is an obviously undisturbed intrafascicular capillary flow. To some extent this is probably a result of the protective properties of the perineurial membrane, constituting a mechanical covering of each fascicle and a diffusion barrier to proteins and many other substances. Another important factor is the "fascicular vascularization" by the vascular plexuses in the perineurium and endoneurium of each fascicle. This special vascularization ensures adequate nutrition of the fascicles even if parts of the epineurium are damaged or resected.

Tension applied to a nerve trunk might cause early compromise of the intraneural microvascular flow. In model experiments we have found that when a distally cut tibial nerve of a rabbit is elongated by tension applied to its distal end, 8 per cent elongation is sufficient to compromise the intraneural venular flow (Lundborg and Rydevik, 1973). At 15 per cent elongation, the intraneural blood flow is completely stopped. Even minimal disturbances in venular flow might be sufficient to build up a stasis in the intraneural vascular bed, thereby starting a vicious circle that can rapidly jeopardize the nutrition of the nerve fibers. Our observations support the view that a large gap in the continuity of peripheral nerve should not be bridged by approximation of the cut ends after extensive mobilization and stretching of the nerve segments.

Microvascular Permeability

An early sign of tissue injury in any organ is the microvascular reactions with increased vascular permeability and the formation of a protein-rich exudate. In a lacerated nerve such an edema may be established in the epineurium as well as in the endoneurium, depending on the quality of the trauma. However, both of these nerve layers are separated by the perineurium, which acts as a diffusion barrier against proteins. This means that, as long as the perineurial barrier is preserved, an epineurial edema cannot spread into the fascicles; on the other hand, an intrafascicular edema cannot be drained outward to the epineurium.

The epineurial vessels normally allow a small amount of protein to pass through their walls, and even a slight injury could induce considerable protein leakage in this layer of the nerve. However, for reasons discussed above, such an edema remains confined to the epineurium. This was illustrated experimentally when an intraneural neurolysis with separation of the individual fascicle bundles was performed in normal rabbit tibial nerves (Rydevik, Lundborg, and Nordborg, 1976). After this procedure there was heavy edema in the epineurium, while the endoneurial vessels were not affected. Three to six weeks postoperatively there was considerable fibrosis in the epineurium of the nerves, while there was little or no fibrosis in the endoneurium.

The mechanisms and consequences of intrafascicular edema formation have been extensively analyzed in model experiments. Normally, the endoneurial blood vessels possess unique permeability properties, constituting a "blood–nerve barrier" corresponding to the blood–brain barrier of the central nervous system. Thus, the fluorescence technique reveals that intravenously injected albumin remains confined to the lumen of the endoneurial capillaries and does not pass into the extravascular space of the endoneurium (see Fig. 58–9A).

However, a heavy trauma to the nerve might cause a rapid leakage of albumin through the vessel walls and an endoneurial edema might occur (Fig. 9B). The perineurial barrier is very resistant to trauma as well as to ischemia, and when its barrier function is preserved the endoneurial edema fluid cannot escape through the perineurium to the epineurium. Such a situation might occur, for example, after longstanding ischemia when the blood flow is restored in the nerve. In experiments where ischemia was induced in a rabbit's hind limb by a pneumatic cuff around the thigh it was demonstrated that the blood–nerve barrier distal to the cuff was not deteriorated even by six hours of ischemia. However, when the blood flow in the nerve was restored after eight hours of ischemia, the barrier was broken down and the albumin was distributed diffusely among the axons in the endoneurial space. In these cases there was no recovery of nerve function, indicating that the edema fluid compromised normal nerve fiber function, or that eight hours of ischemia represented a critical limit for the viability of endothelium cells as well as nerve fibers.

No lymphatic vessels have been demonstrated in the endoneurial space, and if the perineurial barrier is intact the edema fluid can be reabsorbed only via endoneurial vessels. In the fascicles there is free communication in the endoneurial space proximally and distally, and we know that proteins can spread over long distances within these spaces. If the vascular barrier is broken for a long time, and if the endoneurial edema consequently becomes longstanding, one might expect fibroblast invasion and endoneurial scar formation, a situation that might represent an irreversible form of nerve lesion in which attempts at surgical therapy would be useless.

COMMENTS AND CONCLUSIVE REMARKS

By using combinations of various techniques it is possible to achieve considerable information about the structure and function of the intraneural microvascular bed. Perfusion studies on human nerves have revealed an extra- and intrafascicular vascular anatomy closely resembling that of experimental animals. We therefore believe that the intraneural microvascular *flow patterns* in human nerves and animal nerves are essentially the same.

The perineurial membrane normally plays a crucial role in the regulation of the endoneurial milieu by acting as a diffusion barrier to a broad range of substances including proteins (Kristensson and Olsson, 1971; Lundborg et al., 1973). Also, the endoneurial blood vessels constituting a "blood–nerve barrier" are normally impermeable or have a low permeability to proteins. In this way the internal milieu of the fascicles is controlled by the joint action of the two protective barriers — the perineurial membrane and the endothelium of the endoneurial blood vessels. Damage to one or both of these barriers may disturb the intrafascicular environment and might, therefore, interfere with normal nerve function.

The blood–nerve barrier seems to be more susceptible to ischemia and trauma than is the perineurial barrier. For example, while the blood–nerve barrier is deteriorated by eight hours of ischemia, the perineurial barrier is still intact after at least 24 hours of ischemia (Lundborg et al., 1973). In such a situation the "protective function" of the perineurial barrier is reversed and the barrier instead becomes a hindrance to the drainage of the endoneurial edema. A similar situation might occur with certain compression injuries, as the perineurial barrier has also proved to be very resistant to mechanical trauma (see below).

Considering a perfusion pressure in the endoneurial capillaries of about 30 mm Hg, it is obvious that a very slight increase in intrafascicular pressure might obliterate these capillaries, thereby rendering the endoneurial space ischemic. An endoneurial edema might in this way easily jeopardize the intrafascicular vascular perfusion. As discussed by Sunderland (1976), there are reasons to believe that such an endoneurial edema, as long as it is reversible, might constitute the first intermittent symptoms of the carpal tunnel syndrome, an increased tissue pressure and intravenous pressure in the carpal canal being mediated backward into the intrafascicular microvessels. If such an edema becomes longstanding there may be fibroblastic invasion and scar formation, causing the syndrome to move into a more severe and irreversible stage.

The microvascular factor has proved to be also important in acute compression lesions of peripheral nerves. While very high compression has proved to cause mechanical deformation of axons and local demyelination (Fowler, Danta, and Gilliat, 1972), there is now experimental evidence that the first stage of mild compression injury is associated with intraneural microvascular injury and edema formation. Rydevik and Lundborg (1977) have demonstrated in model experiments that when local compression by a "mini cuff" is induced to nerves of experimental animals, 200 to 400 mm Hg for two hours is sufficient to cause permeability disturbances of the endoneurial vessels beneath the edges of the cuff, while the perineurial barrier remains intact. The result is an endoneurial edema under these edges; as the proteins cannot escape through the impermeable perineurium, the edema fluid is bound to the endoneurial space until it is reabsorbed by the intrafascicular vessels.

It appears that a local endoneurial edema might jeopardize the nutritional supply to the nerve fibers by compromising the capillary blood flow within the corresponding area. We know that local ischemia blocks not only impulse transmission but also the fast axoplasmic transport over the corresponding segment (Ochs, 1974). Rydevik et al. have recently demonstrated in model experiments that such a block of fast axoplasmic transport may be induced by a local pressure of only 50 mm Hg applied to a nerve trunk. This may be an anoxic effect, secondary to obliteration of the endoneurial capillaries.

Thus, local changes in intraneural microcirculation and vascular permeability might compromise the energy supply necessary for normal delicate ion and membrane mechanisms in nerve fibers, and can also interfere with the transport of proteins and axoplasmic contents along the axon. It is our belief that this might help to explain the temporary local impairment of nerve conduction sometimes seen in association with compression lesions of peripheral nerves.

REFERENCES

Bateman, J. E.: Trauma to Nerves in Limbs. Philadelphia, W. B. Saunders Co., 1962.

Kristensson, K., and Olsson, Y.: The perineurium as a diffusion barrier to protein tracers. Differences between mature and immature animals. Acta Neuropath. *17*:127, 1971.

Lundborg, G.: Ischemic nerve injury. Experimental studies on intraneural microvascular pathophysiology and nerve function in a limb subjected to temporary circulatory arrest. Scand. J. Plast. Reconstr. Surg. Suppl. 6, 1970.

Lundborg, G., and Rydevik, B.: Effects of stretching the tibial nerve of the rabbit. A preliminary study of the intraneural circulation and the barrier function of the perineurium. J. Bone Joint Surg. *55B*:390, 1973.

Lundborg, G., Nordborg, C., Rydevik, B., and Olsson, Y.: The effect of ischemia on the permeability of the perineurium to protein tracers in rabbit tibial nerve. Acta Neurol. Scand. *49*:287, 1973.

Lundborg, G.: Structure and function of the intraneural microvessels as related to trauma, edema formation and nerve function. J. Bone Joint Surg. *57A*:938, 1975.

Ochs, S.: Energy metabolism and supply of $\sim$ P to the fast axoplasmic transport mechanisms in nerve. Fed. Proc. *33*:1049, 1974.

Olsson, Y.: Studies on vascular permeability in peripheral nerves. 1: Distribution of circulating fluorescent serum albumin in normal, crushed and sectioned rat sciatic nerve. Acta Neuropath. *7*:1, 1966.

Peacock, E. E. Jr., and van Winkle, W. Jr.: Wound Repair. 2nd ed., Philadelphia, W. B. Saunders Co., 1976.

Romeis, B.: Mikroskopische Technique. Munich, Oldenburg, 1948, p. 200.

Rydevik, B., Lundborg, G., and Nordborg, C.: Intraneural tissue reactions induced by internal neurolysis. Scand. J. Plast. Reconstr. Surg. *10*:3, 1976.

Rydevik, B., and Lundborg, G.: Permeability of intraneural microvessels and perineurium following acute, graded experimental nerve compression. Scand. J. Plast. Reconstr. Surg. *11*:179, 1977.

Rydevik, B., McLean, W. G., Sjöstrand, J., and Lundborg, G.: Blockage of axonal transport induced by acute, graded compression of the rabbit vagus nerve. Submitted for publication 1979.

Smith, J. W.: Factors influencing nerve repair. II. Collateral circulation of peripheral nerves. Arch. Surg. *93*:433, 1966.

Steinwall, O., and Klatzo, I.: Double tracer methods in studies on the blood barrier dysfunction and brain edema. In Proc. 17th Congr. Scand. Neurol., Gothenburg, 1964. Acta Neurol. Scand. *41* (suppl. 13,): 1965.

Sunderland, S.: The nerve lesion in the carpal tunnel syndrome. J. Neurol. Neurosurg. Psychiatry *39*:615, 1976.

Waksman, B. H.: Experimental study of diphtheric polyneuritis in the rabbit and guinea pig. III. The blood–nerve barrier in the rabbit. J. Neuropath. Exp. Neurol. *20*:35, 1961.

59

THE APPLICATION OF AXONAL TRANSPORT STUDIES TO PERIPHERAL NERVE PROBLEMS

JOHAN SJÖSTRAND,
W. GRAHAM McLEAN, and
MARTIN FRIZELL

AXONAL TRANSPORT: A DEFINITION

Axonal transport is the process by which material synthesized in cell bodies of central or peripheral neurons is transported to various sites within the axon or dendrites. This material may have a structural or functional role in the nerve cell — it may be neurotransmitters, their precursors, or synthesizing enzymes required for chemical transmission at axon terminals; it may be whole organelles such as mitochondria or smooth endoplasmic reticulum required for normal turnover of those structures within the axon; it may be proteins or glycoproteins to be incorporated in the cell membrane or for construction of intracellular components such as microtubules. Axonally transported material may also include as yet unknown trophic factors necessary for

917

the passage of information from nerve cell body to terminals or between the nerve cell and an adjoining nerve or glial cell or muscle fiber.

The physiology and uses of axonal transport have been the subjects of several reviews (Dahlström, 1971; Jeffrey and Austin, 1973; Cowan and Cuénod, 1975; Heslop, 1975; Lasek, 1975; Lubinska, 1975; Livett, 1976). Two rates of axonal transport of proteins from cell body to terminal have been found — a slow phase moving from 1 to 6 mm per day contains mainly soluble proteins as well as microtubules and neurofilaments, and a rapid phase moving at 40 to 600 mm per day, depending on the nerve concerned, carries all glycoproteins, membrane-bound enzymes, and vesicular material. In addition, a retrograde axonal transport of proteins from terminals to cell bodies occurs.

We still do not know how the axonal transport process works. Two major theories have been advanced, both of which may be operative. In the first (Droz et al., 1974; Markov et al., 1976) glycoproteins and other rapidly moving components are considered to be transported attached to a continuous channel of smooth endoplasmic reticulum, which permits the transfer of the proteins to axonal and synaptic membranes, as is known to occur (Droz, 1973; Cancalon and Beidler, 1975). It is likely that proteins thus incorporated into axolemmal membranes are further transported within the membranes to other sites in the axon (Marchisio et al., 1975).

An alternative means of transport of intracellular materials is through a connection with axonal microtubules. The antimitotic agents colchicine and vinblastine inhibit the axonal transport of noradrenergic vesicles in sympathetic nerves (Dahlström, 1968; Banks et al., 1971) and the inhibition is directly related to a disruption of axonal microtubules. The role of microtubules has been advocated in the "transport filament" hypothesis of Ochs (1974), in which he postulates the existence of filament-like proteins to which synaptic vesicles, mitochondria, and various proteins can attach themselves. The filaments are then transported along the longitudinally aligned microtubules within the axon; the energy required comes from ATP as it is hydrolyzed by a Ca^{++} or Mg^{++} activated ATPase, possibly associated with protein sidearms on the microtubules with which the filaments can interact.

The two theories of the mechanism of axonal transport need not be mutually exclusive. The main evidence for the involvement of smooth endoplasmic reticulum channels concerns the transport of glycoproteins (Markov et al., 1976), while that for microtubule involvement involves noradrenergic vesicles (Banks and Till, 1975).

More detailed information on the transport mechanisms is still lacking. Unanswered questions of particular importance are how the neuron directs its newly synthesized proteins to one of the two or more transport mechanisms, and how, if at all, the nerve cell exerts any control over the rate and amount of transport.

METHODS OF STUDY

There are two main techniques which can be used independently or together to examine the characteristics of axonal transport.

Ligation

Constriction of a nerve results in the accumulation of axonally transported material proximal, and often distal, to the constriction (Weiss and Hiscoe, 1948; Dahlström and Häggendal, 1966). Measurement of the accumulated material (for example, neurotransmitters and enzymes) gives a measure of the rate, amount, and direction of transport.

Radiolabeling

The introduction of radiolabeled amino acids or sugars into nerve cell bodies leads to the axonal transport of detectable waves of radiolabeled proteins or glycoproteins (Ochs et al., 1962; Lasek, 1968). The proteins in the different transport phases can be separated by electrophoresis and identified according to molecular weight (Karlsson and Sjöstrand, 1971a; Willard et al., 1974). Those techniques, along with the use of specific marker enzymes such as horseradish peroxidase, which is taken up by nerve terminals and transported in a retrograde direction toward nerve cell bodies, have found an important application in the study of neuronal connectivity (Cowan and Cuénod, 1975; Lasek, 1975).

The method most commonly used in our laboratories has involved the hypoglossal and vagus nerves of the rabbit. Motor fibers, predominantly myelinated in the hypoglossal nerve and mainly nonmyelinated in the vagus nerve, have their cell bodies in the hypoglossal and dorsal motor nuclei, respectively, of the brain stem.

Male albino rabbits (1.5 to 2.5 kg) are anesthetized with pentobarbitone (36 mg per kg intravenously). The muscles are divided in the neck at the base of the skull, and the fourth ventricle is exposed by removal of the tela choroidea. Small cotton wicks are placed on either side of the aperture to soak up any stray isotope or cerebrospinal fluid. Radioactive leucine (30 μ Ci L-(4,5-^{3}H) leucine, 46 Ci per mmole in 30 μl water; Radiochemical Centre, Amersham, England) is then infused slowly onto the calamus scriptorius over a period of 30 minutes through a fine polythene cannula attached to a Hamilton microsyringe (Miani, 1963). The wound is closed with silk sutures, and the animal is allowed to recover. One main advantage of this method of isotope application is that it permits even radiolabeling of proteins in right and left nerves, since there is an even diffusion of ^{3}H-leucine to the nuclei on both sides of the brain stem. Alterations in the amount of transported proteins in one nerve can be assessed by comparison with its contralateral control.

A second method of isotope application in the vagus nerve is by injection of small volumes of ^{3}H-leucine into the nodose ganglia of the anesthetized rabbit. Nodose ganglia are exposed and 20 μ Ci ^{3}H-leucine in 10 μl of 0.9 per cent NaCl are injected directly into each nodose ganglion through a 30 gauge stainless steel hypodermic needle. The animal is again permitted to recover. The method has the advantages that it is more rapid and less traumatic than injection into the fourth ventricle and that it labels specifically sensory fibers. It has the disadvantage that the labeling of proteins in the two sides of the animal may be uneven owing to variations in the injections.

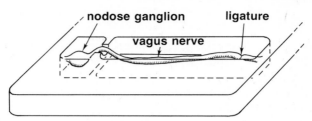

Figure 59–1   The two-compartment perspex chamber for the study of axonal transport in the rabbit vagus nerve/nodose ganglion preparation in vitro. See text for details.

A third technique we have frequently employed is to measure the axonal transport of labeled proteins in sensory fibers of the rabbit vagus nerve in vitro. Cervical vagus nerves with nodose ganglia attached are removed from newly killed rabbits and incubated in a specially constructed two-compartment chamber containing oxygenated medium 199 (Flow, Irvine, Scotland) with the nodose ganglion in the smaller of the two compartments and the remainder of the nerve in the larger (Fig. 59–1). A ligature is tied around the nerve trunk 60 mm from the ganglion and 15 μl (15 μ Ci) ^{3}H-leucine are added to the smaller compartment; that is, to the medium surrounding the ganglion. The chamber, which can take up to eight such nerves, is then incubated for up to 24 hours at 38.5° C in an atmosphere of 95 per cent O_2 to 5 per cent CO_2 at a relative humidity of 96 per cent. After three hours, the medium in the larger compartment is replaced in case of leakage from the compartment containing the isotope, and six hours after the start of the incubation the medium in both compartments is replaced; that is, the isotope is removed. This method has the advantage that known concentrations of drugs may be tested for their effects on the axonal transport mechanism within the axons without their affecting protein synthesis in the cell bodies. An inhibition of axonal transport may be detected as a decrease in the rate or activity of the wave of labeled proteins moving into the axons, or as a decrease in the accumulation of labeled proteins found in the segment of nerve immediately proximal to the ligature.

In all the above methods the nerves are subsequently removed, placed on graph paper, and cut into 5 or 2.5 mm pieces. The pieces are placed individually in 2 ml trichloroacetic acid (TCA) and left overnight at 0 to 4° C to allow precipitation of labeled proteins and diffusion of non-precipitable radioactivity. The TCA is discarded and the tissues are washed once more and finally dissolved in 0.5 ml Soluene (Packard) overnight at room temperature. Ten ml of a toluene based scintillation fluid are added to each dissolved nerve piece in a plastic vial and the radioactivity present is measured in a liquid scintillation counter. Corrections for quenching are made manually or automatically.

The techniques described here are similar to others currently in use. The most common systems are the ventral motor and dorsal sensory fibers of the sciatic nerve of the cat (Ochs, 1972), rat (Karlström and Dahlström, 1973), or frog (Edström and Mattsson, 1972) and the optic nerves of the chick (Marchisio and Sjöstrand, 1972) or rabbit (Karlsson and Sjöstrand, 1971b). Each method provides its own unique information, but the nature of the axonal transport mechanisms in all of the systems is believed to be similar.

RESULTS

Typical Findings

In all the systems discussed, a rapid axonal transport of labeled proteins occurs. This is identified by the shape of the curve of distribution of radiolabeled proteins along the nerve. By measuring the front of the labeled material (that is, the farthest distance that the labeled proteins have moved from the cell bodies at various times after isotope injection), a rate of axonal transport is found. Figure 59–2 shows one such profile for the fast transport in sensory fibers in vivo. The rates of fast transport in the nerves we have studied are similar to those found by other investigators: 400 mm per day and 330 mm per day for both ^{3}H-leucine labeled proteins and ^{3}H-fucose labeled glycoproteins in motor fibers of vagus and hypoglossal nerves, respectively (Sjöstrand, 1969; Frizell and Sjöstrand, 1974a), 330 mm per day for proteins and glycoproteins in sensory vagus nerves in vitro (McLean et al., 1975), and 415 mm per day in vivo (McLean et al., 1976a). Those figures agree with transport rates found in many other nerves (Heslop, 1975).

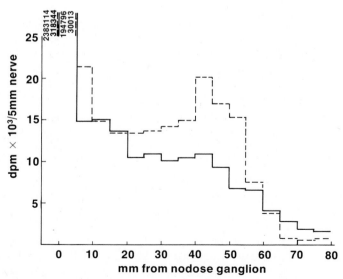

Figure 59–2 The distribution of rapidly-transported (------) and slowly-transported (————) ^{3}H-leucine-labeled proteins in the rabbit vagus nerve *in vivo*. Tritiated leucine was injected into the nodose ganglion; ------ four hours later or ———— 48 hours later the vagus nerve was removed and the protein-bound radioactivity in 5 mm sections of nerve was measured in disintegrations per minute (dpm). The profiles are from individual nerves and represent normal values. In both cases the front of the labeled proteins lies between 60 and 65 mm from the ganglion.

Several hours after injection of ^{3}H-leucine, a wave of labeled proteins is seen to move slowly in the nerve (Fig. 59–2). This later outflow moves at a rate of about 25 mm per day in motor and sensory fibers of the vagus and about 5 mm per day in the hypoglossal nerve (Sjöstrand, 1970, McLean et al., 1976a). The slow transport rate of 25 mm per day in the rabbit vagus is considerably faster than that of slow transport in most other nerves (Heslop, 1975). This makes the vagus a useful nerve for the study of slow transport, since experiments need not be so lengthy, but it must be borne in mind that the mechanism of slow transport in the rabbit vagus may not be identical to that in other nerves. We have found no evidence of the presence of a significant number of proteins transported in the motor vagus at a rate intermediate between fast and slow (McLean et al., 1976b).

In addition to the two rates of anterograde transport, a retrograde axonal transport of proteins occurs in the hypoglossal nerve and in the sensory and motor vagus (Frizell and Sjöstrand, 1974b; McLean et al., in preparation). It is thought that retrograde protein transport represents the return of used material or of breakdown products from nerve terminals to the cell bodies as well as a method for transferring information within the cell.

While the existence of the axonal transport processes is obviously important for the normal functioning of the nerve, it is still unclear to what extent a disruption or reduction of axonal transport is responsible for various peripheral nerve disorders. We present results here which indicate that alterations in axonal transport do occur in situations in which peripheral nerve function would be impaired.

Nerve Regeneration

In a series of experiments, rabbit hypoglossal and cervical vagus nerves were crushed and allowed to regenerate. At various times after the crush, proteins were radiolabeled by application of ^{3}H-leucine or ^{3}H-fucose to the fourth ventricle and the nerves were ligated. The accumulation of rapidly migrating proteins at the ligature on regenerating nerves was compared with that in non-regenerating contralateral control nerves.

The results of the experiments indicate that the changes in axonal transport during nerve regeneration are connected with the success of the regeneration of the nerve. In the hypoglossal nerve, which normally regenerates successfully after crush injury, the slow axonal transport of proteins and the rapid transport of glycoproteins are increased, while the transport of the bulk of rapidly migrating proteins is decreased. In the motor fibers of the vagus, a nerve which regenerates less successfully, the rapid and slow transport of proteins as well as the transport of glycoproteins are decreased (Frizell and Sjöstrand, 1974a and c). The alterations in glycoprotein and slowly migrating protein transport in regenerating nerves may be a result of an alteration in the nerve cell body's capacity to synthesize materials necessary for the construction of new fibers and to move away from the synthesis of material required for normal neurotransmission (Frizell and Sjöstrand, 1974d). It is an interesting question whether or not a general stimulation of axonal transport, as can occur under certain experimental conditions (Edström and Mattsson, 1975; Israel et al., 1975; Wakabayashi, 1976), can improve or accelerate nerve regeneration.

Compression

Compression injury of peripheral nerves occurs in several pathological conditions (Seddon, 1972; Sunderland, 1976). Such injury affects intraneural connective tissue and its blood vessels as well as the nerve fibers. The effects of experimental compression injury on intraneural microcirculation are fully discussed by G. Lundborg in Chapter 58 of this book. In collaboration with G. Lundborg and B. Rydevik, we have studied the effects of experimental nerve compression on axonal transport with a view to determining the extent of recovery of peripheral nerve function after blockade of axonal transport by compression (Rydevik et al., 1979).

Figure 59–3 demonstrates some of the results that have been obtained. Tritium-labeled leucine was injected into rabbit nodose ganglia and two hours later a specially constructed chamber containing an inflatable rubber membrane was placed around the vagus nerve at a distance of about 20 mm from

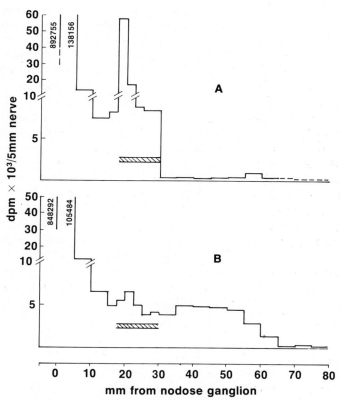

Figure 59–3   The profiles of labeled proteins in rabbit vagus nerves 4 hours after injection of ^{3}H-leucine into the nodose ganglia. In *A*, the nerve was subjected to a pressure of 200 mm Hg for 2 hours, at the zone marked by cross-hatching, 2 hours after isotope injection. A marked accumulation of proteins is seen at the compression zone. In *B*, the nerve was subjected to a pressure of 200 mm Hg for 2 hours, 3 days prior to labeling; i.e., a period of recovery was allowed. A much reduced accumulation of proteins is seen. The results are representative samples from four and seven such experiments in *A* and *B*, respectively.

the ganglion. The chamber was inflated to various known pressures up to 400 mm Hg. The animal was then killed and the profile of radioactive proteins in the nerve was examined as described above.

A pressure as low as 50 mm Hg disrupts axonal transport and causes an accumulation of rapidly migrating labeled proteins proximal to the compression site. The extent of block is less than that found after subjection of the nerve to higher pressures.

In some experiments, nerves were compressed, the animals allowed to recover from anesthesia, and the axonal transport measured at intervals up to 14 days later (Fig. 59–3). Those results indicate that recovery of axonal transport from low pressure block generally occurs within one day, while recovery from a pressure of 400 mg Hg takes longer than three days to occur.

Neurotoxic Effects of Drugs

The systems we have described can be applied usefully to the study of the neurotoxic effects of drugs. The antileukemic agents vinblastine and vincristine are known to have toxic side effects including neuropathy (Casey et al., 1976); they are also potent inhibitors of the formation of neuronal microtubules (Himes et al., 1976) and vinblastine inhibits axonal transport (Banks et al., 1971; Paulson and McClure, 1974; McLean et al., 1975).

We have examined the actions of various agents that are known to have a neurotoxic and particularly a retinotoxic action for their ability to inhibit axonal transport in the rabbit vagus nerve in vitro. These included chloroquine and hydroxychloroquine (Nylander, 1967; Shearer and Dubois, 1967), thioridazine (Zinn, 1975), ethambutol (Roberts, 1974), and clioquinol (Meade, 1975). The results indicated that all the drugs except ethambutol inhibit the accumulation of rapidly transported proteins at a ligature on the vagus nerve (McLean and Sjöstrand, 1977). Thioridazine and clioquinol are inhibitory at a concentration of $10^{-4}M$, while chloroquine and hydroxychloroquine inhibit at $10^{-3}M$. The inhibitory effect of hydroxychloroquine is less than that of chloroquine at the same concentration. While the required concentration of the drugs appears to be relatively high, it should be remembered that, as far as the retinotoxic actions of the drugs are concerned, there is evidence that chloroquine accumulates in the pigment epithelium and thus exists in high concentrations locally (Bernstein et al., 1963). However, a long-term study of the effects on axonal transport of in vivo administered chloroquine has failed to demonstrate inhibitory effects (McLean and Sjöstrand, 1977). The study is continuing with higher doses.

The Diseased State

A final application of axonal transport studies has been the attempt to identify factors that may be at fault in various neurological and muscle disorders. Alterations in axonal transport have been demonstrated in experimental animals with muscular dystrophy and diabetes (Jablecki and Brimijoin, 1974; Komiya and Austin, 1974; Tang et al., 1974; Schmidt, 1975). An obvious cause of neuromuscular dysfunction would be a fault in the axonal transport of neurotransmitter substances. However, the mechanism by which the motor nerve regulates the function and composition of the skeletal muscle cell membrane is still debated. It is likely that trophic factors other than the neurotransmitter acetylcholine are liberated by the nerve to regulate muscle function (for review, see Gutmann, 1976). An alteration in the synthesis and/or axonal transport of any one of these trophic substances may remain undetected by current research techniques and yet may cause profound changes in muscle activity.

FUTURE APPLICATIONS

Within the last decade the nature of axonal transport has been elucidated sufficiently for it to be used with considerable success as a research tool in the study of neuronal connectivity (Cowan and Cuénod, 1975; Livett, 1976), and attempts have been made to identify new neurotransmitter substances on the basis that they will be transported to nerve terminals by axonal transport at a rate or in an amount different from that of other materials (Roberts et al., 1973; Johnson, 1974; Yates and Roberts, 1974).

A major question that has not yet been answered satisfactorily is the extent to which axonal transport may be altered before the nerve starts to function abnormally and, similarly, as we have seen in the case of nerve compression injury, we still require a definition of the relative contributions made by axonal transport blockade and other factors, such as endoneurial edema, to the nerve lesion.

While axonal transport studies have contributed to our widening knowledge of nerve structure and function there has as yet been little clinical application of the manipulation of the axonal transport process. The long list of means by which axonal transport may be inhibited (McClure, 1972) is not matched by the relatively few methods to enhance it, and those to date would appear to have little therapeutic application. The continuing research into the role of transport disorders in nerve or muscle diseases, as well as the basic research into the mechanisms underlying the transport process, will, it is hoped, indicate where and how manipulation of axonal transport can be of clinical importance.

REFERENCES

Banks, P., Mayor, D., Mitchell, M., and Tomlinson, D.: Studies on the translocation of noradrenaline-containing vesicles in post-ganglionic sympathetic neurones *in vitro*. J. Physiol. Lond. *216*:625, 1971.

Banks, P., and Till, R.: A correlation between the effects of anti-mitotic drugs on microtubule assembly *in vitro* and the inhibition of axonal transport in noradrenergic neurons. J. Physiol. *252*:283, 1975.

Bernstein, H., Zvaifler, N., Rubin, M., and Mansour, S. A. M.: The ocular deposition of chloroquine. Inv. Ophthal. *2*:384, 1963.

Cancalon, P., and Beidler, L. M.: Distribution along the axon and into various subcellular fractions of molecules labelled with (^{3}H) leucine and rapidly transported in the garfish olfactory nerve. Brain Res. *89*:225, 1975.

Casey, E. B., Jellife, A. M., Le Quesne, P. M., and Millett, Y. L.: Vincristine neuropathy. Clinical and electrophysiological observations. Brain *96*:69, 1976.

Cowan, W. M. and Cuénod, M.: The Use of Axonal Transport for Studies of Neuronal Connectivity. Amsterdam, Elsevier, 1975.

Dahlström, A.: Effect of colchicine on transport of amine storage granules in sympathetic nerves of rat. Europ. J. Pharmacol. 5:111, 1968.

Dahlström, A.: Axoplasmic transport (with particular respect to adrenergic neurons). Phil. Trans. Roy. Soc. Lond. B. 261:325, 1971.

Dahlström, A., and Häggendal, J.: Studies on the transport and life-span of amine storage granules in a peripheral adrenergic neuron system. Acta. Physiol. Scand. 67:278, 1966.

Droz, B.: Renewal of synaptic proteins. Brain Res. 62:383, 1973.

Droz, B., Di Giamberardino, L., and Koenig, H. L.: Transports axonaux de macromolecules presynaptiques. Actual. Neurophysiol. 10:236, 1974.

Edström, A., and Mattsson, H.: Fast axonal transport in vitro in the sciatic system of the frog. J. Neurochem. 19:205, 1972.

Edström, A., and Mattsson, H.: Small amounts of zinc stimulate rapid axonal transport in vitro. Brain Res. 86:162, 1975.

Frizell, M., and Sjöstrand, J.: The axonal transport of ³H-fucose labelled glycoproteins in normal and regenerating peripheral nerves. Brain Res. 78:109, 1974a.

Frizell, M., and Sjöstrand, J.: Retrograde axonal transport of rapidly migrating proteins in the vagus and hypoglossal nerves of the rabbit. J. Neurochem. 23:651, 1974b.

Frizell, M., and Sjöstrand, J.: The axonal transport of slowly migrating ³H-leucine labelled proteins and the regeneration rate in regenerating hypoglossal and vagus nerves of the rabbit. Brain Res. 81:267, 1974c.

Frizell, M., and Sjöstrand, J.: Transport of proteins, glycoproteins and cholinergic enzymes in regenerating hypoglossal neurons. J. Neurochem. 22:845, 1974d.

Gutmann, E.: Neurotrophic relations. Ann. Rev. Physiol. 38:177, 1976.

Heslop, J. P.: Axonal flow and fast transport in nerves. Adv. Comp. Physiol. Biochem. 6:75, 1975.

Himes, R. H., Kersey, R. N., Heller-Bettinger, I., and Samson, F. E.: Action of the vinca alkaloids vincristine, vinblastine and desacetyl vinblastine amide on microtubules in vitro. Cancer Res. 36:3798, 1976.

Israel, M. A., Kuriyama, K., and Yoshikawa, K.: Effect of ethanol administration on axoplasmic flow in the brain. Neuropharmacology, 14:445, 1975.

Jablecki, C., and Brimijoin, S.: Reduced axoplasmic transport of choline acetyltransferase activity in dystrophic mice. Nature 250:151, 1974.

Jeffrey, P. L., and Austin, L.: Axoplasmic transport. Prog. Neuro. Biol. 5:205, 1973.

Johnson, J. L.: Glutamine in the dorsal sensory neuron. Brain. Res. 69:366, 1974.

Karlsson, J.-O., and Sjöstrand, J.: Characterization of the fast and slow components of axonal transport in retinal ganglion cells. J. Neurobiol. 2:135, 1971a.

Karlsson, J.-O., and Sjöstrand, J.: Characterization of the fast and slow components of axonal on cells. J. Neurochem. 18:749, 1971b.

Karlström, L., and Dahlström, A.: The effect of different types of axonal trauma on the synthesis and transport of amine storage granules in rat sciatic nerve. J. Neurobiol. 4:191, 1973.

Komiya, Y., and Austin, L.: Axoplasmic flow of protein in the scitatic nerve of normal and dystrophic mice. Exp. Neurol. 43:1, 1974.

Lasek, R.: Axoplasmic transport in cat dorsal root ganglion cells as studied with (³H)-L-leucine. Brain Res. 7:360, 1968.

Lasek, R.: Axonal transport and the use of intracellular markers in neuroanatomical investigations. Fed. Proc. 34:1603, 1975.

Livett, B. G.: Axonal transport and neuronal dynamics: contributions to the study of neuronal connectivity. In Porter, R.: International Review of Physiology, Neurophysiology II, Volume 10. Baltimore, University Park Press, 1976.

Lubinska, L.: On axoplasmic flow. Int. Rev. Neurobiol. 17:241, 1975.

McClure, W. O.: Effect of drugs on axoplasmic transport. Adv. Pharmac. Chemother. 10:185, 1972.

McLean, W. G., Frizell, M., and Sjöstrand, J.: Axonal transport of labelled proteins in sensory fibres of rabbit vagus nerve in vitro. J. Neurochem. 25:695, 1975.

McLean, W. G., Frizell, M., and Sjöstrand, J.: Slow axonal transport of labelled proteins in sensory fibers of rabbit vagus nerve. J. Neurochem. 26:1213, 1976a.

McLean, W. G., Frizell, M., and Sjöstrand, J.: Labelled proteins in rabbit vagus nerve between the fast and slow phases of axonal transport. J. Neurochem. 26:77, 1976b.

McLean, W. G., and Sjöstrand, J.: The effects of chloroquine and other retinotoxic drugs on axonal transport of proteins in rabbit vagus merve. Br. J. Pharmac. 60:302P, 1977.

Marchisio, P.-C., Gremo, F., and Sjöstrand, J.: Axonal transport in embryonic neurons. The possibility of a proximo-distal axolemmal transfer of glycoproteins. Brain Res. 85:281, 1975.

Marchisio, P.-C., and Sjöstrand, J.: Radioautographic evidence for protein transport along the optic pathway of early chick embryos. J. Neurocytol. *1*:101, 1972.

Markov, D., Rambourg, A., and Droz, B.: Smooth endoplasmic reticulum and fast axonal transport of glycoproteins, an electron microscope radioautograph study of thick sections after heavy metals impregnation. J. Microsc. Biol. Cell. *25*:57, 1976.

Meade, T. W.: Subacute myelo-optic neuropathy and clioquinol. An epidemiological case-history for diagnosis. Br. J. Prev. Soc. Med. *29*:157, 1975.

Miani, N.: Analysis of the somato-axonal movement of phospholipids in the vagus and hypoglossal nerves. J. Neurochem. *10*:859, 1963.

Nylander, U.: Ocular damage in chloroquine therapy. Acta Ophthalmol. *92*(Suppl.): 1, 1967.

Ochs, S., Dalrymple, D., and Richards, G.: Axoplasmic flow in ventral root nerve fibers of the cat. Exp. Neurol. *5*:349, 1962.

Ochs, S.: Rate of fast axoplasmic transport in mammalian nerve fibres. J. Physiol. (Lond.) *227*:627, 1972.

Ochs, S.: Systems of material transported in nerve fibers (axoplasmic transport) related to nerve function and trophic control. Ann. N.Y. Acad. Sci. *228*:202, 1974.

Paulson, J. C., and McClure, W. O.: Microtubules and axoplasmic transport. Brain Res. *73*:333, 1974.

Roberts, P. J., Keen, P., and Mitchell, J. F.: The distribution and axonal transport of free amino acids and related compounds in the dorsal sensory neuron of the rat, as determined by the dansyl reaction. J. Neurochem. *21*:199, 1973.

Roberts, S. M.: A review of the papers on the ocular toxicity of ethambutol hydrochloride (myambutol) an anti-tuberculosis drug. Am. J. Optom. Physiol. Opt. *51*:987, 1974.

Rydevik, B., McLean, W. G., Sjöstrand, J., and Lundborg, G.: Blockage of axonal transport induced by acute, graded compression of the rabbit vagus nerve. Submitted for publication 1979.

Schmidt, R. E.: Fast and slow axoplasmic flow in sciatic nerve of diabetic rats. Diabetes *24*:1081, 1975.

Seddon, H.: Surgical disorders of peripheral nerves. London, Churchill Livingstone, 1972.

Shearer, R. V., and DuBois, E. L.: Ocular changes included by long-term hydroxychloroquine (Plaquenil) therapy. Am. J. Ophthalmol. *64*:245, 1967.

Sjöstrand, J.: Rapid axoplasmic transport of labelled proteins in the vagus and hypoglossal nerves of the rabbit. Exp. Brain Res. *8*:105, 1969.

Sjöstrand, J.: Fast and slow components of axoplasmic transport in the hypoglossal and vagus nerves of the rabbit. Brain Res. *18*:461, 1970.

Sunderland, S.: The nerve lesion in the carpal tunnel syndrome. J. Neurol. Neurosurg. Psychiatry *39*:615, 1976.

Tang, B. Y., Komiya, Y., and Austin, L.: Axoplasmic flow of phospholipids and cholesterol in the sciatic nerve of normal and dystrophic mice. Exp. Neurol. *43*:13, 1974.

Wakabayashi, M., Araki, K., and Takahashi, Y.: Increased rate of fast axonal transport in methylmercury-induced neuropathy. Brain Res. *117*:524, 1976.

Weiss, P., and Hiscoe, H. B.: Experiments on the mechanism of nerve growth. J. Exp. Zool. *107*:315, 1948.

Willard, M., Cowan, W. M., and Vagelos, P. R.: The polypeptide composition of intra-axonally transported proteins; evidence for four transport velocities. Proc. Nat. Acad. Sci. U.S.A. *71*:2183, 1974.

Yates, R. A., and Roberts, P. J.: Effects of enucleation and intra-ocular colchicine on the amino acids of frog optic rectum. J. Neurochem. *23*:891, 1974.

Zinn, K. M.: Toxicology of the retinal pigment epithelium (thioridazine). Int. Ophthalmol. Clin. *15*:147, 1975.

60

AUTOMATED NERVE FIBER COUNTING IN COMPLEX ANIMAL NERVES

GARY K. FRYKMAN,
VIRCHEL E. WOOD,
and ERNEST L. HALL

Nerve regeneration following repair in humans is often far from ideal except in children. Many investigators have studied experimental animal models in order to define the factors that affect nerve regeneration, especially methods of repair; that is, epineurial, fascicular, or one stitch. Four categories of methods have been used in studying nerve regeneration in experimental animals: functional, electrophysiological, biochemical, and anatomical. A review of these methods reveals that they are often subjective and indirect, and give little quantitative information.

FUNCTIONAL METHODS

Functional studies such as walking pattern and withdrawal to painful stimuli are almost worthless, as the grading systems are subjective and most of the animals have return of all of these functions following nerve repair. (Mayer, Eiken and Nabseth, 1964; Bora, 1967; Cabaud et al., 1976).

928

ELECTROPHYSIOLOGICAL METHODS

One electrophysiological method, nerve conduction velocity, measures only the velocity of fast fibers but does not quantitate the numbers or function of the smaller diameter regenerated axons (Jacobson and Guth, 1965). The comparison of the amplitude of the compound action potential (Orgel and Terzis, 1977) is valid only if the size distribution of axons in the segments of nerves compared is the same. It is known that nerve conduction velocity is impaired in regenerated nerves, both proximal (Cragg and Thomas, 1961) and distal (Cragg and Thomas, 1964) to the injury site. Although reduction in axon diameter is well known in regenerated nerves, it apparently does not entirely account for the reduction in nerve conduction velocity observed (Cragg and Thomas, 1964). Schroder (1972) has suggested this is due to reduction in the ratio of myelin sheath thickness to axon diameter in regenerated nerves.

Electromyograms depend on sampling techniques and measure motor return only (Grabb, Bement, Koepke, and Green, 1970).

BIOCHEMICAL METHODS

Collagen assay (Pleasure, Bora, Lane, and Prockop, 1974) is a very indirect way to measure nerve regeneration. Its relationship to nerve regeneration is not well established. Myelin assays, however, may have a direct relationship to the number of regenerating nerve fibers (Bora, Pleasure, and Didizian, 1976).

ANATOMICAL METHODS

Histologic sections of the sensory end-organs have been studied (Dellon, 1976) but their precise value in assessing nerve regeneration has not yet been determined. Muscle sections depend on sampling techniques and give only a gross subjective estimate of the amount of muscle reinnervation. Comparisons of muscle mass, strength, and efficiency of contraction, however, have some correlation with other methods measuring nerve regeneration (Cabaud, et al., 1976).

The most direct anatomical method is to count the regenerated nerve fibers themselves. One must count axons or Schwann cell units (myelin sheaths), or both (Orgel and Terzis, 1977). The number of Schwann cell units and axons may not always be the same because there are several axons in each myelin tubule, at least in the early period of regeneration (Shawe, 1955).

Previously, others have relied on estimation of the number of nerve fibers present (Wise, Topuzlu, Davis, and Kaye, 1969) or on sampling techniques (Ritter, 1974), both of which are subject to inherent errors due to variability in size, distribution, and location of the nerve fibers. Manually counting all nerve fibers (Cabaud, et al., 1976) in a nerve trunk eliminates these errors. Previous counts have been done on small nerves, such as the recurrent laryngeal nerve of the rabbit, which has about 60 axons (Evans and Murray, 1956). It is easy to count numbers of this magnitude; however, when one is dealing with many thousands or a million or more axons, the magnitude of the task becomes overwhelming.

Most experimental models have dealt with very small nerves, whereas our clinical problem is with larger, more complex nerves. Previous studies have not shown whether large nerves regenerate in the same manner as small nerves. With advances in computer science and image processing fields, methods have been developed to count nerve fibers in cross sections from animal nerves (Potts, et al., 1972; O'Leary, Dunn, and Kumley, 1976). We propose that with an automated counting technique we could have an objective method to compare the number of regenerated nerve fibers following different techniques of nerve repair.

With this preliminary report we present only the method of automated nerve fiber counting (Casey, 1977).

METHOD

Preparation of Nerves

The sciatic nerve of the cat was studied, as it is unbranched for a 3 cm segment distal to the sciatic notch. The nerve was removed from a mongrel cat and placed in paraformaldehyde. Cross sections 1 mm thick were removed from the nerve and stained with osmic acid (which stains the myelin sheaths). The specimens were then embedded in an epoxy resin, Epon 812. Two micron cross sections were cut for mounting on glass slides. The best cross section (Fig. 60–1*A*) was photographed in a grid manner at 66× on 35 mm high contrast copy film transparencies, each frame slightly overlapping the adjacent one. A drawing of the entire nerve cross section was made for later orientation of the numbered transparencies. Figure 60–1*B* shows one frame of a fasciculus from the entire nerve cross section.

For manual counts, an 8 × 10 inch print was made of each frame.

We are counting the stained myelin sheaths (or Schwann cell units), which will be referred to here further as nerve fibers.

A block diagram of the overall scheme of automated counting is given in Figure 60–2.

Digitization

The first step in automated processing is digitization, which converts the film densities of the transparencies into numerical form. A diagram of the digitization process is shown in Figure 60–3. The scanning resolution or number of points per line was determined by considering the average axon sizes. To represent an axon of width 10 microns by 10 points requires a sample spacing of 1 micron between points. This resolution was achieved by the combination of 66 power magnification and digitization of 512 points per line. Each frame was therefore converted into an array of 512 lines with 512 points per line. The gray shade of each point, or pixel (picture element), was retained to an accuracy of 256 gray or density levels. The physical digitization was accomplished using a computer eye made by Spatial Data Systems of Santa Barbara, California. The computer eye consists of a television camera which scans a frame and the

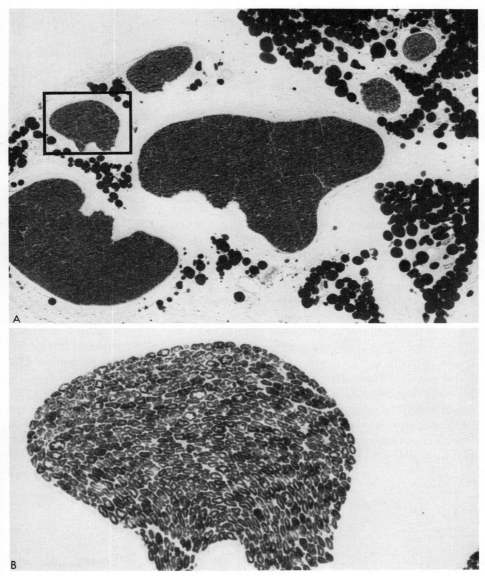

Figure 60–1 Cross sections of a typical nerve. *A*, An entire nerve cross section is shown. *B*, Print of one 35 mm frame taken from *A* at 66 ×.

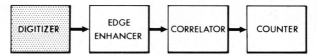

Figure 60–2   Block diagram of the four major steps in processing the 35 mm transparencies by the automated counting system.

electronics which converts the analog video signal to digital form and interfaces to the computer. The video monitor displays the image and allows for focusing and brightness adjustment. The time to digitize a frame is about 20 seconds.

For registration, the adjacent frames of a nerve were made to overlap slightly by a constant, known amount. In the processing, the overlapping lines and columns were deleted.

Segmenting Fascicular Regions

To provide accurate counts, the fascicular regions must be isolated from irrelevant background information such as fat globules. This step was performed in three ways, manually, interactively, and automatically. For manual segmentation, the non-fascicular regions were simply inked off, using a photographic opaque fluid. This method is inexpensive; however, judgment and a high degree of care are required. Since this method was time consuming, an interactive approach was developed. The digitized image was displayed on a monitor and an interactive "joystick" device used to outline the fascicular regions. The background could then be set to black and the resulting segmented image displayed for verification. It is interesting to note that a rough count of the number of axons can be derived by simply dividing the fascicular region area by the size of the average axon. Although the interactive segmentation is simple, it still becomes tedious with a large number of nerves. Therefore, an automated segmentation technique was developed. The automated step was difficult to develop because it is hard to define a criteria based upon brightness or size that differentiates between a fascicular region and a fat globule. The main criteria is that a fascicular region contains axons. Therefore, the matching technique used

Digitizer

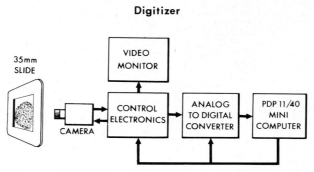

Figure 60–3   Diagram of the digitizer which converts the film image to numerical form for the computer to process.

to locate the axons is also used to locate the global fascicular regions. This technique will be described in a following section.

Image Enhancement

Owing to non-uniformities in the illumination source and response of the film and camera, the average brightness varies across the image, as demonstrated in Figure 60–4*A*. Thresholding assigns the value of white to every pixel with a value above a brightness threshold and black to every pixel below that value. Ideally, the process should segment the image into nerve fibers (white) and background (black). With a nonuniform illumination, thresholding does not produce the ideal response. To overcome this problem, an edge-enhanced image is produced by subtracting the local average brightness from the original image. This process, called unsharp masking, could be accomplished photographically by superimposing a blurred negative over the positive. A simple computer operation is used to produce an equivalent result. This edge-enhanced image can now be thresholded to produce an image in which the nerve fibers are white and the background black, as shown in Figure 60–4*B*.

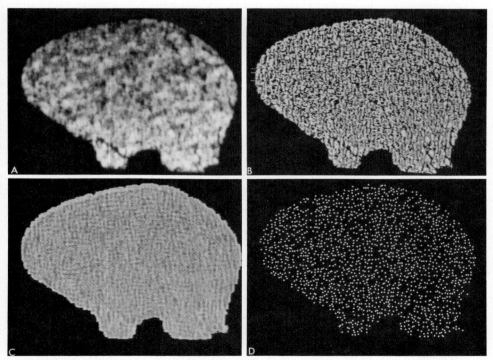

Figure 60–4   Steps in processing frame shown in Figure 60–1*B*. *A*, Original scanned image after digitization. *B*, Result of unsharp masking, which enhances edges of nerve fibers. *C*, Cross-correlation image resulting from template matching. *D*, Result of detecting peaks in the correlation image. These peaks correspond to match points of the template and a matching nerve fiber in the image. Each white dot represents one nerve fiber.

Nerve Fiber Location

Enhancing one of the more prominent features of the nerve fibers is a preprocessing step to counting. In order to count the nerve fiber, the computer must first find it. The method used to locate each nerve fiber is to compare each region of the picture with a reference mask or template of an average nerve fiber. This process is often called template matching. The reference mask was derived by interactively locating and numerically averaging many nerve fibers from several images and then thresholding the template to produce a binary-valued mask, as shown in Figure 60–4C. Nerve fibers are now located at all points in the image that have a high correlation between the reference mask and the region of the image. The computation of this correlation produces a cross-correlation image. A peak in the correlation indicates that a nerve fiber has been found, and its location is determined from the location of the peak. A new image can now be formed by placing the correlation values of the peak into a blank image, as shown in Figure 60–4D. Each bright spot on this new image corresponds to the location of a nerve fiber.

Since the location of a nerve fiber is a decision process, a statistical analysis can be performed to determine a threshold correlation value. If the correlation between the reference mask and the image region is above this correlation threshold, a detection is made and the nerve fiber counted. A further criterion, that the correlation location must be the peak value over a region the size of a nerve fiber, prevents multiple detections of the same fiber. A theoretical analysis of the probabilities of detection and false detection has also been made to characterize the system performance (Casey, 1977).

The data processing is accomplished on a medium speed minicomputer, a PDP 11/40, after development and testing of the algorithms on a larger PDP 10 computer. Both computers are made by Digital Equipment Corporation of Manard, Massachusetts. The programs are written mainly in FORTRAN, with several subroutines written in MACRO-11. The processing time is about five minutes per frame. Because of the binary nature of most of the computations, the total computation time could be greatly reduced with micro computers or special purpose hardware.

RESULTS

Manual Counts

Since manual counting of nerve fibers is the standard by which we compare automated counts, we must first find out how much variation occurs between two trained human counters. We found the difference was 2.24 per cent between the counts of these two individuals in counting over 8100 nerve fibers. This is within the 95 per cent confidence limits that this variation is due to random and not systematic errors.

A source of possible error in our method is the use of multiple frames for a single nerve cross section. Does the amount of overlap of adjacent frames vary enough to unnecessarily exclude some nerve fibers and count others twice? To study this error, two entire nerve cross sections were photographed a second time with the grid on a different axis (90 degress from the first). The count variance was 2.3 per cent in 18,000 nerve fibers in the first nerve cross section and 1.2 per cent in counting 26,000 fibers in the second nerve cross section. These results are again within the 95 per cent confidence limits that these are random errors only.

Manual Counting vs. Automated Counting

The results of comparing the counts on normal nerves are given in Table 60–1. From the table, one can see that the variance between manual and automated counts is greater than the difference between two human counters. However, there is a greater than 90 per cent accuracy when compared to manual counts. This accuracy is sufficient to apply this method to count nerve fibers in almost any size peripheral nerve in a large or small animal. It could be used to study nerve fiber branching in peripheral nerve trunks, and for other applications. Although we have not yet fully applied it, the computer can also generate information on size of nerve fibers.

We believe that further refinements in technique will bring the automated counts closer to the manual standard. However, the time saved has been considerable. It takes one person an eight hour day to count one entire nerve cross section and the computer now takes three hours or less.

Table 60–1 Nerve Fiber Counts

NERVE	MANUAL	AUTOMATED	DIFFERENCE	PER CENT
NN3-P	17,087	15,819	−1258	7.4
NN3-D	16,654	17,871	+1217	7.3
124-P	16,595	17,339	+ 744	4.5
124-D	24,865	24,772	− 93	0.3

Application of Automated Counting to Regenerated Nerves

Since regenerating axons and myelin sheaths are smaller in caliber than normal, slight alterations in the program are necessary in order to apply this method to counting regenerating nerve fibers. Since we are comparing counts proximal and distal to the site of nerve injury, we must demonstrate that the nerve fiber counts remain constant (or at least that the variation is known) across the length of the normal nerve being studied. The number of axons remains constant in the rabbit sciatic nerve for 36 mm, according to Shawe (1955), but some variability was found in human nerve segments by Lavarack, Sunderland and Ray (1951). No studies in cat sciatic nerves were found. We found that the proximal and distal counts 3 cm apart over the sciatic nerve in one cat were 17,087 and 16,654, respectively. The difference of 433 is within random error of counting only.

A second assumption that has been made is that more nerve fibers growing distally means better regeneration. This assumption is strained by the phenomenon of axon sprouting or collateral regeneration. Following nerve section, an axon will sprout many times in order to find empty tubules for distal growth. Previous studies in rabbits have shown that the number of axons found distally does not necessarily equal the number of Schwann cell units, as many myelin sheaths contain up to four axons (Evans and Murray, 1956; Shawne, 1955). The number of distal axons does not remain constant with time, as it was found that the distal nerve fiber count tends to increase with time up to 150 days in rabbit nerves (Evans and Murray, 1956). The number of fibers increases distally as far as 50 mm distal to the nerve section (Shawne, 1955). Nerve fiber counts also increase with laceration compared to crush injury (Evans and Murray, 1956). Thus, there are a number of variables that need to be held constant if one is going to use this method to compare nerve suture techniques.

We are applying this method to compare the number of regenerated nerve fibers in six months following each of three methods of nerve repair: epineurial, fascicular, and one stitch.

SUMMARY

We have developed a new, automated method of counting nerve fibers in cross sections. The stained nerve cross sections from the cat sciatic nerve are photographed and scanned with a video camera, and the images are digitized. The digitized data is then preprocessed by image enhancement techniques. The nerve fibers are located in the digitized image by matching them with a representative mask. Closeness of the match is determined by binary correlation. After the cross section images have been digitized, the system runs automatically.

Using manually counted normal nerves for a standard, the system has been found to be more than 90 per cent accurate.

This technique shows promise for many future applications as a tool to study normal and regenerated nerves.

REFERENCES

Bora, F. W.: Peripheral nerve repair in cats. J. Bone Joint Surg., 49A:659, 1967.

Bora, F. W., Pleasure, D. E., and Didizian, N. A.: A study of nerve regeneration and neuroma formation after nerve suture by various techniques. J. Hand. Surg., 1:138, 1976.

Cabaud, H. E., Rodkey, W. G., McCarroll, H. R., Mutz, S. B., and Neibauer, J. J.: Epineurial and perineurial fascicular nerve repairs: A critical comparison. J. Hand Surg. 1:131, 1976.

Casey, M. E.: Automated particle counting with applications to neurology. Masters Thesis, University of Tennessee, Knoxville, August 1977.

Cragg, B. G., and Thomas, P. K.: Changes in conduction velocity and fiber size proximal to peripheral nerve lesions. J. Physiol. (London) 157:315, 1961.

Cragg, B. G., and Thomas, P. K.: The conduction velocity of regenerated peripheral nerve fibers. J. Physiol. 171:164, 1964.

Dellon, A. L.: Reinnervation of denervated Meissner corpuscles: A sequential histologic study in the monkey following fascicular nerve repair. J. Hand. Surg. 1:98, 1976.

Evans, D. H. L., and Murray, J. G.: A study of regeneration in a motor nerve with a unimodal fiber diameter distribution. Anat. Rec. 126:311, 1956.

Grabb, W. C.: Median and ulnar nerve suture — an experimental study comparing primary and secondary repair in monkeys. J. Bone Joint Surg., 50:964, 1968.

Grabb, W. C., Bement, S. L., Koepke, G. H., and Green, R. A.: Comparison of methods of peripheral nerve suturing in monkeys. Plast. Reconst. Surg., 46:31, 1970.

Hudson, A. R., Morris, J., Weddell, G., and Drury, A.: Peripheral nerve autografts. J. Surg. Res. 12:267, 1972.

Jacobson, S., and Guth, L.: An electrophysiological study of the early stages of peripheral nerve regeneration. Exp. Neurol. *11*:48, 1965.

Lavarack, J. O., Sunderland, S., and Ray, L. J.: The branching of nerve fibers in human cutaneous nerves. J. Comp. Neurol. *94*:293, 1951.

Mayer, R. F., Eiken, O., and Nabseth, D. C.: Nerve regeneration in replanted canine limbs. Am. J. Physiol. *206*:1415, 1964.

O'Leary, D. P., Dunn, R. F., and Kumley, W. E.: On-line computerized entry and display of nerve fiber cross sections using single or segmented histological records. Computers and Biomed. Res., *9*:229, 1976.

Orgell, M. G., and Terzis, J. K.: Epineurial vs perineurial repair, an ultrastructural and electrophysiological study of nerve regeneration. Plast. Reconstr. Surg. *60*:80, 1977.

Pleasure, D., Bora, F., Lane, J., and Prockop, D.: Regeneration after nerve transection: Effect of inhibition of collagen synthesis. Exp. Neurol. *45*:72, 1974.

Potts, A. M., Hodges, D., Shelman, C. B., Fritz, K. J., Levy, N. S., and Mangnall, Y.: Morphology of the primate optic nerve. I. Method and total fiber count. Inves. Ophth. *11*:980, 1972.

Ritter, M. A.: A histological evaluation of peripheral nerve repairs. Clin. Orthop. *103*:279, 1974.

Schröder, J. M.: Altered ratio between axon diameter and myelin sheath thickness in regenerated nerve fibers. Brain Res. *45*:49, 1972.

Shawe, G. D. H.: On the number of branches formed by regenerating nerve fibers. Br. J. Surg. *42*:474, 1955.

Wise, A. J., Topuzlu, C., Davis, P., and Kaye, I. S.: A comparative analysis of macro- and microsurgical neurorrhapy technics. Am. J. Surg. *117*:566, 1969.

61

COORDINATION OF AXON NEUROPHYSIOLOGY AND AXON COUNTING TECHNIQUES IN NERVE REGENERATION

MICHAEL G. ORGEL and
JULIA K. TERZIS

INTRODUCTION

Peripheral nerve regeneration after injury and surgical repair is often incomplete, resulting in distorted sensory and motor function of the denervated part. This problem has been approached both clinically and in the research laboratory. Clinically, improvements in surgical technique have aimed at maximizing axonal regeneration and deleting the greatest obstacle to successful nerve repair, namely, scar at the anastomosis. The introduction of the operating microscope in peripheral nerve surgery (Kurze, 1964; Smith, 1964) has led to more accurate alignment of nerve bundles (Bora, 1967; Goto, 1967; Hakstian, 1968; Grabb, et al., 1970) and tensionless repair with interfascicular nerve grafts when nerve substance is missing (Millesi, 1972). Assessment of peripheral nerve function is currently made by subjective sensory and motor testing and electrophysiological procedures. As the latter become more sophisticated (Terzis et al., 1976), more meaningful data will be obtained; for ex-

938

ample, individual fascicular recordings can now be used intraoperatively to define the problem of the neuroma in continuity (Williams and Terzis, 1976).

The laboratory setting enhances the potential for study of nerve regeneration after injury. Objective electrophysiological studies can be made, and these can be correlated directly with the morphology of the repaired peripheral nerve, something that is rarely available clinically. Many experimental studies have been concerned with this problem (Bora, 1967; Goto, 1967; Grabb et al., 1970). However, the results of nerve regeneration in these various models have been assessed mainly by qualitative or semi-quantitative techniques. Less frequently, assessment has been made by quantitation of the data (Hudson et al., 1972; Bora et al., 1976; Cabaud et al., 1976).

Techniques have been developed in our laboratories that for the first time combine functional (Terzis, 1976) and morphological (Orgel et al., 1972; Orgel and Terzis, 1977) assessment of nerve regeneration. Furthermore, these electrophysiological and anatomical parameters can be quantitated in the same animal model. It is the purpose of this section to describe these techniques and their applicability to the study of peripheral nerve regeneration following injury and repair.

ANIMAL MODEL

The rabbit has been chosen as the experimental animal for all work to date. Reasons for this choice were as follows: This animal has been used in many basic studies concerning cutaneous sensibility and nerve regeneration, and considerable knowledge has been accumulated (Weddell, 1942; Weddell et al., 1955; Guth, 1956); the sciatic nerve of the rabbit is an easily accessible structure with a constant trifascicular pattern that lends itself to experimental work; cost and upkeep are quite reasonable. Serious consideration has been given to a primate model, which more closely corresponds in anatomy and physiology to man; however, lack of primate housing facilities and high costs for purchase and maintenance have made this impractical to date.

METHODS

In the discussions that follow, the techniques used to study nerve regeneration in the rabbit model will first be described and, subsequently, the application of these procedures to specific problems will be considered. In all cases, the various types of nerve repairs to be compared are executed by the same operator. This is necessary to avoid variables in surgical technique. Enough animals are prepared in each study to satisfy statistical analysis of the data. All animals are allowed to survive for the designated periods of study and then randomized for "double blind" study.

Electrophysiological Assessment

This section provides a brief discussion of the compound action potential (CAP), followed by a description of the procedures involved in the electrophysiological assessment of nerve regeneration in the present model.

When a suprathreshold electrical stimulus is applied to a peripheral nerve, a compound action potential (CAP) results which can be recorded with extracellular electrodes. This evoked potential is the algebraic sum of individual fiber action potentials. Although each of the constituent fibers within a nerve trunk obeys the all-or-none law in its response characteristics, the compound potential is a continuously graded response whose amplitude and shape are influenced by changes in the stimulus strength. This results because contributing fibers have different fiber diameters, thresholds of excitation, and conduction velocities. The CAP provides a remarkable amount of information about the functional integrity of the nerve. The mere presence or absence of the CAP is very informative. The size of the CAP is another parameter that provides valuable data, but in relative terms; that is, if it can be compared to another CAP from a normal nerve or single fascicle in the same recording arrangement. The speed of impulse transmission is an accurate measurable quantity that gives an indication of the size of the fibers contributing to the CAP. Since conduction velocity is related to axon diameter, internodal length, and degree of myelination, diseased and immature regenerating axons can be pinpointed by their slower speed of signal transmission. Finally, the shape of CAP offers a qualitative assessment of the functional status of the nerve.

The physiological assessment of the present nerve model involves the following procedures. Under intravenous urethane anesthesia (25 per cent w/v in distilled water; 3 mg per kg body weight until corneal reflex disappeared) the sciatic nerve under study is surgically re-exposed and submitted to electrophysiological recordings (Terzis et al., 1975; Terzis, 1976; Williams and Terzis, 1976). This involves placing platinum stimulating electrodes on the individual fascicles distal to the repair and recording from the corresponding fascicles in the proximal nerve segment. The impulses elicited are amplified $1000 \times$ by a Textronix 122 preamplifier and then introduced into an oscilloscope for visualization of the evoked compound action potential. An S_4 Grass stimulator is utilized for the generation of the electrical pulse. The threshold for stimulation and the responses at different stimulus strengths are accurately determined. Permanent photographic records are obtained with a Grass C_4 oscillographic camera and stored for later analysis of the shape, amplitude, and latency of the evoked signals. The distance between stimulating and recording electrodes is measured at the completion of each recording arrangement to determine the conduction velocity of the compound action potentials. The type of repair in each tested animal (that is, whether epineurial, perineurial or control) is unknown to the examiner. All electrophysiological data are analyzed and tabulated prior to breaking the code.

Morphological Assessment

Although there may be specific histological requirements for individual experiments, the following narrative gives an account of the general procedure followed for morphological study. Upon completion of the electrophysiological studies, the major artery supplying the nerve under consideration is cannulated and locally heparinized. This is followed by perfusion with saline to clear blood cells from the vessels of the nerve, and then perfusion with 3 per cent (cacodylate or phosphate) buffered glutaraldehyde. It has been found that this perfusion technique results in better ultramicroscopic detail than do immersion techniques.

The treated peripheral nerve (Fig. 61–1), including the neuroma and 1 to 2 cm of proximal and distal nerve, is then excised. Only two of the three fascicles are used for the morphological study and these are kept constant throughout the series. In the first, 1 mm transverse incisional biopsies (cut with a razor to avoid crushing) are taken, beginning approximately 1 cm distal to the neuroma. Four to five specimens are removed to ensure an excellent choice of material. This material can be stored in fresh 3 per cent buffered glutaraldehyde at 4° C until processed for ultramicroscopy. The second fascicle is utilized for qualitative study of the longitudinal pattern of recovery. This is accomplished by pinning the rest of the excised nerve to wax to preserve length.

Processing of the transverse biopsies is done by accepted ultramicroscopic technique consisting of post-fixation in osmium tetroxide, dehydration in graduated alcohols, and embedding in an epoxy resin. Care is taken to embed the material "squarely" so that a complete transverse section of the fascicle can be cut on the ultramicrotome. This material is utilized for both light and electron microscopy. For light microscopy, 1 micron sections are counterstained with toluidine blue (Fig. 61–2) (or 1 per cent phenylenediamine if phase

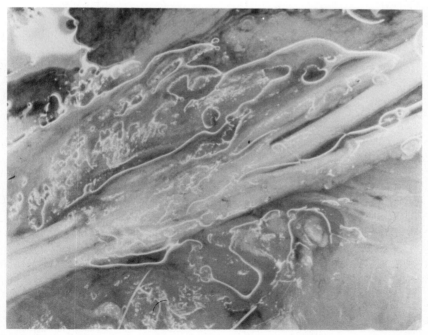

Figure 61–1 Rabbit sciatic nerve after perfusion with 3 per cent buffered glutaraldehyde. Left, proximal — note trifascicular structure. Central, neuroma. Right, distal — transverse biopsies are cut from a fascicle (same in all animals) 1 cm distal to the neuroma.

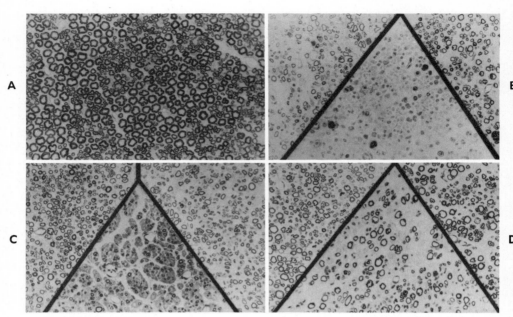

Figure 61–2 Studies under light microscope. *A,* Transverse section of the normal central fascicle of a rabbit's sciatic nerve. *B,* Two month study. The distal stump of the central fascicle of an epineurial repair is demonstrated on the left; of a perineurial repair on the right; and of a control (lacerated, not sutured) in the center. *C,* Four month study. The epineurial repair is on the left, the perineurial repair is on the right, and the control is in the center. *D,* Six month study. The epineurial repair is on the left, the perineurial repair is on the right, and the control is in the center. (Toluidine blue, × 1000.) (From Orgel, M. G., and Terzis, J. K.: Epineurial vs. perineurial repair: An ultrastructural and electrophysiological study of nerve regeneration. Plast. Reconstr. Surg. *60*:80, 1977.)

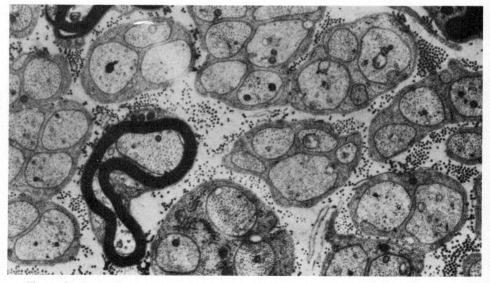

Figure 61–3 Studies under electron microscope. This is a representative area of the normal central fascicle of a rabbit sciatic nerve. Note the myelinated and unmyelinated fibers. (× 10,000).

microscopy is preferred). Preview of this material allows the investigator to choose good areas for electron microscopy. The same blocks are then used to cut ultra thin (silver interference pattern) electron-microscopic sections, which are stained with lead citrate (Fig. 61–3).

Tissue Study

Quantitative study of the total regenerating axonal populations is now possible by utilizing high power light microscopy for study of the myelinated fibers and electron microscopy for study of the unmyelinated fibers (Dyck and Lambert, 1966; Aguayo et al., 1973).

The 1 micron sections are photographed* (see Fig. 61–2) and enlarged 1000 × (so that measurements in millimeters can be translated directly to microns). Care is taken to include all areas of the transverse section and the full perin-eurial perimeter in these photomicrographs. All myelinated fibers in each transverse section are then measured with a Zeiss (TGZ-3) particle size an-alyzer. The total area of each bundle is defined by planimetry. From this data, fiber caliber histograms can be constructed. In addition, the area of each bun-dle occupied by myelinated fibers and the number of myelinated fibers per square millimeter can be calculated (Aguayo, 1975).

Unmyelinated fibers are studied utilizing electronphotomicrographs** (see Fig. 61–3) enlarged 10,000 ×*** (so that measurements in millimeters can be translated directly to tenths of a micron). It is quite difficult with this model to study the total cross-sectional area of a fascicle at 10,000 × magnification, therefore, our electron microscope technique has gradually evolved through-out these experiments. At present, a representative area between grid bars is totally photographed, and this area is defined by planimetry. With this differ-ence in mind, similar histogram construction and calculations, as noted above for myelinated fibers, can be derived for unmyelinated fibers. In addition, the number of unmyelinated fibers per axon–Schwann cell complex and the num-ber of these complexes per square millimeter can be determined.

The derived quantitative data are then submitted to statistical analysis by Students' "t" test or the Mann Whitney "U" test.

Tissue study of a second fascicle is made by postfixation of the remaining nerve in Flemmings' chrome-osmium-acetic solution and embedding it in par-affin. Five micron longitudinal sections (through the proximal stump, neuro-ma, and distal stump of the second fascicle) are counterstained by the modi-fied Weigert method (Gutmann and Sanders, 1943) for qualitative study of axonal organization across the area of repair, amount of regenerating fibers in the distal stump, and amount of scar tissue in the neuroma (Fig. 61–4).

---

*Zeiss Photomicroscope — 1.
**Hitache Electron microscope HU011B.
***Ladd Research, Inc. Grid #5000.

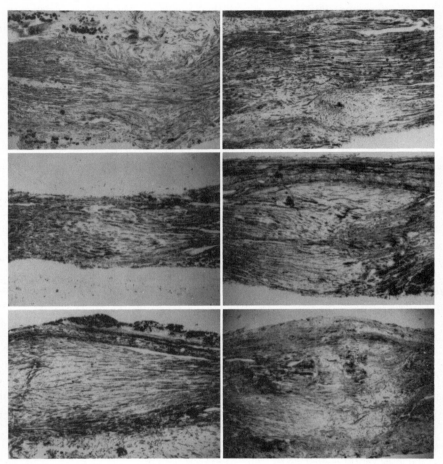

Figure 61–4 Studies of longitudinal (Flemming's) preparations after nerve repairs. In the left column we see the epineurial repairs; in the right column, the perineurial repairs. *Top,* Representative areas from the distal stumps at two months. *Center,* The same at four months. *Bottom,* At five months. There is no consistent pattern or consistent superiority for either method of repair. (From Orgel, M. G., and Terzis, J. K.: Epineurial vs. perineurial repair: An ultrastructural and electrophysiological study of nerve regeneration. Plast. Reconstr. Surg. *60*:80, 1977.)

APPLICATIONS OF THE MODEL TOWARD SOLUTION OF THE PROBLEM

Sensory Nerve Regeneration

MORPHOLOGICAL ASPECTS OF REINNERVATION OF FREE SKIN GRAFTS (Orgel et al., 1972).   Free skin transplants represent pure sensory denervated preparations and have been shown to acquire incomplete function (Moberg, 1958; Mannerfelt, 1962). In this study we investigated the morphological characteristics and sequential course of cutaneous reinnervation of skin grafts in 30 white male rabbits. Full thickness grafts were excised from the left scrotum and were applied to full thickness defects on the dorsolateral aspect of the right ear. The animals were divided into six groups of five, and were studied sequentially from one to six months. Emphasis was placed on the corpuscular nerve endings, fiber caliber, and myelinated and unmyelinated fiber ratios in the grafts, as compared to those in normal skin.

Results

The longitudinal pattern of nerve recovery was surveyed in vivo with the use of methylene-blue as a vital stain. As previously shown (Adeymo and Wyburn, 1957), regenerating nerves were seen to enter the grafts from both the sides and the graft bed, the latter probably being the more significant contributor. No encapsulated nerve endings were found in the grafted skin, al-

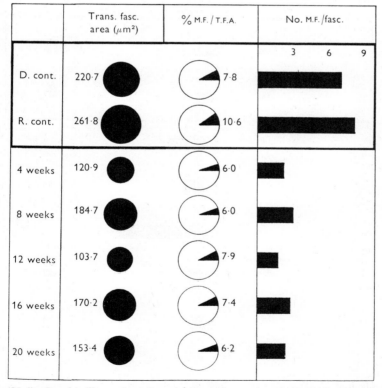

Figure 61–5 Graphic illustration of results from phase microscopy. Trans. Fasc. area = transverse fascicular area. There is a significant decrease in size of nerve bundles in all grafts compared to recipient controls. % M.F./T.F.A. = percentage of myelinated fibers per transverse fascicular area. The area occupied by myelinated fibers in graft nerves is also reduced. No. M.F./fasc. = number of myelinated fibers per fascicle. The number of myelinated fibers is significantly decreased in nerve bundles from grafts. (From Orgel, M., Aguayo, A., and Williams, H. B.: Sensory nerve regeneration: An experimental study of skin grafts in the rabbit. J. Anat. *111*:121, 1972.)

though such corpuscles were abundant in both donor and recipient control skin. In addition, the grafts revealed a greater nerve density than did controls; this was especially notable at 12 to 16 weeks after transplantation.

The quantitative portion of this study (Fig. 61–5) revealed smaller nerve bundles in the skin grafts than in controls, and their contents were dissimilar. The area of each nerve bundle occupied by myelinated fibers was found to be decreased in the grafts. In addition, the absolute number of myelinated fibers per nerve bundle in the grafts was significantly decreased, and this parameter showed no propensity to increase with time. However, the mean caliber of regenerating myelinated fibers was not significantly different in the grafts when compared to normal skin.

Study of the unmyelinated fiber population (Fig. 61–6) revealed a greater number of axons per axon-Schwann cell complex in all grafts compared to

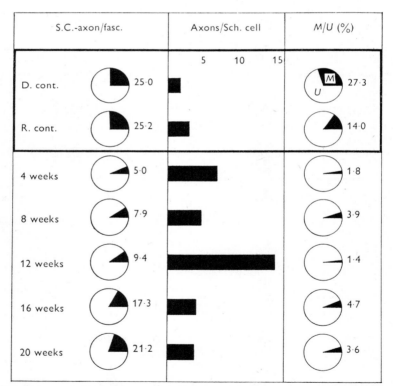

Figure 61–6 Graphic illustration of quantitative results from electron microscopic studies. S.C.-axon/fasc. = Schwann cell–axon complexes (dark) per fascicle. Note the sequential increase of Schwann cell–axon complexes per nerve bundle in the grafts. Axons/Sch. cell = mean number of axons per Schwann cell. There is a significant increase in the number of unmyelinated axons per Schwann cell throughout the study, most marked at 12 weeks. M/U(%) = percentage of fascicle shared by myelinated (M) and unmyelinated (U) fibers. In all grafts there is a significantly larger percentage of unmyelinated fibers (U) than in controls, while that of the myelinated fibers is reduced. (From Orgel, M., Aguavo, A., and Williams, H. B.: Sensory nerve regeneration: An experimental study of skin grafts in the rabbit. J. Anat. *111*:121, 1972.)

control skin. In addition, a relative and absolute increase in unmyelinated fibers was seen in the grafts throughout the study. Again, the mean caliber of regenerating unmyelinated fibers did not significantly differ from the norm.

Discussion

The finding of nerve endings in both normal donor and recipient skin and their absence in the graft is most likely due to the inability of this species to form new terminals. The failure of sensory nerve endings to redevelop in transplanted skin may contribute to diminished sensory function.

Quantitation of phase and electron microscopic findings showed the total number of myelinated fibers per nerve in the grafts to be significantly decreased. The normal ratio of myelinated to unmyelinated fibers seen in control skin was not attained by the grafts, and unmyelinated fibers were increased both relatively and absolutely throughout the study. We suggest that there is a critical balance between myelinated and unmyelinated fibers in nerves of the skin, and that this equilibrium is disrupted following nerve injury.

Functional Aspects of Reinnervation of Free Skin Grafts (Terzis, 1976)

The limited return of sensory capabilities observed in skin transplants in man, along with an absence of physiological documentation of the processes involved in skin graft reinnervation, necessitated this study to provide functional correlation to the morphological analysis. Such functional correlates take advantage either of the electrical activity of afferent fibers that supply normal skin or of regenerating fibers that invade previously denervated skin preparations. Tactile stimuli of sufficient intensity and proper quality delivered to areas of the body surface will evoke a discharge of impulses in the supplying sensory axon. Each sensory fiber terminates in a specified area of skin, known as a peirpheral receptive field, within which application of a mechanical stimulus will result in its excitation. The evoked signals are relayed by the sensory fiber centrally, where conscious appreciation of the sensory experience takes place. An electrode placed at any point in this pathway can sample these electrical signals, and thus detailed analysis of peripheral events can be accomplished.

In this study a technique was introduced in which electrophysiological recordings from individual mechanoreceptors of the skin were obtained following mechanical stimulation, and used to objectively study the sequential course of reinnervation in free skin grafts (Fig. 61–7).

Forty-eight white male rabbits had skin grafts applied as previously described (see Morphological Study). Functional reinnervation was studied at regular intervals for 15 months, and the physiological data obtained from the grafted groups were correlated with the findings of the control group. A detailed description of the electrophysiological procedures is available elsewhere (Terzis, 1976).

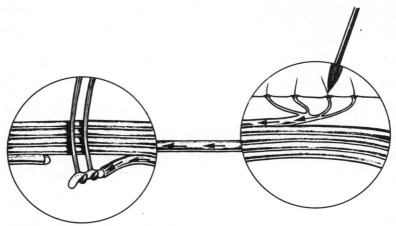

Figure 61-7   Diagrammatic representation of the single unit recording technique. Sharply localized mechanical stimulation of the skin (circle on the right) elicits impulses (arrows) which are mediated in the sensory nerve. A proximal recording electrode (circle on the left) can sample this activity.

Results

There was no evidence of reinnervation prior to three weeks. From three weeks to two months, the sensory fibers entering the skin grafts had slow conduction velocites (6–10 M/sec), indicative of a prevalent unmyelinated fiber population. The majority of regenerating fibers remained unmyelinated

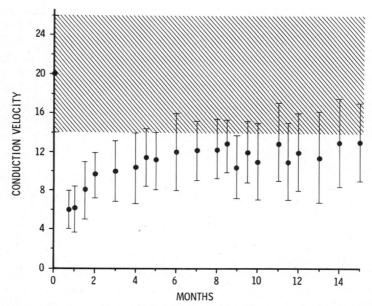

Figure 61-8   Mean conduction velocity (M/sec) versus time (months). The shaded area corresponds to the mean conduction velocity of the control group. The vertical lines depict values from the skin grafted groups at various time intervals.

up to four months. An increasing amount of myelination was acquired by six months, at which time a plateau was reached. Older skin grafts exhibited only a slow transition toward greater afferent fiber myelination and faster conduction velocities. Physiological parameters obtained from normal skin (control group) demonstrated significant differences from the treated groups (P>0.05). Physiologically, normal sensory recovery was not accomplished even after 15 months following skin graft placement (Fig. 61–8).

Discussion

Normal sensory perception is the end result of the afferent input reaching the central nervous system. In the case of cutaneous sensibility, a mechanical stimulus applied to skin causes a local change in the permeability of the sensory receptor (generator potential), which then invades by electrotonic spread the adjacent region of the parent axon, and if threshold is achieved a conducted action potential results. Thus, cutaneous mechanoreceptors are the critical intermediary, transducing sets of external stimuli into patterns of impulses. The spatial distribution and density of the various receptors in the skin also influence sensory awareness. The absence of receptors in skin grafts (Ridley, 1970; Orgel et al., 1972) may explain in part the altered physiological findings observed in this study and detrimentally affect normal sensory perception.

It is known that there is a correlation between the sensations mediated and the diameters of the afferent fibers that mediate this sensory input (Mountcastle, 1968). If the population ratio between myelinated and unmyelinated fibers changes, sensory disturbance is likely. Distortion of the fiber population reinnervating the skin grafts has been documented both ultrastructurally (Orgel, 1972) and electrophysiologically in this study. That this imbalance is due to the inability of the regenerating fibers to make contact with proper sensory receptors is a tempting speculation. The importance of the peripheral influence of the end-organ on its supplying nerve fiber has been stressed by numerous workers (Sanders and Young, 1944; Weiss and Taylor, 1944; Aitken, 1949). The absolute increment in the unmyelinated fiber population throughout both of these studies could reflect lack of such peripheral connections, thus resulting in failure of the regenerating fibers to mature. We suggest that these altered mechanisms may account for the distorted sensory experiences sometimes arising in skin grafts in man.

Epineurial vs. Perineurial Suture

Coordinated Morphology and Electrophysiology (Orgel and Terzis, 1977)

It became apparent after the above studies that coordination of axon physiology and counting techniques in nerve regeneration studies was desirable. The following study was thus conceived and executed in the same animal model.

The repair of lacerated peripheral nerves by suturing the epineurium has been traditional since the 1800's. However, a significant percentage of patients treated by this method do not obtain useful functional results, and other means of nerve repair have been sought. Suture of the perineurium was first advocated in 1917 (Langley and Hashimoto), but this recommendation was largely disregarded, primarily because the technical refinements were not yet available. Since the introduction of the operating microscope in peripheral nerve surgery, interest in perineurial repair has been renewed. However, clinicians have been skeptical about accepting this more laborious technique in the absence of evidence that clearly points to its advantage.

Experimental work comparing the two methods of suture has included subjective assessment of functional return, histological observation, biochemical assay, assessment of nerve conduction and muscle tension, and electromyography (Bora et al., 1967; Goto, 1967; Wise et al., 1969; Grabb et al., 1970; Yamamoto, 1974; Bora et al., 1976; Cabaud et al., 1976). However, the information available has been inadequate to resolve the controversy.

Methods

Forty-eight white male rabbits were divided into six groups of eight animals to be studied sequentially from one to six months after surgery. The left sciatic nerve of each animal was sharply transected 4 cm from the sciatic notch. Three animals in each group underwent an epineurial repair, three a perineurial repair, and two served as controls in which the transected nerve was aligned but not sutured. All the nerve repairs were conducted under the operating microscope utilizing microsurgical techniques. Animals were allowed to survive for their designated period of study and then randomized for "double blind" study.

Results

The longitudinal pattern of recovery was assessed for axonal organization across the suture line, for the number of regenerating fibers present in the distal stump, and for the amount of scar tissue in the neuroma (thus simulating previous studies). These parameters varied considerably over the sequence of the study, and we were unable to determine any consistent pattern or superiority for either method of repair by this technique (see Fig. 61–4).

The remaining portion of this study was based on quantitative data.

Morphology

LIGHT MICROSCOPY. *Myelinated Fiber Study* (Fig. 61–9). Both the epineurial and perineurial repairs showed a significantly greater area of myelinated fiber coverage than did the controls at all periods of study. There was a general trend (seen at specific intervals) toward greater myelinated fiber coverage in the perineurial repairs; this was not statistically significant when comparing all animals in each repair group. In addition, perineurial repairs

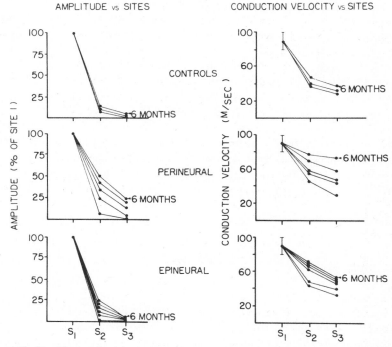

Figure 61–9 Epineurial versus perineurial myelinated fiber study — six month animals. Note the trend toward greater myelinated fiber coverage, and larger number of myelinated fibers per square millimeter in the perineurial repairs. M.F. = myelinated fibers; MEAN CAL = mean caliber.

	% COVER	M.F./SQ.MM.	MEAN CAL.(μ)
NORMAL	20.8	10,584	4.1
CONTROL	6.8	7749	2.9
EPINEUR	11.1	9632	3.3
PERINEUR	12.9	11,535	3.3

	AXONS/S.C.C.	MEAN CAL.(μ)
NORMAL	3.1	0.74
CONTROL	3.0	0.60
EPINEUR	2.3	0.50
PERINEUR	3.1	0.50

Figure 61–10 Epineurial versus perineurial unmyelinated fiber study — five and six month animals. No significant difference in numbers of axons per Schwann cell complex (S.C.C.) or in mean caliber is seen between the repair groups.

Figure 61–11 Electrophysiological results. The amplitude of the action potentials (expressed as a percentage of proximal stump values) and the conduction velocity were measured at three sites. (S_1 = the proximal stump; S_2 = immediately distal to the repair; S_3 = the distal stump.) Note the improvement in the amplitudes and in the conduction velocities with time, and the tendency toward greater electrophysiological return in the perineurial repairs. (From Orgel, M. G., and Terzis, J. K.: Epineurial vs. perineurial repair: An ultrastructural and electrophysiological study of nerve regeneration. Plast. Reconstr. Surg., *60*:80, 1977.)

showed a greater number of myelinated fibers per square millimeter in most study periods, which also became statistically insignificant when comparison was made between all animals in each repair group. The same tendency was seen in larger myelinated fibers in nerves repaired by perineurial suture, which again was not significant when all animals of each group were combined.

ELECTRON MICROSCOPY. *Unmyelinated Fiber Study* (Fig. 61–10). There was no significant difference in the unmyelinated fiber caliber achieved by either repair groups or controls. Similarly, no difference was noted in the number of axons per axon–Schwann cell complex.

ELECTROPHYSIOLOGY. The amplitude of action potentials and conduction velocities was measured at three sites. The first, proximal to the repair, the second, immediately distal to the repair, and the third, in the distal stump. In both repair groups, the functional return (Fig. 61–11) was superior to that in the controls and improved with time. There was a tendency toward greater amplitude and faster conduction velocities in the perineurial repairs.

Discussion

In the perineurial repairs the trend toward larger myelinated fibers, greater area of coverage, and a greater density of fibers was supported by the greater amplitude of the action potentials and faster conduction velocities. However, the results derived from the two types of repairs were not as dissimilar as expected. This was most likely due to the nerve model chosen — only three fascicles were present, and the epineurium was thin and translucent. It was, therefore, quite easy to align the fascicles under the microscope even in the epineurial repairs. It is an important observation that repair of the perineurium led to superior results under these circumstances. It seems reasonable to assume from these findings that a lacerated mixed peripheral nerve in man consisting of multiple fasciculi, an abundance of epineurial connective tissue, and problems with alignment would have a better chance for good functional nerve regeneration after perineurial rather than epineurial repair.

SUMMARY

A laboratory model for the study of nerve regeneration after injury has been presented, and a detailed account of the methodology has been given. Applications of this model toward the solution of two clinically relevant problems have been described. These include nerve regeneration in skin grafts, and epineurial vs. perineurial suture techniques.

This quantitative nerve regeneration model is a dynamic tool of investigation that allows the structural and functional aspects of nerve regeneration to be studied simultaneously for the first time by a critical objective approach. This model will serve as the basis of the study of other traumatic peripheral neuropathies.

REFERENCES

Adeymo, O., and Wyburn, G. M.: Innervation of skin grafts. Transpl. Bull. 4:152, 1957.

Aguayo, A. J., Peyronnard, J. M., and Bray, G. M.: A quantitative ultrastructural study of regeneration from isolated proximal stumps of transected unmyelinated nerves. J. Neuropath. Exper. Neurol. 32:256, 1973.

Aguayo, A. J.: Personal communication, 1975.

Aitken, J. T.: The effect of peripheral connections on the maturation of regenerating nerve fibers. J. Anat. 83:32, 1949.

Bora, F. W.: Peripheral nerve repair in cats. The fascicular stitch. J. Bone Joint Surg. 49A:659, 1967.

Bora, F. W., Pleasure, D. E., and Didizian, N. A.: A study of nerve regeneration and neuroma formation after suture by various techniques. J. Hand Surg. 1:138, 1976.

Cabaud, H. E., Rodkey, W. G., McCarroll, H. R., Mutz, S. B., and Niebauer, J. J.: Epineurial and perineurial fascicular nerve repairs: A critical comparison. J. Hand Surg. 1:131, 1976.

Dyck, P. J., and Lambert, E. H.: Numbers and diameters of nerve fibers and compound action potential of sural nerve; controls and hereditary neuromuscular disorders. Trans. Am. Neurol. Assoc. 91:214, 1966.

Goto, Y.: Experimental study of nerve autografting by funicular suture. Arch. Jap. Chir. 36:478, 1967.

Grabb, W. C., Bement, S. L., Koepke, G. H., and Green, R. A.: Comparison of methods of peripheral nerve suturing in monkeys. Plast. Reconstr. Surg. 46:31, 1970.

Guth, L.: Regeneration in the mammalian peripheral nervous system. Phys. Rev. 36:441, 1956.

Gutmann, E. and Sanders, F. K.: Recovery of fiber numbers and diameters in the regeneration of peripheral nerves. J. Physiol. 101:489, 1943.

Hakstian, R. W.: Funicular orientation by direct stimulation. An aid to peripheral nerve repair. J. Bone Joint Surg. 50A:1178, 1968.

Hakstian, R. W.: Perineurial neurorrhaphy. Orthop. Clin. North Amer. 4:945, 1973.

Hudson, A. R., Morris, J., Weddell, G., and Drury, A.: Peripheral nerve autografts. J. Surg. Res. 12:267, 1972.

Kurze, T.: Microtechniques in neurological surgery. Clin. Neurosurg. 11:128, 1963.

Langley, N. N., and Hashimoto, M.: On the suture of separate nerve bundles in a nerve trunk and on internal plexuses. J. Physiol. 51:318, 1917.

Mannerfelt, L.: Evaluation of functional sensation of skin grafts in the hand area. Brit. J. Plast. Surg. 15:136, 1962.

Millesi, H.: The interfascicular nerve grafting of the median and ulnar nerves. J. Bone Joint Surg. 54A:727, 1972.

Moberg, E.: Objective methods for determining the functional value of sensation in the hand. J. Bone Joint Surg. 40B:454, 1958.

Mountcastle, V. B.: Physiology of sensory receptors. In Mountcastle, V. B.: Medical Physiology. 12th ed., St. Louis, C. V. Mosby Company, 1968.

Orgel, M., Aguayo, A., and Williams, H. B.: Sensory nerve regeneration: An experimental study of skin grafts in the rabbit. J. Anat. 111:121, 1972.

Orgel, M., and Terzis, J. K.; Epineurial vs. perineurial repair: An ultrastructural and electrophysiological study of nerve regeneration. Plast. Reconstr. Surg. 60:80, 1977.

Ridley, A.: A biopsy study of the innervation of forearm skin grafted to the fingertip. Brain 94:547, 1970.

Sanders, F. K., and Young, J. Z.: The role of the peripheral stump in the control of fiber diameter in regenerating nerves. J. Physiol. 103:119, 1944.

Smith, J. W.: Microsurgery of peripheral nerves. Plast. Reconstr. Surg. 34:235, 1964.

Terzis, J. K., Faibisoff, B., and Williams, H. B.: The nerve gap: Suture under tension vs. graft. Plast. Reconstr. Surg. 56:166, 1975.

Terzis, J. K.: Functional aspects of reinnervation of free skin grafts. Plast. Reconstr. Surg. 58:142, 1976.

Terzis, J. K., Dykes, R. W., and Hakstian, R. W.: Electrophysiological recordings in peripheral nerve surgery: A review. J. Hand Surg. 1:52, 1976.

Weddell, G.: Axonal regeneration in cutaneous nerve plexuses. J. Anat. 77:49, 1942.

Weddell, G., Palmer, E., and Pallie, W.: Nerve endings in mammalian skin. Biol. Rev. 30:159, 1955.

Weiss, P., and Taylor, A. C.: Further experimental evidence against "neurotropism" in nerve regeneration. J. Exper. Zool. 95:233, 1944.

Williams, H. B., and Terzis, J. K.: Single fascicular recordings: An intraoperative tool for the management of peripheral nerve lesions. Plast. Reconstr. Surg. 57:562, 1976.

Wise, A. J., Topuzlu, C., Davis, P., and Kaye, I. S.: A comparative analysis of macro- and microsurgical neurorrhapy technics. Am. J. Surg. 117:566, 1969.

Yamamoto, K.: A comparative analysis of the process of nerve regeneration following funicular and epineurial suture for peripheral nerve repair. Arch. Jap. Chir. 43:276, 1974.

62

EVALUATION OF SENSIBILITY BY MICROHISTOLOGICAL STUDIES

MICHAEL E. JABALEY and
A. LEE DELLON

INTRODUCTION

The skin contains the most accessible part of the human nervous system. For this reason, it is not surprising that investigations of cutaneous sensation began as soon as the microscope and histologic staining techniques became available (Jabaley, 1978). The ease of access and minimal donor site deformity plus the quality of microscopic sections that could be obtained from human skin allowed researchers to describe the morphology of nerves in skin and to attempt to relate those findings to function. The broad objective of research in human sensory receptor mechanisms has always been the same: *to correlate those morphological findings at the periphery with the subject's perception of the events which take place there.* The inability to measure sensation precisely has been a persistent obstacle in accomplishing this goal.

The aims of this chapter are 1) to describe the structure of fingertip skin and the terminations of the nervous system within it; 2) to point out those techniques which have been used to obtain such information; 3) to outline the sequence of the events that occur in skin as the result of nerve injury and repair; and 4) to relate these changes to the ultimate goal of treatment: the recovery of useful sensation in the part.

954

Mountcastle has reminded us that the nervous system does not perceive external events directly (Mountcastle, 1975). Instead, the brain receives an abstract picture that is a composite of nerve impulses which originate at the periphery. The development of this topic requires that certain definitions be established. The transformation of external stimuli into conductable impulses is called *transduction* (Loewenstein, 1960). *Sensibility* is the reception or encoding of external stimuli and the transmission of impulses along nerve fibers. In broad terms, sensibility encompasses sight, smell, sound, taste, temperature change, pain, touch-pressure, and movement or change in position. In this chapter, sensibility means the modality of prime importance to the peripheral nerve surgeon — touch-pressure,* that is, the ability to recognize touch, whether moving across the surface or continually applied to a single spot.

In contrast to sensibility, which is primarily a peripheral phenomenon, *sensation* is the central reception and conscious recognition of external stimuli. Sensation involves several facets of central nervous system function, some voluntary and some involuntary. Among these are the orderly reception and integration of impulses from several sources, association with other information (either current or from memory storage), assimilation and interpretation of such data, and, finally, elevation to the conscious level. It may result, at the subject's discretion, in an appropriate response.

The transmission of impulses from skin surface to cerebral cortex requires a chain of three afferent neurons. The cell body of the first order afferent neuron lies in the dorsal ganglion and the other two are in the spinal cord and brain itself. From a practical standpoint, *the peripheral nerve surgeon has access only to the axon of the first order afferent neuron, its receptors, and the skin that contains them.* We will describe only changes that occur at these levels and their importance to the surgeon.

ANATOMY AND PHYSIOLOGY

The glabrous (hairless) skin that occurs on the fingertips, palms, and soles is unique in appearance and familiar to everyone (Cauna, 1954). The surface is characterized by a series of grooves and papillary ridges (Fig. 62–1). The ridges are the initial contact points in touch. The dermis, which is separated from the epidermis by a basement membrane, can be divided arbitrarily into papillary and reticular zones. The epidermis protrudes into the papillary dermis, while the reticular zone is entirely below the lowest level of epidermis. (Unfortunately, the protruding tips of epidermis are also called ridges, and care must be taken to distinguish them from the papillary ridges of the surface.)

There are two types of epidermal ridges: limiting and intermediate. Dermal papillae occupy the spaces between these epidermal ridges. These papillae are closer to the skin surface than is any other portion of the dermis. The highest concentration of nerve endings is also found in the papillary dermis,

---

*Physiologists classify cutaneous sensory receptors as mechanoreceptors (touch-pressure), nociceptors (pain), thermoreceptors (hot or cold), and receptors of motion or position change (as related to joints).

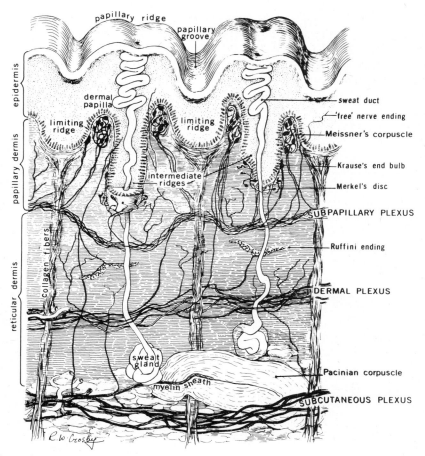

Figure 62–1 The nerves of glabrous skin. Illustration drawn at right angles to the long axis of the papillary ridges. Epidermis is separated by a basement membrane from the papillary dermis and the deeper reticular dermis (left side). There are three plexuses of nerves: subcutaneous, intradermal, and subpapillary. Branches from the plexuses may terminate at any level, but the greatest concentration of endings is in the papillary dermis. Some endings lie "free," others have modified tips and are associated with surrounding cells, and some are encapsulated by a specialized and identifiable structure such as a Meissner corpuscle. In all instances, the role of the tissue surrounding the ending is to condition the stimulus response. Meissner corpuscles occupy characteristic positions in highest reach of papillary dermis and are sensitive to deforming forces on the skin surface. Merkel endings lie about tips of intermediate ridges and respond to ridge movement. Pacinian corpuscles lie in subcutaneous tissue and deep dermis; they respond to high-frequency vibration. A natural stimulus excites several different types of endings simultaneously and produces a message at the cerebral cortex which is a composite of many impulses, each originating at a slightly different location.

especially about the intermediate ridges. These endings arise from three plexuses of nerve fibers: the subpapillary, the intradermal, and the subcutaneous
(Figs. 62–2 and 62–3).

The majority of sensory nerve endings terminate in the dermis, although
some cross the basement membrane and reach the epidermis. The role of those
cells surrounding the nerve endings, whether specialized or not, is to condition
the dynamic response characteristics of the associated fibers (Figs. 62–4 and
62–5). In this respect, each receptor serves as a selective filter, sensitive to
certain forms of energy, indifferent to others (Mountcastle, 1974). For example, the axons of Meissner and the pacinian corpuscles are both of the quickly
adapting type and serve as detectors of transient activity, such as a change
in position or a moving stimulus. When a stimulus is applied, both fibers
respond with a burst of activity, which then subsides quickly. After the initial
response to a stimulus application, the fiber "adapts" and does not fire again
until the stimulus is removed. Quantitative differences in response are due to
the conditioning effect of the corpuscle that surrounds the nerve endings.
Each corpuscle has a unique configuration and each has been shown to be
differentially sensitive to vibrations of different frequencies. Meissner corpus-

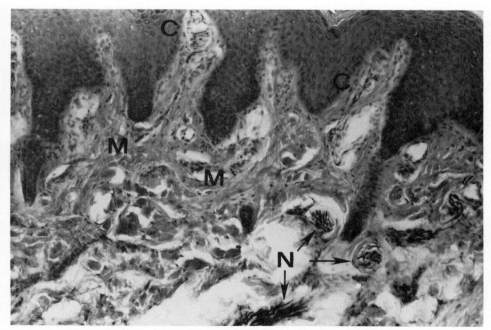

Figure 62–2 Section of epidermis and papillary dermis. Meissner corpuscles (C) lie in characteristic location in papillary dermis. Corpuscle on left is cut through center, corpuscle on right is cut
on tangent. Several endings (M) in vicinity of intermediate ridge may be part of Merkel disk. Large
nerve (N) in lower portion is seen in both longitudinal and transverse section. (Original magnification
100 ×. This and all subsequent photomicrographs were prepared from human tissue by the Winkelmann technique, using silver stains on frozen sections of fingertip skin. They are counterstained with
hematoxylin and eosin.)

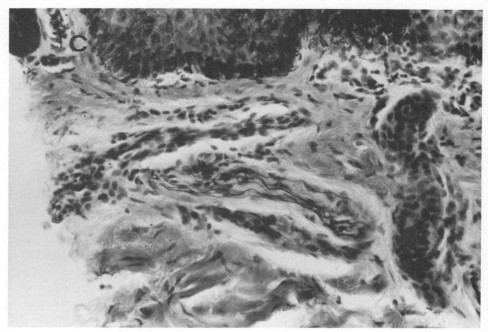

Figure 62–3 Longitudinal section of nerve in usual location in subpapillary plexus contains several fibers of different size. Some may be bound for Meissner corpuscle in upper left of photo (C). (Original magnification 100 ×.)

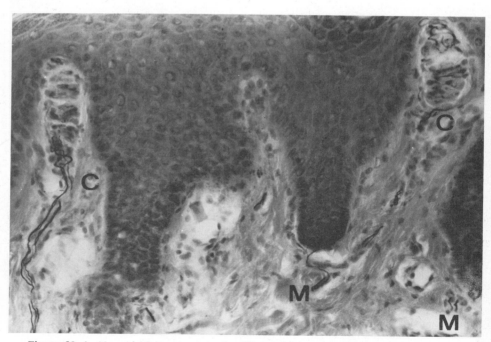

Figure 62–4 Normal Meissner corpuscles (C) may be innervated by as many as seven axons (corpuscle on left has five). Corpuscles have a "fat" appearance and flattened laminar cells (right). Nerve endings with modified tips can be seen at base of intermediate ridges (M). Some of these may be associated with Merkel disk. (Original magnification 200 ×.)

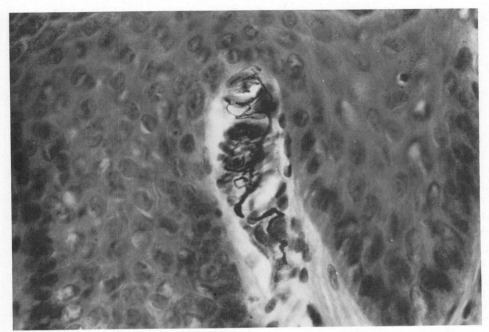

Figure 62–5 A normal Meissner corpuscle. Nerve fibers are of different diameter, several in number, and arranged in typical "coiled spring" configuration. Note proximity to basement membrane and epithelial cells. (Original magnification 400 ×.)

cles respond maximally to stimuli in the range of 30 cycles per second (Hz) while Pacinian corpuscles respond best at about 250 Hz.

Fibers that terminate near Merkel's cells are detectors of both motion and steady states but are especially suited for detection of a constant pressure stimulus. The response generated by these fibers appears to be due to physical deformation of the surrounding skin. The magnitude of response is directly related to the degree of deformation. Skin indentation results in a transient burst of activity on the oscilloscope, which is followed by a continuing measured discharge that persists as long as the stimulus is present. When the stimulus is removed, there is a final volley of increased activity which is similar to the onset response. The Merkel cells and their slowly adapting fibers mediate the perception of the constant touch or pressure.

Individual axons are classified according to fiber diameter and conduction velocity as A, B, and C fibers (a modification of the classification of Erlanger and Gasser). Group A fibers are myelinated and group C fibers are unmyelinated, but both are concerned with sensibility. The fiber population of any sensory nerve is mixed and varies with its ultimate destination. The ratio of C fibers to A fibers may be as high as 5:1 in nerves bound for areas where sensibility is relatively crude, such as the proximal extremity or back, and as low as 1:1 in nerves bound for areas where sensation is most exact, such as the fingertips. Myelinated fibers and their receptors are specifically associated with the more precise aspects of mechanoreception, and sensation is best where they are most concentrated.

Each nerve axon and ending serves an identifiable peripheral field. The impulse generated from a field varies with the location of the stimulus. Response is usually maximal in the center of the field and minimal at the periphery. The sizes of such fields vary but they tend to be smaller where the density of nerves is greater. In areas of high sensory discrimination, such as the fingertips, there is great overlap of fields, and a single stimulus commonly activates several fields and generates impulses in several axons.

Although a laboratory stimulus can purposely be made pure and simple, it is highly unlikely that such a stimulus ever occurs naturally. It would be virtually impossible for a natural stimulus to activate only one nerve ending. For this reason, we must think of the fingertip as a "sensory sheet" containing a variety of receptors, each of which is specific for signaling particular components of a given stimulus. The simple act of grasping an object between the fingertips or stimulating a fingertip with the points of a caliper generates a volley of responses in a large number of nerve axons.

The result of such peripheral activity is the creation of a composite message of multiple impulses, each of a different nature and arising from a slightly different location. The effect is the production of a cerebral cortical picture that is a mosaic of all these impulses. The final picture, of course, is greatly modified by motivation, memory, other sensations, and a variety of undefined factors.

Each individual afferent axon is specific for one of the prime modalities: touch-pressure, heat, cold, position change or movement, or pain. No matter how stimulated, whether naturally or electrically, these axons always produce the same response; that is, they are modality-specific. The intensity of the response may vary with the intensity of the stimulus but there is no crossover to other modalities; that is, mechanoreceptors do not become thermoreceptors. This factor is of practical importance in nerve repair where crossing over of axons at the site of suture may occur.

SPECIFIC HISTOLOGIC TECHNIQUES

Structure-Function Studies

The only end-organs that are large enough to identify and whose axons can be used for single-unit recordings are the pacinian corpuscle, the Iggo touch-corpuscle or touch-dome in the cat, and the Merkel-rete papilla of the raccoon. It is not presently possible to record directly from the Meissner corpuscle because of its size and location. It appears that tattoo marking of skin under magnification (Burgess and Horch, 1974) prior to nerve manipulation and india-ink marking of skin (Munger, Pubols, and Pubols, 1971) after peripheral field recording and prior to punch biopsy of the field are acceptable techniques for structure-function correlation. This approach is currently being employed and is providing useful information.

Tissue Preparation

The method of tissue fixation must be consistent with the experimental design. Histochemical techniques and vital dyes give beautiful histologic pictures, but the tissue must be stained shortly after it is obtained. These techniques are satisfactory if a single observation is to be made. If longitudinal studies are desired in which several biopsies are taken at different times but fixed and sectioned concurrently, then techniques employing nerve and connective tissue stains on formalin-fixed tissue are more satisfactory.

Staining Techniques

Nerve stains are myriad and are almost unique to every laboratory. For this reason, it is best to use a technique with which one's histologist is already experienced. Nearly all stains employ silver ions to stain axons and may or may not use a counterstain for other structures. Consistency is essential if true morphologic change is to be distinguished from artifact. In our hands, the Winkelmann, Azzopardi, and Bielchowsky methods have been most satisfactory although equally valid observations have been made with other techniques (Winkelmann and Schmit, 1957).

Connective tissue stains are valuable for observations on the non-neural corpuscle components. Although haematoxylin and eosin are readily available (and therefore less expensive), we prefer the discrimination given by special stains. The Masson trichrome stain, which stains axoplasm pink and lamellar structures blue, has been useful in the study of the Meissner corpuscle. Myelin stains can be used to differentiate between myelinated and nonmyelinated axons.

Vital dyes have given excellent results (Miller, Ralston, and Kasahara, 1958) and are recommended for use in animals. The use of methylene blue is limited by the fact that the tissue must be perfused with the dye prior to fixation. The enzyme cholinesterase is present in different forms in sensory end-organs. One such form, nonspecific cholinesterase, has been used to identify Meissner corpuscles following nerve sections because the enzyme itself can be stained. Although this technique reproducibly labels sensory end-organs, it is misleading unless one wishes only to identify the presence of a corpuscle (Winkelmann, 1960; Wong and Kanagasuntheram, 1971). Meissner corpuscles accept the stain after denervation, after axonal degeneration, and even after the corpuscle structure itself has begun to atrophy. Furthermore, application of a cholinesterase inhibitor fails to change sensation in the fingertip, so the functional significance of a cholinesterase-positive corpuscle is unclear (Hurley and Koelle, 1958).

ANIMAL EXPERIMENTS

Although Waller described the axon consequences of cranial nerve division in 1859, it has only been within the last decade that the effects of nerve division upon sensory endings have been explored. Previous experimental attempts to define the fate of denervated sensory end-organs were either byproducts of studies originally designed to determine donor or recipient site dominance in skin grafts, misadventures with "skin regeneration," or isolated observations after nerve division. The time lag is not surprising when one considers that motor function, not sensory function, preoccupied investigators for the past century and that histologic precision and reproducibility are *still* difficult to achieve when studying sensory corpuscles. For example, as recently as 1912 one observer catalogued 34 discrete types of sensory endings in the human fingertip. Most authors in the early twentieth century estimated the number of sensory endings to be about 12, but there was little agreement about classification or structure-function relationships. Improvements in techniques of tissue handling, embedding, sectioning, and staining have resulted in more uniform material for evaluation and a better understanding of morphology.

In 1960, Winkelmann summarized both his own work and that of several contemporaries, and helped clarify receptor morphology (Winkelmann, 1960). In this work the sensory endings in human distal glabrous skin are defined and illustrated, and their evolution from subprimate mammals is described. This work and that of others (Cauna, 1954, 1960; Miller, Ralston, and Kasahara, 1958; Weddell, Palmer and Pallie, 1955) has contributed to the clarification of the morphology of cutaneous receptors and their function.

An active investigator of the 1930's was J. Boeke of the Netherlands (Boeke, 1940). His experiments were typical of many in which skin grafts were exchanged between dissimilar areas to determine the fate of identifiable end-organs. Boeke's model was the duck, whose bill contains the characteristic corpuscles of Herbst and Grandry. He exchanged skin grafts between the bill and foot and concluded that new end-organs "regenerated" in bill skin placed on the foot but not in the foot skin on the bill. These studies were interpreted as demonstrating 1) the dominance of the graft over the recipient site in determining reinnervation patterns and 2) the potential of skin for "regeneration" of end-organs. Similar studies with guinea pig snouts and pig snouts were conducted by other investigators who reached opposite conclusions, however.

A present day interpretation of such studies is that sensory organs that are transplanted within a skin graft undergo denervation and subsequent atrophy. If the skin is transplanted to a recipient site that contains the appropriate types of sensory axons, these fibers may re-enter the graft and reinnervate the already present and atrophic end-organs.

Another type of investigation of "regeneration" of end organs of skin of the duck bill or monkey paw has also been performed. Units of skin are excised, "new and regenerated" skin forms, is subsequently biopsied, and the biopsies are interpreted as showing regenerated end-organs. In retrospect, it is likely that these studies of "regenerated" skin were actually biopsies of adjacent normal tissue which had been passively drawn into the area as a spontaneously healing wound contracted. Although it is possible that some species, such as the mole and duck, may form de novo end-organs with nerve regeneration, it seems unjustified to extrapolate these findings to primates.

More recently, Lowenstein and his associates have combined neurophysiologic and morphologic techniques to study sensory receptor population (Schiff and Loewenstein, 1972). They chose the pacinian corpuscle and its single, quickly adapting nerve fiber to study the fate of the encapsulated end-organs following nerve division. In one experiment, they denervated the pacinian corpuscles of the cat mesentery by dividing the inferior mesenteric nerve. They observed that the axon within each corpuscle degenerated and that mechanical stimulation of the denervated corpuscle failed to initiate an impulse in the more proximal, degenerated axon. "Reunion" of the divided inferior mesentric nerve resulted in reinnervation of the pacinian corpuscle and return of the normal transducer mechanism. Since the experiments were of short duration, no long-term observations were made upon the fate of the denervated lamellar corpuscle.

In a subsequent experiment, Schiff and Loewenstein "united" the hypogastric nerve (the hypogastric nerve goes to the bladder, which contains no pacinian corpuscles) to the distal end of a cut inferior mesenteric nerve (Schiff and Loewenstein, 1972). After a period of recovery, they observed restoration of transducer potential in 23 of 64 pacinian corpuscles studied. Although this study is sometimes quoted as demonstrating that end-organs are not specific for a given type of sensory axon, it is also possible to interpret the results as simply demonstrating that among the hypogastric nerve fibers reinnervating corpuscles, about one third were quickly adapting. Those corpuscles which were reinnervated by these fibers had their transducer capability restored and became functional. An analogous situation may occur in humans if the proximal radial nerve is used to innervate the median nerve at the wrist when the proximal median nerve has been irreparably damaged. Although there are no pacinian corpuscles on the dorsum of the hand, there are quick adapting fibers in the radial nerve that presumably innervate hair follicles. These fibers can probably reinnervate the pacinian corpuscles of the fingertips and restore the transducer capability, thus restoring some measure of mechanoreception.

Burgess and Horch have applied neurophysiologic and morphologic techniques to study the effects of denervation and reinnervation of sensory endorgans in the cat hind limb touch dome, a receptor for slowly adapting fibers in hairy skin (Burgess et al., 1974). Following denervation, they found that the Merkel cells, the touch corpuscles present in the touch-dome base, atrophy, and that the entire touch dome ultimately flattens and is indistinguishable from the surrounding skin. Following nerve regeneration into the hindlimb, touch domes not only reappeared but were found at locations which coincided with their original positions. This occurred in a statistically significant number of instances and Burgess and Horch postulated a trophic factor to account for this reinnervation; some neurohumoral substance attacts the regenerating axon sprouts to dermal-epidermal regions capable of forming touch domes.

Dellon studied the remaining sensory end-organ in the distal glabrous skin, the Meissner corpuscle (Dellon, Witebsky, and Terrill, 1975; Dellon, 1976). In two experiments in primates, denervated Meissner corpuscles were found to undergo progressive degeneration of the axon terminals and atrophy of the lamellar corpuscular structure. Following interfascicular nerve repair, the atrophic Meissner corpuscles were reinnervated, and their appearance then returned to normal. No new Meissner corpuscles were noted to form; that is, no *de novo* corpuscles were identified.

In summary, it appears that in primate fingertips the sensory end-organs responsible for touch are the Merkel disc (a slowly adapting transducer mediating constant touch and pressure), the Meissner corpuscle (a quickly adapting transducer, sensitive to low-frequency vibration and mediating touch movements) and the pacinian corpuscle (a quickly adapting transducer, sensitive to high frequency vibrations and mediating touch movements). Denervation of these sensory end-organs results in the well-recognized wallerian degeneration of their axon terminals and atrophy of their non-neural components, the corpuscles.

It appears that the Merkel cell, being most dependent upon trophic influences, atrophies quickest. The Meissner corpuscle, which contains more extensive supporting structural components may require up to nine months to atrophy into a small amorphic mass. Although no studies exist regarding the long-term effects of denervation upon the pacinian corpuscle, it is likely that, given enough time, even this dense onion-like lamella structure will also undergo atrophy. Thus, a practical consideration of prime importance to the peripheral nerve surgeon is the timing of operation and the ability (or inability) of these specialized organs to recover function following reinnervation.

HUMAN EXPERIMENTS

In contrast to the extensive research effort devoted to peripheral nerve suture and axon regeneration, relatively few reports have dealt with the status of human nerve endings and receptors at the skin level, their fate with denervation, and their potential for reinnervation or regeneration (Jabaley and Bryant, 1976). In 1975, Jabaley and associates performed clinical testing, fingertip biopsies, and histologic evaluation in 17 patients with nerve injuries between the elbow and palm in an effort to examine these questions (Jabaley et al., 1976). Since some patients had injuries to more than one nerve, 26 separate sensory nerve territories were evaluated. The interval from nerve injury to repair averaged 24 months. The level of sensory recovery was estimated by the patient's subjective opinion, performance of objective tests, and functional usage of the parts supplied by the repaired nerve.

The battery of objective tests was designed specifically to test perception of vibratory stimuli of varying frequencies and a pressure stimulus applied in both a movable and constant fashion. These tests were felt to measure the function of specific types of fiber-receptor systems. Functional testing included Moberg's pick-up test, object identification, and two-point discrimination.

3.5 millimeter circular skin biopsies were obtained from the index or little fingers. They were fixed in formalin, serially cut into 20 micron sections, and stained for nerve tissue by the silver impregnation method of Winkelmann. All sections were then counterstained with hematoxylin and eosin and submitted to five observers as unknowns for interpretations.

We should emphasize that the fixing, sectioning, and staining of nerve tissue can result in a variable interpretation. Such factors as pH, temperature, timing, and age of both the fixatives and the stains can influence appearance. Normally occurring structures may be distorted, overstained, or understained. Worse yet, silver may precipitate and mask shapes and may lead to completely erroneous interpretations. These factors are responsible in part for some changes which have been previously described in skin and have led to identification and classification of structures which may not always exist. Careful examination of an entire biopsy specimen cut into serial sections will minimize errors and confusion due to artifact.

Observers were asked to classify each section as containing no nerve, occasional nerve (the presence of *any* clearly identifiable fibers), or abundant nerve (amount and appearance which could not be distinguished from normal). They were also asked to note the character of identifiable corpuscles (Figs. 62–6 through 62–8). *A striking finding was that all patients with a technically satisfactory nerve suture had some identifiable return of nerve fibers to the level of the reticular dermis and that approximately two thirds had return to the highest level of the papillary dermis.* In some patients, the volume of nerve was sparse, while in others it could not be distinguished from normal.

Clinical testing of the patients indicated that everyone had recovered some degree of measurable sensation. The level of function was quite variable, however, and ranged from poor to excellent. *No significant correlation was found between the presence of identifiable nerve and receptors in the biopsy and the patient's functional performance.* The lack of correlation between function and presence of nerve in fingertip skin suggest that factors other than simple nerve regeneration influence the eventual use of a reinnervated part.

In a technically satisfactory nerve repair, the proximal axons are stimulated naturally to sprout and grow. They find their way into the distal Schwann cell system and follow the distal sheaths to their terminations. Eventually, many axons appear to regain function as sensory receptors. Questions that cannot be answered are: do axons find their way to the same receptors to which they were originally united? (This seems highly unlikely.) Do they find their way to the same type of receptors? (This may be more likely.) Can they find their way to completely different types of receptors? (This also seems likely.) Can normal transducer function be restored by a completely foreign receptor which has been reunited with a regenerating axon? (Perhaps a previous Meissner fiber can reinnervate a pacinian corpuscle and vice versa, as suggested earlier).

To summarize this data: 1) axons clearly regenerate to the skin level following successful nerve repair, 2) they reinnervate receptors that were present prior to injury and have not arisen *de novo,* and 3) these receptors can function as transducers and code external stimuli into transmittable nerve impulses.

The critical question from the standpoint of useful sensation and functional use of the part has to do with the sensory cortical representation of peripheral events. The work of Paul, Goodman, and Merzenich (1974) suggests that cortical distortion of the peripheral stimulus occurs in laboratory animals even in carefully performed nerve suture under ideal conditions. When one extrapolates from this finding to the clinical setting, where wounds are greater in magnitude, delays in treatment are unavoidable, other structures are sometimes injured, obligatory gaps and tension may be introduced, and nerve grafts are sometimes used, then cortical distortion may be amplified many times.

We can speculate about nerve repair as follows: the high density of nerve fibers normally found in the fingertips permits them to perform precise tasks with comparative ease. As is the case with other organs such as the liver or kidney, it is likely that a small percentage of these nerve fibers could still supply sufficient sensory input for normal use *provided their central connections are appropriate and undistorted.*

Following nerve repair and axon regrowth to terminal receptors, a usable (interpretable) cortical picture will result and useful function will follow *if mis-*

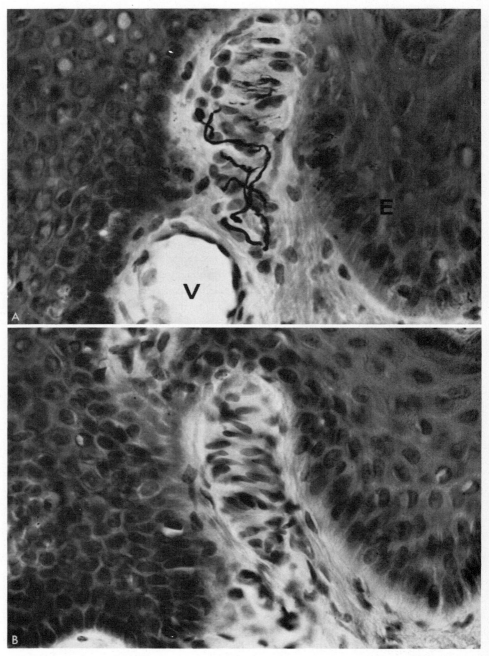

Figure 62–6 *A,* Normal Meissner corpuscle. Flattened laminar cells contrast sharply with rounder epidermal cells (E). Nerve axons are sharply defined. A capillary (V) is seen below corpuscle. (Original magnification 400 ×.) *B,* Denervated Meissner corpuscle. Wallerian degeneration has occurred and no axons are seen. In other respects, corpuscle still appears normal. Size, shape, and appearance have changed very little. (Original magnification 400 ×.)

Illustration continued on the opposite page.

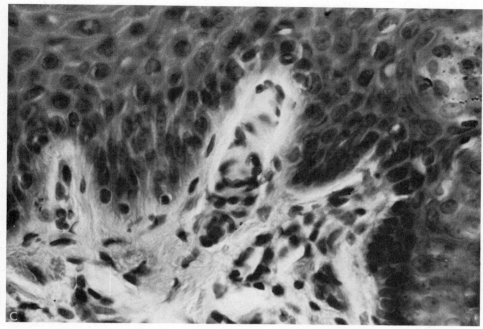

Figure 62–6 *Continued.* *C*, Effect of longstanding denervation. After several months, the corpuscle is still present, but its size is smaller, and significant atrophy has occurred. Corpuscles do not disappear but atrophy is progressive and at some point becomes irreversible. Thereafter, it is unlikely that function can be re-established even if successful reinnervation occurs (original magnification 400 ×.)

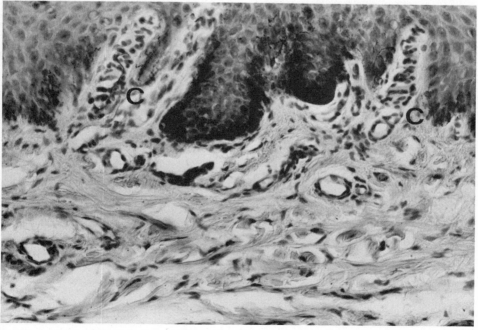

Figure 62–7 Effect of reinnervation. Two corpuscles (C) can be seen. The one on the left has been successfully reinnervated while the one on the right remains denervated. (100 × Magnification.)

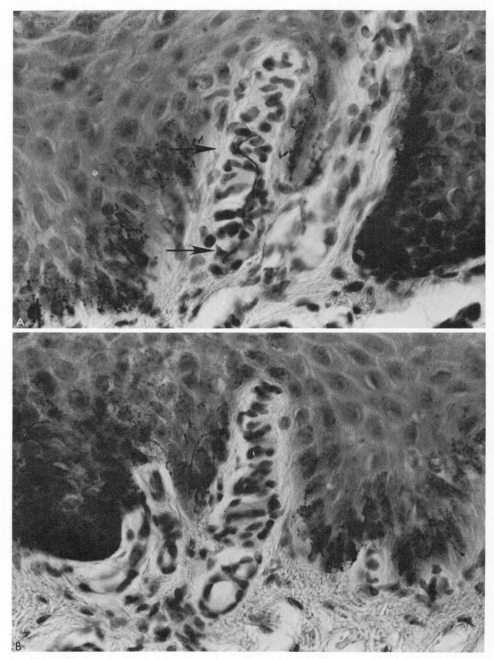

Figure 62–8   *A*, Enlargement of Figure 62–7, left. Axon can be seen to extend from the base of the corpuscle (arrow) to over half its length. It can be seen to branch at its termination (original magnification 400 ×). *B*, Enlargement of Figure 62–7, right. Corpuscle is atrophic and remains denervated. If growing axons return to such a corpuscle, function may return. With time, corpuscle may become an amorphous mass, virtually unidentifiable. Such a corpuscle is unlikely to recover function even if reinnervated. (Original magnification 400 ×.)

direction of regenerating axon sprouts at the site of nerve suture can be held to an acceptable level.

It is now clear that the level of function following nerve repair can be further improved by a re-education program even in those patients whose initial result may appear satisfactory (Dellon, Curtis, and Edgerton, 1974) (see Chapter 47, on Re-Education of Sensation). In some patients who perform poorly after nerve suture, the cause may be an unacceptable level of cortical distortion and misrepresentation due to axonal crossover at the suture line — i.e., the signal generated at the periphery is reaching the brain but not in an easily usable form. Re-education can be an important adjunct in the rehabilitation of such patients, and if successful, may be preferable to reoperation.

REFERENCES

Boeke, J.: The Problems of Nervous Anatomy. London, Oxford Press, 1940, p. 12.

Burgess, P. R., English, K. B., Horch, K. W., and Stensaas, L. J.: Patterning in the regeneration of type I cutaneous receptors. J. Physiol. *236*:57, 1974.

Cauna, N.: Nerve supply and nerve endings in Meissner's corpuscles. Am. J. Anat. *99*:315, 1956.

Cauna, N.: Nature and functions of the papillary ridges of the digital skin. Anat. Rec. *119*:449, 1954.

Dellon, A. L.: Reinnervation of denervated Meissner corpuscles. J. Hand Surg. *1*:98, 1976.

Dellon, A. L., Curtis, R. M., and Edgerton, M. T.: Reeducation of sensation in the hand after nerve injury and repair. Plast. Reconstr. Surg. *53*:297, 1974.

Dellon, A. L., Witebsky, F. G., and Terrill, R. E.: The denervated Meissner corpuscle. Plast. Reconstr. Surg. *56*:182, 1975.

Hurley, H. J., and Koelle, G. B.: The effect of inhibitions of non-specific cholinesterase in human volar skin. J. Invest. Derm. *31*:243, 1958.

Jabaley, M. E.: Recovery of sensation in flaps and skin grafts. *In* Tubiana, R. (ed.): The Hand, Philadelphia, W. B. Saunders Company (*in* press, 1979).

Jabaley, M. E., Burns, J. E., Orcutt, B. A., and Bryant, W. M.: Comparison of histologic and functional recovery after peripheral nerve repair. J. Hand Surg. *1*:119, 1976.

Jabaley, M. E., and Bryant, W. M.: The effect of denervation and reinnervation on encapsulated receptors in digital skin. *In* Marchac, D. (ed.): Transactions of VI International Congress of Plastic and Reconstructive Surgery. Paris, 1976, p. 103.

Loewenstein, W. R.: Biological transducers. Scientific American, *203*:98, 1960.

Miller, M. R., Ralston, H. J., and Kasahara, M.: The pattern of cutaneous innervation of the human hand. Am. J. Anat. *102*:183, 1958.

Mountcastle, V. B.: Sensory receptors and neural encoding: Introduction to sensory processes. *In* Mountcastle, V. B., (ed.): Medical Physiology, St. Louis, C. V. Mosby Company, 1974, p. 285.

Mountcastle, V. B.: The view from within: Pathways to the study of perception. Johns Hopkins Med. J. *136*:109, 1975.

Munger, B. L., Pubols, L. M., and Pubols, B. H.: The Merkel-rete papilla: A slowly-adapting sensory receptor in mammalian glabrous skin. Brain Res. *29*:47, 1971.

Paul, R. L., Goodman, H., and Merzenich, M.: Alteration in mechanoreceptor input to Brodmann's areas 1 and 3 of the postcentral hand area of Macaca mulatta after nerve section and regeneration. Brain Res. *39*:1, 1972.

Schiff, I., and Loewenstein, W. R.: Development of a receptor on a foreign nerve fiber in a pacinian corpuscle. Science *177*:712, 1972.

Weddell, G., Palmer, E., and Pallie, W.: Nerve endings in mammalian skin. Biological Reviews of the Cambridge Philosophical Society *30*:159, 1955.

Winkelmann, R. K., and Schmit, R. W.: A simple silver method for nerve axoplasm. Proc. Mayo Clin. *32*:217, 1957.

Winkelmann, R. K.: Nerve Endings in Normal and Pathologic Skin. Springfield, Ill., C. C Thomas Co., 1960.

Wong, W. C., and Kanagasuntheram, R.: Early and late effects of median nerve injury on Meissner's and pacinian corpuscles of the hand of the Macaque. J. Anat. *109*:135, 1971.

63

PRIMATE LABORATORY MODELS FOR PERIPHERAL NERVE REPAIR

DAVID G. KLINE

Scarcity of primates for biomedical research in recent years due to embargoes on exportation, primarily from India but also from Africa, is a reality. Realization of this has stimulated more stateside efforts to improve primate reproductivity, primarily in the seven primate centers (Goodwin, 1970). Unfortunately, the demand for these animals on the part of investigators is still greater than the supply. In any case, primates are expensive to buy, even more expensive to keep properly over a long period of time, and at times can be difficult to handle, especially when compared to the relative ease of purchasing and caring for rats, hamsters, rabbits, cats, and dogs. There is little question that many valuable observations concerning the anatomy, physiology, and neurochemistry of the peripheral nervous system and its central and more peripheral connections have been, and will continue to be, made in lower phylum non-primate animals (Guttman, 1948). Nonetheless, studies made in lower animals of the pathophysiology of nerve injury and techniques for its repair have found limited application to the human, giving the primate some degree of pre-eminence as a research animal in this field.

Other factors besides species of animal are perhaps of even more importance in evaluating experimental results. If crude or ineffective end points are

970

used to measure regeneration or the potential for it, interpretation of results and subsequent application to the human will be difficult despite correct selection of species for experimental study. Carefully prepared experimental repairs will not provide useful information if inadequate measurements of function are made. It is almost axiomatic that basic research concerned with nerve injury or repair and intended for application to humans should not only be done in a carefully selected species of animal but should also include thorough measurements of regeneration and subsequent function if it is to be useful.

The following is a review of papers published in English over the last two decades which concerned peripheral nerve regeneration and repair in primates and which seemed to have some clinical application. A portion of the references was obtained from an off-line bibliographic citation list (Medlars) supplied by the National Library of Medicine and dated December 30, 1977.

SPECIES RESPONSE TO NERVE INJURY

Ramon y Cajal in 1928 suggested that species as well as age of animal determines the rate of reinnervation of the distal musculature after neural severance but did not supply data to support this concept. Studies were published in 1964 which were designed to answer part of the question of whether or not there was a species response to nerve injury (Kline et al., 1964a, 1964b). Nerves were left to regenerate after removal of a 1 cm segment, which with retraction resulted in a 2 to 3 cm gap. Also studied was crush as well as suture after removal of a segment of nerve. Injuries and repairs were made in dogs, rhesus monkeys, baboons, and chimpanzees. Resultant neuromas were graded for a number of gross and histologic characteristics including neuroma size, degree of connective tissue proliferation, degree of axonal spanning of the injury site, amount of axonal disorganization at the repair site, degree of distal tubular collapse secondary to endoneurial proliferation, and axonal counts. The axonal counts were done without regard to size distribution by using an ocular square grid of 100 squares under a magnification of 970X. Ten squares in each field were counted and the average of these counts was multiplied by the number of squares containing axons in each field. Full cross sections were counted and matched and compared with the calculated counts, and variation was only in the neighborhood of 3.5 per cent. Nonetheless, determination of distal counts without regard to fiber distribution and formation of a distal to proximal ratio was a crude index of regeneration by today's standards. Histology was evaluated by Masson, Bodian, and Luxol fast blue staining techniques. Canines did especially well in bridging the gaps left without repair. Axonal and connective tissue organization in these animals was good and recovery of some distal muscular contraction was invariable even though the gap was left unrepaired. The rhesus monkey did well but not as well as the dog and was more comparable to the baboon and chimpanzee. Primates formed relatively large and disorganized neuromas and did not span the injury gap with mature axons as had the dog. The degree of connective tissue and axonal disorganization of sutured nerves was greater in the higher primates such as chimpanzee and baboon than in the dog and rhesus monkey. Decreased variability among species was seen with a crushing injury where distortion of the connective tissue framework of the nerve secondary to the original injury was less than with severance and suture. Injured and repaired nerves were electrically stimulated looking for distal muscle function, and threshold values favored the lower phylum animal, the dog.

Our own unpublished experience, as well as that of others, with animals such as frogs, rats, guinea pigs, cats, and rabbits indicates that response of these lower phylum animals to injury is even more positive in terms of effective regeneration than that of the dog, let alone a primate or human. Nonetheless, such lower phylum animals are repeatedly used for experimental studies in nerve repair, and the reader is asked to believe that regenerative results gained in the rat, rabbit, guinea pig, or dog are obtainable in man if the same technique or techniques are used.

EFFECT OF INJURY ON NERVE IN PRIMATE MODELS

Primates have been used by a number of investigators to study conductive properties in presumably intact nerves so that such observations can be transferred to man (McLeod, 1967). In addition, peripheral neuropathies due to acrylamide (Hopkins and Gilliatt, 1971) and other toxic agents (McLeod, 1969), as well as mechanical compression (Gilliatt et al., 1975; Sunderland, 1974) or response to cold (Beazley et al., 1974), and infection (Dastur and Razzok, 1971) have also been studied in primates. In addition, Paul, Goodman, and Merzenich (1972) used the rhesus monkey to study alterations in the mechanoreceptor input to brain after section and regeneration of the median nerve. Similar studies of the brain's response to peripheral alteration due to cord lesions have also been done in other primates (Guth, 1974).

Boyle removed short segments of the facial nerve of rhesus monkeys just rostral to the stylomastoid foramen (Boyle, 1966). Astonishingly, seven of nine animals showed some peripheral evidence of regeneration by three months. Where longer segments were removed, regeneration was poor and crossover which was looked for from the trigeminal nerve did not occur. Study of injection injury as well as crush and catgut ligation of the facial nerve indicated some spontaneous recovery, suggesting that moderate injury to this nerve is reversible by regeneration unaided by other cranial nerves. Unfortunately, only histologic techniques were used for evaluation in this relatively early study using primates.

Lehman and Hayes (1967) studied chimpanzee nerves which had epineurial suture with or without a variety of silicone wrappers placed around the repair site. They were interested in the factors leading to axonal and connective tissue disorganization in neuromas in continuity. It was pointed out that loss of perineurium with disappearance of fascicular architecture is always a feature of traumatic degeneration and that swelling and subsequent disorganization associated with regeneration extended centrally to the point where the perineurium was preserved. They, therefore, advanced the argument that tubulation by restraining swelling would promote longitudinal regeneration. Needed for more thorough study of this thesis as well as others concerning regeneration and techniques of repair in primates were relatively objective in vivo measurements of regeneration.

Studies reported in 1968 and 1969 delineated the usefulness of nerve action potential recording across an injury such as crush or severance and suture in evaluating early and significant axonal regeneration through the lesion and on into the distal stump (Kline and DeJonge, 1968). Nerve action potentials could be recorded weeks before there was evoked EMG or muscle action potential evidence of recovery. In an adequately regenerating nerve, a large number of axons of sufficient maturity to conduct an NAP penetrated well into the distal stump weeks before motor end-plate reconstruction could be recorded by EMG (Kline and Hackett, 1968; Kline et al., 1969). In addition, the presence and form of the NAP's could be related in a semiquantitative fashion to axonal distributions as to both size and number at the distal stump recording sites. Ability to record an NAP from the distal stump depended on the presence of moderate and/or large diameter axons and the degree of their myelination. Such a technique for in vivo NAP recording without killing the nerve made serial electrical evaluation of relatively early regeneration of the nerve itself a possibility. More recent experiments indicate that under some circumstances similar reliable NAP information can be recorded non-invasively in the primate as well as the human (Kline et al., 1973).

Nerve action potential and evoked EMG recording was then used to evaluate fractional injuries to nerve (Kline et al., 1970a, 1970b). Injuries were created in a controlled fashion using the evoked electrical data to permit reduction in amplitude of evoked responses by a reproducible percentage. The same electrophysiologic tests were then used to restudy the injury for a period of time thereafter. After determining baseline evoked NAP and EMG amplitude and conduction velocity, nerves were partially injured using evoked studies to approximate the degree of injury, a 25 per cent injury would reduce evoked NAP amplitude by 25 per cent. Follow-up studies revealed that not only would NAP amplitude decrease further with time but so would the conduction velocity even though it was constant immediately after the injury. Partial laceration was associated with the most apparent progression of injury, while crush was next, and then blood injection. Although initial loss of NAP amplitude was produced by saline injection, this change was reversible and conduction velocity changes were insignificant. It appeared that presence of injured neural tissue or extravasation of blood, or both, were responsible for extension of the original injury. As will be seen later, attempts to modify extension of such an injury by treatment with steroids were unsuccessful.

A similar model for evaluating neural function was combined with vascular injections to study the effect of mobilization on regeneration of injured primate nerves (Kline et al., 1972). Three types of injury were used — partial crush, complete crush, and severance and suture. Nerve on one side was injured and repaired with mobilization of the nerve from buttock to lower leg regions along with sacrifice or killing of the collateral vessels. Nerve on the other side was injured and/or repaired in the same fashion but not mobilized and collateral vessels were left intact. Nerves on both sides had baseline electrical studies performed on them. The same electrical studies were then repeated at an interval of one to 52 weeks later and extremities were then perfused with a Micropaque (25 per cent) and gelatin (8 per cent) mixture. Mobilized and injured nerves kept electrical and histological pace with those not injured but mobilized. Patterns of revascularization were identical in both groups except in the early weeks after injury, when a larger quantity of both collateral and intraneural vessels were seen in the non-mobilized nerves than in those mobilized.

Although NAP studies, especially when coupled with evoked EMG studies, were valuable for assessing regeneration in the early weeks to months after injury, an improved measure of late function appeared necessary to supplement these laboratory studies. As a result, muscle power has been measured in each of our laboratory experiments in primates over the last five years. In order to do this, a holding apparatus was constructed. The most recent model is made of stainless steel and Plexiglas. The holding apparatus includes a hinged footplate attached by wire to a strain gauge mounted on a metal bar. A tibial pin is placed and then clamped to vertical bars, which in turn are adjustable and can be fixed to longitudinal runners. Deformation of the strain gauge mounted on the bar produces signals which are modulated by a wheatstone bridge, recorded on the DC channel of a differential amplifier, and displayed on an oscilloscope. Muscle contraction is thus measured by a modified isometric technique. Single stimuli, supramaximal to threshold and applied by bipolar electrodes directly to the nerve, result in single twitch plantar flexion while trains of stimuli, 200 to 400 cycles per second, result in tetanic contraction. Both of these tests give some idea of maximal and thus, admittedly, unrefined muscle power. Nonetheless, these muscle power tests when combined with NAP and EMG data give a relatively thorough picture of the electrophysiologic function of the axon to motor endplate to muscle function. These techniques were then used in a lengthy study to verify the phenomenon of extension or progression of injury in partially lacerated primate nerves (Hudson and Kline, 1975; Kline et al., 1975). Muscle tension data corroborated the earlier reports of progression found on evoked NAP and EMG studies, and when combined with both light and electron microscopic studies suggested that progression of the original injury was due to an ongoing process of partial degeneration including axonotmesis and demyelinating changes in the intermediate zone adjacent to the laceration, with transient changes in the peripheral zone being due to edema shown by electron microscopy as an increase in protein-like substance. Reversibility of loss was due primarily to regenerative reconstruction in the intermediate as well as peripheral zones with little or no recovery occurring in the more neurotmetic zone of laceration.

REPAIR EXPERIMENTS IN PRIMATES

Earlier experiments than those reporting species response to injury used primates to study repair methods (Weiss, 1943). For example, Tarlov (1948) utilized primates as well as other animals to study plasma clot suture and use of threads to span gaps, while Matson, Alexander, Weiss, and Woods studied the use of catgut, silk, or nylon thread to bridge such gaps and to provide a scaffolding for downgrowth of regenerating axons (Alexander et al., 1948). Histologic techniques were used to evaluate results in both of these sets of experiments.

Wrapping or Entubulation

In 1964, chimpanzees were used to study resorbable wrappers made of reconstituted and irradiated but tanned bovine collagen (Kline, 1964). Peroneal nerves repaired end-to-end on one side were compared to those on the other side repaired in the same fashion, but wrapped with collagen. Repaired nerves were re-exposed at intervals up to eight months post injury and graded for gross and histologic characteristics as well as response to simple nerve stimulation, much as in the species response studies. Other monkeys had collagen film wrapped around intact nerves so that characteristics of resorbability could be studied. It was found that resorption time for the collagen could be altered by variation in the tanning process but that some epineurial and perineurial inflammatory infiltrates resulted, and a few areas of fascicular damage occurred in the wrapped and otherwise intact nerves. Wrapped and repaired nerves had less disorganization and axonal carry through was more orderly and concentrated than seen in the non-wrapped control nerves. Delayed rechallenge with collagen did not give a heightened response of inflammation but acute rechallenge did. Thresholds for response to stimulation favored wrapped nerves, but this was by present standards a very crude electrophysiologic evaluation.

Ducker and Hayes (1968) then used a large group of dogs and a smaller group of chimpanzees to study the value of Silastic entubulation for repaired nerves. They found that Silastic was tolerated well over a three year period of followup. An internal tube diameter of 2½ to 3 times the diameter of the nerve was felt best. Other data reported in this paper concerned work in dogs which determined the ideal thickness and length for Silastic tubes and the suture material to be used. Again, the end points used for measurement were primarily histologic. A grading system similar to that reported earlier was used for degree of scarring, neuroma formation, axonal spanning, axonal diameter, degree of axonal disorganization, and connective tissue proliferation. Epineurial repair was compared to millipore wrap, irradiated collagen wrap, Silastic wrap, and Silastic entubulation (Ducker, 1968). Again, a thin Silastic tube seemed to give the best result based on the histologic criteria mentioned.

Nerve Grafts in Primates

Ducker and Hayes (1968, 1970) also studied whole nerve homografts in dogs as well as chimpanzees. It was found that, in chimps, grafts were successful up to 4.5 centimeters in length if pretreated by degeneration and irradiation. Unsuccessful grafts were replaced by fibrous stria, vascularized spaces, and some fat cells in their distal reaches. Histologic observations were the main determinants of regeneration, although muscle was stimulated and chronaxie values were determined to provide some assessment of regeneration into and subsequent reconstruction of the axon to motor end-plate to muscle relationship.

Ashley et al. (1967) placed irradiated homografts in both median and ulnar nerves in 11 rhesus monkeys and four Japanese apes. Evaluation was primarily electromyographic. All but three grafts which were lengthy survived. Controls were not ideal in this experiment and consisted only of intact nerves.

Pollard, Gye, and McLeod (1971) used both rats and rhesus monkeys to assess the effect of immunosuppressive agents on experimental allografts that had been freeze-dried and irradiated. Animals in the treated group received azathioprine placed intraperitoneally for 48 hours prior to graft repair. The five primates so treated had evidence of regeneration while four of six not treated did not. Parameters studied were histologic and included density and diameter of myelinated fibers distal to the repair sites and internodal length studied in single teased fibers. Conduction velocities were determined by stimulating the nerves presumably proximal to the graft and recording muscle action potentials from the thenar musculature. The electrical data favored use of immunosuppressive agents when homografts were placed.

EFFECT OF STEROIDS ON PRIMATE NERVE REGENERATION

Graham et al. (1973) used adult squirrel monkeys to evaluate transection of the ulnar nerve at the level of the wrist and the tibial at the level of the ankle. After primary suture on both sides, the repair site on one side was injected with triamcinolone, while that of the opposite limb had saline injection. Transected and repaired radial nerves were treated in the same fashion, although the control side received the inactive base of triamcinolone rather than the drug itself. Histologic studies were used to evaluate results. The authors concluded that those nerves receiving steroid injections in the neighborhood of the repair site had decreased scar in and around the repair and less axonal disorganization. It appeared to them that axonal growth was denser and axons larger in diameter on the treated side than on the non-treated side. It should be stressed that functional electrical studies were not included.

A partial laceration model similar to that reported earlier was used to see if a short-term, high-dosage regimen of a dexamethasone series steroid would abort or change the progressive nature of the lesion (Kline et al., 1971). Animals with partially lacerated nerves were also treated with saline injections as a control. Primates were begun on injections of either saline or dexamethasone immediately postoperatively. This was continued every six hours for a five-day period. Uninjured but mobilized nerves served as a further control. Although the epineurium appeared thickened, NAP conduction velocities and amplitudes were maintained in this control group of nerves despite re-exposure of the nerve at both two and eight weeks. Evaluation of electrophysiologic as well as histologic data in the primates with partially lacerated nerves failed to show any significant difference between steroid-treated and saline-treated groups.

PRIMARY VS. SECONDARY REPAIR IN PRIMATES

Grabb (1968) studied both sharply and bluntly sectioned distal wrist level median and ulnar nerves in rhesus monkeys. Primary repair was compared to secondary repair carried out three weeks after transection. Regeneration was assessed by serial electromyographic sampling of muscle activity, particularly in

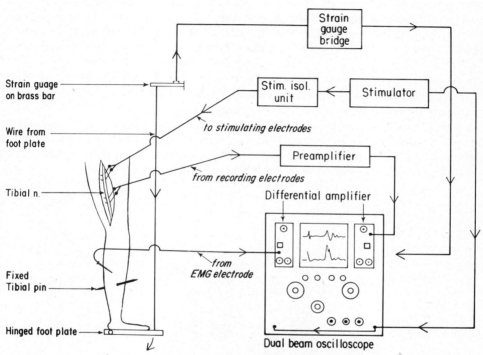

Figure 63-1 Experimental model for investigation of primate peripheral nerve regeneration in use at Louisiana State University Medical Center in New Orleans. After operative exposure of tibial nerve, leg is placed into muscle tension measuring apparatus with foot on hinged plate, as shown in Figure 63-2, tibial pin fixed to frame of apparatus, and wire from foot plate to strain gauge mounted on a brass bar. Stimulating and recording electrodes are placed about tibial nerve, and electromyographic electrode is placed in the gastrocnemius muscle. Nerve stimulation displaces foot plate, pulls rigid wire, and deforms brass bar. Strain gauge signals are modulated by Wheatstone bridge and then recorded on DC channel differential amplifier and displayed on an oscilloscope. Nerve action potentials (NAP) and muscle action potentials (MAP) are recorded by distal electrodes. NAP's are processed by Grass P5 preamplifier and then by AC channeled differential amplifier. (Reprinted with permission of the Journal of Neurosurgery.)

the thenar and hypothenar eminence in response to proximal stimulation of the nerve. Evoked electromyographic or muscle action potential responses were graded and it appeared that, using this type of end point, those animals with primary repair had a higher grade of reinnervation than those repaired secondarily.

Stimulated by Grabb's 1968 experiment, primate tibial nerves were transected with bottleglass after baseline evoked NAP, EMG, and muscle power studies had been obtained (Kline et al., 1975; Kline and Hackett, 1975). Nerve on one side was then repaired primarily, while that on the other side was repaired secondarily several weeks later. At the same post-repair intervals, extending from 12 to 52 weeks, evoked NAP's, EMG, and muscle power studies were repeated and results were matched with light histologic study of the repair site and distal stump of the nerve. In 14 of the 20 instances, primary repair was ahead with better functional values even at one year post injury. Experience with a series of 15 rhesus monkeys who had crush and then resection and repair primarily on one side matched against a secondary resection and repair again favored primary repair, although differences were not as significant as they had been with the bluntly lacerating injury. Of great importance in both of these experimental series, examination of the histologic patterns of regeneration alone failed to identify the regenerative leaders (Figs. 63–1 through 63–5).

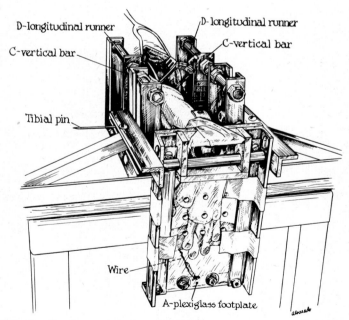

Figure 63–2   Details of a portion of muscle tension apparatus which provides fixation of the leg and placement of foot. Heel of animal was taped into triangular slot and sole was placed flat on Plexiglass footplate (A) and positioned in relation to holes on the plate. Pin (B) was drilled through tibia and clamped to vertical bars (C), which are adjustable on longitudinal runners (D). Slotted fittings for base vertical bars were numbered, as were all of the settings, so that position of limb in relation to tibial pin and footplate could be reproduced. Exposure of the tibial nerve at the level of the thigh is also shown. (Reprinted with permission of the Journal of Neurosurgery.)

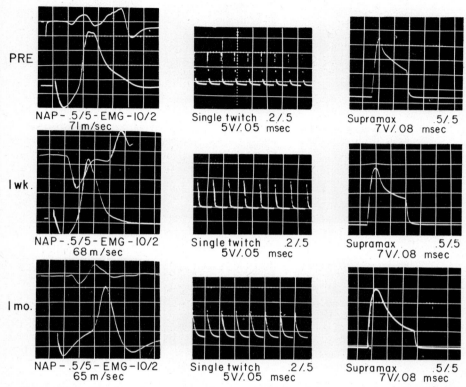

PRE

NAP - .5/5 - EMG - 10/2
71 m/sec

Single twitch   .2/.5
5V/.05 msec

Supramax   .5/.5
7V/.08 msec

I wk.

NAP - .5/5 - EMG - 10/2
68 m/sec

Single twitch   .2/.5
5V/.05 msec

Supramax   .5/.5
7V/.08 msec

I mo.

NAP - .5/5 - EMG - 10/2
65 m/sec

Single twitch   .2/.5
5V/.05 msec

Supramax   .5/.5
7V/.08 msec

Figure 63-3 Tracings from a control, nonlacerated but mobilized nerve just before initial operation, one week, and four weeks later. Traces in left column show evoked nerve action potentials below and muscle action potentials above. The downward deflection preceding each NAP on this subsequent figure is due to shock artifact which was difficult to minimize because of the relatively short distance between stimulating and recording electrodes. Traces in the center column are those of single twitch or contraction and response to relatively brief (0.05 msec) but supramaximal (5V) stimulus at a rate of two per second. Traces in the right column show muscle contraction in response to a tetanic burst of supramaximal (7V and .08 msec) stimuli. Oscilloscope settings for NAP's were 0.5V with prior preamplification by a Grass P5 preamplifier and 0.5 msec per division on the grid, while for EMG or MAP they were 10 millivolts and 2 msec per division. Single twitches were recorded at 0.2 millivolt and 0.5 sec per division while supramaximal or tetanic traces are recorded at 0.5 millivolt and 0.5 sec per division. Owing presumably to repeated mobilization, single twitch amplitude was reduced by 13.5 per cent and 15.0 per cent at one and four weeks after initial exposure. Tetanic strength, however, was maintained. Conduction velocity had decreased mildly by 4.2 per cent at one week and 8.5 per cent at four weeks. (Reprinted with permission of the Journal of Neurosurgery.)

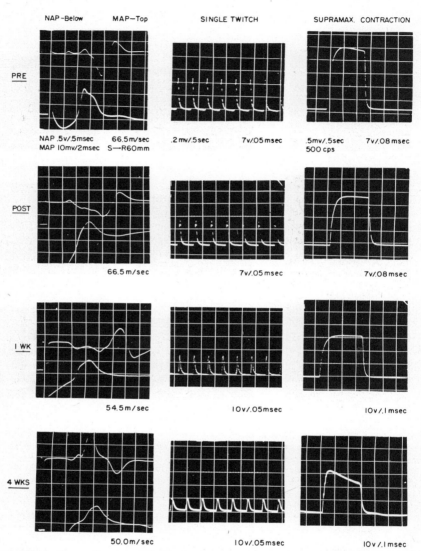

Figure 63–4 Traces from partially lacerated tibial nerve. The tracings show the evoked NAP's and single twitch as well as tetanic contraction prior to laceration, 15 minutes after laceration (post), and at one and four weeks post injury. Losses of function measured at one and four weeks following laceration are greater than those recorded from the control limb. Thus, single twitch was reduced by another 21.0 per cent and 41.9 per cent at one and four weeks following the 15 minute post injury traces while tetanic contraction values were reduced by another 12.5 and 12.5 per cent, respectively. Stimulating to recording distance for NAP's was 60 millimeters. Stimulus parameters are listed under each of the muscle power recordings. (Reprinted with permission of the Journal of Neurosurgery.)

Figure 63–5 Light and electron microscopic examination of a partially lacerated major fasciculus reveals three zones of injury. The lacerated zone shows neurotmetic change with subsequent scar, while the adjacent or intermediate zone shows changes of partial degeneration and is the area of the nerve most responsible for progression of partial injury while the zone most peripheral to the laceration shows changes in the ground substance. Progression is due to ongoing changes in the intermediate and peripheral zones, while the relatively early recovery is due to reversal of changes in these zones. Some, although only a small amount of, regeneration occurs through the lacerated or neurotmetic zone and does account for a small degree of functional recovery. (Reprinted with permission of the Journal of Neurosurgery.)

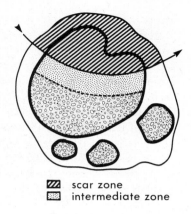

▨ scar zone
▨ intermediate zone

FASCICULAR AND INTERFASCICULAR GRAFT REPAIR IN PRIMATES

In 1970, Grabb and associates compared epineurial with perineurial or fascicular repair once again in the distal median and ulnar nerves of rhesus monkeys. An integrated electromyogram was used, and the author felt that data provided by this technique favored fascicular repair, although, when electrical attempts were made to match fascicles more accurately, the results in this series were no better than those found with a similar and less complicated fascicular repair. The EMG alone has limitations, for it is a sampling technique and values derived depend on needle placement as well as the thoroughness of the examiner, and this must be kept in mind when assessing the data in this experiment. Other electrophysiologic studies such as NAP recording were combined with axonal counts to study the same question in a thorough fashion but with lower phylum animals such as rabbits (Orgel and Terzis, 1977).

Vasconez, Mathes, and Grau (1976) used primate median and ulnar nerves at the wrist level to study end-to-end epineurial repair after a segment of the nerve had been excised and replaced with interfascicular sural nerve grafts. This repair was compared with direct replacement of the excised segment of nerve, which was used as a whole nerve graft. Animals were observed in their cages for degree of hand function. It should be noted that such observations must have been difficult, especially since it appeared that both median and ulnar nerves had lesions in the same limb. Methodology as delineated in the published article was not clear to this reviewer. Did the authors compare one type of repair done in the ulnar nerve with the same repair done in the median nerve? If so, data might not be valid. Each nerve was stimulated proximal to the repair to check for distal muscle contraction. Electromyography studies utilizing electrodes placed in the abductor pollicis brevis for the median repairs and in the first dorsal interosseus muscle for the ulnar repairs were used. These authors apparently studied gaps up to 20 millimeters in length and concluded that fascicular repair by use of grafts was more successful than end-to-end repair and that surgical heroics to close long gaps were contraindicated. A report of the same study published in *Surgical Forum* showed faster conduction in nerves with end-to-end interfascicular repair than in the intrafascicular graft repairs, although comparison of evoked muscle action potentials revealed no significant differences (Mathes et al., 1975). Biopsies were studied histologically and the authors found similar axonal growth in both groups. Full return of function was noted in every case in which a nerve segment had been excised and the gap was less than 15 millimeters (only three animals were studied with gaps over 15 millimeters; i.e., 20 millimeters). All nerves had what was felt to be full contraction in response to direct nerve stimulation. This latter observation points out, perhaps, the incongruity of using such distal segments of nerves for study even in primates because relatively rapid recovery is almost ensured and this bears little similarity to man.

The first phase of a five-year study of different repair methods involving a colony of 60 rhesus monkeys has recently been published (Bratton et al., 1979; Hudson et al., 1979). In one group of animals, transected tibial nerve on one side was repaired by a fascicular technique and thus under mild tension while that on the other side was repaired by interposition of short interfascicular grafts and thus under no tension. In another group of primates, a segment of nerve was resected and one side was repaired by an end-to-end epineurial technique where tension was moderate while that on the other side was repaired by interposition of interfascicular grafts so that tension was minimal. Evoked nerve and muscle action potentials and muscle strength in response to stimulation were recorded prior to and post-injury. Electrophysiologic and histologic data indicated that those nerves repaired end-to-end had in the early months post-repair regeneration superior to that recorded in nerves with grafts, provided that distraction had not occurred. By one year, however, regeneration was comparable in both groups. Use of autogenous interfascicular grafts offers no advantage over end-to-end repair except where the latter cannot be achieved, and then the use of short interfascicular grafts will work.

Primate experiments that compare fascicular with epineurial repair await publication. Data from these experiments indicate that regeneration is superior in those nerves repaired by an epineurial technique, especially at four and six months following suture.

STUDIES OF SENSORY REINNERVATION IN THE PRIMATE

In the last three decades, a large literature comparing and evaluating various sensory end-organs studied under a variety of circumstances, particularly the Meissner's corpuscles and pacinian bodies, has developed and some of these studies have been done in rhesus monkeys or other primates, such as the stumptail monkey or the loris or lemur, which is closely related to Old World monkeys (Krishanamurti et al., 1973; Miller and Ruserles, 1976; Wong and Kanagasuntheram, 1971). For example, in a relatively early study in primates, Winkelmann (1962) used the frozen silver technique to detect axoplasm, a diazo-coupling technique for alkaline phosphatase, and a thiocholine technique for cholinesterase. If done carefully and thoroughly, skin biopsies in a field of altered innervation can be very valuable in assessing end-input sensory function. For example, a recent study by Dellon (1976) showed that Meissner's corpuscles do not regenerate de novo in the monkey as they appear to do in some other, lower phylum animals. Rather, the Meissner's corpuscles contract with degeneration due to nerve injury and then with distal re-input of axons re-expand.

Chacha et al. (1977) studied transfer of the superficial radial or the dorsal cutaneous branch of the ulnar nerve to the median nerve, as suggested by Sunderland (1974) and reported successful sensory reinnervation by 35 to 40 weeks in eight monkeys. The authors correctly chose to study Meissner's corpuscles by microscopy as well as histochemical measurement of cholinesterase. Regenerated nerve fibers in conjunction with the Meissner's corpuscles were seen.

It should be noted that two-point discrimination and sensory conduction velocities have been compared in 19 patients at a point five years following nerve suture (Almquist and Eeg-Olofsson, 1970). Good two-point discrimination did not necessarily correspond with good conduction velocity in these late regenerative studies. However, sensory nerve action potential recording remains a valid index of earlier sensory regeneration. Certainly, the sensory fibers of the limb that has absent or markedly depressed sensory conduction months after repair have not regenerated as quickly as those of the limb with good sensory conduction. Thus, this type of study should not be discarded experimentally let alone clinically when evaluating relatively early regeneration.

CURRENT PRIMATE MODEL IN USE IN OUR LABORATORY

The following experimental model is currently in use in our laboratory to evaluate injury and repair to primate nerve:

1. Adult primates five or more years of age are used. Animals are ready for use after a 90-day period of quarantine with intermittent testing for tuberculosis. Limbs of the animals are inspected to assure absence of significant scars, atrophy, or ulceration. The animal is squeezed as gently in his cage as possible and tranquilized using phencyclidine. The dose is usually 1 to 2 cc IM. Once the animal is tranquilized he is removed from his cage and an intravenous line, usually a butterfly needle, is placed and he is given intravenous pentobarbital, 20 to 25 mg per kg.

2. Nerves are exposed using sterile, sharp technique with preservation of longitudinal and subepineurial blood supply. Baseline electrical studies are made by placing bipolar stimulating and recording electrodes well on either side of the intended lesion or repair site. Care is taken to place an EMG needle deep into muscle in the innervational field of the nerve to be studied so that evoked muscle action potentials can be coupled with evoked nerve action potentials. The animal is fixed in our primate frame, a tibial pin is placed, and baseline single twitch and supramaximal tetanic contraction studies are carried out. Differential amplifiers, oscilloscope, and Polaroid camera are used to make multiple photographs for each physiologic test. All wounds are carefully sutured closed (Figs. 63–1 and 63–2).

3. Postoperatively, the animal's clinical function is observed periodically as he moves about in his cage.

4. At a predetermined interval post-injury or repair, the evoked NAP and EMG studies and determinations of muscle power are repeated (Figs. 63–3 and 63–4).

5. After gross inspection of the lesion and notation of its characteristics, in vivo fixation is carried out, usually using glutaraldehyde after pretreatment with hyaluronidase. Further fixation in glutaraldehyde and then sectioning under the microscope for both EM and light histologic studies are done. Those specimens intended for light histologic studies are placed in 10 per cent formalin. Currently used as a routine are Masson's trichrome, Bodian, and Luxol fast blue staining techniques. Those specimens intended for EM studies are placed in buffered sodium bicarbonate, then 10 per cent osmium tetroxide, and then dehydrated and begun on the final processing steps for EM study (Fig. 63–5).

6. One may wish to study sensory end organs as well as sensory nerve action potentials, and biopsy of skin or muscle or both may be necessary. We have had no personal experience with such skin biopsies but have had experience with sensory conduction studies.

7. If possible, the life of the animal should be preserved, since unrelated studies may sometimes be conducted, especially on the more central nervous system.

8. Axon counts by size can now be done electronically using a planographic technique. Such data can be used to construct histograms, which can then be correlated with the electrical data. More classic evaluation of axonal organization, connective tissue proliferation, and degree of myelination by light as well as electron microscopic study can complement the histograms.

REFERENCES

Alexander, E., Woods, R. P., and Weiss, P.: Further experiments on bridging long nerve gaps in monkeys. Proc. Soc. Exp. Biol. Med. 68:380, 1948.

Almquist, E., and Eeg-Olofsson, O.: Sensory-nerve-conduction velocity and two-point discrimination in sutured nerves. J. Bone and Joint Surg. 52A:791, 1970.

Ashley, F. L., Murphey, J. E., Morgan, S. C., Balch, C. R., Conover, N. A., Galloway, D. V., and Cross, L.: Axon growth through irradiated median and ulnar nerve homografts in primates. Plast. Reconstr. Surg. 42:313, 1967.

Beazley, R. M., Bayley, D. H., and Ketcham, A. S.: The effect of cryosurgery on peripheral nerves. J. Surg. Res. 16:231, 1974.

Boyle, W. F.: Facial nerve paralysis. An experimental investigation of facial nerve regeneration in monkeys. Laryngoscope 76:1921, 1966.

Bratton, B. R., Hudson, A. R., and Kline, D. G.: Experimental interfascicular nerve grafting. J. Neurosurg. 51:323, 1979.

Cajal, R. y: Degeneration and Regeneration of the Nervous System. R. M. May (Trans.), London, Oxford University Press, Vol. 2, 1928.

Chacha, P. B., Krishnamurte, A., and Soin, K.: Nerve transfer in monkeys: Experimental sensory reinnervation of the median nerves. J. Bone Joint Surg. 59A:386, 1977.

Dastur, D. K., and Razzok, Z. A.: Degeneration and regeneration in teased nerve fibers, I-Leprous neuritis. Acta Neuropathol. 18:286, 1971.

Dellon, A. L.: Reinnervation of denervated Meissner corpuscles: A sequential histologic study in the monkey following fascicular repair. J. Hand Surg. 1:98, 1976.

Ducker, T. B.: Peripheral nerve injuries: A comparative study of anatomical and functional results following primary repair in chimpanzees. Military Med. 133:298, 1968.

Ducker, T. B., and Hayes, G. J.: Experimental improvements in the use of Silastic cuff for peripheral nerve repair. J. Neurosurg. 28(6):582, 1968a.

Ducker, T. B., and Hayes, G. J.: Irradiated Wallerian degenerated homografts in dogs and chimpanzees. Surg. Forum 19:444, 1968b.

Ducker, T. B., and Hayes, G. J.: Peripheral nerve grafts: Experimental studies on the dog and chimpanzees. J. Neurosurg. 32:236, 1970.

Gilliatt, R. W., Fowler, J. J., and Rudge, P.: Peripheral neuropathy in baboons. Adv. Neurol. *10*:253, 1975.

Goodwin, W. J.: Current use of non-human primates in biomedical research. Lab. Anim. Care *20*:229, 1970.

Grabb, W. C.: Median and ulnar nerve suture: An experimental study comparing primary and secondary repair in monkeys. J. Bone Joint Surg. *50*:964, 1968.

Grabb, W. C., Bement, S. C., and Koepke, G. H.: Comparison of methods of peripheral nerve suturing in monkeys. Plast. Reconstr. Surg. *46*:31, 1970.

Graham, W. P., Pataky, P. E., Calabretta, A. M., Munger, B. L., and Buda, M. J.: Enhancement of peripheral nerve regeneration with triamcinolone after neurorrhaphy. Surg Forum *24*:457, 1973.

Guth, L.: Axonal regeneration and functional plasticity in central nervous system. Exp. Neurol. *45(3)*:606, 1974.

Guttman, E.: Effects of delay in innervation on recovery of muscle after nerve lesions. J. Neurophysiol. *11*:279, 1948.

Hopkins, A. P., and Gilliatt, A. W.: Motor and sensory nerve conduction velocity in the baboon: Normal values and changes during acrylamide neuropathy. J. Neurol. Neurosurg. Psychiatry *34(4)*:415, 1971.

Hudson, A. R., and Kline, D. G.: Progression of partial injury to peripheral nerve: II – Light and electron microscopy studies. J. Neurosurg. *42*:15, 1975.

Hudson, A. R., Hunter, D., Kline, D. G., and Bratton, B. R.: Histologic studies of experimental interfascicular graft repairs. J. Neurosurg. *51*:333, 1979.

Kline, D. G., Hayes, G. J., and Morse, A. S.: A comparative study of response of species to peripheral nerve injury. I. Severance. J. Neurosurg. *21*:968, 1964a.

Kline, D. G., Hayes, G. J., and Morse, A. S.: A comparative study of response of species to peripheral nerve injury. II. Crush and severance with primary suture. J. Neurosurg. *21*:980, 1964b.

Kline, D. G.: The use of resorbable wrapper for peripheral nerve repair. J. Neurosurg. *21*:737, 1964.

Kline, D. G., and DeJonge, B. R.: Evoked potentials to evaluate peripheral nerve injuries. Surg. Gynecol. Obstet. *127*:1239, 1968.

Kline, D. G., and Hackett, E. R.: Early evaluation of nerve injuries by evoked potentials and electromyography. Surg. Forum *19*:442, 1968.

Kline, D. G., and Hackett, E. R.: Reappraisal of timing for exploration of civilian peripheral nerve injuries. Surgery *78*:54, 1975.

Kline, D. G., Hackett, E. R., Davis, G., and Myers, B.: The effect of mobilization on the blood supply and regeneration of injured nerves. J. Surg. Res. *12*:254, 1972.

Kline, D. G., Hackett, E. R., and LeBlanc, H. J.: The value of primary repair for bluntly transected nerve injuries: Physiologic documentation. Surg. Forum *25*:436, 1974.

Kline, D. G., Hackett, E. R., and May, P. R.: Evaluation of nerve injuries by evoked potentials and electromyography. J. Neurosurg. *31*:128, 1969.

Kline, D. G., Hackett, E. R., and May, P. R.: Partial nerve laceration evaluated by evoked potentials. J. Surg. Res. *10*:81, 1970a.

Kline, D. G., Hackett, E. R., and May, P. R.: Electrophysiologic studies of fractional nerve injuries. *In*: Current Topics in Surgical Research. New York, Academic Press, 1970b, Vol. 2, p. 205.

Kline, D. G., Happel, L. J., Bratton, B. R., and Hackett, E. R.: Computerized non-invasive recording of nerve action potentials in primates and humans with injured nerves (Abstract). EEG Clin. Neurophys. *34*:807, 1973.

Kline, D. G., Hudson, A. R., Hackett, E. R., and Bratton, B. R.: Progression of partial injury to peripheral nerve: I — Periodic measurements of muscle contraction strength. J. Neurosurg. *42*:1, 1975.

Kline, D. G., May, P. R., Hackett, E. R., McGarry, P. R., and Hill, C. W.: Dexamethasone treatment of partially injured nerves. *In*: Current Topics in Surgical Research. New York, Academic Press, Vol. 2, 1970. p. 173.

Krishanamurti, A., Kanagasuntheram, K., and Viz, S.: Failure of reinnervation of pacinian corpuscles after nerve crush. Acta Neuropathol. *23(4)*:338, 1973.

Lehman, R. A., and Hayes, G. J.: Degeneration and regeneration in peripheral nerve. Brain *90(2)*:285, 1967.

Mathes, S. J., Vasconez, L. O., and Gray, G. K.: Direct fascicular repair and interfascicular nerve grafting of median and ulnar nerves in rhesus monkeys. Surg. Forum *26*:545, 1975.

McLeod, J. G.: Conduction velocity and fibre diameter of median and ulnar nerves of the baboon. J. Neurol. Neurosurg. Psychiatry *30*:240, 1967.

McLeod, J. G., and Penny, R. J.: Vincristine neuropathy: An electrophysiological and histological study. J. Neurol. Neurosurg. Psychiatry *32*:297, 1969.

Miller, S. H., and Ruserles, I.: Changes in primate pacinian corpuscles following volar pad excision and skin grafting: A preliminary report. Plast. Reconstr. Surg. *57(5)*:627, 1976.

Orgel, M. G., and Terzis, J. K.: Epineurial vs perineurial repair. J. Plast. Reconstr. Surg. *60*:80, 1977.

Paul, R. L., Goodman, H., and Merzenich, M.: Alternatives in mechanoreceptor input to Brodmann's areas 1 and 3 of the postcentral hind area of *macaca mulatta* after nerve section and regeneration. Brain Res. *37(1)*:1, 1972.

Pollard, J. D., Gye, R. S., and McLeod, J. G.: An assessment of immunosuppressive agents in experimental peripheral nerve transplantation. Surg. Gynecol. Obstet. *132*:839, 1971.

Rudge, P., Ochoa, J., and Gilliatt, R. W.: Acute peripheral nerve compression in the baboon. J. Neurol. Sci. *23(3)*:403, 1974.

Sunderland, S.: The restoration of median nerve function after destructive lesions which preclude end-to-end repair. Brain *97*:1974.

Tarlov, I. M., Baernstein, W., and Bermon, D.: Nerve regeneration: A comparative experimental study following suture by clot and thread. J. Neurosurg. *5*:62, 1948.

Vasconez, L., Mathes, S. S., and Grau, G.: Direct fascicular repair and interfascicular nerve grafting of median and ulnar nerves in rhesus monkeys. Surg. Forum *26*:545, 1975.

Weiss, P.: Functional nerve regeneration through frozen dried nerve grafts in rats and monkeys. Proc. Soc. Exp. Biol. Med. *54*:277, 1943.

Winkelmann, R. K.: Effect of sciatic nerve section on enzymatic reacting of sensory end organs. J. Neuropathol. Exp. Neurol. *21*:655, 1962.

Wong, W. C., and Kanagasuntheram, R.: Early and late effects of median injury in Meissner's and pacinian corpuscles of the hand of the macaque. J. Anat. *109(1)*:135, 1971.

Name Index

Index

Note: Page numbers in *italic* type refer to illustrations;
page numbers followed by (t) refer to tables.